ANAESTHESIA

ANAESTHESIA

EDITED BY

WALTER S. NIMMO
BSc, MD, FRCP, FRCA, FANZCA, FFPM
Chief Executive and Chairman
Inveresk Clinical Research Ltd
Edinburgh

DAVID J. ROWBOTHAM
MD, MRCP, FRCA
Senior Lecturer
University Department of Anaesthesia
Leicester Royal Infirmary

GRAHAM SMITH
BSc, MD, FRCA
Professor and Head
University Department of Anaesthesia
Leicester Royal Infirmary

IN TWO VOLUMES
VOLUME 2

SECOND EDITION

OXFORD

BLACKWELL SCIENTIFIC PUBLICATIONS
LONDON EDINBURGH BOSTON
MELBOURNE PARIS BERLIN VIENNA

First published 1989
Reprinted 1989, 1990
Four Dragons edition 1990
Second edition 1994

Set by Setrite Typesetters, Hong Kong
Printed and bound in Great Britain
at The Alden Press, Oxford

DISTRIBUTORS

Marston Book Services Ltd
PO Box 87
Oxford OX2 0DT
(*Orders*: Tel: 0865 791155
          Fax: 0865 791927
          Telex: 837515)

USA
Blackwell Scientific Publications, Inc.
238 Main Street
Cambridge, MA 02142
(*Orders*: Tel: 800 759-6102
                 617 876-7000)

Canada
Times Mirror Professional Publishing, Ltd
130 Flaska Drive
Markham, Ontario L6G 1B8
(*Orders*: Tel: 800 268-4178
                 416 470-6739)

Australia
Blackwell Scientific Publications Pty Ltd
54 University Street
Carlton, Victoria 3053
(*Orders*: Tel: 03 347-5552)

A catalogue record for this title
is available from the British Library

ISBN 0-632-03244-8

Library of Congress
Cataloging in Publication Data

Anaesthesia/edited by Walter S. Nimmo,
   David J. Rowbotham, Graham Smith. — 2nd ed.
      p.   cm.
   Includes bibliographical references
   and index.
   ISBN 0-632-03244-8
   1. Anesthesiology.   I. Nimmo, W.S.
II. Rowbotham, David J.   III. Smith, G. (Graham)
   [DNLM: 1. Anesthesia.
WO 200 A5287 1994]
RD81.A542   1994
617.9'6 — dc20

Contents

List of Contributors

A. P. ADAMS MB, PhD, FRCA, *Professor of Anaesthesia, Department of Anaesthesia, United Medical School of Guy's and St Thomas' Hospitals, London SE1 9RT, UK*

A. R. AITKENHEAD MD, FRCA, *Professor of Anaesthesia, Department of Anaesthesia, University Hospital, Queen's Medical Centre, Clifton Boulevard, Nottingham NG7 2UH, UK*

E. N. ARMITAGE DRCOG, FRCA, *Consultant Anaesthetist, Department of Anaesthesia, Brighton General Hospital, Brighton BN2 3EW, and Royal Alexandra Hospital for Sick Children, Elm Grove, Brighton BN1 3JN, UK*

A. J. ASBURY MBChB, PhD, FRCA, *Senior Lecturer in Anaesthesia, Department of Anaesthesia, University of Glasgow, Western Infirmary, Dumbarton Road, Glasgow G11 6NT, UK*

P. J. F. BASKETT BA, MBBCh, BAO, FRCA, *Chairman of the European Resuscitation Council, and Consultant Anaesthetist, Department of Anaesthesia, The Royal Infirmary and Frenchay Hospital, Bristol BS16 1LE, UK*

D. R. BEVAN MA, MB, MRCP, FRCA, *Professor of Anaesthesia and Head, Department of Anaesthesia, The University of British Columbia, Vancouver General Hospital, Vancouver, BC V5Z 4E3, Canada*

S. BENNETT FRCA, *Staff Anaesthetist, Department of Cardiothoracic Anaesthesia and Surgery, University of Umea, S901–85 Umea, Sweden*

C. E. BLOGG MBBS, DObstRCOG, FRCA, *Consultant Anaesthetist, Nuffield Department of Anaesthetics, University of Oxford, Radcliffe Infirmary, Oxford OX2 6HE; Clinical Lecturer, University of Oxford, Oxford, UK; and Associate Professor, Department of Anesthesiology, University of Texas Southwestern Medical Center, 5323 Harry Hines Boulevard, Dallas, TX 75235–9068, USA*

J. B. BOWES MB, FRCA, *Formerly Consultant Anaesthetist, Department of Anaesthesia, Bristol Royal Infirmary, Upper Maudlin Street, Bristol BS2 8HW, UK*

W. C. BOWMAN BPharm, PhD, DSc, FIBiol, FPS, FRSE, FRCA, *Professor, Department of Physiology and Pharmacology, University of Strathclyde, Royal College, 204 George Street, Glasgow G1 1XW, UK*

D. P. BRAID MBChB, FRCA, *Formerly Consultant Anaesthetist, Department of Anaesthesia, University of Glasgow, Western Infirmary, Dumbarton Road, Glasgow G11 6NT; and Formerly Honorary Senior Clinical Lecturer, Glasgow Dental School, University of Glasgow, Glasgow G11 6NT, UK*

B. R. BROWN JR MD, PhD, FRCA, *Head, Department of Anesthesiology, University of Arizona College of Medicine, Tucson, AZ 85724, USA*

F. P. BUCKLEY MB, FRCA, *Associate Professor, Department of Anesthesiology, University of Washington School of Medicine, Seattle, WA 98195, USA*

K. BUDD MBChB, FRCA, *Consultant Anaesthetist, Department of Anaesthesia, Bradford Royal Infirmary, Duckworth Lane, Bradford, West Yorkshire BD9 6RJ, UK*

A. M. BURNS MRCP, FRCA, *Senior Registrar in Anaesthetics and Intensive Care, John Farman Intensive Care Unit, Addenbrooke's Hospital, Hills Road, Cambridge CB2 2QQ, UK*

T. N. CALVEY BSc, MD, PhD, *Honorary Senior Research Fellow, Department of Anaesthesia, University of Liverpool, Royal Liverpool Hospital, Prescot Street, Liverpool L69 3BX, UK*

I. T. CAMPBELL MD, FRCA, *Senior Lecturer in Anaesthesia, Department of Anaesthesia, University of Manchester, Withington Hospital, Nell Lane, West Didsbury, Manchester M20 8LE, UK*

G. R. D. CATTO MD, DSc, FRCP, *Professor of Medicine and Therapeutics, Department of Medicine, University of Aberdeen, Aberdeen Royal Infirmary, Foresterhill, Aberdeen AB9 2ZB, UK*

W. A. CHAMBERS MD, FRCA, *Consultant Anaesthetist, Department of Anaesthetics, University of Aberdeen, Aberdeen Royal Infirmary, Foresterhill, Aberdeen AB9 2ZB, UK*

C. R. CHAPMAN PhD, *Professor of Anesthesiology, Department of Anesthesiology, University of Washington School of Medicine, Seattle, WA 98195, USA*

J. E. CHARLTON MBBS, FRCA, *Consultant in Pain Management and Anaesthesia, Department of Anaesthesia, Royal Victoria Infirmary, Queen Victoria Road, Newcastle upon Tyne NE1 4LP, UK*

M. J. COUSINS MBBS, MD, FRCA, FANZCA, *Professor of Anesthesia and Head, Department of Anesthesia and Pain Management, University of Sydney, Royal North Shore Hospital, St Leonards, NSW 2065, Australia*

B. G. COVINO (The Late) PhD, MD, *Formerly Professor of Anesthesia, Department of Anesthesia, Brigham and Women's Hospital, Harvard Medical School, 75 Francis Street, Boston, MA 02115, USA*

A. J. CUNNINGHAM MD, FRCPC, *Professor of Anaesthesia, Department of Anaesthesia, Royal College of Surgeons in Ireland, Professorial Unit, Beaumont Hospital, Dublin 9, Ireland*

J. M. DAVIES MSc, MD, FRCPC, *Professor of Anaesthesia, Department of Anaesthesia, University of Calgary, Foothills Hospital, 1403−29th Street NW, Calgary, Alta T2N 2T9, Canada*

G. DOLAN MRCP, MRCPath, *Consultant Haematologist, Department of Haematology, University Hospital, Queen's Medical Centre, Clifton Boulevard, Nottingham NG7 2UH, UK*

D. J. R. DUTHIE MD, FRCA, *Consultant Anaesthetist, Department of Anaesthesia, Papworth Hospital NHS Trust, Papworth Everard, Cambridgeshire CB3 8RE, UK*

D. L. EDBROOKE MBChB, FRCA, *Consultant Anaesthetist, Department of Anaesthesia, Central Sheffield University Hospital, Glossop Road, Sheffield S10 2JF, UK*

F. R. ELLIS PhD, FRCA, *Professor of Anaesthesia, Academic Unit of Anaesthesia, St James's University Hospital, Becket Street, Leeds LS9 7TF, UK*

I. K. FARQUHAR FRCA, *Lecturer in Anaesthesia, Department of Anaesthesia, University Hospital, Queen's Medical Centre, Clifton Boulevard, Nottingham NG7 2UH, UK*

J. P. H. FEE PhD, FRCA, *Senior Lecturer in Anaesthesia, Department of Anaesthetics, The Queen's University of Belfast, Belfast BT9 7BC; and Consultant Anaesthetist, Department of Anaesthetics, Musgrave Park Hospital, Stockmans Lane, Belfast BT9 7JB, and Royal Victoria Hospital, Grosvenor Road, Belfast BT12 6BA, UK*

D. FELL MBChB, FRCA, *Consultant Anaesthetist, University Department of Anaesthesia, Leicester Royal Infirmary, Infirmary Square, Leicester LE1 5WW, UK*

W. FITCH BSc, MBChB, PhD, FRCA, FRCP, *Professor of Anaesthesia, Department of Anaesthesia, University of Glasgow, Glasgow Royal Infirmary, 8−16 Alexandra Parade, Glasgow G31 2ER, UK*

P. FOËX MD, FRCA, *Professor of Anaesthesia, Nuffield Department of Anaesthetics, University of Oxford, Radcliffe Infirmary, Oxford OX2 6HE, UK*

M. L. FONTES MD, *Clinical Instructor, Department of Anesthesia, University of California, San Francisco, CA 94143, USA*

C. D. FORBES BSc, MD, MRCP, *Professor of Medicine, Department of Medicine, Ninewells Hospital, Dundee DD1 9SY, UK*

A. H. GIESECKE MD, *Jenkins Professor of Anesthesia and Chairman, Department of Anesthesiology, University of Texas Southwestern Medical Center, 5323 Harry Hines Boulevard, Dallas, TX 75235-9068, USA*

I. S. GRANT MRCP, FRCPE, FFARCSI, *Consultant Anaesthetist and Medical Director, Intensive Therapy Unit, Western General Hospital, Edinburgh EH4 2XU, UK*

J. GREIFF MBChB, FRCA, *Research Fellow, University Department of Anaesthesia, Leicester Royal Infirmary, Infirmary Square, Leicester LE1 5WW, UK*

G. M. HALL PhD, FRCA, *Professor of Anaesthesia, Department of Anaesthesia, St George's Hospital, Blackshaw Road, London SW17 0QT, UK*

M. J. HALSEY BSc, PhD, *Nuffield Department of Anaesthetics, University of Oxford, Radcliffe Infirmary, Oxford OX2 6HE, UK*

C. D. HANNING BSc, MBBS, FRCA, *Senior Lecturer, University Department of Anaesthesia, Leicester Royal Infirmary, Infirmary Square, Leicester LE1 5WW, UK*

D. J. HATCH MBBS, FRCA, *Portex Professor of Anaesthesia, Hospital for Sick Children, Great Ormond Street, London WC1N 3JH, UK*

D. E. HOLLAND BSc, MRCP, FRCA, *Consultant Anaesthetist, Department of Anaesthetics, Southmead Hospital, Southmead, Bristol BS10 5NB, UK*

J. N. HORTON MB BS, FRCA, *Consultant Anaesthetist, Anaesthetics Service Centre, University Hospital of Wales, Heath Park, Cardiff CF4 4XW, UK*

K. HOUGHTON MB ChB, DRCOG, FRCA, *Consultant Anaesthetist, Department of Anaesthesia, Torbay Hospital, Lawes Bridge, Torquay, Devon TQ2 7AA, UK*

C. J. HULL MB ChB, FRCA, *Professor of Anaesthesia, Department of Anaesthesia, Royal Victoria Infirmary, Queen Victoria Road, Newcastle upon Tyne NE1 4LP, UK*

J. M. HUNTER MB ChB, FRCA, *Senior Lecturer in Anaesthesia, University of Liverpool, PO Box 147, Liverpool L69 3BX, UK*

A. INNES MB, MRCP, *Senior Registrar in Renal and General Medicine, Nottingham City Hospital, Hucknall Road, Nottingham NG5 1PB, UK*

J. L. JENKINSON MB ChB, FRCA, *Consultant Anaesthetist, Department of Clinical Neurosciences, Western General Hospital, Crewe Road, Edinburgh EH4 2XU; and Part-time Senior Lecturer, Department of Anaesthetics, University of Edinburgh, Edinburgh EH8 9YL, UK*

M. J. JONES FRCA, MRCP, *Consultant Anaesthetist, Department of Anaesthesia, Glenfield General Hospital, Groby Road, Leicester LE3 9QP, UK*

R. M. JONES MD, FRCA, *Professor of Anaesthesia, Department of Anaesthesia, St Mary's Hospital Medical School, Praed Street, London W2 1NY, UK*

G. N. C. KENNY MD, BSc, MB ChB, FRCA, *Senior Lecturer in Anaesthesia, Department of Anaesthesia, University of Glasgow, Glasgow Royal Infirmary, 8–16 Alexandra Parade, Glasgow G31 2ER, UK*

S. W. KRECHEL MD, *Associate Professor of Anaesthesia, University of Missouri–Columbia, Department of Anesthesiology, 1 Hospital Drive, Columbia, MO 65212, USA*

J. A. LANGTON MB BS, FRCA, *Senior Lecturer, University Department of Anaesthesia, Leicester Royal Infirmary, Infirmary Square, Leicester LE1 5WW, UK*

I. McA. LEDINGHAM MB ChB, MD, FRCS, FRCP, FIBiol, FRSE, *Dean, Faculty of Medicine and Health Sciences, Department of Emergency and Critical Care Medicine, The United Arab Emirates University, Jameah, PO Box 17666, Al Ain, UAE*

E. S. LIN BSc, MB ChB, MRCP, FRCA, *Consultant Anaesthetist, Department of Anaesthesia, Glenfield General Hospital, Groby Road, Leicester LE3 9QP, UK*

L. LOH MB BS, FRCA, *Consultant Anaesthetist, Nuffield Department of Anaesthetics, University of Oxford, Radcliffe Infirmary, NHS Trust, Oxford OX2 6HE, UK*

G. L. LUDBROOK MB BS, FANZCA, *NH and MRC Research Scholar, Department of Anaesthesia and Intensive Care, University of Adelaide, Adelaide, SA 5000, Australia*

W. McCAUGHEY MD, FRCA, FFARCSI, *Consultant Anaesthetist, Craigavon Area Hospital, Craigavon, Co. Armagh BT63 5QQ; and Lecturer in Anaesthesia, Department of Anaesthetics, The Queen's University of Belfast, Belfast BT9 7BL, UK*

D. B. L. McCLELLAND MB ChB, PhD, FRCP, *Director, South-East Regional Scottish National Blood Transfusion Service, Department of Transfusion Medicine, Royal Infirmary of Edinburgh, Lauriston Place, Edinburgh EH3 9YW, UK*

K. J. McGRATH MB, FFARCSI, *Acting Professor of Anesthesiology, Department of Anesthesiology, University of Washington School of Medicine, Seattle, WA 98195, USA*

P. J. McKENZIE MD, FRCA, *Consultant Anaesthetist, Nuffield Department of Anaesthetics, University of Oxford, John Radcliffe Hospital, Headington, Oxford OX3 9DU, UK*

L. R. McNICOL FRCA, *Consultant Anaesthetist, Department of Anaesthesia, Royal Hospital for Sick Children, Yorkhill, Glasgow G3 8SJ; and Honorary Clinical Senior Lecturer, University of Glasgow, Glasgow G11 6NT, UK*

H. J. McQUAY MD, FRCA, *Clinical Reader in Pain Relief, Oxford Regional Pain Relief Unit, Churchill Hospital, Headington, Oxford OX3 7LJ; and Nuffield Department of Anaesthetics, University of Oxford, Oxford, UK*

D. T. MANGANO MD, PhD, *Professor of Anesthesia and Vice-Chairman, Department of Anesthesia, Veterans Affairs Medical Center, 4150 Clement St, San Francisco, CA 94121, USA*

B. E. MARSHALL MD, FRCP, FRCA, *Professor of Anesthesia, Department of Anesthesia, University of Pennsylvania, 3400 Spruce Street, Philadelphia, PA 19104-4283, USA*

L. E. MATHER ASTC, MSc, PhD, FANZCA, *Professor of Anaesthesia and Analgesia, Department of Anaesthesia and Pain Management, University of Sydney, Royal North Shore Hospital, St Leonards, NSW 2065, Australia*

M. MORGAN MB BS, DA, FRCA, *Reader in Anaesthetic Practice, Royal Postgraduate Medical School, and Honorary Consultant Anaesthetist, Department of Anaesthesia, Hammersmith Hospital, Du Cane Road, London W12 0HS, UK*

R. S. NEILL MD, BAO, FFARCSI, *Formerly Consultant Anaesthetist, Department of Anaesthesia, University of Glasgow, Glasgow Royal Infirmary, 8–16 Alexandra Parade, Glasgow G31 2ER, UK*

R. A. NELSON MB, MRCP, FRCA, *Senior Registrar in Anaesthesia, Mersey Region, UK; and Research Fellow, Division of Clinical Pharmacology, Vanderbilt University, Nashville, TN 37232-6602, USA*

A. F. NIMMO MB ChB, FRCA, *Senior Registrar, Department of Anaesthesia, Royal Infirmary of Edinburgh, Lauriston Place, Edinburgh EH3 9YW, UK*

W. S. NIMMO BSc, MD, FRCP, FRCA, FANZCA, FFPM, *Chief Executive and Chairman, Inveresk Clinical Research Ltd, Research Park, Rickarton, Edinburgh EH14 4AP, UK*

D. O' FLAHERTY MD, *Department of Anesthesiology, University of Texas Southwestern Medical Center, 5323 Harry Hines Boulevard, Dallas, TX 75235-9068, USA*

A. J. OGILVY FRCA, *Lecturer in Anaesthesia, University Department of Anaesthesia, Leicester Royal Infirmary, Infirmary Square, Leicester LE1 5WW, UK*

G. R. PARK MD, FRCA, *Director of Intensive Care and Consultant in Anaesthesia, John Farman Intensive Care Unit, Addenbrooke's Hospital, Hills Road, Cambridge CB2 2QQ, UK*

J. E. PEACOCK MB ChB, FRCA, *Senior Lecturer in Anaesthesia, Department of Surgical and Anaesthetic Sciences, University of Sheffield, Royal Hallamshire Hospital, Sheffield S10 2JF, UK*

I. POWER MD, FRCA, *Senior Lecturer in Anaesthesia, Department of Anaesthesia, University of Wales College of Medicine, Cardiff CF4 4XN, UK*

L. F. PRESCOTT MD, FRCP, FRCPE, FFPM, FRSE, *Professor of Clinical Pharmacology, Clinical Pharmacology Unit, Royal Infirmary of Edinburgh, Lauriston Place, Edinburgh EH3 9YW, UK*

D. S. PROUGH MD, *Professor of Anesthesia and Chairman, Rebecca Terry White Chair, Department of Anesthesiology, University of Texas Medical Branch, Suite 2A, Route E-91, Galveston, TX 77555-0591, USA*

C. S. REILLY MD, FRCA, *Professor of Anaesthesia, Department of Anaesthesia, University of Sheffield Medical School, Beech Hill Road, Sheffield S10 2RX, UK*

S. REIZ MD, PhD, *Professor of Anaesthesiology, Department of Anaesthesiology, University of Umea, S901-85 Umea, Sweden*

D. J. ROWBOTHAM MD, MRCP, FRCA, *Senior Lecturer in Anaesthesia, University Department of Anaesthesia, Leicester Royal Infirmary, Infirmary Square, Leicester LE1 5WW, UK*

D. ROYSTON FRCA, *Consultant in Cardiothoracic Anaesthesia, Department of Anaesthesia, Harefield Hospital, Harefield, Middlesex UB9 6JH, UK*

W. B. RUNCIMAN BSc, MB BCh, FRCA, PhD, FHKCA, *Professor of Anaesthesia and Head, Department of Anaesthesia and Intensive Care, Royal Adelaide Hospital, North Terrace, Adelaide, SA 5000, Australia*

J. W. SEAR MA, BSc, PhD, MB BS, FRCA, *Clinical Reader in Anaesthetics, Nuffield Department of Anaesthesia, University of Oxford, John Radcliffe Hospital, Headington, Oxford OX3 9DU, UK*

J. F. SEARLE MB BS, FRCA, *Consultant Anaesthetist, Department of Anaesthesia, Royal Devon and Exeter Hospital, Barrack Road, Exeter EX2 5DW, UK*

P. S. SEBEL MB BS, PhD, FFARCSI, *Professor of Anesthesiology, Department of Anesthesiology, Emory University School of Medicine, Crawford W. Long Hospital, Atlanta, GA 30365, USA*

K. H. SIMPSON FRCA, *Consultant Anaesthetist and Senior Clinical Lecturer, Department of Anaesthesia, St James's University Hospital, Becket Street, Leeds LS9 7TF, UK*

P. J. SIMPSON MD, FRCA, *Consultant Anaesthetist, Department of Anaesthesia, Frenchay Hospital, Bristol BS16 1LE; and Senior Clinical Lecturer in Anaesthetics, University of Bristol, Bristol BS8 1TH, UK*

M. SIVAKUMARAN MB BS, LRCP, LRCS, MRCP, *Senior Registrar in Haematology, Department of Haematology, Phase III Building, Leicester Royal Infirmary, Infirmary Square, Leicester LE1 5WW, UK*

J. R. SKOYLES BSc, MB BS, FRCA, *Senior Registrar in Anaesthetics, University Department of Anaesthetics, Leicester Royal Infirmary, Infirmary Square, Leicester LE1 5WW, UK*

G. SMITH BSc, MD, FRCA, *Professor of Anaesthesia and Head, University Department of Anaesthesia, Leicester Royal Infirmary, Infirmary Square, Leicester LE1 5WW, UK*

I. SMITH BSc, MB BS, FRCA, *Senior Registrar in Anaesthesia, Midlands Anaesthetic Training Scheme, Birmingham, UK*

A. A. SPENCE MD, FRCP, FRCA, *Professor of Anaesthetics and Head, Department of Anaesthesia, Royal Infirmary of Edinburgh, Lauriston Place, Edinburgh EH3 9YW, UK*

S. J. THOMAS MD, *Department of Anesthesiology, ST-1052, New York Hospital, Purnell Medical School, 525 East 68th Street, New York, NY 10021, USA*

J. G. TODD MB ChB, FRCA, *Consultant Anaesthetist, Department of Anaesthesia, University of Glasgow, Western Infirmary, Dumbarton Road, Glasgow G11 6NT, UK*

G. T. TUCKER PhD, *Professor of Clinical Pharmacology, Department of Medicine and Pharmacology, Section of Pharmacology and Therapeutics, University of Sheffield, Royal Hallamshire Hospital, Glossop Road, Sheffield S10 2JF, UK*

D. A. B. TURNER MB BS, FRCA, *Consultant Anaesthetist, University Department of Anaesthesia, Leicester Royal Infirmary, Infirmary Square, Leicester LE1 5WW, UK*

R. G. TWYCROSS MA, DM, FRCP, *Consultant Physician, Sir Michael Sobell House, Churchill Hospital, Headington, Oxford OX3 7LJ; and Macmillan Clinical Reader in Palliative Medicine, University of Oxford, Oxford, UK*

J. L. VINCENT MD, *Professor of Intensive Care Medicine, Clinical Director, Department of Intensive Care, Erasme University Hospital, Route de Lennik 808, B-1070 Brussels, Belgium*

D. WEATHERILL BSc, MB ChB, PhD, FRCA, *Senior Lecturer in Anaesthetics, Department of Anaesthetics, Royal Infirmary of Edinburgh, Lauriston Place, Edinburgh EH3 9YW, UK*

D. C. WHITE MB BS, FRCA, *Consultant Anaesthetist, Department of Anaesthesia, Northwick Park Hospital, Watford Road, Harrow, Middlesex HA1 3UJ, UK*

M. WHITE BSc, PhD, MB ChB, FRCA, *Staff Anaesthesiologist, Department of Anaesthesiology, University Hospital Leiden, PO Box 9600, 2300 RC Leiden, The Netherlands*

P. F. WHITE PhD, MD, FRCA, *Professor and Holder of the McDermott Chair in Anesthesiology, Department of Anesthesiology and Pain Management, University of Texas Southwestern Medical Center, 5323 Harry Hines Boulevard, Dallas, TX 75235-9068, USA*

J. A. W. WILDSMITH MD, FRCA, *Consultant Anaesthetist and Senior Lecturer, Department of Anaesthesia, Royal Infirmary of Edinburgh, Lauriston Place, Edinburgh EH3 9YW, UK*

S. M. WILLATTS FRCA, *Consultant Anaesthetist in Charge of Intensive Therapy Unit, Department of Anaesthetics, Bristol Royal Infirmary, Upper Maudlin Street, Bristol BS2 8HW, UK*

J. K. WOOD FRCP, FRCPE, FRCPath, *Consultant Haematologist, Department of Haematology, Phase III Building, Leicester Royal Infirmary, Infirmary Square, Leicester LE1 5WW, UK*

M. WOOD MB ChB, FRCA, *Professor of Anesthesiology and Associate Professor of Clinical Pharmacology, Division of Clinical Pharmacology, Vanderbilt University, Nashville, TN 37232-6602, USA*

D. L. WRAY MD, *Assistant Professor of Anesthesiology, Department of Anesthesiology, New York Hospital — Cornell Medical Center, New York, NY 10021, USA*

I. H. WRIGHT MRCP, FRCA, *Senior Registrar in Anaesthetics, South Western Regional Training Scheme, Bristol Royal Infirmary, Upper Maudlin Street, Bristol BS2 8HW, UK*

Preface

To the Second Edition

The first edition of this book was designed primarily for the anaesthetist preparing for the final part of the then FFARCS (now FRCA) examination but was also intended to provide a comprehensive source of reference for the established consultant anaesthetist. To a large extent, these aims were successful as shown by our own knowledge of the reading material of anaesthetists in training and by the sales of the text worldwide in a market which has become more competitive in the last 5 years. The success of the first edition has encouraged us to proceed with this second edition.

As scientific knowledge continues to expand, the knowledge required of the anaesthetist also increases, at times rapidly. This accounts for the relatively short interval between the appearance of this edition and the first. Also, in spite of our efforts to contain the extent of information presented, there has been a considerable increase in size of this edition. It comprises not merely an update of previous chapters, but also several new contributions, which were suggested by our own discussions and by readers of the first edition.

The basic organization of the book remains unchanged; sections are devoted to the scientific basis of clinical practice, the clinical practice of anaesthesia and its equipment, local anaesthesia, acute and chronic pain, and intensive care. There are many new authors and each chapter reflects the knowledge, insight and experience of recognized experts in their fields. To help with the increased work-load, we have co-opted a third editor, Dr David Rowbotham, to join the editorial team. His help has been invaluable in reflecting the opinion of the younger generation of examiners for the FRCA diploma.

The first section has been expanded considerably. New chapters include those concerned with non-steroidal anti-inflammatory drugs, gastric emptying and postoperative nausea and vomiting, depth of anaesthesia and awareness, anaesthetic equipment, statistics and clinical trials. Several chapters in the first edition had a wide remit and many have been divided into more specific and detailed chapters. For example, there are now individual chapters dealing with intravenous anaesthetic agents, volatile agents, anaesthetic gases, haematology, hepatic function, neuromuscular blocking drugs, and delivery systems for intravenous drugs.

In the second section mortality/morbidity and audit of anaesthesia are given more prominence in this edition, but the general structure remains the same. All chapters have been updated and many have been expanded.

We have retained the basic structure of the third section on local anaesthesia, as this proved to be particularly popular in the first edition. It is with great regret that we have to report the death of one of the most distinguished contributors to the first edition. Dr Ben Covino was an internationally acknowledged expert in the field of local anaesthesia, a pre-eminent researcher and much sought after world-wide as a stimulating lecturer. His chapter in the first edition was truly outstanding and we are grateful to Mrs L. Covino for allowing Dr J.A.W. Wildsmith to update this work.

The modifications and expansion of the fourth section, dealing with acute and chronic pain, reflect the rapid advances occurring within the specialty. An overview of all the common conditions seen in the pain clinic is given with detailed examination of the assessment of acute and chronic pain, psychological considerations and management of each type of chronic pain. Material on acute pain has been expanded considerably and there is a new chapter on analgesia in children.

All chapters covering aspects of intensive care in the final section have been carefully revised and updated. They include medical, surgical and pharmacological aspects as well as the relationship to anaesthesia of this important discipline.

Textbooks of this type represent major works of effort and organization. We are grateful to all our contributors, many of whom are international authorities in their respective fields, and all have been generous with their time in either revising their previous chapters or producing new ones. As with the first edition, the timely return of their chapters is reflected by the contemporary nature of many of the references quoted in this work. We continue to be grateful to our publishers, Blackwell Scientific Publications, and, in particular, to Miss Clare Brownhill. We also thank Drs J. Haycock, A. Ogilvy, J. Skoyles, M. Mushambi and S. Graham, and the other proof-readers, for proof-reading the text.

It may not be possible to provide within a single text *all* the knowledge required for the anaesthetist but we see a clear need for modern anaesthetic practice to be *summarized* in one text, particularly for those studying for examinations. Of the textbooks on anaesthesia currently available, we believe that this text covers the broadest range of material examined in postgraduate anaesthetic diplomas and also provides a current, readable and authoritative work for anaesthetists. If it continues to enjoy the same success as the first edition, then the efforts of the contributors, editors and publishers will have been well expended.

Walter S. Nimmo, David J. Rowbotham
1993   *and Graham Smith*

To the First Edition

Over the past decade there have been dramatic changes in the practice of anaesthesia. This is manifest not only in the practical administration of anaesthetics, but also by the progressive migration of anaesthetists into areas of medical practice outside the immediate operating room environment. Thus, the provision of obstetric analgesic services has been extended, involvement of anaesthetists in intensive care continues to expand steadily and there has emerged a new specialty of intractable pain, in which anaesthetists play a predominant role. In addition, in some countries, and especially in the UK, there has been a renaissance in local analgesic techniques which has stimulated research into this area.

As may be expected, these changes have been associated with alterations in training requirements. There has been an accompanying change in format of postgraduate examinations, at least in those con-

ducted by the Faculty of Anaesthetists of the Royal College of Surgeons of England.

This book was conceived at a time, we believe, when there was no single major textbook of anaesthesia which reflected these developments in anaesthetic practice and which provided a broad and balanced account appropriate for the new examinations.

This text was designed primarily therefore for anaesthetists preparing for the new final part of the FFARCS examination. Our aim was to provide for the first time, within a single work, virtually all the anaesthetic information required by a candidate with a sound knowledge of medicine and surgery. In attempting to achieve this objective, it follows that the text should be valuable also for all tutors and supervisors of trainee anaesthetists, and established consultants requiring a comprehensive and readily available source of reference.

Anaesthesia teaching has standards which are judged on a world stage and this work is intended to fill a gap in available texts for trainees in other English speaking nations — a glance at the list of contributors illustrates our attempts to recruit a truly international team.

The text is in five main sections for ease of reference. Section I, *The Application of Scientific Principles to Clinical Practice*, serves as a reminder to trainees of their basic science knowledge and is intended to place this information into clinical perspective. Section II is the largest section and is devoted to all aspects of *General Anaesthesia* including the design of operating rooms, and current recommendations in 1989 on handling patients with AIDS or hepatitis. This is a core section for examination preparation and it is divided into 33 chapters for ease of reading, study or reference. *Local Anaesthesia* is described in detail in Section III; this comprehensive review of all relevant aspects of the subject is unique in this type of textbook. Section IV is devoted to the management of *Acute and Chronic Pain* and once again the subject matter is detailed and comprehensive with practical — in addition to theoretical — advice. The last section contains 11 chapters describing *Intensive Care* and includes medical, surgical and anaesthetic aspects of this important field of knowledge.

The text has been prepared by a team of experts, many of whom are international authorities. Some contributors are drawn from non-anaesthetic disciplines and many are practising currently outside the UK. The majority of our authors are from the UK, but in their writing they reflect the best of practice in all countries of the world. We are grateful for the excellence of their contributions and the timely return of their chapters so that the book appears very soon after submission of manuscripts in an attempt to be as contemporary as possible. For the rapid typesetting, we are grateful to our publishers and in particular to Peter Saugman, Edward Wates and Emmie Williamson at Blackwell Scientific Publications. We are also grateful to Drs Sue Coley, Rhian Lewis, Boyd Meiklejohn, Robin Mitchell and Malcolm Parsloe for proof-reading.

The text is offered by the editors as an attempt to facilitate preparation for examinations, teaching, ward rounds or theatre sessions, or simply for the caring anaesthetist to remain contemporary in his knowledge. It represents a major effort of organization and study and also some satisfaction obtained by collaboration with distinguished men and women. If the contributors think the effort worthwhile and the reader finds the text as useful as the editors have found the project stimulating, all will be well.

Walter S. Nimmo and
1988 *Graham Smith*

Anaesthesia for Orthopaedic Surgery

P.J. McKENZIE

Modern techniques in orthopaedic surgery can do much to improve the quality of life, perhaps the most notable example being joint replacement procedures. Regional anaesthesia is often suitable for many orthopaedic operations on the limbs but general anaesthesia is still frequently employed, either as the sole technique or in combination with regional analgesia.

Anaesthetic problems may be inherently associated with the surgical procedure or may result from associated disease processes. In addition, consideration should be given to the relative advantages and disadvantages of general and regional techniques.

Hip replacement

Most patients presenting for these procedures are elderly and suffering from osteoarthritis or rheumatoid arthritis. The latter can present special problems which are discussed later in the chapter.

Joint replacement in many centres is performed in a 'clean-air enclosure' (Charnley, 1972) which, while minimizing infection risk, can create difficulties for the anaesthetist in terms of access to the patient and communication with the surgical team. The velocity of air flow causes an appreciable cooling effect which may be up to 10 times that expected in a normal operating theatre. Elderly patients are particularly susceptible. Patients should breathe warmed and humidified anaesthetic gases and should be placed on a warming water circulation mattress. In addition to monitoring patient temperature, the temperature of the mattress should be monitored independently by a thermistor probe, as some types of mattress are not completely reliable as regards temperature control and this can lead to skin burns, particularly where skin condition and perfusion are impaired. Intravenous fluids should be warmed and the patient covered with a 'space' blanket.

Limited access must be taken into account and extensions to intravenous giving sets are useful. Monitoring should include end-tidal carbon dioxide to detect air embolism at the time of prosthesis insertion and to avoid hypocapnia in elderly patients. In addition to the other routine monitors, pulse oximetry and temperature measurement are important. Some anaesthetists use direct intra-arterial pressure monitoring during hip replacement because of the profound changes in arterial pressure which can accompany insertion of the prostheses and cement (see below). Non-invasive automatic measurement of arterial pressure offers an increasingly popular alternative.

Insertion of prostheses

Total hip replacement consists of insertion of acetabular and femoral prostheses which are commonly secured with polymethylmethacrylate cement. Hemiarthroplasty procedures are also carried out where the femoral component only is replaced, with or without cement as appropriate (e.g. Thompson's prosthesis). This type of procedure is usually carried out as an emergency after subcapital fracture of the femur.

The insertion of prostheses may be associated with decreases in arterial pressure and arterial oxygen tension (Modig et al., 1975). Problems seem to occur more commonly with insertion of the femoral component and when cement is used. There is considerable debate as to the mechanism of the changes but it seems likely that a combination of factors is involved.

The liquid monomer which is a component of the cement, is known to cause hypotension and tachycardia if allowed to enter the circulation. When mixed with the powdered methylmethacrylate, an exothermic reaction occurs as the cement sets. Thus, the cement may be responsible for the decrease in arterial pressure if any remaining monomer is forced into the circulation.

Air embolus occurring when the prosthesis is impacted has been demonstrated (Michel, 1980) but venting of the medullary cavity may not reliably prevent it. Medullary contents can also be forced into the circulation and lead to fat embolus and thromboplastin release resulting in pulmonary microembolization (Modig et al., 1975).

Combinations of these factors lead to peripheral vasodilatation and decreases in arterial pressure.

Decreases in arterial oxygen tension are associated with increased pulmonary vascular resistance and pulmonary venous admixture. The reduction in Pao_2 seems to recover after about 30 min, whereas the changes in arterial pressure are usually transient but occasionally severe and can lead to cardiac arrest. Patients having Thompson's hemi-arthroplasty seem to be at particular risk.

Substantial blood loss can occur during hip replacement and postoperative losses may equal intraoperative loss. Extradural and subarachnoid anaesthesia are associated with reduced intraoperative bleeding as are techniques of general anaesthesia employing induced hypotension. However, although these techniques certainly achieve worthwhile reductions in blood loss, overall blood-loss reduction is less dramatic, as postoperative losses are substantial. For example, Keith (1977) found mean overall blood loss was 743 ml after hip replacement under extradural anaesthesia, 986 ml after general anaesthesia with halothane and 1168 ml after a neuroleptanaesthesia technique. The total blood loss associated with halothane and extradural anaesthetics were not statistically significantly different. Thorburn and colleagues (1980) found mean total blood loss using subarachnoid block to be 1001 ml, which was significantly less than the value of 1504 ml when general anaesthesia with intermittent positive-pressure ventilation (IPPV) and relaxants was used.

Ketanserin, a selective serotonin S2-receptor antagonist, has been shown to reduce intraoperative blood loss very significantly (van Ee et al., 1991). Mean blood loss was 894 ml with placebo and 454 ml with ketanserin.

Anaesthetic technique

The preoperative visit and premedication are carried out as usual and proposed procedures discussed. Clearly, if regional anaesthesia is planned this should be discussed and explained fully to the patient.

The evidence for the relative merits of general and regional techniques is reviewed in more detail by McKenzie and Loach (1986).

Regional techniques

Regional anaesthesia is a very suitable technique for hip replacement and is often combined with sedation by propofol infusion. Spinal and extradural anaesthesia reduce intraoperative blood loss and there is some evidence that elderly patients suffer less mental deterioration when hip replacement is carried out under extradural analgesia compared with general anaesthesia (Hole et al., 1980). However, Hughes and colleagues (1988) found little change in memory after spinal or general anaesthesia and indeed found 'an inexplicable but significant decrease in the ability to recognize words after spinal anaesthesia'.

An obvious advantage of a continuous extradural technique is to provide analgesia into the postoperative period although patient-controlled analgesia (PCA) is also highly effective.

Deep vein thrombosis

The most accurate method of detection of deep vein thrombosis (DVT) is ascending contrast venography (Browse, 1978). The incidence of DVT has been shown by venography to be significantly reduced when spinal anaesthesia is used, being 29% compared with 53% after general anaesthesia (Thorburn et al., 1980). This study was the first to show an effect of regional anaesthesia on DVT but was not randomized. A more recent randomized study (Davis et al., 1989) using impedance plethysmography and fibrinogen uptake test combined in some cases with venography, found the DVT incidence to be 13% after spinal and 27% after general anaesthesia — a significant difference.

Extradural anaesthesia has also been shown to be associated with a reduction in DVT (Modig et al., 1983). This study, using venography, found an incidence of DVT of 77% after general anaesthesia compared with 40% after extradural anaesthesia. (These figures are derived from the raw data in figures in the paper and are not actually stated in the text or tables.) (Chi-square analysis with Yates' correction yields $p < 0.01$.) A more detailed appraisal of the subject of DVT and anaesthesia is available (McKenzie, 1991).

Hip replacement was associated with an overall mortality at 90 days after operation of 11 deaths per 1000 operations and 23 : 1000 at one year in a study of 11 607 procedures carried out in the Oxford region, England, during 1976–85 (Seagroatt et al., 1991). This large study found ischaemic heart disease was the single most common ascribed underlying cause of death (7.7 : 1000). However, DVT and pulmonary embolism accounted for only 0.8 deaths per 1000 operations, both figures being the total over the year following operation.

It is thus important to remember that reduction of DVT incidence does not indicate that total mortality is reduced (Mitchell, 1979) and no study, to the author's knowledge, has shown that regional anaesthesia improves overall outcome in hip replacement. Any such study would have to have a huge number of patients and a very rigorous protocol.

Many surgeons use prophylactic anticoagulation, a policy which many authorities feel is a contraindication to extradural and spinal anaesthesia. Some authorities have felt subarachnoid block to be safe when low-dose heparin is employed as the method of prophylaxis. A compromise used in some centres is to withhold anticoagulants until the second postoperative day and then to start warfarin.

General anaesthesia

Light general anaesthesia may be used to supplement local analgesia. Techniques may include spontaneous ventilation with nitrous oxide in oxygen and a trace of volatile agent or infusion of propofol either as sedation (see above) or anaesthesia if appropriate. This may preserve the advantages of a regional technique while making the procedure tolerable when the patient is in an uncomfortable position.

If general anaesthesia alone is used, a technique using controlled ventilation and muscle relaxants is best in view of the considerable manipulation of the affected limb that is required. Some degree of induced hypotension may be valuable if thought to be safe for the particular patient.

In all patients, care should be taken to avoid hypovolaemia at the time of prosthesis insertion and a raised inspired oxygen tension is important at this time and for at least 30 min afterwards whether regional or general anaesthesia is employed. Some authorities feel that nitrous oxide should be withdrawn 10 min before prosthesis insertion (Loach, 1983) to avoid the expansion of any air entering the circulation. Clearly, oxygen saturation should be closely monitored in all cases. If profound hypotension occurs associated with prosthesis insertion, this should be treated with intravenous fluids, and judicious use of an α-agonist vasopressor such as methoxamine in 2-mg increments. This particular drug is especially useful in the patient with ischaemic heart disease as it has no inotropic effect and indeed has mild β-blocking action. Thus, it should not increase myocardial oxygen demand while improving

oxygen supply. However, bradycardia is a relatively frequent occurrence and judicious pretreatment with glycopyrronium or atropine is worth considering.

Knee replacement

Knee replacement is an increasingly common procedure. Much of what is described above about hip replacement applies also to knee replacement. However, many, but by no means all such procedures are carried out under tourniquet. Obviously, this reduces intraoperative blood loss to a minimum but postoperative blood losses can be significant.

Tourniquets have been shown not to increase the risk of DVT (Angus et al., 1983). As with hip replacement, extradural anaesthesia has been shown to be associated with a significant reduction in DVT incidence in comparison with general anaesthesia, with incidences of 18% and 59% respectively (Jørgensen et al., 1991). The procedure is particularly painful postoperatively and even more so if bilateral. PCA or continued extradural analgesia are particularly desirable.

If performed under general anaesthesia, these procedures do not usually require muscle relaxation and a technique using the laryngeal mask airway and spontaneous ventilation may be used.

Elective spinal surgery

For many procedures, the most common example being laminectomy, patients are in the prone position. It is extremely important that the patient is positioned to minimize venous engorgement. The abdomen should not be compressed. The legs are often dependent.

Although regional anaesthesia is employed in some centres (Silver et al., 1976), general anaesthesia is the most common technique. In view of the position and length of the procedure, a technique with controlled ventilation is the most appropriate. Tracheal tubes must be particularly carefully secured and of a non-kinking design (armoured, for example). A throat pack helps to ensure a seal if the cuff fails. The eyes must be taped and protected. Care must be taken to avoid high, mean intrathoracic pressures leading to raised venous pressure. If the legs are dependent, peripheral pooling may lead to reduction in arterial pressure.

Surgery for the correction of scoliosis

Scoliosis is abnormal lateral curvature of the spine. It

is usually idiopathic but may be the result of congenital deformities or associated with a large variety of other conditions. Of particular concern to the anaesthetist are patients with muscular dystrophies.

Procedures for the correction of scoliosis and kyphoscoliosis can be associated with major difficulties for the anaesthetist. The topic is excellently reviewed by Schofield (1983).

Careful preoperative assessment is required and often involves the opinion of cardiologists and respiratory physicians. Severe deformities are associated with marked derangement of respiratory function. Interpretation of respiratory function tests is made difficult by the fact that standing height is reduced, leading to underestimation of pulmonary restriction. Norms can be calculated by reference to arm span. Respiratory function tests may show a restrictive pattern with substantial reduction in vital capacity (VC) and total lung volume (TLV). Arterial hypoxaemia is also usual in severe deformities due to ventilation : perfusion ($\dot{V} : \dot{Q}$) inequality. An obstructive component is unusual.

If respiratory function is substantially impaired, elective ventilation may be required for several days after operation. Surgical correction of scoliosis seems mainly to arrest deterioration in lung function rather than improve it, although small improvements in arterial oxygenation and physiological deadspace have been shown. Patients with long-standing disease have pulmonary hypertension and can progress to right heart failure.

Children with muscular dystrophy are of particular concern from the cardiac point of view. Ellis (1974) feels that the anaesthetist should assume that all children with muscular dystrophy have myocardial involvement. The patient should be assessed by an experienced cardiologist. Significant cardiomyopathy is common. During anaesthesia these children are prone to arrhythmias, venous congestion and sudden cardiac arrest.

Clearly, the risks of the procedure must be balanced against the physical, psychological and cosmetic benefits.

The most common surgical procedures include Harrington instrumentation which may be preceded by Dwyer's instrumentation. Harrington rods are inserted from a posterior approach, with the patient prone. Dwyer's procedure involves shortening the convex portion of the curve by an anterior approach. This is usually performed with the patient in a lateral position and often involves a transthoracic approach.

Intubation may be difficult because of deformity and the use of a 'polio' blade may be necessary.

Blood loss may be profuse and arterial and central venous pressure monitoring is mandatory. Occasionally, where there is concern about cardiac function, the insertion of a balloon-tipped, flow-directed pulmonary artery catheter may be advisable.

In patients with myotonic dystrophy, suxamethonium should not be used as it can result in elevation of serum potassium concentration and myotonic spasm. Other muscle relaxants should be used with caution.

Wake-up test

The surgeon may request a 'wake-up' test of cord function after distraction of the spine is applied. Various methods are possible and the reader is referred to the text by Schofield (1983). A recommended technique is to use opioid premedication and then balanced anaesthesia with droperidol, increments of fentanyl, nitrous oxide and muscle relaxant. Increments of intravenous agents are withheld for about 30 min before wake-up, minute ventilation is decreased and 100% oxygen is given just prior to wake-up. A peripheral nerve stimulator is useful to check recovery of neuromuscular function. Occasionally a small dose of naloxone is required. If repeated wake-up is required, nitrous oxide may be turned on and off as required. The wake-up test may be used less frequently in future as the technique of spinal evoked potentials is becoming an accepted alternative.

During posterior spinal fusion, a pneumothorax may occur if the parietal pleura is breached.

Repair of fractured neck of femur

Although strictly speaking, this topic might be considered under 'trauma', the history of trauma may be minimal and the fracture may be pathological. The incidence of this condition has increased out of proportion to the increase in numbers of elderly people in the population and indeed, Boyce and Vessey (1985) found the true incidence in Oxford had doubled over a period of 30 years. Surgical repair of fractured neck of femur has thus become one of the most common orthopaedic procedures.

The condition mainly affects elderly people and the ratio of females to males is approximately 2 : 1. Patients frequently suffer from a variety of chronic medical conditions and are receiving multiple medications. A common feature of patients with femoral neck fracture is hypovolaemia and dehydration, which may be inadequately corrected by junior house surgeons because of fear of fluid overload. Elderly people have an impaired thirst mechanism and quite commonly are taking regular diuretic medication. There is bleeding and extravasation at the fracture site. In addition, patients often lie immobile for some time before help arrives. The final insult to fluid balance is to be fasted before anaesthesia — sometimes more than once, if cancelled from the theatre list to make way for very urgent trauma! Dehydration is very difficult to assess in elderly patients, but serum urea and electrolyte concentrations, urine output, skin turgor and dryness of the tongue are pointers, together with a careful history.

There is considerable debate about the ideal time for surgery, but between 12 and 24 h after the fracture would seem optimum, allowing time for resuscitation, investigations and cross-matching of blood. Postponement should only be for a really pressing reason which can be corrected rapidly, for example, severe hypokalaemia. An active chest infection is an indication to proceed as it tends to worsen with the patient immobile and in pain. General anaesthesia in this situation can allow effective bronchial suction and flexible bronchoscopy if necessary.

Patients with fractured neck of femur tend to be somewhat hypoxaemic when presenting for surgery. After general anaesthesia there is a further deterioration in Pao_2 (Wishart et al., 1977; McKenzie et al., 1980). This can result in severe desaturation if patients are allowed to breathe room air, particularly in the period between 5 and 10 min after nitrous oxide is discontinued (McKenzie, 1984). Early postoperative hypoxaemia has been shown to be significantly associated with confusion in patients after hip fracture repair (Berggren et al., 1987). Supplementary oxygen should thus be given *continuously* for at least 6 h after general anaesthesia, most importantly including the period during transfer from theatre to the recovery room. Patients having 'pin and plate' internal fixation procedures under spinal anaesthesia do not show any changes in Pao_2. However, especially in patients having primary hip prosthesis procedures, it is wise to administer added oxygen as reductions in Pao_2 can occur on insertion of the prosthesis (see under 'Hip replacement', p. 1029) and in association with hypotension resulting from blood loss.

Although there is a clinical impression that postoperative confusional states are less frequent when these procedures are carried out under spinal rather than general anaesthesia, this has not been confirmed by controlled studies (Riis et al., 1983; Bigler et al., 1985; Berggren et al., 1987). Berggren and colleagues

found that a history of mental depression and the use of anticholinergic drugs were the predominant risk factors for postoperative confusion and that confused patients had significantly more complications and an almost four-fold increase in length of hospital stay.

Spinal anaesthesia can present difficulties and disadvantages particularly to those inexperienced in its use in elderly patients with hip fracture. Positioning for lumbar puncture can be intensely painful for the patient and requires skilled help. Analgesic doses of ketamine, 20–30 mg, are useful. Lumbar puncture can be difficult, time-consuming and occasionally impossible. The operative procedure can outlast the block. As there is often covert hypovolaemia, arterial pressure may decrease dramatically and profoundly as the block becomes established.

Anecdotal reports exist of cardiac arrest at the time of prosthesis insertion under spinal anaesthesia. The explanation is probably that of a patient with some degree of hypovolaemia being subjected to hypotension and hypoxaemia simultaneously.

Mortality in the short term is less when spinal anaesthesia is employed (McLaren et al., 1978; McKenzie et al., 1984) but the advantage is short lived and long-term outcome is identical (McKenzie et al., 1984; Valentin et al., 1986; Davis et al., 1987). The reason for the reduction in short-term mortality is thought to be caused by reduction in thromboembolism consequent upon the reduction in incidence of DVT which has been demonstrated in this type of patient when spinal anaesthesia is used (McKenzie et al., 1985). The incidence of DVT detected by venography was found to be 76.2% after general anaesthesia for repair of femoral neck fracture compared with 40% after spinal anaesthesia. The major reason for this finding is probably reduced stasis consequent upon vasodilatation and increased limb blood flow, also associated with substantial reductions in blood viscosity (Drummond et al., 1980). General anaesthesia in contrast has been shown to reduce blood flow in the deep veins (Clark & Cotton, 1968; Kemble, 1971) and to increase blood viscosity if haematocrit remains constant (Drummond et al., 1980).

General anaesthesia

Meticulous attention to detail is probably the key to good results. When general anaesthesia is chosen, the author would recommend omitting premedication except when analgesia is required. After preoxygenation, intravenous induction with etomidate, 0.2–0.3 mg/kg, is preceded by fentanyl, 50–100 µg, to reduce the pressor response to intubation. Controlled ventilation should be adjusted to avoid hypocapnia. A low concentration of volatile agent is added. A short-acting non-depolarizing relaxant should be given only if required and then in low dose. Techniques using the laryngeal mask airway with spontaneous ventilation may also be used in suitable patients.

It has been suggested that controlled ventilation in the patient having repair of hip fracture is associated with an increase in postoperative mortality (Spreadbury, 1980). However, a randomized study comparing controlled and spontaneous ventilation techniques of general anaesthesia (Coleman *et al.*, 1988) has shown that this is not so. Careful attention was paid to ensure no residual neuromuscular block (atracurium was used if necessary and in low dose) and continuous supplementary oxygen was given after operation. Mortality rates were low for this category of patient and not significantly different between the groups up to 6 months after operation.

On balance, the author would choose general anaesthesia for the majority of patients having repair of fractured neck of femur with special attention to the points mentioned above, especially regarding postoperative oxygenation. Spinal anaesthesia can be extremely useful in certain patients, especially those with significant respiratory disease but is not a technique for the inexperienced anaesthetist. Unfortunately, postoperative chest infection is not prevented by spinal anaesthesia.

Medical conditions associated with orthopaedics

Certain conditions which present problems to the anaesthetist are associated with orthopaedic conditions.

Rheumatoid arthritis

Rheumatoid arthritis is a relatively common condition with systemic as well as joint involvement.

Airway problems may occur leading to difficult or impossible intubation. A previous anaesthetic with successful intubation should not obviate special caution about airway management. Instability of the upper cervical spine and erosion of the odontoid peg can lead to atlantoaxial subluxation. Preoperative radiographs should be taken of the cervical spine. Flexion of the neck is best avoided. The temporomandibular joint may be involved with resultant restricted mouth opening. The cricoarytenoid joints

of the larynx may also be affected and in extreme cases result in severe airway compromise. Awake intubation under local anaesthesia or the use of a fibre-optic laryngoscope may be considered.

The lumbar spine is usually spared, making spinal or extradural analgesia an option, although positioning of the patient for the block may prove difficult.

Respiratory problems may include rheumatoid nodules in the lungs and interstitial pulmonary fibrosis. Chest expansion may also be limited.

There may be anaemia, leucocytopenia or thrombocytopenia. Preoperative blood transfusion may be necessary. Amyloid may affect the kidneys.

A wide variety of drugs have been used in the treatment of rheumatoid arthritis. Prolonged use of steroids may have occurred necessitating added steroid cover for major surgery. Steroids also reduce resistance to infection and may produce multiple other problems including hypertension, hypokalaemia, osteoporosis and skin atrophy. The widespread use of non-steroidal anti-inflammatory drugs (NSAIDs) carries risks of gastrointestinal bleeding.

Haemophilia

Although haemophilia is uncommon in the population, the condition often gives rise to orthopaedic complications. Haemophilia A (the most common by far) is caused by deficiency of Factor VIII. Haemophilia B (or Christmas disease) is due to Factor IX deficiency. Von Willebrand's disease occurs in both sexes and consists of Factor VIII deficiency and platelet abnormalities.

Assessment of the haemophiliac patient must involve the Haemophilia Centre, which arranges for cover with appropriate factor.

Unfortunately, a large percentage of haemophiliacs now are HIV-positive and must be screened for this and also hepatitis B surface antigen (HBsAg) before surgery.

Extradural and spinal anaesthesia are contraindicated but some forms of local block may be safe (e.g. Bier's block).

Intramuscular injections are contraindicated although they have been given when the patient is fully 'covered' with Factor VIII. PCA by the intravenous route is ideal, or sublingual buprenorphine may be adequate.

Ankylosing spondylitis

Ankylosing spondylitis is a chronic and progressive disease. Problems for the anaesthetist arise mainly from involvement of the cervical spine leading to fixation either in the erect position 'poker spine' or flexed. In addition, there is a restrictive ventilatory defect (Zorab, 1962). Aortic regurgitation and cardiomyopathy may occur (Loach, 1983).

Intubation may be extremely difficult but may not be necessary for many procedures as the airway may be satisfactory with a face mask anaesthetic (Loach, 1983) or laryngeal mask airway. Possible solutions where tracheal intubation is mandatory include: awake intubation with local analgesia; either blind or with a fibre-optic laryngoscope, blind nasal or fibre-optic intubation under inhalation anaesthesia; intubation through a laryngeal mask airway; retrograde intubation using a wire threaded via the cricothyroid membrane (Blogg & Ward, 1983) and, as a last resort, tracheostomy. The reader is referred to Latto and Rosen (1985).

The alternative of regional anaesthesia may be hazardous if local anaesthetic toxicity occurs, as rapid intubation may be impossible. Spinal or extradural anaesthesia is probably impossible. Brachial plexus block via the interscalene or supraclavicular route may lead to phrenic nerve block or pneumothorax and may result in respiratory failure in patients with little reserve.

References

Angus P.D., Nakielny R. & Goodrum D.T. (1983) The pneumatic tourniquet and deep venous thrombosis. *Journal of Bone and Joint Surgery* **65B**, 336–9.

Berggren D., Gustafson Y., Eriksson B., Bucht G., Hansson L.I., Reiz S. & Winblad B. (1987) Postoperative confusion after anesthesia in elderly patients with femoral neck fractures. *Anesthesia and Analgesia* **66**, 497–504.

Bigler D., Adelhoj B., Petring O.U. & Pederson N.O. (1985) Mental function and morbidity after acute hip surgery during spinal and general anaesthesia. *Anaesthesia* **40**, 672–6.

Blogg C.E. & Ward M.E. (1983) Difficult tracheal intubation: improvements in trans-laryngeal guide wire technique. *Postgraduate Medical Journal* **59**, 612.

Boyce W.J. & Vessey M.P. (1985) Rising incidence of fracture of the proximal femur. *Lancet* **i**, 150–1.

Browse N. (1978) Diagnosis of deep-vein thrombosis. *British Medical Bulletin* **34**, 163–7.

Charnley J. (1972) Postoperative infection after total hip replacement with special reference to air contamination in the operating room. *Orthopaedics and Related Research* **87**, 167–87.

Clark C. & Cotton L.T. (1968) Blood-flow in deep veins of leg. Recording technique and evaluation of methods to increase flow during operation. *British Journal of Surgery* **55**, 211–14.

Coleman S.A., Boyce W.J., Cosh P.H. & McKenzie P.J. (1988) Outcome after general anaesthesia for repair of fractured neck of femur: a randomised trial of spontaneous versus controlled ventilation. *British Journal of Anaesthesia* **60**, 43–7.

Davis F.M., Woolner D.F., Frampton C., Wilkinson A., Grant A., Harrison R.T., Roberts M.T.S. & Thadaka R. (1987) Prospective, multi-centre trial of mortality following general or spinal anaesthesia for hip fracture in the elderly. *British Journal of Anaesthesia* **59**, 1080–8.

Davis F.M., Laurenson V.G., Gillespie W.J., Wells J.E., Foate J. & Newman E. (1989) Deep vein thrombosis after total hip replacement. A comparison between spinal and general anaesthesia. *Journal of Bone and Joint Surgery (Britain)* **71** (2), 181–5.

Drummond A.R., Drummond M.M., McKenzie P.J., Lowe G.D.O., Smith G., Forbes C.D. & Wishart H.Y. (1980) The effects of general and spinal anaesthesia on red cell deformability and blood viscosity in patients undergoing surgery for fractured neck of femur. In *Haemorheology and Diseases* (Eds Stolz J.F. & Drouin P.) pp. 445–51. Paris, Doin Editeurs.

Ellis F.R. (1974) Neuromuscular disease and anaesthesia. *British Journal of Anaesthesia* **46**, 603–12.

Hole A., Terjesen T. & Breivik H. (1980) Epidural versus general anaesthesia for total hip arthroplasty in elderly patients. *Acta Anaesthesiologica Scandinavica* **24**, 279–87.

Hughes D., Bowes J.B. & Brown M.W. (1988) Changes in memory following general or spinal anaesthesia for hip arthroplasty. *Anaesthesia* **43** (2), 114–17.

Jørgensen L.N., Ràsmussen L.S., Nielsen P.T., Leffers A. & Albrecht-Beste E. (1991) Antithrombotic efficacy of continuous extradural analgesia after knee replacement. *British Journal of Anaesthesia* **66**, 8–12.

Keith I. (1977) Anaesthesia and blood loss in total hip replacement. *Anaesthesia* **32**, 444–50.

Kemble J.V.H. (1971) The effect of surgical operation on leg venous flow measured with radioactive hippuran. *Postgraduate Medical Journal* **47**, 773–6.

Latto I.P. & Rosen M. (1985) In *Difficulties in Tracheal Intubation*. London, Baillière Tindall.

Loach A.B. (1983) In *Anaesthesia for Orthopaedic Patients*, London, Edward Arnold.

McKenzie P.J. (1984) Anaesthesia for repair of fractured neck of femur. A comparison of spinal and general anaesthesia. M.D. thesis, University of Glasgow.

McKenzie P.J. (1991) Editorial: Deep venous thrombosis and anaesthesia. *British Journal of Anaesthesia* **66**, 4–7.

McKenzie P.J. & Loach A.B. (1986) Local anaesthesia for orthopaedic surgery. *British Journal of Anaesthesia* **58**, 779–89.

McKenzie P.J., Wishart H.Y., Dewar K.M.S., Gray I. & Smith G. (1980) Comparison of the effects of spinal anaesthesia and general anaesthesia on postoperative oxygenation and perioperative mortality. *British Journal of Anaesthesia* **52**, 49–54.

McKenzie P.J., Wishart H.Y. & Smith G. (1984) Long-term outcome after repair of fractured neck of femur. Comparison of subarachnoid and general anaesthesia. *British Journal of Anaesthesia* **56**, 581–5.

McKenzie P.J., Wishart H.Y., Gray I. & Smith G. (1985) Effects of anaesthetic technique on deep vein thrombosis. A comparison of subarachnoid and general anaesthesia. *British Journal of Anaesthesia* **57**, 853–7.

McLaren A.D., Stockwell M.C. & Reid V.T. (1978) Anaesthetic techniques for surgical correction of fractured neck of femur. *Anaesthesia* **33**, 10–14.

Michel R. (1980) Air embolism in hip surgery. *Anaesthesia* **35**, 858−62.

Mitchell J.R.A. (1979) Can we really prevent postoperative pulmonary emboli? *British Medical Journal* **i**, 1523−4.

Modig J., Busch C., Olerud S., Saldeen T. & Waernbaum G. (1975) Arterial hypotension and hypoxaemia during total hip replacement: the importance of thromboplastic products, fat embolism and acrylic monomers. *Acta Anaesthesiologica Scandinavica* **19**, 28−43.

Modig J., Borg T., Karlstrom G., Maripuu E. & Sahlstedt B. (1983) Thromboembolism after total hip replacement: role of epidural and general anaesthesia. *Anesthesia and Analgesia* **62**, 174−80.

Riis J., Lomholt B., Haxholdt O., Kehlet H., Valentin N., Danielsen U. & Dyrberg V. (1983) Immediate and long-term mental recovery from general versus epidural anaesthesia in elderly patients. *Acta Anaesthesiologica Scandinavica* **27**, 44−9.

Schofield N. McC. (1983) Anaesthesia for spinal disorders. In *Anaesthesia for Orthopaedic Patients* (Ed. Loach A.B.). London, Edward Arnold.

Seagroatt V., Tan H.S., Goldacre M., Bulstrode C., Nugent I. & Gill L. (1991) Elective total hip replacement: incidence, emergency readmission rate, and postoperative mortality. *British Medical Journal* **303**, 1431−5.

Silver D.J., Dunsmore R.H. & Dickson C.M. (1976) Spinal anesthesia for lumbar disc surgery. *Anesthesia and Analgesia* **55**, 550−4.

Spreadbury T.H. (1980) Anaesthetic techniques for surgical correction of fractured neck of femur. A comparative study of ketamine and relaxant anaesthesia in elderly women. *Anaesthesia* **35**, 208−14.

Thorburn J., Louden J.R. & Vallance R. (1980) Spinal and general anaesthesia in total hip replacement: frequency of deep vein thrombosis. *British Journal of Anaesthesia* **52**, 1117−21.

Valentin N., Lomholt B., Jensen J.S., Hejgard N. & Kreiner S. (1986) Spinal or general anaesthesia for surgery of the fractured hip? *British Journal of Anaesthesia* **58**, 284−91.

van Ee R., & van Oene J.C. (1991) Effect of ketanserin on intraoperative blood loss during total hip arthroplasty in elderly patients under general anaesthesia. *British Journal of Anaesthesia* **66**, 496−9.

Wishart H.Y., Williams T.I.R. & Smith G. (1977) A comparison of the effect of three anaesthetic techniques on postoperative arterial oxygenation in the elderly. *British Journal of Anaesthesia* **49**, 1259−63.

Zorab P.A. (1962) The lungs in ankylosing spondylitis. *Quarterly Journal of Medicine* **31**, 267−80.

Anaesthesia for Plastic Surgery

C.E. BLOGG

Patients who present for plastic surgery range from neonates to the elderly. The majority of the plastic surgery is superficial, involving only the body surface tissues and so does not result in major tissue trauma.

General principles

Tissue perfusion versus blood loss. There is a need for a balance in trying to achieve the two goals of minimizing blood loss and yet achieving adequate tissue perfusion in potentially threatened skin or pedicle flaps.

Bleeding. When venous pressure is increased during coughing, straining, hiccuping or vomiting, increased bleeding and venous congestion result, so blood loss is increased. The viability of skin grafts and flaps may be impaired if blood accumulates under the flap. The use of such measures as induced hypotension, positioning, controlled ventilation with avoidance of hypercapnia, local vasoconstrictors (e.g. adrenaline) or tourniquets for peripheral limb surgery can all reduce blood loss. These are particularly valuable during operations on highly vascular areas.

Multiple procedures. Several operations may be required to complete the correction of lesions in plastic surgery. The risks of repeated use of some drugs, e.g. halothane, needs to be considered carefully (Blogg, 1986; Emmanuel, 1988).

Immobility of grafted or transposed tissue is necessary postoperatively. Adequate postoperative analgesia and, in some cases application of splints or plaster casts help to maintain immobility. Patient-controlled analgesia is particularly valuable.

Congenital abnormalities require correction to allow function to develop normally or to improve cosmetic appearance. For functional development, the timing of surgery may be critical, for example, finger grasp should be achieved at 6 months of age. Many patients have multiple congenital abnormalities which may influence anaesthetic management and should be sought at the preoperative visit.

Cosmetic/aesthetic surgery. Cosmetic or aesthetic surgery is rarely urgent but whilst the lesion carries no threat to life, it may have great psychological importance to the patient (Schmidt-Tinteman, 1978).

Congenital lesions

Cleft palate and cleft lip

Surgical management of these children differs; cleft lips may be repaired in the neonatal period both to restore function and to improve the appearance early to enhance the bonding process between mother and baby. In the majority of plastic surgery units, cleft lips are repaired at 3 months of age when 4.5 kg body weight and a haemoglobin of 10 g/litre have been achieved. Babies with Treacher Collins and Pierre Robin's syndromes may present extreme difficulty in intubation due to micrognathia and cleft palate. Retrograde wire intubation techniques may be necessary (Ramsay & Salyer 1981; Blogg & Ward, 1985). Preliminary fixation of the tongue to the mandible may even be required to relieve corpulmonale secondary to airway obstruction caused by glossoptosis (Wexler *et al.*, 1979). Positive upper respiratory tract bacterial cultures contraindicate surgery.

Preparation for anaesthesia includes cessation of milk feeds for 4 h with unlimited clear oral fluids being given up to 2 h before induction. Premedication comprises atropine, 0.02 mg/kg, to dry oral secretions and thus facilitate placement of the surgical gag and reduce the vagotonic effects of suxamethonium.

Opioid analgesic premedication may depress respiration and is best avoided in babies who require gaseous induction of anaesthesia. Preoperative opioids are rarely used even for babies of 6 months of age or older with normal upper airway anatomy and never for those with an abnormality which is likely to pose difficulty in intubation or ventilation. Promethazine, 3–4 mg/kg orally, provides adequate drying of secretions and sedation.

ECG and pulse oximetry (Sp_{O_2}) monitoring is begun before induction of anaesthesia. Inhalation induction with halothane or isoflurane in oxygen ensures that spontaneous ventilation is maintained even if the anatomy of the airway is abnormal. Manual ventilation with a mask and paediatric breathing system may be difficult if a close fit between mask and face cannot be achieved. When anaesthesia is sufficiently deep, an intravenous infusion is set up. Suxamethonium, 1.5 mg/kg i.v., preceded by atropine, is the agent of choice to produce rapid neuromuscular block. Injection of suxamethonium directly into the muscle of the tongue can be used if intravenous access cannot be achieved readily. A laryngoscope with a C-section blade 'bridges' the palatal defect when intubating the infant. Alternatively, the palatal gap can be filled by a gauze pack. Kink-resistant, precurved, non-cuffed tracheal tubes of predetermined length are used (e.g. RAE tube) with a throat pack. Manual ventilation with an Ayre's T-piece system (Ayre, 1956; Jackson Rees & Owen Thomas, 1966) ensures that each breath is felt by the ventilating hand and any change in compliance is detected immediately. The surgeon usually places a gag to fix the tube centrally along the tongue and to hold the mouth open. Continuous listening through a precordial stethoscope placed on the left side of the chest ensures that if the tube is pushed into the right main bronchus, the loss of breath sounds is readily detectable by the anaesthetist. A small condenser–humidifier in the breathing system helps to retain heat and moisture. Heat loss can be minimized by swaddling the baby in warmed covers with a heat-reflecting outer layer. The ambient temperature in the operating room should be maintained between 22–24°C despite the likely discomfort for the operating room staff. Maintenance of anaesthesia with nitrous oxide and halothane is usual. Measurement of expired carbon dioxide in respired gases aids in maintaining slight hypocapnia and the early detection of disconnection. Long-acting neuromuscular blocking drugs are rarely necessary.

Perioperative analgesia is produced principally by infiltration with lignocaine 0.5% solution containing adrenaline, 1:200 000, and dramatically reduces bleeding. Topical cocaine or adrenaline can also be used to reduce blood loss. Fentanyl, 1.0 μg/kg i.v., can be used to supplement anaesthesia.

General principles of paediatric anaesthesia apply — maintenance intravenous fluids are infused and blood loss is replaced when necessary. The threshold for transfusion is an anticipated blood loss likely to exceed 10% of blood volume. Blood loss is, however, difficult to estimate as much may be absorbed by the throat packs and not seen by the anaesthetist. A calibrated trap in the suction tubing reduces the uncertainty (Herbert et al., 1990).

At the end of the procedure, the patient is awakened on the operating table, to be near to assistance, as well as intubation and suction facilities. The surgeon may be asked to place a tongue stitch to pull the tongue forward in infants who have had palatal closure operations. The tracheal tube is left in place until the infant attemps to cry and is vigorous. Following extubation, the child is nursed in the tonsil position.

Postoperative care is focused initially on ensuring that added oxygen is effectively given until the child is fully awake and can maintain a clear airway. Paracetamol suppositories, 60–120 mg, placed on arrival in the recovery room are helpful in achieving analgesia during the early recovery period. Many babies become content when restored to their mothers and can be fed 2 h postoperatively.

Palatoplasty operations and revision of the cleft palate or lip repairs are commonly needed in older children. The same general principles apply as in infants.

Syndactyly

Syndactyly is often associated with other congenital lesions; there are often cardiac, palatal or other skeletal defects. Hand defects are first operated on at around 6 months of age to achieve a useful grasp, and defects of the foot are corrected after one year when walking is likely to begin.

It is difficult to monitor the patient and to gain venous access as several limbs may need to be operated upon simultaneously. However, the jugular veins are accessible and the ECG, pulse oximetry and auscultation of heart sounds through an oesophageal stethoscope can be used.

Hypospadias

This is the commonest congenital abnormality in males, and occurs in approximately 1:300 births. Surgical fashions vary in the urgency for correcting hypospadias but complete correction is expected by the age of approximately 4 years. The usual principles of paediatric anaesthesia are followed but analgesia can be enhanced by either penile or caudal block. Some surgeons prefer to place the penile block themselves and choose to avoid caudal blocks to reduce the potential for the patient requiring catheterization until bladder sensation returns.

Bupivacaine 0.25% without adrenaline in a dose of 0.5 ml/kg (maximum 2 mg/kg) is usually adequate for caudal block. For penile block, plain solutions of bupivacaine or lignocaine should be used (1–4 mls), injected 1 cm from the midline on one side deep to Buck's fascia (Soliman & Tremblay, 1978) at the base of the penis and slightly caudal and inferior to the inferior border of the pubis. Subcutaneous infiltration on the ventral surface of the penis may also be required. Adequate and early analgesia is vital to prevent the child becoming distressed in the postoperative period which would increase the risk of haematoma in the penis.

Bat ears

Children tend to present at around puberty for correction of this common problem. The incidence of postoperative vomiting may be as high as 80% for which conventional antiemetic drugs, even in combination, appear to have little effect. Local anaesthesia by a combination of preoperative EMLA cream, block of the great auricular nerve and infiltration is satisfactory for older children and eliminates the possibility of emesis.

Skin lesions and skin grafting

Congenital skin blemishes range from the small benign dermatofibroma to huge pigmented hairy naevi, which are not only unsightly but may eventually become malignant.

Infiltration with lignocaine and adrenaline at the excision site reduces blood loss and the need for deep anaesthesia or postoperative analgesia. Preoperative EMLA cream allows split-thickness skin grafts to be taken painlessly (Goodacre et al., 1988) and is preferable to injected lignocaine. Skin grafts are commonly taken from the thigh and appropriate blocks of the lateral cutaneous nerve of thigh, iliofemoral/ilioinguinal and femoral nerves before the start of surgery should remove the pain and discomfort at the donor sites in the immediate postoperative period.

Skin lesions in adults may be malignant, e.g. malig-nant melanoma, squamous or basal-cell carcinoma. It is unwise to use regional block if injection of local anaesthetic is required into an area containing the lymphatics draining from the lesion, and so supra-clavicular or interscalene block is preferable to axillary brachial block. Similarly, lumbar epidural or spinal block are more suitable than femoral nerve block for lower limb procedures.

Where skin has actually been lost, skin cover is necessary. This can be achieved by the use of flaps of skin based on vascular pedicles, which are moved into new positions. Perfusion and viability of the flaps are adversely affected by many factors (Daniel & Kerrigan, 1979) including pain, cold, increased endogenous catecholamines and reduced perfusion pressure (despite the inevitable surgical sympathetic block resulting from disruption of the nerves accompanying the blood vessels). It is important that the vascular pedicles are not compressed in the postoperative period and that the tissue can be inspected easily to assess its perfusion and viability. Skin-expansion techniques, by which a plastic bag is inserted under normal skin adjacent to the lesion and then gradually expanded by injected saline over several weeks or months, have revolutionized the potential for electively achieving skin cover. Expanders may interfere with the airway if inserted to the neck and should be deflated before attempting intubation.

Cosmetic surgery

Breast augmentation or reduction

During augmentation mammoplasty, a silastic bag containing a silicon gel is placed under the skin or, preferably, deep to pectoralis major. A small skin incision is used, and the dissection is continued through this restricted aperture; thus, it is difficult to reach blood vessels to achieve haemostasis. After mastectomy operations, an expandable prosthesis can be inserted and then gradually expanded over several weeks, then removed and replaced by a permanent prosthesis at a second operation.

In breast operations, it is important that the patient's arms are positioned accurately to ensure symmetry. Venous access may require cannulation of a leg or foot vein. The large blood loss associated with operations to reduce breast size, especially if both breasts are operated on simultaneously, can be limited by the use of moderate induced hypotension.

The benefits of surgery to change breast size appear to be related to the psychological need for change rather than the physical alteration achieved (Schmidt-Tintemann, 1978).

Rhinoplasty

The success of this operation is put at risk from bleeding. Preoperative application of cocaine solution 4% or cocaine paste vasoconstricts the nasal mucosa. Infiltration with adrenaline-containing local anaesthetic solution also reduces bleeding and permits the use of light general anaesthesia. Fifteen degrees of head-up tilt further reduces bleeding by promoting venous drainage. A precurved, cuffed oral tracheal tube (e.g. RAE) intrudes minimally into the surgical field. Throat packs are necessary to prevent blood passing into the oesophagus. An oral airway should be inserted before extubation to ensure an adequate airway as the nasal route is usually obstructed by surgical packs.

Liposuction

Liposuction is now used for removing unsightly fat from a wide range of sites — buttocks to eyelids, and can often be achieved on a day-case basis.

Reconstructive surgery

Free flaps and reimplantation surgery

Improvements in surgical techniques of anastomosis of small blood vessels and nerves allow innervated, vascularized tissue to be separated from one part of the body and then joined to existing structures elsewhere, to provide skin cover, tissue bulk or bony support. There is little published information on the anaesthetic factors which influence the viability of the transplanted tissue (Robins, 1983; MacDonald, 1985). Decrease in temperature results in vasoconstriction and must be prevented by reducing heat loss (by raising ambient temperature and conserving heat and moisture in expired gases). External heat can be supplied from warming blankets and blood-warming devices to warm intravenous fluids. Adequate tissue perfusion must be maintained. Blood pressure should be kept near normal whilst peripheral vascular resistance should be reduced (to improve blood flow) by the use of systemic vasodilators. Such drugs include α-adrenergic blockers and direct-acting vasodilators, e.g. isoflurane, hydrallazine, or infusions of nitroglycerine or nitroprusside. Thymoxamine, 40 mg orally, followed by infusion, 5 mg/h, has been also recommended (Robins, 1983).

Central venous pressure must be maintained near normal despite blood loss and vasodilatation.

Fluid balance is important and should be controlled by measurement of central venous pressure and urine output.

Plasma osmotic pressure should be maintained near normal by infusing warmed colloid solutions to replace modest blood loss. Dextran 70 may be useful in preventing venous thrombosis by inhibiting platelet aggregation and increasing fibrinolytic enzyme activity. If colloid infusion of more than 500 ml is required, preparations of hydroxyethyl starch or modified gelatins should be used. Haemodilution to a haematocrit value of 35% to reduce viscosity is accepted practice in some centres. Perioperative antithrombotic therapy with aspirin is commonly used (Salemark, 1991). Dexamethasone, 0.1 mg/kg, given prior to separation of the flap may reduce intracellular oedema. Normocapnia is likely to optimize perfusion by avoiding the vasoconstriction. Regional local anaesthetic techniques produce sympathetic block and vasodilatation and so have achieved popularity. However, grafted vessels are necessarily already sympathectomized and the effects of sympathectomy are principally seen in improved venous drainage. Some limb lesions can be managed entirely under continuous regional anaesthesia if the surgery is swift, uncomplicated and limited to one limb. Preoperative intravenous regional guanethidine block may produce prolonged sympathetic block (Davies, 1976). Studies in animals suggest that perioperative calcium-channel blocking agents (e.g. nifedipine) may benefit flap perfusion (Pal et al., 1991).

Monitoring of all accessible variables (ECG, Sp_{O_2}, systemic and central venous blood pressures, skin and core temperatures, end-expired carbon dioxide, blood loss, urine output) becomes increasingly important as the duration of surgery increases, bringing further problems in attempting to maintain the anaesthetist's concentration as fatigue progresses. Maintenance of the anaesthetist's concentration may be a problem as some operations may last as long as 20 h.

At present, there is no reliable method of predicting the viability of a tissue flap, but transcutaneous oxygen pulse oximetry (Lindsey et al., 1991) or pH electrodes, temperature probes and intravascular injection of fluorescent dyes are sometimes used to supplement clinical signs. When flaps are buried and inaccessible, implanted monitoring such as Doppler flowmeters and impedance monitors can be useful (Manktelow & Ahn, 1991).

Tissue expanders have recently reduced the need

for free-flap surgery providing there is no urgency for the treatment. Although anaesthesia is then required for two surgical procedures, the morbidity of these brief procedures is considerably reduced.

Craniofacial reconstruction

Many patients who present for reconstruction of the face and head have major congenital abnormalities and the largely cosmetic correction may be initiated within 6 months of birth. The airway may be compromised either by the procedure or the lesion itself. Forward planning and anticipation of difficulty in intubation is essential. Awake intubation or gaseous induction of anaesthesia is preferable if difficulty in intubation is expected. The anaesthetist should examine the patient and review the X-ray films, computerized axial tomograms and nuclear magnetic resonance imaging to discover other skeletal malformations around the region of the airway. Difficulties in intubation may be overcome by use of a fibreoptic laryngoscope, light wands or retrograde insertion of a wire through the larynx or trachea or intubation through a laryngeal mask airway. Elective or emergency tracheostomy may be necessary. A kink-resistant tracheal tube is used and must be securely fastened. Access to the airway may be difficult and in some procedures, e.g. frontal advancement, it may be necessary to change the tube from oral to nasal (or vice versa) in the middle of the operation (Fergusson *et al.*, 1983). Close liaison with the surgeons is vital.

Blood loss may be considerable (Uppington & Goat, 1987) and, particularly whilst bony dissection is in progress, can be reduced by induced hypotension and posture. Direct arterial blood pressure monitoring, central venous cannulation and continuous urinary drainage assist in the management of the blood replacement and fluid losses. Osmotic dehydration agents, modest drainage of cerebral spinal fluid (<5 ml/minute), corticosteroids and controlled ventilation to achieve hypocapnia are necessary to control brain volume for intracranial procedures. The procedure may take many hours and so careful positioning and protection of pressure points are required. Heat conservation is helped by warming blankets, a humidifier in the breathing system and warm coverings for the patient surrounded by metallized reflective plastic sheeting.

Postoperative care is directed to maintenance of a clear airway, adequate fluid and blood replacement and observation of the state of consciousness in case intracranial bleeding occurs.

References

Ayre P. (1956) The T-piece technique. *British Journal of Anaesthesia* **28**, 520–3.

Blogg C.E. (1986) Halothane hepatitis: the problem revisited and made obsolete. *British Medical Journal* **292**, 1691–2.

Blogg C.E. & Ward M.E. (1985) Difficult tracheal intubation. Improvements in translaryngeal guide wire techniques. *Postgraduate Medical Journal* **59**, 69.

Daniel R.K. & Kerrigan C.L. (1979) Skinflaps: an anatomical and hemodynamic approach. *Clinics in Plastic Surgery* **6**, 181–200.

Davies K.H. (1976) Guanethidine sympathetic blockade: its value in reimplantation surgery. *Lancet* **i**, 876–7.

Emmanuel E.R. (1988) Multiple anaesthetics for a malignant hyperthermia susceptible patient. *Anaesthesia* **43**, 666–70.

Fergusson D.J.M., Barker J. & Jackson I.T. (1983) Anesthesia for craniofacial osteotomies. *Annals of Plastic Surgery* **10**, 333–8.

Goodacre T.E.E., Sanders R., Watts D.A. & Stoker M. (1988) Split-skin grafting using topical local anaesthesia (EMLA): a comparison with infiltrated anaesthesia. *British Journal of Plastic Surgery* **41**, 533–8.

Herbert K.J., Eastley R. & Milward T.M. (1990) Assessing blood loss in cleft lip and palate surgery. *British Journal of Plastic Surgery* **43**, 497–8.

Jackson Rees G. & Owen Thomas J.B. (1966) A technique for pulmonary ventilation with a nasotracheal tube. *British Journal of Anaesthesia* **38**, 901–6.

Lindsey L.A., Watson J.D. & Quaba A.A. (1991) Pulse oximetry in postoperative monitoring of free muscle flaps. *British Journal of Plastic Surgery* **44**, 27–9.

MacDonald D.J.F. (1985) Anaesthesia for microvascular surgery. A physiological approach. *British Journal of Anaesthesia* **57**, 904–12.

Manktelow R.T. & Ahn D.S. (1991) Monitoring free muscle transfer. *Microsurgery* **12**, 367–72.

Pal S., Khazanchi R.K. & Moudgil K. (1991) An experimental study of the effect of nifedipine on ischaemic skin flap survival in rats. *British Journal of Plastic Surgery* **44**, 299–301.

Ramsay M.A.E. & Salyer K.E. (1981) The management of a child with a major airway abnormality. *Plastic and Reconstructive Surgery* **67**, 668–70.

Robins D.W. (1983) The anaesthetic management of patients undergoing free flap transfer. *British Journal of Plastic Surgery* **36**, 231–4.

Salemark L. (1991) International survey of current microvascular practices in free tissue transfer and replantation surgery. *Microsurgery* **12**, 308–11.

Schmidt-Tinteman U. (1978) Psychophysical and psychosocial aspects of mammaplasty. *Chirurgia Plastica (Berlin)* **4**, 103–7.

Soliman M.G. & Tremblay N.A. (1978) Nerve block of the penis for postoperative pain relief in children. *Anesthesia and Analgesia* **57**, 495–8.

Uppington J.W. & Goat V.A. (1987) Anaesthesia for major craniofacial surgery: a report of 23 cases in children under four years of age. *Annals of the Royal College of Surgeons of England* **69**, 175–8.

Wexler M.R., Kaplan H., Abu-Dalu K. & Rousso M. (1979) A dynamic fixation of the base of the tongue to the mandible using de-epithelized tongue flap in the Pierre Robin Syndrome. *Chirurgia Plastica (Berlin)* **4**, 297–301.

Anaesthesia for Abdominal and Major Vascular Surgery

A.J. CUNNINGHAM

Associated covert or overt coronary artery disease is the critical factor that influences early and late mortality after surgical attempts to correct occlusive or aneurysmal disease of the aorta, occlusive or ulcerative disease of the carotids or occlusive disease of the lower extremities. These surgical procedures may involve aortic cross clamping, major intravascular fluid shifts, endogenous catecholamine and stress hormone responses, respiratory dysfunction, incisional pain and temperature fluctuations. These multiple and cumulative physiological changes in the intraoperative and postoperative period may adversely affect outcome by inducing significant changes in myocardial oxygen supply/demand balance.

Atherosclerosis is commonly associated with arterial aneurysmal and occlusive disease. Patients presenting for major vascular surgery tend to be elderly and relatively inactive physically with a high incidence of coexisting hypertension, diabetes, chronic obstructive lung disease, renal impairment and endocrine dysfunction.

The major determinants of outcome after vascular surgery are the patient's age, degree of coronary artery disease, status of the left ventricle, presence and extent of coexisting disease states (especially cardiovascular) and surgical considerations (occlusive/aneurysmal disease) (Table 50.1).

Recent advances in the management of patients presenting for major vascular surgery include new insights into the pathogenesis of aortic aneurysm formation, an expanded number of preoperative screening tests for perioperative myocardial ischaemia and infarction and more sophisticated intraoperative techniques to assess haemodynamic function and to detect myocardial ischaemia. Outcome data, especially after carotid endarterectomy, from large prospective multicentre studies are now available. The objectives of this chapter are to highlight the clinical

characteristics of the patient population presenting for major vascular surgery; to assess the non-invasive techniques currently available for preoperative risk factor identification; and to outline the considerations surrounding intraoperative anaesthetic management and the principles of postoperative care.

Abdominal aortic reconstruction

Graft replacement therapy for abdominal aortic aneurysm (AAA) was introduced by Du Bost and associates in 1952 (Dubost et al., 1952). The early mortality (within 30 days of surgery) has declined from 10–18% in the 1950s and 1960s to 1–6% in the past decade (Cunningham, 1989a). In marked contrast, 30-day death rates may approach 70% in patients with ruptured aneurysms, depending on the severity of the haemodynamic abnormality at the time of surgery (Johansen et al., 1991). The increasing incidence of abdominal aortic aneurysms in the UK population, the tendency for familial predisposition, the rate of change in size of AAA and the relative risk of rupture are issues of increasing clinical interest.

Pathogenesis of abdominal aortic disease

Aneurysms and occlusive disease of the abdominal aorta are associated with atherosclerosis in over 90%

Table 50.1 Outcome after abdominal aortic surgery

Patient's age
Coexisting disease states
Associated coronary artery disease
Surgical considerations
   Occlusive/aneurysmal disease
   Elective/emergency surgery
   Surgical practice
   Institution, i.e. teaching/community

of patients. Other processes that may require surgical intervention include fibromuscular disease, embolic phenomenon and traumatic injury. Atherosclerotic occlusive disease may begin in childhood or early adolescence as a fatty streak with subsequent progression over the next decades to fibrous plaque formation and ultimately the development of complicated lesions (Ross, 1986). Progression of the atherosclerotic process may depend on genetic predisposition, diet, gender, smoking, diabetes and hyperlipidaemia (Lowdon & Isaacson, 1991).

Fatty streaks are minimally elevated intimal lesions composed of lipid-laden macrophages, smooth-muscle, elastin and collagen fibres. A fibrous plaque may develop within the intima of the artery. Fibrous plaques are accumulations of degenerated foam cells which form a necrotic centre and are covered by a thick layer of proliferated smooth muscle cells. With time, increasing lipid deposition, core haemorrhage and calcium deposition all expand the plaque to produce complicated lesions which may be associated with ischaemia, embolization or thrombosis of the abdominal/pelvic organs or the lower extremities. The cellular response in the evolution of atherosclerosis thus involves macrophage migration from blood to intima, intimal macrophage lipid accumulation, smooth-muscle cell migration from media to intima, intimal smooth-muscle cell proliferation, lipid-laden macrophage necrosis and organic calcium precipitation (Ross, 1990).

Familial predisposition

The tendency for AAAs to occur in families and the potential for screening high-risk individuals has been the subject of recent reports in the literature. In a 9-year prospective study of 542 consecutive patients undergoing elective AAA resection, Darling and colleagues (1989) found that 82 (15.1%) patients had a first-degree relative with an aneurysm compared to nine (1.8%) of a control group of 500 patients of similar age and sex without aneurysmal disease. A positive female marker, i.e. identification of a family with AAAs and a female member with an aneurysm — was strongly correlated with risk of rupture. A Canadian retrospective study of 305 families noted a positive history of an affected, first-degree relative in 34 (11%) families (Cole et al., 1989). Siblings of patients with an affected first-degree relative may represent a high-risk group that may benefit from a screening programme for early detection and elective management of AAA.

In a study pertaining to AAAs among first-degree relatives of 91 patients, Webster and colleagues (1991a) reported the relative risk of developing an AAA was 3.97 for fathers, 4.03 for mothers, 9.92 for brothers and 22.93 for sisters. An ultrasound study, by the same authors, of first-degree relatives of patients with AAA reported 5:20 men (25%) and 2:29 women (6.9%) over 55 years had previously undiagnosed AAA (Webster et al., 1991b). Early detection and treatment of aneurysms may be of paramount importance in reducing the morbidity and mortality rates in patients not diagnosed until rupture occurs. Siblings >55 years of patients with known aneurysms represent a high-risk group. Ultrasound screening programmes in this population may be cost-effective in the detecting of a previously unknown aneurysm for elective resection, serial observation or patient risk-factor modification by blood pressure control or drug therapy, i.e. β-adrenergic blockers to retard or prevent aneurysm growth.

Aneurysms of the abdominal aorta occur with atherosclerosis or connective tissue disorders. Detailed biochemical investigation of the changes in the smooth muscle cells, elastin and collagen components of the aortic media have been undertaken by Powell and Greenhalgh (1989). These authors noted that the elastin content of aneurysms was lower than in normal aortas. This was associated with an increase in elastase activity in the aneurysm tissues. The authors also noted that patients with a family history of aortic aneurysm had a decrease in the content of Type III collagen in the media of the aorta.

A genetic basis for aneurysm formation is the subject of continuing laboratory investigation (Tilson, 1989). Recent studies refer to substitution in the Type III procollagen gene on chromosome 2 and genes for haptoglobin α-chain on chromosome 16. The ultimate hope is that a specific gene abnormality or abnormalities will be identified that will permit earlier detection of individuals likely to have aneurysms before aneurysm formation actually begins.

Surgical indications and outcome studies

Recent UK data (Fowkes et al., 1989) suggests that there has been a steady progressive increase in deaths attributed to AAAs. Age-standardized AAA mortality rates have revealed a 20-fold increase from 2.4 to 47.1:100 000 for men and an 11-fold increase from 2.0 to 22.2:100 000 for women from 1950 to 1984. This dramatic increase may reflect greater prevalence of aortic aneurysm formation as well as advances in diagnostic techniques. Greater use of abdominal ultrasonography and computed tomographic scanning, even in the absence of specific aneurysm screening programmes, have increased the identification of previously unrecognized aneurysms. Many of these aneurysms are relatively small (<5 cm diameter) and the relative indications for surgery in these cases has been the subject of spirited editorial comment (Crawford & Hess, 1989).

Previous case-series from referral centres have indicated that the mean rate of expansion for small aneurysms is approximately 0.4–0.5 cm per year (Bernstein & Chan, 1984). In contrast, community-based screening studies in Oxford (Collin et al., 1989) and Munich (Kremer et al., 1984) have found considerably lower median rates of expansion for small aneurysms (0.13 and 0.22 cm per year, respectively). Recent population-based studies have provided new insights into the natural course of abdominal aortic disease. Nevitt and colleagues (1989) in a follow-up study of 370 residents of Rochester, Minnesota in whom an aneurysm was initially diagnosed from 1951 to 1984, noted that the diameter of the aneurysm increased by a median of 0.21 cm per year. Only 24% had a rate of expansion of 0.4 cm or more per year. The data suggested that, for aneurysms less than 5 cm in diameter, the risk of rupture was considerably lower than had been previously reported. In a study designed to examine the influence of various clinical parameters on aneurysm expansion and subsequent outcome in 73 patients with small (<6 cm diameter) AAAs initially selected for non-operative management, the need for subsequent aneurysm resection was predicted by younger age at diagnosis and larger initial aneurysm size (Cronenwett et al., 1990). Final aneurysm size was predicted by initial size, duration of follow-up, and both systolic and diastolic pressure.

Outcome

The extensive multicentre prospective study of 666 patients undertaken by Johnston and Scobie (1988) defined current North American standards for the investigation, management, morbidity and mortality for elective AAA resection and identified the clinical variables most likely to predict adverse outcome. Patients without clinical evidence of coronary artery disease had an 0.8% mortality rate from cardiac disease compared with 6.2% if any stigmata of coronary disease were present.

Numerous studies have documented long-term survival for patients who have undergone elective aneurysm resection comparable with life expectancy and quality of life of the general population. Rohren and colleagues (1988) noted no discernible differences in life style, degree of independence or productivity when 65 patients who survived ruptured AAA resection were compared with 100 who underwent elective resection. The degree of specialization of the surgeon and the pre-existing health of the patient may be the most important determinants of survival after ruptured AAA resection. Citing experience over 10 years in managing 243 patients with ruptured aneurysms, Ouriel and colleagues (1990) claimed the most significant factors affecting survival were preoperative systolic blood pressure, presence of chronic obstructive lung disease and history of chronic renal insufficiency. The absolute number of cases referred to an individual surgeon or institution may influence outcome. Members of the Cleveland Vascular Society operating on more than 25 aneurysms per year had substantially better results (mortality 2.9%) than those dealing with 10 to 25 per year (mortality 15.9%) (Campbell, 1991). While North American studies have failed to show differences, a recent report from the north of England has described substantial differences between district and teaching hospitals (Guy et al., 1990). Variations in referral patterns and intensive care staffing and facilities may have contributed to differences in outcome.

Preoperative risk assessment and management

The high prevalence of coexisting coronary artery disease, hypertension, chronic obstructive pulmonary disease, diabetes and renal impairment in relatively elderly patients presenting for abdominal aortic surgery is well documented. Myocardial infarction is responsible for 40–70% of the mortality associated with abdominal aortic surgery (Jamieson et al., 1982). A previous myocardial infarct, based on history and documented by electrocardiogram and/or enzyme changes have been reported in 40–50% of this patient population, while 50–60% have hypertension, 10–20% have angina and 10–15% have signs of congestive cardiac failure at the time of admission (Cunningham, 1989a) (Table 50.2). Recent (<6 months) myocardial infarction and current congestive heart failure have been consistently associated with an increased risk of perioperative cardiac complications (Mangano, 1990). The value of other historical predictors, e.g. angina, hypertension, old infarct and diabetes mellitus is still unresolved. Some of these conditions are of importance to the extent that they correlate with the presence of coronary artery disease

Table 50.2 Abdominal aortic surgery — coexisting disease states

Disease states	(%)
Heart disease	
Previous myocardial infarct	40–50
Angina	10–20
Congestive heart failure	10–15
Hypertension	50–60
Chronic obstructive pulmonary disease	25–50
Diabetes mellitus	9–12
Renal impairment	5–17

The range of coexisting disease (%) reported in association with abdominal aortic surgery. (Data from Cunningham, 1989a)

or congestive cardiac failure, while some appear to provide independent information regarding risk.

A thorough evaluation of the current cardiovascular status is essential. History, physical examination and routine ECG may identify a low-risk patient subgroup. Patients without previous myocardial infarction, angina, diabetes, congestive heart failure and with a normal resting ECG have been reported to be at very low risk (<1%) for major perioperative cardiac complications (Johnston, 1989). The choice among subsequent diagnostic tests is complicated by the inability of vascular surgery patients to exercise, thus limiting the usefulness of standardized exercise tolerance tests and exercise thallium tests.

The objectives of the various multifactorial risk index analyses and invasive and non-invasive tests are to identify high-risk patients, to determine the current functional status of the coronary circulation and myocardial function and to control factors associated with increased morbidity and mortality following anaesthesia and surgery.

Clinical assessment

Landmark epidemiological investigations by the Framingham group identified factors that increased the probability that an individual will develop coronary artery disease (Kannel, 1990). These risk factors include a family history of heart disease, smoking, hypertension, obesity, hypercholesterolaemia, and ECG left ventricular hypertrophy. Although each of these factors is an independent correlate of the eventual risk of developing coronary artery disease, their independent association with perioperative cardiac

complications and major vascular surgery is unknown.

A history of prior myocardial infarction (MI) has consistently been reported to be a major risk factor for perioperative cardiac morbidity (Jamieson *et al.*, 1982). In studies prior to 1983, a risk of death or recurrent infarction was reported to be about 30% in patients having surgery within 3 months of an MI and about 15% in patients having surgery between 3 and 6 months after an infarct (Steen *et al.*, 1978).

More recently, lower reinfarction rates (attributed to more intensive monitoring and treatment in the intraoperative and postoperative period), have been reported in patients who have had surgery within 3 months of infarction (Rao *et al.*, 1983). The risk of reinfarction or death may be influenced less by whether the infarction was associated with a Q-wave (rather than the cardiac functional status before infarction), the presence of left ventricular failure at the time of infarction, and subsequent ventricular ectopy and an ejection fraction less than 0.40 after infarction (The Multicentre Post-infarction Research Group, 1983). Shah and colleagues (1990) studied 275 patients with prior myocardial infarction and assessed the relation between infarction/surgery-time interval and perioperative myocardial reinfarction. The urgency of operation and aortic or vascular procedures were the only variables that approached, but failed to achieve statistical significance. Rivers and colleagues (1990) reported on 30 patients requiring urgent or emergency vascular procedures in the first 6 weeks after a myocardial infarction (median 11 days). There were three cardiac-related deaths and two non-fatal reinfarctions.

The independent importance of stable angina as a preoperative risk factor is controversial, with the weight of data suggesting an increase in risk but not to the extent associated with a recent MI. Although data on outcome of vascular surgery in patients with unstable angina is limited, the assumption is that unstable angina carries a far higher risk than stable angina (Goldman, 1991).

Hypertension is a common finding in patients presenting for major vascular surgery. Most studies of cardiac risk in non-cardiac surgery have not found hypertension to be a major independent predictor of cardiac events, especially after controlling for pre-existing coronary disease or left ventricular failure (Goldman & Caldera, 1979). Asymptomatic hypertensive patients [with diastolic pressures below 14.6 kPa (110 mmHg) and systolic pressures below 23.9 kPa (180 mmHg)], however, are more likely to develop perioperative blood pressure lability. Cardiac arrhythmias are associated with more extensive coronary artery disease and left ventricular dysfunction. In the perioperative period, a history of frequent premature ventricular contractions, and a rhythm, other than sinus on the preoperative ECG have been associated with an increased risk of cardiac complications. These arrhythmias appear to be markers of the severity of the underlying cardiac disease (Rivers *et al.*, 1990).

Multivariate risk-factor analysis

In 1977, Goldman and colleagues proposed a cardiac risk index (CRI) to estimate the probability of a life-threatening complication (ventricular tachycardia, cardiogenic pulmonary oedema and/or myocardial infarction) or death during or following non-cardiac surgery. Nine independent statistically significant factors were noted, and each was assigned a points score based on its importance in a multivariate analysis.

The most significant prognostic factors were signs of congestive cardiac failure, recent myocardial infarction, arrhythmias and age greater than 70 years. Jeffrey and colleagues (1983) reported that the CRI underestimated the risk in 99 patients undergoing aortic aneurysm surgery but it still stratified patients into high-, moderate- and low-risk groups. The CRI assigns a low score to the type of surgery being performed, which may fail to reflect the profound haemodynamic derangements associated with aortic vascular surgery. The Goldman CRI may correlate with long-term survival inpatients undergoing elective abdominal aortic surgery. Recent data highlighted the adverse survival associated with CRI Classes III—IV status, cardiac and cerebrovascular disease, and renal impairment in long-term follow-up studies (White *et al.*, 1988). Goldman used the multifactorial CRI to estimate the probability of cardiac complications in patients having AAA surgery. By multiplying the prior odds of complications by the likelihood ratio for each class, the approximate risk of major cardiac complications increased from 3% in Class I to 75% in Class IV patients (Goldman, 1987).

The advantages of multivariate risk-factor analysis are that the methods utilize standard clinical ECG and X-ray findings, are inexpensive and are widely applicable to patient populations. The disadvantages are that individual asymptomatic patients with significant coronary artery disease may not be detected.

Acute myocardial infarction and other complications of ischaemic heart disease account for 60—70% of perioperative mortality and 35—70% of all late deaths following AAA resection. In a comprehensive literature review, including cumulative analysis of 4642 patients reported in six large series, perioperative cardiac events (myocardial infarction, ischaemia, arrhythmia or congestive heart failure) averaged 1.7% in patients without, compared with 11% in patients with clinically evident coronary artery disease (Hertzer *et al.*, 1987). Given the documented impact of ischaemic heart disease on the mortality and morbidity associated with AAA repair, it is imperative that the potentially high-risk cardiac patient be identified before surgery. Patients at high risk are typically older with known coronary artery disease (typical angina or previous MI) with symptoms or signs of left ventricular dysfunction (history of congestive heart failure, rates, S3 gallop or jugular venous distension). A decision to proceed with laboratory testing should be made only after the risk of non-cardiac surgery and the patient's clinical-risk profile have been considered. Preoperative laboratory testing is useful in stratifying risk in patients at medium or high clinical risk (Eagle & Boucher, 1989).

Non-invasive assessment

In 1984, the first of a series of studies addressed the prognostic value of specialized preoperative cardiac testing. Exercise stress testing, ambulatory electrocardiographic monitoring, radionuclear and dipyridamole thallium imaging were all evaluated over the next 6 years and were advocated for use in patients undergoing major vascular surgery. The results are, however, preliminary and the efficacy/cost-effectiveness of these procedures remains controversial.

Exercise testing

The classical ECG manifestation of ischaemia on exercise stress testing is ST-segment depression, which is indicative of subendocardial ischaemia. ST-segment elevation may represent transmural ischaemia or regional wall motion abnormality associated with a previously infarcted area (Sheffield, 1988). Arrhythmias, in the absence of chest pain or ECG evidence of ischaemia, are not considered a positive result for ischaemia. The absence of a rise in blood pressure or an absolute fall in systolic blood pressure, implies significant myocardial dysfunction, which may be secondary to ischaemic heart disease.

ECG-monitored exercise testing has been proposed as a cost-effective, easily applicable means of screening for asymptomatic coronary artery disease in patients presenting for major vascular surgery. Cutler and colleagues (1981) noted that 30% of patients with no previous history of myocardial infarction or angina and with a normal ECG will manifest an ischaemic event during or following exercise. Proponents of exercise testing claim that an ischaemic response — defined as 1 mm or greater ST-segment depression, arrhythmia or intractable angina — is a useful predictor of perioperative cardiac complications. Patients able to achieve greater than 85% of their predicted maximum heart rate at high, maximal oxygen uptake may represent a low-risk group for major vascular surgery. The ability of vascular surgery patients to participate in exercise studies may be hampered by claudication, arthritis and amputation, while digitalis, diuretic and β-blocking agent administration may cause difficulties of ECG interpretation. In addition, limited sensitivity and low specificity have been reported for exercise testing. False-positive tests may be encountered in patients with repolarization abnormalities, i.e. Wolffe−Parkinson−White syndrome. The advent of more sensitive and specific screening tests of cardiac performance have relegated the importance of exercise testing in the preoperative assessment of major vascular surgery patients.

Ambulatory ECG monitoring

Continuous 24-h ambulatory ECG monitoring, utilizing both inferior and lateral leads, has become a valid and reproducible technique to detect myocardial ischaemia (Cohn, 1988). Recent data indicates that the majority of myocardial ischaemic episodes are silent and are not associated with chest discomfort, exercise or increases in heart rate (Knight *et al.*, 1989). Preliminary evidence suggests that ischaemia detected by ambulatory monitoring independently predicts the risk of cardiac events in patients with stable and unstable angina pectoris. Recent data suggest that preoperative ambulatory ECG monitoring used to detect episodes of myocardial ischaemia is a useful assessment of cardiac risk in patients undergoing major vascular surgery (Pasternack *et al.*, 1989); in particular, the absence of myocardial ischaemia during monitoring indicates a very low operative risk.

Ambulatory ECG monitoring has been prospectively evaluated by Raby and colleagues (1989) in 176 consecutive patients undergoing elective vascular surgery to determine the value of preoperative ischaemia to predict a postoperative cardiac event. Of the 32 patients with ischaemia before surgery (mostly silent), 12 had postoperative cardiac events. Only one postoperative event occurred among 144

patients who did not have preoperative ischaemia (sensitivity of preoperative ischaemia was 92%; specificity 88%; predictive value of positive result 38%; predictive value of negative result 99%). Pasternack and colleagues (1989) studied 200 major vascular surgery patients and showed the occurrence of silent myocardial ischaemia and angina were the only significant predictors of perioperative myocardial infarction. Continuous ambulatory ECG in the perioperative period has been used to monitor 108 patients with known cardiovascular disease undergoing non-cardiac surgery (McHugh *et al.*, 1991). The mean duration of ischaemic ST segments was increased significantly in those patients with treated hypertension. Preoperative ischaemia and postoperative systolic arterial pressure were significant correlates with postoperative myocardial ischaemia.

Because of the high incidence of coronary heart disease in patients undergoing major vascular surgery, ambulatory ECG monitoring may offer the appropriate combination of sensitivity and specificity to make it part of the routine preoperative evaluation of this patient population (Fig. 50.1). Perioperative

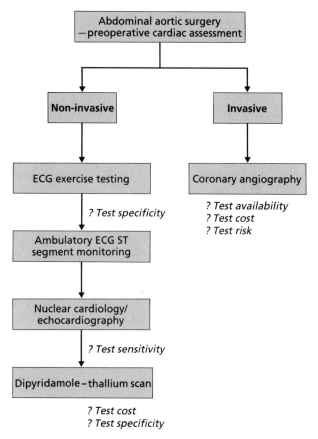

Fig. 50.1 Abdominal aortic surgery — preoperative cardiac assessment.

monitoring for silent myocardial ischaemia may non-invasively identify those patients undergoing major vascular surgery who are at increased risk for perioperative myocardial infarction, permitting implementation of timely preventive measures in selected patients. Such Holter monitoring may have several advantages over other laboratory tests, including lower costs and wider availability. The major drawbacks with ambulatory ECG monitoring is the fact that 10% or more of patients have underlying ECG abnormalities that limit or preclude the interpretation of ST segment depression.

Nuclear cardiology and echocardiography

The use of ejection fraction (EF), the ratio of stroke volume (SV) to ventricular end-diastolic volume (EDV) has become well accepted as a clinically useful quantitative measurement of left ventricular performance. Although EF is clearly afterload-dependent, and arguably preload-dependent, the measurement of left ventricular EF, in the absence of valvular incompetence, is easily performed as a 'first-pass' or multigated equilibrium scanning technique. Combined with reasonable clinical judgement, the use of left ventricular EF has become established as a good clinical estimate of left ventricular function (Robotham et al., 1991).

The initial application of cardiac radionuclide assessment (RNA) to patients presenting for major vascular surgery was optimistic. Resting RNA determination of left ventricular ejection fraction (LVEF) was reported to predict perioperative myocardial infarction rates in patients presenting for abdominal aortic aneurysm resection and lower limb revascularization. No patients with LVEF >56% sustained perioperative MIs (Pasternack et al., 1985). Kazmers and colleagues (1988) reported a cumulative mortality rate of 50% in patients with LVEF <35% compared with 14% in those with LVEF >35% over a 20.2 ± 11.9-month study period.

In recent years, the value of preoperative resting LVEF in predicting left ventricular performance during elective aortic surgery has been questioned. Preoperative knowledge of LVEF, as determined by multiple unit gated acquisition angiography (MUGA) scan, did not predict the haemodynamic performance during abdominal aortic surgery (Grant et al., 1990). Recent data suggest that resting ejection fraction is a poor predictor of perioperative myocardial infarction in patients undergoing major vascular surgery (Franco et al., 1989).

RNA may not be sufficiently sensitive to discriminate patients with normal coronary arteries from those with significant coronary artery disease. Preoperative exercise radionuclide scanning may prove more informative in patients with coronary artery disease. Exercise RNA testing may better predict perioperative mortality rate and suggest further cardiac evaluation. An LVEF of less than 50% at rest with abnormal myocardial contractility and/or an increase of LVEF of less than 5% following exercise should suggest surgical deferral pending coronary angiography (Jain et al., 1985).

Two-dimensional echocardiography can provide an accurate qualitative assessment of left ventricular wall motion and ejection fraction. The accuracy of two-dimensional echocardiography for estimating left ventricular function sometimes obviates the need for the somewhat more precise, but generally more expensive, measurements that can be obtained by radionuclide ventriculography. In addition, Doppler echocardiography may provide accurate estimates of valvular regurgitation and intracardiac shunts.

Dipyridamole—thallium scanning

Preoperative exercise stress testing is an additional objective means of functional assessment before major vascular surgery. The primary limitation of exercise stress testing cardiovascular assessment in this patient population is the patient's inability to undergo adequate physical exertion. Such limited exercise performance, in turn, substantially reduces the sensitivity of stress testing and hence its potential prognostic value. Non-physiological stress testing by means of dipyridamole—thallium-201 scintigraphy (DTS) offers an alternative evaluation of the patient unable to exercise because of vascular, orthopaedic, neurological or other general medical limitations.

Dipyridamole, an antiplatelet vasodilator, should increase blood flow in normal coronary arteries, but not in stenotic arteries that are not able to dilate or infarcted myocardium. Segments of stenotic coronary arteries will have lower concentrations of thallium-201 (cold spot) isotope after dipyridamole infusion. A redistribution or reversible thallium defect on delayed imaging 2–4 h later indicates myocardial ischaemia, whereas the presence of a persistent defect suggests the presence of infarction.

Two groups of investigators have found that reversible defects seen on preoperative thallium scanning can identify those patients undergoing major vascular surgery who are at high risk of adverse cardiac outcomes (Eagle et al., 1987; Leppo et al., 1987). Sensitivities in excess of 85% in detecting significant coronary disease were reported. The current role of DTS in the preoperative evaluation of patients undergoing major vascular surgery has been the subject of recent comprehensive investigations and reviews. The early studies were unblinded and uncontrolled. Mangano and colleagues (1991) re-evaluated DTS as a preoperative screening test for perioperative ischaemia and infarction. In a prospective blinded study of 60 patients undergoing major vascular surgery, the sensitivity of DTS for perioperative ischaemia and adverse outcome ranged from 40–54%. The authors suggested that changes in clinical management, i.e. surgery cancelled or modified, the use of invasive monitoring, nitroglycerine therapy and longer ICU stay may have biased earlier studies. Pohost (1991) in an accompanying editorial, challenged the conclusions of Mangano's provocative study by questioning the exclusion criteria and outcome parameters used in the study. The editorial concluded with an unqualified 'yes' to the question posed 'Dipyridamole–thallium test – is it useful for predicting coronary events after vascular surgery?'

The major problem with DTS is its relative lack of specificity (50–80%) and its low predictive value of 15–50% (identifying the presence of coronary abnormalities) because of the large number of false positives. Such patients may be referred for unnecessary invasive testing and revascularization, which may increase patient risk (Zellner et al., 1990; Strawn & Guernsey, 1991). In a population with a relatively low predicted event rate, a screening test should have, in addition to high sensitivity, sufficient specificity and positive predictive value to minimize the number of false positives.

Combining clinical markers and preoperative dipyridamole–thallium imaging was evaluated by Eagle and colleagues (1989) in 200 patients undergoing major vascular surgery. Logistic regression identified five clinical predictors (advanced age, angina, diabetes, Q-waves and history of ventricular ectopic activity) and two dipyridamole–thallium predictors of postoperative events. Of patients with none of the clinical variables, only 3.1% had ischaemic events in contrast with 50% ischaemic events in patients with three or more clinical markers. The multivariate model, using both clinical and thallium variables, showed significantly higher specificity at equivalent sensitivity levels compared with models using clinical or thallium variables alone. The majority of DTS studies reported have used the intravenous form of the drug, which is still not available in the US for general use. Encouraging reports have been recently published on the use of oral DTS as a

screening test to identify cardiac complications following major vascular surgery (Mackaroun et al., 1990).

Tischler and colleagues (1991) evaluated the role of dipyridamole echocardiography in predicting major cardiac events among 109 unselected patients undergoing elective major vascular surgery. A positive test was defined as development of new regional-wall-motion abnormalities or worsening of pre-existing wall-motion abnormalities. The reported sensitivity and specificity of dipyridamole echocardiography for predicting cardiac events was 88 and 98% – significantly higher than reported with DTS. In addition, the test may be performed in 20 min.

To improve specificity, Lette and colleagues (1989) and Levinson and colleagues (1990) recently developed semiquantitative scoring systems that combine dipyridamole-induced reversible ventricular dilatation with scintigraphic indices for severity and extent of reversible perfusion defects. Determining the extent of redistribution by dipyridamole–thallium-201 allowed patients to be classified into intermediate and high-risk subgroups. Patients with greater number of coronary territories showing thallium-201 redistribution are at higher risk for ischaemic cardiac complications. In contrast, when the extent of the thallium redistribution is limited, the adverse cardiac event risk is low.

Invasive assessment

Coronary angiography

Routine coronary angiography to determine the presence and severity of severe coronary artery disease has been recommended for all patients under consideration for elective vascular reconstruction at the Cleveland Clinic since 1978. Those found to have severe, correctable coronary artery disease were advised to undergo myocardial revascularization before major vascular surgery. This, and other institutions performing routine coronary angiography prior to abdominal vascular surgery reported that, of those patients considered clinically and electrocardiographically free of coronary artery disease, 15–30% have greater than 70% stenosis of one or more vessels (Hertzer et al., 1984). Following the initiation of a policy of routine coronary angiography, early encouraging reports highlighted low mortality rates in patients having elective aortic reconstruction following myocardial revascularization. However, recent Cleveland Clinic studies report a 5.7% mortality rate among 70 coronary artery bypass grafts (CABG) in patients with infrarenal aortic aneurysms. The incidence of aneurysm rupture after cardiac surgery was 2.9% and mortality rates for aneurysm repair after bypass grafting was 1.8%. Routine preoperative coronary angiography was not associated with obvious clinical benefits at the Cleveland Clinic and is no longer standard practice (Beven, 1986).

Coronary angiography, while the most specific and sensitive assessment of coronary artery disease, may not be a widely applicable screening test for all patients scheduled for aortic vascular surgery because of inherent risk, cost and manpower implications.

The selective application of coronary angiography in patients with positive preoperative non-invasive screening for coronary artery disease may be a safer and more cost-effective means of lowering perioperative mortality.

Preoperative evaluation and clinical management

Preoperative evaluation of patients undergoing major vascular surgery involves evaluation, diagnosis and risk factor stratification. Aggressive medical management, further cardiac evaluation and a modification or avoidance of the planned operative approach may be required if significant coronary artery disease and impaired myocardial function is detected on preoperative clinical evaluation and screening tests. An algorithm for patient management and surgical selection is suggested in Fig. 50.2. Patients may be divided into four classes.

Class I. Patients with no angina, previous myocardial infarct, congestive heart failure, cerebrovascular disease or diabetes and with a normal resting ECG may proceed to surgery with the expectation of very

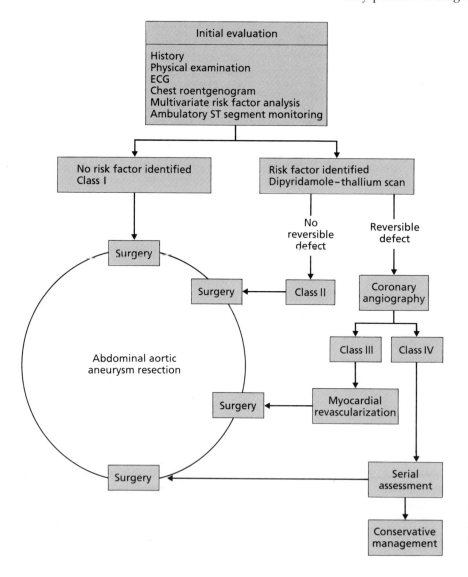

Fig. 50.2 Algorithm for patient management and surgical selection — abdominal aortic aneurysm resection.

low cardiac risk (Johnston & Scobie, 1988). Raby and colleagues (1989) noted a high negative predictive value (99%) with preoperative ambulatory ECG monitoring for ischaemia in such unselected patients undergoing major vascular surgery.

Class II. Patients with abnormalities on routine clinical evaluation but no myocardial redistribution on DTS should also proceed to surgery with the expectation of low perioperative cardiac morbidity. DTSs are most useful in stratifying patients who by clinical evaluation are in a moderate-risk group (Eagle *et al.*, 1989). Patients without redistribution have low cardiac complication risk.

Class III. Patients with clinical coronary disease and extensive myocardial segments and coronary territories showing thallium redistribution are at higher risk for ischaemic cardiac complications. For these patients, with high clinical-risk profiles and abnormal DTS, coronary angiography and myocardial revascularization before major vascular surgery may be warranted. This approach has been reported to reduce significantly the risk of perioperative infarction during the subsequent abdominal aortic surgery (Hollier *et al.*, 1984).

Class IV. Myocardial revascularization may not be possible in patients with diffuse small-vessel coronary artery disease and poor left ventricular function. For such high cardiac-risk patients, a conservative policy of serial 3-monthly ultrasound or CT assessment may be adopted, with selective resection of rapidly expanding aneurysms or if symptoms develop (Bernstein & Chan, 1984).

Haemodynamic changes with aortic cross-clamping and unclamping

The haemodynamic consequence of aortic cross-clamping will be influenced by the preoperative coronary circulation and myocardial function, the site of cross-clamp application, the intravascular volume, the anaesthetic technique and agents employed and the surgical pathology, i.e. the collateral circulation around the site of occlusion (Cunningham, 1989a). Aortic cross-clamping reduces or abolishes blood flow to the pelvis and lower extremities distal to the clamp. The anticipated consequences of an abrupt aortic cross-clamping include an increased impedance to ventricular ejection (afterload), a decreased venous return (preload) and decreased velocity and shortening of myocardial muscle fibres (Sonnenblick & Downing, 1963).

Experimental studies with isolated papillary muscle as well as the intact heart have shown that the velocity and extent of systolic myocardial fibre shortening are inversely related to the force generated by the muscle fibre during systole (Clark & Stanley, 1991). For the intact left ventricle, the stress developed in the myocardium during systole represents the ventricular afterload. As defined by Laplace's relation (pressure = 2 tension/radius), the principal determinants of afterload are the ventricular radius and systolic intraventricular pressures.

Venous return is decreased due to exclusion of the venous system in the pelvis and lower extremities from effective perfusion pressure (Attia *et al.*, 1976). Left ventricular end-systolic volume is increased by the same volume that stroke volume declines. The left ventricular end-diastolic volume is determined by the relative reduction in venous return and the increased end-systolic volume. Left ventricular filling pressures are usually unchanged or slightly reduced in patients with adequate coronary circulation and ventricular function. The haemodynamic consequences of aortic cross-clamping have been evaluated also in extensive clinical studies. Clinical reports have consistently demonstrated a 15–35% reduction in stroke volume and cardiac index, coupled with an increased arterial blood pressure and up to 40% increase in systemic vascular resistance (Cunningham, 1989a).

Myocardial function

The patient's preoperative cardiac status and myocardial reserve may exert a profound influence on the haemodynamic responses to aortic cross clamping. Very different responses to cross-clamping in patients with and without coronary artery disease have been observed (Attia *et al.*, 1976; Gooding *et al.*, 1980). Patients with impaired myocardial contractility and ischaemic heart disease developed signs of acute left ventricular decompensation and pump failure after infrarenal aortic cross clamping. These adverse outcomes may be manifested by significant reductions in stroke volume and cardiac output, an acute rise in pulmonary artery occlusion pressure (PAOP), and ECG or echocardiographic signs of myocardial ischaemia.

Extensive evaluations of left ventricular function during aortic cross-clamping have been reported using systolic time intervals, nuclear ventriculography and two-dimensional transoesophageal echocardiography. Kalman and colleagues (1986), using perioperative nuclear ventriculography, demonstrated impaired myocardial performance (the relationship between cardiac index and end-diastolic volume index) and systolic function (the relationship between systolic blood pressure and the systolic volume index) suggesting impaired myocardial contractility following cross-clamping. The haemodynamic consequences of aortic cross-clamping may vary greatly depending on the site of clamp application. Roizen and colleagues (1984), using two-dimensional transoesophageal echocardiographic studies, reported significant increases in left-ventricular end-systolic and end-diastolic volumes, decreases in ejection fraction and frequent wall-motion abnormalities with clamping at the supracoeliac level. Ryan and colleagues (1991) reported no significant changes in echocardiographic LVEF after infrarenal aortic cross-clamping. The extent of collateral circulatory changes in patients with aortoiliac occlusive disease has been proposed as the mechanism for a different haemodynamic response to aortic cross-clamping compared to patients with abdominal aortic aneurysms (Cunningham et al., 1989). Gelman and colleagues (1988) have shown that, in the absence of an acute rise in PAOP, reduction in cardiac output after aortic cross-clamping may not represent cardiac failure but rather a physiological adaptation to the reduction in total body oxygen consumption (Vo_2).

In summary, the pathophysiological consequences of aortic cross-clamping may include acute left ventricular strain or failure; myocardial ischaemia; hypoperfusion of the kidneys, spinal cord and intestine; and the accumulation of acid metabolites in the tissues below the clamp.

Aortic unclamping

During infrarenal aortic cross-clamping, the lower extremities and pelvis undergo ischaemic vasodilatation and vasomotor paralysis. Although systemic vascular resistance and arterial blood pressure decrease following unclamping, the consequent changes in cardiac output are dependent on the intravascular volume at the time of cross-clamp release. The magnitude and direction of the cardiac output changes, and the increased blood flow to the lower extremities and pelvis may cause diversion of flow from the coronary, renal and hepatic vascular beds.

Two postulates have been advanced to account for the reduction in blood pressure commonly observed following declamping (Clark & Stanley, 1991). Older data suggest that myocardial depression is caused by the wash-out of acid, acid metabolites, myocardial depressant and vasoactive substances from the ischaemic pelvis and extremities when blood flow is restored (Lim et al., 1969; Brant et al., 1970). This hypothesis has been largely discredited in recent years. Transoesophageal echocardiographic studies suggest that reactive hyperaemia in the newly revascularized areas decreases total vascular resistance, venous return and blood pressure (Roizen et al., 1984). Unclamping hypotension probably results from hypovolaemia (pooling of blood in capacitance vessels). Prevention of unclamping hypotension and maintenance of a stable cardiac output is achieved best by volume loading to a pulmonary artery occlusion wedge which is 0.53–0.8 kPa (4–6 mmHg) higher than the baseline value prior to induction of anaesthesia (Cunningham et al., 1989). When the PAOP is increased to a level that ensures optimal ventricular performance (the more horizontal portion of the Starling curve), cardiac output may change little after declamping.

The kidney

Abdominal aortic surgery exerts profound effects on renal blood flow and function. Aortic dissection, surgical manipulation, infrarenal aortic cross-clamping, reductions in cardiac output and blood pressure may all contribute to produce a consistent reduction in renal cortical blood flow, glomerular filtration rate and urine output. Aortic cross-clamping is associated with renin release and an elevated plasma concentration of renin and angiotensin following surgery (Cunningham, 1989a).

Inconclusive experimental and human studies have been published on the effects of infrarenal aortic cross-clamping on renal perfusion and intrarenal blood-flow distribution. Using xenon-wash-out techniques to measure the distribution of intrarenal blood flow, Abbott and colleagues (1973) demonstrated decreased cortical blood flow during aortic cross-clamping. Gamulin and colleagues (1984) demonstrated profound and sustained alterations in renal haemodynamics using Cr EDTA and I-145 Hippuran clearance techniques. Despite stable cardiovascular variables, infrarenal aortic cross-clamping was associated with a 38% decrease in renal blood flow and a 75% increase in renal vascular resistance. However, microsphere renal studies have demonstrated no change in the distribution of renal blood flow if adequate intravascular volume and a stable cardiac output are maintained. Failure to standardize species and study methods, cardiovascular variables and intravenous hydration, have complicated comparisons of published data.

Despite improvements in patient selection, anaesthetic management and surgical techniques, a 0.2–3% incidence of acute renal failure following elective surgery has been reported. This complication is more frequent in patients with ruptured aneurysms who sustain significant hypotension and those in whom suprarenal aortic cross-clamping is required (Stein et al., 1972). Despite aggressive management, mortality rates approaching 25% may follow renal failure (McCoombs & Roberts, 1979). Diminished preoperative renal function, advanced age, iodinated contrast material injection, inadequate balanced salt replacement of the extracellular fluid deficit caused by angiography, mechanical bowel preparation and fasting, may all contribute to impaired renal function following surgery.

Predisposing causes of acute renal failure following aortic vascular surgery include hypotension, large volumes of blood transfusion, atheromatous plaque embolization to renal arteries, intravascular myoglobin and other by-products of muscle ischaemia, and suprarenal aortic cross-clamping with normothermic ischaemic time. Recently, it was suggested that infusion of verapamil into the renal arteries just before reperfusion may be beneficial (Miller & Myers, 1987). Albert and colleagues (1984) have shown that, although intraoperative urine output does not predict the level of postoperative renal function, renal insufficiency is unlikely if urine output remains at or above 60 ml/h. The role of diuretic therapy to improve renal perfusion or minimize nephrotoxic effects is controversial. Mannitol, an osmotic diuretic, may be beneficial in preserving renal function in aortic surgery when transient hypovolaemia develops. High-dose mannitol, 12.5–50 g, may improve renal cortical flow, may reduce renal cell swelling following total ischaemia and, in the presence of a contracted intravascular volume, may prevent sludging of cellular debris in the renal tubules. Combinations of mannitol, frusomide, 5–50 mg, and infusions of low-dose dopamine, $1-3\,\mu g \cdot kg^{-1} \cdot min^{-1}$, have been advocated to prevent renal dysfunction during aortic vascular surgery (Paul et al., 1986). However, much of the data supporting the proposed benefit of these measures come from animal experiments in which deliberate extracellular fluid expansion was not employed.

A preoperative balanced salt solution infusion to replace extracellular fluid deficit associated with fasting, angiography and bowel preparation, mannitol, 12.5 g, before aortic cross-clamping coupled with aggressive and prompt intraoperative hydration and blood loss replacement, will best ensure adequate urine output and normal renal function following abdominal aortic surgery.

The spinal cord

Paraplegia is an uncommon but devastating consequence of thoracic, thoracoabdominal or even abdominal aortic reconstructive surgery. The blood supply to the spinal cord is derived from a single anterior spinal artery and paired posterior spinal arteries that span the length of the spinal cord. The spinal arteries receive collateral blood flow along their course, including branches of the vertebral artery, multiple segments of the intercostal and lumbar arteries and the internal iliac arteries. The artery of Adamkiewicz, or greater radicular artery, which usually originates from an intercostal branch between T8 and L2, provides the major blood flow to the anterior spinal artery and distal spinal cord (Wadouh et al., 1984).

Spinal cord damage or untoward events associated with aortic vascular surgery may follow translumbar abdominal aortography during the surgical intervention. In an extensive review of 3164 procedures with temporary occlusion of the abdominal aorta, Szilagri and colleagues (1978) reported a 0.25% incidence of spinal cord damage following abdominal aortic surgery, and a 0.01% incidence following translumbar aortography. The incidence of spinal cord damage was 10 times more prevalent in ruptured, compared to unruptured, aneurysms and no spinal cord damage was associated with surgery for aortoiliac occlusive disease. The most common neurological deficits noted were complete flaccid paraplegia with dissociated sensory loss.

The expected incidence of lower limb neurological events vary according to the extent and cause of the aneurysm. Patients with most or all of the descending thoracic abdominal aorta down to the renal arteries are classified as Type I; most or all of the descending and most or all of the abdominal aorta, Type II; half or less of the descending thoracic aorta and most or all of the abdominal aorta, Type III; and the upper half or all the abdominal aorta, Type IV. Modern surgery for repair of thoracoabdominal aortic aneurysms involves left thoracoabdominal incision, circumferential division of the hemidiaphragm, one-lung anaesthesia, heparinization and extraperitoneal aortic surgery. Impressive 30-day mortality rates of 5% were recently reported from the Brigham and Womens Hospital (Golden et al., 1991). Spinal cord ischaemia, however, remains an unresolved source of morbidity.

Various methods to prevent paraplegia after thoracoabdominal aortic surgery have included surface hypothermia, temporary atriofemoral or femorofemoral pump bypass, cardiopulmonary bypass with or without profound hypothermia, reattachment of intercostal and lumbar arteries, somatosensory and motor evoked potential monitoring, cerebrospinal fluid (CSF) drainage and the use of a variety of drugs including steroids, oxygen free-radical scavengers and mannitol (Hollier & Moore, 1990). Spinal cord ischaemia and paraplegia following thoracoabdominal aortic aneurysm resection have been attributed variously to increased CSF pressure associated with hypertension proximal to the cross-clamp, the site and duration of cross-clamp application, intraoperative hypotension and accidental permanent interruption of critical lower-intercostal and lumbar arteries. A significant reduction in the incidence of neurological damage has recently been reported with CSF drainage in the canine model (Bower et al., 1989). Decreasing CSF pressure should, in theory, enhance spinal cord blood flow by increasing spinal cord perfusion pressure, the difference between peripheral arterial pressure and CSF pressure. However, recent conflicting experimental studies have reported no relationship between spinal cord damage and arterial blood pressure, intracranial or intraspinal pressure.

Crawford and colleagues (1990), in a prospective randomized series of 98 patients with Type I and Type II thoracoabdominal aneurysms, reported that the methods of treatment, including reattachment of the intercostal and lumbar arteries, temporary atriofemoral bypass during aortic occlusion and CSF drainage did not significantly reduce the incidence of neurological deficits. Aortic clamp times in this series of patients with Type I aneurysms varied from 17–79 min (median 36 min), and Type II aneurysms varied from 29–109 min (median 54 min). The incidence of paraplegia increased from 7–55% with increase in clamp time.

Prolonged clamp time with inadequate flow or failure to implant critical intercostal arteries may result in paraplegia. Preoperative identification of critical intercostal arteries may facilitate rapid intercostal reimplantation and thus reduce cord ischaemia time. Williams and colleagues (1991) recently supported the validity of this concept in a study of 47 patients who underwent selective catheterization of the middle- and lower-thoracic intercostal and upperlumbar arteries to define the origin of the artery of Adamkiewicz. Svensson and colleagues (1991) described a rapid method of intraoperative identification of those arteries that supply the spinal cord by the use of an intrathecal platinum electrode to detect the hydrogen in solution that had been injected into the aortic ostia. A pilot study in eight patients showed that the technique can be used to identify rapidly segmental arteries supplying the spinal cord, to determine if distal perfusion is supplying the spinal cord with blood flow and if reattached segmental arteries are patent. An experimental technique of directly measuring the oxygen tension of the spinal cord surface in pigs has been described recently (Wadough et al., 1990). The limitations of intraoperative somatosensory and motor evoked potential monitoring of anterior spinal cord function are well known and the risk:benefit assessment in this patient population has yet to be established.

The intestine

In the majority of AAA resections, the inferior mesenteric artery, the primary arterial supply of the descending and sigmoid colon, is sacrificed. Following inferior mesenteric artery ligation, collateral flow from the splenic flexure to mid-rectum should come from the mid-colic branch of the superior mesenteric artery and from the haemorrhoidal branches of the hypogastric vessels. Ischaemic colitis is a well-recognized complication of abdominal aortic surgery. Prospective studies employing postoperative endoscopic examinations suggest that the true incidence of ischaemic colitis following elective abdominal aortic surgery may be as high as 6% (Ernst et al., 1976). Improper inferior mesenteric artery ligation, operative trauma to the colon, hypotension and low cardiac output states, failure to restore hypogastric arterial flow and congenital absence of communicating collaterals between mesentric and systemic vessels have all been implicated in the etiology of ischaemic colitis.

Prophylactic measures against stress ulceration should be employed routinely because of the established association between abdominal aortic aneurysm and peptic ulceration and the complications of gastrointestinal bleeding and peptic ulceration associated with elective resection (Crowson et al., 1984).

Anaesthetic management

The objectives of anaesthetic management include: an intensive preoperative assessment of risk factors and management of coexisting disease states; the utilization of monitoring techniques to detect promptly signs of myocardial ischaemia and impaired myocardial contractility; maintenance of adequate intravascular volume, optimal cardiac output and tissue oxygenation; avoidance or prompt pharmacological amelioration of untoward haemodynamic or metabolic changes associated with aortic clamping and unclamping; and intensive postoperative care.

Monitoring

Extensive monitoring of patients presenting for aortic vascular surgery is mandatory. Standard monitoring practice should include the patient's exposed extremity to check colour, capillary filling and radial pulse palpation; continuous electrocardiographic display (lead II for arrhythmia detection and a precordial V_5 lead to detect ST-segment changes associated with myocardial ischaemia); oesophageal stethoscope with thermal probe for heart/breath sounds auscultation and temperature monitoring; pulmonary gas-exchange monitoring with oximetry and capnography; neuromuscular function monitoring and bladder catheterization for urine output determination. Direct intra-arterial blood pressure monitoring is now virtually standard practice to permit beat-to-beat recognition of arterial pressure and any adverse haemodynamic response to aortic clamping procedures and for frequent blood gas determinations (Table 50.3).

Preload

The choice of invasive haemodynamic monitoring during abdominal aortic surgery has become a topic of controversy. Some authors have recommended the routine use of a pulmonary artery catheter in all patients undergoing abdominal aortic reconstructive surgery. Attia and colleagues (1976) claimed that the left ventricular filling pressure should be monitored in all patients with severe coronary artery disease because of the lack of correlation between central venous pressure and PAOP. Whittemore and colleagues (1980) hypothesized that an improved operative mortality rate might be associated with close monitoring of cardiac performance and attention to fluid management. Isaacson and colleagues (1990), in a recent prospective controlled and randomized study of 100 patients which excluded those with uncompensated cardiopulmonary or renal disease, reported no statistically significant difference between the groups monitored with central venous pressure catheter and pulmonary artery catheter with regard to morbidity (perioperative cardiac, pulmonary or renal sequelae) mortality rate, duration of intensive care, postoperative stay or cost of hospitalization. Similar observations were reported by Tuman and colleagues (1989) in a study of 1094 consecutive patients undergoing coronary artery surgery. No significant differences were noted in any outcome variable in any group of patients with similar quantitative risk classification managed with or without

Table 50.3 Abdominal aortic surgery — intraoperative monitoring techniques

ECG	Lead 11 — rhythm
	CM 5 — ischaemia
Stethoscope	
Temperature	
Urine output	
Neuromuscular function	
Blood pressure	Indirect — automated
	Direct — intra-arterial
Ventilation	End-tidal CO_2
Oxygenation	Pulse oximetry
Preload	CVP and/or PAOP
Supplementary techniques	
Pulmonary artery catheter	PAOP
	Cardiac output
	Systemic vascular resistance
	Mixed venous O_2 saturation
Transoesophageal echocardiography	Preload
	Ejection fraction
	Myocardial ischaemia
	Ventricular wall stress

pulmonary catheters. Moreover, marked variability has been observed in physicians' understanding of pulmonary artery catheter application and assessment of data (Iberti *et al.*, 1990).

Pulmonary artery catheterization may still be beneficial in many patients presenting for abdominal aortic surgery to optimize intravenous fluid administration and to detect adverse haemodynamic or ischaemic changes associated with aortic cross-clamping and release. Although changes in central venous pressure (CVP) predict the magnitude and direction of PAOP changes accurately in the majority of patients, there exists a group of patients in whom there is no substitute for left-sided filling pressure measurement (Mangano, 1980). Because fewer haemodynamic derangements follow aortic cross-clamping in patients with aorto-occlusive disease and good collateral vascularization compared with AAA patients, CVP may closely reflect the balance between intravascular volume, venous capacitance and left ventricular function in this patient population if no significant coronary artery disease or ventricular dysfunction is apparent (Cunningham *et al.*, 1989).

Myocardial performance

Pulmonary artery catheterization may be indicated in patients with a history of previous myocardial infarction, angina pectoris or signs of cardiac failure; in patients demonstrating diminished ejection fraction or abnormal ventricular-wall motion on preoperative resting or exercise radionuclide or echocardiographic studies; and in patients with evidence of redistribution on dipyridamole−thallium imaging. In addition to measurement of PAOP, pulmonary artery catheterization facilitates calculation of derived cardiac indices (stroke volume, cardiac index, left ventricular stroke work index), systemic and pulmonary vascular resistance and intrapulmonary shunt. The appearance of an abnormal V-wave of the PAOP trace may indicate the onset of myocardial ischaemia before surface ECG ST-segment changes occur (Kaplan & Wells, 1981).

The incorporation of intraoperative trans-oesophageal two-dimensional echocardiography (TOE) into anaesthetic practice has provided a practical means of estimating left ventricular dimensions and myocardial performance in addition to the detection of wall motion abnormalities. A short-axis cross-sectional view of the left ventricle may provide an excellent qualitative assessment of left ventricular filling volumes, global ventricular contractility and regional ventricular function.

TOE has been extensively used to measure left ventricular end-diastolic area as an approximation of left ventricular end-diastolic volume. Typically, endocardial and epicardial borders at end-diastole and end-systole are traced. End-diastole is indicated by the peak of the ECG R-wave and end-systole is defined as the smallest endocardial area (Leung *et al.*, 1989).

Left ventricular ejection fraction is determined by the calculation

$$\frac{\text{(end-diastolic area} - \text{end-systolic area)} \times 100}{\text{(end-diastolic area)}}$$

In situations such as abdominal aortic surgery, with the potential for alterations in left ventricular compliance, TOE may provide a better estimate of left ventricular volume than PAOP. TOE may provide an assessment of left ventricular end-systolic wall stress (ESWS), which is directly related to afterload (a function of arterial blood pressure, internal diameter of the ventricle and myocardial wall thickness).

Recent studies have compared measurements of intraoperative cardiac output by TOE and pulsed-wave Doppler monitoring of pulmonary and mitral valve flow with measurements obtained by thermodilution. These studies demonstrate only a modest correlation between thermodilution and TOE estimates of cardiac output derived from pulsed-wave Doppler imaging across the pulmonary artery and little, if any, relationship with flow across the mitral valve (Muhiudeen, 1991). More encouraging results were observed in a comparative study of bio-impedance and thermodilution measurements of cardiac output during abdominal aortic surgery (Sullivan *et al.*, 1991).

Myocardial ischaemia

Intraoperative myocardial ischaemia may be precipitated by increases in myocardial oxygen demand caused by tachycardia, hypertension and sympathetic responses, or by decreased myocardial oxygen supply caused by external factors such as hypotension, tachycardia and hypoxaemia, or by internal factors such as acute coronary thrombosis and spasm (Mangano, 1990). Intraoperative myocardial ischaemia may be detected by ECG ST-segment changes (V5 most consistently), PAOP changes and V-wave development, or segmental wall-thickening changes detected by TOE or cardiokymography (Leung *et al.*, 1989). The earliest physiological changes following experimental coronary ligation are changes in myocardial wall thickening, followed by changes in the endocardial ECG and the surface ECG (Battler *et al.*, 1980). Since 1985, a number of important outcome studies in patients undergoing cardiac and non-cardiac surgery have highlighted the dynamic role of intra-operative ischaemia predicting perioperative cardiac morbidity. Smith and colleagues (1985) noted that 24:50 patients studied had new regional wall motion abnormalities (RWMA) whereas only six had ST-segment changes. This was the first study to demonstrate the greater sensitivity (abnormal wall motion or thickening when ischaemia or infarction is present) of TOE for the intraoperative detection of myocardial ischaemia. Segmental wall motion and thickening changes detected by TOE may be the most sensitive indicators of ischaemia and preliminary data suggested that such intraoperative changes may predict patient outcome (Gewertz *et al.*, 1987).

More recently, however, the relationship between RWMA and postoperative cardiac outcome in non-cardiac surgery has been questioned. London and colleagues (1990) reported that although RWMAs were more common in patients undergoing aortic vascular surgery, 40% of these episodes occurred randomly (with no apparent relation to clinical or haemodynamic events) and that persistent RWMAs resolved without evidence of infarction. Leung and colleagues (1990) studied the relationship between RWMAs and indices of myocardial oxygen supply and demand. In this study, RWMAs most often were not triggered by acute increases in myocardial oxygen demand, suggesting that a primary decrease in myocardial oxygen supply is the important mechanism.

The question of specificity of RWMAs remains (Thys, 1987). How often are the RWMAs observed clinically caused by factors other than ischaemia? Considerable heterogeneity of ventricular contraction has been demonstrated in patients without evidence of ischaemic heart disease. The question of the effects of ventricular loading conditions and inotropism on RWMA during abdominal aortic vascular surgery is of major interest. Buffington and Coyle (1991) systematically examined the effects of preload and afterload of RWMA in controlled and ischaemic myocardium. Systolic ventricular wall thickening increased with increasing left atrial pressure under control conditions, whereas it did not change with increasing left atrial pressure in the postischaemic myocardium. The magnitude of systolic wall thickening decreased with increasing afterload in the control and post-ischaemic myocardium. The authors concluded that the postischaemic myocardium had a diminished response to increases in preload and that the response

to changes in afterload was unchanged by ischaemia and reperfusion.

Anaesthetic technique

No single anaesthetic agent or technique is ideal for all patients presenting for aortic vascular surgery. Controversy abounds concerning: (i) use of regional plus general anaesthesia; (ii) use of inhalation versus opioid anaesthesia; and (iii) use of isoflurane in patients with coronary artery disease. The anaesthetic agents and techniques chosen should ensure a smooth induction of anaesthesia, a favourable cardiovascular dose-response relationship which preserves the delicate myocardial oxygen supply/demand balance, adequate muscle relaxation with intraoperative analgesia and amnesia. The choices of anaesthetic technique include nitrous oxide/oxygen with incremental volatile agent or opiate supplementation; opiate−oxygen or an opiate−oxygen−volatile agent combination with or without regional anaesthesia (Cunningham, 1989b) (Table 50.4).

Only limited data are available in the literature on cardiac performance during aortic vascular surgery. A 'balanced' nitrous oxide−oxygen−relaxant technique (Falk *et al.*, 1981) and a nitrous oxide−oxygen−relaxant−volatile agent technique (Bush *et al.*, 1977) have been associated with depressed ventricular performance following induction of anaesthesia which persisted following cross-clamp application. Friesen and colleagues (1986), using high-dose fentanyl (100 μg/kg) oxygen−relaxant anaesthetic technique, reported an unacceptably high incidence of hyperdynamic circulatory responses to surgical stimuli before, during and after aortic cross-clamping. A technique of intermittent bolus administration of high-dose fentanyl (total dose 125 μg/kg) and sufentanil−oxygen−relaxant (total dose 25 μg/kg) required supplementation with volatile agents to achieve haemodynamic stability (Crosby *et al.*, 1990).

A combination of an opiate (fentanyl, 30 μg/kg, induction with maintenance infusion) with the volatile agent halothane (Moffit *et al.*, 1985) or enflurane (Moffit *et al.*, 1986) in oxygen maintained reduced myocardial contractility, unchanged systemic vascular resistance and preserved myocardial oxygenation in patients with good left ventricular function undergoing coronary artery bypass grafting. A combined high-dose fentanyl−oxygen−isoflurane anaesthetic technique maintained a stable cardiac index, a left ventricular stroke work index and a systemic vascular resistance during the cross-clamp period, and was not associated with hyperdynamic circulatory

Table 50.4 Abdominal aortic surgery — guidelines for anaesthetic management

1	*Preoperative hydration*	Maintenance of intravenous fluids overnight	
2	*Premedication*	Benzodiazepine ± opiate	
3	*General anaesthesia*	*Ventricular function*	
		Satisfactory	*Impaired*
	Induction	Barbiturate	Opiate
	Maintenance	N20/02	O$_2$
		Opiate	Opiate
		Volatile agent	Volatile agent
	Ventilation	Controlled normocapnia	
	Nitroglycerine	Myocardial ischaemia	
		Hypertension >20% baseline arterial pressure	
4	*Intravenous fluid management*		
	Crystalloid infusion ± colloid	PAOP 1.33–2 kPa (10–15 mmHg) Urine output >60 ml/h	
	Blood	Loss >15% estimated blood volume	
	Mannitol	Urine output <60 ml/h +PAOP >2 kPa (15 mmHg)	
5	*Postoperative management*		
	Mechanical ventilation Homeostasis	Cardiac and respiratory	
	Regional anaesthesia	Postoperative analgesia	

responses previously reported with unsupplemented fentanyl–oxygen technique (O'Sullivan *et al.*, 1989). A combined opiate–oxygen–volatile anaesthetic technique may be the technique of choice for aortic aneurysm resection in high-risk patients, since it ensures a hypodynamic circulation with preservation of myocardial oxygenation. However, the requirement for prolonged postoperative ventilation is a major disadvantage of this technique.

Theoretically, isoflurane should be the volatile anesthetic agent of choice for aortic vascular surgery (Gelman *et al.*, 1984). Despite its direct myocardial depressant effects, isoflurane administration is associated with preserved cardiac output due to increased heart rate and reduced systemic vascular resistance. Unfortunately, in patients with coronary artery disease, isoflurane administration may be deleterious if a vasodilatory or coronary-steal effect is produced. The coronary arteriolar vasodilating properties of isoflurane are now well documented in experimental and clinical studies. However, the clinical implications of isoflurane-induced coronary arteriolar dilatation in patients with coronary artery disease remains controversial.

A number of recent studies have attempted to modify the adverse haemodynamic effects and prevent myocardial ischaemia on aortic cross-clamp and release. The ability of the angiotensin I-converting enzyme inhibitor, captopril, 25 mg, given orally, to prevent perioperative adverse haemodynamic effects was studied in 10 patients (Kataja *et al.*, 1989). Oral captopril increased the risk of hypotension and bradycardia after induction of anesthesia and did not prevent postoperative hypertension compared with the 10 control patients. In a double-blind placebo-controlled study, 5 µg/kg oral clonidine given 90 min before surgery did not decrease the amount of alfentanil, the principal anaesthetic drug, when haemodynamic parameters were used as end-points for dosing but decreased the need for supplemental droperidol administration (Engelman *et al.*, 1989). However, the alpha-2 agonist was associated with lower heart rates and fewer episodes of tachycardia. An infusion of clonidine, 7 µg/kg, was associated with reduced concentrations of vasoactive hormones noradrenaline, adrenaline and vasopressin and more stable cardiovascular homeostasis (fewer episodes of tachycardia and hypertension) compared with a control group after abdominal aortic surgery (Quintin *et al.*, 1991).

Mesenteric traction during aortic surgery may produce facial flushing, reduced mean arterial pressure and systemic vascular resistance, with increased heart rate and cardiac index. In a recent study, the inhibition by ibuprofen of 6-keto-prostaglandin-F$_{1\alpha}$ and its associated haemodynamic changes, confirmed the hypothesis that prostacyclin is the mediator of the mesenteric traction response in abdominal aortic surgery (Hudson *et al.*, 1990). Although increased 6-keto $PGF_{1\alpha}$, attributed to mesenteric traction, was reported by Galt and colleagues (1991), subsequent elevations in thromboxane B_2 were not detected in the placebo group or ibuprofen group when physiological volume loading and extradural/general anaesthesia was employed.

The prophylactic or specific use of vasodilatory agents to prevent haemodynamic changes associated with surgical interventions during aortic vascular surgery remains controversial. Nitroglycerine therapy may maintain normal transmural distribution of blood flow and may facilitate endocardial perfusion by decreasing ventricular wall tension secondary to preload reduction (Hummel *et al.*, 1982). The balance of evidence currently available would support the administration of $1-2\,\mu g \cdot kg^{-1} \cdot min^{-1}$ nitroglycerine infusion if hypertension, impaired myocardial contractility and tissue oxygenation or signs or myocardial ischaemia develop following aortic cross-clamp application. This therapy should decrease arterial pressure, systemic vascular resistance and myocardial oxygen consumption. Intravenous dobutamine infusion may also be administered to sustain myocardial function if evidence of impaired contractility develops following aortic cross-clamping.

Intraoperative fluid and blood transfusion therapy

Patients undergoing abdominal aortic surgery usually experience major functional extracellular fluid and blood loss. Functional extracellular fluid loss into a non-functional or 'third-space' may follow extensive tissue trauma, manipulation, exposure and surgical retraction. Sequestration of fluid within the lumen wall of the intestine and formation of major retroperitoneal oedema account for most of the fluid shift from the circulation. The issue of whether a crystalloid or colloid intravenous fluid regimen better preserves circulatory homeostasis and renal function during major vascular surgery has not been resolved. Restoration of normal intravascular and interstitial fluid volumes is a primary objective in intravenous fluid administration. Larger volumes of crystalloid solution will be required to restore the intravascular volume compared with colloid solutions (Skillman *et al.*, 1975). Advocates of a crystalloid regimen claim greater urine output and a reduction in the incidence of oliguric renal failure following abdominal aortic surgery. However, intraoperative urine output failed to predict postoperative renal insufficiency in

patients undergoing aortic reconstruction (Albert *et al.*, 1984). Conflicting data have been published showing improved postoperative respiratory function following colloid administration. A combination of balanced salt and colloid solutions, guided by appropriate CVP monitoring, will ensure adequate intravascular volume, optimal cardiac output, satisfactory renal and end-organ blood flow, and minimal extravascular losses into the pulmonary interstitium and traumatized tissues.

A balanced salt solution, with or without a colloid solution should be infused in volumes sufficient to maintain a PAOP of 1.33–1.9 kPa (10–15 mmHg) during the cross-clamp period and to ensure a urine output greater than 60 ml/h. If urine output is unsatisfactory, despite PAOP measurement of 1.9 kPa (15 mmHg) or greater, diuretic therapy with mannitol or frusemide should be considered. Low-dose dopamine, 2 μg/kg, following surgery has been reported to increase renal blood flow significantly and also glomerular filtration rate, urine output and sodium excretion. The PAOP should be increased to 0.4–0.6 kPa (3–5 mmHg) above the preoperative value before cross-clamp release, to prevent hypotension and cardiac-output reduction following aortic unclamping.

The techniques currently available to minimize homologous blood transfusion during elective aortic vascular surgery include multiple predeposit autologous collection, storage and retransfusion; immediate preoperative phlebotomy, haemodilution and autologous transfusion; intraoperative blood salvage and reinfusion. Intraoperative autotransfusion may be an economical method of reducing homologous blood transfusions significantly. Initial reports (Brewster *et al.*, 1979) suggested a 40–50% avoidance of homologous blood transfusions, which has increased up to 80% in recent studies (Hallett *et al.*, 1987). The initial application of autotransfusion was complicated by haemolysis and coagulation disorders, air and fat emboli, platelet and leucocyte microaggregation and sepsis (Duncan *et al.*, 1974). Technological advances have virtually eliminated the significant problems of air and particulate embolization. No significant haemolysis or coagulopathies have been noted with autotransfusion techniques in recent studies. Because autotransfused blood is, in essence, a preparation of washed, packed red blood cells suspended in saline solution without platelets and clotting factors, fresh frozen plasma and platelet concentrate transfusion may be necessary. By providing fresh warm blood with optimal pH and 2,3-diphosphoglycerate content, autotransfusion may prevent some of the adverse cardiovascular effects associated with extensive transfusion of stored homologous blood.

Reduction or elimination of homologous blood transfusion during abdominal aortic surgery may be achieved by careful surgical technique, higher threshold for transfusion and the routine use of autotransfusion. Early encouraging reports have highlighted the relative safety of a simple, disposable, autotransfusion system for the intraoperative collection and reinfusion of shed blood (Duchateau et al., 1990).

Regional anaesthesia

Growing interest in regional anaesthesia for abdominal aortic surgery have been stimulated by reports suggesting improved operative outcome. Postoperative analgesia provided by extradural local anaesthetics and/or opioids combined with 'light' general anaesthesia reduced operative mortality and postoperative morbidity due to myocardial infarction, congestive cardiac failure and infection compared with a group receiving general anaesthesia and postoperative parenteral opioids (Yeager et al., 1987).

Proponents of regional anaesthesia claim reduction in volatile anaesthetic and narcotic requirements in the intraoperative period and significant alleviation of postoperative pain. Elevations in skin temperature, increased graft blood flow and reduced muscle blood flow have been reported (Cousins & Wright, 1971). Recent studies have evaluated the physiological changes associated with regional anaesthesia. Blomberg and colleagues (1990), in a study of patients with severe coronary artery disease, showed that regional cardiac sympathetic block with high thoracic extradural anaesthesia significantly increases the diameter of stenotic but has no effect on non-stenotic epicardial coronary artery segments. The authors postulated that extradural-induced dilatation of stenotic segments of large coronary arteries without causing any changes in the tone of the coronary resistance vessels may be valuable when thoracic extradural anaesthesia is used to control pain in patients with coronary artery disease. A recent randomized, double-blind, placebo-controlled study noted less pain and systemic and opiate requirement, lower plasma norepinephrine levels and fewer hypertensive episodes requiring treatment in the group given 6 mg morphine sulphate in the extradural space, compared with a control group (Breslow et al., 1989).

Despite the well known and accepted advantages of regional anaesthesia alone, or in combination with general anaesthesia and tracheal intubation, these techniques have not been adopted universally, partly due to the lingering controversy surrounding extradural catheters and anticoagulant therapy. However, the use of combined general anaesthesia and continuous lumbar extradural anaesthesia for major aortic vascular surgery has increased during the past decade. This technique has been associated with greater total perioperative fluid volume administration and reduced left ventricular function compared with general anaesthesia alone (Blunt et al., 1987). The merits of combined regional and general anaesthetic techniques, compared with conventional general anaesthesia alone for aortic vascular surgery, must await the publication of more extensive clinical investigations (McPeak, 1987). The first definitive study to examine the isolated effects of primary anaesthetic technique per se on postoperative outcome was a recent large population study by Baron and colleagues (1991). A total of 173 patients scheduled for abdominal aortic surgery were randomized to receive either 'balanced' general anaesthesia or thoracic extradural anaesthesia in combination with light general anaesthesia. The study, which focused on intraoperative techniques, demonstrated that thoracic extradural anaesthesia, combined with light general anaesthesia, had no influence on cardiac and respiratory function after abdominal aortic surgery. The authors contended that postoperative extradural analgesia rather than intraoperative extradural anaesthesia was responsible for any reduction in postoperative cardiac and respiratory complications.

Postoperative management

Patients recovering from aortic vascular surgery are at risk of developing cardiac, respiratory and renal failure in the immediate postoperative period. Close monitoring of the patient's intravascular volume status, temperature, respiratory and renal function will be required in addition to assessment of graft patency and lower extremity blood flow. Provision of adequate analgesia is also a priority.

The postoperative respiratory deficit is primarily restrictive with decreased functional residual capacity and pulmonary compliance. Pre-existing obstructive defects are compounded by altered secretions, impaired cough and mucociliary clearance, atelectasis and postoperative pulmonary infections (Falk et al., 1981). In these situations, intermittent mandatory ventilation in the immediate postoperative period may be indicated. Coexisting cardiac and respiratory disease is common in this mainly elderly patient population. An extended midline incision, abdominal distension following extracellular fluid sequestration, bed rest in the supine position, abdominal pain requiring narcotic administration, large volumes of blood and electrolyte infusion, and hypothermia following prolonged procedures may all preclude early weaning and tracheal extubation. A slow emergence from anaesthesia reduces the likelihood of agitation, shivering and cardiorespiratory instability in the early postoperative period.

Recent attention has focused on the relationship between postoperative ischaemic episodes and perioperative cardiac morbidity. Haemodynamic stress may be precipitated by painful emergence from anaesthesia, fluid shifts, temperature changes and alterations in respiratory function. Marked changes occur in plasma-catecholamine concentrations, ventricular function and coagulation following major vascular surgery, especially in patients with pre-existing cardiac disease. Postoperative patients may have heart rate increases of 25—50% over intraoperative values and postoperative ischaemia typically is silent (Wong et al., 1988).

Mangano and colleagues (1990) have recently documented the impact of early postoperative ischaemia on adverse cardiac outcome in high-risk patients undergoing non-cardiac surgery. Postoperative myocardial ischaemia occurred in 41% of the 474 men monitored and this event was associated with a 2.8-fold increase in the odds of all adverse cardiac outcomes. Daily clinical evaluation, serial ECGs and cardiac enzymes should be performed to detect postoperative cardiac morbidity. Pharmacological control of heart rate and postoperative pain relief should be utilized to reduce postoperative myocardial ischaemia and improve patient outcome.

Influence of surgical technique

The standard surgical approach for abdominal aortic reconstruction has been a vertical or horizontal incision with a transperitoneal approach. Reports in the 1960s advocated a transverse flank incision with retroperitoneal approach for high-risk patients with severe cardiac and respiratory compromise (Sharp & Donovan, 1987). The retroperitoneal approach for elective AAA resection may be associated with significantly better perioperative oxygenation and preservation of lung volumes compared with the transabdominal approach (Sicard et al., 1987). The retroperitoneal approach may better preserve dia-

phragmatic contractility. The right lateral decubitus position required for the retroperitoneal approach has not been associated with significant haemodynamic changes following aortic cross-clamping and release.

Recent comparative studies of transperitoneal and retroperitoneal techniques have provided conflicting outcomes. Gregory and colleagues (1989) reported significantly shorter operating time, shorter ileus, fewer cardiac complications and shorter hospital stay in the retroperitoneal compared with the transperitoneal patients. Cambria and colleagues (1990) noted identical respiratory morbidity and similar indices of postoperative recovery, e.g. hospital-stay complication rate, metabolic and gastrointestinal function with the two surgical approaches. Shepherd and colleagues (1991) claimed that the retroperitoneal approach facilitated proximal abdominal aortic exposure and anastomosis, especially in large pararenal aneurysms or in situations unfavorable to a transabdominal approach.

Peripheral vascular surgery of the lower limb

Peripheral vascular surgery of the lower limb may be elective (in the case of claudication treatment, ischaemic rest pain or ulceration and gangrene) or acute in the case of thromboembolic lower-limb arterial occlusion (Roizen, 1989).

Lower-limb vascular reconstructive procedures are generally categorized as either inflow or outflow procedures. Inflow reconstruction involves bypass of the obstruction in the aortoiliac segment, whereas outflow procedures are those performed below the inguinal ligament to bypass femoropopliteal or distal obstructions.

A prosthetic graft, reversed saphenous vein, or in situ saphenous vein originating in the common femoral and extending to the popliteal and tibial arteries may be used to bypass obstructive lesions. Prosthetic bypasses, especially when extended below the knee, have lower patency rates (Leather et al., 1991). Reversed saphenous vein bypassing involves stripping of the vessel from the common femoral vein to the level of the distal anastomosis, ligation and division of the branches, reversal of the vein's direction and tunnelling from the femoral artery to the distal vessel. Improved patency rates have been reported with in situ compared with reversed saphenous vein bypass. In situ procedures involve dissection of the vein and ligation of its branches, end-to-side anastomosis of vein to common femoral artery, lysis of obstructing valves with cutters or valvutomes and distal end-to-side anatomosis at the distal end.

Acute lower-limb arterial occlusion may be caused by thrombosis of a stenotic or ulcerated atherosclerotic vessel or embolism caused by cardiac arrhythmia, myocardial infarction or ventricular aneurysm. These patients may be critically ill and embolectomy/ thrombectomy may be associated with significant blood and fluid loss. Extensive monitoring and local anaesthetic infiltration of the groin are common practice. If blood flow is not restored with passage of Fogarty catheters, a more complex reconstructive procedure may be required. Patients presenting for peripheral vascular surgery tend to be elderly with high cardiac risk, i.e. prevalence of diabetes mellitus, hypertension, history of angina and previous myocardial infarction, and signs of compensated/ uncompensated congestive heart failure. Cardiac death (myocardial infarction, major arrhythmia and left ventricular failure) account for 40–60% of early postoperative deaths (Hertzer et al., 1984).

In an analysis of six studies totalling approximately 4500 patients, Hertzer (1987) claimed that perioperative cardiac events occurred in 16% of patients with clinical evidence of coronary artery disease and in only 1.7% of patients without coronary artery disease. Jain and colleagues (1985) used first-pass RNA at rest and exercise to measure global left ventricular function (ejection fraction) and to identify individuals with exercise-induced myocardial ischaemia. Of 78 patients presenting for peripheral surgery, 53 had abnormal RNA studies. In this patient population, diabetics may have an increased morbidity (congestive heart failure and myocardial infarction) and subsequent mortality. Nesto and colleagues (1990) reported that 57% of a series of 30 diabetics presenting for peripheral vascular surgery had abnormal DTSs. Furthermore, diabetic patients may manifest myocardial ischaemia and infarction more often than non-diabetic patients.

Thirty eight percent of 50 patients undergoing peripheral vascular surgery had episodes of myocardial ischaemia, mostly silent, in a series reported by McCann and Clements (1989). Ischaemia was more prominent in the postoperative rather than the preoperative and intraoperative period. Tachycardia was often associated with ischaemia. Significantly more cardiac-related morbidity and death occurred in patients who were documented to have had silent myocardial ischaemia. A number of important issues and controversies, i.e. the prevalence of coronary artery disease in patients with peripheral vascular disease, the impact of coronary artery disease on outcome after peripheral vascular surgery, the effect of coronary artery bypass surgery on prognosis, preoperative evaluation and management strategies — were recently addressed by Gersh and colleagues (1991) in a comprehensive review.

The duration and complexity of peripheral vascular procedures are determined by surgical skill, the quality of the saphenous vein and the patency and size of the distal outflow vessels. The nature and complexity of the monitoring required will depend on the patients pre-existing cardiorespiratory status. Major blood loss and intraoperative haemodynamic changes are unusual. However, the procedures are frequently lengthy. Berlauk and colleagues (1991), in a prospective controlled randomized study, assessed whether optimizing haemodynamic performance with a pulmonary artery catheter 12 h before surgery (fluid loading, afterload reduction, and/or inotropic support to predetermined end points) would improve outcome in 89 patients undergoing lower limb vascular surgery. Patients managed with a pulmonary artery catheter had significantly fewer adverse intraoperative events, less postoperative cardiac morbidity and less early graft thrombosis. The mortality rate was 9.5% in the control group and 1.5% in the pulmonary artery catheter group.

A regional technique, usually intraoperative local anaesthetic solution with opioids for postoperative pain relief, is a common technique if no established contraindications are present. Bladder catheterization, because of the duration of surgery; supplemental oxygen administration; temperature preservation and good hydration, to prevent peripheral vasoconstriction, are all part of good perioperative anaesthetic management.

Carotid endarterectomy

Cerebral blood flow, which normally is approximately $50\,\text{ml}\cdot100\,\text{g}^{-1}\cdot\text{min}^{-1}$, is provided to the circle of Willis by the right and left internal carotids and the vertebrobasilar arteries. Therefore, even complete occlusion of one of these arteries may not cause cerebral ischaemia if there is sufficient collateral blood flow. However, partial occlusion of an internal carotid artery by an atheromatatus stenosis or an ulcerated plaque may produce emboli that lodge in arteries distal to the circle of Willis, causing an ipsilateral transient ischaemic event. The likelihood of a future stroke will be significant if there has been preceding ischaemic strokes, transient ischaemic attacks or retinal infarctions. The degree of carotid stenosis, expressed as a percentage reduction in the diameter of the relevant artery, may be mild (less than 30%), moderate (30–69%), or severe (70–99%).

Recent community-based UK studies have established that each year 42:100 000 of the population sustain a transient ischaemic attack (TIA) and about 200:100 000 have a completed stroke (Dennis et al., 1989). These data are similar to earlier North American and European community-based studies. About 80% of TIAs are in the carotid artery territory; the remainder are in the vertebrobasilar distribution or they are of uncertain vascular distribution. Of interest, 40% of strokes subsequent to TIAs occur in a vascular territory different to that of the incident TIA. The incidence of TIAs increases sharply with advancing age. In middle age, men are more likely to suffer a TIA (odds ratio 2.6) but the male predominance declines in elderly people.

Dennis and colleagues (1990) evaluated the prognosis of a TIA over a mean follow-up of 3.7 years in 184 patients drawn from a community-based study of approximately 105 000 persons. Patients who suffered a TIA has a 13-fold excess risk of stroke during the first year and a seven-fold excess risk over the following 7 years compared with a population without TIAs. Occurrence of a TIA also indicated that these patients were more likely to have coronary artery disease, so their overall risk of death, stroke or MI is about 10% annually.

Indications for surgery and outcome studies

The role of carotid endarterectomy in the management of patients with cerebrovascular disease has been the subject of continuous controversy since Eastcott and colleagues from St Mary's Hospital, London reported the first successful internal carotid reconstruction in 1954. The causes of the persistent controversy has centred on the lack of data concerning the natural course and progression of carotid artery disease; the lack of compelling scientific evidence to prove the benefits of carotid endarterectomy, especially in patients with asymptomatic stenosis or bruit; the possible benefits of conservative management and finally, the widely publicized reports of overliberal indications for carotid surgery.

Carotid endarterectomy has been considered, until recent times, to be a well-established, frequently performed operation directed towards the treatment of cerebral vascular disease and the prevention of stroke. Classical indications for surgery have included symptomatic patients with transient ischaemic attacks and completed stroke. Indications for surgery

were subsequently extended to patients with acute strokes. Initial reports of high mortality associated with surgery for acute stroke were highlighted and attention then focused on the role of surgical intervention in asymptomatic carotid disease (Table 50.5).

The number of carotid endarterectomies performed in the US has risen dramatically from 15 000 in 1971 to a peak of 107 000 in 1985, with a subsequent decline to 87 000 in 1987. These figures do not include procedures performed in Veteran Administration Hospitals. Up to 40% of these procedures have been performed in asymptomatic patients with carotid bruits or varying degrees of stenosis. Barnett (1990) claims that the US figures are 27 times those of the UK and seven times those of neighbouring Canada. Carotid endarterectomy has become the third commonest procedure in North America.

In the early 1980s it was perceived that large-scale controlled randomized trials were needed to assess the benefits of carotid endarterectomy and to determine the level of perioperative risk at which the procedure becomes acceptable. A major stimulus for these investigations was the report by Winslow and colleagues (1988) concerning the appropriateness of carotid endarterectomy, as judged by a multidisciplinary national expert panel, in a random sample of 1302 medicare patients in three geographical areas in 1981. Only 35% of patients had the procedure for appropriate reasons, 32% for equivocal reasons and 32% had surgery for inappropriate reasons. After carotid endarterectomy, 9.8% of patients had a major complication (stroke with residual deficit or death within 30 days of surgery). A survey of academic and larger medical centres in the same year revealed a more comforting 6.4% perioperative morbidity and mortality rate.

Several large-scale trials of carotid endarterectomy, including the European Carotid Surgery Trial (ECST), which began in 1981, and the North American Symptomatic Carotid Endarterectomy Trial (NASCET), which began in 1988, have already issued

Table 50.5 Carotid endarterectomy — indications for surgery

Established
Transient ischaemic attacks
Completed strokes
Symptomatic/asymptomatic patients with high-grade stenosis (70–99%)

Speculative
Selected patients with:
   Asymptomatic bruit
   Low-/moderate-grade stenosis

Table 50.6 Carotid endarterectomy — morbidity and mortality

Operative mortality	Operative morbidity
Perioperative myocardial infarction	*Perioperative stroke*
	Pre-existing neurological
Angina	deficit
MI < 6 months	Frequent TIAs
Congestive heart failure	Neurological deficits
Hypertension	secondary to multiple
Chronic obstructive	cerebral infarctions
pulmonary disease	Uncontrolled hypertension
	Pre- and postoperative

preliminary reports. To assess the natural history of carotid disease and the efficacy of surgical intervention, four large-scale multicentre controlled trials of carotid endarterectomy are in progress or nearing completion. Two trials are sponsored by the National Institute of Neurological and Communicative Disorders and Stroke (NINCDS) and two are sponsored by the Veterans Administration. The multiplicity of biological variables associated with elderly patients, with coexisting medical pathology, presenting for major vascular surgery has proved a major difficulty in obtaining sound data (Table 50.6). Biological variables include the patient's age, coexisting disease states, the extent of the neurological symptoms (the symptomatic patient may be at more risk than the asymptomatic and the patient with lateralizing hemispheric symptoms may be at more risk than one with amaurosis fugax); the collateral circulation (the contralateral carotid, the vertebrobasilar system, the carotid siphon and the intracerebral vessels), and the size/morphology of the carotid plaque.

The ECST, the largest randomized trial of any surgical procedure to date, is a multinational trial of carotid endarterectomy for patients who, after a carotid territory non-disabling ischaemic stroke, transient ischaemic attack, or retinal infarct, are found to have a stenotic lesion in the ipsilateral carotid artery (ECST Collaborative Group, 1991). Over the past 10 years, 2518 patients have been randomized and the mean follow-up was almost 3 years. For the 776 patients with 'severe' (70–99%) stenosis, the immediate risks of surgery were significantly outweighed by the later benefits. Although 7.5% had a stroke or died within 30 days of surgery, over the next 3 years the risks of ipsilateral ischaemic was an extra 2.8% for surgery-allocated patients compared with 16.8% for controls (treated with stopping smoking, hypertension control, and, in recent years, the use of aspirin as an antithrombotic agent). In contrast, for those with mild carotid stenosis (less than 30%)

any benefits of surgery were outweighed by the risks (2.3% death or disabling stroke).

Results very similar to those in the ECST study have been made public in a 'Clinic Alert' from NASCET (NINCDS, 1991). After randomizing over 1000 patients between surgery and non-surgery over a mean follow-up of about 2 years, statistically definitive results have emerged from NASCET in patients with 70–99% stenosis among whom (as in ECST) surgery involved a 30-day mortality risk of a few percent, followed by avoidance of most ipsilateral carotid territory ischaemic strokes. In NASCET, as in ECST, the results for patients with moderate 30–69% stenosis on the prerandomized angiogram remained unclear, so in both studies randomization of such patients continues.

The implications for the UK of the ECST study was addressed in an accompanying editorial (Editorial, 1991). An increase of three- to five-fold in the number of carotid endarterectomies per annum in the next decade is anticipated. The reported incidence of asymptomatic carotid bruits in the population over 40–50 years is 4–5%. In addition, 10–20% of patients scheduled for coronary artery bypass grafting or other vascular surgery may have an asymptomatic carotid bruit. A more sophisticated screening process for patients with TIAs will be required. The detection of a carotid bruit by auscultation is insufficiently sensitive. Duplex ultrasonography should be most cost-effective in that it would exclude from further angiography 80% of patients with TIAs whose stenosis is insufficient to warrant further evaluation or surgical intervention. Cranial computerized tomography (CT) scanning has become more common to exclude alternative causes of cerebral symptoms and to identify silent infarcts. It is presumed that this information might alter the timing of surgical intervention, predict outcome and select patients for non-operative therapy. Recent data suggests that routine CT scanning did not reveal unsuspected pathology, did not influence surgical decisions and was not cost-effective (Martin *et al.*, 1991).

In addition, a number of other strategies may be effective in reducing the stroke from carotid lesions. Collins and colleagues (1990) summarized evidence from several major prospective, observational, epidemiological studies which indicate that anti-hypertensive therapy associated with a long-term reduction of 0.66–0.8 kPa (5–6 mmHg) in mean diastolic blood pressure was associated with about 35–40% less strokes. The Antiplatelet Triallists' Collaboration Report (1988) on 31 randomized trials of antiplatelet treatment suggested a reduced vascular mortality of 15% and non-fatal vascular event reduction of 30%. In men who were at high risk for cardiovascular events, intensive lipid-lowering therapy with hydroxymethylglutaryl CoA reductase inhibitors reduced the frequency of progression and increased the frequency of regression of coronary lesions (Brown *et al.*, 1990).

Anaesthetic technique

Recent large-scale follow-up studies have identified the impact of cardiac risk on perioperative long-term mortality in patients undergoing carotid endarterectomy. To identify patients undergoing carotid endarterectomy who were at increased risk of cardiac events and death, Mackey and colleagues (1990) followed 614 patients who underwent carotid endarterectomy for up to 15 years following surgery. Patients were divided into two groups: Group 1 had overt coronary artery disease and Group 2 were without overt coronary artery disease. Thirty-day mortality was 1.5% in those with overt coronary artery disease and 0% in those without overt coronary artery disease. Five-, 10- and 15-year survival for those without coronary artery disease was 68.4%, 44.9% and 36.4% compared with 86.4%, 72.3% and 54.3%, respectively for those with overt coronary artery disease. Overt coronary artery disease was associated with diminished 30-day late survival. Myocardial infarction was the most frequent cause of death in all groups. Patients with overt coronary artery disease were at highest risk for late cardiac events and death.

Judging by the number of reports published in the past decade, interest in the use of local or regional anaesthesia for carotid surgery appears to be growing. The major advantages claimed by proponents of local or regional anaesthesia is that the conscious patient may undergo repeated neurological evaluation and a sensitive assessment of cerebral function may be obtained during carotid occlusion. Regional anaesthesia may render intraluminal shunting unnecessary, thereby reducing the technical difficulties — intimal dissection, air and thromboembolism — associated with the procedure. A trial of carotid artery occlusion varying from 30s to 4 min has been reported to safely avoid intraluminal shunting in 82—96% of patients studied.

Regional anaesthesia

C2, C3 and C4 roots emerge from their intervertebral foramina and pass out to the respective transverse processes before splitting into ascending and descending branches, which form the superficial and deep cervical plexus. The traditional approach to the deep cervical plexus block involves placing needles at the transverse process of C2, C3 and C4 (Youngberg & Gold, 1991). The C2 transverse process can usually be palpated inferior to the mastoid process. C3 and C4 transverse processes may be more difficult to palpate. A 1.5—2 in needle is injected perpendicular to all planes and is advanced till paraesthesias are elicited and/or the transverse process is located. After careful aspiration, 4—8 ml of local anaesthetic is injected per needle location.

The accepted contraindications to regional technique include clotting abnormalities or bleeding diatheses, anticoagulant therapy, infection at the site of needle insertion and limited patient co-operation or refusal. Because the vertebral artery lies posterior to the transverse process in the transverse foramen, an intra-arterial injection with rapid seizure activity and loss of consciousness is a possibility. Intrathecal or extradural anaesthesia is a possibility if the needle should pass through the intervertebral foramen and enter the extradural space or dura. An inadvertent high spinal block would require immediate haemodynamic and ventilatory support. A unilateral phrenic nerve palsy, commonly associated with deep cervical plexus block, is seldom of major clinical significance. In addition to the combination of superficial and deep cervical plexus block, infiltration along the posterior border of the sternocleidomastoid muscle to block cutaneous nerves is required. Supplementary infiltration of the carotid sheath may be performed. Patient anxiety remains a factor limiting the use of regional anaesthesia. Early studies claimed a lower incidence of perioperative MI, a decreased incidence of major blood pressure fluctuations in the perioperative period and reduced costs because of shorter intensive care unit (ICU) and hospital stay. Perioperative blood pressure stability has been using general and regional techniques with greatly differing results. Corson and colleagues (1986) reported that perioperative blood pressure was unstable for a longer period of time after general anaesthesia compared with cervical plexus block. Vasoactive drugs were required for significantly longer periods in the general anaesthetic group. Muskett and colleagues (1986) noted no differences in operative time, anaesthetic time, maximum or minimum blood pressures, postoperative haemodynamic data or the requirement for or duration of intravenous pressor or antihypertensive medications. In marked contrast, Gableman and colleagues (1983) found higher intraoperative pressure in the regional group, with 39% of the cases requiring intravenous antihypertensives or pressor drugs compared with only 15% for the general anaesthetic group. Major variations in study design including retrospective versus prospective, observational versus intervention, and methodological differences including selection criteria, outcome analysis and lack of randomization have all inhibited valid comparisons.

Prospective randomized studies have been reported recently comparing regional and general anaesthesia for carotid endarterectomy. No significant differences in the incidence of death, myocardial infarction, stroke or transient ischaemic attacks were noted while regional anaesthesia proved to be superior to general anaesthesia in terms of cost-effectiveness, i.e. shorter ICU and hospital stays (Takolander *et al.*, 1990).

General anaesthesia

The objectives of general anaesthesia are to provide perioperative haemodynamic stability, to ensure adequate coronary and cerebral blood flow and to provide satisfactory oxygenation and ventilation. Compared to regional anaesthesia, general anaesthesia provides more scope to manipulate Pa_{CO_2} and Pa_{O_2}. Changes in both Pa_{CO_2} and Pa_{O_2} produce alterations in cerebral blood flow (CBF) that are most likely mediated by fluctuations in the pH surrounding the smooth muscles of cerebral arterioles. Hypoxaemia [a reduction in Pa_{O_2} below 8 kPa (60 mmHg)] is associated with maximum cerebral blood flow. CBF increases $1-2\,\mathrm{ml}\cdot 100\,\mathrm{g}^{-1}\cdot\mathrm{min}^{-1}$ for each 0.133 kPa (1 mmHg) increase in Pa_{CO_2} over the range from 3.3−13.3 kPa (25−100 mmHg). Hypercapnia, a possible consequence of opioid or major tranquillizer administration with a regional anaesthetic technique, may produce an undesirable 'steal' effect by shunting blood away from ischaemic areas (which are already maximally vasodilated) during carotid cross-clamp. However, relative normocapnia, which can best be provided with general anaesthesia, is preferred to extreme hypocapnia because vessels in marginal areas of perfusion may undergo vasoconstriction and convert an area of relative ischaemia to one of frank ischaemia.

There exists a body of data which suggests that, relative to halothane or enflurane, isoflurane is the volatile agent of choice because it may offer a degree of cerebral protection for transient incomplete regional ischaemia during carotid endarterectomy (Messick *et al.*, 1987). Isoflurane has the theoretical advantage that, unlike halothane or enflurane, at 2 minimum alveolar concentration (MAC), an isoelectric EEG is obtained with a reduction in cerebral metabolic oxygen demand (CMRO$_2$) similar to barbiturate therapy. Moreover, a critical CBF of $20\,\mathrm{ml}\cdot 100\,\mathrm{g}^{-1}\cdot\mathrm{min}^{-1}$ for halothane, $15\,\mathrm{ml}\cdot 100\,\mathrm{g}^{-1}\cdot\mathrm{min}^{-1}$ for enflurane compared with a $10\,\mathrm{ml}\cdot 100\,\mathrm{g}^{-1}\cdot\mathrm{min}^{-1}$ for isoflurane and nitrous oxide at normocapnia prevailed until EEG signs of cerebral ischaemia appeared. Michenfelder and colleagues (1987) in a retrospective analysis of data from the Mayo Clinic, reported that the incidence of EEG ischaemic changes was significantly less (18%) during isoflurane anaesthesia than during either enflurane (26%) or halothane (25%) anaesthesia. This difference occurred despite the fact that preoperative risk status was higher in the patients given isoflurane. There was, however, no difference in neurological outcome between the three anaesthetics.

General anaesthesia provides the additional advantage that active physiological and pharmacological brain protection measures can be readily initiated if EEC evidence of cerebral ischaemia develops during or after cross-clamp application or release. The pathophysiological changes associated with a cerebral ischaemic insult and the various pharmacological management strategies available were outlined by Murdoch and Hall (1990a,b) in a comprehensive two-part review. Ischaemia, whether focal or global in nature, produces a sequence of intracellular events leading to increased cell permeability to water and ions including calcium ions. There is loss of cellular integrity and function, with increased production of prostaglandins, oxygen free radicals and intracellular acidosis with lactate accumulation. Hyperglycaemia may exacerbate these ischaemic events.

Neuroprotective agents may exert their effect by reducing CMRO$_2$, increasing cerebral oxygen delivery, or by altering ongoing pathological processes (Table 50.7). Hypothermia provides neuroprotection by reducing the CMRO$_2$ necessary for synaptic transmission and the components for cellular metabolism and cell membrane integrity while barbiturates reduce the CMRO$_2$ for synaptic transmission only. Lignocaine, like hypothermia, may reduce CMRO$_2$ by affecting both cellular metabolic processes. The mechanism of action of calcium channel entry blocking agents may be due to improved blood flow as opposed to altering abnormal calcium ion fluxes. Agents like ketamine and MK-801 may prevent abnormal calcium ion fluxes or glutamate accumulation through their competitive interaction with N-methyl-D-aspartate (NMDA) receptors. Agents

Table 50.7 Carotid endarterectomy — cerebral protection

Increased cerebral perfusion pressure
Induced mild systemic hypertension

Increased cerebral/collateral blood flow
$Paco_2$ adjustments

Increased cerebral ischaemia tolerance (CMR O_2)
Hypothermia
Barbiturates
Isoflurane

Speculative
Calcium ion entry blockers
NMDA-receptor agonists

possibly worthy of further investigation include corticosteroids, free-radical scavengers and prostaglandin inhibitors.

The conflicting priorities of cerebral protection using pharmacologic blood-pressure support and myocardial well-being were highlighted by Smith and colleagues (1988) when they noted an alarming incidence of myocardial ischaemia in patients who received phenylephrine to maintain blood pressure during isoflurane or halothane anaesthesia as compared with patients who were lightly anaesthetized. The major cause of cerebral dysfunction following carotid endarterectomy is thromboembolism rather than blood flow reduction while the major cause of morbidity results from myocardial dysfunction. Smith and colleagues (1988) advocate EEG monitoring to indicate when blood pressure may be safely decreased and TOE to monitor myocardial well-being when arterial blood pressure is being pharmacologically augmented.

Cerebral function monitoring

Monitoring during carotid endarterectomy is directed mainly at the cardiovascular system and the CNS. The surgical procedure is not associated with major blood loss or fluid shifts but profound fluctuations in heart rate and blood pressure may follow surgical manipulation of the carotid baroreceptors and carotid cross-clamp and release. Numerous techniques have been used in an attempt to monitor the adequacy of cerebral perfusion, particularly when the ipsilateral common carotid is clamped. The results of these measurements in some cases have formed a basis for the decision to insert an intraluminal shunt.

Surgical opinion has divided between routine shunting, no shunting and shunt bypass based on the detection of intraoperative cerebral ischemia. Similar overall outcome in series reported by advocates in each of these three groups has led to controversy regarding the need for monitoring or bypass shunting.

Early techniques for monitoring the adequacy of cerebral perfusion have included determination of jugular venous oxygen saturation, assessment of neurological status during a trial period of carotid occlusion under regional anaesthesia and measurement of pressure in the internal carotid artery (stump pressure).

An internal carotid stump pressure of <6.7 kPa (50 mmHg) was hypothesized to represent adequate collateral circulation through the circle of Willis or the external carotid circulation. However, in practice, stump pressure does not correlate with clinical signs if cerebral ischaemia, measured regional cerebral blood flow or EEG changes.

The clinical value of continuous monitoring of transconjunctival oxygen tension ($Pcjo_2$) to assess cerebral perfusion is limited because of large interindividual variations in basal $Pcjo_2$ readings and $Pcjo_2$ changes during carotid artery clamp do not allow for early and accurate recognition of impending cerebral ischaemia (Kresowik *et al.*, 1991).

The EEG signals recorded from the scalp are generated by excitatory and inhibitory postsynaptic potentials that summate in the pyramidal cells in the cerebral cortex. The standard scalp recorded EEG — classically described by four basic rhythms or frequencies, i.e. delta (δ) (1–4 Hz), theta (θ) (4–8 Hz), alpha (α) (8–13 Hz) and beta (β) (13–30 Hz) — has proved a sensitive monitoring device during carotid endarterectomy but its specificity is limited by the similar changes associated with hypothermia, hypotension and general anaesthetic agents. Cerebral ischaemia is associated with a reduction or slowing of high-frequency activity and the development of new or augmented activity in the θ and δ range.

The use of EEG monitoring equipment is expensive, cumbersome, difficult to interpret and time consuming. Notwithstanding claims from Sundt and colleagues (1981) from the Mayo Clinic that no patient has emerged from anaesthesia with a neurologic deficit that was not predicted by the EEG, recent reports have questioned the impressive sensitivity of EEG monitoring in detecting perioperative cerebral ischaemia. Kresowik and colleagues (1991), in a retrospective analysis of 458 consecutive carotid endarterectomies performed under general anaesthesia, reported that five of 10 patients with immediate strokes and all five patients with immediate transient deficits had no ischaemic EEG changes during the procedure.

The traditional EEG is plotted on a strip chart as voltage against time. Data are interpreted using pattern-recognition skills that depend on the expertise of the observer. To facilitate intraoperative use by anaesthesia staff with limited EEG interpretation experience, EEG signal processing techniques include fewer recording channels, data compression and colour-coded displays to facilitate feature extraction and trend recognition.

The most common forms of processed EEGs are the cerebral function monitor (CFM), the compressed spectral array (CSA), the density spectral array (DSA) and aperiodic analysis techniques. The CMF filters the EEG input from a single channel to remove frequencies below 2 Hz and above 15 Hz and the average peak voltage is displayed on a strip chart recorder.

Processed EEG signal utilizing fast Fourier analysis to produce a CSA has been developed to simplify the recognition and interpretation of EEG changes during anaesthesia. The CSA presents the power spectrum analysis in the form of a graph of relative power (amplitudes squared) versus frequency. The frequencies with greater power are presented as hills at that frequency, whereas valleys represent frequencies with less power. The DSA is displayed in dot-matrix form, the larger dots signify areas of high activity and the small ones low activity. Several studies have indicated that these systems are reliable indicators of significant alterations of cerebral blood flow. Templehoff and colleagues (1989) assessed the reliability of two-channel monitoring of both CSA and simultaneous unprocessed EEG in predicting the requirement for intraluminal shunting in 100 patients undergoing carotid endarterectomy. A correlation between total cumulative ischaemic EEG time and postoperative neurological examination was demonstrated and the two-channel monitoring of both CSA and unprocessed EEG simultaneously proved a reliable indicator of the need for bypass shunting.

The processed EEG Lifescan Monitor (Neurometrics) obtains the EEG signal from a two bipolar-channel, five-lead system which uses aperiodic analysis to display the processed EEG in graphical form on a high-resolution screen. Silbert and colleagues (1989) compared processed EEG with awake neurological assessment in detecting cerebral ischaemia in 70 patients undergoing carotid endarterectomy under cervical plexus block. The manifestations of ischaemia consist of loss of high-frequency activity and the development of new or augmented low-frequency activity, both best demonstrated by frequency edge line. Of the six patients demonstrating neurological signs on cross-clamping, five dis-

played simultaneous EEG changes and one was detected after retrospective analysis of the processed EEG recording. Another four patients displayed EEG changes indicative of ischaemia but unassociated with neurological signs. The authors claimed the presence of false negatives, possible false positives and technical errors associated with a processed EEG made this technique less reliable than a neurological assessment for the detection of cerebral ischaemia.

Case reports have highlighted the value of processed EEG in suggesting the need for hyperventilation to reverse EEG ischaemic changes which failed to respond to maintenance of blood pressure and the detection of shunt occlusion in the absence of other systemic changes.

Regional blood flow reduction to specific brain areas may cause functional neurological changes despite the presence of a satisfactory global perfusion, as determined by the EEG. Placement of electrodes in the frontomastoid configuration, as with the various processed EEG monitoring devices, allows portions of the brain perfused by the middle cerebral artery to remain unmonitored rendering the technique less sensitive in detecting localized ischaemia.

Transcranial Doppler (TCD) ultrasonography permits monitoring of the direction and velocity of blood flow in the horizontal segment of the middle cerebral artery and other proximal branches of the circle of Willis. Hence TCD has been advocated as a supplementary monitoring technique to increase the sensitivity of processed EEG monitoring during carotid endarterectomy.

Halsey and colleagues (1989) reported the relationship between regional cerebral blood flow and mean velocity in the middle cerebral artery, determined by TCD during 31 carotid endarterectomies. The relation between rCBF and mean velocity was dependent on the rCBF. If rCBF was less than $20 \, \text{ml} \cdot 100 \, \text{g}^{-1} \cdot \text{min}^{-1}$ the correlation was strong but if rCBF was greater than $20 \, \text{ml}/100 \, \text{g}$, the correlation weakened.

To test the hypothesis that TCD was a useful intraoperative technique monitoring to detect cerebral ischaemia, Bass and colleagues (1989) prospectively used the technique to study patients undergoing carotid endarterectomy. The authors reported a 27% incidence of technical difficulty, primarily because of probe position difficulties, and normal TCD data in one patient (1.2%) who sustained an operative stroke. The authors concluded that TCD was not a useful routine monitor to detect intraoperative cerebral ischaemia during carotid endarterectomy.

There is no concensus as to the most appropriate

monitor to detect cerebral ischaemia during carotid endarterectomy. Somatosensory-evoked potential monitoring (SSEP) offers the potential advantages over EEG monitoring of being technically easier to perform and interpret and provides information specific to the sensory cortex, an area supplied by the middle cerebral artery that is placed at risk during carotid cross-clamp. Lam and colleagues (1991) recently compared conventional EEG with SSEP in 64 consecutive patients undergoing carotid endarterectomy under general anaesthesia. The authors concluded that although SSEP and EEG are both associated with a considerable false-positive rate, no new neurologic deficits were observed in patients with unchanged SSEP.

Postoperative management

In addition to neurological deficits, the immediate postoperative period may be associated with a variety of complications including wound haematoma and upper-airway obstruction; carotid body and baro-receptor dysfunction and cranial nerve damage due to recurrent laryngeal, superior laryngeal, hypoglossal and marginal mandibular nerve injury.

Major fluctuations in blood pressure are commonly observed. Hypertension following carotid endarterectomy, especially in patients with poorly controlled blood pressure, was associated with an increased incidence of postoperative neurological deficits in a retrospective evaluation by Assidao and colleagues (1982) of 166 patients undergoing carotid endarterectomy. The aetiology of hypertension has been the focus of recent investigation. The mechanism, to date, is uncertain but is likely to involve a number of perioperative factors. Various authors have implicated exacerbations of preoperative hypertension, carotid sinus dysfunction, and elevated cerebral renin or norepinephrine concentrations.

Conclusion

This review includes analysis of recent data concerning major vascular surgery involving the carotid artery and the abdominal aorta.

Recent data have highlighted the dramatic increases in the past four decades of deaths attributable to AAAs and community-based screening studies have provided new insights into the natural course and progression of abdominal aortic disease. Also, recent data suggest that the median rate of expansion of small aneurysms were slower than previously reported and the risk of rupture in aneurysms <5 cm

in diameter were lower than previously predicted. The tendency for AAAs to occur in families is of interest, and prospective screening studies have noted that patients with familial aneurysms are more likely to be women. A genetic basis for aortic aneurysm formation is the subject of continuing laboratory investigation.

Recent extensive prospective multicentre studies of AAA patients have defined the current North American standards for the investigation and management of these patients and have supported the aggressive lifelong approach to the management of coronary artery disease in this patient population. Given the documented impact of ischaemic heart disease on the morbidity/mortality associated with AAAs, the relative merits of preoperative non-invasive investigations have been the subject of recent investigations. Ambulatory ECG monitoring may offer the appropriate combination of sensitivity and specificity to make it part of the routine preoperative evaluation in this patient population.

The value of DTS as a preoperative screening test for perioperative myocardial ischaemia has been questioned. Recent data suggests that semiquantitative DTS analysis may improve its specificity. In younger patients, without cardiac symptoms or obvious risk factors, the anticipated perioperative cardiac morbidity is low (<1%), which does not justify extensive mandatory screening tests. DTS and other preoperative tests may be more helpful in stratification of patients at immediate risk (one or more clinical risk variables) who comprise most of the patient population.

Recent interest has focused on the role of pulmonary artery catheters in the management of patients undergoing abdominal aortic reconstruction. Pulmonary artery monitoring, compared with CVP, was not associated with improved patient outcome in a recent prospective randomized study. The relationship between echocardiographic RWMAs and postoperative cardiac outcome has been questioned. Such changes were considered sensitive indicators of myocardial ischaemia but many of these episodes occur randomly and may not be associated with increases in myocardial oxygen demand. The specificity of RWMAs in indicating myocardial ischaemia has been investigated under varying preload and afterload conditions.

Paraplegia is an uncommon but devastating consequence of thoracic and thoracoabdominal aortic reconstruction. Recent inconclusive studies have addressed the potential of CSF drainage and intercostal artery reimplantation to minimize this complication. Conflicting reports have been published comparing retroperitoneal and transabdominal surgical approach in terms of morbidity and cost-effectiveness.

Growing interest in regional anaesthesia for AAA has been stimulated by a report of improved operative outcome. However, recent data highlight the dilemma of acceptance of the basic concept of nociceptive block as a prerequisite for improved postoperative morbidity with lack of scientific documentation of benefits with extradural anaesthesia and analgesia. The first definitive study to examine the isolated effects of primary anaesthetic technique on postoperative outcome showed that thoracic extradural anaesthesia added to 'light' general anaesthesia was not associated with improved outcome compared with 'balanced' general anaesthesia.

The surgical indications for carotid endarterectomy have been clarified with the publication of extensive European and North American studies. For symptomatic patients with 'severe' (70–99%) stenosis, the immediate risks of surgery are considerably outweighed by later benefits in terms of reduced rates of disabling stroke. Outcome following surgery may be influenced more by the presence or absence of ischaemic heart disease and by surgical considerations, primarily the numbers of procedures performed annually by the individual surgeon rather than the status of the institution involved.

Judging by the number of reports published in the last decade, interest in the use of local or regional anaesthesia for carotid surgery appears to be growing. Recent prospective randomized studies comparing general with regional anaesthesia have noted no significant differences in the incidence of death, myocardial infarction, stroke, or transient ischaemic attacks but regional anaesthesia proved superior in terms of cost-effectiveness. Surgical opinion remains divided between routine shunting, no shunting and shunt bypass based on the detection of intraoperative cerebral ischaemia.

Various processed EEG signals have been developed to simplify the detection and interpretation of EEG changes during anaesthesia. However, some investigators have claimed that the presence of false negatives, possible false positives and technical errors associated with processed EEG make this monitoring technique less reliable than awake neurological assessment for the detection of cerebral ischaemia. Similar observations have been made concerning transcranial Doppler assessment of middle cerebral artery blood flow.

The conflicting priorities of cerebral protection, using pharmacological blood pressure support and myocardial oxygen supply/demand imbalance have been recently highlighted and TOE has been advocated to detect subtle myocardial ischaemia associated with pharmacologic augmentation of systolic blood pressure.

References

Abbott W.M., Cooper J.D. & Austen W.G. (1973) The effect of aortic clamping and declamping on renal blood flow distribution. *Journal of Surgical Research* **14**, 385–92.

Albert R.A., Roizen M.F. & Hamilton W.K. (1984) Intraoperative urine output does not predict postoperative renal function in patients undergoing abdominal aortic revascularization. *Surgery* **95**, 707–11.

Antiplatelet Trialists' Collaboration (1988) Secondary prevention of vascular disease by prolonged antiplatelet treatment. *British Medical Journal* **296**, 320–31.

Assidao C.B., Donegan J.H., Whitesell R.C. & Kalbfleisch J.H. (1982) Factors associated with perioperative complications during carotid endarterectomy. *Anesthesia and Analgesia* **61**, 631–7.

Attia R.R., Murphy J.D., Snider M., Lappas D.G., Darling R.C. & Lowenstein E. (1976) Myocardial ischemia due to infrarenal aortic cross clamping during aortic surgery in patients with severe coronary artery disease. *Circulation* **53**, 961–4.

Barnett H.J.M. (1990) Symptomatic carotid endarterectomy trials. *Stroke* **21**, 111–15.

Baron J.F., Bertrand M., Barre E., Godet G., Mundler O., Coriat P. & Viars P. (1991) Combined epidural and general anesthesia versus general anesthesia for abdominal aortic surgery. *Anesthesiology* **75**, 611–18.

Bass A., Krupski W.C., Schneider P.A., Otis S.M., Dilley R.B. & Bernstein E.F. (1989) Intraoperative transcranial Doppler: limitations of the method. *Journal of Vascular Surgery* **10**, 549–53.

Battler A., Froelicher V.F., Gallagher K.P., Kemper W.S. & Ross J. (1980) Dissociation between regional myocardial dysfunction and ECG changes during ischemia in the conscious dog. *Circulation* **62**, 735–44.

Berlauk J.F., Abrams J.H., Gilmour I.J., O'Connor R., Knighton D.R. & Cerra F.B. (1991) Preoperative optimization of cardiovascular hemodynamics improves outcome in peripheral vascular surgery. *Annals of Surgery* **214**, 289–97.

Bernstein E.F. & Chan E.L. (1984) Abdominal aortic aneurysm in high risk patients. Outcome of selective management based on size and expansion rate. *Annals of Surgery* **200**, 255–62.

Beven E.G. (1986) Routine coronary angiography in patients undergoing surgery for abdominal aortic aneurysm and lower extremity occlusive disease. *Journal of Vascular Surgery* **3**, 682–4.

Blomberg S., Emanuelsson H., Kvist H., Lamm C., Ponten J., Waagstein F. & Ricksten S.E. (1990) Effects of thoracic epidural anesthesia on coronary arteries and arterioles in patients with coronary artery disease. *Anesthesiology* **73**, 840–7.

Bower T.C., Murray M.J. & Gloviezki P. (1989) Effects of thoracic aortic occlusion and cerebrospinal fluid drainage on regional spinal cord blood flow in dogs: correlation with neurologic outcome. *Journal of Vascular Surgery* **9**, 135−44.

Brant B., Armstrong R.P. & Vetto R.M. (1970) Vasodepressor factor in declamp shock production. *Surgery* **67**, 650−3.

Breslow M.J., Jordan D.A., Christopherson R., Rosenfeld B., Miller C.F., Lanley D.F., Beattie C., Traystman R.J. & Rogers M.C. (1989) Epidural morphine decreases postoperative hypertension of attenuating sympathetic nervous system hyperactivity. *Journal of the American Medical Association* **261**, 3577−81.

Brewster D.C., Ambrosino J.J. & Darling R.C. (1979) Intra-operative autotransfusion in major vascular surgery. *American Journal of Surgery* **137**, 507−12.

Brown G., Albers J.J. & Fisher L.D. (1990) Regression of coronary disease as a result of intensive lipid-lowering therapy in men with high levels of apolipoprotein B. *New England Journal of Medicine* **323**, 1289−98.

Buffington C.W. & Coyle R.J. (1991) Altered load dependence of postischemic myocardium. *Anesthesiology* **75**, 464−74.

Bunt T.J., Manczuk M. & Warley K. (1987) Continuous epidural anaesthesia for aortic surgery: thoughts on peer review and safety. *Surgery* **101**, 706−14.

Bush H.L., Logerfo F.W. & Weisel R.D. (1977) Assessment of myocardial performance and optimal volume loading during elective abdominal aortic aneurysm resection. *Archives of Surgery* **112**, 1302−6.

Cambria R.P., Brewster D.C. & Abbott W.M. (1990) Trans-peritoneal versus retroperitoneal approach for aortic reconstruction: a randomized prospective study. *Journal of Vascular Surgery* **11**, 314−25.

Campbell W.B. (1991) Mortality statistics for elective aortic aneurysms. *European Journal of Vascular Surgery* **5**, 111−13.

Clark N.J. & Stanley T.H. (1991) Anesthesia for vascular surgery. In *Anesthesia* 3rd edn. (Ed. Miller R.D.) pp. 1693−1736. Churchill Livingstone, New York.

Cohn P.F. (1988) Silent myocardial ischemia. *Annals of Internal Medicine* **109**, 312−17.

Cole C.W., Barber G.G., Bouchard A.G., McPhail N.V., Roberge C., Waddell W. & Wellington J.L. (1989) Abdominal aortic aneurysm: consequences of a positive family history. *Canadian Journal of Surgery* **32**, 117−20.

Collin J., Araujo L. & Walton J. (1989) How fast do very small abdominal aortic aneurysms grow? *European Journal of Vascular Surgery* **3**, 15−17.

Collins R., Peto R., MacMahon S., Herbert P., Fiebach N.H., Eberlain K.A., Godwin J., Quisalbash N., Taylor J.O. & Hennekens C.H. (1990) Blood pressure, stroke and coronary artery disease. *Lancet* **335**, 827−38.

Corson J.D., Chang B.B., Leopold P.W., DeLeo B., Shah D.M., Leather R.P. & Karmody A. (1986) Perioperative hypertension in patients undergoing carotid endarterectomy: shorter duration under regional block anesthesia. *Circulation* **74** (Suppl. 1), 1−4.

Cousins M.J. & Wright C.J. (1971) Graft, muscle, skin blood flow after epidural block in vascular surgery procedures. *Surgery Gynecology Obstetrics* **133**, 59−65.

Crawford E.S. & Hess K.R. (1989) Abdominal aortic aneurysm. *New England Journal of Medicine* **321**, 1040−2.

Crawford E.S., Svensson L.G., Hess K.R., Shenaq S.S., Coselli J.S., Safi H.J., Mohindra P.K. & Rivera V. (1990) A prospective randomized study of cerebrospinal fluid drainage to prevent paraplegia after high-risk surgery on the thoracoabdominal aorta. *Journal of Vascular Surgery* **13**, 36−46.

Cronenwett J.L., Sargent S.K. & Wall M.H. (1990) Variables that affect the expansion rate and outcome of small abdominal aortic aneurysms. *Journal of Vascular Surgery* **11**, 260−9.

Crosby E.T., Miller D.P., Hamilton P.P., Martineau R.J., Bouchard A. & Wellington J. (1990) A randomized double blind comparison of fentanyl and sufentanil-O_2 anesthesia for abdominal aortic surgery. *Journal of Cardiothoracic Anesthesiology* **4**, 168−76.

Crowson M., Fielding J.W.L., Black J., Ashton F. & Stanley G. (1984) Acute gastrointestinal complications of infrarenal aortic aneurysm repair. *British Journal of Surgery* **71**, 205−8.

Cunningham A.J. (1989a) Anaesthesia for abdominal aortic surgery − a review (Part I). *Canadian Journal of Anaesthesia* **36**, 426−44.

Cunningham A.J. (1989b) Anesthesia for abdominal aortic surgery − a review (Part II). *Canadian Journal of Anaesthesia* **36**, 568−77.

Cunningham A.J., McDonald N., Keeling F., O'Toole D.P. & Bouchier-Hayes D. (1989) The influence of collateral vascular-isation on haemodynamic performance during aortic vascular surgery. *Canadian Journal of Anaesthesia* **36**, 44−50.

Cutler B.S., Wheeler H.B., Paraskos J.A. & Cardullo P.A. (1981) Applicability and interpretation of electrocardiographic stress testing in patients with peripheral vascular disease. *American Journal of Surgery* **141**, 501−5.

Darling R.C. III, Brewster D.C., Darling R.C., La Muraglia G.M., Monclure A.C., Cameria R.P. & Abbott W.M. (1989) Are familial abdominal aortic aneurysms different? *Journal of Vascular Surgery* **10**, 39−43.

Dennis M.S., Bamford J.M., Sandercock P.A.G. & Warlow C.P. (1989) Incidence of transient attacks in Oxfordshire, England. *Stroke* **20**, 333−9.

Dennis M.S., Bamford J.M., Sandercock P.A.G. & Warlow C.P. (1990) The prognosis of transient ischaemic attacks in the Oxford Community Stroke Project. *Stroke* **21**, 848−53.

Dubost C., Allary M. & Oeconomos N. (1952) Resection of an aneurysm of the abdominal aorta: Re-establishment of the continuity by a preserved human arterial graft with results after five months. *Archives of Surgery* **64**, 405−8.

Duchateau J., Nevelsteen A., Suy R., Demeyere R., Van Decrean J., Goossens M., Bogaerts M., Arnot J. & Vermycen J. (1990) Autotransfusion during aortic-iliac surgery. *European Journal of Vascular Surgery* **4**, 349−54.

Duncan S.E., Edwards W.H. & Dale W.A. (1974) Caution regard-ing autotransfusion. *Surgery* **76**, 1024−30.

Eagle K.A. & Boucher C.A. (1989) Cardiac risk of non-cardiac surgery. *New England Journal of Medicine* **321**, 1330−2.

Eagle K.A., Singer D.E., Brewster D.C., Darling R.C., Mulley A.G. & Boucher C.A. (1987) Dipyridamole-thallium scanning in patients undergoing vascular surgery. *Journal of the American Medical Association* **257**, 2185−9.

Eagle K.A., Coley C.M., Newell J.B., Brewster D.C., Darling C., Strauss H.W., Guiney T.E. & Boucher C.A. (1989) Combining clinical and thallium data optimizes preoperative assessment of cardiac risk before major vascular surgery. *Annals of Internal Medicine* **110**, 859−66.

Editorial (1991) Operating to prevent stroke. *Lancet* **337**, 1255–6.

Engelman E., Lipszyc M., Gilbert E., Bellens B., Van Romphey A. & de Rood M. (1989) Effects of clonidine on anesthetic drug requirements and hemodynamic response during aortic surgery. *Anesthesiology* **71**, 178–87.

Ernst C.B., Hagihara P.F., Daugherty M.E., Sachatello C.R. & Griffen W.O. (1976) Ischemic colitis incidence following abdominal aortic reconstruction: a prospective study. *Surgery* **80**, 417–21.

European Carotid Surgery Triallists' Collaborative Group (1991) MRC European Carotid Surgery Trial: interim results for symptomatic patients with severe (70–99%) or with mild (0–29%) carotid stenosis. *Lancet* **337**, 1235–43.

Falk J.L., Rackow E.C., Blumenberg R., Gelfand M. & Fein I.A. (1981) Hemodynamic and metabolic effects of abdominal aortic cross clamping. *American Journal of Surgery* **142**, 174–7.

Fowkes F.G.R., MacIntyre C.C.A. & Ruckley C.V. (1989) Increasing incidence of aortic aneurysms in England and Wales. *British Medical Journal* **298**, 33–5.

Franco C.D., Goldsmith J., Veith F.J., Ascer E., Wengerter E.R., Calligaro K.D. & Gupta S.K. (1989) Resting gated pool ejection fraction: a poor predictor of perioperative myocardial infarction in patients undergoing vascular surgery for infrainguinal bypass grafting. *Journal of Vascular Surgery* **10**, 656–61.

Friesen R.M., Thomson I.R. & Hudson R.J. (1986) Fentanyl oxygen anaesthesia for abdominal aortic surgery. *Canadian Anaesthetists' Society Journal* **33**, 719–22.

Gableman C.G., Gann D.S., Ashworth C.J. & Carney W.I. (1983) One hundred consecutive carotid reconstructions: local versus general anesthesia. *American Journal of Surgery* **145**, 477–82.

Galt S.W., Bech F.R., McDaniel M.D., Dain B.J., Yeager M.P., Schneider J.R., Walsh D.B., Zwolak R.M. & Cronenwett J.L. (1991) The effect of ibuprofen on cardiac performance during abdominal aortic cross-clamping. *Journal of Vascular Surgery* **13**, 876–84.

Gamulin Z., Forster A., Morel D., Simonset F., Aymon E. & Favre H. (1984) Effect of infrarenal aortic cross clamping on renal hemodynamics in humans. *Anesthesiology* **61**, 394–9.

Gelman S., Fowler K.G. & Smith L.R. (1984) Regional blood flow during isoflurane and halothane anesthesia. *Anesthesia and Analgesia* **63**, 557–65.

Gelman S., McDowell H. & Varner P.D. (1988) The reason for cardiac output reduction after aortic cross clamping. *American Journal of Surgery* **155**, 578–81.

Gersh B.J., Rihal C.S., Rook T.W. & Ballard D.J. (1991) Evaluation and management of patients with both peripheral vascular and coronary artery disease. *Journal of the American College of Cardiology* **18**, 203–14.

Gewertz B.L., Kremser P.C., Zarins C.K., Smith J.S., Ellis J.E., Feinstein S.B. & Roizen M.F. (1987) Transesophageal echocardiographic monitoring of myocardial ischemia during vascular surgery. *Journal of Vascular Surgery* **5**, 607–13.

Golden M.A., Donaldson M.C., Whittemore A.D. & Mannick J.A. (1991) Evolving experience with thoracoabdominal aortic aneurysm repair at a single institution. *Journal of Vascular Surgery* **13**, 792–7.

Goldman L. (1987) Multi-factorial index of cardiac risk in non-

cardiac surgery — a 10-year status report. *Journal of Cardiothoracic Anesthesia* **1**, 237–44.

Goldman L. (1991) Cardiac risk assessment in patients with atherosclerotic vascular disease. In *Vascular Anesthesia* 1st edn. (Ed. Kaplan J.A.) pp. 1–20. Churchill Livingstone, New York.

Goldman L. & Caldera D.L. (1979) Risk of general anesthesia and elective operation in the hypertensive patient. *Anesthesiology* **50**, 285–9.

Goldman L., Caldera D.L. & Nussbaum S.R. (1977) Multi-factorial index of cardiac risk in new cardiac surgery procedures. *New England Journal of Medicine* **297**, 845–50.

Gooding J.M., Archie J.P. & McDowell H. (1980) Hemodynamic response to infrarenal aortic across clamping in patients with and without coronary artery disease. *Critical Care Medicine* **8**, 382–5.

Grant R.P., Morgan C., Page M.S., Malm D.N., Huckel V. & Jenkins L.C. (1990) Dipyridamole–thallium myocardial scanning in the preoperative assessment of patients undergoing abdominal aortic aneurysmectomy. *Canadian Journal of Anaesthesia* **37**, 409–15.

Gregory R.T., Wheeler J.R. & Synder S.D. (1989) Retroperitoneal approach to aortic surgery. *Journal of Cardiovascular Surgery* **30**, 185–9.

Guy A.J., Lambert D., Jones N.A.G. & Chamberlain J. (1990) After the Confidential Enquiry into Perioperative Deaths — aortic aneurysm surgery in the northern region. *British Journal of Surgery* **77**, 344–5A.

Hallett J.W., Popovsky M. & Ilstrup D. (1987) Minimizing blood transfusions during abdominal aortic surgery: recent advances in rapid autotransfusion. *Journal of Vascular Surgery* **5**, 601–6.

Halsey J.H., McDowell H.A., Gelman S. & Morawetz R.B. (1989) Blood velocity in the middle cerebral artery and regional cerebral blood during carotid endarterectomy. *Stroke* **20**, 53–8.

Hertzer N.R. (1987) Basic data concerning associated coronary disease in peripheral vascular patients. *Annals of Vascular Surgery* **1**, 616–20.

Hertzer N.R., Beven E.G. & Young J.R. (1984) Coronary artery disease in peripheral vascular patients. A classification of 1000 coronary angiograms and results of surgical management. *Annals of Surgery* **199**, 223–33.

Hertzer N.R., Loop F.D., Beven E.G., O'Hara P.J. & Krajewski L.P. (1987) Surgical staging for simultaneous coronary and carotid disease: a study including prospective randomization. *Journal of Vascular Surgery* **12**, 615–20.

Hollier L.H., Plate G. & O'Brien P.C. (1984) Late survival after abdominal aortic repair: influence of coronary artery disease. *Journal of Vascular Surgery* **1**, 290–9.

Hollier L.H. & Moore W.M. (1990) Avoidance of renal and neurologic complications following thoracoabdominal aortic aneurysm repair. *Acta Chirurgica Chir Scandinavica Supplementum* **555**, 129–35.

Hudson J.C., Wurm W.H., O'Donnell J.F., Kane F.R., Mackey W., Su Y.F. & Watkins W.D. (1990) Ibuprofen pretreatment inhibits prostacyclin release during abdominal exploration in aortic surgery. *Anesthesiology* **72**, 443–9.

Hummel B.W., Raess D.H., Gernertz B.L., Wheeler H.T. & Fry W.J. (1982) Effect of nitroglycerin and aortic occlusion on myocardial blood flow. *Surgery* **92**, 159−65.

Iberti T.J., Fisher E.P., Leibowitz A.B., Panacek E.D., Silverstein J.H., Albertson T.E. & the Pulmonary Artery Catheter Study Group (1990) *Journal of the American Medical Association* **204**, 2928−32.

Isaacson E.J., Lowdon J.D., Berry A.J., Smith R.B., Knos G.B., Weitz F.I. & Ryan K. (1990) The value of pulmonary artery and central venous monitoring in patients undergoing abdominal aortic reconstructive surgery: a comparison study of two selected, randomized groups. *Journal of Vascular Surgery* **12**, 754−60.

Jain K.M., Patel K.D., Doctor U.S. & Peck S.L. (1985) Preoperative cardiac screening before peripheral vascular operation. *American Surgeon* **51**, 77−81.

Jamieson W.R.E., Janusz M.T., Miyagishima R.T. & Gerein A.N. (1982) Influence of ischemic heart disease on early and late mortality after surgery for peripheral occlusive vascular disease. *Circulation* **66** (Suppl. 1), 92−7.

Jeffrey C.C., Kunsman J., Cullen D.C. & Brewster D.C. (1983) A prospective evaluation of cardiac risk index. *Anesthesiology* **58**, 462−4.

Johansen K., Kohler T.R., Nicholls S.C., Zierler R.E., Clowes A.W. & Kazmers A. (1991) Ruptured abdominal aortic aneurysm: The Harbourview experience. *Journal of Vascular Surgery* **13**, 240−7.

Johnston K.W. (1989) Multicenter prospective study of non-ruptured abdominal aortic aneurysm. Part II. Variables predicting morbidity and mortality. *Journal of Vascular Surgery* **9**, 437−47.

Johnston K.W. & Scobie T.K. (1988) Multicenter prospective study of non-ruptured abdominal aortic aneurysms. Populations and operative management. *Journal of Vascular Surgery* **7**, 69−81.

Kalman P.G., Wellwood M.R. & Weisel R.D. (1986) Cardiac dysfunction during abdominal aortic operation: the limitations of pulmonary wedge pressures. *Journal of Vascular Surgery* **3**, 773−9.

Kannel W.B. (1990) Contribution of the Framingham study of preventive cardiology. *Journal of the American College of Cardiology* **15**, 206−11.

Kaplan J.A. & Wells P.H. (1981) Early diagnosis of myocardial ischemia using the pulmonary artery catheter. *Anesthesia and Analgesia* **60**, 789−93.

Kataja J.H.K., Kaukinen S. & Vinamaki O.U.K. (1989) Hemodynamic and hormonal changes in patients pretreated with captopril for surgery of the abdominal aorta. *Journal of Cardiothoracic Anesthesia* **3**, 425−32.

Kazmers A., Cerqueria M. & Ziefler R.E. (1988) The role of preoperative radionuclide ejection fraction in direct abdominal aortic aneurysm repair. *Journal of Vascular Surgery* **8**, 128−36.

Knight A.A., Hollenberg M. & London M.J. (1989) Myocardial ischemia in patients awaiting coronary artery bypass grafting. *American Heart Journal* **117**, 1189−95.

Kremer H., Weigold B., Dobrinski W., Schreiber M.A. & Zollner N. (1984) Sonographisce Verlaufsbeobachtungen von Bauchaorten-Aneurysmen. *Clinics Wochenscur* **62**, 1120−5.

Kresowik T.F., Worsey J., Khoury M.D., Krain L.S., Shamma A.R., Sharp W.J., Stern J.A. & Corson J.D. (1991) Limitations of electroencephalographic monitoring in the detection of cerebral ischemia accompanying carotid endarterectomy. *Journal of Vascular Surgery* **13**, 439−43.

Lam A.M., Manninen P.H., Ferguson G.G. & Nantau W. (1991) Monitoring electrophysiologic function during carotid endarterectomy: a comparison of somatosensory evoked potentials and conventional electroencephalogram. *Anesthesiology* **75**, 15−21.

Leather R.P., Shah D.M. & Karmody A.M. (1981) Infrapopliteal arterial bypass for limb salvage: increased patency and utilization of the saphenous vein used *in-situ*. *Surgery* **90**, 1000−9.

Leppo J., Plaja J., Gionet M., Tumolo J., Paraskos J.A. & Cutler B.S. (1987) Non-invasive evaluation of cardiac risk before elective vascular surgery. *Journal of the American College of Cardiology* **9**, 269−76.

Lette J., Waters D., Lapointe J., Gagnon A., Picard M., Cering M. & Kerouac M. (1989) Usefulness of the severity and extent of reversible perfusion defects during thallium−dipyridamole imaging for cardiac risk assessment before non-cardiac surgery. *American Journal of Cardiology* **64**, 276−81.

Leung J.M., Schiller N.B. & Mangano D.T. (1989) Transesophageal echocardiographic assessment of left ventricular function. *International Journal of Cardiac Imaging* **5**, 63−70.

Leung J.M., O'Kelly B.F., Mangano D.T. & the SPI research group (1990) Relationship of regional wall motion abnormalities to hemodynamic indices of myocardial oxygen supply and demand in patients undergoing CABG surgery. *Anesthesiology* **73**, 802−14.

Levinson J.R., Boucher C.A., Coley C.M., Guiney J.E., Strauss W. & Eagle K. (1990) Usefulness of semiquantitative analysis dipyridamole−thallium-201 redistribution for improving risk stratification before vascular surgery. *American Journal of Cardiology* **66**, 406−10.

Lim R.C., Bergentz S.F. & Lewis D.H. (1969) Metabolic and tissue blood flow changes resulting from aortic cross clamping. *Surgery* **65**, 304−10.

London M.J., Tubau J.F., Wong M.G., Layug E., Hollenberg M., Krupski W.C., Rapp J.H., Besuner W.S. & Mangano D.T. (1990) The 'natural history' of segmental wall motion abnormalities in patients undergoing non-cardiac surgery. *Anesthesiology* **73**, 644−55.

Lowdon J.D. & Isaacson I.J. (1991) Anesthesia for patients with diseases of peripheral arteries and veins. In *Vascular Anesthesia* (Ed. Kaplan J.A.) pp. 395−416. Churchill Livingstone, New York.

Mackaroun M.S., Shuman-Jackson N., Rippley A., Schreiner D. & Arvan S. (1990) Cardiac risk in vascular surgery. The oral dipyridamole−thallium stress test. *Archives of Surgery* **125**, 1610−13.

Mackey W.C., O'Donnell T.F. & Callow A.D. (1990) Cardiac risk in patients undergoing carotid endarterectomy: impact on perioperative and long term mortality. *Journal of Vascular Surgery* **11**, 226−34.

Mangano D.T. (1980) Monitoring pulmonary artery pressure in coronary artery disease. *Anesthesiology* **53**, 364−70.

Mangano D.T. (1990) Perioperative cardiac morbidity. *Anesthesiology* **72**, 153−84.

Mangano D.T., Browner W.S., Hollenberg M., London M.J., Tubau J.F., Tateo I.M & the SPI group (1990) Association of perioperative myocardial ischemia with cardiac morbidity and mortality in men undergoing non-cardiac surgery. *New England Journal of Medicine* **323**, 1781–8.

Mangano D.T., London M.J., Tubau J.F., Browner W.S., Hollenberg M., Krupski W., Layug E.L. & Massie B. (1991) Dipyridamole thallium-201 scintigraphy as a preoperative screening test. A re-examination of TTS predictive potential. *Circulation* **84**, 493–502.

Martin J.D., Valentine J., Myers S.I., Rossi M.B., Patterson C.B. & Clagett G.P. (1991) Is routine CT scanning necessary in the preoperative evaluation of patients undergoing carotid endarterectomy? *Journal of Vascular Surgery* **14**, 267–70.

McCann R.L. & Clements F.M. (1989) Silent myocardial ischemia in patients undergoing peripheral vascular surgery: incidence and association with perioperative cardiac morbidity and mortality. *Journal of Vascular Surgery* **9**, 583–7.

McCoombs P.R. & Roberts B. (1979) Acute renal failure following resection of abdominal aortic aneurysm. *Surgery, Gynecology and Obstetrics* **148**, 175–8.

McHugh P., Gill N.P., Wyld R., Nimmo W.S. & Reilly C.S. (1991) Continuous ambulatory ECG monitoring in the preoperative period: relationship of preoperative status and outcome. *British Journal of Anaesthesia* **66**, 285–91.

McPeak B. (1987) Inference, generalizability and a major change in anesthetic practice. *Anesthesiology* **66**, 723–4.

Messick J.M., Casement B., Sharbrough F.W., Milde L.N., Michenfelder J.D. & Sundt T.M. (1987) Correlation of regional cerebral blood flow (rCBF) with EEG changes during isoflurane anesthesia for carotid endarterectomy: Critical rCBF. *Anesthesiology* **66**, 344–9.

Michenfelder J.D., Sundt T.M., Fode N. & Sharbrough F.W. (1987) Isoflurane when compared to enflurane and halothane decreases the frequency of cerebral ischemia during carotid endarterectomy. *Anesthesiology* **67**, 336–40.

Miller D.C. & Myers B.D. (1987) Pathophysiology and prevention of acute renal failure associated with thoraco-abdominal or abdominal-aortic surgery. *Journal of Vascular Surgery* **5**, 518–22.

Moffitt E.A., McIntyre A.J. & Glenn J.J. (1985) Myocardial metabolism and haemodynamic responses with fentanyl-halothane anaesthesia for coronary patients. *Canadian Anaesthetist's Society Journal* **32**, 86S.

Moffitt E.A., McIntyre A.J. & Barker R.A. (1986) Myocardial metabolism and hemodynamic responses with fentanyl-enflurane anesthesia for coronary artery surgery. *Anesthesia and Analgesia* **65**, 46–52.

Muhiudeen I.A., Kuecherer H.F., Lee E., Cahalan M.K. & Schiller N.B. (1991) Intraoperative estimation of cardiac output by transesophageal pulsed doppler echocardiography. *Anesthesiology* **74**, 9–14.

Multicenter Post-infarction Research Group (1983) Risk stratification and survival after myocardial infarction. *New England Journal of Medicine* **309**, 333–6.

Murdoch J. & Hall R. (1990a) Brain protection: physiological and pharmacological considerations. Part I: The physiology of brain injury. *Canadian Journal of Anaesthesia* **37**, 663–71.

Murdoch J. & Hall R. (1990b) Brain protection: physiological and pharmacological considerations. Part II: The physiology of brain injury. *Anaesthesia* **37**, 762–77.

Muskett J., McGreevy J. & Miller M. (1986) Detailed comparison of regional and general anesthesia for carotid endarterectomy.

American Journal of Surgery **152**, 691–3.

National Institute of Neurological Disorder and Stroke (NINCDS) (1991) *Clinical Alert*: benefit of carotid endarterectomy for patients with high grade stenosis of the internal carotid artery. February.

Nesto R.W., Watson X.S., Kowalchuk G.J., Zarich S.W., Hill T., Lewis S.M. & Lane S.E. (1990) Silent myocardial ischemia and infarction in diabetics with peripheral vascular disease: assessment by dipyridamole thallium-201 scintigraphy. *American Heart Journal* **120**, 1073–7.

Nevitt M.P., Ballard D.J. & Hallett J.W. (1989) Prognosis of abdominal aortic aneurysms. A population-based study. *New England Journal of Medicine* **321**, 1009–14.

O'Sullivan K., O'Toole D.P., Bouchier-Hayes D. & Cunningham A.J. (1989) Left ventricular function during aortic aneurysm resection — influence of anesthetic technique. *Anesthesia and Analgesia* **68**, 217S.

Ouriel K., Geary K., Green R.M., Fiore W., Geary J.E. & De Weese J.A. (1990) Factors determining survival after ruptured aortic aneurysm: the hospital, the surgeon and the patient. *Journal of Vascular Surgery* **11**, 493–6.

Pasternack P.F., Imperato A.M., Riles T.S. & Bauman F.G. (1985) The value of radionuclide angiogram in the prediction of perioperative myocardial infarction in patients undergoing lower extremity revascularization procedures. *Circulation* **72** (Suppl. II), 13–17.

Pasternack P.E., Grossi E.A., Baumann F.G., Riles T.S., Lamparello P.J., Giangola G., Primis L.K., Mintzer R. & Imparato A.M. (1989) The value of silent myocardial ischemia monitoring in the prediction of perioperative myocardial infarction in patients undergoing peripheral vascular surgery. *Journal of Vascular Surgery* **10**, 617–25.

Paul M.D., Mazar C.D., Byrick R.J., Rose D.K. & Goldstein M.B. (1986) Influence of mannitol and dopamine on renal function during elective infrarenal aortic clamping in man. *American Journal of Nephrology* **6**, 427–34.

Pohost G.M. (1991) Dipyridamole thallium test. Is it useful for predicting coronary events after vascular surgery? *Circulation* **84**, 931–2.

Powell J. & Greenhalgh R.M. (1989) Cellular, enzymatic and genetic factors in the pathogenesis of abdominal aortic aneurysms. *Journal of Vascular Surgery* **9**, 297–304.

Quintin L., Roudot F., Roux C., Macquin I., Basmaciogullari A., Guyene T., Vaubourdolle M., Viale J.P., Bonnet F. & Chignone M. (1991) Effect of clonidine on the circulation and vasoactive hormones after aortic surgery. *British Journal of Anaesthesia* **66**, 108–15.

Raby K.F., Goldman L. & Creager M.A. (1989) Correlation between preoperative ischemia and major cardiac events after peripheral vascular surgery. *New England Journal of Medicine* **321**, 1296–1300.

Rao T.L.K., Jacobs K.H. & El-Etr A.A. (1983) Re-infarction following anesthesia in patients with myocardial infarction. *Anesthesiology* **59**, 499–505.

Rivers S.P., Scher L.A., Gupta S.K. & Veith F.J. (1990) Safety of peripheral vascular surgery after recent acute myocardial infarction. *Journal of Vascular Surgery* **11**, 70–6.

Robotham J.L., Takata M., Berman M.L. & Harasawa Y. (1991) Ejection fraction revisited. *Anesthesiology* **74**, 172–83.

Rohren M.J., Cutler B.S. & Wheeler H.B. (1988) Long-term

survival and quality of life following ruptured abdominal aortic aneurysm. *Archives of Surgery* **123**, 1213–17.

Roizen M.F., Beaupre P.N., Albert R.A. & Kremer P. (1984) Monitoring with two-dimensional transesophageal echocardiography. *Journal of Vascular Surgery* **1**, 300–5.

Roizen M.F. (1989) Anesthesia for vascular surgery. In *Clinical Anesthesia* (Eds Barash P.G., Cullen B.F. & Stoelting R.K.) pp. 1015–47. Lippincott, Philadelphia.

Ryan T., Maguire M., Bouchier-Hayes D. & Cunningham A.T. (1991) Left ventricular function during transesophageal echocardiographic assessment of abdominal aortic aneurysm resection. *British Journal of Anaesthesia* **67**, 204P–5P.

Ross R. (1986) The pathogenesis of atherosclerosis — an update. *New England Journal of Medicine* **314**, 488–500.

Ross R. (1990) Atherosclerotic coronary heart disease. In *The Heart* (Eds Hurst J.W., Schlant R.C. & Rackney C.V.) p. 877. McGraw-Hill, New York.

Shah K.B., Kleinman B.S., Sami H., Patel J. & Rao T.L.K. (1990) Re-evaluation of perioperative myocardial infarction in patients with prior myocardial infarction undergoing noncardiac operations. *Anesthesia and Analgesia* **71**, 231–5.

Sharp W.V. & Donovan D.L. (1987) Retroperitoneal approach to the abdominal aorta: revisited. *Journal of Cardiovascular Surgery* **28**, 270–3.

Sheffield L.T. (1988) Exercise stress testing. In *Heart Disease* 3rd edn. (Ed. Braunwald E.) p. 224. W.B. Saunders, Philadelphia.

Shepard A.D., Tollefson D.F.J., Reddy D.J., Evans J.R., Elliott J.P. & Smith R.F. (1991) Left flank retroperitoneal exposure: a technical aid to complex aortic reconstruction. *Journal of Vascular Surgery* **14**, 283–91.

Sicard G.A., Freeman M.B., Vander Woude J.C. & Anderson C.B. (1987) Comparison between the transabdominal and retroperitoneal approach for reconstruction of the infrarenal abdominal aorta. *Journal of Vascular Surgery* **5**, 19–27.

Silbert B.S., Koumoundouros E., Davies M.J. & Cronin K.D. (1989) Comparison of processed electroencephalogram and awake neurological assessment during carotid endarterectomy. *Anaesthesia in Intensive Care* **17**, 298–304.

Skillman J.J., Restall S. & Salzman E.W. (1975) Randomized trial of albumin vs. electrolyte solutions during abdominal aortic operations. *Surgery* **78**, 291–302.

Smith J.S., Cahalan M.K., Benefiel D.J., Byrd B.F., Lurz F.W., Shapiro W.A., Roizen M.F., Bouchard A. & Schiller N.B. (1985) Intraoperative detection of myocardial ischemia in high-risk patients: electrocardiography versus two-dimensional transesophageal echocardiography. *Circulation* **72**, 1015–21.

Smith J.S., Roizen M.F., Cahalan M.K., Benefiel D.J., Beaupre P.N., Sohn Y.J., Byrd B.F., Schiller N.B., Stoney R.J., Ehrenfeld W.K., Ellis J.F. & Aronson S. (1988) Does anesthetic choice make a difference? Augmentation of systolic blood pressure during carotid endarterectomy: effects of phenylephrine versus light anesthesia and isoflurane versus halothane on the incidence of myocardial ischemia. *Anesthesiology* **69**, 846–53.

Sonnenblick E.H. & Downing S.E. (1963) Afterload as a primary determinant of ventricular performance. *American Journal of Physiology* **204**, 604–10.

Steen P.A., Tinker J.H. & Tarhan S. (1978) Myocardial infarction after anesthesia and surgery. *Journal of the American Medical Association* **239**, 2566–70.

Stein M., James P.M., Kelly J., Browne D., Suircliffe A.C. & Patterson W.B. (1972) Renal protection during aortic cross clamping. *Annals of Surgery* **38**, 681–8.

Strawn D.J. & Guernsey J.M. (1991) Dipyridamole thallium scanning in the evaluation of coronary artery disease in elective abdominal aortic surgery. *Archives of Surgery* **126**, 880–4.

Sullivan P.J., Martineau R.J., Hull K.A. & Miller D.R. (1991) Comparison of bioimpedence and thermodilution measurements of cardiac output during aortic surgery. *Canadian Journal of Anaesthesia* **38**, 78S.

Sundt T.M., Scarbrough F.W., Piepgras D.G., Kearns T.P., Messick J.M. & O'Fallon W.M. (1981) Correlation of cerebral blood flow and electroencephalographic changes during carotid endarterectomy: results of surgery and hemodynamics of cerebral ischemia. *Mayo Clinical Proceedings* **56**, 533–43.

Svensson L.G., Patel V., Robinson M.F., Ueda T., Roehm J.O.F. & Crawford E.S. (1991) Influence of preservation of perfusion of intraoperative identified spinal cord blood supply on spinal motor evoked potentials and paraplegia after aortic surgery. *Journal of Vascular Surgery* **13**, 355–65.

Szilagri D.E., Hagemann J.H., Smith R.F. & Elliott J.P. (1978) Spinal cord damage in surgery of the abdominal aorta. *Surgery* **83**, 38–56.

Takolander R., Bergqvist D., Hulthen U.L., Johansson A. & Katzman P.L. (1990) Carotid artery surgery. Local versus general anesthesia as related to sympathetic activity and cardiovascular effects. *European Journal of Surgery* **4**, 265–70.

Templehoff R., Modica P.A., Grubb R.I., Rich K.M & Holtmann B. (1989) Selective shunting during carotid endarterectomy based on two channel computerized electroencephalographic/compressed spectral array analysis. *Neurosurgery* **29**, 339–44.

Thys D.M. (1987) The intraoperative assessment of regional myocardial performance: Is the cart before the horse? *Journal of Cardiothoracic Anesthesia* **1**, 273–5.

Tilson M.D. (1989) Status of research on abdominal aortic aneurysm disease. *Journal of Vascular Surgery* **9**, 367–9.

Tischler M.D., Lee T.H., Hirsh A.T., Lord C.P., Goldman L., Creager M.A. & Lee R.T. (1991) Prediction of major cardiac events after peripheral vascular surgery using dipyridamole echocardiography. *American Journal of Cardiology* **68**, 593–7.

Tuman K.J., McCarthy R.J., Spiess B.D., DaValle M., Humpland S.J., Dabir R. & Ivankovich A.D. (1989) Effect of pulmonary artery catheterization on outcome in patients undergoing coronary artery surgery. *Anesthesiology* **70**, 199–206.

Wadouh F., Lindemann E.M. & Arndt C.F. (1984) The arteria radicularis magna anterior as a decisive factor influencing spinal cord damage during aortic occlusion. *Journal of Thoracic Cardiovascular Surgery* **88**, 1–10.

Wadouh F., Wadouh R., Hartman M. & Crisp-Lindgren N. (1990) Prevention of paraplegia during aortic operations. *Annals of Thoracic Surgery* **50**, 543–52.

Webster M.W., St Jean P.L., Steed D.L., Ferrell R.E. & Majumder P.P. (1991a) Abdominal aortic aneurysm: results of a family study. *Journal of Vascular Surgery* **13**, 366–72.

Webster M.W., Ferrell R.E., St Jean P.L., Majumder P.P., Fogel S.R. & Steed D.L. (1991b) Ultrasound screening of first-degree relatives of patients with an abdominal aortic aneurysm. *Journal of Vascular Surgery* **13**, 9–14.

White G.H., Advani S.M. & Williams R.A. (1988) Cardiac risk index as a predictor of long-term survival after repair of abdominal aortic aneurysm. *American Journal of Surgery* **156**, 103–6.

Whittemore A.D., Clowes A.W., Hechtman H.B. & Mannick J.A. (1980) Aortic aneurysm repair. Reduced operative mortality associated with maintenance of optimal cardiac performance. *Annals of Surgery* **192**, 414–21.

Williams G.M., Perler B.A., Burdick J.F., Osterman F.A., Mitchell S., Merine D., Drenger B., Parker S.D., Beattie C. & Reitz B.A. (1991) Angiographic localization of spinal cord blood supply and its relationship to postoperative paraplegia. *Journal of Vascular Surgery* **13**, 23–35.

Winslow C.M., Solomon D.H., Chassin M.R., Kosecoff J., Merrick N.J. & Brook R.H. (1988) The appropriateness of carotid endarterectomy. *New England Journal of Medicine* **318**, 721–7.

Wong M.G., Wellington Y.C., London M.J., Layung E. & Mangano D.F. (1988) Prolonged postoperative myocardial ischemia in high risk patients undergoing non-cardiac surgery. *Anesthesiology* **69**, 56A.

Yeager M.P., Glass D.D., Neff R.K. & Brinck-Johnsen T. (1987) Epidural anesthesia and analgesia in high risk surgical patients. *Anesthesiology* **66**, 729–36.

Youngberg J.A. & Gold M.D. (1991) Carotid Artery Surgery: Perioperative anesthetic considerations. In *Vascular Anesthesia* (Ed. Kaplan J.A.) pp. 333–61. Churchill Livingstone, New York.

Zellner J.L., Elliott B.M., Robinson J.G., Hendrix G.H. & Spicer K.M. (1990) Preoperative evaluation of cardiac risk using dobutamine–thallium imaging in vascular surgery. *Annals of Vascular Surgery* **4**, 238–43.

Anaesthesia and Diabetes

J.N. HORTON

The anaesthetist may become involved in the management of diabetic patients in a variety of circumstances in the operating theatre, the intensive care unit and the ward (Table 51.1). Fortunately, the subject is regularly reviewed (Milaskiewicz & Hall, 1992).

Diabetes is a condition of protean aetiology characterized by a diminution in action of insulin, produced in varying degrees by failure of production or diminished effectiveness. It has been customary to classify diabetes into types which distinguish between age of onset and insulin dependence. However the terms 'juvenile onset' and 'maturity onset', while convenient and still used widely, are now obsolete. An alternative classification based on insulin dependence alone is also rather unsatisfactory as individuals may vary in their requirements from time to time, and a non-insulin-dependent patient may, under some circumstances, become insulin dependent.

Table 51.2 shows a much-simplified version of the exhaustive classification produced by the National Diabetes Data Group (1979). For working purposes there are two groups likely to be encountered in anaesthetic practice. Type I diabetics develop the disorder commonly before the age of 30 and have limited or absent endogenous insulin function, therefore usually requiring frequent injections of insulin to survive. They are prone to ketoacidosis. Type II diabetics are usually older, often obese, and while secreting insulin more or less normally, display insulin resistance frequently. While they may develop hyperosmolar coma, ketoacidosis is unlikely in this group.

Occurrence of diabetes

Diabetes is rare in early childhood whilst in older children there are peaks of incidence at approximately 6 and 12 years of age. The incidence increases gradually in early adult life but after approximately 40 years, there is a sharp increase, which is when the main incidence of Type II diabetes is found. In Western populations (but not always in other races) women are affected more commonly, possibly because of obesity, parity and the effects of the menopause.

Twenty percent of diabetics have an affected close relative. There is a very significant association between early Type I diabetes and certain HLA antigen markers and with the presence of cell-surface antibodies which react specifically with pancreatic island beta cells (Leslie & Pyke, 1991).

The incidence of diabetes in the population varies

Table 51.1 Involvement of the anaesthetist in the management of the diabetic patient

Primary care of the patient with coma produced by:
Diabetic ketoacidosis

Hyperosmolality

Hypoglycaemia

Intercurrent conditions causing coma, including respiratory failure in grossly obese patients and intracranial haemorrhage or thrombosis

Surgery in the diabetic patient
Identification of undiagnosed diabetes

Assessment of the diabetic patient requiring surgery in the future

Elective surgery for diabetes-induced conditions

Elective surgery for other conditions

Emergency surgery for diabetes-induced conditions or for other conditions
  With mild or stable diabetes
  With disturbances of diabetes causing hyperglycaemia, ketoacidosis and, occasionally, coma

Table 51.2 Simplified classification of diabetes. (Data from National Diabetes Data Group, 1979)

	Other names	Aetiological features
Type I	Insulin-dependent juvenile onset	Associated with HLA types and islet-cell antibodies either at diagnosis or persistently
Type II	Non-insulin-dependent maturity onset	May be related to obesity Aetiology various; may be different in obese and non-obese
Other types Pancreatic disease	Secondary diabetes	Chronic pancreatitis Pancreatic calcification (alcohol-associated) Pancreatectomy Haemochromatosis Malnutrition Cassava consumption
Hormonal		Cushing's syndrome Glucagonoma Acromegaly Thyrotoxicosis Phaeochromocytoma
Drug induced		Diuretics Psychoactive agents Catecholamines Analgesics
Insulin receptor abnormalities		Congenital lipodystrophy Acanthosis nigrans Autoimmune insulin receptor antibodies
Genetic syndromes		Glycogen storage disease Huntingdon's chorea Dystrophia myotonica Down's syndrome Prader−Willi syndrome
Gestational diabetes		

widely from race to race and in different societies. In Western countries the prevalence of diagnosed diabetes in the general population is approximately 1.2%. It is remarkable that in some races, e.g. Alaskan Eskimos, the condition is almost unknown, whereas an incidence of 50% is claimed for certain North American Indian tribes. What is of more importance to the anaesthetist is the incidence in the surgical population. In the Cardiff hospitals in 1992, this was 2.8%.

Fifty percent of diabetics require surgery for a diabetes-related condition at some time after diagnosis (Byyny, 1980) (Table 51.3). Twenty-five percent of diabetics requiring surgery are diagnosed initially on admission, either following routine ward urine testing or because they are admitted in diabetic ketosis precipitated by an acute surgical condition.

Surgery in diabetics is generally said to carry a higher mortality than in non-diabetics, principally because of myocardial disease and infection. Morbidity is also generally assumed to be high for the same reasons, and because of the high incidence of obesity, renal disease, delayed wound healing and difficulties in control of the blood glucose level over the perioperative period. Nevertheless, controlled studies (Hjortrup *et al.*, 1985) have found that there was no difference in the incidence of complications between diabetic and non-diabetic patients.

Table 51.3 Diabetic conditions requiring surgical intervention

Infections	Typically perianal, ischiorectal, soft tissue
Gangrene	Usually foot or leg. Excision of decubitus ulcers, especially in obese patients; vascular surgery; amputation
Eyes	Cataract, retinal surgery for retinopathy, vitrectomy for complications of retinopathy
Cardiac	Operations for ischaemic heart disease; vein grafts; cardiac transplantation
Curative	Pancreas transplants (at present experimental)
Renal	Transplantation for nephropathy Operations to alleviate neuropathic bladder
Pregnancy	Extradural block to avoid blood glucose fluctuations; forceps delivery and Caesarean section are required more frequently in diabetic than in non-diabetic mothers
'Rarities'	Somatostatinoma Glucagonoma Insulinoma

Biochemical basis of diabetes
(Alberti & Hockaday, 1987)

The hyperglycaemia of diabetes results from: (i) a reduced rate of removal of glucose from the blood by the peripheral tissues; and (ii) an increased rate of release of glucose from the liver into the circulation. In both instances the cause is the ineffectiveness or failure of production of endogenous insulin. The basis of this can be understood best by a consideration of metabolic processes in the normal healthy person.

At times of food intake and absorption, an excess of foodstuff substrates is available, which passes to the liver in the portal circulation. The liver takes up some 60–80% of a typical 100 g 'package' of carbohydrates, storing some as glycogen for future use, and converting the remainder to fatty acids and triglycerides which are recirculated to adipose tissues as very-low-density lipoproteins. These are taken up in the adipose tissues and stored as fatty acids. The remainder of the glucose is taken up by other tissues, including muscle, where it is used as an energy substrate or stored as glycogen. Absorbed amino acids are also taken up, primarily by the liver and later by other tissues, and used in part for oxidation but mainly for protein synthesis. Fats are transported directly from the gastrointestinal mucosa to the adipose tissues and stored as fatty acids.

In fasting conditions, the obligatory carbohydrate requirements are obtained from the liver by glycogenolysis and, as glycogen reserves become depleted, by gluconeogenesis from lactate, pyruvate, amino acids and glycerol. As starvation progresses there is an inhibition of tissue glucose oxidation and an increasing dependence on fatty acids from adipose store tissues. These are taken up by muscles (up to 90% of their energy requirements being obtained from this source) and liver where they are utilized in the production of acetyl coenzyme A (acetyl CoA). The liver converts the acetyl CoA to the ketone bodies acetoacetate and 3-hydroxy-butyrate through the 3-hydroxymethyl-glutaryl-CoA pathway. These are taken up by other tissues which are able to use them as energy substrates in the citric acid cycle at a rate which depends on their availability.

These processes are finely regulated by a group of hormones (Table 51.4) of which insulin is the prime anabolic and anticatabolic member. The main effects of insulin are seen in the liver, muscle and adipose tissues (Table 51.5). In the liver, insulin controls

Table 51.4 Hormones affecting metabolism. (Data from Alberti & Thomas, 1979)

	Anabolic effects			Catabolic effects				
	Glyco-genesis	Lipogenesis	Protein synthesis	Glyco-genolysis	Gluco-neogenesis	Lipolysis	Ketogenesis	Proteolysis
Insulin	++	++	++	−	− −	− −	− −	− −
Glucagon	−	−	0	+	++	(+)	+	0
Cortisol	±	±	− −	±	+	+	(+)	++
Catecholamines	−	0	0	++	++	++	+	0
Growth hormone	0	0	++	0	+	(+)	(+)	0
Thyroid hormone	0	0	+?	0	+	+	(+)	+

0 no effect; − inhibitory effect; − − major inhibitory effect; + stimulatory effect; ++ major stimulatory effect; ± stimulation if insulin present otherwise inhibitory; (+) important only if insulin absent.

Table 51.5 Effects of insulin in tissues. (Data from Alberti & Hockaday, 1987)

Effects	Tissue
Carbohydrate metabolism	
Increased	
Glucose transport	Muscle, fat
Glucose phosphorylation	Liver, muscle, fat
Glycogenesis	Liver, muscle
Glycolysis	Liver, muscle, fat
Pentose phosphate pathway	Liver, fat
Decreased	
Glycogenolysis	Liver, muscle
Gluconeogenesis	Liver
Lipid metabolism	
Increased	
Fatty acid synthesis	Liver
Triglyceride synthesis	Liver, fat
VLDL formation	Liver
Lipoprotein degradation	Fat
Decreased	
Lipolysis	Fat, ?liver, ?heart, ?muscle
Fatty acid oxidation	Liver, muscle
Ketogenesis	Liver
Lipoprotein degradation	Muscle
Protein metabolism	
Increased	
Amino acid transport	Liver, muscle, etc.
Protein synthesis	Liver, muscle, etc.
Decreased	
Protein degradation	Liver, muscle, etc.
Ureagenesis	Liver
Electrolyte metabolism	
Increased	
Potassium transport	All cells
Phosphate entry	All cells
Decreased	
Sodium uptake	All cells

hepatic glucose production by action on phosphorylase, pyruvate carboxylase, phosphenol pyruvate carboxykinase and fructose 1,6-diphosphatase. The overall effects are reductions in hepatic glycogenolysis and gluconeogenesis. Insulin also stimulates glucokinase activity to promote the phosphorylation of glucose. This facilitates glycogen and lipid synthesis and inhibits ketogenesis. Overall, therefore, insulin decreases hepatic production of glucose and ketone bodies and promotes the storage of glycogen in the liver and lipids in other tissues. In muscle, glucose transport is enhanced and glucose-6-phosphate and glycogen synthesis are increased. Insulin also has a major effect on muscle protein metabolism to increase amino acid transport and decrease protein breakdown. Additionally, there is an important effect on muscle cell membranes in promoting the transfer of potassium and phosphate into the cell. In adipose tissues, insulin causes inhibition of lipolysis and hence reduction in ketogenesis.

In the diabetic subject these processes are disturbed to an extent which depends on the degree of deficiency of insulin. In partial deficiency (Type II and less severe cases of Type I diabetes) there is no tendency to increase ketogenesis although hyperlipidaemia, hyperglycaemia and glycosuria are invariably found. In severe Type I diabetes there is uncontrolled glycogenolysis, gluconeogenesis, lipolysis and protein breakdown. These changes are accompanied by an increased secretion of hormones which oppose the actions of insulin, namely glucagon, growth hormone and catecholamines. The secretion of the latter is enhanced by the presence of infection or by severe acidaemia causing haemodynamic disturbances. Ketogenesis is increased by further glucagon secretion, and the excess of ketones results in severe acidaemia. Hyperglycaemia is exacerbated by the inability of muscle and adipose tissue to take up glucose. The well-known symptoms of glycosuria, polyuria, dehydration, hyperosmolality and coma are the results of these metabolic disturbances.

Metabolic response to anaesthesia and surgery

It might be expected that the hormonal and endocrine changes accompanying anaesthesia and surgery would have an effect on the metabolic changes described above. Indeed, both before and during the procedure there are increases in the secretion of catecholamines (initially noradrenaline and later adrenaline), adrenocorticotrophic hormone, cortisol and cyclic adenosine monophosphate, in addition to less important increases in growth hormone and thyroid-stimulating hormone. There are marked decreases in insulin secretion and sensitivity to insulin, probably as a consequence of increased circulating catecholamines. As a result, blood glucose concentrations increase both in diabetic and non-diabetic patients.

Overall, there is a catabolic response to surgery which is more severe if prolonged metabolic disturbances result, and insulin, combined with enteral or parenteral sources of calories and nitrogen is therefore essential for adequate anabolism following surgery. Anaesthesia, unless accompanied by unusual stresses such as hypoxaemia has, *per se*, relatively little effect on metabolism, and indeed there is evidence that preoperative anxiety has a greater effect. Nevertheless, nearly all general anaesthetics cause an elevation of the blood glucose which is substantially greater than that resulting from local or regional anaesthesia.

These responses to surgery and anaesthesia are exaggerated in diabetics. Although there are well-proven increases in blood glucose and inhibition of effectiveness of insulin with most volatile agents, the choice of the anaesthetic drugs is of less importance than an appreciation of the overall effects of illness, surgery and subsequent recovery. Despite a reduced calorie intake during surgery and hence a relatively reduced insulin requirement, Type I diabetics need a modification of their exogenous insulin supply to accommodate the increased catabolism resulting from the changes described above. In both Type I and Type II diabetics, demand may outstrip availability, resulting in greater impairment of muscle glucose utilization and accelerated gluconeogenesis. Hyperglycaemia and hyperosmolality are therefore risks requiring careful monitoring in all Type I and many Type II diabetics during and after surgery.

Complications of diabetes

These are listed in Table 51.6. Apart from those which may require surgery, certain complications may present specific anaesthetic hazards.

Renal disease

This is usually in the form of: (i) nodular glomerulosclerosis (Kimmelstiel–Wilson lesion); (ii) chronic pyelonephritis and pyelitis; and (iii) secondary lesions resulting from hypertension and atherosclerosis.

As far as anaesthesia is concerned, these can be grouped together as 'diabetic nephropathy' and identified by routine renal function tests (blood urea and serum creatinine) which should be carried out on all diabetic patients before anaesthesia.

Renal disease due to diabetes is frequently associated with refractory hypertension. Generalized microvascular disease (including ischaemic heart disease) may be assumed to be present in most cases of established diabetic nephropathy. Patients with

Table 51.6 The chronic complications of diabetes. (Data from Alberti & Hockaday, 1987)

Complication	Possible causes
Macroangiopathy (atherosclerosis, myocardial disease)	Hyperlipidaemia Hyperinsulinaemia ? Hyperglycaemia ? Increased growth hormone levels ? Platelets and other vascular factors
Microangiopathy (retinopathy, neuropathy, capillary basement-membrane thickening)	Hyperglycaemia Protein (basement membrane) Hormonal factors, e.g. growth hormone Insulin deficiency
Neuropathy	Sorbitol accumulation Deficient myoinositol Myelin glycosylation Hyperglycaemia
Diabetic cataract	Hyperglycaemia Protein glycosylation
Collagen change	

diabetic nephropathy are frequently treated with angiotensin converting enzyme inhibitors, but these are unlikely to cause significant problems during anaesthesia.

Careful control of intraoperative changes in blood pressure and of fluid balance is particularly important in diabetics as lack of control has been found to be associated with a high incidence of postoperative renal failure (Charleson *et al.*, 1989).

Diabetic neuropathy

This affects all types of neuronal axons. Peripheral neuropathy with arterial disease is a common cause of gangrene, and of trophic changes requiring surgery, especially in obese and immobile patients, and those with long-standing diabetes. A rare complication requiring surgery is Charcot's neuroarthropathy.

Autonomic neuropathy is a relatively common complication which may affect as many as 60% of diabetics. Autonomic nerves may be affected at any site, but of particular relevance to anaesthesia are the possibilities of gastric stasis and cardiovascular disturbances. The latter may be asymptomatic but cardiorespiratory arrest during and shortly after anaesthesia is a well-documented occurrence (Page & Watkins, 1978) and may be related to the increased incidence of sleep apnoea in patients with diabetic autonomic neuropathy (Rees *et al.*, 1981). There are two aspects of autonomic cardiovascular neuropathy which are of concern in anaesthesia:

1 Involvement of the sympathetic vasomotor fibres, which may abolish or diminish the vasoconstrictive response to a reduction in cardiac output. This presents a particular hazard following the introduction of intermittent positive-pressure ventilation or during haemorrhage.

2 Cardiac involvement, either of the cardiac vagal fibres or of the conducting system of the heart. In view of the seriousness of this complication, it is important to look for evidence of cardiovascular autonomic neuropathy in all severe diabetics, particularly if there is a history of fainting, postural hypotension, diarrhoea, urinary retention, or evidence of cardiac arrhythmias. Two tests which are of value in this assessment are:

(a) The arterial pressure and heart-rate changes in response to the Valsalva manoeuvre. In patients with autonomic disturbance there is lack of 'overshoot' of arterial pressure immediately after the end of the manoeuvre, and little alteration in heart rate during and after the test. In addition, normal sinus arrhythmia may be absent.

(b) The effect of a change of posture on the heart rate as measured by the R–R interval on the ECG. Normally, if a subject stands up from the lying position, his/her heart rate increases rapidly then declines again; the R–R interval 15 beats after standing up should be approximately 1.2 times that after 30 beats. In diabetic neuropathy the ratio is likely to be no more than 1.04.

Coronary artery disease

The most common single cause of death in diabetics is coronary artery occlusion. The incidence is much higher in diabetics than in non-diabetics and the risk of death from ischaemic heart disease is particularly high in females. Approximately 10% of all diabetics between the ages of 50 and 70 have diagnosed coronary artery disease. In addition to the usual precautions to be taken with any patient with coronary artery disease undergoing surgery, it should be remembered that thiazide diuretics, calcium-channel blockers, and particularly beta blockers, may affect insulin release and activity, and alterations in dosage of these drugs may need a reappraisal of the patient's insulin requirements. In addition, the myocardium may be affected directly (diabetic cardiomyopathy).

Proliferative retinopathy

Retinopathy in one form or another is present in 70% of cases of more than 15 years' duration. The proliferative form carries special risk during anaesthesia, as sudden hypertensive episodes may precipitate vitreous haemorrhage. A similar risk exists with high intraocular venous pressure such as may occur as a result of therapeutic positive end-expiratory pressure.

Treatment of diabetes

Treatment is based on increasing the availability of insulin to the tissues, either by the more effective supply or use of endogenous insulin, or by the use of exogenous insulin.

Many Type II diabetics may be kept free of hyperglycaemia and glycosuria solely by careful control of diet to ensure a negative energy balance. If adequately controlled by diet alone, these patients present few problems of control during surgery. Other diabetics require either insulin or oral hypoglycaemic drugs. Insulin is required by most Type I diabetics and by many Type II diabetics, in whom careful control is necessary over a prolonged period to avoid complications. Although the majority of patients receive, or self-administer, insulin by subcutaneous injection, a few patients receive a continuous infusion of subcutaneous insulin [a particularly convenient method in suitable patients (Dunnett, 1985)], or rarely by the intramuscular, intravenous or intraperitoneal route. Most diabetics are able to carry out home testing of their blood glucose concentrations and adjust their dosage accordingly. Developments in treatment which are at present little more than experimental are the 'artificial pancreas', which delivers insulin automatically in response to a negative feedback signal based on continuous blood glucose measurement, and pancreatic transplantation, which although technically feasible, is accompanied by major difficulties of immunosuppression. Pancreatic transplantation may, however, halt the progression of diabetic neuropathy (Kennedy *et al.*, 1990).

In the UK, insulins are standardized to contain 100 IU/ml, but a wide range of degrees of purity, source, and length of action is available. These are summarized in Fig. 51.1. Human insulin is used widely although it is not clear if it has significant advantages over highly purified porcine insulin.

Oral hypoglycaemic agents may be classified into (i) sulphonylureas; and (ii) biguanides.

1 Sulphonylureas act by stimulating insulin release and increasing the number of functional insulin receptors, so potentiating the effects of endogenous insulin, and by increasing the sensitivity of the beta cells in the islets of Langerhans to the stimulating effects of glucose, increase the output of insulin.

2 Biguanides act by inhibiting absorption of carbohydrates from the gut, increasing the uptake of glucose in peripheral tissues, and reducing hepatic gluconeogenesis. They are liable to cause a number of side-effects, including weakness, gut malabsorption and lactic acidosis. Metformin is the only biguanide currently available in the UK. It may be used alone or in combination with sulphonylureas in patients who have some endogenous insulin production.

The oral hypoglycaemic agents available in the UK are listed in Table 51.7. Chlorpropamide and gliclazide have half-lives of sufficient length to have significant hypoglycaemic effect on the day following administration. It is therefore possible to render a patient hypoglycaemic by normal preoperative starvation, especially if insulin is given in addition. Patients on these long-acting agents should therefore have their blood glucose concentrations monitored carefully before and during anaesthesia.

There are a number of drug interactions involving antidiabetic agents which may be significant if changes are made to concurrent drug therapy preoperatively. These are summarized in Table 51.8.

Preparation of the diabetic patient for anaesthesia and surgery

This is determined by the type of diabetes, the nature and length of the operation and the urgency of the procedure.

As far as possible (dictated by clinical rather than administrative considerations) all diabetics, except those controlled by diet alone, should be admitted to hospital for surgery 48 h before operation for assessment and stabilization. 'Day case' surgery is contraindicated in all insulin-controlled diabetics and most of those on oral hypoglycaemic drugs. Overall physical assessment should include a search for evidence of diabetic renal involvement, autonomic neuropathy, retinopathy and heart disease.

If the patient is taking insulin, his/her regimen should be reviewed, preferably by the patient's regular diabetologist. Stability is demonstrated by the need for only minor variations in dosage on the basis of home testing of glucose concentrations in blood or urine, lack of hypoglycaemic attacks and a glycosylated haemoglobin concentration below 10%. The blood glucose concentration should be measured

Table 51.7 Oral hypoglycaemic agents available in the UK

Type	Half-life (h)
Suphonylureas	
Tolbutamide	7*
Chlorpropamide	40
Glibenclamide	8
Gliclazide	15
Glipizide	6
Gliquidone	3*
Tolazamide	7*
Biguanides	
Metformin	18

* Rarely used in the UK.

at regular intervals after admission; a fasting level of 4−8 mmol/litre, increasing to 14 mmol/litre postprandially, indicates satisfactory control (Shamoon, 1983).

Most diabetics receiving insulin are stabilized readily by attention to their dosage, diet and general health. There is, however, a group (approximately 5%) of 'brittle' diabetics, mainly children and young adults, who suffer recurrent attacks of hypoglycaemia or ketoacidosis and are difficult to control. In many cases the cause can be traced to non-compliance with diet, inappropriate dosage or timing or emotional or social causes. Nevertheless, it should be remembered that the instability may be a result of infection or organic disease (Table 51.9). Whatever the cause, the advice and assistance of an experienced diabetologist is essential in preoperative management.

There is a difference of opinion as to the best way of managing patients who are taking oral hypoglycaemic agents. Many authors recommend the withdrawal of sulphonylureas on the day of operation and, if long-acting, on the previous day as well. For minor surgery of short duration with little perioperative debility, this is probably satisfactory for most patients although the blood glucose concentration should be monitored throughout this time. There is evidence, however, that a more satisfactory control can be achieved by converting the patient's treatment to insulin for the perioperative period, particularly if the surgery is complex or prolonged. This is particularly important in intercurrent conditions which are associated with resistance to the effects of insulin (Table 51.9) (Alberti & Hockaday, 1987). Management then follows one of the plans outlined below for insulin-dependent diabetics. In view of the increased

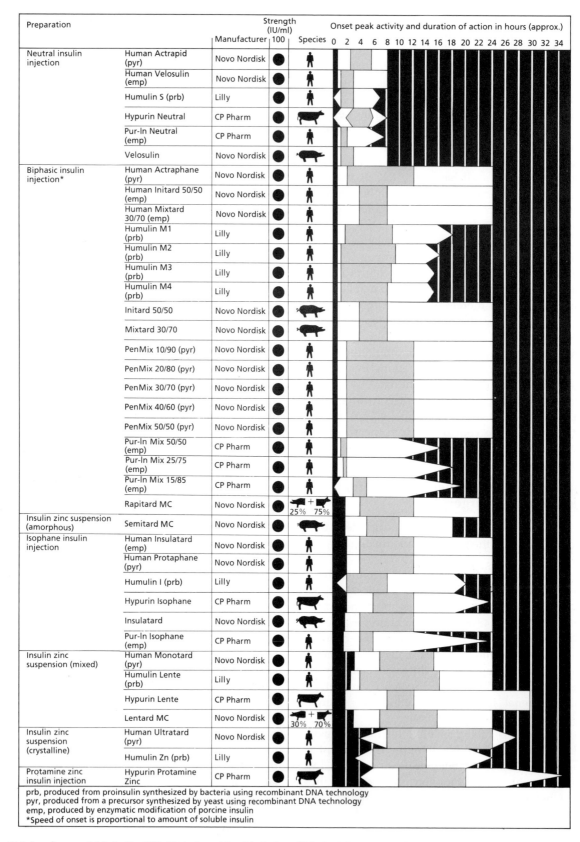

Fig. 51.1 Insulins available in the UK. (Data from Monthly Index of Medical Specialities (MIMS), May 1993, which is regularly updated.)

Table 51.8 Possible drug interactions with antidiabetic drugs. (Data from Logie *et al.*, 1976)

Drug group	Interaction with	Hypoglycaemic effect
Insulin, oral hypoglycaemics	*Drugs influencing glucose metabolism*, e.g. Salicylates Beta-adrenoceptor blocking drugs Adrenergic neurone blockers Monoamide-oxidase inhibitors Clonidine	Potentiated
	Diuretics Glucocorticoids Oestrogens Sympathomimetics Barbiturates Calcium-channel blockers Lithium	Antagonized
Sulphonylureas	*Drug-metabolizing microsomal enzyme inhibitor agents*, e.g. Coumarin anticoagulants Monoamine-oxidase inhibitors	Potentiated
	Displacement from plasma protein drug binding sites, e.g. Clofibrate Phenylbutazone Sulphonamides	Potentiated

insulin requirement during severe metabolic stress, this would seem appropriate management.

Diabetics controlled adequately on diet alone require no special preoperative measures.

Management of diabetes during anaesthesia and surgery

If the patient is well controlled in the preoperative period, and the surgery is planned electively, the preferred method of control during the perioperative period is based on continuous infusion of glucose and insulin. This has developed from techniques for the management of acute diabetic ketoacidosis. There are two main methods of administration:

1 Continuous infusion of dextrose over the perioperative period (starting on the morning of operation and continuing until the patient is taking normal oral nutrition postoperatively) with appropriate doses of insulin added to the infusion bag. The regimen recommended by Alberti and Hockaday (1987) is shown in Table 51.10. This involves the addition of insulin to an infusion bag of dextrose. Continuous-infusion techniques with insulin and dextrose in the same

Table 51.9 Insulin requirements during surgery in insulin-resistant states. (Data from Alberti & Hockaday, 1987)

	Intravenous requirements	
	units/g dextrose	units/500 ml dextrose 10%
Normal	0.3	15
Obesity	0.4−0.6	20−30
Liver disease	0.5−0.6	25−30
Serious infection	0.5−0.8	25−40
Steroid therapy	0.5−0.8	25−40
Cardiopulmonary bypass	0.8−1.2	40−60

Table 51.10 Insulin infusion regimen for pre- and postoperative management of diabetes during surgery. (Data from Alberti & Hockaday, 1987)

---

1 Add 16 units short-acting insulin (soluble, Actrapid) + 10 mmol potassium chloride to 500 ml dextrose 10%
2 Run 25—50 ml through infusion tubing before attaching to patient
3 Infuse at 100 ml/h
   If there is need to limit fluids, use double amounts of insulin and potassium chloride in dextrose 20% and infuse at 50 ml/h

---

If blood glucose is greater than 10 mmol/litre, increase insulin by 4 units/500 ml; check blood glucose 2 h later; increase by further 4-unit increments as necessary. If blood glucose is less than 5 mmol/litre, decrease insulin by 6 units/500 ml; check blood glucose 2 h later; decrease by further 4-unit decrements as necessary.

Table 51.11 Regimen for management of the diabetic patient who requires insulin before, during and after surgery. (Regimen used in the University Hospital of Wales)

---

1 Long and intermediate-acting insulins discontinued 24 h preoperatively and patient controlled on short-acting insulins instead
2 When first meal missed, start intravenous dextrose 5%, 1 litre 8-hourly, and separate infusion soluble insulin 1—3 units/h (50 units soluble insulin in 50 ml normal saline delivered by syringe pump). Adjust insulin rate according to hourly blood glucose measurements to keep level between 7 and 10 mmol/litre (4—7 mmol/litre in pregnancy)
3 Check blood glucose at induction and during operation. Frequency of sampling and rate adjustment will determine tightness of control
4 Check potassium level and add potassium chloride to dextrose infusion if required (13 mmol/litre dextrose solution)

---

container have the advantage that in the event of failure of the infusion there is no risk of the patient receiving insulin without dextrose.

2 Alternatively, insulin can be administered intravenously in a more concentrated form from a continuously slow-running motor-driven syringe (Leslie & Mackay, 1978). Thus, the rate of delivery can be controlled independently of the dextrose solution. It is preferable to administer the insulin through a separate intravenous cannula to obviate the unnoticed sequestration of insulin in the dextrose infusion tubing if the cannula becomes blocked. This danger can be avoided by the use of a one-way valve in the dextrose infusion line. With a technique involving a syringe pump it is essential that the pump is reliable and operated by staff who are trained in its use.

With continuous-infusion techniques, hypokalaemia may occur frequently because of the effect of insulin on potassium transfer into cells. For this reason, the routine addition of 13 mmol potassium chloride (KCl) to each litre of dextrose is recommended. Techniques involving continuous infusion are widely used and are to be recommended for all Type I and many Type II diabetics. The regimen used in the University Hospital of Wales is outlined in Table 51.11 as an example of the practical use of such a method.

Many regimens have claimed success on the basis of blood glucose measurements alone. While this may be satisfactory for routine control, the true efficacy of a management regimen can be assessed fully only by measurement of blood ketones, pyruvate, lactate and non-esterified fatty acid levels, and a study of the effect on protein catabolism and

serum potassium and other electrolyte concentrations. A further difficulty in assessment of claims of efficacy has been the paucity of comparison with other techniques and the lack of standardization of the type of surgery and the anaesthetic agents and techniques used. Although most authorities have tended to advocate regimens of continuous insulin and dextrose (Thomas et al., 1984), a note of caution in claims for superiority for this technique has been made (Hall, 1984). Furthermore, a survey in one UK health region showed that continuous infusion techniques were by no means universally preferred (Dunnet et al., 1988).

Monitoring of blood glucose levels

Laboratory methods of measurement of blood glucose by the glucose oxidase method are rapid and accurate but entail sending a sample of blood to the laboratory, with subsequent delay. Bedside tests, utilizing test strips which are read visually or by a portable meter, are readily available and are of sufficient accuracy for routine management.

Control of the diabetic for emergency surgery

Approximately 5% of operations on diabetics are emergency procedures resulting from infection or vascular insufficiency. The time available for assessment and stabilization is short and in many instances it is the surgically remediable condition which makes the diabetic state difficult to control. The patient may be hyperglycaemic and ketoacidotic with the attendant problems of hyperosmolality, electrolyte imbalance and coma. Occasionally, a patient with acute ketoacidosis may have clinical features similar to those of an 'acute abdomen'.

It is essential that ketoacidosis and hyperosmolality are corrected before anaesthesia is induced. The mortality from ketoacidosis is as high as 30%, particularly in elderly patients. The reasons for this high mortality are, regrettably, errors of management as well as the condition itself and its precipitating cause. Treatment (Alberti & Hockaday, 1987) must be prompt and aggressive and carried out under the direct advice of an experienced diabetologist:

1 Measurement of blood glucose, serum sodium, potassium, phosphate, and arterial pH, Pco_2, Po_2 and base deficit should be obtained. Direct arterial pressure, central venous pressure and ECG monitoring should be established.

2 Insulin should be given, initially as a bolus of 6 units intravenously and then approximately 6 units/h by infusion according to the blood glucose concentration measured every 30 min.

3 A rapid infusion of saline should be started. If the initial measurement of serum sodium is greater than 145 mmol/litre this should be 0.45% sodium chloride, otherwise 0.9% should be used. One litre should be given in the first 15−30 min and then a further 2 litres in 1−2 h, depending on the rate of decrease in serum osmolality. Although there may be urgency to correct the fluid deficit and proceed with surgery, caution must be exercised in the use of hypo-osmolar solutions and the too-rapid correction of pH and osmolality as ketoacidotic patients may develop paradoxical intracerebral acidosis and cerebral oedema during treatment. Furthermore, large volumes of infused fluids may result in adult respiratory distress syndrome.

When the blood glucose concentration decreases to 10−15 mmol/litre, the fluid may be changed to dextrose 5% and the patient managed by the convential continuous glucose−insulin regimen.

4 Potassium chloride should be given by infusion of 13−26 mmol in 500 ml 0.9% saline, and the rate adjusted to keep the plasma concentration within the normal range (3.5−5.5 mmol/litre). There is likely to be a considerable extracellular potassium deficit and it is therefore important to give adequate quantities, bearing in mind that much of the infused potassium is transferred into the interior of the cells by the action of insulin. Caution is necessary if renal failure is present. Estimations of serum potassium concen-

tration should be made hourly and a rapid reduction anticipated. Alterations in the T-wave of the ECG are also of value in the assessment of potassium requirements.

5 The administration of bicarbonate is usually unnecessary and is likely to cause further hypokalaemia and a shift of the oxygen−haemoglobin dissociation curve to the left, impairing oxygen release to the tissues. In most cases bicarbonate solutions should not be given unless the arterial pH is less than 6.9.

6 The stomach should be aspirated and a nasogastric tube left in place on free drainage as gastric stasis is likely.

7 Appropriate antibiotics should be given, and the use of low-dose, subcutaneous, low-molecular-weight heparin is advisable in patients who are comatose, obese or hyperosmolar, to combat the risk of deep-vein thrombosis.

8 Disseminated intravascular coagulopathy is a recognized, although uncommon, complication of diabetic ketoacidosis.

The diabetic patient for emergency surgery who is not unduly hyperglycaemic and has no evidence of ketoacidosis presents fewer problems. In most cases (including Type II diabetics on oral hypoglycaemic drugs) a continuous insulin−glucose regimen should be commenced, bearing in mind that higher or lower doses than usual of insulin may be required, depending on the extent of insulin or food taken recently.

Anaesthetic management of the diabetic patient

It has been noted already that, although most anaesthetic agents cause hyperglycaemia, the choice of agent is of comparatively little importance compared with adequate assessment, stabilization and monitoring of the diabetic state. The usual intravenous induction agents have negligible effect on the blood glucose concentration although ketamine may cause significant hyperglycaemia (Shamoon, 1983). Fentanyl, and presumably other opioids appear to cause less substrate mobilization than halothane, possibly by inhibition of release of cortisol and growth hormone. Extradural and spinal analgesia also have minimal effects on blood glucose concentrations and are to be recommended for the very frequent operations on the lower limb in diabetic patients. This has the added advantage of an awake patient in whom incipient hypoglycaemia can be detected more readily. Although there may be theoretical objections to the use of regional blocks in patients with diabetic neuro-pathy, these are used extensively in practice without problems.

There are certain additional points concerning anaesthesia in the diabetic patient which require particular attention:

1 Gastric atony is not infrequent, especially in associ-ation with autonomic neuropathy and diabetic ketoacidosis. The normal period of preoperative star-vation is not reliable, and if necessary a rapid-sequence induction technique should be used, even in elective cases. Gastric atony is relieved only par-tially by metoclopramide or domperidone (Mulhall & O'Fearghail, 1984). However, the antibiotic erythro-mycin may, through its action as a motilin agonist, aid gastric emptying in these patients (Janssens *et al.*, 1990).

2 Hypoxaemia and hypercapnia aggravate hyper-glycaemia by stimulating catecholamine release. Additionally, there is evidence that 25% of diabetics have impaired sensitivity to hypoxaemia or decreased ventilatory response to hypercapnia (Williams *et al.*, 1984).

3 The anaesthetic technique chosen should ensure a rapid return to consciousness to obviate the masking of hyperglycaemic or hypoglycaemic coma.

4 Hypertensive episodes during anaesthesia, e.g. during tracheal intubation and in light anaesthesia, may precipitate vitreous haemorrhage in patients with proliferative retinopathy, and measures should be taken in such patients to avoid sudden increases in arterial pressure.

5 The tendency of diabetic patients who suffer changes in mean arterial pressure and fluid imbalance to develop postoperative renal failure has been noted. Unfortunately, diabetic patients who are hyperten-sive preoperatively are more likely to develop intra-operative falls in blood pressure, particularly if elderly or in negative fluid balance (Charleson *et al.*, 1990).

6 Diabetic autonomic neuropathy affecting the cardiovascular system constitutes a considerable hazard during and after anaesthesia. If there is evidence of autonomic neuropathy, continuous and close monitoring of the cardiovascular system by ECG and intra-arterial pressure measurement should commence before the induction of anaesthesia and continue into the postoperative period. Meticulous fluid balance and the availability of antiarrhythmic drugs are essential.

7 Hartmann's solution (compound lactate solution, Ringer's lactate) should be avoided in diabetics, as infused lactate is rapidly converted to glucose with resulting hyperglycaemia.

8 Induced hypotension has additional hazards in severe diabetes and should be used with care. Dia-betics are particularly prone to cerebrovascular and cardiac disease. Ganglion-blocking agents, though now not commonly used, may block sympathetically-mediated hepatic gluconeogenesis with the possi-bility of hypoglycaemia. The use of beta blockers is associated with a normal insulin response but a slower recovery from hypoglycaemia if it occurs. This effect is less with cardioselective drugs such as metoprolol. Very close monitoring of the blood glu-cose concentration is therefore necessary when arterial pressure is deliberately reduced, and direct-acting vasodilators such as sodium nitroprusside, glyceryl trinitrate, halothane and isoflurane, are to be preferred if the technique is used.

9 Although abnormalities of transmission across the neuromuscular junction can occur in diabetics (Schiller & Rahamimoff, 1989), the clinical response to neuromuscular blocking drugs is normal. Care should be taken to position the electrodes of the neuromuscular block monitor over a nerve known not to be affected by diabetic neuropathy. The use of suxamethonium in extensive diabetic neuropathy is inadvisable because of excessive potassium release from denervated muscle.

Considerations in special circumstances

Cardiopulmonary bypass

The association of ischaemic heart disease and dia-betes suggests that patients for coronary artery sur-gery are frequently diabetics. The fluid used to prime the bypass machine contains a considerable quantity of dextrose (typically 1.5 litres of 5% solution), which mixes with the patient's circulating intravascular volume. This and the insulin resistance caused by surgery and light anaesthesia, causes substantial hyperglycaemia requiring additional insulin when cardiopulmonary bypass is first established. This is usually followed by a gradual decline during surgery. Frequent measurements of blood glucose and the adjustment of the rate of infusion of insulin are required.

Renal transplantation

This is carried out frequently on diabetic patients who develop irreversible renal failure as a result of diabetic nephropathy. There are reports of serious hyperkalaemia associated with hyperglycaemia in such patients, and especially careful control of the blood glucose concentration, with frequent measurements of the serum potassium concentration, is essential. These patients are particularly likely to have retinopathy. Chlorpropramide, normally long-acting, is excreted mainly unchanged through the kidney, and is therefore likely to have an especially long action in patients with renal failure. Insulin is metabolized in the kidney as well as in the liver and a reduction in insulin requirements might therefore be expected postoperatively.

Anaesthesia in the diabetic parturient

The frequency of previously diagnosed diabetes in women at term is approximately 0.3%. Additionally, there is an incidence of so-called gestational diabetes of 0.8%. The success of pregnancy in the diabetic mother depends in considerable measure on good antenatal care. Developments in the management of this and of delivery have resulted in a much reduced perinatal mortality.

The fetus *in utero* is, because of lack of active glucose-6-phosphatase, unable to produce glucose either by glycogenolysis or by gluconeogenesis, and is dependent on maternal glucose which diffuses freely across the placenta. The fetal blood glucose concentration therefore follows the maternal concentration closely and the fetus is at risk when there is maternal hypoglycaemia. Maternal hyperglycaemia stimulates fetal insulin production, so subsequent maternal control with insulin may result in fetal hypoglycaemia. Maintenance of a normal blood glucose concentration throughout labour, including any operative procedures under regional or general anaesthesia, is therefore essential if fetal hypoglycaemia is to be avoided.

During labour, the diabetic mother is managed best by a regimen of continuous intravenous insulin and glucose as described previously. This can be continued if an operative delivery becomes necessary. After delivery it is likely that the insulin requirements will fall sharply.

Until recently, elective Caesarian section at 35–37 weeks' gestation was the preferred management of the diabetic parturient. More recently it has been found that careful home monitoring of blood glucose levels and improved techniques for assessing fetal well-being have allowed a higher proportion of spontaneous deliveries at term, and a lower proportion of operative interventions (Murphy et al., 1984).

Extradural analgesia during labour and for Caesarian section is to be recommended, other factors being equal, as it reduces the stress response, controls blood pressure in pre-eclampsia, and improves placental blood flow. However, it has been pointed out that in the non-pre-eclamptic diabetic, placental blood flow is pressure dependent and maternal arterial pressure must therefore be strictly maintained (Crawford, 1984). A reduced volume of local analgesic agent may be required to produce extradural block in diabetic compared with non-diabetic mothers (Bromage, 1978).

For a variety of reasons, the preferred method of anaesthesia for Caesarian section and other operative procedures in diabetic mothers is spinal or extradural block. Gastric atony, always present in obstetric patients, is a particular risk in diabetics. The hyperglycaemic response to regional block is minimal compared with most general anaesthetic techniques. The mother, being awake, can take food by mouth soon afterwards and therefore return sooner to her pre-pregnancy diabetic control regimen. Nevertheless, fetal acidosis is more likely if regional block is used unless very careful control of maternal blood glucose, arterial pressure and the avoidance of excessive glucose infusions are observed. Additionally, the operation may be difficult technically if the baby is large. Whatever technique is used, there is an increased risk of aortocaval compression because of hydramnios and large baby.

In addition to macrosomia, the neonate of the diabetic mother is more likely to have cardiac and other congenital abnormalities. In particular, respiratory distress syndrome is more common in the infants of diabetic mothers because of lack of pulmonary surfactant.

Acknowledgement

The author would like to acknowledge the advice and assistance of Dr K. Peters, Consultant Physician, University Hospital of Wales.

References

Alberti K.G.M.M. & Hockaday T.D.R. (1987) Diabetes mellitus. In *Oxford Textbook of Medicine* (Eds Weatherall D.J., Ledingham J.G.G. & Warrell D.A.) pp. 9.51–9.101. Oxford University Press, Oxford.

Alberti K.G.M.M. & Thomas D.J.B. (1979) The management of diabetes during surgery. *British Journal of Anaesthesia* **51**, 693–703.

Bromage P.R. (1978) Complications and contraindications. In *Epidural Analgesia* (Ed. Bromage P.R.) pp. 654–715. W.B. Saunders, Eastbourne.

Byyny R.L. (1980) Management of diabetes during surgery. *Postgraduate Medicine* **68** (4), 191–202.

Charleson M.E., Mackenzie C.R., Gold J.P., Ales K.L. & Shires G.T. (1989) Postoperative renal dysfunction can be predicted. *Surgery, Gynecology, and Obstetrics* **169** (4), 303–9.

Charleson M.E., Mackenzie C.R., Gold J.P. Ales K.L., Tomkins M. & Shires G.T. (1990) Preoperative characteristics predicting intraoperative hypotension and hypertension among hypertensives and diabetics undergoing noncardiac surgery. *Annals of Surgery* **212** (1), 66–81.

Crawford J.S. (1984) *Principles and Practice of Obstetric Anaesthesia* 5th edn. pp. 360–1. Blackwell Scientific Publications, Oxford.

Dunnett S.R. (1985) Insulin infusion pump. *British Medical Journal* **291**, 1808–9.

Dunnet J.M., Holman R.R., Turner R.C. & Sear J.W. (1988) Diabetes mellitus and anaesthesia. A survey of the perioperative management of the patient with diabetes mellitus. *Anaesthesia* **43**, 538–42.

Hall G.M. (1984) Diabetes and anaesthesia – a promise unfulfilled? *Anaesthesia* **39**, 627–8.

Hjortrup A., Sørensen C., Dyremose E., Hjortsø N.C. & Kehlet H. (1985) Influence of diabetes mellitus on operative risk. *British Journal of Surgery* **72**, 783–5.

Janssens J., Peeters T.L., Ventrappen J., Tack J., Urbain M., Muls E. & Bouillon R. (1990) Improvement of gastric emptying in diabetic gastroparesis by erythromycin. *New England Journal of Medicine* **322**, 1028–31.

Kennedy W.R., Navarro X., Goetz F.C., Sutherland D.E.R. & Najarian J.S. (1990) Effects of pancreatic transplantation on diabetic neuropathy. *New England Journal of Medicine* **322**, 1031–7.

Leslie R.D.G. & Mackay J.D. (1978) Intravenous insulin infusion in diabetic emergencies. *British Medical Journal* **2**, 1343–4.

Leslie R.D.G. & Pyke D.A. (1991) Escaping insulin dependent diabetes. *British Medical Journal* **302**, 1103–4.

Logie A.W., Galloway D.B. & Petrie J.C. (1976) Drug interactions and long-term antidiabetic therapy. *British Journal of Clinical Pharmacology* **3**, 1027–32.

Milaskiewicz R.M. & Hall G.M. (1992) Diabetes and anaesthesia: the past decade. *British Journal of Anaesthesia* **68**, 198–206.

Mulhall P.B. & O'Fearghail M. (1984) Diabetic gastroparesis. Case report and review of the literature. *Anaesthesia* **39**, 468–9.

Murphy J., Peters J., Morris P., Hayes T.M. & Pearson J.F. (1984) Conservative management of pregnancy in diabetic women. *British Medical Journal* **288**, 1203–5.

National Diabetes Data Group (1979) Classification and diagnosis of diabetes mellitus and other categories of glucose intolerance. *Diabetes* **28**, 1039–57.

Page M. McB. & Watkins P.J. (1978) Cardiorespiratory arrest and diabetic autonomic neuropathy. *Lancet* **i**, 14–16.

Rees P.J., Prior J.G., Cochrane G.M. & Clark T.J.H. (1981) Sleep apnoea in diabetic patients with autonomic neuropathy. *Journal of the Royal Society of Medicine* **74**, 192–5.

Shamoon H. (1983) Influence of stress and surgery on glucose regulation in diabetes: pathophysiology and management. In *Endocrinology and the Anaesthetist* (Ed. Oyama T.) pp. 95–122. Elsevier, Amsterdam.

Schiller Y. & Rahamimoff R. (1989) Neuromuscular transmission in diabetes: response to high-frequency activation. *Journal of Neuroscience* **9** (11), 3709–19.

Thomas D.J.B., Platt H.S. & Alberti K.G.M.M. (1984) Insulin-dependent diabetes during the peri-operative period. An assessment of continuous glucose–insulin–potassium infusion, and traditional treatment. *Anaesthesia* **39**, 629–37.

Williams J.G., Morris A.I., Hayter R.C. & Ogilvie C.M. (1984) Respiratory responses of diabetics to hypoxia, hypercapnia, and exercise. *Thorax* **39**, 529–34.

Anaesthesia for Pituitary and Adrenal Disease

D. WEATHERILL

Anaesthesia and surgery are associated with a 'stress' response that is detectable as a series of endocrine and metabolic events and that depends, at least in part, on functions of the pituitary and adrenal glands. For example, there are alterations in the secretion of cortisol from the adrenal cortex influenced by control from the anterior pituitary and changes in function within the efferent sympathetic nervous system including changes in the rate of secretion of catecholamines from the adrenal medulla. Thus, patients with disease of these endocrine glands may exhibit unusual responses to anaesthesia and surgery.

Depending on the severity of the endocrine dysfunction, disease of the pituitary or adrenal glands may be associated with an anatomical or physiological abnormality that may be of immediate concern to the anaesthetist during the perioperative period; examples are anatomical abnormalities of the airway in patients with acromegaly, osteoporosis associated with Cushing's syndrome, or disturbances of body fluids and electrolytes, and cardiovascular dysfunction in patients with severe adrenocortical insufficiency. Irrespective of the nature of the endocrine disturbance, surgery of the pituitary and adrenal glands may present particular anaesthetic problems because of the need for surgery to be performed at specific anatomical locations with attendant potential perioperative surgical difficulties. The demands presented by pituitary and adrenal disease continue to increase as improvement in endocrinological diagnostic techniques provides an increasing number of patients for endocrine surgery (Weatherill & Spence, 1984).

This chapter attempts to define those aspects of diseases of the pituitary and adrenal glands that are of significance to the anaesthetist.

Pituitary gland

The anatomy of the anterior and posterior lobes of the pituitary gland and their structural and functional relationships with the hypothalamus provide a basis for an understanding of the separate endocrine functions of the two lobes. Despite these functional differences, diseases of both lobes are considered together here because disease processes do not necessarily respect anatomical or functional divisions. The anterior lobe of the pituitary contains secretory cells that produce adrenocorticotrophic hormone (ACTH), thyroid-stimulating (thyrotrophic) hormone (TSH), prolactin (PRL), growth hormone (GH), the gonadotrophins, luteinizing hormone, follicle-stimulating hormone and some other cleavage molecules referred to generically as melanocyte-stimulating hormone. The release of these hormones from the anterior pituitary is controlled in turn by a complex series of molecules which are synthesized within neurones in the hypothalamus (release and release-inhibitory hormones) and are carried to the pituitary through the hypophyseal portal vessels within the pituitary stalk (Harris, 1972). In contrast, the hormones secreted from the posterior pituitary, antidiuretic hormone (ADH) and oxytocin, are synthesized within hypothalamic neurones whose axons pass down through this pituitary stalk to the posterior lobe and are released from nerve endings within the gland.

Recently, a vast neuroendocrinological literature has accumulated as a result of the biochemical and physiological study of the functions of the hypothalamic neurones involved in these control processes and in the links between CNS and pituitary endocrine functions (Reichlin, 1985). Of particular interest to anaesthetists are studies of the neurotransmitter mechanisms involved in the neuroendocrine pathway from the hypothalamus to the pituitary and modification of control of this pathway by drugs. For example, many investigations have attempted to identify the effects of endogenous and exogenous opioids (Huang & McCann, 1983) and anaesthetic agents (Sheward & Fink, 1991) in the control of pituitary endocrine function; conversely, other investigations have sought to determine the influence of endocrine responses on the effects of drugs acting on the CNS (Kasson & George, 1983).

Pathophysiology

Consideration of the pathophysiology of the pituitary should include disease processes affecting the hypothalamus and connections between the hypothalamus and the pituitary, as both may be associated with pituitary endocrine dysfunction. Causes of pituitary disease have been described by Scheithauer (1984a,b, 1985) and include benign neoplasm (e.g. anterior pituitary adenomas, craniopharyngioma, meningioma), malignant neoplasm arising usually from secondary spread (e.g. direct invasion from leukaemia or lymphomatous infiltration of the meninges, or metastatic deposits from carcinoma of breast or lung), inflammatory diseases (e.g. sarcoidosis), rarely infection (viral or bacterial) and vascular lesions (e.g. ischaemia secondary to hypovolaemia). The majority of these pathological processes are associated with a reduction in pituitary secretory activity leading most extremely to panhypopituitarism. Primary adenomas of the anterior pituitary, providing probably the commonest indication for primary surgery of the pituitary, are associated with a wide range of clinical syndromes determined largely by cell type and growth behaviour. Thus, adenomas composed of actively secreting cells are accompanied by clinical features associated with hypersecretion of one or, less commonly, two of the anterior pituitary hormones, whereas adenomas containing cells with little secretory activity may remain silent or be accompanied by clinical features arising from tumour extension. Suprasellar expansion of these 'macroadenomas' may cause compression of the pituitary stalk, interference with hypothalamic function, visual field disturbances, involvement of other cranial nerves, and may be associated only rarely with a significant increase in intracranial pressure. Pituitary stalk and hypothalamic involvement together with direct compression of adjacent normal pituitary tissue may lead to varying degrees of pituitary hypofunction.

Hypopituitarism

The anaesthetic management of patients with hypopituitarism should take account of the secondary effects of the disease particularly on thyroid and adrenocortical function, and any disorders of posterior pituitary function involving ADH secretion. The preoperative preparation of patients is governed by the severity of the endocrine dysfunction especially in relation to fluid and electrolyte balances and distributions, and cardiovascular function. Choice of anaesthetic drugs and techniques, and the administration of these, should take account of the clinical features; adrenocortical insufficiency is described later in this chapter and hypothyroidism in Chapter 53.

Anterior pituitary adenomas

The most common actively secreting anterior pituitary adenomas in decreasing order of reported frequency of presentation for neurosurgery are PRL-, GH-, ACTH- and mixed GH-PRL-secreting tumours (Scheithauer, 1984a; Wilson, 1984); the majority of these tumours present clinically in adult life as hyperprolactinaemia, acromegaly, or hyperadrenocorticism (Cushing's disease). Pituitary adenomas may occur in association with other endocrine neoplasm of the parathyroid glands and pancreatic islet cells (multiple endocrine neoplasia syndrome, Type I). Patients with PRL-secreting tumours and hyperprolactinaemia may present with a variety of clinical features that include amenorrhoea, galactorrhoea, infertility and signs of local tumour extension. Anaesthetic management of these patients should be appropriate for the specific surgical procedure to be undergone (usually pituitary microsurgery) but signs of other endocrinopathy should be sought, namely of hyposecretion of one or more of the other pituitary hormones.

The anaesthetic management of patients with tumours secreting excessive quantities of ACTH (Cushing's disease) is considered later in this chapter.

Acromegaly

The anaesthetic management of patients with acromegaly may be complicated by a variety of clinical features including abnormalities of the upper airway, hypertension, congestive cardiac failure, glucose intolerance and diabetes mellitus. The upper airway in acromegaly may be affected by a number of changes: development of prognathism, enlargement of the tongue, hypertrophy within the mucosa of the pharynx, changes within the structure of the larynx and narrowing of the larynx. These are accompanied by changes of voice, dyspnoea on exertion or even dyspnoea at rest. In relation to anaesthesia, the changes within the pharynx may predispose to airway obstruction in the unconscious patient (Whitwam et al., 1973) and difficulty with laryngoscopy (Burn, 1972; Southwick & Katz, 1979); laryngeal narrowing may cause difficulty with tracheal intubation (Hassan et al., 1976) and severe postoperative respiratory obstruction (Kitahata, 1971) may be associated with the development of pulmonary oedema (Goldhill et al., 1982; Singelyn & Scholtes, 1988). Thus the airway should be assessed carefully preoperatively and elective tracheostomy considered where there is marked airway involvement (Kitahata, 1971; Burn, 1972; Southwick & Katz, 1979). Whelan and colleagues (1982) have recommended medical treatment to reduce plasma concentrations of GH for a period of at least 12 months before non-urgent surgery (e.g. corrective maxillofacial surgery) but it is not clear if such therapy would reduce airway difficulties.

It is apparent from the above that disease affecting the pituitary may provide a wide range of problems to the anaesthetist, with complex endocrine and metabolic disturbances, depending in part on whether or not the patient presents for pituitary (Frohman, 1991) or non-endocrine surgery, and specific dysfunction of many organs. The management of endocrine disorders requires careful preoperative assessment particularly with respect to thyroid function and function of the hypothalamic—pituitary—adrenal axis (HPA). Some consider that patients presenting for pituitary surgery should receive corticosteroid supplementation therapy over the perioperative period (Coté & Rouillard, 1977; Messik et al., 1978; Daughaday, 1985), although this might not be required by some patients undergoing selective microsurgery of the pituitary (Teasdale, 1983; Hout et al., 1988), and complicates the postoperative biochemical assessment of HPA function (Beyer et al., 1985). Other potential postoperative endocrine abnormalities include development of hypothyroidism and transient or permanent diabetes insipidus, both requiring hormone replacement therapy.

Adrenal cortex

The adrenal cortex is composed of three anatomical layers demonstrable histologically: an outer zona glomerulosa, an intermediate zona fasciculata, and an inner zona reticularis. These layers differ from each other with respect to histological cell type, cellular arrangement and relationship to blood supply. There are functional differences, the zona glomerulosa secreting mineralocorticoid hormones and the zona fasciculata and zona reticularis secreting glucocorticoid and adrenocorticoid sex hormones.

Pathophysiology

Diseases of the adrenal cortex discussed here include tumours of the cortex which secrete either mineralocorticoid or glucocorticoid hormones, destruction of adrenocortical tissue by a variety of disease processes including autoimmune disease, infection, malignant infiltration and secondary dysfunction of the adrenal cortex with structural change arising from abnormalities of control by trophic or secretogogue hormones, e.g. hypopituitarism, ACTH-secreting adenoma (Cushing's disease), ectopic ACTH secretion, secondary hyperaldosteronism (see Neville & O'Hare, 1982, for a review of the pathology of the adrenal cortex). Some of these pathological features are discussed further below under the separate descriptions of adrenocortical hypersecretion and insufficiency.

The stress response

The responses of the adrenal cortex to stress and trauma including anaesthesia and surgery have been studied in detail during the last 60 years and are described fully in Chapter 30. Observation of an increase in the plasma concentration of corticosteroids during anaesthesia and surgery (Franksson & Gemzell, 1954; Sandberg et al., 1954) was followed by the measurement of an increase in the rate of secretion of cortisol from the adrenal gland in response to surgery (Hume et al., 1962). The plasma concentration of cortisol increases rapidly after induction of anaesthesia and commencement of surgery and remains elevated for a variable period after operation, and the magnitude and duration of this response has been related to the magnitude of the surgical stimulus (Plumpton et al., 1969a). These changes in plasma concentration of cortisol are associated also with an increase in the plasma concentration of ACTH (Hume & Egdahl, 1959; Oyama & Takiguchi, 1970).

Both general anaesthesia and surgical stimulation may be involved in the initiation of the cortisol response. The administration of sedative or tranquillizer drugs as premedication may reduce an increase in plasma concentration of cortisol associated with preoperative 'stress' (Oyama et al., 1969). Induction of anaesthesia using an intravenous agent, e.g. thiopentone, followed by introduction of an inhalation technique, may be associated with a small increase in the plasma concentration of cortisol but a solely inhalation induction may be accompanied by a greater response (Oyama et al., 1968). Differences between the magnitudes of the responses seen using different inhalation agents have also been described (Oyama, 1980). The intravenous induction agent etomidate causes direct inhibition of cortisol synthesis within the adrenal cortex and may modify the plasma cortisol response to anaesthesia and surgery to a variable extent dependent on the magnitude of the surgical stimulus (Duthie et al., 1985; Sear, 1985).

In addition to the increase in the rate of cortisol secretion during anaesthesia and surgery, there occurs an increase in the rate of secretion of aldosterone (Hume et al., 1962) and in the plasma concentration of aldosterone (Cochrane, 1978; Oyama et al., 1979; Moore et al., 1985). This response persists for 24 h after lower abdominal surgery. The response may occur after inhalation induction of anaesthesia and is increased further following surgical stimulation; the mechanism of the response is not known but may involve changes in plasma concentrations of ACTH and renin, the latter response possibly occurring secondary to alterations of cardiovascular function (Robertson & Michelakis, 1972).

The metabolic consequences of these adrenocortical responses to anaesthesia and surgery have not been identified. Whereas some of the metabolic changes that have been observed in patients undergoing surgery (hyperglycaemia, protein breakdown, water and sodium retention) may be stimulated by the administration of corticosteroids to normal patients, relationships between particular endocrine changes and specific responses have not been identified. Thus, the hyperglycaemic response during upper abdominal surgery may be abolished in the presence of a cortisol response (Buckley et al., 1982) and conversely, the cortisol response may be inhibited without reduction of the hyperglycaemic response (Moore et al., 1985); sodium and water retention accompanying anaesthesia and surgery are not dependent on an increase in plasma aldosterone concentration (Cochrane, 1978; Brandt et al., 1979). The role of corticosteroids in the maintenance of cardiovascular homeostasis, apart from the effects of these hormones on renal regulation of water and electrolyte excretion, have been investigated [e.g. interaction between corticosteroids and the cardiovascular responses to changes in catecholamine concentrations (Kehlet et al., 1974)], and corticosteroid involvement in fluid shifts occurring within the body in response to haemorrhage (Barton & Passingham,

1982) has also been studied. The ability to dissociate specific endocrine and metabolic responses associated with anaesthesia and surgery and the ability of patients to withstand surgery after inhibition of some of the endocrine responses by regional anaesthesia or high-dose opioid anaesthesia (Hall, 1985) have made more elusive the significance of both the corticosteroid and metabolic responses to anaesthesia and surgery, particularly in relation to patient morbidity.

Adrenocortical insufficiency

The first description of primary adrenocortical insufficiency by Addison in 1855 was of a clinical syndrome that included anaemia, asthenia, gastrointestinal symptoms, hypotension, weight loss and pigmentation associated with a 'diseased condition of the suprarenal capsules' (widely referred to as Addison's disease). Subsequent investigations of the pathological processes affecting the adrenal cortex and correlation between these and functional disturbances of the gland have led to a better understanding of the complex array of diseases included under the term primary adrenocortical insufficiency. Early in this century the most common cause of Addison's disease was bilateral destruction of the adrenal gland by tuberculosis but this is now an uncommon cause in Europe, although it may remain common in some other parts of the world (Neville & O'Hare, 1982). Today the most common cause is an idiopathic, organ-specific autoimmune adrenalitis (idiopathic Addison's disease) and this may be associated with other autoimmune disease (hypothyroidism, diabetes mellitus, pernicious anaemia). Other rarer causes of destruction of the adrenal glands include amyloid infiltration, metastatic carcinoma, protozoal and fungal infections, and haemorrhage into the adrenal glands (Waterhouse—Friderichsen syndrome) associated with septicaemia, cardiac failure or use of anticoagulant therapy. These processes probably occur frequently without sufficient disruption of adrenal cortical tissue to produce adrenocortical endocrine dysfunction; however, significant impairment of adrenocortical function may not be uncommon in patients with renal amyloid associated, for example, with chronic inflammatory diseases including rheumatoid arthritis (Danby et al., 1990).

Secondary adrenocortical insufficiency occurs as a result of inadequate secretion of ACTH and may be caused by any disease process affecting the hypothalamus or pituitary, as described above. The commonest type of adrenocortical insufficiency arises in patients receiving corticosteroid therapy with consequent hypothalamic-pituitary suppression of ACTH secretion. Topical, aerosol, oral or parenteral administration of steroid therapy may all cause adrenocortical insufficiency (Feiwel *et al.*, 1969; Choo-Kang *et al.*, 1972).

The clinical features of adrenocortical insufficiency depend on the nature of the disease process and vary from a chronic condition as described by Addison to an acute condition with collapse; the features of the condition depend also on the pattern of corticosteroid hyposecretion (Burke, 1985). Thus, patients with hypopituitarism and consequent failure of secretion of ACTH may show features of hypothyroidism in addition to signs of hyposecretion of glucocorticoids, although mineralocorticoid secretion may be affected also, not necessarily as a result of a direct effect of lack of ACTH on the adrenal cortex but possibly by involvement of the renin–angiotensin system.

The clinical sequelae of glucocorticoid hyposecretion include weight loss, hypoglycaemia, fatigue, hypotension, vomiting, hyponatraemia, muscle weakness and anaemia, but, as Burke (1985) has shown, the clinical features shown by individual patients may be very variable and may depend particularly on whether the glucocorticoid hyposecretion is acute or chronic. Isolated mineralocorticoid hyposecretion is rare, this usually accompanying glucocorticoid deficiency; the consequences of mineralocorticoid lack in relation to cardiovascular and fluid and electrolyte physiological mechanisms may complicate further the clinical picture of adrenocortical insufficiency. Once the presence of adrenocortical dysfunction has been suspected, a variety of biochemical tests are available to determine the nature of the pathology and, as a consequence, treatment can be aimed at restoring normal fluid and electrolyte balance, and maintaining appropriate corticosteroid hormone replacement therapy with either cortisol or cortisone and, where required, fludrocortisone (Cullen *et al.*, 1980; Liddle, 1982; Williams & Dluhy, 1983).

In relation to anaesthesia, the variety of presentations of adrenocorticoid insufficiency complicates diagnosis, and the biochemical and metabolic consequences of the disease complicate the administration of anaesthesia; the anaesthetic management of patients with acute adrenocortical insufficiency has been described by Smith and Byrne (1981) and Hertzberg and Shulman (1985). The commonest encounter of the anaesthetist with patients at risk of developing adrenocortical insufficiency is with those receiving or having recently received corticosteroid

therapy either as hormone replacement therapy or as therapy for a non-endocrine disease.

A series of reports of 'collapse' in the immediate postoperative period in patients receiving steroid therapy (e.g. Fraser *et al.*, 1952; Lewis *et al.*, 1953) aroused suspicion of acute adrenocortical insufficiency stimulated by stress of surgery, and consequently high-dose corticosteroid cover was recommended widely for the perioperative management of patients requiring steroid therapy (Bayliss, 1958). However, very few of these reports included measurement of associated low plasma concentrations of corticosteroids (Sampson *et al.*, 1961, 1962; Jasani *et al.*, 1968) and consequently the involvement of adrenocortical insufficiency in the reported collapse has been questioned (Mattingly & Tyler, 1965; Cope, 1966; Plumpton *et al.*, 1969a). More recently, the observation that some patients may withstand major surgical procedures after inhibition or abolition of the cortisol response to surgery by a variety of anaesthetic techniques (Hall, 1985) has obscured further the significance of adrenocortical insufficiency developing in patients receiving steroid therapy. Measurements of responses of plasma concentrations of cortisol during surgery in patients receiving steroid therapy have shown considerable variation, from absent to normal responses (Plumpton *et al.*, 1969a; Kehlet & Binder, 1973). Preoperative biochemical tests (the insulin-hypoglycaemia test of HPA function and the ACTH stimulation test of adrenocortical function) may be used to identify patients who are unable to produce a cortisol response to stress but such testing is necessarily elaborate and despite impairment of the cortisol response patients may withstand surgery without steroid supplementation therapy. In a large group of patients Kehlet and Binder (1973) observed a relatively high incidence of perioperative hypotension but were able to relate this to a low plasma concentration of cortisol in only one patient.

The observation that some patients do require steroid supplementation therapy during the perioperative period and the possible adverse effects of excessive corticosteroid administration, e.g. the unknown significance of the endocrine and metabolic responses to anaesthesia and surgery, retardation of healing, increased susceptibility to infection, and incidence of gastrointestinal haemorrhage (Diethelm, 1977), have stimulated attempts to rationalize steroid supplementation regimens by defining a safe minimum dosage. This is important when viewed against a variety of proposed dosage schemes (Plumpton *et al.*, 1969b; Kehlet, 1975; Diethelm, 1977; Black &

Montgomery, 1982; Liddle, 1982; Williams & Dluhy, 1983) that recommend a total dose of hydrocortisone on the day of surgical procedure for adult patients ranging from 25–600 mg.

Attempts have been made to produce supplementation regimens that mimic the normal cortisol response, taking into account the magnitude of the surgical stimulus. Thus Plumpton and colleagues (1969b) found that appropriate plasma concentrations of cortisol could be achieved by administering hydrocortisone, 100 mg i.v., during induction of anaesthesia for patients undergoing minor surgery and continuing with hydrocortisone, 100 mg i.m., every 6 h for 3 days for major surgery. Using estimations of daily rates of secretion of cortisol, Kehlet (1975) suggested a lower dosage (hydrocortisone, 25 mg i.v.) during induction of anaesthesia and thereafter an infusion of 100 mg/24 h until resumption of gastrointestinal function; this schedule has been used successfully in a small group of patients by Symreng and colleagues (1981).

Lower-dose regimens than those used earlier may provide adequate cortisol concentrations in the perioperative period. However, a number of problems remain, particularly in relation to the identification of those patients who require steroid supplementation and especially amongst patients who have discontinued steroid therapy. The level of inhibition of HPA function by corticosteroid therapy at a central (hypothalamic or pituitary) or peripheral (adrenocortical) site may be important and the significance of frequency, duration and dosage of therapy requires identification (Hodges, 1984). For patients receiving continuing corticosteroid therapy for treatment of a non-endocrine disease process, the maintenance of appropriate steroid concentrations also provides a further problem distinct from the imitation of a normal response to the stress of the perioperative period.

Adrenocortical hypersecretion of glucocorticoid hormones

Cushing's syndrome arises from a chronic increase in the plasma concentration of glucocorticoids as a result usually of either administration of exogenous steroid therapy or an excessive secretion of glucocorticoids. Causes of excessive secretion are classified into those associated with elevated plasma concentrations of ACTH (ACTH dependent) and those associated with primary adrenocortical tumours and primary adrenal hypersecretion with consequently low plasma concentrations of ACTH (non-ACTH

dependent). The ACTH-dependent type usually shows excessive release of ACTH from the pituitary and bilateral adrenocortical hyperplasia (Cushing's disease) but up to 20% involve ectopic secretion of ACTH from, for example, oat cell bronchial carcinomas or carcinoid tumours (Neville & O'Hare, 1982). The non-ACTH-dependent type involves either adrenocortical adenomas, that are usually small, or larger carcinomas that may require extensive surgical resection (Jensen et al., 1991). The most common cause of Cushing's syndrome arising from excessive glucocorticoid secretion is pituitary hypersecretion (60–70%), whilst primary adrenal tumours provide only 20–30% (Orth & Liddle, 1971).

The clinical features of Cushing's syndrome are well known: central obesity, muscle-wasting, osteoporosis, thinning and bruising of the skin, hirsutism, psychiatric disturbance, amenorrhoea, susceptibility to infection, glucose intolerance and hypertension. Glucose intolerance is common, and 20–30% of patients develop frank diabetes mellitus (Soffer et al., 1961; Ross et al., 1966; Welbourn et al., 1971; Ernest & Ekman, 1972). Hypertensive disease is often severe (Ernest & Ekman, 1972) and may be associated with congestive cardiac failure. Many patients exhibit hypokalaemia (Welbourn et al., 1971).

A variety of biochemical and radiological techniques have been used to determine the site of the primary pathology in patients with Cushing's syndrome (Cullen et al., 1980; Nelson, 1980; Howlett et al., 1985) and hence to define appropriate therapy. The treatment of patients with pituitary-dependent disease has changed with the advent of transsphenoidal hypophysectomy so that now radiotherapy or bilateral adrenalectomy tend to be considered only where pituitary microsurgery is likely to fail or has in fact failed (Howlett et al., 1985; Burke et al., 1990; Atkinson, 1991). As a consequence, patients with Cushing's syndrome may present for a variety of surgical procedures that include hypophysectomy, removal of adrenal tumours, and surgical treatment of tumours causing ectopic ACTH secretion, in addition to any other surgical treatment.

Preoperative management of patients may require treatment of hypertension and congestive cardiac failure, diabetes mellitus and hypokalaemia (Black & Montgomery, 1982). Specific medical therapy has been used preoperatively to reduce plasma concentrations of cortisol, and this has been recommended especially for patients with severe disease (Howlett et al., 1985). Drugs used include metyrapone which causes a direct inhibition of adrenocortical synthesis of cortisol, and drugs that act centrally to inhibit

ACTH release (bromocriptine and cyproheptadine). The use of this chemotherapy is controversial (Teasdale, 1983; Atkinson, 1991).

Descriptions of the anaesthetic management of patients with Cushing's syndrome show that a wide range of anaesthetic drugs has been used (Stephen, 1977; Maddi & Gabel, 1980; Black & Montgomery, 1982). The neuroanaesthetic management of patients undergoing hypophysectomy is described in Chapter 41. Specific problems to be anticipated in patients undergoing adrenal surgery include the need for careful movement and positioning of patients with osteoporosis and a fragile skin, cardiovascular instability in hypertensive patients with potential electrolyte disturbances aggravated during the surgical procedure by caval compression, direct handling of the adrenal glands or surgical haemorrhage, and the possibility of trauma to the pleura and development of pneumothorax. A high incidence of thromboembolic sequelae has been reported following adrenal surgery (Blichert-Toft et al., 1972; Ernest & Ekman, 1972).

Patients with Cushing's syndrome require corticosteroid supplementation therapy during and after surgery and greater supplementation may be required than in other conditions (James, 1970; Black & Montgomery, 1982). A variety of glucocorticoid schedules has been used for both hypophysectomy and adrenalectomy (Besser & Edwards, 1972; Ernest & Ekman, 1972; Tyrell et al., 1978; Black & Montgomery, 1982; Teasdale, 1983); a total adult dose of hydrocortisone, 300 mg, given throughout the day of surgery is probably adequate. Subsequent postoperative steroid replacement therapy is related to the nature of the disease process and surgical procedure; patients following bilateral adrenalectomy require mineralocorticoid replacement, but many patients following pituitary microsurgery or unilateral adrenalectomy will go on to develop normal adrenocortical function at some time after operation. Thus, the requirement for steroid replacement therapy should be assessed biochemically (Teasdale, 1983; Burke et al., 1990). After pituitary surgery, chronic deficiencies in secretion of ACTH, TSH, gonadotrophin and ADH are not uncommon (Burke et al., 1990).

Adrenocortical hypersecretion of mineralocorticoid hormones

Primary adrenocortical hypersecretion of aldosterone may arise from a benign adenoma within the cortex in 75–80% of patients, or from bilateral adrenocortical hyperplasia in approximately 20% of patients; adrenocortical carcinoma causing hypersecretion of aldosterone is rare (Brown et al., 1972; Nelson, 1980; Neville & O'Hare, 1982). Conn (1955) first described the syndrome of hypertension, hypokalaemia and metabolic alkalosis associated with low plasma concentrations of renin and usually with the presence of a solitary adrenocortical adenoma. Subsequently, this was distinguished from the syndrome with bilateral cortical hyperplasia (see Neville & O'Hare, 1982) and, since then, considerable emphasis has been given to the diversity of disease processes involved in the associations between corticosteroid secretory dysfunction and hypertension in terms of both histopathological and biochemical features (Biglieri et al., 1990; Biglieri, 1991; Connell & Fraser, 1991; Melby, 1991; Ulick, 1991).

Hypertension in primary hyperaldosteronism is of varying severity and may be responsible for approximately 1% of hypertensive disease (Brown et al., 1972). The magnitude of potassium depletion and hypokalaemia is variable and may depend on sodium intake but can be severe and associated with muscle weakness. Metabolic alkalosis may be in part a consequence of potassium depletion (Williams, 1976) and may cause tetany and paraesthesiae. Impairment of glucose tolerance occurs in many patients (Streeten et al., 1973) and has been related to the effects of potassium depletion on insulin secretion (Conn, 1965). Renal dysfunction with polyuria may be related to chronic potassium depletion and hypertensive disease.

Identification of the adrenocortical pathology is important in determining appropriate treatment and a variety of biochemical and radiological techniques have been developed to locate unilateral tumours or identify bilateral hyperplasia. Treatment of unilateral adenoma is by surgical removal but the treatment of choice for bilateral adrenocortical hyperplasia is medical as, in this condition, bilateral adrenalectomy fails to effect a useful correction of hypertensive disease. Drugs that have been used in treatment include spironolactone and amiloride and, in patients with bilateral hyperplasia, the use of angiotensin-converting enzyme inhibitors has been investigated (Ferriss et al., 1975; Melby, 1985).

Reports of the anaesthetic management of patients with primary hyperaldosteronism (Garlington & Bailey, 1958; Gangat et al., 1976; Matsuki et al., 1976; Shipton & Hugo, 1982a) and reviews (Finch, 1969; Shipton & Hugo, 1982b) suggest that whilst a wide variety of anaesthetic agents has been used, few anaesthetic complications have been observed.

Specific medical treatment (aldosterone antagonism) has been use preoperatively to assist correction of potassium depletion and metabolic alkalosis (Brown *et al.*, 1972); specific antihypertensive therapy may also be required (Biglieri, 1976). Anaesthetic management should take account of the presence of hypertensive disease, persistent potassium depletion (and interaction with the actions of neuromuscular-blocking drugs), metabolic alkalosis (and its potential aggravation by hyperventilation), and glucose intolerance. Additionally, any of the intraoperative problems during adrenal surgery, as noted above, should be anticipated. Postoperative care demands attention to fluid and electrolyte balances especially with respect to administration of appropriate amounts of potassium. Mineralocorticoid replacement may be required temporarily but glucocorticoid replacement should be required only if both adrenal glands have been mobilized or removed (Shipton & Hugo, 1982b).

Hypersecretion of aldosterone may occur in some patients as a secondary consequence of elevation of plasma concentrations of renin in a variety of conditions, e.g. cardiac, renal and hepatic failure, frequently with oedema, and may show some features of primary aldosteronism. The anaesthetic management of a patient with tertiary hyperaldosteronism (with hyperreninaemia, hypokalaemia, metabolic alkalosis, and without hypertension) has been described by Abston and Priano (1981).

Adrenal medulla

The adrenal medulla is embryologically and functionally distinct from the adrenal cortex. It is composed of chromaffin tissue and is considered frequently as a component of the efferent sympathetic nervous system. The medulla secretes catecholamines, predominantly adrenaline, into a local vascular system that is perfused at least in part with blood draining from the sinusoids of the adrenal cortex (Coupland & Selby, 1976). This anatomical relationship is of interest in view of many attempts that have been made to identify a physiological role of adrenal corticosteroids in the regulation of the secretory function of the medulla (Weinkove & Anderson, 1985). The responses of the sympathetic nervous system during anaesthesia and surgery have received much interest during the last 50 years as investigations of activity in efferent sympathetic nerve fibres, of autonomic reflex effects studied by observation of effector organ responses, or more recently of plasma concentrations of catecholamines (Derbyshire & Smith, 1984).

Phaeochromocytoma

The majority of disease processes affecting the adrenal medulla are associated with disease of adjacent adrenocortical tissue, and often the clinical features are those of associated adrenocortical dysfunction. One notable exception is the development of a catecholamine-secreting tumour of chromaffin tissue (phaeochromocytoma). This is an uncommon tumour occurring usually within the adrenal medulla, but it may develop at a large number of extra-adrenal sites and rarely occurs bilaterally. The majority of phaeochromocytomas are benign. The tumour may be associated occasionally with medullary carcinoma of the thyroid as a component of a multiple endocrine neoplasia syndrome, or with neurofibromatosis (Melicow, 1977; Modlin *et al.*, 1979; Hartley & Perry-Keene, 1985).

Clinical features attributable to chronic hypersecretion of catecholamines include hypertension and a triad of symptoms: headache, sweating and palpitations. Other features include malaise, weight loss, glucose intolerance that may lead on to development of diabetes mellitus, and psychiatric disturbances. The symptoms and the hypertension may occur paroxysmally; some patients remain normotensive between paroxysms although a majority show a maintained hypertension with superimposed elevations of blood pressure. It is uncommon for phaeochromocytoma to be associated with hypotension (Modlin *et al.*, 1979; Bravo & Gifford, 1984). Cardiac failure may be secondary to hypertension or occur in association with a specific cardiomyopathy (Hull, 1986; Sardesai *et al.*, 1990).

A variety of biochemical techniques have been developed to aid diagnostic identification of pathological hypersecretion of catecholamines. These include measurements of plasma concentrations of catecholamines (Brown *et al.*, 1981; Collste *et al.*, 1986) and their responses to the administration of clonidine (Bravo & Gifford, 1984) and measurements of the rate of urinary excretion of the metanephrines and hydroxymethyl mandelic acid (Bravo & Gifford, 1984; Manu & Runge, 1984). Localization of the tumour has involved a number of techniques including differential sampling of caval blood (Collste *et al.*, 1986), computerized tomography (CT), magnetic resonance imaging (Sheps *et al.*, 1990) and ^{131}I-meta-iodobenzylguanidine (MIBG) scintigraphy (Ackery *et al.*, 1984; Gough *et al.*, 1985; Shapiro *et al.*, 1985). Combined use of CT and MIBG techniques has been used to locate phaeochromocytomas at either adrenal or extra-adrenal sites (Koizumi *et al.*, 1986).

The treatment of choice for phaeochromocytoma

is surgical removal after a period of medical therapy titrated accurately to control the paroxysmal effects of the disease. Such therapy has involved attempts to inhibit catecholamine synthesis using α-methyltyrosine (Perry *et al.*, 1990) or, more commonly, attempts to suppress the responses to hypersecretion of catecholamines, particularly by producing α-adrenergic block using phenoxybenzamine or prazosin followed by β-adrenergic block where necessary to control arrhythmias. A number of reports of series of elective surgical treatment of phaeochromocytomas (Remine *et al.*, 1974; Modlin *et al.*, 1979) suggest that the introduction of this method of medical management has been associated with a reduction in mortality related to surgical removal. However, there remains, in addition, a number of patients with undiagnosed phaeochromocytomas who represent a particular at-risk group during anaesthesia and surgery.

In addition to the direct and immediate effects of hypersecretion of catecholamines, cardiovascular instability during anaesthesia and surgery in patients with phaeochromocytoma has been attributed to an anticipated reduction in blood volume associated with chronic elevation of plasma concentrations of catecholamines, and the occurrence of vasodilatation immediately after tumour removal and consequent catecholamine withdrawal. However, the significance of a reduction in blood volume in patients with phaeochromocytoma has been questioned (Sjoerdsma *et al.*, 1966; Tarazi *et al.*, 1970) and the use of phenoxybenzamine during preoperative preparation may be associated in itself with an increase in blood volume (Stenstrom & Kutti, 1985); accordingly, prophylactic administration of intravenous fluid to patients undergoing removal of phaeochromocytoma (Desmonts & Marty, 1984; Hull, 1986) may be undesirable in the absence of direct determination of blood volume.

The choice of individual anaesthetic agents and techniques for patients with phaeochromocytoma is determined by the need for prevention of stimulation of catecholamine release either from the tumour or from other adrenergic sites, and of exacerbation of the effects of any released catecholamines. There are reports of the use of a very wide variety of anaesthetic drugs and combinations of agents in patients with phaeochromocytoma. However, a recent review (Hull, 1986) lists some commonly used drugs that may be avoided rationally and this list includes droperidol, the administration of which may be associated with increases in arterial pressure (Sumikawa *et al.*, 1983); atropine; suxamethonium; histamine-releasing, competitive, neuromuscular-blocking drugs; and histamine-releasing opioids. Amongst the volatile anaesthetic agents, enflurane and isoflurane are associated less with myocardial sensitization to the arrhythmogenic effects of catecholamines than halothane (Eger, 1981).

The administration of anaesthesia, and anaesthetic and surgical manoeuvres, should be conducted to minimize stimulation of autonomic responses to tracheal intubation and surgery (Desmonts & Marty, 1984). Cardiovascular function should be monitored very carefully, particularly with respect to changes in heart rate and in arterial pressure (especially during induction of anaesthesia and during surgical mobilization of the tumour) and to avoidance of hypovolaemia as a result of surgical haemorrhage or the effect of reduction of plasma concentrations of catecholamines after removal of the tumour. Hypertension intraoperatively is usually controlled using sodium nitroprusside or phentolamine. Arrhythmias have been controlled using β-adrenergic antagonists, although, in patients with cardiac failure, antiarrhythmic local anaesthetic agents may be preferable (Desmonts & Marty, 1984; Hull, 1986). Marked hypoglycaemia may follow tumour removal (Channa *et al.*, 1987).

References

Abston P.A. & Priano L.L. (1981) Bartter's syndrome: anesthetic implications based on pathophysiology and treatment. *Anesthesia and Analgesia* **60**, 764–6.

Ackery D.M., Tippett P.A., Condon B.R., Sutton H.E. & Wyeth P. (1984) New approach to the localization of phaeochromocytoma. Imaging with iodine-131-meta-iodobenzylguanidine. *British Medical Journal* **288**, 1587–91.

Atkinson A.B. (1991) The treatment of Cushing's syndrome. *Clinical Endocrinology* **34**, 507–13.

Barton R.N. & Passingham B.J. (1982) Early responses to hemorrhage in the conscious rat: effects of corticosterone. *American Journal of Physiology* **243**, R416–23.

Bayliss R.I.S. (1958) Surgical collapse during and after corticosteroid therapy. *British Medical Journal* **2**, 935–6.

Besser G.M. & Edwards C.R.W. (1972) Cushing's syndrome. *Clinics in Endocrinology and Metabolism* **1**, 451–90.

Beyer H.S., Bantle J.P., Mariash C.N., Steffes M.W., Seljeskog E.L. & Oppenheimer J.H. (1985) Use of dexamethasone–adrenocorticotrophin test to assess the requirement for continued glucocorticoid replacement therapy after pituitary surgery. *Journal of Clinical Endocrinology and Metabolism* **60**, 1012–18.

Biglieri E.G. (1976) A perspective on aldosterone abnormalities. *Clinical Endocrinology* **5**, 399–410.

Biglieri E.G. (1991) Spectrum of mineralocorticoid hypertension. *Hypertension* **17**, 251–61.

Biglieri E.G., Irony I. & Kater C.E. (1990) Adrenocortical forms of human hypertension. In *Hypertension: Pathophysiology, Diagnosis and Management* (Eds Laragh J.H. & Brenner B.M.)

p. 1609. Raven Press, New York.

Black G.W. & Montgomery D.A.D. (1982) Adrenal disease. In *Medicine for Anaesthetists* (Ed. Vickers M.D.) p. 451. Blackwell Scientific Publications, Oxford.

Blichert-Toft M., Bagerskov A., Lockwood K. & Hasner E. (1972) Operative treatment, surgical approach and related complications in 195 operations upon the adrenal glands. *Surgery, Gynecology and Obstetrics* **135**, 261–6.

Brandt M.R., Olgaard K. & Kehlet H. (1979) Epidural analgesia inhibits the renin and aldosterone response to surgery. *Acta Anaesthesiologica Scandinavica* **23**, 267–72.

Bravo E.L. & Gifford R.W. (1984) Pheochromocytoma: diagnosis, localization and management. *New England Journal of Medicine* **311**, 1298–303.

Brown J.J., Fraser R., Lever A.F. & Robertson J.I.S. (1972) Aldosterone: physiological and pathophysiological variations in man. *Clinics in Endocrinology and Metabolism* **1**, 397–449.

Brown M.J., Allison D.J., Jenner D.A., Lewis P.J. & Dollery C.T. (1981) Increased sensitivity and accuracy of phaeochromocytoma diagnosis achieved by use of plasma–adrenaline estimation and a pentolinium suppression test. *Lancet* **i**, 174–7.

Buckley F.P., Kehlet H., Brown N.S. & Scott D.B. (1982) Postoperative glucose tolerance during extradural analgesia. *British Journal of Anaesthesia* **54**, 325–31.

Burke C.W. (1985) Adrenocortical insufficiency. *Clinics in Endocrinology and Metabolism* **14**, 947–76.

Burke C.W., Adams C.B.T., Esiri M.M., Morris C. & Bevan J.S. (1990) Transsphenoidal surgery for Cushing's disease: does what is removed determine the endocrine outcome? *Clinical Endocrinology* **33**, 525–37.

Burn J.M.B. (1972) Airway difficulties associated with anaesthesia in acromegaly. *British Journal of Anaesthesia* **44**, 413–14.

Channa A.B., Mofti A.B., Taylor G.W., Mekki M.O. & Sheikh M.H. (1987) Hypoglycaemic encephalopathy following surgery on phaeochromocytoma. *Anaesthesia* **42**, 1298–301.

Choo-Kang Y.F.J., Cooper E.J., Tribe A.E. & Grant I.W.B. (1972) Beclomethasone diproprionate by inhalation in the treatment of airways obstruction. *British Journal of Diseases of the Chest* **66**, 101–6.

Cochrane J.P.S. (1978) The aldosterone response to surgery and the relationship of this response to postoperative sodium retention. *British Journal of Surgery* **65**, 744–7.

Collste P., Brismar B., Alveryd A., Bjorkhem I., Hardstedt C., Svensson L. & Ostman J. (1986) The catecholamine concentration in central veins of hypertensive patients — an aid not without problems in locating phaeochromocytoma. *Acta Chirurgica Scandinavica* **530** (Suppl.), 67–71.

Conn J.W. (1955) Primary aldosteronism, a new clinical syndrome. *Journal of Laboratory and Clinical Medicine* **45**, 3–17.

Conn J.W. (1965) Hypertension, the potassium ion and impaired carbohydrate tolerance. *New England Journal of Medicine* **273**, 1135–43.

Connell J.M.C. & Fraser R. (1991) Adrenal corticosteroid synthesis and hypertension. *Journal of Hypertension* **9**, 97–107.

Cope C.L. (1966) The adrenal cortex in internal medicine — Part I. *British Medical Journal* **2**, 847–53.

Coté J. & Rouillard M. (1977) Considerations anesthesiques sur l'hypophysectomie trans-sphenoidale: étude rétrospective. *Canadian Anaesthetists' Society Journal* **24**, 275–81.

Coupland R.E. & Selby J.E. (1976) The blood supply of the mammalian adrenal medulla: a comparative study. *Journal of Anatomy* **122**, 539–51.

Cullen D.R., Reckless J.P.D. & McLaren E.H. (1980) Clinical disorders involving adrenocortical insufficiency and overactivity. In *General Comparative and Clinical Endocrinology of the Adrenal Cortex* vol. 3 (Eds Chester Jones I. & Henderson I.W.) p. 57. Academic Press, London.

Danby P., Harris K.P.G., Williams B., Feehally J. & Walls J. (1990) Adrenal dysfunction in patients with renal amyloid. *Quarterly Journal of Medicine* **76**, 915–22.

Daughaday W.H. (1985) The anterior pituitary. In *William's Textbook of Endocrinology* 7th edn. (Eds Wilson J.D. & Foster D.W.) p. 568. W.B. Saunders, Philadelphia.

Derbyshire D.R. & Smith G. (1984) Sympathoadrenal responses to anaesthesia and surgery. *British Journal of Anaesthesia* **56**, 725–39.

Desmonts J.M. & Marty J. (1984) Anaesthetic management of patients with phaeochromocytoma. *British Journal of Anaesthesia* **56**, 781–9.

Diethelm A.G. (1977) Surgical management of complications of steroid therapy. *Annals of Surgery* **185**, 251–63.

Duthie D.J.R., Fraser R. & Nimmo W.S. (1985) Effect of induction of anaesthesia with etomidate on corticosteroid synthesis in man. *British Journal of Anaesthesia* **57**, 156–9.

Eger E.I. II (1981) Isoflurane: a review. *Anesthesiology* **55**, 559–76.

Ernest I. & Ekman H. (1972) Adrenalectomy in Cushing's disease. A long-term follow-up. *Acta Endocrinologica* **160** (Suppl.), 5–41.

Feiwel M., James V.H.T. & Barnett E.S. (1969) Effect of potent topical steroids on plasma-cortisol levels of infants and children with eczema. *Lancet* **i**, 485–7.

Ferriss J.B., Brown J.J., Fraser R., Haywood E., Davies D.L., Kay A.W., Lever A.F., Robertson J.I.S., Owen K. & Peart W.S. (1975) Results of adrenal surgery in patients with hypertension, aldosterone excess and low plasma renin concentration. *British Medical Journal* **i**, 135–8.

Finch J.S. (1969) Primary aldosteronism. Review of the anaesthetic experience in sixty patients. *British Journal of Anaesthesia* **41**, 880–3.

Franksson C. & Gemzell C.A. (1954) Blood levels of 17-hydroxy-corticosteroids in surgery and allied conditions. *Acta Chirurgica Scandinavica* **106**, 24–30.

Fraser C.G., Preuss F.S. & Bigford W.D. (1952) Adrenal atrophy and irreversible shock associated with cortisone therapy. *Journal of the American Medical Association* **149**, 1542–3.

Frohman L.A. (1991) Therapeutic options in acromegaly. *Journal of Clinical Endocrinology and Metabolism* **72**, 1175–81.

Gangat Y., Triner L., Baer L. & Puchner P. (1976) Primary aldosteronism with uncommon complications. *Anesthesiology* **45**, 542–4.

Garlington L.N. & Bailey P.J. (1958) Primary hyperaldosteronism: anesthetic experience with two cases. *Anesthesiology* **19**, 661–4.

Goldhill D.R., Dalgleish J.G. & Lake R.H.N. (1982) Respiratory problems and acromegaly. *Anaesthesia* **37**, 1200–3.

Gough I.R., Thompson N.W., Shapiro B. & Sisson J.C. (1985)

Limitations of 131 I-MIBG scintigraphy in locating pheochromocytomas. *Surgery* **98**, 115—20.

Hall G.M. (1985) The anaesthetic modification of the endocrine and metabolic response to surgery. *Annals of the Royal College of Surgeons* **67**, 25—9.

Harris G.W. (1972) Humours and hormones. *Journal of Endocrinology* **53**, ii—xxii.

Hartley L. & Perry-Keene D. (1985) Phaeochromocytoma in Queensland — 1970—83. *Australia and New Zealand Journal of Surgery* **55**, 471—5.

Hassan S.Z., Matz G.J., Lawrence A.M. & Collins P.A. (1976) Laryngeal stenosis in acromegaly: a possible cause of airway difficulties associated with anesthesia. *Anesthesia and Analgesia* **55**, 57—60.

Hertzberg L.B. & Shulman M.S. (1985) Acute adrenal insufficiency in a patient with appendicitis during anesthesia. *Anesthesiology* **62**, 517—19.

Hodges J.R. (1984) The hypothalamo-pituitary-adrenocortical system. *British Journal of Anaesthesia* **56**, 701—10.

Hout W.M., Arafah B.M., Salazar R. & Selman W. (1988) Evaluation of the hypothalamic—pituitary—adrenal axis immediately after pituitary adenomectomy: is perioperative steroid therapy necessary? *Journal of Clinical Endocrinology and Metabolism* **66**, 1208—12.

Howlett T.A., Lees L.H. & Besser G.M. (1985) Cushing's syndrome. *Clinics in Endocrinology and Metabolism* **14**, 911—45.

Huang X.Y. & McCann S.M. (1983) Interaction of atropine with naloxone to alter anterior pituitary hormone secretion. *American Journal of Physiology* **245**, E502—7.

Hull C.J. (1986) Phaeochromocytoma. Diagnosis, preoperative preparation and anaesthetic management. *British Journal of Anaesthesia* **58**, 1453—68.

Hume D.M. & Egdahl R.H. (1959) The importance of the brain in the endocrine response to injury. *Annals of Surgery* **150**, 697—712.

Hume D.M., Bell C.C. & Bartter F. (1962) Direct measurement of adrenal secretion during operative trauma and convalescence. *Surgery* **52**, 174—87.

James M.L. (1970) Endocrine disease and anaesthesia. *Anaesthesia* **25**, 232—52.

Jasani M.K., Freeman P.A., Boyle J.A., Reid A.M., Diver M.J. & Buchanan W.W. (1968) Studies of the rise in 11-hydroxycorticosteroids (11-OHCS) in corticosteroid-treated patients with rheumatoid arthritis during surgery: correlations with the functional integrity of the hypothalamo—pituitary—adrenal axis. *Quarterly Journal of Medicine* **61**, 407—21.

Jensen J.C., Pass H.I., Sindelar W.F. & Norton J.A. (1991) Recurrent or metastatic disease in select patients with adrenocortical carcinoma. *Archives of Surgery* **126**, 457—61.

Kasson B.G. & George R. (1983) Endocrine influences on the actions of morphine. III Responses to hypothalamic hormones. *Neuroendocrinology* **37**, 416—20.

Kehlet H. (1975) A rational approach to dosage and preparation of parenteral glucocorticoid substitution therapy during surgical procedures. *Acta Anaesthesiologica Scandinavica* **19**, 260—4.

Kehlet H. & Binder C. (1973) Adrenocortical function and clinical course during and after surgery in unsupplemented glucocorticoid-treated patients. *British Journal of Anaesthesia* **45**, 1043—8.

Kehlet H., Nikki P., Jaattela A. & Takki S. (1974) Plasma catecholamine concentrations during surgery in unsupplemented glucocorticoid-treated patients. *British Journal of Anaesthesia* **46**, 73—7.

Kitahata L.M. (1971) Airway difficulties associated with anaesthesia in acromegaly. *British Journal of Anaesthesia* **43**, 1187—90.

Koizumi M., Endo K., Sakahara H., Nakashima T., Nakano Y., Nakao K. & Torizuka K. (1986) Computed tomography and 131 I-MIBG scintigraphy in the diagnosis of pheochromocytoma. *Acta Radiologica: Diagnosis* **27**, 305—9.

Lewis L., Robinson R.F., Yee J., Hacker L.A. & Eisen G. (1953) Fatal adrenal cortical insufficiency precipitated by surgery during prolonged continuous cortisone treatment. *Annals of Internal Medicine* **39**, 116—26.

Liddle G.W. (1982) Adrenal Cortex. In *Textbook of Medicine* 16th edn. (Eds Wyngaarden J.B. & Smith L.H.) p. 1225. W.B. Saunders, Philadelphia.

Maddi R. & Gabel R.A. (1980) Anesthetic considerations for adrenalectomy. In *Contemporary Anesthesia Practice. Anesthesia and the Patient with Endocrine Disease* (Ed. Brown B.R.) p. 1. F.A. Davis Co., Philadelphia.

Manu P. & Runge L.A. (1984) Biochemical screening for pheochromocytoma. Superiority of urinary metanephrines measurements. *American Journal of Epidemiology* **120**, 788—90.

Matsuki A., Baba S., Kudo T. & Oyama T. (1976) Enflurane anaesthesia for removal of aldosterone producing adenoma. *Anaesthesist* **25**, 72—5.

Mattingly D. & Tyler C. (1965) Plasma 11-hydroxycorticoid levels in surgical stress. *Proceedings of the Royal Society of Medicine* **58**, 1010—12.

Melby J.C. (1985) Diagnosis and treatment of primary aldosteronism and isolated hypoaldosteronism. *Clinics in Endocrinology and Metabolism* **14**, 977—95.

Melby J.C. (1991) Diagnosis of hyperaldosteronism. *Endocrinology and Metabolism Clinics of North America* **20**, 247—55.

Melicow M.M. (1977) One hundred cases of pheochromocytoma at the Columbia-Presbyterian Medical Center 1926—1976. A clinicopathological analysis. *Cancer* **40**, 1987—2004.

Messik J.M., Laws E.R. & Abboud C.F. (1978) Anesthesia for transsphenoidal surgery of the hypophyseal region. *Anesthesia and Analgesia* **57**, 206—15.

Modlin M., Farndon J.R., Shepherd A., Johnston I.D.A., Kennedy T.L., Montgomery D.A.D. & Welbourn R.B. (1979) Phaeochromocytoma in 72 patients: clinical and diagnostic features, treatment and long term results. *British Journal of Surgery* **66**, 456—65.

Moore R.A., Allen M.C., Wood P.J., Rees L.H. & Sear J.W. (1985) Perioperative endocrine effects of etomidate. *Anaesthesia* **40**, 124—30.

Nelson D.H. (1980) *The Adrenal Cortex: Physiological Function and Disease.* W.B. Saunders, Philadelphia.

Neville A.M. & O'Hare M.J. (1982) *The Human Adrenal Cortex. Pathology and Biology — An Integrated Approach.* Springer-Verlag, Berlin.

Orth D.N. & Liddle G.W. (1971) Results of treatment in 108 patients with Cushing's syndrome. *New England Journal of Medicine* **285**, 241—7.

Oyama T. (1980) Influence of general anesthesia and surgical stress on endocrine function. In *Contemporary Anesthesia Practice. Anesthesia and the Patient with Endocrine Disease* (Ed. Brown B.R.) p. 173. F.A. Davis Co., Philadelphia.

Oyama T. & Takiguchi M. (1970) Plasma levels of ACTH and cortisol in man during anesthesia and surgery. *Anesthesia and Analgesia* **49**, 363–6.

Oyama T., Shibata S., Matsumoto F., Takiguchi M. & Kudo T. (1968) Effects of halothane anaesthesia and surgery on adrenocortical function in man. *Canadian Anaesthetists' Society Journal* **15**, 258–66.

Oyama T., Kimura K., Takazawa T. & Takiguchi H. (1969) An objective evaluation of tranquillizers as preanaesthetic medication: effect on adrenocortical function. *Canadian Anaesthetists' Society Journal* **16**, 209–16.

Oyama T., Taniguchi K., Jin T., Satone T. & Kudo T. (1979) Effects of anaesthesia and surgery on plasma aldosterone concentration and renin activity in man. *British Journal of Anaesthesia* **51**, 747–52.

Perry R.R., Keiser H.R., Norton J.A., Wall R.T., Robertson C.N., Travis W., Pass H.I., Walther M.M. & Linehan W.M. (1990) Surgical management of pheochromocytoma with the use of metyrosine. *Annals of Surgery* **212**, 621–8.

Plumpton F.S., Besser G.M. & Cole P.V. (1969a) Corticosteroid treatment and surgery. 1. An investigation of the indications for steroid care. *Anaesthesia* **24**, 3–11.

Plumpton F.S., Besser G.M. & Cole P.V. (1969b) Corticosteroid treatment and surgery. 2. The management of steroid care. *Anaesthesia* **24**, 12–18.

Reichlin S. (1985) Neuroendocrinology. In *Williams Textbook of Endocrinology* 7th edn. (Eds Wilson J.D. & Foster D.W.) p. 492. W.B. Saunders, Philadelphia.

Remine W.H., Chong G.C., Van Heerden J.A., Sheps S.G. & Harrison E.G. (1974) Current management of pheochromocytoma. *Annals of Surgery* **179**, 740–8.

Robertson D. & Michelakis A.M. (1972) Effect of anesthesia and surgery on plasma renin activity in man. *Journal of Clinical Endocrinology and Metabolism* **34**, 831–6.

Ross E.J., Marshall-Jones P. & Friedman M. (1966) Cushing's syndrome: diagnostic criteria. *Quarterly Journal of Medicine* **59**, 149–92.

Sampson P.A., Brooke B.N. & Winstone N.E. (1961) Biochemical confirmation of collapse due to adrenal failure. *Lancet* **i**, 1377.

Sampson P.A., Winstone N.E. & Brooke B.N. (1962) Adrenal function in surgical patients after steroid therapy. *Lancet* **ii**, 322–5.

Sandberg A.A., Eik-Nes K., Samuels L.T. & Tyler F.H. (1954) The effects of surgery on the blood levels and metabolism of 17-hydroxycorticosteroids in man. *Journal of Clinical Investigation* **33**, 1509–16.

Sardesai S.H., Mourant A.J., Sivathandon Y., Farrow R. & Gibbons D.O. (1990) Phaeochromocytoma and catecholamine induced cardiomyopathy presenting as heart failure. *British Heart Journal* **63**, 234–7.

Scheithauer B.W. (1984a) Surgical pathology of the pituitary: the adenomas. Part I. *Pathology Annual* **19** (Part 1), 317–74.

Scheithauer B.W. (1984b) Surgical pathology of the pituitary: the adenomas. Part II. *Pathology Annual* **19** (Part 2), 269–329.

Scheithauer B.W. (1985) Pathology of the pituitary and sellar region: exclusive of pituitary adenoma. *Pathology Annual* **20** (Part 1), 67–155.

Sear J. (1985) Etomidate and adrenocortical synthesis in man. *British Journal of Anaesthesia* **57**, 1265–6.

Shapiro B., Sisson J.C., Eyre P., Copp J.E., Dmuchowski C. & Beierwaltes W.H. (1985) 131-I-MIBG — a new agent in diagnosis and treatment of pheochromocytoma. *Cardiology* **72**, (Suppl. 1), 137–42.

Sheps S.G., Jiang N.-S., Klee G.G. & van Heerden J.A. (1990) Recent developments in the diagnosis and treatment of pheochromocytoma. *Mayo Clinic Proceedings* **65**, 88–95.

Sheward W.J. & Fink G. (1991) Effects of corticosterone on the secretion of corticotrophin-releasing factor, arginine vasopressin and oxytocin into hypophysial portal blood in long-term hypophysectomized rats. *Journal of Endocrinology* **129**, 91–8.

Shipton E.A. & Hugo J.M. (1982a) An aldosterone-producing adrenal cortical adenoma. *Anaesthesia* **37**, 933–6.

Shipton E.A. & Hugo J.M. (1982b) Primary aldosteronism and its importance to the anaesthetist. *South African Medical Journal* **62**, 60–3.

Singelyn F.J. & Scholtes J.L. (1988) Airway obstruction in acromegaly: a method of prevention. *Anaesthesia and Intensive Care* **16**, 491–4.

Sjoerdsma A., Engelman K., Waldmann T.A., Cooperman L.H. & Hammond W.G. (1966) Pheochromocytoma: current concepts of diagnosis and treatment. *Annals of Internal Medicine* **65**, 1302–26.

Smith M.G. & Byrne A.J. (1981) An Addisonian crisis complicating anaesthesia. *Anesthesia* **36**, 681–4.

Soffer L.J., Iannaccone A. & Gabrilove J.L. (1961) Cushing's syndrome. A study of fifty patients. *American Journal of Medicine* **30**, 129–46.

Southwick J.P. & Katz J. (1979) Unusual airway difficulty in the acromegalic patient — indications for tracheostomy. *Anesthesiology* **51**, 72–3.

Stenstrom G. & Kutti J. (1985) The blood volume in pheochromocytoma patients before and during treatment with phenoxybenzamine. *Acta Medica Scandinavica* **218**, 381–7.

Stephen C.R. (1977) Anesthesia for adrenal surgery. *Urologic Clinics of North America* **4**, 319–26.

Streeten D.H.P., Dalakos T.G., Souma M., Fellerman H., Clift G.V., Schletter F.E., Stevenson C.T. & Speller P.J. (1973) Studies of the pathogenesis of idiopathic oedema: the role of postural changes in plasma volume, plasma renin activity, aldosterone secretion rate and glomerular filtration rate in the retention of sodium and water. *Clinical Science* **45**, 347–73.

Sumikawa K., Matsumoto T., Amenomori Y., Hirano H. & Amakata Y. (1983) Selective actions of intravenous anesthetics on nicotinic- and muscarinic-receptor-mediated responses of the dog adrenal medulla. *Anesthesiology* **59**, 412–16.

Symreng T., Karlberg B.E., Kagedal B. & Schildt B. (1981) Physiological cortisol substitution of long-term steroid-treated patients undergoing major surgery. *British Journal of Anaesthesia* **53**, 949–54.

Tarazi R.C., Dustan H.P., Frohlich E.D., Gifford R.W. & Hoffman G.C. (1970) Plasma volume and chronic hypertension. *Archives of Internal Medicine* **125**, 835–42.

Teasdale G. (1983) Surgical management of pituitary adenoma. *Clinics in Endocrinology and Metabolism* **12**, 789–823.

Tyrell J.B., Brooks R.M., Fitzgerald P.A., Cofoid P.B., Forsham

P.H. & Wilson C.B. (1978) Cushing's disease. Selective trans-sphenoidal resection of pituitary microadenomas. *New England Journal of Medicine* **298**, 753–8.

Ulick S. (1991) Two uncommon causes of mineralocorticoid excess. Syndrome of apparent mineralocorticoid excess and glucocorticoid-remediable aldosteronism. *Endocrinology and Metabolism Clinics of North America* **20**, 269–76.

Weatherill D. & Spence A.A. (1984) Anaesthesia and disorders of the adrenal cortex. *British Journal of Anaesthesia* **56**, 741–9.

Weinkove C. & Anderson D.C. (1985) Interactions between adrenal cortex and medulla. In *Adrenal Cortex* (Eds Anderson D.C. & Winter J.S.D.) p. 208. Butterworth, London.

Welbourn R.B., Montgomery D.A.D. & Kennedy T.L. (1971) The natural history of treated Cushing's syndrome. *British Journal of Surgery* **58**, 1–16.

Whelan J., Redpath T. & Buckle R. (1982) The medical and anaesthetic management of acromegalic patients undergoing maxillo-facial surgery. *British Journal of Oral Surgery* **20**, 77–83.

Whitwam J.G., Tunbridge W.M.G. & Fuller W.I. (1973) Management of patients for yttrium-90 implantation of the pituitary gland. *British Journal of Anaesthesia* **45**, 1121–9.

Williams G.D. & Dluhy R.G. (1983) Diseases of the adrenal cortex. In *Principles of Internal Medicine* 10th edn. (Eds Petersdorf R.G., Adams R.D., Braunwald E., Isselbacher K.J., Martin J.B. & Wilson J.D.) p. 634. McGraw-Hill, New York.

Williams G.H. (1976) Aldosterone, potassium and acidosis. *New England Journal of Medicine* **294**, 392–3.

Wilson C.B. (1984) A decade of pituitary microsurgery. *Journal of Neurosurgery* **61**, 814–33.

Anaesthesia for Thyroid and Parathyroid Disease

P. S. SEBEL

Anatomy

The thyroid gland, which normally weighs 20–25 g, lies behind the strap muscles of the neck and anterior to the larynx and trachea. It consists of an isthmus, which overlies the second to fourth tracheal rings, connecting two pear-shaped lateral lobes. The lateral lobes extend from the thyroid cartilage to the fifth or sixth tracheal ring, inferiorly. Behind the thyroid, in the groove between the trachea and oesophagus, lies the recurrent laryngeal nerve which supplies all the intrinsic laryngeal muscles except the cricothyroid muscle. This is supplied by the external branch of the superior laryngeal nerve which lies deep to the upper pole of the thyroid. The thyroid gland consists of a large number of follicles which are lined with cuboidal epithelial cells. These follicles are filled with colloid, the main constituent of which is thyroglobulin, a glycoprotein.

Enlargement of the thyroid can potentially compress the trachea causing difficulty in respiration. Downward enlargement of the gland into the thoracic inlet (retrosternal goitre) may be associated also with impaired respiration. Carcinoma of the thyroid may invade and erode the trachea, oesophagus or even the carotid sheath.

There are four parathyroid glands. They are the size of small peas and ochre in colour. The superior glands lie posterior to the apex of each thyroid lobe whereas the inferior parathyroids are related to the bases. Approximately 10% of inferior parathyroid glands are aberrant, lying posterior to the pretracheal fascia or in the superior mediastinum related to the thymus.

Physiology

The main hormones secreted by the thyroid gland are iodine containing amino acids, thyroxine (T_4) and triiodothyronine (T_3) (Ganong, 1985). The euthyroid range for T_4 is 55–150 nmol/litre and for T_3, 1.4–3.5 nmol/litre. Reverse triiodothyronine (RT_3), which is inactive, and other compounds are secreted by the thyroid also.

T_3 is more active than T_4; however, very little T_3 is produced by the thyroid, most of it being formed from T_4 in the tissues. Thyroid-stimulating (thyrotrophic) hormone (TSH) is secreted from the anterior pituitary and controls thyroid hormone synthesis by a negative feedback control mechanism. TSH secretion is stimulated also by thyrotrophic-releasing hormone, arising from the hypothalamus. Long-acting thyroid stimulator (LATS) is an IgG immunoglobulin which has effects similar to those of TSH on thyroid cells. There are probably other thyroid stimulators, including LATS protector.

The physiological effects of thyroid hormones are related to stimulation of oxygen consumption (Ganong, 1985). Increased secretion causes an increase in basal metabolic rate (BMR) of up to 100%; nitrogen excretion is increased and body weight decreases. Muscle weakness may be associated with the increase in nitrogen excretion and thyrotoxic myopathy may result. There may be an associated increase in body temperature.

This results in a decrease in peripheral resistance because of a consequent increase in skin blood flow, but cardiac output, arterial pressure and heart rate increase as a result of direct actions of thyroid hormones and catecholamines on the myocardium. Myocardial sensitivity to catecholamines is increased because thyroid hormones increase the number of β-receptors.

Congenital absence of thyroid hormones may produce cretinism, a syndrome characterized by mental retardation. This is probably not an effect on oxygen/glucose metabolism but a direct effect on the brain.

There are three hormones associated principally

with bone and calcium metabolism. Parathormone, secreted by the parathyroid glands, stimulates osteoclasts causing mobilization of calcium, increases phosphate excretion by an action on renal tubules and increases calcium absorption in the small intestine.

Calcitonin, secreted primarily by the thyroid gland, inhibits bone resorption, and dehydroxycholecalciferol, formed from vitamin D, increases calcium absorption from the digestive tract (Ganong, 1985).

Parathormone is necessary for life. If the parathyroid glands are removed, there is a progressive decrease in the serum calcium concentration associated with an increase in neuromuscular excitability, which is followed by hypocalcaemic tetany. Hypoparathyroidism occurs most commonly after subtotal thyroidectomy when the parathyroids are removed inadvertently and symptoms may develop any time up to several weeks postoperatively.

Hyperparathyroidism, occurring either as a result of a parathyroid adenoma or generalized hyperplasia, is associated with an increase in plasma and urinary calcium concentrations, renal stones, hypertension and bone pain.

Effects of anaesthesia and surgery

Induction of anaesthesia with diethyl ether or halothane produces increased plasma concentrations of T_4, whereas a thiopentone/nitrous oxide/curare sequence produces a reduction in T_4 concentration (Oyama et al., 1969). Surgical stimulation results in a further increase in T_4 concentrations in the volatile groups, but not in the thiopentone group.

With isoflurane anaesthesia, plasma T_4 concentration tends to increase as with ether and halothane, but remains within the normal range (Oyama et al., 1975a), whereas Althesin anaesthesia produces a decrease similar to that of thiopentone (Oyama et al., 1975b).

Anaesthesia with halothane (Oyama et al., 1969) or isoflurane (Oyama et al., 1975a) results in an increase in plasma T_4 concentration, whereas a thiopentone/ nitrous oxide/curare sequence produces a reduction in T_4 concentration (Oyama et al., 1969). In a study comparing general anaesthesia with thiopentone/ pethidine/pancuronium/nitrous oxide, with extradural anaesthesia, a significant difference in TSH secretion was found, being increased in the general anaesthetic group, but unchanged in the extradural group (Noreng et al., 1987). Both groups of patients had reductions in plasma T_3 and T_4 concentrations and T_3 bindings were unchanged during surgery.

High-dose fentanyl anaesthesia probably does not affect the thyroid hormone response to surgical stress (Imberti et al., 1988). After cardiac surgery under high-dose fentanyl/oxygen anaesthesia, all patients had an increase in T_3 parallel with an increase in RT_3, which is biologically inactive.

Assessment of thyroid function

The most useful laboratory tests of thyroid function are radioimmunoassay of T_4, which is affected by alterations in thyroxine binding, and the T_4 determination which measures metabolically active T_4. T_3 measurement is necessary in cases of thyrotoxicosis when normal T_4 concentrations are found. The cause may be T_3 thyrotoxicosis. Serum TSH may be measured also. The normal range is below 5 milliunits/litre and values in excess of 40 milliunits/ litre may occur when gross thyroid insufficiency is present.

Radioiodine uptake by the thyroid gland is a useful adjunct investigation, being increased in thyrotoxicosis and decreased in hypothyroidism.

Thyroid scans after tracer doses of radioactive iodine or technetium help to define an autonomous toxic nodule or a carcinoma (Rains & Ritchie, 1984). Other non-specific tests are sometimes helpful: an increased serum cholesterol concentration being indicative of hypothyroidism; the Achilles tendon reflex is rapid in hyperthyroidism and the relaxation time is prolonged in hypothyroidism. Tests such as the BMR and protein-bound iodine have been largely superseded.

Diseases of thyroid and parathyroids

Simple goitre

This may occur in patients living in areas where iodine is lacking. Thyroid function tests are usually normal. Surgery is indicated if there are signs of compression of the trachea or other structures in the neck.

Hypothyroidism

Primary hypothyroidism occurs in approximately 1:5000 births. Until recently it was thought that congenital absence of the thyroid was associated with the physical changes of cretinism. However, few hypothyroid infants detected through screening have the characteristics of cretinism (Greer, 1987). Although primary hypothyroidism, which is caused by a defect in the thyroid structure or thyroid hormone synthesis, is the most common cause of hypothyroidism, secondary hypothyroidism may occur (caused by pituitary failure) and tertiary hypothyroidism (probably caused by inadequate TSH secretion as a result of inadequate TRH). The symptoms of myxoedema or hypothyroidism occurring in the adult are fatigue, cold intolerance, dry skin, constipation and hoarseness. Clinical findings include bradycardia, hypothermia, periorbital oedema, dry skin and a goitre.

There is a reduced BMR and, in general, reduced ability to increase core temperature. The myxoedematous patient is therefore at risk of developing intraoperative and postoperative hypothermia (Murkin, 1982). It is possible that acute postoperative hypothyroidism may occur. One patient was reported to have developed acute hypothyroidism 12 days after emergency oversewing of a gastric ulcer. Although the patient was treated with T_3, she died, with severe hypotension (Mogensen & Hjortso, 1988).

Myocardial function is depressed. Pre-ejection period is increased and left ventricular ejection fraction decreased. Cardiac output may be reduced markedly as a result of both bradycardia and reduced stroke volume (Murkin, 1982). Myxoedema does not usually cause heart failure directly but the depression of myocardial function renders the heart unable to respond effectively to further stress.

Myxoedema affects the respiratory system also. There may be a reduction in maximum breathing capacity and a reduction in carbon monoxide transfer factor. Both hypoxic and hypercapnic ventilatory drives may be depressed markedly. Associated with myxoedema is a reduction in plasma volume by as much as 25%.

Hypothyroidism in elderly patients may be associated with pericardial effusion. The cardiac silhouette may be massively enlarged because of fluid accumulation. The effusion usually disappears during the first few weeks of therapy, tamponade is very unusual and pericardiocentesis is almost never indicated.

Treatment of hypothyroidism is simple and effective using synthetic laevothyroxine as the treatment of choice. Treatment should be carried out cautiously in the presence of heart disease, as angina or infarction may be precipitated.

The end-stage of untreated or neglected myxoedema is myxoedema coma, with hypothermia, hypotension and hypoventilation with associated hypoxia and hypercapnia. The syndrome may be precipitated by infection or exposure to cold. In addition to ventilatory and cardiac support, specific treatment comprises laevothyroxine and hydrocortisone in addition to ventilatory and cardiac support. Active warming should be avoided (Camargo & Kolb, 1986).

Hyperthyroidism

The commonest causes of hyperthyroidism or thyrotoxicosis, are Graves' disease (primary hyperthyroidism), toxic nodular goitre and thyroiditis. The occurrence of hyperthyroidism, or thyrotoxicosis, implies that the thyroid gland is unresponsive to TSH. The pathogenesis, however, remains unclear and may involve autoantibodies binding to TSH receptors on the thyroid cell membrane. LATS and LATS protector may be the immunoglobulins involved.

Thyrotoxicosis is most common in women aged 20–40 years. The clinical features vary considerably, especially in elderly patients. A history of weight loss with good appetite is common as are weakness, sweating, heat intolerance and nervousness. There is usually a diffuse goitre but this may be absent, particularly in elderly patients, who may present without hypermetabolic signs.

There may be marked muscle wasting, especially in the shoulders and the legs, periodic paralysis may occur and myasthenia gravis occasionally occurs in conjunction with Graves' disease.

Thyrotoxic patients have quickness of speech and movement with some degree of tremor, which may be gross. The eyes appear bright and staring and there is usually some degree of exophthalmos. The degree of exophthalmos correlates poorly with the degree of thyrotoxicosis. The bright-eyed look of the thyrotoxic patient results from lid retraction. There is usually associated conjunctivitis and the external ocular muscles may be paralysed, leading to diplopia. Exophthalmos is a result of oedema and deposition of fat and mucopolysaccharide. If exophthalmos and lid retraction are severe, the lids cannot cover the cornea and dangerous ulceration may result. Eye changes often do not revert after successful treatment of the underlying thyrotoxicosis. Steroids and local β-blocking drugs appear ineffective, methyl cellulose drops may provide some relief, but lateral tarsorraphy is indicated if the cornea is endangered.

Thyrotoxic patients may complain of an irregular, rapid pulse and ECG features may include tachycardia and atrial fibrillation. Elderly patients, in particular, may present in cardiac failure, which is unresponsive to treatment with digitalis.

Treatment of thyrotoxicosis is aimed at controlling

excess secretion of thyroid hormones. Graves' disease may be characterized by long periods of remission in many patients. The first line of treatment is with antithyroid drugs such as propylthiouracil or methimacole or carbimazole which inhibit thyroid hormone synthesis. All act by blocking intrathyroid synthesis of T_3 and T_4. Propylthiouracil also decreases the conversion of T_4 to T_3 in the periphery. When the patient is euthyroid, treatment may be stopped. Up to 25% of patients may maintain a lasting remission. Some centres consider subtotal thyroidectomy as the most effective method of controlling hormone excretion. Before thyroidectomy, it is necessary for the patient to be adequately prepared and rendered euthyroid. The three main lines of treatment are the antithyroid drugs, beta blockers and iodine. In the older age group, radioactive iodine (^{131}I) is a suitable method of destroying overactive thyroid tissue. There is a high incidence of hypothyroidism after radio-iodine treatment and there exists the possibility of carcinogenicity from this type of treatment.

Even with effective treatment, the thyroid remains vascular and hyperplastic, rendering surgery difficult. Toxic reactions to thiouracils are rare, but include rash and agranulocytosis.

Even when the patient is euthyroid, the gland may remain vascular and hyperplastic, which may make surgery difficult. Approximately 10–20 days before surgery, oral iodine therapy is commenced. This is reputed to maintain euthyroid status and reduce the vascularity of the gland. The mechanism of action of iodine is unclear but may relate to the excess of substrate provided, thereby reducing blood supply to the gland.

Propranolol, 80–240 mg/day, is often used in the preparation of the hyperthyroid patient, either alone or in combination with conventional therapy. Pre-operative propranolol therapy is associated with good cardiovascular stability during surgery (Trench et al., 1978). Propranolol reverses rapidly the catecholamine-mediated features of thyrotoxicosis especially tremor and tachycardia. Propranolol is contraindiciated when asthma is present and should not be used when the patient is in cardiac failure.

Thyroid storm

With current therapy, thyroid storm or thyrotoxic crisis has, fortunately, become a rare event. It occurs primarily in undiagnosed or incompletely treated hyperthyroid patients or those with intercurrent infection, immediately after subtotal thyroidectomy or occasionally after radioactive-iodine therapy. The syndrome is characterized by fever, delirium, CNS irritability, and cardiac arrhythmias, which may be life-threatening. The most effective treatment is with large doses of propranolol given intravenously in combination with rehydration and antithyroid therapy.

General resuscitative measures are indicated also: administration of oxygen, sedation, cooling and careful electrolyte balance. Steroids were used previously in the treatment of thyroid storm.

In the perioperative period, thyrotoxic crisis may produce a syndrome similar to that of malignant hyperthermia and indeed the two have been confused (Peters et al., 1981). Thyroid storm presenting under general anaesthesia had been assumed to be malignant hyperthermia and has been treated with dantrolene (Bennet & Wainwright, 1989). As both syndromes have similar presentations and skeletal muscle abnormality, it is not unreasonable to use intravenous dantrolene in the treatment of thyroid storm, and it has been used as a treatment of thyroid storm where conventional therapy has failed (Christensen & Nissen, 1987).

Hypoparathyroidism

This is seen most commonly after subtotal thyroidectomy, when all the parathyroid glands are removed. After removal of a parathyroid adenoma or occasionally after thyroidectomy, transient hypoparathyroidism may occur.

The symptoms of hypoparathyroidism are those of increased neuromuscular irritability. Acute presentation may begin with paraesthesiae and progress to tetany with muscle cramps, CNS irritability, carpopedal spasms, dyspnoea, wheezing and laryngeal stridor, which may be fatal. Convulsions may occur.

In the early stages, diagnosis may be helped by tapping the facial nerve near the angle of the jaw to produce facial muscle contraction (Chvostek's sign) and application of tourniquet above systolic arterial pressure produces carpopedal spasm (Trousseau's sign).

There is also a genetic defect, idiopathic hypoparathyroidism or pseudohypoparathyroidism, where the parathyroids are present and may be hyperplastic but the renal tubules are insensitive to parathormone. It is associated with short stature, mental retardation, cataracts and defective nails and teeth.

The diagnosis of hypoparathyroidism is distinguished from tetany resulting from metabolic alkalosis by the finding of an abnormally low serum calcium concentration. The serum phosphorus is raised, which does not occur with other forms of hypocalcaemic tetany (rickets, osteomalacia and acute pancreatitis). Parathyroid hormone concentrations are reduced in postoperative hypoparathyroidism but normal or raised in the congenital syndrome.

Treatment of acute hypocalcaemic tetany is to ensure a clear airway and to administer 10–20 ml calcium chloride 10% or gluconate 10% intravenously until the tetany stops. Serum calcium concentration should be maintained in the lower part of the normal range. If it is maintained at too high a level, irreversible tissue calcification may occur. Calcium salts should be given orally when the acute attack is controlled and may be sufficient on their own for treatment of transient postoperative hypoparathyroidism.

Primary hyperparathyroidism

The commonest cause of primary hyperparathyroidism (up to 80%) is an adenoma of one of the four parathyroid glands, with suppression of the other three. Fifteen to 20% are caused by hypertrophy and hyperplasia of all four glands, and 2% by carcinoma. The three types cannot be distinguished biochemically. The presentation of hyperparathyroidism is related to renal or urinary tract involvement, skeletal problems and/or those related to the direct effects of hypercalcaemia. Renal stones are probably the commonest method of presentation.

Hypercalcaemia produces polydipsia, polyuria, hypertension, duodenal ulcer, uraemia, anorexia and constipation. Some patients are asymptomatic, diagnosis being made as a result of biochemical screening with elevation of serum and urinary calcium concentrations and decreased concentrations of serum and urinary phosphate. With earlier diagnosis, the skeletal manifestations of hyperparathyroidism are less common; they include back pain and joint pain and may progress to pathological fractures. The classic X-ray feature is of subperiosteal resorption of bone, especially from the proximal phalanges. Other organ systems may become involved. There may be a distinctive proximal myopathy, with fatiguability and proximal muscle weakness. Peptic ulcer and anaemia may exist in conjunction with hyperparathyroidism. Patients may present with hypercalcaemic crisis with accompanying anuria (Schou & Knudsen, 1988). This is conventionally treated with fluids, electrolytes, mithramyacin, calcitonin, etidronate and prednisolone. Continuous arteriovenous haemofiltration may be used when the hypercalcaemia is refractory to conventional treatments (Schou & Knudsen, 1988).

Diagnosis is achieved by finding a high serum calcium concentration in the presence of a low phosphate with high parathormone concentrations. Hypercalcaemia in the presence of normal parathormone hormones is indicative also of hyperparathyroidism as the hypercalcaemia should suppress parathormone. Electrocardiography may demonstrate a decreased QT interval. The distinction between hyperplasia and adenoma may be helped by computerized tomography (CT) scan or technetium–thallium scanning, but the results are not always consistent with the findings at surgery. Frozen section is needed to obtain a final diagnosis.

Treatment of a parathyroid adenoma is by surgical excision. There may be multiple adenomata or, in the case of a single adenoma, the other three glands may be suppressed. The adenoma may be ectopic, occurring in the mediastinum. In the case of hyperplasia, current practice is to remove all four glands and to transplant a small amount of parathyroid tissue into the forearm. Thus, if hyperplasia recurs, re-exploration is avoided. The sternocleidomastoid muscle has also been recommended (Lando et al., 1988) as this involves only one operation site.

In patients unsuitable for surgery, or in mild cases, medical management may be appropriate: a high fluid intake produces dilute urine and reduces the risk of calculus production. Oral phosphates may be used if renal function is good, but there is some risk of ectopic calcification. Long-term administration of propranolol may lower both calcium and parathormone concentrations in primary hyperparathyroidism.

There are other types of hyperparathyroidism: secondary hyperparathyroidism occurs after persistently low serum calcium concentrations (usually from vitamin D deficiency). Although parathormone concentrations are increased, serum calcium concentrations are always decreased. Tertiary hyperparathyroidism occurs when a parathyroid gland becomes autonomous after secondary hyperparathyroidism and an adenoma develops. The diagnosis and treatment is the same as for primary hyperparathyroidism, and the diagnosis is established if there is a history of low serum calcium concentration. Pseudo-hyperparathyroidism is said to occur when parathormone-like substances are secreted by tumours which do not arise from the parathyroid glands (Fletcher, 1977).

Anaesthesia for thyroid surgery

Preoperative assessment

At the preoperative visit, the anaesthetist should determine that thyroid function has been controlled adequately and that the patient is clinically euthyroid. Tremor, tachycardia (especially during sleep), and undue anxiety are clinical signs that suggest the patient is thyrotoxic. There is a greater risk of the uncontrolled thyrotoxic developing postoperative thyroid storm (Mercer & Eltringham, 1985) and therefore surgery should be postponed until adequate control is achieved. In addition to routine clinical examination, the neck should be examined and the position of the trachea noted. Any deviation of the trachea or possible compression from an enlarged thyroid gland may cause problems with tracheal intubation. Particularly, if the patient has been thyrotoxic, preoperative management should be directed towards producing a well-sedated, calm patient. The anaesthetic procedure should be explained and the patient reassured strongly.

A strongly sedative premedication is to be preferred to reduce anxiety and tachycardia. Benzodiazepines have been recommended (Mercer & Eltringham, 1985) but the preference of this author is to use an appropriate dose of papaveretum and hyoscine. Atropine should be avoided because of the risk of producing unwanted tachycardia. Beta blockers should be continued and the current maintenance dose of beta blocker should be given with the premedication. If the patient is taking digitalis, this should be given also with the premedication.

It is important to establish before surgery that vocal-cord movement is intact and the laryngeal nerves have not been damaged. It is therefore appropriate to carry out indirect mirror laryngoscopy in all patients before surgery to check that both vocal cords move correctly and especially to check if abduction occurs during deep inspiration.

Preoperatively, in addition to a chest X-ray, an X-ray of the thoracic inlet is appropriate to exclude retrosternal thyroid extension. A well-centred view of the neck is also appropriate so that the outline of the trachea can be seen and any deviation on compression should alert the anaesthetist to a possibly difficult intubation. CT scanning of the neck may also be indicated.

In addition to preoperative thyroid function tests, a full blood count and serum urea and electrolyte concentrations should be obtained. Blood should be grouped and cross-matched. A preoperative ECG should be obtained.

Anaesthetic technique

Before induction of anaesthesia, a large intravenous cannula should be inserted into an appropriate vein. An extension and three-way tap added to the giving set is useful as access to the arm is limited. Baseline measurement of arterial pressure should be made and the ECG monitored continuously. If a difficult tracheal intubation is not expected, the patient's lungs should be preoxygenated and anaesthesia induced with an appropriate intravenous induction agent, e.g. thiopentone. The anaesthetist should check that the lungs can be inflated manually before administering a neuromuscular blocking agent to facilitate tracheal intubation. An opioid and/or benzodiazepine may be given at the time of induction.

As neck manipulation or extension may occur during the procedure, a disposable flexometallic tracheal tube is preferable. The tracheal tube should be taped firmly in place and the eyes lubricated and taped closed. Eye care is especially important in the exophthalmic patient.

If the lungs cannot be ventilated manually, an inhalation agent should be introduced and an attempt made to visualize the larynx during spontaneous ventilation. If this fails, the patient should be allowed to wake up and intubation performed using a flexible fibre-optic laryngoscope or bronchoscope. Similarly, if tracheal intubation is obviously going to be difficult, a fibre-optic intubation should be considered *ab initio* (Wei *et al.*, 1988).

The patient should be positioned on the table with the head resting on a head-ring and a small sand bag placed between the scapulae. The neck should be extended fully and a small amount of head-up tilt of the table should reduce venous oozing, although at a risk of allowing air embolism to occur.

As the anaesthetist has limited access to the patient, in addition to ECG and arterial pressure measurements, a pulse oximeter and oesophageal stethoscope are useful. Indirect arterial pressure measurements are usually sufficient, although an indwelling arterial cannula should be considered when the patient is in heart failure or there are signs of cardiovascular instability. Minimal monitoring standards are obligatory (Chapter 35).

Maintenance of anaesthesia

Although spontaneous ventilation (Atkinson *et al.*, 1977) was originally proposed as a suitable method for anaesthetizing patients with thyroidectomy, it appears that there are no disadvantages to intermittent positive-pressure ventilation (IPPV) (Mercer & Eltringham, 1985). This author considers that this method is most appropriate for maintenance of anaesthesia.

In all events, coughing and straining during surgery should be avoided. This author favours the use of IPPV with a muscle relaxant of intermediate duration of action because it enables carbon dioxide concentrations to be controlled and the intrathoracic pressure is higher, thus making air embolus less likely. It allows also rapid return of consciousness at the end of surgery. Of the volatile agents, isoflurane is probably the most appropriate agent to use, as it produces a smaller increase in T_4 concentrations than halothane. If the surgeon intends to infiltrate the field with adrenaline, again isoflurane is the most appropriate agent, because isoflurane does not increase adrenaline-induced arrhythmias (Eger, 1981).

It is important at the end of surgery, when spontaneous respiration is adequate, to remove the tracheal tube under direct vision. The vocal cords should be visualized and the surgeon reassured if both cords are moving equally, because the recurrent laryngeal nerves are then intact. In the unlikely event of both nerves being damaged, the vocal cords are fixed in adduction, and the tracheal tube should be left *in situ* during the early postoperative period.

Regional anaesthesia

It is possible to produce satisfactory analgesia for thyroid or parathyroid surgery by using bilateral deep and superficial cervical plexus blocks or bilateral superficial blocks alone using bupivacaine with adrenaline (Saxe *et al.*, 1988). The indications for regional anaesthesia are patient preference and/or associated cardiopulmonary disease. In some cases regional anaesthesia is not successful.

Postoperative management

The patient should be nursed in the head-up position. Stitch cutters or clip removers should be immediately available in the event of sudden haemorrhage. The patient should be made comfortable, adequate analgesia and antiemetic therapy given as required, and oxygen should be administered via a face-mask. Continuation of beta blockers into the postoperative period is dependent on the degree of cardiovascular stability present.

Complications

Haemorrhage. This may occur suddenly in the early postoperative period and may be life-threatening. Immediate removal of sutures or clips is required. If there is evidence of tracheal obstruction, tracheal intubation should be performed immediately.

Laryngeal oedema. This is an uncommon occurrence, but may appear on the second or third postoperative day (Atkinson *et al.*, 1977). If there is marked stridor, a temporary (5 days) tracheostomy may be used.

Tracheal collapse. This is extremely rare except when tracheal cartilage has been removed during resection of an extensive thyroid malignancy. Immediate tracheal intubation is required and reconstructive surgery may be necessary.

Nerve injury. Recurrent laryngeal nerve injury is serious only when permanent injury to both cords results in bilateral vocal cord adduction. Either a permanent tracheostomy or reconstructive surgery to widen the glottis is required. If the recurrent laryngeal nerve on one side only is damaged, the other vocal cord compensates usually and no further intervention is necessary.

If the superior laryngeal nerve is damaged, cricothyroid paralysis may produce a change in voice. Sensory damage to the nerve may result in difficulty in swallowing. Further treatment is not usually required after superior laryngeal nerve damage.

Thyrotoxic crisis. With adequate preparation, this has become an uncommon postoperative complication. It occurs particularly in the uncontrolled thyrotoxic and is manifest by tachycardia, hypertension, hyperthermia, delirium and CNS irritability. Treatment is with propranolol, rehydration and antithyroid drugs.

Hypocalcaemic tetany. This occurs after radical thyroidectomy when the parathyroid glands have been removed also and may occur in the early postoperative weeks. Acute treatment is with intravenous calcium solutions, but for long-term therapy oral calcium and vitamin D are given.

Anaesthetic consideration in hypothyroidism

In the treated myxoedematous patient, who has been rendered euthyroid by thyroxine treatment, elective or emergency anaesthesia should not present a problem.

In the untreated, overtly myxoedematous patient, elective surgery should be postponed until the patient is euthyroid. If possible, emergency surgery should be delayed to allow for at least 48 h of thyroid replacement (Murkin, 1982). There is an increased incidence of adrenocortical insufficiency in association with hypothyroidism, so steroid supplementation is recommended in the untreated hypothyroid patient requiring surgery.

Chronic hypothyroidism is associated with a reduction in the circulating blood volume (up to 1 litre) and therefore any anaesthetic induction agent should be used with caution, in small doses. In addition to arterial pressure monitoring, either central venous pressure or pulmonary capillary wedge pressure should be monitored as an indication of fluid balance.

The most appropriate anaesthetic technique in uncontrolled hypothyroidism is to use nitrous oxide/opioid/oxygen with minimum volatile or intravenous anaesthetic with IPPV. Either vecuronium or atracurium are appropriate agents to use to produce neuromuscular block.

Anaesthetic supplements should be used with caution as the volatile agents are likely to produce profound hypotension even in low doses and opioids are likely to be associated with prolonged respiratory depression and delayed recovery from anaesthesia (Kim & Hackman, 1977).

Whatever anaesthetic technique is used, the possibility of delayed recovery should be considered and arrangements made for possible postoperative admission to an intensive therapy unit and for postoperative ventilatory support.

During anaesthesia and in the postoperative period, hypothermia may be exacerbated. Therefore, core temperature should be monitored continuously and the operating theatre environment and the patient should be kept warm. All intravenous fluids should be warmed and respiratory gases should be warmed and humidified.

Myxoedema is associated with reduced free-water excretion and hyponatraemia may occur (Shalev et al., 1979). Therefore saline-containing intravenous fluids should be used and the plasma sodium concentration should be monitored carefully.

Anaesthesia and hyperparathyroidism

With adequate preoperative preparation, patients with hyperparathyroidism do not present a problem. The anaesthetic technique for parathyroidectomy is similar to that for thyroidectomy. Patients with severe hypercalcaemia may vomit severely with consequent dehydration and chloride depletion (Fletcher, 1977). Correction of the dehydration and restoration of normal electrolyte balance are necessary before surgery.

References

Atkinson R.S., Rushman G.B. & Lee J.A. (1977) *A Synopsis of Anaesthesia* 8th edn. p. 563. Wright, Bristol.

Bennett M.H. & Wainwright A.P. (1989) Acute thyroid crisis on induction of anaesthesia. *Anaesthesia* **44**, 28–30.

Carmago C.A. & Kolb F.O. (1986) *Current Medical Diagnosis and Treatment* (Eds Krupp M.A., Chatton M.J. & Tierney L.M.) pp. 693–763. Lange, California.

Christensen P.A. & Nissen L.R. (1987) Treatment of thyroid storm in a child with dantrolene. *British Journal of Anaesthesia* **59**, 523.

Eger E.I. (1981) Isoflurane — a review. *Anesthesiology* **55**, 559–76.

Fletcher P.F. (1977) *Thyroid and Parathyroid Disease in Medicine for Anaesthetists* 1st edn. (Ed. Vickers M.D.) p. 513. Blackwell Scientific Publications, Oxford.

Ganong W.F. (1985) *Review of Medical Physiology* 12th edn. Lange, California.

Greer M.A. (1987) Disorders of the thyroid. In *Internal Medicine* 2nd edn. (Eds Stein J.H. & Kohler P.O.) pp. 1918–40. Little Brown, Boston.

Imberti R., Maira G., Confortini M.C., Preseglio I., Domenegati E. (1988) Effect of fentanyl-oxygen anesthesia during cardiac surgery on serum thyroid hormones. *Acta Anaesthesiologica Belgica* **39**, 217–22.

Kim J.M. & Hackman L. (1977) Anesthesia for untreated hypothyroidism: report of 3 cases. *Anesthesia and Analgesia* **56**, 299–302.

Lando M.J., Hoover L.A., Zuckerbraun L. & Goodman D. (1988) Autotransplantation of parathyroid tissue into sternocleidomastoid muscle. *Archives of Otolaryngology, Head and Neck Surgery* **114**, 557–60.

Mercer D.M. & Eltringham R.J. (1985) Anaesthesia for thyroid surgery. *Ear Nose and Throat Journal* **64**, 375–8.

Mogensen T. & Hjortso N.-C. (1988) Acute hypothyroidism in a severely ill surgical patient. *Canadian Journal of Anaesthesia* **35**, 74–5.

Murkin J.M. (1982) Anesthesia and hypothyroidism: a review of thyroxine, physiology, pharmacology and anesthetic implications. *Anesthesia and Analgesia* **61**, 371–83.

Noreng M.F., Jensen P. & Tjellden N.U. (1987) Peri- and postoperative changes in the concentration of serum thyrotropin under general anaesthesia, compared to general anaesthesia with epidural analgesia. *Acta Anaesthesiologica Scandinavica* **31**, 292–4.

Oyama T., Shibata S., Matsuki A. & Kudo T. (1969) Serum endogenous thyroxine levels in man during anaesthesia and surgery. *British Journal of Anaesthesia* **41**, 103–8.

Oyama T., Latto P., Holaday D.A. & Chang H. (1975a) Effect of isoflurane anaesthesia and surgery on thyroid function in man. *Canadian Anaesthetist's Society Journal* **22**, 474–7.

Oyama T., Maeda A., Jin J., Satone T. & Kudo M. (1975b) Effect of althesin (CT-1341) on thyroid–adrenal function in man. *British Journal of Anaesthesia* **47**, 837–40.

Peters K.R., Nance P. & Wingard D.W. (1981) Malignant hyperthyroidism or malignant hyperthermia? *Anesthesia and Analgesia* **60**, 613–15.

Rains A.J.H. & Ritchie H.D. (1984) *Bailey and Love's Short Practice of Surgery* 19th edn. p. 611. H.K. Lewis, London.

Saxe A.W., Brown E. & Hamburger S.W. (1988) Thyroid and parathyroid surgery performed with patient under regional anesthesia. *Surgery* **103**, 415–20.

Schou H. & Knudsen F. (1988) Continuous arteriovenous hemofiltration — a new treatment in hypercalcemic crisis. *Blood Purification* **6**, 227–9.

Shalev O., Naparstek Y., Brezis M. & Ben-Yishai D. (1979) Hyponatraemia in myxedema: a suggested therapeutic approach. *Israel Journal of Medical Sciences* **15**, 913–16.

Trench A.J., Buckley F.P., Drummond G.B., Arther G.R. & Scott D.B. (1978) Propranolol in thyrotoxicosis — cardiovascular changes during thyroidectomy in patients pre-treated with propranolol. *Anaesthesia* **33**, 535–9.

Wei W.I., Siu K.F., Lau W.F. & Lam K.H. (1988) Emergency endotracheal intubation under fiberoptic endoscopic guidance for malignant laryngeal obstruction. *Otolaryngology, Head and Neck Surgery* **98**, 10–13.

Inherited Metabolic Diseases and Anaesthesia

K.H. SIMPSON AND F.R. ELLIS

Metabolic problems may be inherited or acquired, and are often the result of defective enzyme structure or function. Enzymes are protein catalysts which control and mediate biochemical reactions. The 'one gene, one enzyme' hypothesis implies that each metabolic step is controlled by one enzyme which is the product of a particular gene. Inborn errors of metabolism are defects caused by interruption of the metabolic process because of an absent or defective enzyme. Some genetic abnormalities result in a defective polypeptide rather than a defective enzyme, and this could be thought of as a 'one gene, one polypeptide' hypothesis.

Inborn errors of carbohydrate metabolism

Glucose problems

Glucose-6-phosphate dehydrogenase deficiency

There are many variants of glucose-6-phosphate dehydrogenase (G6PD) which have lower activity than the normal enzyme. Patients with low enzyme activity cannot increase the rate of oxidation of glucose in the presence of oxidative agents, for example some drugs. Low G6PD activity in red blood cells leads to oxidation of haemoglobin to methaemoglobin and oxidation of red cell membranes, causing haemolysis.

Inheritance. Sex linked, fully expressed in males and homozygous females. There is variable expression in heterozygous females, who are genetic mosaics.

Incidence. Very common, varies with ethnic origin, affecting 35% Sardinians and Sephardic Jews, 13% of Negroes and 1–3% of Caucasians.

Manifestations. Patients with G6PD deficiency may experience haemolysis when exposed to oxidative agents or during infections. Anaemia, jaundice, splenomegaly and abdominal or loin pain may occur. The degree of haemolysis depends upon the type of enzyme problem. Severe haemolysis may cause renal failure.

Anaesthetic problems (Smith & Snowdon, 1987). Adequate fluid intake should be ensured and oxidative drugs should be avoided to prevent haemolysis (Table 54.1). If haemolysis occurs, good urine output should be maintained. Red cell transfusion may be necessary to treat severe anaemia. G6PD deficiency should always be considered in patients with postoperative jaundice.

Galactosaemia

Inability to metabolize galactose causes products of incomplete metabolism to accumulate in blood, tissues and urine.

Galactose-1-phosphate uridyl transferase deficiency

Inheritance. Autosomal recessive.

Table 54.1 Some agents to avoid in patients with glucose-6-phosphate dehydrogenase deficiency

Fava (broad) beans	Sulphonamides
Paracetamol	Antimalarial drugs
Chloramphenicol	Prilocaine
Nitrofurantoin	Vitamin K
Penicillin	Quinidine
Probenecid	Methylene blue
Streptomycin	Isosorbide dinitrate
Nalidixic acid	Sodium nitroprusside
Isoniazid	

Incidence. One in 40 000 births.

Manifestations. Symptoms usually begin shortly after birth, and include vomiting, diarrhoea, failure to thrive, hepatosplenomegaly, cirrhosis, ascites, jaundice, proteinuria, aminoaciduria, cataracts and mental retardation. The disease is fatal if untreated.

Galactokinase deficiency

Inheritance. Autosomal, probably recessive.

Incidence. One in 500 000 births.

Manifestations. Galactose accumulates, resulting in cataracts.

Anaesthetic problems (Jackson, 1973). The treatment of galactosaemia involves dietary restriction. A patient whose diet is properly managed should present no problems. In recently diagnosed infants, perioperative hypoglycaemia, metabolic acidosis, electrolyte problems and hepatic and renal impairment require careful management.

Pentosuria

Xylitol dehydrogenase deficiency

Inheritance. Autosomal recessive.

Incidence. One in 2000—5000 of the Jewish population.

Manifestations. Patients have asymptomatic excretion of xylose in urine.

Anaesthetic problems. None, but may be misdiagnosed diabetic.

Fructose problems

Essential fructosuria
Fructokinase deficiency.

Inheritance. Autosomal recessive.

Incidence. One in 130 000 births.

Manifestations. Asymptomatic.

Anaesthetic problems. None, but may be misdiagnosed diabetic.

Hereditary fructose intolerance

Abnormal fructose-1-phosphate aldolase.

Inheritance. Autosomal recessive.

Incidence. Unknown.

Manifestations. Patients are asymptomatic unless fructose or sorbitol is ingested, when sweating, dizziness and emesis result. Dehydration and coma may occur. After fructose ingestion hypoglycaemia develops rapidly in children. Persistent fructose administration may cause failure to thrive and the stigmata of liver impairment. Adults show anxiety and dyspepsia.

Anaesthetic problems (Jackson, 1973). A patient who is well controlled by diet should not present any difficulty. Blood glucose must be monitored perioperatively and intravenous glucose should be given. Preparations containing fructose or sorbitol must be avoided. In newly diagnosed infants, hypoglycaemia, vomiting and dehydration may occur. Renal and hepatic impairment may be present, but are usually reversible.

Fructose-1,6-diphosphatase deficiency

Inheritance. Uncertain.

Incidence. Very rare.

Manifestations. Glucose availability is impaired during starvation or stress because the liver cannot produce glucose from fructose, lactate, glycerol or alanine. Infants present in the first 6 months of life with vomiting, failure to thrive, hypotonia, jaundice, hepatosplenomegaly, ascites and bleeding. Metabolic problems include hypoglycaemia, hypophosphataemia, lactic acidosis, abnormal liver function and loss of amino acids, sugars, uric acid and protein in the urine. Mental development remains normal despite fructose intake.

Anaesthetic problems (Jackson, 1973; Hashimoto *et al.*, 1978). Dietary restriction of fructose, sucrose, sorbitol and glycerol may be used in management. A fructose-free diet should be taken for 24—48 h before surgery and glucose should be infused perioperatively. Lactated Ringer's (Hartmann's) solution should be avoided. There is a tendency to hypoglycaemia and lactic acidosis, therefore intraoperative monitoring of

Table 54.2 Classification of glycogen storage diseases

Type	Enzyme defect	Eponym	Main effects
O	UPDG-glycogen transferase		Liver
Ia	Glucose-6-phosphatase	Von Gierke	Liver
IIa,b	Lysosomal alpha-2,4-glucosidase	Pompe	Muscle
IIIa,b,c,d	Amylo-1,6-glucosidase and/or oligo-1,4 to 1,4-glucantransferase	Cori, Forbe	Liver
IV	Amylo-1,4 to 1,6-transglucosylase	Anderson	Liver
V	Muscle phosphorylase	McArdle	Muscle
VI	Liver phosphorylase	Hers	Liver
VII	Phosphofructokinase	Thompson	Muscle
VIII	Phosphohexosisomerase	Tarin	Muscle
IX	Liver phosphorylase kinase		Liver
X	Muscle phosphorylase kinase		Muscle
XI	Phosphoglucomutase		Liver
XII	Cyclic 3',5'-AMP-dependent kinase		Liver

blood glucose, arterial blood gases and acid—base status is required.

Pyruvate problems

Pyruvate dehydrogenase deficiency

A defect in the enzymes of the pyruvate dehydrogenase complex results in accumulation of lactate and pyruvate in blood and tissues.

Inheritance. Unknown.

Incidence. Rare.

Manifestations. Three enzyme defects have been identified — E1, E2 and E3.
E1 Progressive neurological problems occur which are not affected by dietary restrictions.
E2 Neurological problems and lactic acidosis occur. The lactic acidosis may be precipitated by a high carbohydrate intake.
E3 Lactic acidosis, lethargy, optic atrophy, laryngeal stridor and ventilatory problems occur.

Anaesthetic problems (Dierdorf & McNiece, 1983). A high carbohydrate intake must be avoided before surgery. Lactate-containing fluids must not be given perioperatively. Care should be taken to reduce factors which cause acidosis such as sepsis, hypercapnia and hypothermia. Postoperatively, patients should be carefully monitored for ventilatory problems.

Glycogen storage diseases

Liver glycogen is used to maintain blood glucose, and muscle glycogen stores are used to respond to the demands of exercise. Enzyme defects in the metabolic pathways of glycogen result in liver and muscle disease, and Cori's original classification of four diseases has now been extended to thirteen (Table 54.2). The inheritance is autosomal recessive, except for Type IX, which is sex-linked. Diagnosis is made by liver or muscle biopsy and enzyme studies. Hepatic disease is treated by continuous intragastric feeding, total parenteral nutrition and, sometimes, by portocaval shunting (Casson, 1975). Liver transplantation may be used in some cases. There is no specific therapy for muscle disease, but exercise should be avoided. Patients with glycogen storage diseases may present serious problems to the anaesthetist (Cox, 1968; Jackson, 1973; Brown *et al.*, 1975).

Liver glycogenoses

Type O

This form of glycogen storage disease results in an inadequate rate of glycogen synthesis and hypoglycaemia. The other forms of liver glycogenoses are often indistinguishable clinically, showing mild to severe hypoglycaemia and hepatomegaly.

Type I (Von Gierke's disease)

This is the commonest of the glycogenoses and involves impairment of the ability to mobilize liver glycogen in response to demand. Energy requirements have to be met by fat metabolism, and ketosis may result. Hypoglycaemia and lactic acidosis occur during the first year of life and may lead to convulsions. Children present with pallor, accumulation of subcutaneous fat, short stature, xanthomata, distended abdomen and enlarged liver and kidneys. Increased susceptibility to infection and bleeding disorders due to platelet dysfunction are common. The condition may not be symptomatic until after puberty, when patients may suffer from gout.

Anaesthetic problems (Bevan, 1980; Ellis, 1980). Stress may provoke hypoglycaemia, lactic acidosis, keto-acidosis and circulatory collapse. Careful monitoring is required. Abdominal distension may cause ventilatory problems. Hyperventilation should be avoided as respiratory alkalosis causes release of lactate, which the patient cannot metabolize. Continuous preoperative intragastric and intravenous feeding should be used to maintain blood glucose and reduce the risk of acidosis. Lactated intravenous fluids should be avoided. Correction of biochemical abnormalities reduces the bleeding diathesis.

Type III

This is difficult to distinguish clinically from Type I, although the illness is milder, with less hypoglycaemia, and a better prognosis. Cardiac problems do not usually occur, although a progressive cardiomyopathy has been described. Treatment includes frequent feeding with a high-protein low-fat diet and avoidance of strenuous exercise.

Anaesthetic problems. The problems are the same as with Type I, but of a milder degree. Preoperative fasting should be minimized and any infection treated prior to surgery. Blood glucose and acid–base status should be monitored. Cardiodepressant drugs must be used with care.

Type IV

Rare and usually fatal by the second year of life.

Anaesthetic problems. Severe liver disease and wasting alter drug distribution and metabolism.

Type VI (Hers' disease)

This disease often results in death before puberty due to liver cirrhosis and portal hypertension. Patients have splenomegaly, which is not a feature of any of the other glycogenoses.

Anaesthetic problems. Liver impairment and hypoglycaemia.

Muscle glycogenoses

Problems occur during exercise when there is inadequate mobilization of muscle glycogen. Vigorous exercise is associated with cramp, weakness and, occasionally, myoglobinuria. The condition presents in childhood in all cases except Type VIII.

Type V (McArdle's disease)

This disease is manifest by inability to perform strenuous exercise and sensitivity to ischaemia, which causes cramps, weakness and muscle damage. Glucose infusion relieves symptoms rapidly. Muscle contractures may develop. Muscle wasting may occur in older patients. There is no associated cardiac problem. Myoglobinuria can occur and has occasionally caused renal failure.

Anaesthetic problems (Ellis, 1980; Coleman, 1984). Suxamethonium should be avoided as it may cause myoglobinuria and renal damage. Regional anaesthesia may be preferable in some cases (Samuels & Coleman, 1988). Heat loss should be minimized as it leads to postoperative shivering and muscle damage. Temperature monitoring is essential. Pyrexia should be prevented as a hypermetabolic state is undesirable. The use of a tourniquet is contraindicated as it may cause ischaemic damage and muscle atrophy. Automatic blood-pressure-recording devices should be used with caution. Glucose, fructose or lactose should be infused as a perioperative energy source. It has been suggested that infusion of 50% glucose, at the end of surgery, may improve muscle function and decrease the major risk of respiratory failure. Substrate infusion should continue for 24 h after surgery.

Type IIa (Pompe's disease)

This is a severe glycogen storage disease, which is seen in infants who seem normal for the first few months of life. Children commonly present with feeding difficulties. Blood glucose is normal. There is generalized deposition of glycogen with muscle flaccidity, areflexia, enlarged tongue, neurological problems and increased susceptibility to chest infections. Myocardial involvement is an important feature of the disease. Death occurs during the first year of life, usually due to respiratory failure. Sudden death may occur due to obstructive cardiomyopathy.

Type IIb

This disease is due to a defect in the same enzyme as Type IIa, but does not result in cardiac involvement. Children show severe muscular dystrophy or myopathy but survive longer than those with Type IIa.

Anaesthetic problems (McFarlane & Soni, 1986; Rosen & Broadman, 1986). The same considerations apply as with Type V. Oxygenation may be difficult due to macroglossia and compression of the lungs by the large heart. High inspired-oxygen concentrations should be used from the outset. Heart failure may be precipitated by drugs which depress cardiac function or increase afterload in patients with Type IIa disease who may have congestive or obstructive cardiac failure. Careful monitoring of cardiovascular status is vital. Temperature monitoring is mandatory. Suxamethonium is contraindicated, because of the risk of muscle damage. If a muscle relaxant is needed, vecuronium is probably suitable. Muscle weakness may necessitate postoperative ventilatory support. Regional anaesthesia has been suggested for surgery on the lower limbs, however caudal or extradural anaesthesia has not been described in these patients. Lumbar plexus or brachial plexus block may be more appropriate.

Lipid storage diseases

Glycosphingolipidosis (Fabry's disease)

Deficiency of the lysosomal enzyme α-galactosidase-A, leads to progressive deposition of neutral glycosphingolipids in viscera and tissue fluids.

Inheritance. X-linked, fully manifest in the male. Some heterozygous females have attenuated disease.

Incidence. One in 40 000 births.

Manifestations. Males have telangectasia, decreased sweating, sparse hair, corneal opacities, tortuous retinal and conjunctival vessels, severe pain, paraesthesia, angina, cardiomegaly, heart failure and renal problems with hypertension. Some females have corneal clouding and, very rarely, the full syndrome.

Anaesthetic problems. Pain is often the most debilitating feature of the disease and crises produce burning in the palms and soles. Pain sometimes responds to carbamazepine or phenytoin. Chronic paraesthesia of the hands and feet may occur, therefore local blocks should perhaps be avoided. The other features

of the disease are treated symptomatically. Some patients respond to steroids. Attacks of abdominal and flank pain may simulate appendicitis or renal colic, therefore the anaesthetist may be faced with a patient needing emergency surgery. Cardiovascular and renal problems require management. Dialysis or renal transplantation may be necessary.

Glucosyl ceramide lipidosis (Gaucher's disease)

Deficiency of β-glucosidase causes accumulation of glucocerebrocides in the reticular endothelial cells. Patients also have elevated plasma acid phosphatase. Three syndromes have been described.

Chronic non-neuropathic form

Inheritance. Autosomal recessive.

Incidence. Commonest.

Manifestations. Patients may present at any age with hepatomegaly, hypersplenism, portal hypertension, bone lesions, limb pain, skin pigmentation and bleeding secondary to thrombocytopenia. Chest infection is the commonest cause of death.

Acute infantile neuropathic form

Inheritance. Autosomal recessive.

Incidence. Rare.

Manifestations. The disease is seen in infancy. Patients have severe neurological abnormalities such as cranial nerve and extrapyramidal lesions with strabismus, head retroflexion and spastic extremities. Thrombocytopenia, splenomegaly and chronic cough are common. Respiratory complications usually cause death within 3 years.

Subacute juvenile neuropathic form

Inheritance. Autosomal.

Incidence. Rare.

Manifestations. The signs of illness begin at any time during childhood and combine the features of the chronic form of the disease with slowly progressive neurological deterioration.

Anaesthetic problems. The course of the disease is protracted, with multiorgan involvement. Splenectomy may be indicated to reduce anaemia. Bleeding problems often contraindicate regional anaesthesia. There is no specific treatment for the illness. Enzyme replacement therapy and bone marrow transplantation have been used. There is a high risk of postoperative chest infection.

Sphingomyelin lipidosis (Niemann–Pick disease)

There are several disorders characterized by extensive tissue deposition of sphingomyelin. There are two main groups.

Sphingomyelinase-deficient disorders

Tissue sphingomyelin concentrations of 10–100 times normal.

Acute neuropathic form (Type A)

Inheritance. Autosomal recessive.

Incidence. Unknown.

Manifestations. The illness presents before 6 months of age with abdominal enlargement, diffuse pulmonary infiltration, physical and mental retardation. The disease progresses to a vegetative state, with death occurring before the fourth year.

Non-neuropathic form (Type B)

Inheritance. Autosomal recessive.

Incidence. Uncertain.

Manifestations. Patients display purely visceral involvement. The nervous system is spared. Although chronic chest infections and hypersplenism occur, lifespan can be normal.

Indeterminate forms of sphingomyelin storage (Types C or D)

These are a heterogeneous group of patients with similar clinical signs, but normal or only slightly deficient sphingomyelinase activity, with an increase of only one- to two-fold in tissue sphingomyelin. Children appear normal for a few years and then develop hepatosplenomegaly and later neurological problems including seizures, behavioural problems and mental retardation. There is no specific treatment.

Anaesthetic problems. Drugs such as diethyl ether and cyclopropane increase fat metabolism and, in theory, should be avoided. However, stress-stimulated catecholamine production has such a profound effect on fat metabolism that anaesthetic drug effects are overshadowed. Perioperative intravenous glucose is recommended to prevent fat mobilization due to hypoglycaemia. Hypercapnia, hypoxia and hypothermia should be avoided as they increase fat metabolism. Regional techniques may reduce fat mobilization, but their use in the presence of neurological problems requires careful consideration.

Inborn errors of amino acid and purine metabolism

Maple syrup urine disease

A block in oxidative decarboxylation of branched-chain amino acids to fatty acids results in the accumulation of leucine, isoleucine, alloisoleucine, valine and their α-keto acids in blood and urine.

Inheritance. Autosomal recessive.

Incidence. One in 100 000–300 000.

Manifestations. Patients are normal at birth, but apnoeic attacks, hypotonia, failure to feed and hypoglycaemia occur during the first weeks of life. Mental retardation, seizures and death supervene. A milder form of the disease can present later, after the introduction of protein into the diet or following an infection.

Anaesthetic problems (Delaney & Gal, 1976). Dietary restriction of leucine, isoleucine and valine is needed before neurological damage occurs. Catabolism of endogenous proteins due to preoperative fasting, anaesthesia, surgery, blood in the gut, postoperative starvation, emesis and infection, all act to elevate amino acid concentrations. Breakdown of endogenous proteins can be reduced by limiting starvation and providing intravenous glucose. Hypoglycaemia and acidosis can occur, probably due to high plasma leucine concentrations. Perioperative monitoring of blood glucose and acid–base status is essential. The anaesthetic technique chosen is less important than careful observation and provision of carbohydrate substrate. Postoperative nutrition must be maintained, parenterally if necessary, to reduce catabolism. Infections should be treated early, and may prove fatal.

Hyperphenylalaninaemias

As hydroxylation of L-phenylalanine to tyrosine is a complex reaction involving several genes, there are several hyperphenylalaninaemia variants.

Classic phenylketonuria

Classic phenylketonuria (PKU) is due to almost complete absence of phenylalanine hydroxylase, which causes excess phenylalanine to accumulate in blood, cerebrospinal fluid and urine. Metabolism via minor pathways results in renal excretion of phenylpyruvic acid. Disturbances of tyrosine and tryptophan metabolism diminish the formation of catecholamines, serotonin and melanin.

Inheritance. Autosomal recessive.

Incidence. One in 10 000—20 000 births are homozygotes.

Manifestations. Mental retardation occurs by mid-infancy. Children have microcephaly, hypertonicity, seizures, psychotic behaviour, dysphagia, emesis, eczema, a mousy odour, pale skin and growth retardation. PKU is usually detected by neonatal screening. Children with plasma phenylalanine concentrations exceeding 0.85 mmol/litre require treatment. Dietary restriction is used to maintain low blood phenylalanine levels until the age of 8—10 years.

Hyperphenylalaninaemic variants

These are independent autosomal recessive variants, which must be recognized to avoid inappropriate genetic counselling and therapy.

Anaesthetic problems (Jackson, 1973). Severely affected individuals may be mentally retarded and may be sensitive to CNS depressant drugs. Patients are prone to seizures, especially during recovery from anaesthesia, and should not have hyperventilation or be given epileptogenic agents. The patient's temperature should be monitored as pyrexia may precipitate convulsions. Patients often have deficient catecholamine production and denervation hypersensitivity. An increased response to exogenous catecholamines may occur, therefore these should be avoided. Abnormal catecholamine metabolism may result in hypoglycaemia, which increases protein catabolism and elevates phenylalanine concentrations. Fasting should be minimized and blood glucose should be measured and corrected regularly. If patients require parenteral nutrition, solutions low in phenylalanine must be used.

Alcaptonuria

Absent homogentisic acid oxidase causes accumulation of homogentisic acid from metabolism of phenylalanine and tyrosine.

Inheritance. Autosomal recessive.

Incidence. One in 200 000 births.

Manifestations. The condition is benign until middle life when pigmentation of connective tissues and degenerative arthritis of the hips, knees, shoulders and spine occurs. Cardiovascular disease is common, including heart-valve problems and peripheral vascular disease. Dietary restriction to achieve a low enough intake of phenylalanine, and tyrosine to prevent illness is impossible. There is no specific therapy, but large doses of ascorbic acid have been used to reduce pigment formation.

Anaesthetic problems. Cardiovascular manifestations of the disease may require attention. Cervical spine problems may lead to difficulty with intubation. Care must be taken when positioning patients with joint disease, who often need orthopaedic surgery.

Cystinuria

A specific enzyme defect has not been identified in this inherited disorder of amino acid transport across the cells of the gut and kidney.

Incidence. Common, 1 : 2000—15 000 births.

Inheritance. Autosomal recessive.

Manifestations. The illness may present in childhood or even in old age. It is characterized by precipitation of cystine crystals in the urine. Infection, obstruction, renal calculi and renal failure may occur.

Anaesthetic problems (Jackson, 1973). Dietary restrictions, liberal fluid intake and drugs, e.g. D-penicillamine and pyridoxine have been used to reduce excretion and increase the solubility of cystine. Alkalinization of the urine was practised, but may create more problems than it solves, especially in patients with poor renal function. Dehydration and reduction in perioperative urine output may cause kidney-stone formation. A high-volume urine output must be maintained using intravenous fluids. Diuretics may be required if urine output is low.

Homocystinuria

Several genetic disorders lead to homocystinuria. The most common is a deficiency of cystathionine β-synthetase, which converts methionine to cysteine.

Inheritance. Autosomal recessive.

Incidence. One in 200 000–300 000 births. Five times more common in Ireland.

Manifestations. Excess quantities of homocystine and methionine accumulate in the blood and are excreted in urine. Some patients have a tendency to hypoglycaemia, secondary to increased insulin production. Patients have weakened collagen. Ectopia lentis is seen in 90% of affected individuals. Retinal detachment, optic atrophy and cataracts are common. Other manifestations include osteoporosis, scoliosis, pectus excavatum, genu valgum, lax ligaments, lengthened extremities and a high arched palate. Fifty to 80% of patients are mentally retarded. Seizures may occur. Death commonly follows thromboembolism. This may be due to abnormal collagen in blood vessels or activation of clotting factors by homocystine. A low-methionine diet, and high-dose pyridoxine may be helpful in some cases. Folate stores must always be replenished prior to treatment. Mental retardation is more likely to occur if treatment is delayed.

Anaesthetic problems (Crook *et al.*, 1971; Brown *et al.*, 1975). Anaesthesia and surgery carry a bad prognosis. Patients commonly present for ophthalmic surgery. Pyridoxine should be given before surgery. Patients may pose an intubation problem, and chest deformity may lead to ventilatory difficulties. The main problems are hypoglycaemia and thrombosis. Blood glucose should be measured regularly and hypoglycaemia must be corrected promptly. Aspirin and dipyridamole have been used to decrease platelet adhesiveness. These measures contraindicate nerve blocks near major blood vessels and spinal anaesthesia. Cardiac output and peripheral blood flow should be kept as high as possible during anaesthesia. Blood viscosity should be reduced by avoiding dehydration and giving intravenous fluids (dextran 70 has been advocated). Limb movements during surgery, calf massage and antiembolus stockings have been recommended. Early postoperative ambulation is important. Deaths in the postoperative period are common.

Lesch–Nyhan syndrome

This condition is caused by abnormal purine metabolism due to absence of hypoxanthine-guanine phosphoribosyltransferase. It results in excessive purine production and increased concentrations of uric acid in blood and tissues.

Inheritance. Sex-linked recessive, only affects males.

Incidence. 5.2 cases per million male births.

Manifestations. Patients are mentally retarded and often have spastic limbs and seizures. Arthritis is common. Renal stones occur and may lead to obstructive renal failure. Patients often die of renal failure by the age of 20.

Anaesthetic problems (Larson & Wilkins 1985). Careful assessment of preoperative renal function is essential. Anaesthesia should be planned with this in mind. Self-mutilation is common in this condition and damage to the face and mouth may lead to difficulty with the airway. Careful positioning of the patient is necessary because of limb spasticity and joint problems. Aspiration of gastric contents is a particular hazard and adequate precautions should be taken to prevent this. Patients do not have an adrenergic pressor response to stress. There is a reduction in monoamine oxidase activity and exogenous catecholamines should be used in reduced doses and with care.

Connective tissue disorders

The mucopolysaccaridoses

A lysosomal defect causes deficiency of enzymes needed to degrade mucopolysaccharides which accumulate in connective tissue throughout the body. Ten lysosomal enzyme deficiencies have been demonstrated. A classification system of the mucopolysaccaridoses (MPS) has evolved according to clinical features and enzyme abnormalities. However, it is not clear how each clinical feature relates to a specific enzyme defect.

Hurler's syndrome

Hurler's syndrome (MPS IH) is a condition caused by lack of lysosomal α-L-iduronidase, which normally degrades the side chains of chondroitin sulphate and heparatin sulphate. These mucopolysaccarides are deposited in the tissues in which they normally occur.

Inheritance. Autosomal recessive.

Incidence. One in 100 000 births.

Manifestations. Children may appear normal at birth. The disease becomes evident after a few months of life and progresses during childhood. The head is enlarged with coarse features, a broad nose, thick lips, large tongue and relatively small mandible. The teeth are widely separated. Airway obstruction causes a perpetually open mouth and noisy breathing. The laryngeal and tracheobronchial cartilages are abnormal. The skin is ridged and grooved with nodular thickening and the extremities are covered with thick hair. Corneal clouding and progressive mental retardation occur. There are many skeletal abnormalities including large skull with hydrocephalus, short neck, atlantoaxial instability, short stature and joint deformities. Kyphosis may cause restrictive airways disease and chest infection is common. Cardiomegaly, ischaemic heart disease and heart valvular lesions are common. Hepatosplenomegaly occurs. Umbilical and inguinal hernias may require surgery. Death before 10 years of age is common, usually due to cardiorespiratory problems.

Scheie's syndrome

Scheie's syndrome (MPS IS) is a rare variant of Hurler's syndrome and is caused by deficiency of α-L-iduronidase. (It used to be defined as MPS V.)

Inheritance. Autosomal recessive.

Incidence. One in 500 000.

Manifestations. Patients develop joint stiffness, skin pigmentation, retinal degeneration, glaucoma, corneal clouding, valvular heart lesions especially aortic regurgitation, hernias and nerve entrapment. They are of normal height and do not have gargoyle-like faces. They have normal intelligence and survive into adulthood.

Hurler's/Scheie's syndrome

Inheritance. Recessive.

Incidence. One in 115 000 births.

Manifestations. Features are intermediate between Hurler's and Scheie's syndromes, and it is defined as MPS I(HS). Micrognathia is common and patients are often mentally retarded.

Hunter's syndrome

Hunter's syndrome (MPS II) is caused by deficiency of iduronate sulphatase.

Inheritance. X-linked recessive (one-third of cases are mutations).

Incidence. One in 70 000−150 000 births.

Manifestations. The condition is similar to Hurler's syndrome but may be less severe and more slowly progressive. Patients appear normal at birth. Coarsening of features begins at about 2 years of age. Patients develop grotesque features, stiff joints, nodular thickening of the skin, hepatosplenomegaly and deafness. Patients are often of normal intelligence. Corneal clouding does not occur. Cardiac enlargement, pulmonary hypertension and heart failure are common. Lymphoid tissue in the larynx often causes partial upper airway obstruction. Chest deformity occurs within pectus excavation and sometimes kyphoscoliosis. Death usually occurs before the age of 15.

Sanfilippo's syndrome

There are two variants of Sanfilippo's syndrome (MPS III), which are clinically indistinguishable:
1 heparine-N-sulphatase deficiency;
2 N-acetyl-α-glucosaminidase deficiency.

Inheritance. Autosomal recessive.

Incidence. Less than 1 : 100 000.

Manifestations. This is the mildest MPS. Patients appear normal at birth. Mental retardation and minor somatic changes develop during childhood. These include hypertrichosis, stiff joints and minimal coarsening of facial features, but no corneal clouding. There are no cardiac or skeletal problems or hepatosplenomegaly. Dementia may occur in late childhood and death usually occurs before 20 years of age.

Morquio's syndrome

Morquio's syndrome (MPS IV) is caused by hexosamine-6-sulphatase deficiency.

Inheritance. Autosomal recessive.

Incidence. Rare.

Manifestations. Patients have a short nose, prominent maxilla, widely spaced teeth with defective enamel. Corneal opacities and hearing problems are common. Dwarfism, osteoporosis, lax joints and kyphoscoliosis occur. Distortion of the chest leads to severe respiratory problems. Patients have normal intelligence. Absence of the odontoid process and atlantoaxial instability may result in spinal cord compression. Cardiac problems are common, especially aortic incompetence. Patients do not often survive beyond 30 years of age.

Maroteaux–Lamy syndrome

Three forms of Maroteaux–Lamy syndrome (MPS VI) syndrome are all characterized by a deficiency of aryl sulphatase B.

Inheritance. Autosomal recessive.

Incidence. Rare.

Manifestations. Patients appear normal at birth and later develop a coarse facial appearance. They have normal intelligence. Corneal clouding and severe skeletal deformities, including growth retardation and kyphoscoliosis occur. Chest infections and chronic respiratory problems are common. Hepatosplenomegaly, anaemia and thrombocytopenia may occur. Hypoplasia of the odontoid peg can lead to atlantoaxial instability. Death usually occurs by the age of 30 due to respiratory failure.

Anaesthetic problems (King *et al.*, 1984; Herrick & Rhine, 1988). Many of the problems associated with

MPS require surgery, e.g. hernias, eye problems, bony deformities and nerve entrapment. The perioperative death rate is approximately 20%. Airway maintenance and intubation may be difficult in Hurler's, Hunter's, Morquio's and Maroteaux–Lamy syndromes. Inelasticity of the tissues and anatomical abnormalities of the head, neck and tracheobronchial tree are present. Therefore appropriate precautions must be taken to deal with airway problems. Instability of the cervical spine may lead to neurological damage in some patients. Great care must be taken during intubation and positioning of patients and a cervical collar or plaster cast may be needed. Abdominal distension and hepatosplenomegaly may cause difficulty with ventilation. Careful preoperative assessment of cardiorespiratory function is essential. Endocarditis is a risk in patients with heart-valve defects and antibiotic cover is mandatory. Cardiac failure must be corrected prior to surgery. Cardiac depressant drugs should be used cautiously. Obstructive airways disease and pulmonary congestion predispose to postoperative chest infection. Techniques which avoid ventilatory depression should be chosen. Maintenance of hydration, humidification of anaesthetic gases and postoperative chest physiotherapy are recommended. Patients should be positioned carefully if they have joint problems.

Marfan's syndrome

This condition is caused by a generalized disorder of connective tissue. Abnormalities of collagen and elastin have been implicated.

Inheritance. Autosomal dominant (15% of cases are mutations).

Incidence. One in 10 000–50 000 births.

Manifestations. Patients have long, thin extremities, arachnodactyly, pectus excavatum, pectus carinatum and a high arched palate. The latter feature is not specific to Marfan's syndrome but may be seen in congenital myopathy, myotonic dystrophy and homocystinuria. Weakness of ligaments, flat feet, recurrent joint dislocation, subluxation of the lens, tremor of the iris, retinal detachment, severe myopia and glaucoma may be present. Kyphoscoliosis, and cystic disease of the lungs may occur. Progressive diffuse dilatation of the proximal aorta with aortic and mitral regurgitation are common. Aortic dilatation may compress the trachea. The commonest causes of death are heart failure, cardiac arrhythmias, pulmonary problems and dissection of the aorta.

Anaesthetic problems (Verghese, 1984; Wells & Podolakin, 1987). Mortality is high (5−15%) after surgery. Bony abnormalities of the face and palate could theoretically cause intubation difficulties. However, in practice, this is not usually a problem. Severe chest deformities may lead to ventilatory embarrassment and spontaneous pneumothorax. Patients are at risk from bacterial endocarditis and require antibiotic prophylaxis. A myopathy has been reported, so the use of muscle relaxants should be monitored carefully.

Porphyria

Porphyrins are tetrapyrrole pigments in which four monopyrroles are linked by carbon bridges to form a ring. The various porphyrins differ only in the structure of their side chains, whose sequential arrangement determines the isomer type (numbered from I to IV). Porphyrins are components of several haem proteins (haemoglobin, myoglobin, cytochromes) and the enzymes catalase and tryptophan pyrrolase, which are concerned with oxidation, electron transport and hydroperoxidation. Only protoporphyrin IX (a III isomer) has physiological functions. It serves as the prosthetic group for haemoglobin and other haem proteins (Fig. 54.1). The other porphyrins are metabolic byproducts which have escaped from the haem synthetic pathway by oxidation of the reduced porphyrinogens. The rate of porphyrin and haem synthesis is regulated by aminolaevulinic acid (ALA) synthetase activity (Fig. 54.1). The inhibition of this enzyme by haem and other products of the reaction normally prevents the overproduction of haem and the accumulation of metabolic intermediates. Haem formation is active in the erythroid tissue of bone marrow and liver. Small amounts of porphyrins and their precursors are normally excreted in urine and bile from these sources.

The porphyrias are a group of diseases caused by inherited defects or acquired dysfunction of enzyme systems or control mechanisms in porphyrin metabolism and haem synthesis (Dean, 1971). The diseases are characterized by excessive secretion of one or more porphyrins, porphyrinogens or porphyrin precursors in the urine and/or faeces. A relationship exists between the biochemical lesion and the symptoms (Table 54.3). Although enzyme defects are present in many tissues, the erythrocytes and the liver manifest most of the derangements. Therefore porphyrias are classified as erythropoietic or hepatic. Patients with porphyria can present serious anaesthetic problems (Sumner, 1975; Mustajoki & Heinonen, 1980).

Erythropoietic porphyria

In erythropoietic porphyria (EP) excess porphyrins accumulate in red blood cells and bone marrow.

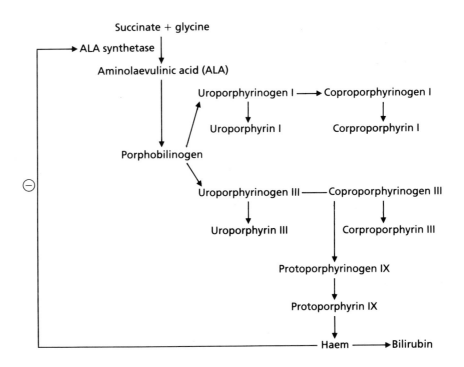

Fig. 54.1 Haem synthesis.

Table 54.3 Relationship between the biochemical lesion and symptoms in porphyria

Defect	Effect	Disease
ALA, PBG alone	Acute demyelination	AIP
Porphyrins alone	Photosensitivity	EP
ALA, PBG, porphyrins	Acute demyelination and photosensitivity	HCP,PV

AIP, acute intermittent porphyria; ALA, aminolaevulinic acid; EP, erythropoietic porphyria; HCP, hereditary coproporphyria; PBG, porphobilinogen; PV, porphyria variegata. See also Fig. 54.1.

Uroporphyria

Inheritance. Autosomal recessive.

Incidence. Rare.

Manifestations. There is faulty conversion of porphobilinogen (PBG) to uroporphyrinogen III in the maturing erythroid cells. The urine contains uroporphyrin I and coproporphyrin I, and turns red on standing. The faeces contain excess urobilinogen, but excretion of ALA and PBG are normal. The disease is manifest just after birth, when excess porphyrins in the tissues cause photosensitivity and severe mutilation. Hypertrichosis and erythrodontia are always present. Haemolytic anaemia with splenomegaly may occur. There are no nervous or gastrointestinal manifestations. The disease progresses slowly and death results from infection or severe anaemia. Therapy includes avoidance of sunlight, treatment of anaemia and splenectomy in some cases.

Protoporphyria

Inheritance. Autosomal dominant.

Incidence. Uncertain.

Manifestations. This variant is due to deficiency of ferrochelatase which inserts iron into protoporphyrin IX. There is increased protoporphyrin in erythrocytes and normoblasts. Urinary ALA, PBG and uroporphyrin concentrations are normal, but the faecal protoporphyrin concentration is increased. Biochemical stigmata may occur in the absence of signs and symptoms or may be manifest in childhood with skin sensitivity. The disease usually runs a benign course, with skin changes and sometimes a mild haemolytic anaemia. The liver is sometimes diseased and biliary stasis, cholelithiasis, portal inflammation, ductal proliferation and fibrosis may occur. Cirrhosis and hepatic failure may occur in some patients. Treatment includes avoidance of sunlight and administration of β-carotene to decrease photosensitivity. Cholestyramine has been used to facilitate removal of protoporphyrin from the liver in patients with hepatic problems.

Anaesthetic problems (Jackson, 1973). The EPs do not cause abdominal or neurological symptoms. Airway maintenance may be difficult because of extensive facial scarring. Anaesthetic drugs do not precipitate EPs. Anaemia and liver disease require consideration when planning the anaesthetic technique.

Hepatic porphyria

Excess porphyrin is produced by the liver. These conditions pose problems for the anaesthetist (Jackson, 1973).

Acute intermittent porphyria

Inheritance. Autosomal dominant.

Incidence. Acute intermittent porphyria (AIP) is the commonest form of porphyria, 1 : 100 000 births.

Manifestations. AIP is due to deficiency of uroporphyrinogen I synthetase in the liver and red blood cells. The condition is diagnosed by enzyme assay in erythrocytes. Functional expression of the enzyme disorder appears limited to the liver, although the effects of the deficiency are widespread. Bone marrow porphyrin content is normal, but the liver has high concentrations of porphyrin precursors. Reduction of haem synthesis stimulates augmented activity of ALA synthetase, and increased formation and excretion of ALA and PBG. Urinary ALA and PBG concentrations are elevated, even in the absence of symptoms (latent porphyria). The urine is normal colour when voided, but turns red after standing in sunlight or boiling with acid, due to the formation of porphobilin. PBG is colourless, but produces a red colour when combined with Ehrlich's aldehyde reagent (the colour cannot be extracted by chloroform, unlike urobilinogen). Faecal porphyrins are normal, except in the rare instance when urine porphyrins are markedly elevated.

The disease usually presents between the ages of

15 and 60 with slightly more females affected than males. Gastrointestinal and nervous system symptoms can be vague, so that the condition may remain undiagnosed for years. Photosensitivity is not a feature of the disease, but pigmentation can occur during an attack. Periodic attacks of nausea, vomiting and colicy abdominal pain occur, which can lead to surgical intervention. Severe constipation may also be a presenting complaint. Neuritis, painful extremities, autonomic neuropathy, paraplegia or bulbar palsy may occur, leading to respiratory distress requiring ventilation. Autonomic disturbance may cause hypertension and tachycardia. Seizures and motor disturbances may occur. Patients may present with psychiatric problems including psychosis. The death rate is high.

Anaesthetic problems. An acute exacerbation of AIP may be precipitated by low carbohydrate intake, infection, alcohol, pregnancy, menstruation and lead exposure. Prolonged preoperative fasting must be avoided. Hepatic iron overload may trigger an attack in susceptible individuals. A detailed preanaesthetic evaluation must include cardiovascular and neurological examination. Regional anaesthetic techniques are probably contraindicated in AIP, as neurological complications may be ascribed to them.

Various drugs may trigger an attack of AIP by increasing ALA synthetase activity (Table 54.4). All these agents are metabolized by microsomal liver enzymes which contain haem proteins. The response of an individual to a porphyrogenic drug is very unpredictable. Attacks are often irreversible and untreatable. Thus, avoidance of precipitating causes and drugs is vital. Prevention remains the primary approach. Opinions about drugs capable of precipitating AIP have been based on clinical experience. Animal models have been developed to assess porphyrogenicity in which a sensitizing drug is used in conjunction with the drug under test (Blekkenhorst *et al.*, 1980). It is possible to predict the safety of drugs in terms of these tests but, the ultimate evaluation must remain clinical. Symptomatic treatment of acute attacks is required, including liberal intravenous glucose to suppress activity of ALA synthetase.

Hereditary coproporphyria

Inheritance. Autosomal dominant.

Incidence. Rare (only 30 cases reported).

Table 54.4 Drugs to be avoided in hepatic porphyria, and those which may be administered safely

Drugs which may precipitate acute episodes in hepatic porphyria

Alcohol	Methyldopa
Alcuronium	Metoclopramide
Aminopyrine	Metronidazole
Amitriptyline	Metyrapone
Antipyrene	Nickethamide
All barbiturates	Oestrogen/oral contraceptives
All benzodiazepines	Pentazocine
Chlormethiazole	Phenoxybenzamine
Chlorpropamide	Phenylbutazone
Cimetidine	Phenytoin
Clonidine	Piritramide
Cocaine	Prochlorperazine
Ergometrine	Spironolactone
Erythromycin	Steroids
Glutethimide	Sulphanomides
Griseofulvin	Theophylline
Hydralazine	Tolbutamide
Meprobamate	

Drugs which may be given safely in hepatic porphyria

Anticoagulants	Lignocaine*
Aspirin	Neostigmine
Atropine	Nitrous oxide
Bupivacaine	Opioids
Buprenorphine	Oxytocin
Cephalosporins	Pancuronium*
Chloral hydrate	Paracetamol
Chlorpromazine	Paraldehyde
Cyclopropane	Pentolinium
Diethyl ether	Phenoperidine
Disopyramide	Phentolamine
Droperidol	Procaine
Enflurane*	Promazine
Etomidate*	Promethazine
Gallamine	Propanidid
Halothane*	Propofol†
Heparin	Propranolol
Hyoscine	Sodium valproate
Isoflurane	Suxamethonium
Ketamine*	Tubocurarine
Labetolol	

* Some conflicting evidence; † Weir & Hodkinson, 1988; Meissner *et al.*, 1989.

Manifestations. Hereditary coproporphyria is caused by partial deficiency of coproporphyrinogen oxidase leading to excessive excretion of ALA and PBG in the urine and high levels of coproporphyrin in the urine and faeces. Some individuals are symptomatic, or exhibit only photosensitivity. The disease can be latent, with only abnormal porphyrin excretion.

Anaesthetic problems. Acute attacks are manifest similarly to AIP and may be precipitated by the same conditions and drugs, which must be avoided (Table 54.4). Intravenous glucose is probably the most effective form of therapy.

Porphyria variegata (porphyria cutanea tarda hereditaria)

Inheritance. Autosomal dominant.

Incidence. Low worldwide (common in South Africa).

Manifestations. Porphyria variegata may be due to a defect in the conversion of protoporphyrin IX to haem, and is usually manifest between 10 and 30 years of age. There is increased secretion of coproporphyrin and protoporphyrin in the faeces at all times but asymptomatic latent phases can occur. During acute attacks there is increased urinary excretion of ALA and PBG. There is excessive skin fragility to mechanical trauma and pigmentation in exposed areas, but this is less severe than seen in EP. Photosensitivity is infrequent, but the distribution of the lesions suggests that sunlight is important in pathogenesis. It used to be thought that the condition was purely cutaneous, but any or all manifestations of AIP may occur. As long as the liver remains capable of excreting porphyrins in the bile, the patient remains asymptomatic. If this capacity is impaired, then increased bilirubin, porphyrinaemia, porphyrinuria and cutaneous lesions may result. When there is gross disturbance of liver function, ALA and PBG appear in the urine, and all the manifestations of AIP occur.

Anaesthetic problems. Treatment is as for AIP, including glucose and avoidance of precipitating conditions and drugs (Table 54.4).

Porphyria cutanea tarda

Inheritance. Autosomal dominant.

Incidence. Unknown.

Manifestations. Porphyria cutanea tarda is due to partial deficiency of uroporphyrinogen decarboxylase, and can be diagnosed by erythrocyte enzyme assay. In addition to the enzyme deficiency, liver injury (including siderosis or alcoholic disease), is present. There is excess hepatic synthesis and urinary excretion of uroporphyrin I. Urinary ALA and PBG concentrations are not increased, and faecal porphyrin concentrations are normal or only slightly elevated. In the absence of a liver problem, the enzyme defect does not seem to result in the clinical syndrome. The disease remains latent until precipitated by hepatic parenchymal iron overload. The condition has been described in males aged 40–70 with alcoholic cirrhosis, hepatic adenomas or systemic lupus erythematosis. Toxins such as polychlorinated phenols and hexachlorobenzene have been implicated as precipitating factors. Photosensitivity, pigmentation, hypertrichosis and liver manifestations occur, but there are no gastrointestinal or neurological problems.

Anaesthetic problems. Treatment includes phlebotomy, chelating agents and abstinence from alcohol. Liver dysfunction should be considered during anaesthesia. Triggering conditions and drugs must be avoided. Chloroquine is no longer recommended as it produces hepatic necrosis in the presence of excessive liver porphyrins.

Malignant hyperthermia

It is now recognized that malignant hyperthermia (MH) occurs in individuals who have inherited, as an autosomal dominant characteristic, a structural abnormality of either the sarcolemma or the sarcoplasmic reticulum (SR). It is likely that such a defect is caused by an abnormal protein structure in the membrane.

Recently, a gene on the long arm of chromosome 19 has been shown to be the likely candidate gene for MH. Specifically, the RYR gene has been implicated. This gene encodes for the protein controlling the ryanodine receptor which is associated with one of the important calcium channels in the SR. This is a conceptually satisfying explanation of the inheritance of MH as it is known that the MH episode is due to an uncontrolled calcium release into the sarcoplasm.

However, the genetics of MH seems to be potentially more complex. Recently, a number of MH families have been shown to have no linkage with chromosome 19. Thus these 'non-chromosome 19' families exhibit the type of heterogeneity which delays the development of a DNA-based method for detecting MH susceptibility (MHS). (For a discussion of these developments see Ellis, 1992.)

From the numerous case reports of MH, it seems that skeletal muscle is especially involved in the disease process. There is no good evidence that other tissues are implicated, though there is some experimental work which suggests that both white and red blood cells are abnormal in MHS individuals.

Signs of a malignant hyperthermia

In an acute episode of MH, there are two groups of abnormalities.

Hypermetabolism

The stimulation of metabolic processes appears to be out of central control. The increased metabolism results in a marked rise in oxygen utilization and demand. This causes an increased cardiac output (tachycardia) and decreased saturation of arterial blood when the oxygen supply system begins to fail. Cyanosis may become evident and at this stage metabolic acidosis occurs. The grossly elevated carbon dioxide production causes respiratory acidosis, especially in patients receiving mechanical ventilation. Spontaneously breathing subjects may keep the carbon dioxide within normal limits initially by hyperventilating. The increased metabolism causes an increase in body temperature which presumably is most marked in the affected skeletal muscles. Liver metabolism increases with the elevation of lactate production by muscle. The increase in body temperature can be very rapid.

Abnormal muscle function

Serum creatine kinase (CK) can become grossly elevated during an acute episode of MH and the CK derives from damaged muscle cells following muscle contracture, which is usually a part of the syndrome. The increase in CK is associated with hyperkalaemia and myoglobinaemia, which presumably have a similar pathogenesis.

Presentation

The full classical presentation is becoming increasingly rare as anaesthetists learn to recognize the early changes and take appropriate action. A much commoner presentation is as an aborted attack, which by its nature can only be suggestive of MH and not fully diagnostic. The earliest possible sign which comes into this category is muscle spasm following suxamethonium — this often involves only the masseter muscles (masseteric muscle spasm).

Other conditions which can mimic the early states of MH includes myotonic muscle disease such as myotonia congenita and other muscle diseases such as Duchenne dystrophy, in which greatly elevated serum CK and potassium are found. Causes of non-MH hypermetabolism include phaeochromocytoma and psychological stress. Attempts have been made to link MH with other conditions such as sudden infant death syndrome, and a variety of muscle or metabolic diseases such as thyroid disease. None of these has been substantiated and, as explained earlier, it seems that MH is a distinct genetic entity and not a 'rag-bag' of conditions, as some have suggested.

Incidence and mortality

The observed incidence of MH amongst the anaesthetized population varies considerably from 1 : 6000 in Japan to 1 : 200 000 in the UK. There is no evidence that the incidence varies in different races or ethnic groups, though in small communities in which inbreeding has occurred, if the MH gene(s) is/are present, MHS may be comparatively common. We estimated that 1 : 300 of the population of a small Yorkshire town was MHS. For the disease to be expressed, a genetically predisposed individual must be exposed to a trigger agent for long enough. The trigger agents include all inhalation anaesthetic vapours and probably suxamethonium. Only a proportion of anaesthetized subjects receive these anaesthetic agents, and so the observed incidence of MH does not reflect the number of susceptible patients undergoing anaesthesia. A higher incidence is found in patients having surgery for trauma or ENT problems, but this is probably because these patients receive the trigger agents more commonly as part of their anaesthetic regimen. The mortality figures for MH in the UK remained at about 24% throughout the 1970s and the early 1980s. However, there has been a marked improvement recently and this has coincided with more routine use of pulse oximetry and capnography — though most anaesthetists are nowadays more aware of the presentation of MH than a decade ago.

Screening

When a family has been identified as MHS, members should be investigated by muscle biopsy and *in vitro* screening using the halothane and caffeine contracture tests (IVCT). Because of the dominant inheritance of MHS, parents, siblings and children of known cases of MHS carry a 0.5 probability for inheriting the susceptibility to the disease.

Treatment

If MH is considered a possible diagnosis, administration of trigger agents should be stopped and surgery terminated. Heart rate, arterial pressure and body temperature should be recorded every 5 min and pulse oximetry and end-tidal capnography displayed continuously. Arterial blood gas tensions, pH, serum potassium and CK should be measured. The ECG should be observed for arrhythmias and evidence of hyperkalaemia. The first voided urine should be tested for myoglobin, and CK should be checked after 6, 12 and 24 h. Specific therapy includes dantrolene sodium (1−10 mg/kg), which lowers intracellular ionic calcium and glucocorticoids, which stabilize cell membranes. The calcium-channel blockers do not seem to be particularly useful as they seem to be effective largely on the plasma-membrane calcium channels. Supportive therapy is designed to control hyperkalaemia (insulin/dextrose, ion exchangers, etc.) and acidosis, and to reduce the likelihood of obstructive renal failure from intense myoglobinaemia using a forced diuresis. Surface cooling is useful in young, thin individuals.

If MH is detected early, termination of the trigger agents is usually all that is required. If a significant degree of metabolic derangement has occurred, dantrolene is necessary, though if severe acidosis and marked muscle contractures have developed, dantrolene may be ineffective — muscle contractures may severely inhibit muscle blood flow.

Reversal of MH signs with dantrolene is not pathognomonic for MH. Any cause of cellular hypermetabolism is likely to be reversed with dantrolene.

Anaesthesia for malignant hyperthermia susceptibility

Anaesthesia should not be a problem if MH trigger agents are avoided. Opioids, all local anaesthetics, non-depolarizing relaxants and nitrous oxide are apparently safe, as are atropine and neostigmine. Phenothiazines should be avoided, though it is likely that reports of reactions to these drugs similar to MH are probably examples of the neuroleptic malignant syndrome (NMS) and not MH. The relationship between NMS and MH has been clarified recently by Krivosic-Horber (1987) and using the IVCT, it is now clear that the muscle abnormality associated with MH does not occur in NMS.

References

Bevan J.C. (1980) Anaesthesia for Von Gierke's disease. *Anaesthesia* **35**, 699−702.

Blekkenhorst G.H., Harrison G.G., Cook E.S. & Eales L. (1980) Screening of certain anaesthetic agents for their ability to elicit acute porphyric phases in susceptible patients. *British Journal of Anaesthesia* **52**, 759−62.

Brown B.R., Walson P.D. & Taussing L.M. (1975) Congenital metabolic diseases of pediatric patients: anaesthetic implications. *Anesthesiology* **43**, 197−209.

Casson H. (1975) Anaesthesia for portocaval bypass in patients with metabolic disease. *British Journal of Anaesthesia* **47**, 969−75.

Coleman P. (1984) McArdle's disease. Problems of anaesthetic management for Caesarean section. *Anaesthesia* **39**, 784−7.

Cox J.M. (1968) Anaesthesia and glycogen-storage disease. *Anaesthesiology* **29**, 1221−5.

Crook J.W., Towers J.F. & Taylor W.H. (1971) Management of patients with homocystinuria requiring surgery under general anaesthesia. *British Journal of Anaesthesia* **43**, 96−9.

Dean G. (1971) *The Porphyrias, A Story of Inheritance and Environment* 2nd edn. Pitman Medical, London.

Delaney A. & Gal T.J. (1976) Hazards of anaesthesia and operation in maple syrup urine disease. *Anesthesiology* **44**, 83−6.

Dierdorf S.F. & McNiece W.L. (1983) Anaesthesia and pyruvate dehydrogenase deficiency. *Canadian Anaesthetist's Society Journal* **30**, 413−16.

Ellis F.R. (1980) Inherited muscle disease. *British Journal of Anaesthesia* **52**, 153−63.

Ellis F.R. (1992) Detecting susceptibility to malignant hyperthermia. (Editorial) *British Medical Journal* **304**, 791−2.

Hashimoto Y., Watanabe H. & Satou M. (1978) Anesthetic management of a patient with hereditary fructose-1,6-diphosphate deficiency. *Anesthesia and Analgesia* **57**, 503−6.

Herrick I.A. & Rhine E.J. (1988) The mucopolysaccharidoses and anaesthesia: a report of clinical experience. *Canadian Anaesthetist's Society Journal* **35**, 67−73.

Jackson S.H. (1973) Genetic and metabolic disease: inborn errors of metabolism. In *Anaesthesia and Uncommon Disease* (Eds Katz J. & Kadis D.H.) pp. 1−31. W.B. Saunders Co., Philadelphia.

King D.H., Jones R.M. & Barnett M.B. (1984) Anaesthetic considerations in mucopolysaccharidoses. *Anaesthesia* **39**, 126−31.

Krivosic-Horber R., Adnet P., Guevart D., Theunynck D. & Lestavel P. (1987) Neuroleptic malignant syndrome and malignant hyperthermia. *British Journal of Anaesthesia* **59**, 1554−6.

Larson L.O. & Wilkins R.G. (1985) Anaesthesia and the Lesch−Nyhan syndrome. *Anesthesiology* **63**, 197−99.

McFarlane H.J. & Soni N. (1986) Pompe's disease and anaesthesia. *Anaesthesia* **41**, 1219−24.

Meissner P.N., Hift R.J. & Harrison G.G. (1989) Propofol and porphyria. *Anaesthesia* **44**, 612−3.

Mustajoki P. & Heinonen J. (1980) General anaesthesia in 'inducible' porphyria. *Anaesthesiology* **53**, 15−20.

Rosen K.R. & Broadman L.M. (1986) Anaesthesia for diagnostic muscle biopsy in an infant with Pompe's disease. *Canadian Anaesthetist's Society Journal* **33**, 790−4.

Samuels T.A. & Coleman P. (1988) McArdle's disease and Caesarean section. *Anaesthesia* **43**, 161–2.

Smith C.L. & Snowdon S.L. (1987) Anaesthesia and G6PD deficiency. A case report and review of the literature. *Anaesthesia* **42**, 281–8.

Sumner E. (1975) Porphyria in relation to surgery and anaesthesia. *Annals of the Royal College of Surgeons* **56**, 81–8.

Verghese C. (1984) Anaesthesia in Marfan's syndrome. *Anaesthesia* **39**, 917–22.

Weir P.M. & Hodkinson B.P. (1988) Is propofol a safe agent in porphyria? *Anaesthesia* **43**, 1022–4.

Wells D.G. & Podolakin W. (1987) Anaesthesia and Marfan's syndrome: case report. *Canadian Anaesthetists Society Journal* **34**, 311–14.

Further reading

Ellis F.R. & Heffron J.J.A. (1985) Clinical and biochemical aspects of malignant hyperpyrexia. In *Recent Advances in Anaesthesia and Analgesia* vol. 15 (Eds Atkinson R.A. & Adams A.P.) Churchill Livingstone, Edinburgh.

Pollard B.J. & Harrison M.J. (1989) *Anaesthesia for Uncommon Diseases*. Blackwell Scientific Publications, Oxford.

Wyngaarden J.B. & Smith L.H. (Eds) (1988) *Cecil's Textbook of Medicine* 17th edn. pp. 1130–203. W.B. Saunders Co., Philadelphia.

Anaesthesia and Miscellaneous Diseases

J.E. PEACOCK

Some diseases are encountered in anaesthetic practice very rarely and all cannot be included in a book of this nature. The reader is referred to other texts for specific details of those problems not mentioned here (see Further reading). In this chapter, four main areas are discussed: endocrine neoplasia within the gastrointestinal system, muscle diseases, connective tissue and skin disorders, and drug abuse and anaesthesia.

The medical aspects of individual diseases are discussed in addition to anaesthetic management.

Neuroendocrine tumours within the gastrointestinal tract

The physiological control of the gastrointestinal system is now accepted as having its basis in the regulatory peptides. Bayliss and Starling first demonstrated the existence of secretin in 1902 and this was followed by the discovery of gastrin in 1905 by Edkins. However, most of the work on regulatory peptides has occurred since the 1960s with the development of radioimmunoassay (RIA). There has been a great increase in the number of peptides identified (O'Dorisio, 1986). Before the development of RIA, the neuroendocrine tumours were diagnosed on the basis of a clinical syndrome resulting from the effects of the peptides with possible improvement after removal of the tumour. Carcinoid was described first in 1888, although the endocrine nature of the tumour was not recognized until the period around 1950.

Most of the syndromes are a result of secretion of a single peptide, although many of the tumours secrete more than one peptide. Histologically, the tumours arise from the diffuse endocrine system. The normal cells have been grouped together as the amine, precursor uptake and decarboxylation (APUD) system although their specific origin is controversial (Walter & Israel, 1987). This includes:

1 The chromaffin cells of the adrenal medulla and paravertebral sympathetic plexuses.
2 The argentaffin cells of the gastrointestinal tract which secrete 5-hydroxytryptamine.
3 Pancreatic islet cells.
4 Thyroid C-cells.
5 Parathyroid cells.
6 Melanocytes.

Problems of the adrenal medulla and sympathetic plexuses, and thyroid and parathyroid are described elsewhere in Chapters 52 and 53. Most of the tumours to be discussed here are derived from the argentaffin or pancreatic islet cells.

The tumours are of an extremely variable nature. Some are benign adenomata whereas other are malignant and metastasize, although they all tend to be slow growing. As a result they are often identified only when the full syndrome is apparent and metastatic deposits may be present already. Then complete removal may not be possible in spite of recent advances in scanning techniques for localization of the tumours. The exception to this is the tumour found as an incidental finding, e.g. appendiceal carcinoid. Most of the tumours are single but some may occur as part of the multiple endocrine neoplasia (MEN) syndrome. In this situation, the tumour may be one of several endocrine tissues affected at the same time. Three familial syndromes are recognized (all autosomal dominant) in which different combinations of endocrine involvement exist (Walter & Israel, 1987) (Table 55.1).

Carcinoid syndrome

'Carcinoid' was the name given in 1909 by Oberndorfer (as 'Karzinoide') to describe a tumour that 'resembled carcinoma' but was of a benign nature. Carcinoid tumours may have different patterns of peptide secretion. They have been classified accord-

Table 55.1 Multiple endocrine neoplasia

MEN I	Parathyroid glands: hyperparathyroidism Pancreas (islet cell tumours): Zollinger—Ellison syndrome or hyperinsulinism
MEN II	Thyroid gland: medullary carcinoma Parathyroid glands: hyperparathyroidism Phaeochromocytoma
MEN III	Thyroid gland: medullary carcinoma Multiple neuromata within the CNS

Table 55.2 Common symptoms associated with carcinoid syndrome: 1—3 are the most common

Organ	Symptom
Skin	Flushing (1) Telangiectasia Cyanosis
Gastrointestinal tract	Diarrhoea (2) Pain (3)
Cardiovascular	Pulmonary stenosis Tricuspid regurgitation
Respiratory	Asthma (wheeze)

ing to their embryological origin to try and distinguish these (Williams & Sandler, 1963).

Foregut carcinoids include respiratory and pancreatic tumours and mainly secrete serotonin. *Midgut* carcinoids include ileal and appendiceal tumours. *Hindgut* tumours include colonic and rectal carcinoids. The latter two groups secrete many peptides. Those which produce the syndrome tend to secrete kinins when there are widespread metastases.

The carcinoid syndrome appears only when there is sufficient release of peptide from the tumour into the peripheral circulation. Usually this implies widespread metastases (especially to the liver) for midgut carcinoids to produce symptoms, although foregut tumours may bypass the portal circulation and show symptoms much earlier.

Symptoms

Symptoms may be related to a number of systems and are listed in Table 55.2. Flushing is the most common symptom with increased duration as the disease progresses but may or may not be associated with hypotension or hypertension during the flush. Diarrhoea may be episodic and watery with associated cramps, and borborygmi and malabsorption with steatorrhoea may also be present but is not common. Cardiac symptoms result from subendocardial fibrosis resulting in tricuspid regurgitation and pulmonary stenosis. Bronchoconstriction may occur and may be severe in the presence of cardiac disease.

Classically, the cause of carcinoid is the peptide serotonin [5-hydroxytryptamine (5-HT)]. This is the cause of many of the symptoms including the diarrhoea and has been the basis of pharmacological therapy. However, serotonin antagonists such as methysergide, cypropheptadine and ketanserin may have no effect on flushing. Kallikrein production and conversion to bradykinin is now thought to be the cause of flushing (Creutzfeldt & Stockmann, 1987).

The diagnosis of carcinoid is made by finding elevated concentrations of 5-hydroxyindoleacetic acid (5-HIAA) in the urine. One must be careful to exclude spurious elevations resulting from serotonin-containing food and drugs (e.g. phenothiazines).

Anaesthesia

The subject of anaesthesia for carcinoid has been reviewed by Déry (1971) and Mason and Steane (1976). Further pharmacological advances have occurred since that time with the availability of ketanserin and the manufacture of the drug octreotide, which is a somatostatin analogue (Dollery, 1991).

The major problems for the anaesthetist are listed in Table 55.3 but are primarily fluid and electrolyte balance, arterial pressure control and bronchospasm. The mixture of possible effects is related to the two peptides and these may be controlled by adequate preoperative preparation (Maton *et al.*, 1983). Fluid and electrolyte imbalance should be corrected preoperatively. Serotonin antagonists which have been shown to be effective include methysergide, cyproheptadine and, most recently, ketanserin (Fischler *et al.*, 1983; Casthely *et al.*, 1986; Houghton & Carter, 1986; Solares *et al.*, 1987). Effects of bradykinin may

Table 55.3 Anaesthetic problems in carcinoid

1 The possibility of marked flushing, vasodilatation, and hypotension associated with bradykinin release, or
2 The possibility of marked hypertension associated with serotonin release
3 Bronchoconstriction
4 Fluid and electrolyte imbalance in the presence of severe diarrhoea
5 Delayed recovery, hypoproteinaemia and hyperglycaemia

be controlled by a perioperative infusion of aprotinin (Maton *et al.*, 1983). Most recently, the aforementioned somatostatin analogue, octreotide, has been investigated for its effects in carcinoid. Somatostatin itself reduces the flush in carcinoid (Frolich *et al.*, 1978) and octreotide may control peptide secretion. Octreotide is effective in gastrinoma and insulinoma (Tsai *et al.*, 1986) and has been used in the preoperative preparation of a patient with carcinoid syndrome (Roy *et al.*, 1987). Since that time, other reports have become available on its successful preoperative use (Watson *et al.*, 1990; McCrirrick & Hickman, 1991). Marsh and colleagues (1987) described the emergency use of the analogue to control the extremely severe hypotension in a patient undergoing laparotomy. There was an impressive response to the drug. Personal experience with octreotide in the management of carcinoid has resulted in reliable control of arterial pressure changes even during anaesthesia for removal of hepatic secondaries.

Should hypertension occur perioperatively, it may be controlled by intravenous administration of cyproheptadine or ketanserin. Hypotension may be more of a problem but should probably not be treated with catecholamines as this may increase peptide release further and exacerbate the situation. Aprotinin infusion has been used to combat hypotension although octreotide is probably now the drug of choice. Hughes and Hodkinson (1989) reported the use of ketanserin to control the hypertensive response after octreotide at the time of induction. Smooth control of arterial pressure was achieved by an infusion of ketanserin with no evidence of hypotension after the administration of octreotide.

A large number of studies have proposed a varied list of drugs as part of the preoperative preparation in the carcinoid syndrome. These have included:
1 Cyproheptadine or ketanserin orally to control symptoms of excessive (5-HT) excretion.
2 An aprotinin infusion commenced or available before induction to control the symptoms of bradykinin.
3 An oral benzodiazepine as premedicant.
4 Methyl prednisolone to block the synthesis of prostaglandins which may be released or involved in the action of bradykinin (Parry *et al.*, 1986).

Personal experience in carcinoid syndrome has resulted in the following guidelines: octreotide subcutaneously 1 h prior to induction after a test dose if not already part of maintenance therapy; oral benzodiazepine to control anxiety. Additional doses of octreotide should be available to control any hypotensive response but has not been required in over 20 cases. Parenteral forms of ketanserin or cyproheptadine may be used to control hypertensive responses or the agents commonly employed during anaesthesia.

Anaesthesia should be induced by drugs which do not cause serotonin or histamine release. A fentanyl/benzodiazepine induction has been recommended because of its haemodynamic stability (Solares *et al.*, 1987) although most drugs have been used. Intubation of the trachea should be conducted to avoid a hypertensive response. Suxamethonium should *not* be used as it may precipitate hormone release. A competitive neuromuscular-blocking drug which does not release histamine or produce hypotension should be used, e.g. vecuronium or pancuronium. Morphine should be avoided as it may release histamine or serotonin and precipitate bronchospasm.

Maintenance of anaesthesia should avoid myocardial depression. The synthetic potent opioids are used frequently as part of the anaesthetic regimen. Regional anaesthesia may be contraindicated as the hypotension may precipitate release of bradykinin but has been used for postoperative analgesia. Monitoring may include pulse, ECG, direct arterial pressure, central venous pressure, electrolytes, blood sugar concentrations and arterial blood gas tensions. Intensive observations should continue into the postoperative period.

Gastrinoma

Gastrin is secreted normally by the G-cells of the gastric antrum. It stimulates secretion of acid from the gastric parietal cells. However, gastrinomas arise from islet cells in the pancreas. They result in hypersecretion of gastric acid which results in severe peptic ulceration. This syndrome of pancreatic islet-cell tumour and peptic ulceration was reported originally in 1955 by Zollinger and Ellison (ZE syndrome) with isolation of gastrin from a tumour by Gregory and Tracey. Approximately 25% of ZE patients have MEN I. Epigastric pain is the most common symptom but weight loss, nausea and vomiting, haematemesis and melaena and severe diarrhoea may occur also. Diarrhoea may be a result of large gastric volumes entering the intestine, steatorrhoea, with failure of pancreatic enzymes in an acid pH or acid enteritis.

Diagnosis is by analysis of gastric output and serum concentrations of gastrin. Approximately 60% of gastrinomas are malignant (Townsend & Thompson, 1986) but they are usually small. As a result, metastases may be present at diagnosis. Surgery may be indicated to resect the tumour in case of malignancy and to control symptoms although medical control of symptoms is possible usually with H$_2$-receptor antagonists. Omeprazole blocks the sodium−potassium hydrogen-ion pump and is also effective.

Anaesthesia

Anaesthesia is straightforward provided there is adequate preoperative preparation. Possible problems are related to fluid and electrolyte balance or additional hormone abnormalities if MEN exists. The only specific requirement is prophylaxis against aspiration of large volumes of gastric acid. Adequate H$_2$-block and neutralization of any acid present usually suffices.

Insulinoma

The main symptoms of insulinoma are related to the neurological consequences of hypoglycaemia. Hypoglycaemia occurring during fasting or exercise may be the presenting complaint but the diagnosis must be distinguished from other causes (Kaplan *et al.*, 1987). In the absence of MEN and the secretion of other peptides, the anaesthetic problems of insulinomas relate to the maintenance of normal blood sugar. Various regimens have been suggested regarding the methods and agents to be used. Hargadon and Ormston (1963) suggested that inhalation agents should be avoided because of hyperglycaemic and hypotensive effects. Hyperglycaemia may be unwanted, as removal of the tumour tends to produce such a response when excess insulin is no longer secreted. Hyperglycaemia itself has been used to detect complete removal of tumour (which may be multiple), but this has now been shown to be unreliable (Muir *et al.*, 1983). Colella and Vandam (1972) suggested the use of diethyl ether, making use of its hyperglycaemia effects and avoiding glucose infusions. Automatic glucose analysers such as the Biostater with feedback to an intravenous glucose infusion or insulin have been recommended (Karam *et al.*, 1979).

Muir and colleagues (1983) came to the conclusion that glucose infusion should be commenced preoperatively with frequent estimations of blood glucose to maintain blood sugar concentrations between 10 and 15 mmol/litre. The use of such a regimen ensures that hypoglycaemia is avoided and is the safest option available. Serum potassium concentrations should be measured also. With adequate preoperative concentrations and avoiding exogenous insulin, maintaining normoglycaemia avoids large changes in potassium concentrations.

Glucagonoma

The glucagonoma syndrome is again related to an islet-cell tumour of the pancreas. Physiologically, glucagon promotes a catabolic response from carbohydrate metabolism. This results in hyperglycaemia and may be confused easily with diabetes mellitus. Although hyperglycaemia is the main biochemical abnormality, the syndrome includes skin rashes and possible vitamin deficiencies (Wood & Bloom, 1984; Bloom & Polak, 1987a).

The skin changes consist of a necrolytic migratory erythematous rash, angular stomatitis and painful glossitis. These may result in referral to a dermatologist. Mild diabetes, a normochromic normocytic anaemia, weight loss and a tendency to thrombosis are part of the syndrome. The tumours are often large and may be malignant. They may be part of MEN and secrete other peptides. Surgical removal results in cure of the diabetes and resolution of the rash.

Anaesthesia

From the physiological and pharmacological actions of glucagon, it could be expected that myocardial or metabolic problems may occur. Nicoll and Catling (1985) described a case of anaesthesia for removal of glucagonoma. Benzodiazepine premedication was used and anaesthesia was induced using fentanyl and thiopentone. Alcuronium was given for muscle paralysis. The lungs were ventilated with nitrous oxide in oxygen and anaesthesia was maintained by bolus doses of fentanyl intravenously and low inspired concentrations of halothane. No problems were encountered and the patient made a good recovery. No treatment was required for hyperglycaemia although all dextrose-containing solutions were avoided. Plasma glucagon concentrations were measured at different times during anaesthesia and surgery and showed considerable increases during and after manipulation of the tumour but failed to reach pharmacologically active concentrations.

Intensive monitoring of the patient is advised during tumour manipulation in anticipation of possible glucagon or other peptide activity. However, the effects seen in the case presented were minimal.

VIPoma

VIPoma is a result of synthesis and release of

vasoactive intestinal peptide from a tumour that usually (90%) occurs within the pancreas (Friesen, 1987; Krejs, 1987). Previously known as diarrhoe-ogenic syndrome or Vermer Morrison syndrome (amongst other titles), the major effect is to produce severe watery diarrhoea. Volumes may exceed 3 litres/day and result in dehydration and hypokalaemia. This may produce weakness or hypotension and may be accompanied by flushing (in the absence of raised 5-HIAA concentrations). It is associated with severe hypochlorhydria or achlorhydria, which prevents peptic ulceration. Hypercalcaemia and hypomagne-saemia may be present also. The tumour may be malignant and produce metastases or be part of MEN and be associated with the secretion of other hormones.

Problems for the anaesthetist may be severe dehydration, acidosis and hypokalaemia. Adequate preoperative preparation is essential although pre-operative control of diarrhoea may be achieved by the use of somatostatin analogue. Once the patient is hydrated adequately, anaesthesia may continue according to the general requirements of the patient.

Somatostatinoma

Secretion of excess of somatostatin tends to produce inhibition of all other gut hormones. As a result, somatostatin-secreting tumours tend to cause weight loss, malabsorption, diabetes, gallstones and hypo-chlorhydria (Bloom & Polak, 1987b; Friesen, 1987). The tumours grow slowly and are often large at the time of presentation. Any problems for the anaesthe-tist are related to a malnourished patient rather than to any peptide release and there are no specific requirements.

Ectopic hormone secretion

All the above tumours could be included in this category as they may produce peptides at abnormal sites. Classically, the description relates to the ectopic adrenocorticotrophic (ACTH) syndrome with secretion of ACTH from a non-adrenal tumour (Chahal & O'Shea, 1984). Such a tumour may be an oat-cell carcinoma of the bronchus although bronchial adenomas may be involved in the carcinoid syn-drome. The symptoms produced relate to the hor-mone/peptide secreted from the tumour, and management is indicated according to the relevant hormone. Thus, ACTH-secreting tumours are man-aged according to the scheme described for Cushing's syndrome (see Chapter 52). Other hormones secreted

in an ectopic fashion include: parathormone (see Chapter 53), melanocyte-stimulating hormone and other hormones from within the APUD system (see above).

Muscle diseases

There are a large number of neuromuscular diseases which present a formidable challenge to the anaes-thetist. Some of the particular diseases and the longer-term problems relating to intensive care are discussed elsewhere (Chapter 88). The general dilemmas seen with neuromuscular dysfunction and anaesthesia are discussed and related to the specific difficulties associated with myasthenia gravis, the muscular dys-trophies, periodic paralysis and multiple sclerosis.

Presentation

A patient with muscular disease may present in one of two categories: as a patient with a hitherto unknown disease exposed by an adverse response to anaesthesia, or, alternatively, as a patient with a recognized diagnosis. Many muscular diseases may have gone unnoticed, even by the patient and presen-tation occurs not infrequently following anaesthetic difficulties such as prolonged neuromuscular block or prolonged respiratory depression. Abnormal response to one of the muscle relaxants is plainly the most likely cause of postoperative weakness but many of the agents used during anaesthesia also have an effect on neuromuscular function. Other abnormal responses include the potential for malignant hyper-thermia (MH) in some cases of muscular dystrophy and the effect of suxamethonium on abnormally innervated muscle resulting in massive release of potassium. Hyperkalaemia in response to the admin-istration of suxamethonium after spinal cord injury (Stone et al., 1970) or major burns (Tolmie et al., 1967) is well recognized but also applies to hemiplegia after cerebrovascular accident (Cooperman et al., 1970) and probably to denervation as a result of polyneuropathy (Nicholson, 1971; Fergusson et al., 1981).

Although a specific abnormal muscle response is the most likely presentation, other systems may also be affected. Muscular diseases have a multiplicity of systemic manifestations that must be assessed. Car-diac involvement is not an uncommon feature of many disorders and may result in heart failure or arrhythmias. In those patients who already have evi-dence of generalized muscular disease, the symptoms are almost invariably accompanied by some degree of respiratory impairment with inability to cough effectively and occult infection. Physical abnormalities of the chest wall and airway may also present problems in addition to the abnormal pharmacodynamic response to the anaesthetic agents.

Myasthenia gravis

First described by Willis in 1672, myasthenia gravis is characterized by weakness and fatigue that varies during the day and is made worse by exercise. The condition affects, most commonly, the ocular muscles causing ptosis and diplopia but cranial nerve involvement may result in facial weakness, dysarthria and dysphagia. Where limb muscle groups are affected, proximal muscles are more often involved than distal and upper limb more often than lower. Respiratory weakness is unusual unless a myasthenic or cholinergic crisis supervenes. The incidence is approximately 3 : 100 000 with a 3 : 1 preponderance of females in the younger age groups (10−40 years). In older patients there is a more-or-less equal sex incidence. As with many autoimmune diseases, there are associations with other conditions which include thymitis, thymoma and thyrotoxicosis. Until the advent of anticholinesterase therapy in the 1930s, the disease had a very high mortality. Although not curative, long-term medication may now control the symptoms of the disease.

Pathophysiology

Although the factor which induces the onset of the disease is unknown the basic defect which causes the weakness is a decrease in the number of available acetylcholine receptors on the postsynaptic membrane of the neuromuscular junction. Also there is an abnormal response to acetylcholine at the surviving receptors with a tendency to produce a variety of depolarizing and non-depolarizing blocks. Humoral autoimmune processes are involved with T-helper lymphocytes also playing a part. It was noted that there was a factor in the plasma globulin of myasthenic patients which inhibited the binding of α-bungarotoxin, which normally binds irreversibly to acetylcholine receptors. Circulating antiacetylcholine receptor antibodies are found in 90% of cases and identification is a reliable diagnostic sign. However, there seems to be little relationship between antibody titres and severity of the disease and antibodies are not detectable in all patients. The lifespan of receptors is shortened from 7 days to 1 day but the precise pathway by which the antibodies produce a loss of receptors remains unclear. However, it is clear that the thymus gland has an important part to play in the disease process. Fifteen percent of sufferers have a thymoma and 60% of the remainder have thymitis. As a result the most common reason for an individual to present for anaesthesia is for thymectomy which may result in remission or improvement in 60−80% of patients but sometimes after a delay of several years.

Diagnosis

Diagnosis is confirmed by a classical decrease in single-twitch height and a decreasing response to tetanic or repeated stimuli on electromyography. Edrophonium 2 mg preceded by atropine, followed by further doses if no response has occurred in 30 s produces full return of muscle power. Symptoms due to cholinergic effects may occur in normal individuals or treated myasthenics.

Myasthenia gravis has been classified according to the muscle groups involved and the degree of weakness (Osserman & Genkins, 1971). Although usually occurring in adult patients, myasthenia may also occur in paediatric patients; 20% of infants of myasthenic mothers may have transient symptoms due to transplacental passage of maternal antibodies (neonatal) or it may arise at 2−3 months of age (congenital). Muscle weakness may be precipitated by drugs such as antibiotics (aminoglycosides), infection, electrolyte abnormalities, pregnancy or surgical stress.

Treatment

There are four main avenues of treatment: anticholinesterases, immunosuppression, plasmapheresis and thymectomy. Neostigmine and pyridostigmine are the anticholinesterase drugs usually used to treat myasthenia. The drugs increase the amount of acetylcholine at the neuromuscular junction by reducing its hydrolysis. Pyridostigmine is usually used as it is longer acting and has fewer muscarinic side-effects than neostigmine. The potential problem of anticholinesterase drugs is for excessive treatment to result in muscle weakness known as cholinergic crisis. The association of weakness with sweating, colic, lacrimation and fasciculation after edrophonium (Tensilon) confirms the diagnosis of cholinergic crisis, but can be difficult to distinguish clinically from myasthenia which is improved by edrophonium. This may be especially confusing as both conditions may be present in different muscle groups at the same time. Treatment of cholinergic crisis is supportive with withdrawal of cholinergic therapy, maintenance of the airway and support of ventilation as necessary. Cholinergic symptoms may be treated by atropine as indicated.

Immunosuppression using steroids, azathioprine or cyclosporin or plasmapheresis to reduce the amount of circulating antibody may also be used. The problem with immunosuppressive therapy is that side-effects may occur and withdrawal tends to worsen the disease. Thymectomy is usually recommended in patients with resistant disease although one study found that patients treated surgically had a better outcome than those treated medically. The response to surgery may be varied with some patients demonstrating a marked improvement very rapidly so that drug therapy is no longer needed whilst others may respond very slowly and may only be improved by management with lower doses of cholinesterase drugs. Management differs between centres but early surgery is now considered to be the treatment of choice in many patients.

Anaesthesia

Preoperative preparation of the myasthenic patient involves assessment of associated diseases in addition to estimation of the degree of impairment of muscular function. For elective surgery, optimization of preoperative muscle function is required and therefore anticholinesterase therapy should be continued up to the time of operation. Careful assessment of respiratory function including blood-gas analysis and treatment of infection will minimize the need for postoperative ventilation. It is sensible to avoid sedative or respiratory depressant premedicants in case of preoperative deterioration. The use of regional anaesthetic techniques is appropriate provided that higher thoracic blocks which may precipitate respiratory failure are avoided. These may also be of value in the postoperative period for analgesic purposes (Burgess & Wilcosky, 1989).

The actual methods used during general anaesthesia vary but intubation and ventilation are always necessary. Intravenous or inhalation anaesthetic agents can be used but the latter do have an appreciable effect on neuromuscular function. Whereas inhalation agents alone have minimal effect on twitch height in normal patients they can produce marked, but variable reductions in myasthenic patients. Nilsson and colleagues (1989) and Nilsson and Müller (1990) showed larger effects with isoflurane (55% reduction) on train-of-four ratio compared with equal minimum alveolar concentrations of halothane (33% reduction). Despite the larger effect of isoflurane, it may still be the agent of choice as it is excreted more rapidly than halothane. The effects of the inhalation agents on neuromuscular function imply that specific muscle relaxants and their potential complications can often be avoided.

The problems associated with the use of muscle relaxants in myasthenia gravis are not only related to the relative sensitivity of the patients to the non-depolarizing drugs. Myasthenic patients have been shown to be resistant to suxamethonium (Eisenkraft et al., 1988) with the ED_{50} and ED_{95} levels being twice that of normal patients. However there are clinical reports where suxamethonium has been used effectively and without problems (Baraka & Tabboush, 1991). The additional complicating factor is that there are also reports of non-depolarizing type of block occurring after suxamethonium (Wainwright & Brodrick, 1987). It is clear that if rapid intubating conditions are required then larger doses of suxamethonium should be used than normal (1.5–2.0 mg/kg).

The effects of the non-depolarizing muscle relaxants are more clear. All the drugs in this category produce an increase in the degree of block compared with normal patients. In addition, some drugs may also produce a block of longer duration than normal although duration of block is proportional to the amount of drug administered and it may be difficult to compare truly equipotent doses. For these reasons some authors have recommended that muscle relaxants are not used in myasthenic patients. Vecuronium and atracurium are the shorter-acting non-depolarizing muscle relaxants in present use although the newer agents may have a place when they become available. Both agents have been used in several studies in myasthenia gravis. Vecuronium doses required are 50% lower than in normal patients (Eisenkraft et al., 1990) but with considerable variation between individuals. Atracurium dose requirements are also reduced being one-fifth of those normally recommended (Bell et al., 1984), again with marked difference between patients.

It is apparent that the use of non-depolarizing muscle relaxants differs between centres. Some use the properties of the inhalation agents to avoid the use of muscle relaxants completely whereas others choose to use the specific effects of relaxants in an attempt to improve the quality of recovery. None of the studies has demonstrated problems with reversal of the above two agents but there may be theoretical advantages to atracurium because of the mechanism of metabolism. Whatever technique is used, monitoring of neuromuscular function with continuous train-of-four is mandatory.

Postoperative care

Historically, patients with myasthenia gravis underwent elective ventilation postoperatively, often with a tracheostomy. With the advent of improved anaesthetic drugs which have less effect in the postoperative period, in the majority of patients the trachea is extubated early in the recovery period. Further improvements in the management of postoperative pain may also minimize the need for delayed extubation. Other factors which help in the management of such patients is the recommencement of anticholinesterase drugs as soon as possible after surgery. Prediction of those cases which require elective mechanical ventilation is more difficult. Leventhal and colleagues (1980) showed that the greatest risk factors were the duration of myasthenia, respiratory disease, dose of pyridostigmine and vital capacity. The intensive care management of myasthenic patients is discussed elsewhere (see Chapter 88).

Myasthenic syndrome

This syndrome was first described by Eaton and Lambert in 1957 and complicates approximately 1% of bronchogenic carcinomas. Almost all cases are older males and the diagnosis may predate the diagnosis of the primary malignancy by several years. Unlike myasthenia gravis patients, the muscles most commonly affected in the syndrome tend to be the proximal muscles of the limbs with the legs rather than the arms being more commonly affected. Involvement of the bulbar muscles is rare but there are similar associations with thyroid disease, polyarteritis, dermatomyositis and systemic lupus erythematosus (SLE). The major difference is an improvement in power with exercise and the anticholinesterases are ineffective. There is weakness and an aching pain in the muscles and the tendon reflexes are depressed. Electromyography shows low-voltage twitches with tetanic stimulation producing a progressive increase in twitch height with post-tetanic facilitation.

The anaesthetic considerations are similar to those of myasthenia gravis with the exception that there is sensitivity to suxamethonium in addition to the non-depolarizing muscle relaxants. Anticholinesterases may be used to reverse any block but the likelihood for prolonged mechanical ventilation should be borne in mind.

Muscular dystrophies

There are several familial diseases characterized by increasing muscular weakness from atrophy of the muscle. The innervation of the muscle is normal but there is increasing degeneration of muscle and replacement with fibrous tissue. Many of the diseases are classified according to clinical similarities and known by various eponyms.

Duchenne muscular dystrophy

This X-linked recessive disorder is the most severe and yet the most common form of progressive muscular dystrophy and commences in males between the ages of 2 and 5 years. The first muscles to be affected are the proximal muscles, especially of the pelvis; and hence the difficulty in standing up from a supine position and the characteristic waddling gait. They classically use their arms to assist in standing by walking up their legs (Gowers' sign). The proximal atrophy produces the appearance of paradoxical hypertrophy, particularly affecting the calves and hence the alternative name of pseudohypertrophic muscular dystrophy. Deterioration is progressive and most are unable to walk by the age of 10 and death frequently occurs by 20 years of age. Contractures and kyphoscoliosis occur, the latter producing a restrictive ventilatory defect with reduced vital capacity. Respiratory weakness and difficulty in swallowing may lead to pneumonia, which is the most common cause of death. Cardiac involvement is common in the form of cardiomyopathy with arrhythmias and reduced contractility.

Other forms of muscular dystrophy include *Becker muscular dystrophy* which occurs later in life, is less severe and cardiomyopathy does not occur. *Limb-girdle muscular dystrophy* is autosomal recessive, appears to affect the upper body first, and involves the legs when the individual is around 30 years of age when a wheelchair may be required. Cardiac involvement is variable. *Fascioscapulohumeral muscular dystrophy* is an autosomal dominant disease which is compatible with a normal life span.

Anaesthesia

Anaesthesia for patients with muscular dystrophy has been described with a large number of agents. The main areas for concern are the preoperative condition of the patient with the potential for cardiac and respiratory impairment and the response to the neuromuscular-blocking drugs. It is now recognized that patients with Duchenne muscular dystrophy are more likely to have MH (Boltshauser *et al.*, 1980; Brownell *et al.*, 1983) and may have an abnormal response to suxamethonium which may be MH-negative (Breuckling & Mortier, 1990). There have been a number of reports of cardiac arrest or rhabdomyolysis associated with anaesthesia in these patients in addition to a number of reports of patients who have had no abnormal response. The choice of anaesthetic agents should be based on avoidance of respiratory and cardiac depressant drugs. Inhalation and intravenous drugs have been used for induction of anaesthesia without complication although halothane induction alone has been reported to produce rhabdomyolysis and cardiac arrest from MH (Kelfer *et al.*, 1983) and should probably be avoided. Vecuronium has been used without complication (Buzello & Huttarsch, 1988) although the recovery time was longer than normal and neuromuscular transmission was allowed to recover spontaneously. This is important as Buzello and colleagues (1982) had previously reported a tonic response to neostigmine as seen by a marked increase in baseline tension.

In addition the possibility of late-onset problems should also be considered. Smith and Bush (1985) reported six cases of delayed respiratory depression and muscle weakness after suxamethonium. All patients had uneventful anaesthesia with recovery of muscle function to preoperative levels. However, inadequate ventilation was apparent 5–36 h after anaesthesia. Five of the six patients died as a result of cardiac arrest, which was presumed to be related to cardiomyopathy. The actual mechanism for the above events was unclear, but observation should be carried out for longer periods than normal.

Dystrophia myotonica

The characteristic response of the myotonias is persistent contraction either as inability to relax after voluntary use, or in response to mechanical stimulation of a muscle. Although the myotonia is the classical response which can be elicited by percussion of muscles or may be precipitated by cold, these patients also show considerable weakness and atrophy. Inherited as an autosomal dominant with variable penetrance, there is an incidence of 5 : 100 000 which may be an underestimate due to misdiagnosis or patients not seeking medical attention. Although the primary symptoms are related to muscle dysfunction, it is a systemic disease associated with cataracts, frontal balding, gonadal atrophy, various endocrine disorders, cholelithiasis and intellectual changes. The typical features also include facial weakness, pharyngeal dystrophy with nasal speech and difficulty in swallowing, delayed gastric emptying due to poor smooth-muscle motility, cardiomyopathy and cardiac conduction disorders. Weakness of respiratory muscles also occurs and patients often die of cardiorespiratory failure.

The disease is due to an abnormality of calcium metabolism in skeletal, smooth and cardiac muscle. There is a failure of calcium ATPase to return calcium from the sarcoplasmic reticulum following depolarization of the muscle membrane. This allows continued contraction following stimulation and the typical myotonia. There are also characteristic changes in the muscle histology which eventually progress to include necrosis and fibrosis associated with myopathy (Buxton, 1980).

Anaesthesia

The disease may be unrecognized at presentation for anaesthesia which may unmask the diagnosis. Complications associated with anaesthesia may be related to the severity of the disease or the response to drugs. The classical dilemma is the response to suxamethonium which, although variable may induce severe myotonia. Several cases have been reported where generalized myotonia has resulted from the administration of suxamethonium. A typical response includes generalized spasm followed by a jaw clamped shut and a rigid abdomen. Intubation and ventilation may prove impossible until relaxation occurs. Mitchell and colleagues (1978) demonstrated a rise in baseline muscle tension with a smaller-than-anticipated decrease in twitch height after even a small dose of suxamethonium. Similarly, the response to anticholinesterases is unpredictable as they have been used successfully to reverse non-depolarizing block (Blumgart *et al.*, 1990) but alone, neostigmine has also resulted in myotonia (Buzello *et al.*, 1982). Myotonia may also be precipitated by shivering associated with cold, halothane and extradural anaesthesia. Since the underlying abnormality is of the muscle rather than the nerves or the neuromuscular junction, this muscle activity is not suppressed by general or regional anaesthesia. Direct infiltration of local anaesthetic suppresses the abnormal muscle action and this may be used to avoid myotonia at the operation site or elsewhere (Cope & Miller, 1986).

The response to non-depolarizing muscle relaxants is also variable. Some reports have indicated a normal response (Mitchell *et al.*, 1978), whereas others have suggested increased sensitivity (Azar, 1984). Although myotonia is the classical sign, the response to the non-depolarizing agents may depend upon the severity of the dystrophic wasting associated with the disease and the size of the dose of non-depolarizing agent. Nightingale and colleagues (1985) reported the use of atracurium in a severe case of myotonia 'without sensitivity'. However, intubation was achieved after 10 mg atracurium when the $T_4 : T_1$ ratio was 0. The true response to these drugs is not clear as it is difficult to distinguish between the neuromuscular effects of induction agents, inhalation agents and non-depolarizing muscle relaxants.

Unexpectedly, there may also be a sensitivity to thiopentone (Aldridge, 1985). There have been numerous occasions when thiopentone has been used without complication but a number of authors have described cases where prolonged apnoea followed its use. Whether the cases described were due to respiratory depression or laryngeal myotonia and airway obstruction is uncertain. The response appears to be idiosyncratic, so that an intravenous induction agent should be given in the smallest possible dose. Induction may alternatively be achieved by the use of an inhalation agent but respiratory weakness may still be a problem and cardiac conduction defects may also result in heart block.

Complications due to the severity of the disease are usually associated with cardiorespiratory failure and may appear after the end of an uncomplicated case (Moore & Moore, 1987). Preoperative preparation includes assessment of the patient for evidence of respiratory failure, pulmonary infection and cardiac involvement. Chest infection may arise as a result of atrophic respiratory weakness and inability to cough effectively or be due to myotonia. Alternatively, aspiration may occur with pharyngeal involvement. It has been proposed that respiratory control is also altered with decreased ventilatory response to hypercapnia. However, it is probable that the reduction in response is primarily due to weakness and fatigue of muscles rather than altered responsiveness of the central and peripheral chemoreceptors.

The choice of anaesthetic technique depends upon the type of surgery proposed but small doses of induction agent and neuromuscular-blocking drugs should be used. Suxamethonium should be avoided and the non-depolarizing agents may not be required if weakness is clinically apparent, although atracurium may be the agent of choice because of its method of degradation and adequate neuromuscular monitoring is essential. Neither spinal anaesthesia nor neuromuscular block can guarantee prevention of myotonia, which can be modified by injecting local anaesthetic in the muscle itself. Controlled ventilation is recommended, but extubation should be delayed until ventilation is clearly adequate. Analgesia is required to encourage an adequate cough but respiratory depression should be avoided. Local anaesthetic techniques may offer advantages. Despite the problems of myotonia, patients continue to present for anaesthesia for investigation of sterility, cataracts and biliary surgery.

Congenital myotonia

Congenital dystrophia myotonica is a form of the disease which presents in infants. Older children may present with a mild form of the adult disease but neonates may present with difficulty in breathing, have a typical 'tent-shaped' mouth and mental retardation is usually present. Although weakness is present, myotonia does not occur in babies (Bray & Inkster, 1984) and cardiac abnormalities are not significant. Gradual improvement occurs in the first decade before the adult syndrome develops with the appearance of myotonia.

Familial periodic paralysis

The sporadic appearance of weakness with familial inheritance can be of three main types: hypokalaemic, normokalaemic and hyperkalaemic, although similarities can exist with other conditions.

Hypokalaemic periodic paralysis

Inherited as an autosomal dominant the disorder tends to appear more commonly in males and can occur sporadically without family history. Classically, it presents in the second decade with flaccid paralysis occurring after a meal high in carbohydrate content. Cold, exercise, emotional stress, hypokalaemia, liquorice, glucocorticoids or insulin may all predispose to or precipitate attacks. The paralysis is usually most profound in proximal muscles but with sparing of muscles of respiration and laryngeal reflexes. However, an attack may be so severe as to cause death from respiratory failure. During attacks, there is a profound decrease in serum potassium with associated cardiac arrhythmias. Symptoms may become apparent when the serum potassium concentration falls to 3 mmol/litre with severe weakness occurring between 2 and 2.5 mmol/litre. The muscles cannot be excited even by direct electromyographic stimulation though tendon reflexes are usually preserved.

Treatment is aimed at preventing hypokalaemia. Potassium supplements, acetazolamide which causes a metabolic acidosis and spironolactone which antagonizes aldosterone-induced urinary loss, all maintain serum potassium concentrations. The exact mechanism is uncertain but no additional potassium is excreted. It appears that extracellular potassium enters the muscle cells which alters the membrane potential and causes inexcitability during attacks.

Anaesthetic experiences in a family were presented by Horton in 1977. Preparation for anaesthesia includes avoidance of carbohydrate load in addition to control of potassium concentrations. During elective surgery the problems associated with changes in potassium concentrations are infrequent. However it is usually recommended that dextrose-containing solutions are avoided, the use of muscle relaxants minimized and neuromuscular monitoring used with measurement of potassium concentrations. The most important aspect of the intraoperative care is to monitor temperature and maintain normothermia. A more significant problem has been the management of the disease during extracorporeal bypass for cardiac surgery. It is recognized that potassium concentrations can vary markedly during bypass due to a number of factors including the use of insulin and dextrose containing cardioplegia, hypothermia and rewarming, bicarbonate to correct metabolic acidosis and the use of diuretics. Lema and colleagues (1991) following comments from Rollman and Dickson (1985) presented a case of hypothermic bypass without complication. Although it has been recommended that the use of muscle relaxants be avoided (Melnick *et al.*, 1983), Bashford (1977) described a normal response to D-tubocurarine and Rooney and colleagues (1988) reported the successful use of atracurium in a case without muscular weakness postoperatively. In addition to attention to the particular agents and techniques used which may produce a normal intraoperative course, it is also important to maintain adequate observation and monitoring in the postoperative period when late effects may become apparent.

Normokalaemic periodic paralysis

This condition occurs in early childhood. Attacks are precipitated by stresses similar to those provoking hypokalaemic periodic paralysis but the attacks are very severe, prolonged and respiratory and laryngeal muscular involvement is the rule. Despite normokalaemia, cardiac arrhythmias are common. Treatment is essentially supportive, although administration of sodium may be of benefit.

Hyperkalaemic periodic paralysis

The precipitating factors for this condition are almost

the opposite to those for hypokalaemic periodic paralysis. Attacks accompany hunger, exercise and administration of potassium. The attacks are frequently short-lived (less than 1 h) and occur during the day. Weakness occurs soon after exercise and involves limb, trunk and facial muscles and is accompanied with massive outpouring of potassium from affected muscle. This results in hyperkalaemia with associated ECG changes. Myotonia may also occur although respiratory involvement is rare. Hyperkalaemia is treated by dextrose and insulin with sodium replacement. Anaesthetic problems include prolonged paralysis, which may be precipitated by preoperative starvation. This may be remedied by intravenous hydration with dextrose solutions. The use of muscle relaxants is probably not recommended. Suxamethonium may induce potassium release and induce myotonia. Although non-depolarizing agents are probably safe, reversal with neostigmine may also induce myotonia. For this reason, atracurium would be the agent of choice, leaving the neuromuscular function to recover spontaneously.

Multiple sclerosis

Multiple sclerosis is an example of demyelinating disease of the CNS. The disease is acquired most commonly in young adults between 15 and 40 years in temperate climates. Genetic factors are involved in the aetiology with theories of viral infection resulting in altered immune responses. Small rises in temperature (0.5°C) have also been implicated in the production of additional neurological signs. Symptoms relate to the area of demyelination within the CNS. Lesions of the cerebellar region cause disturbance of gait, the optic-nerve visual changes and the spinal-cord sensory and motor changes. Urinary incontinence and sexual impotence may be early symptoms. Later problems include spasticity and tremor. Classically, symptoms occur over a few days and then gradually improve after a stable period of a few weeks. The intermittent nature of the disease would suggest that biochemical changes cause any initial problems before demyelination occurs. Intermittent exacerbation with remission but gradual progression of symptoms may lead to chronic disability and orthopaedic problems which require surgery.

Anaesthesia

Preoperative assessment should take account of the progress of the disease including any recent relapse. The effect of additional stress from surgery may exacerbate the symptoms of multiple sclerosis whatever anaesthetic technique is utilized. As a result of the above changes and the intermittent nature of the disease, postoperatively, exacerbations may be blamed on the anaesthetic drugs used. Evidence of any infection should be sought because of the potential for exacerbation with pyrexia. The degree of spasticity and muscle atrophy should be carefully assessed in association with any kyphoscoliosis to ensure adequate ventilation can be maintained and any muscle relaxants are used in appropriate dosages. Respiratory function testing may be required if major degrees of impairment are thought to be present. There is increased platelet aggregation with multiple sclerosis so that prophylaxis against deep vein thrombosis should be considered and an increased incidence of epilepsy may alter the choice of anaesthetic agents used.

The choice of anaesthetic technique lies between general anaesthesia and regional anaesthesia. General anaesthesia is most commonly selected as there is concern that local anaesthetics may cause exacerbations of the disease. Jones and Healey (1980) reviewed several reports and concluded that spinal anaesthesia should be avoided in multiple sclerosis as complications may result. However Crawford and colleagues (1981) reported the successful use of extradural anaesthesia in more than 50 cases of multiple sclerosis without complication. The lower concentrations of local anaesthetic with the extradural route may be the reason for this relative safety.

Although general anaesthesia is usually chosen, the drugs used should be selected with care. Methohexitone and enflurane should probably not be used because of the association with epilepsy. As with other neuromuscular diseases, care should be exercised with the use of depolarizing muscle relaxants as hyperkalaemic responses have been observed in multiple sclerosis with large masses of atrophic muscle. The non-depolarizing muscle relaxants should also be used with care as atrophy may reduce the dose requirement of the drugs. Corticosteroids have been used to minimize the extent of any relapse after surgery, and antipyretics have been given prophylactically to prevent any rise in body temperature. As with all patients with muscle weakness, careful observation should be carried out in the postoperative period to detect any changes in muscle function.

Skin and connective tissue disorders

Many of the skin diseases are rare in their association with anaesthesia and there are few reports regarding their management in the anaesthetic literature. The connective tissue disorder which is well documented is rheumatoid disease and this is discussed separately. However, there are many similarities between the different skin and connective tissue disorders. Many connective tissue disorders involve more than one system. The presence of cardiac or respiratory impairment may be more pertinent to the anaesthetic management than the external manifestations.

Problems associated with the skin

Many skin diseases may cause abnormal *skin fragility*, which may result in blister formation or bullae. Epidermolysis bullosa is an inherited disorder of varying degree of severity. Minor trauma may result in blister formation which may progress to scar formation. All mucosal surfaces are at risk and this includes the airway. Patients in whom the diagnosis has been made preoperatively may be on steroid therapy to minimize the effects of trauma. Reports of cases presenting during anaesthesia (Lee & Nagel, 1975; Pratilas & Biezunski, 1975) highlight the potential problems of the disease. Profuse bleeding resulted from bullae induced by minor trauma and the patient was observed for delayed respiratory obstruction. Pemphigus and pemphigoid are similar diseases where there is bullous formation at different sites within the skin. Toxic epidermal necrolysis and Stevens−Johnson syndrome are two other diseases which may result in skin damage after minimal trauma.

The anaesthetic implications are multiple. Simple monitoring, e.g. automatic arterial pressure measurements, may cause skin damage in severe cases. Minor trauma to the airway with an oro- or nasopharyngeal airway or after tracheal intubation may result in skin damage. This may lead to ulceration with an increased risk of infection, loss of fluid, bleeding as described or scar formation in the longer term. Other causes of skin damage include: adhesive tape used to secure intravenous infusions; pressure from external sources such as inadequately protected arm supports; and even face masks when applied with firm pressure. If generalized skin disruption occurs (e.g. in Stevens−Johnson syndrome) temperature, and more importantly, fluid homeostasis may be disrupted. All care should be continued into the postoperative period.

Long-term scarring of the skin may result in difficulty in two major areas — obtaining intravenous access and intubation of the trachea. Scleroderma is recognized to produce more scarring than many skin disorders. This characteristically results in a small 'fish' mouth because of skin contracture with severe limitation in jaw movement and well-recognized problems at intubation of the trachea. Superficial veins may be particularly difficult to see and central venous cannulation may be required. Some of the problems with scleroderma in anaesthesia are described by Younker and Harrison (1985).

Systemic problems associated with connective tissue disease

In addition to problems associated directly with the skin, patients may have complications caused by therapy or generalized involvement.

Corticosteroid therapy

Patients with active skin or connective tissue disease may be prescribed steroids. Chronic therapy is associated with many problems. There may be local effects in the skin (e.g. bruising and fragile veins) and systemic effects seen in Cushing's syndrome. Connective tissue disorders where steroid therapy may be used include SLE, polyarteritis nodosa, dermatomyositis, sarcoidosis and rheumatoid arthritis.

Visceral involvement

Although often considered to be superficial disease, these disorders may have widespread effects on visceral function (e.g. polyarteritis nodosa, which produces generalized end-organ disease). All the major organs may be involved to some degree according to the specific disease.

Cardiac involvement occurs with sarcoid, polyarteritis nodosa, SLE and rheumatoid arthritis and may consist of left ventricular enlargement, congestive cardiac failure or angina pectoris. Scleroderma may produce primary heart disease or congestive cardiac failure as a result of pulmonary hypertension.

Respiratory disease may take a number of forms. Rheumatoid arthritis and scleroderma may result in pulmonary fibrosis, whereas sarcoid shows evidence of granulomatous changes or hilar enlargement. All reduce pulmonary compliance and may eventually end in respiratory failure. Changes in oesophageal motility and incoordination of swallowing resulting in aspiration of food material may give rise to chronic lung infection with dermatomyositis.

Muscle disease is most apparent in dermatomyositis where specific weakness may occur. There is increased sensitivity to neuromuscular-blocking drugs, whereas in other diseases there may be generalized debility and malaise without weakness.

Renal disease is often present in SLE, polyarteritis nodosa and rheumatoid arthritis (as amyloid). This may progress to end-stage renal failure or cause altered drug excretion.

Other evidence of generalized disease may be anaemia which may follow from any chronic disease. This may be marked and require treatment before surgery.

Anaesthesia

The choice of anaesthetic regimen is directed towards the specific requirements of the surgeon and the state of the patient. Attention to detail is necessary (e.g. specific care may need to be taken in positioning and protection of the skin). General or regional anaesthesia may be acceptable except in cases of scleroderma where unpredictable spread and prolonged duration of action of local anaesthesia may occur (Thomson & Conklin, 1983).

Rheumatoid arthritis

This chronic, progressive symmetrical polyarthropathy affects some 2% of the population, with a 3 : 1 female preponderance. Onset can be at any age, but it occurs commonly in the 30s. The disease is characterized by proliferative inflammation of the synovium with subperiosteal erosion of affected joints. Synovial invasion of the articular surface occurs producing destruction of the joint. Healing occurs by fibrosis, both in the joint and in the surrounding ligaments producing characteristic deformities. Extra-articular manifestations of the disease are very common and include congestive cardiac failure, angina, diffuse pulmonary fibrosis, pleural effusions, pulmonary granulomata and fibrotic nodules in the lung (Caplan's nodules). The disease is chronic, mutilating and debilitating. Normocytic, normochromic anaemia is the rule and infection is common. Some 20% of sufferers develop renal amyloidosis with additional renal problems due to vasculitis. Pulmonary function is made worse by involvement of the costovertebral joints, which produces a restrictive ventilatory defect. Rheumatoid nodules can occur, typically on the extensor surface of the arms, but they may occur anywhere, including the myocardium.

Additional problems may arise due to the drugs used in the medical management of the disease. Pain, stiffness and inflammation are treated using non-steroidal anti-inflammatory drugs such as salicylates which may result in gastrointestinal haemorrhage and impair platelet function making any anaemia worse. Steroids may still be used although they are not considered first-line treatment and produce their well-known side-effects. Gold salts are effective at reducing the inflammation but may produce additional renal damage leading to nephrotic syndrome, bone-marrow depression and exfoliative dermatitis. Penicillamine may also produce a similar picture but a myasthenic type state may also occur.

Anaesthesia

These patients may have considerable deformities which require surgical correction and particularly joint replacement surgery and an individual may undergo repeated anaesthetics. In addition to the associated pathology already mentioned deformities and nodules may cause problems in transport and positioning for surgery and identification of the anatomy for regional anaesthesia may be very difficult. The skin may be atrophic due to the disease and steroid therapy. However, probably the most important area is the potential for a difficult intubation. Airway problems are not uncommon (Table 55.4).

Accurate preoperative assessment is of prime importance. Clinical examination should be aimed at identifying any limitation of neck extension or subluxation and radiological examination should include flexion–extension views. Jaw opening should be specifically assessed and changes in the voice should alert the anaesthetist to laryngeal involvement. The cricoarytenoid joint is not infrequently involved and may produce a narrowed airway (Phelps, 1966).

Cardiovascular assessment should include clinical examination and ECG and chest X-ray with additional tests such as echocardiography for conduction, pericardial and valvular abnormalities as

Table 55.4 Airway problems in rheumatoid arthritis

1 *Temporomandibular joint*: involvement limiting the degree of mouth opening
2 *Cervical spine arthritis*: may be severe in as many as 50% of cases. Neck mobility may be limited with the potential for atlantoaxial subluxation and cord compression
3 *Laryngeal synovial joints*: may result in airway narrowing
4 *Mandibular hypoplasia*: from chronic disease in the young and steroid therapy

indicated. Laboratory tests should include blood count and electrolyte measurements with possible assessment of clotting and pulmonary function tests.

At first glance, regional techniques would appear to be attractive for orthopaedic procedures. Some of the typical problems are described by Hodgkinson (1981). However, deformities may alter landmarks and make the performance of nerve blocks difficult. Spinal (intrathecal or extradural) anaesthesia may be difficult due to rigidity of the back, calcified ligaments and narrow interspaces.

General anaesthesia may be difficult because of uncertainties with the airway. Intravenous induction and the use of muscle relaxants cannot be recommended unless it can be guaranteed that the airway can be secured. The options for achieving intubation without vigorous flexion or extension vary between centres but include: inhalation induction and blind nasal intubation; or direct laryngoscopy and intubation with the patient breathing spontaneously or fibre-optic laryngoscopy and intubation under local or general anaesthesia. With the advent of fine, flexible laryngoscopes, awake intubation under local anaesthesia with or without sedation must be recommended, except in children.

In addition to meticulous care being required with positioning, all drugs should be used with caution. Cardiac and renal function may be limited resulting in myocardial depression or prolonged action of drugs and impaired oxygenation due to anaemia or respiratory disease requires high-inspired oxygen concentrations and controlled ventilation. Postoperative care requires adequate analgesia and appropriate oxygen therapy. (See specific chapters for details of anaesthesia in diseases of particular systems.)

Drug abuse and anaesthesia

Increasingly, the chances are that a patient presenting for anaesthesia is taking regularly or has taken substances which alter the patient's response to anaesthesia or may modify the management of anaesthesia and the recovery period. Within the USA it is well recognized that substance abuse is related to violence and trauma but in the UK, it is also a significant problem (Wood & Soni, 1989). The number of drugs used illegally is increasing, the use of alcohol is widespread and patients are commonly dependent on sedative drugs. Patients may present with trauma in an acutely drug-intoxicated state, or may present for elective surgery when the problems of chronic use and withdrawal may arise. In addition to the problems during resuscitation and anaesthesia, the

Table 55.5 Problems and definitions associated with drug addiction

---

1 *Addiction*: Compulsive need to take a drug
2 *Dependence*: May be psychological or physical. Effects of habitual and repeated exposure
3 *Tolerance*: Increased quantities of drug required to produce observed effects
4 *Withdrawal*: Physical and psychological effects which may be life-threatening when drug is not available
5 *Acute overdose*: Severe effects seen with excessive doses
6 *Pathological effects*: Secondary to metabolic and nutritional effects

---

problems of withdrawal in the recovery period will be discussed.

It is commonly recognized that the effects of acute overdose may be life-threatening but the consequences of acute withdrawal, especially in a severely traumatized postoperative patient, may be similarly severe. The problems and definitions associated with drug addiction are listed in Table 55.5. The mechanisms by which tolerance develops are increased rates of metabolism due to stimulation of liver enzymes so that less drug is available and reduced responsiveness of receptors as they adapt to the continual presence of drug. Cross-tolerance may also occur with other drugs and hence the old adage that 'alcoholics require more anaesthetic' and the difficulty in assessing anaesthetic and analgesic requirements in the chronic user. However, the additive effects of depressant drugs seen immediately after acute use may indicate the need for reduced doses. The effects of acute withdrawal vary with the drug in question but will relate to the physiological effects of the drug and the elimination half-life of the drug as to when symptoms will begin to appear.

Specific drugs

Alcohol

Alcoholism continues to be prevalent in today's society and despite attempts to reduce the incidence of drinking and driving, acutely intoxicated victims of accidents continue to require treatment. In the acutely intoxicated patient, lack of co-operation makes therapeutic procedures more difficult. The risk of vomiting is high and aspiration may have already occurred. In the severe case, respiratory depression may add to the problems of recovery and oxygenation and prevents respiratory compensation for metabolic acidosis. Marked vasodilatation may cause increased heat loss and reduce the ability to

compensate for blood loss and there may be a chronic reduction in the plasma volume. The rapid preoperative assessment required in emergencies should also look for the problems associated with chronic alcoholism, including hypoglycaemia and withdrawal (Edwards & Mosher, 1980).

Chronic alcoholism results in a wide range of pathological changes. There may be reduced stress responses, impaired defence mechanisms, bone marrow depression, electrolyte and fluid imbalance, hypoglycaemia, liver disease, cardiomyopathy, peripheral or autonomic neuropathy, drug tolerance and acute withdrawal syndrome (Edwards, 1985). Preoperative assessment should permit full evaluation of the extent of such changes in an individual. The extensive metabolic and pathological effects are discussed in greater depth in Edwards and Mosher (1980). Anaesthesia traditionally has involved larger doses of drugs because of enzyme induction and tolerance but these may not be the only changes and it may not always be a safe assumption. Large doses of induction agents may result in marked hypotension in cardiomyopathy and in hypoalbuminaemia with reduced protein binding. Cirrhosis may alter the metabolism of non-depolarizing muscle relaxants. Alcoholics are more prone to hypoxia and cerebral damage, especially in the withdrawal syndrome. Specific anaesthetic techniques should be modified according to the state of individual patients and their surgery.

The withdrawal syndrome produces tremor, sweating, vomiting and muscular weakness and may start within 8h of abstinence. The patient becomes agitated and hostile and may suffer hallucinations. Delerium tremens is more serious but does not occur in all patients. It may not occur for several days but is characterized by extreme disorientation, hallucinations and hyperthermia and is usually preceded by grand mal seizures. Management of the patient may be impossible unless alcohol is allowed or drugs given to prevent symptoms and progression to serious effects. Chlormethiazole or benzodiazepines are effective intravenously or orally if applicable but should be used to produce anxiolysis and sedation without loss of protective reflexes. Tissue hypoxia is a feature and oxygen should be administered.

Opioids

Opioids are frequently abused and may be administered by a number of routes including intravenous, nasal and sublingual. Although well absorbed from the gastrointestinal tract, this route is not commonly used as extensive metabolism reduces the effects of the drug. With parenteral administration, many of the problems of intravenous users are infective in origin; cellulitis, abscesses, thrombophlebitis and septic arthritis. Transmission of hepatitis or human immunodeficiency virus (HIV) may lead to more serious sequelae. Tolerance to the analgesic, euphoric and sedative effects may occur with cross-tolerance between the opioids.

Withdrawal produces sympathetic effects of hypertension, tachycardia, sweating with tremors, flushes and muscle and bone discomfort as withdrawal progresses. Severe abdominal cramps and muscle spasms will occur but are not life-threatening. Clonidine is now used to relieve such symptoms by its alpha-2 agonist effects.

Anaesthesia should involve adequate preoperative medication to allay anxiety and an equivalent dose of opioid drug should continue to be given to avoid withdrawal. Anaesthesia may be maintained with volatile agents rather than the large doses of opioids which would be required. However, mixed agonists/ antagonists should not be used as they produce the problems associated with withdrawal. Regional anaesthetic techniques which reduce the need for postoperative analgesia may help in the management of such patients. One of the problems of opioids is that patients may manage to maintain their own supplies with resultant overdose when medical prescriptions are also given. Treatment of overdose depends on the symptoms produced but is readily reversed by antagonists.

Cocaine

The use of cocaine varies between centres but is generally increasing and is widespread through the USA. It is most commonly inhaled nasally and may result in septal ulceration, or it may be smoked in a highly purified form as 'crack' when it has been removed from its hydrochloride and the speed of onset of the 'free-base' is equivalent to intravenous administration. This may also produce an increased problem of accelerated dependence and the potential for withdrawal. One of the problems in the USA is the presentation of acute overdosage with cocaine. Patients present with acute anxiety or psychosis and signs of sympathetic stimulation consisting of hypertension, tachycardia and skin pallor. This progresses to seizures and ventricular arrhythmias, with respiratory failure, unconsciousness and circulatory failure (Dollery, 1991). The toxic effects may be alleviated by propranolol. As with other addictive drugs, depen-

dence, tolerance and withdrawal effects occur. Withdrawal results in profound depression (including suicide), tremor, muscle pains and EEG changes and may also occur in the newborn. Cocaine also has drug interactions with monoamine oxidase inhibitors as it potentiates catecholamines. Sudden death is more likely in those with reduced plasma cholinesterase activity as the drug is partly metabolized by this route.

Barbiturates and benzodiazepines

Addiction and dependence to these drugs may be related to medical prescription for sedation and anxiolysis or to substance abuse in young adults. Physical dependence and withdrawal may occur but is less severe and more delayed with benzodiazepines due to slower elimination and production of active metabolites. However potentially life-threatening effects may be seen with withdrawal due to grand mal seizures or cardiovascular collapse. Cross-tolerance may occur with anaesthetic drugs resulting in awareness if inadequate doses are used and enzyme induction may occur with the barbiturates but not the benzodiazepines.

References

Neuroendocrine tumours

Bloom S.R. & Polak J.M. (1987a) Glucagonoma syndrome. *American Journal of Medicine* 82 (Suppl. 5B), 25–35.

Bloom S.R. & Polak J.M. (1987b) Somatostatin. *British Medical Journal* 295, 288–90.

Casthely P.A., Jablons M., Griepp R.B., Ergin M.A. & Goodman K. (1986) Ketanserin in the preoperative and intraoperative management of a patient with carcinoid tumour undergoing tricuspid valve replacement. *Anesthesia and Analgesia* 65, 809–11.

Chahal P. & O'Shea J.P. (1984) Ectopic ACTH syndrome. *Hospital Update* 10, 263–76.

Colella J.J. & Vandam L.D. (1972) Diethyl ether anaesthesia for a patient with hyperinsulinism. *Anesthesiology* 37, 354–6.

Creutzfeldt W. & Stockmann F. (1987) Carcinoids and carcinoid syndrome. *American Journal of Medicine* 82 (Suppl. 5B), 4–16.

Déry R. (1971) Theoretical and clinical considerations in anaesthesia for secreting carcinoid tumours. *Canadian Anaesthetists' Society Journal* 18, 245–63.

Dollery C. (1991) *Octreotide. Therapeutic Drugs* vol. 2. pp. 1–4. Churchill Livingstone, Edinburgh.

Fischler M., Dentan M. & Westerman M.N. (1983) Prophylactic use of ketanserin in a patient with carcinoid syndrome. *British Journal of Anaesthesia* 55, 920.

Friesen S.R. (1987) Update on the diagnosis and treatment of rare neuroendocrine tumours. *Surgical Clinics of North America* 67, 379–93.

Frolich J.C., Bloomgarden Z.T., Oates J.A., McGuigan J.E. & Rabinowitz D. (1978) The carcinoid flush. *New England Journal of Medicine* **299**, 1055—7.

Hargadon J.J. & Ormston T.O.G. (1963) Anaesthesia for excision of islet-cell tumour of the pancreas. *British Journal of Anaesthesia* **35**, 807—10.

Houghton K. & Carter J.A. (1986) Peri-operative management of carcinoid syndrome using ketanserin. *Anaesthesia* **41**, 596—9.

Hughes E.W. & Hodkinson B.P. (1989) Carcinoid syndrome: the combined use of ketanserin and octreotide in the management of an acute crisis during anaesthesia. *Anaesthesia and Intensive Care* **17**, 367—9.

Kaplan E.L., Arganini M. & Kang S.J. (1987) Diagnosis and treatment of hypoglycaemic disorders. *Surgical Clinics of North America* **67**, 395—410.

Karam J.H., Lorenzi M., Young C.W., Burns A.D., Prosser P.R., Grodsky G.M., Galante M. & Forsham P.H. (1979) Feedback-controlled dextrose infusion during surgical management of insulinomas. *American Journal of Medicine* **66**, 675—80.

Krejs G.J. (1987) VIPoma syndrome. *American Journal of Medicine* **82** (Suppl. 5B), 37—47.

Marsh H.M., Martin J.K., Kvols L.K., Gracey D.R., Warner M.A., Warner M.E. & Moertel C.G. (1987) Carcinoid crisis during anaesthesia: successful treatment with a somatostatin analogue. *Anesthesiology* **66**, 89—91.

Mason R.A. & Steane P.A. (1976) Carcinoid syndrome: its relevance to the anaesthetist. *Anaesthesia* **31**, 228—42.

Maton P.N., Camilleri M., Allison D.J., Hodgson H.J.E. & Chadwick V.S. (1983) Role of hepatic arterial embolisation in the carcinoid syndrome. *British Medical Journal* **287**, 932—5.

McCrirrick A. & Hickman J. (1991) Octreotide for carcinoid syndrome. *Canadian Journal of Anaesthesia* **38**, 539—40.

Muir J.J., Endres S.M., Offord K., van Heerden J.A. & Tinker J.H. (1983) Glucose management in patients undergoing operation for insulinoma removal. *Anesthesiology* **59**, 371—5.

Nicoll J.M.V. & Catling S.J. (1985) Anaesthetic management of glucagonoma. *Anaesthesia* **40**, 152—7.

O'Dorisio T.M. (1986) Gut endocrinology: clinical and therapeutic impact. *American Journal of Medicine* **81** (Suppl. 6B), 1—7.

Parry T., Perera J. & Hammond J.E. (1986) Anaesthesia and gastric carcinoid. *Anaesthesia* **41**, 1265—6.

Roy R.C., Carter R.F. & Wright P.D. (1987) Somatostatin, anaesthesia and the carcinoid syndrome. *Anaesthesia* **42**, 627—32.

Solares G., Glanco E., Pulgar S., Diago C. & Ramos F. (1987) Carcinoid syndrome and intravenous cyproheptadine. *Anaesthesia* **42**, 989—92.

Townsend C.M. & Thompson J.C. (1986) Gastrinoma. *Surgical Clinics of North America* **66**, 695—712.

Tsai S.-T., Eckhauser F.E., Thompson N.W., Strodel W.E. & Vinik A.I. (1986) Perioperative use of long-acting somatostatin analogue in patients with endocrine tumours of gastroenteropancreatic axis. *Surgery* **100**, 788—95.

Walter J.B. & Israel M.S. (1987) *General Pathology* 6th edn. pp. 484—6. Churchill Livingstone, Edinburgh.

Watson J.T., Badner N.H. & Ali M.J. (1990) The prophylactic use of octreotide in a patient with ovarian carcinoid and valvular heart disease. *Canadian Journal of Anaesthesia* **37**, 798—800.

Williams F.D. & Sandler M. (1963) The classification of carcinoid tumours. *Lancet* **i**, 238—9.

Wood S.M. & Bloom S.R. (1984) Glucagonoma syndrome. *Hospital Update* **10**, 573—9.

Muscle diseases

Aldridge L.M. (1985) Anaesthetic problems in myotonic dystrophy. *British Journal of Anaesthesia* **57**, 1119—30.

Azar I. (1984) The response of patients with neuromuscular disorders to muscle relaxants: a review. *Anesthesiology* **61**, 173—87.

Baraka A. & Tabboush Z. (1991) Neuromuscular response to succinylcholine—vecuronium sequence in three myasthenic patients undergoing thymectomy. *Anesthesia and Analgesia* **72**, 827—30.

Bashford A.C. (1977) Case report: anesthesia in familial hypokalemic periodic paralysis. *Anesthesia Intensive Care* **5**, 74—5.

Bell C.F., Florence A.M., Hunter J.M., Jones R.S. & Utting J.E. (1984) Atracurium in the myasthenic patient. *Anaesthesia* **39**, 961—8.

Blumgart C.H., Hughes D.G. & Redfern N. (1990) Obstetric anaesthesia in dystrophia myotonica. *Anaesthesia* **45**, 26—9.

Boltshauser E., Steinmann B., Meyer A. & Jerusalem F. (1980) Anaesthesia-induced rhabdomyolysis in Duchenne muscular dystrophy. *British Journal of Anaesthesia* **52**, 559.

Bray R.J. & Inkster J.S. (1984) Anaesthesia in babies with congenital dystrophia myotonica. *Anaesthesia* **39**, 1007—11.

Breuckling E. & Mortier W. (1990) Anesthesia in neuromuscular diseases. *Acta Anaesthesiologica Belgica* **41**, 127—32.

Brownell A.K.W., Paasuke R.T., Elash A., Fowlow S.B., Seagram C.G.F., Diewold R.J. & Friesen C. (1983) Malignant hyperthermia in Duchenne muscular dystrophy. *Anesthesiology* **58**, 180—2.

Burgess F.W. & Wilcosky B. (1989) Thoracic epidural anesthesia for transsternal thymectomy in myasthenia gravis. *Anesthesia and Analgesia* **69**, 529—31.

Buxton P.H. (1980) Pathology of muscle. *British Journal of Anaesthesia* **52**, 139—51.

Buzello W. & Huttarsch H. (1988) Muscle relaxation in patients with Duchenne's muscular dystrophy. *British Journal of Anaesthesia* **60**, 228—31.

Buzello W., Krieg N. & Schlickewei A. (1982) Hazards of neostigmine in patients with neuromuscular disorders. *British Journal of Anaesthesia* **54**, 529—34.

Cooperman L.H., Strobel G.E. & Kennell E.M. (1970) Massive hyperkalemia after administration of succinylcholine. *Anesthesiology* **32**, 161—4.

Cope D.K. & Miller J.N. (1986) Local and spinal anesthesia for Caesarean section in a patient with myotonic dystrophy. *Anesthesia and Analgesia* **65**, 687—90.

Crawford J.S., James F.M., Nolte H., Van Steenberge A. & Shah J.L. (1981) Regional anaesthesia for patients with chronic neurological disease and similar conditions. *Anaesthesia* **36**, 821.

Eisenkraft J.B., Book W.J., Mann S.M., Papatestas A.E. & Hubbard M. (1988) Resistance to succinylcholine in myasthenia gravis: a dose—response study. *Anesthesiology* **69**, 760—3.

Eisenkraft J.B., Book W.J. & Papatestas A.E. (1990) Sensitivity to vecuronium in myasthenia gravis: a dose—response study.

Canadian Journal of Anaesthesia **37**, 301–6.

Fergusson R.J., Wright D.J., Willey R.F., Crompton G.K. & Grant I.W.B. (1981) Suxamethonium is dangerous in polyneuropathy. *British Medical Journal* **282**, 298–9.

Horton B. (1977) Anesthetic experiences in a family with hypokalemic familial periodic paralysis. *Anesthesiology* **47**, 308–10.

Jones R.M. & Healy T.E.J. (1980) Anaesthesia and demyelinating disease. *Anaesthesia* **35**, 879–84.

Kelfer H.M., Singer W.D. & Reynolds R.N. (1983) Malignant hyperthermia in a child with Duchenne muscular dystrophy. *Pediatrics* **71**, 118–19.

Lema G., Urzua J., Moran S. & Canessa R. (1991) Successful anesthetic management of a patient with hypokalemic familial periodic paralysis undergoing cardiac surgery. *Anesthesiology* **74**, 373–5.

Leventhal S.R., Orkin F.K. & Hirsh R.A. (1980) Prediction of the need for postoperative mechanical ventilation in myasthenia gravis. *Anesthesiology* **53**, 26–30.

Melnick B., Chang J.L., Larson C.E. & Bedger R.C. (1983) Hypokalemic familial periodic paralysis. *Anesthesiology* **58**, 263–5.

Mitchell M.M., Ali H.H. & Savarese J.J. (1978) Myotonia and neuromuscular blocking agents. *Anesthesiology* **49**, 44–8.

Moore J.K. & Moore A.P. (1987) Postoperative complications of dystrophia myotonica. *Anaesthesia* **42**, 529–33.

Nicholson M.J. (1971) Circulatory collapse following succinylcholine: report of a patient with diffuse lower motor neuron disease. *Anesthesia and Analgesia* **50**, 431–7.

Nightingale P., Healy T.E.J. & McGuinness K. (1985) Dystrophia myotonica and atracurium. *British Journal of Anaesthesia* **57**, 1131–5.

Nilsson E. & Müller K. (1990) Neuromuscular effects of isoflurane in patients with myasthenia gravis. *Acta Anaesthesiologica Scandinavica* **34**, 126–31.

Nilsson E., Paloheimo M., Müller K. & Heinonen J. (1989) Halothane-induced variability in the neuromuscular transmission of patients with myasthenia gravis. *Acta Anaesthesiologica Scandinavica* **33**, 395–401.

Osserman K.E. & Genkins G. (1971) Studies in myasthenia gravis — review of a 20 year experience in over 1200 patients. *Mount Sinai Journal of Medicine* **38**, 497–537.

Rollman J.E. & Dickson C.M. (1985) Anaesthetic management of a patient with hypokalemic familial periodic paralysis for coronary artery bypass surgery. *Anesthesiology* **65**, 526–7.

Rooney R.T., Shanahan E.C., Sun T. & Nally B. (1988) Atracurium and hypokalemic familial periodic paralysis. *Anesthesia and Analgesia* **67**, 782–3.

Smith C.L. & Bush G.H. (1985) Anaesthesia and progressive muscular dystrophy. *British Journal of Anaesthesia* **57**, 1113–18.

Stone W.A., Beach T.P. & Hamelberg W. (1970) Succinylcholine — danger in the spinal-cord-injured patient. *Anesthesiology* **32**, 168–9.

Tolmie J.D., Joyce T.H. & Mitchell G.D. (1967) Succinylcholine danger in the burned patient. *Anesthesiology* **28**, 467–70.

Wainwright A.P. & Brodrick P.M. (1987) Suxamethonium in myasthenia gravis. *Anaesthesia* **42**, 950–7.

Skin and connective tissue disorders

Hodgkinson R. (1981) Anesthetic management of a parturient with severe rheumatoid arthritis. *Anesthesia and Analgesia* **60**, 611–12.

Lee C. & Nagel E. (1975) Anesthetic management of a patient with recessive epidermolysis bullosa dystrophica. *Anesthesiology* **43**, 122–4.

Phelps J.A. (1966) Laryngeal obstruction due to cricoarytenoid arthritis. *Anesthesiology* **27**, 518–22.

Pratilas V. & Biezunski A. (1975) Epidermolysis bullosa manifested and treated during anesthesia. *Anesthesiology* **43**, 581–3.

Thompson J. & Conklin K.A. (1983) Anesthetic management of a pregnant patient with scleroderma. *Anesthesiology* **59**, 69–71.

Younker D. & Harrison B. (1985) Scleroderma and pregnancy. *British Journal of Anaesthesia* **57**, 1136–9.

Drug abuse and anaesthesia

Dollery C. (1991) *Cocaine. Therapeutic Drugs* vol. 1, pp. C330–3. Churchill Livingstone, Edinburgh.

Edwards R. (1985) Anaesthesia and alcohol. *British Medical Journal* **291**, 423–4.

Edwards R. & Mosher V.B. (1980) Alcohol abuse, anaesthesia and intensive care. *Anaesthesia* **35**, 474–89.

Wood P.R. & Soni N. (1989) Anaesthesia and substance abuse. *Anaesthesia* **44**, 672–80.

Further reading

Katz J. & Steward D.J. (1987) *Anesthesia and Uncommon Pediatric Diseases*. W.B. Saunders, Philadelphia.

Katz J., Benumof J. & Kadis L.B. (1981) *Anesthesia and Uncommon Diseases. Pathophysiologic and Clinical Considerations* 2nd Ed. W.B. Saunders, Philadelphia.

Stoelting R.K., Dierdorf S.F. & McCammon R.L. (1988) *Anesthesia and Co-existing Disease* 2nd Ed. Churchill Livingstone, New York.

Anaesthetic Management of the Obese Patient

F.P. BUCKLEY

The definition of obesity is related usually to the individual's ideal body weight (IBW) taken from insurance companies' tables or derived from indices relating height to weight such as body mass index (BMI)*. Obesity is usually defined as beginning at IBW plus 20% or a BMI more than 28. Approximately 1–15% of adults in the UK (Rosenbaum et al., 1985) and the USA (Van Itallie, 1985) fall within this group. The massively obese, usually termed the morbidly obese (MO), are those who weigh more than IBW plus 45 kg, have a BMI in excess of 35, and constitute some 1–2% of the population. Mild obesity has minor implications for the patient's health and anaesthetic management, whereas MO has major implications for both health and anaesthetic management.

Obesity is associated with a wide variety of physiological and pathological abnormalities which may affect anaesthetic management (Fisher et al., 1975). The data on the pathological and physiological abnormalities found in obese patients and their implications for anaesthetic management discussed in this chapter have come primarily from studies of MO patients. The reader is cautioned to keep this in mind when applying the recommendations in this chapter to the management of those who are obese, but who are not MO. It is likely that obese patients who have not reached the heroic proportions of the MO will have physiological and pathological abnormalities similar to the MO, but probably to a lesser degree. The majority of the reports of anaesthetic management of the MO patient have concerned patients without evidence of clinically significant disease, other than obesity.

The presence of cardiovascular, respiratory or metabolic disease may produce further pathophysiological changes which may impair function further

and be associated with a high incidence of perioperative complications (Buckley et al., 1983).

Pathophysiology of obesity and preoperative evaluation

The magnitude of any physiological/pathological abnormalities associated with obesity depends to some extent on the anatomical distribution of body fat. Obese patients may be classified into those with android obesity (primarily truncal), with a waist : hip circumference ratio of greater than 0.9 in men or 0.7 in women, or gynaecoid obesity (primarily affecting hip, buttocks and thighs). Fat in the android distribution is metabolically more active than fat in the gynaecoid distribution and is associated with a greater increase in oxygen consumption ($\dot{V}o_2$). The MO with fat in the android distribution have more metabolic complications, and a higher incidence of mortality from ischaemic heart disease than gynaecoid MO. Further, evidence that the regional distribution of body fat has pathophysiologic significance is emerging, the MO with a high proportion of intra-abdominal fat have a high incidence of cardiovascular disease (Peiris et al., 1989) and left ventricular dysfunction (Nakajima et al., 1989).

Respiratory evaluation [Farebrother, 1979; Luce, 1980; Vaughan, 1982a (Fig. 56.1)]

While fat is not as metabolically active as muscle it does have a metabolic oxygen requirement and, as extra work is necessarily expended in moving parts or all of an obese body, $\dot{V}o_2$ and carbon dioxide output ($\dot{V}co_2$) in the obese patient are raised in comparison with non-obese patients. (Basal metabolic rate, being related to body surface area is usually within the range of normality.) Because of the necessity to move body-wall fat, the work of

---

* $BMI = \dfrac{weight\ (kg)}{height^2\ (m)}$. A 70-kg, 1.7-m male has a BMI of 26.

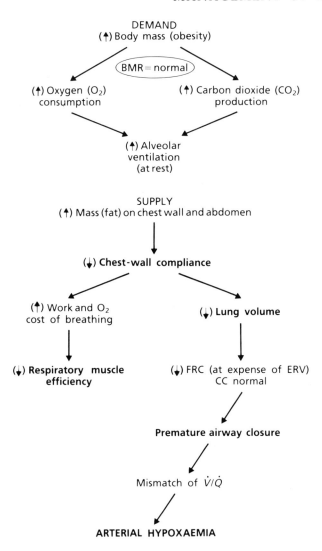

Fig. 56.1 Pulmonary dysfunction in the MO patient represented as a supply–demand imbalance leading to arterial hypoxaemia at rest. BMR, basal metabolic rate. (Redrawn from Vaughan, 1982a.)

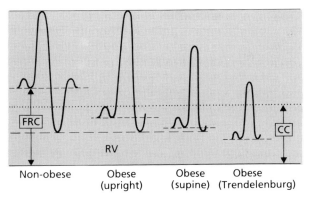

Fig. 56.2 The effect of body position on lung volumes in the MO patient. (Redrawn from Vaughan, 1982a.)

breathing is raised and, with the need for an increased minute volume of ventilation ($\dot{V}_E$) to maintain normocapnia, leads to an increased oxygen cost of breathing. Oxygen consumption during exercise increases more sharply in the obese patient than in normals, as does the oxygen cost of breathing during exercise; the latter implies respiratory muscle inefficiency.

The high oxygen cost of breathing results largely from the fact that total respiratory compliance in the obese patient may be as little as 30% normal. Such changes can be simulated in normals by mass-loading the lower thorax and upper abdomen. This reduction in total compliance is primarily a function of a

reduction in chest-wall compliance, lung compliance remaining essentially normal. Total compliance may be reduced further by lying down, presumably as a consequence of the additional chest-wall and abdominal load. The mass-loading of the thorax and abdomen produces effects upon other pulmonary volumes (Fig. 56.2). Residual volume remains normal but expiratory reserve volume (ERV) and functional residual capacity (FRC) are often reduced, even in the upright position. FRC may be reduced to the extent that it may fall within the range of closing capacity (CC), leading to alveolar closure in the upright position with ventilation : perfusion ($\dot{V}:\dot{Q}$) mismatch or a frank right–left shunt resulting in arterial hypoxaemia, even in the upright position (Table 56.1). On lying down FRC may fall further within CC with a consequent worsening of Pao_2. The effect of fat in the android distribution versus gynaecoid distribution upon respiratory parameters has not been studied.

Despite a low Pao_2, the majority of obese patients maintain a sufficient $\dot{V}_E$ to maintain normocapnia and a normal response to carbon dioxide challenge and hypoxaemia. However, with worsening obesity and time, some patients progress to fall within a group in whom $Paco_2$ increases and who rely then on hypoxic drive for respiration. This is termed the obesity hypoventilation syndrome (OHS) and is associated often with sleep apnoea, daytime hypersomnolence and potential or overt upper airway difficulties. At the worst end of the spectrum is the Pickwickian syndrome (obesity, hypersomnolence, hypoxia, hypercapnia, right ventricular failure and polycythaemia) described originally by Burwell and colleagues (1956).

Clinical history should concentrate on finding

Table 56.1 Mean values of preoperative respiratory measurements in MO patients

Author	Anaesthetic	Number	Mean age (years)	Mean weight (kg)	Mean height (cm)	Mean sitting Pa_{O_2} (mmHg)	FRC % predicted	ERV % predicted
Vaughan *et al.* (1974)	GA	20	30	144	168	74		
Fox (1975)	GA	13		137			50	26
Hedenstierna & Santesson (1976)	GA	10	41	134	169	74		
Anderson *et al.* (1977)	GA	37	38	130	168	79		
Hamm & Koehler (1979)	GA	21	34	145	163			
Gelman *et al.* (1980)	GA	17	39	137		85		
	TEB	21	36	149		79		
Fox *et al.* (1981)	GA and TEB	110	35	135		78		
Buckley *et al.* (1983)	GA	28	38	125	167	81	65	
	TEB	42	40	129	166	79	67	

GA, general anaesthesia; TEB, thoracic extradural block.

symptoms reflecting the previously mentioned abnormalities, i.e. dyspnoea on exertion, orthopnoea, symptoms suggestive of sleep apnoea syndrome and episodes of upper respiratory obstruction, especially if associated with anaesthesia and surgery. Physical examination should be thorough and it may be worthwhile measuring hip and waist circumferences and calculating the hip : waist circumference ratio as the android group may have an increased incidence of respiratory problems. Chest X-rays should be obtained and scrutinized. In young patients, routine tests such as forced vital capacity, forced expiratory volume in 1 s ($FEV_{1.0}$) and peak expiratory flow-rate are likely to be within normal limits. Such tests, however, may be helpful in identifying unsuspected respiratory disease. Arterial blood-gas measurements in the sitting and supine positions should be considered as useful indices of respiratory disease, to exclude OHS and may provide useful guidelines for perioperative oxygen administration. More detailed evaluations such as specific lung volumes (FRC, ERV) or $\dot{V}:\dot{Q}$ scans probably do not contribute much to routine preoperative evaluation. Given the degree of respiratory compromise often suffered by obese patients, it is important that their respiratory status is brought to an optimal state before embarking upon anaesthesia and surgery.

Cardiovascular evaluation (Reisin & Frolich, 1981; Vaughan, 1982a; Alexander, 1985)

Obesity is nearly always accompanied by alterations in haemodynamic status. Circulating blood volume, plasma volume and cardiac output increase proportionately with increasing weight and $\dot{V}_{O_2}$. Cerebral and renal blood flows approximate to those in normals, but splanchnic blood flow is approximately 20% higher than in normals. Much of the remainder of the increase in cardiac output is directed to fat stores. Blood flow to fat averages between $2-3\,\text{ml} \cdot 100\,\text{g tissue}^{-1} \cdot \text{min}^{-1}$ when at rest. Thus, for a patient 50 kg above IBW, fat accounts for 1.5−2 litres of extra cardiac output. Further portions of the increase in cardiac output go to muscle and skin, both of which may be increased in quantity in the obese patient.

Systemic arteriovenous oxygen content difference [$(a-v)C_{O_2}$] is usually normal or slightly raised in obese patients and thus the increase in cardiac output parallels the increase in $\dot{V}_{O_2}$, but cardiac index (being related to body surface area) is within the normal range. Pulse rate is usually normal and thus, to maintain an increased cardiac output, stroke volume increases. Direct arterial pressure measurements reveal severe hypertension in 5−10% of obese patients and moderate hypertension in 50% of patients. Cardiac output increases faster in response to exercise than in non-obese patients and is often associated with an increase in left ventricular end-diastolic pressure and pulmonary capillary wedge pressure. Changes in $\dot{V}o_2$ (raised 11%), cardiac output (raised 35%) and pulmonary artery pressure (raised 30%) similar to those seen during exercise have been reported when moving MO patients from the sitting to the standing position in the perioperative period; such changes are likely to occur in the postoperative period (Paul et al., 1976). Pulmonary hypertension may result often from a thickening of the small pulmonary arteries resulting in an increase in right ventricular afterload. In patients with OHS, chronic hypercapnia and hypoxia may lead to pulmonary vasoconstriction which, superimposed on the pre-existing effects of obesity, may produce severe left ventricular or biventricular failure.

Obesity is associated with changes in left ventricle size and function. Moderately obese (50% > IBW), normotensive patients with no evidence of coronary artery disease have been shown to have normal left ventricle function but raised pre- and afterload (Corrello & Gittens, 1987). However, the effects of obesity greater than moderate upon left ventricle function is somewhat unclear. The moderately MO (around 45 kg > IBW) with an increased left ventricle wall thickness (presumably compensatory in response to the extra cardiac work) have been reported to have a normal left ventricular response to exercise, whereas similar patients, without increased left ventricle wall thickness, do not (Alexander, 1985). The latter group is likely to manifest a degree of cardiac decompensation in response to cardiac stress. With increasing weight the very MO (170% > IBW) show a progressive increase in left ventricle wall thickness and a progressive decrease in left ventricular response to exercise (Alper et al., 1989).

Evaluation should seek to confirm the presence of the above-mentioned abnormalities. A history of dyspnoea on exercise and orthopnoea should be sought. Physical examination should be directed specifically towards evidence of hypertension and left or right ventricular failure. It is useful to check for sites of venous access and it is worthwhile performing an Allen's test to ensure ulnar artery patency. An ECG should be obtained in all patients and chest X-rays scrutinized for increases in cardiac diameter and for evidence of pulmonary congestion. Suspicions of heart disease or systemic or pulmonary congestion should lead to further studies such as exercise ECG, echocardiography, ejection frac-

tions and pulmonary artery catheterization. In patients who have evidence of either the OHS or the Pickwickian syndrome and in very obese patients, it is imperative to obtain a cardiological opinion and to consider sophisticated investigations. As with patients with respiratory abnormalities, it is important to optimize cardiovascular function before submitting the patient to anaesthesia and surgery.

Endocrine and metabolic evaluation

In order to maintain a stable weight, obese patients have to maintain a greater than normal caloric intake. But, as with $\dot{V}o_2$, when this caloric intake is related to body surface area it is similar to non-obese patients (Leibel & Hirsch, 1985). Glucose tolerance is impaired frequently in the obese patient, with pancreatic islet hypertrophy and hyperinsulinaemia, irrespective of the state of carbohydrate tolerance. This is reflected in a high incidence of diabetes mellitus. Abnormal serum lipid profiles are frequently found and are associated with an increased incidence of ischaemic heart disease.

Preoperative evaluation should include a fasting blood sugar and urine test for ketones. Should gross carbohydrate intolerance or frank diabetes be found, control of these abnormalities should be achieved prior to either elective or emergency surgery.

Gastrointestinal evaluation

Obese patients have an increased incidence of hiatus hernia and show a linear increase in intra-abdominal pressure with increasing weight. At the time of induction of anaesthesia, 90% of MO patients have a gastric fluid volume in excess of 25 ml and a gastric fluid pH of less than 2.5 (Vaughan et al., 1975). These figures are generally accepted as indicative of a special risk of causing pneumonitis should such fluid be regurgitated and reach the airway. As both volume of gastric contents and intra-abdominal pressure increase with pregnancy, the pregnant obese patient is particularly at risk for aspiration pneumonitis.

Liver fat content is increased in approximately 90% of the MO and appears to relate to the duration of obesity rather than its degree. The degree of hepatic fatty infiltration may not be reflected by abnormalities in the usual clinical biochemical investigations. The incidence of hepatic dysfunction is increased in the obese patient and is particularly high in those patients who have undergone intestinal bypass operations. The effect of gastric partitioning operations upon hepatic function in not known. A history characteristic of a hiatus hernia and a history or evidence of hepatic dysfunction should be sought preoperatively and liver function tests should be obtained.

Airway management

Airway management and tracheal intubation in the obese patient may be difficult for a variety of reasons. Cervical spine and atlanto-occipital flexion may be limited by numerous chins and by thoracic and breast fat. Extension of these joints may be limited by low cervical and upper thoracic fat pads and mouth opening may be restricted by numerous chins. Fleshy cheeks, a large tongue and copious flaps of soft palatal, pharyngeal or supralaryngeal soft tissue may narrow the airway and impede laryngoscopy. Moreover, the larynx tends to occupy the 'infantile' position being 'high and anterior'.

A history of airway difficulties during previous anaesthetics should be obtained from the patient or from previous anaesthetic records. Symptoms suggestive of an obstructive sleep apnoea syndrome, which is common in the MO (Wittels & Thompson, 1990), such as excessive nocturnal snoring, with or without apnoeic episodes, and daytime hypersomnolence should also be sought, as they imply potential mechanical airway obstruction when the level of consciousness is decreased. Patients with such a history and those presenting for operations (tracheostomy, palatoplasty) designed to alleviate such conditions must be scrutinized especially closely as they often present formidable airway difficulties. These difficulties may include large tonsils, excessive soft palate tissue, large base-of-tongue area and multiple folds of pharyngeal tissue (Chung & Crags, 1980; Thawley, 1985). The patient should be examined carefully with particular emphasis upon the possible difficulties enumerated above. Such an examination should be undertaken by the person who is going to perform the intubation. Lateral soft-tissue X-rays of the neck in the neutral and extended positions, computerized tomography (CT) scans of the pharynx and hypopharynx, X-ray cinematography (Norton & Brown, 1990) and consultations with ENT surgeons for indirect or direct laryngoscopy may be helpful in delineating airway difficulties.

Psychology of the obese patient
(Wadden & Stunkard, 1985)

Large surveys of obese patients in the USA and Europe have failed to reveal an increased incidence of psychopathology among the obese population in general, when compared with the normal population. There is some evidence for an increased incidence of psychopathology among the MO. These findings notwithstanding, obese patients have the reputation among the medical profession of being 'difficult'. Specific instances are that they are intolerant of discomfort and inconvenience, are non-compliant with suggested treatments, are difficult to handle on an interpersonal basis and given to resorting to outbursts of anger and/or hysteria. It is not certain if such behavioural characteristics are inherent in the obese patient or are a reaction to the prejudices, discriminations, attitudes and behaviours towards obese people by the 'thin-thinking population'. There is evidence that obese people suffer from such prejudice and discriminations from an early age, and in a variety of situations — academic, social, vocational and financial. Obese people are characterized as ugly, slothful, self-indulgent, lacking in self-control and self-esteem, and being prone to despondence, depression and self-consciousness.

The author's bias is that the reported behaviour of obese patients is a consequence of their interactions with the non-fat population, and physicians specifically. Experience with a large number of MO patients who were to undergo gastric stapling operations was that MO patients were interested in their management, compliant with suggestions on management regimens and conducted themselves in a normal fashion throughout the perioperative period (Buckley et al., 1983). Such a group of patients is highly selected and motivated as they have elected to undertake a very dramatic course of action in an attempt to remedy their obesity. Thus, their behaviour may not reflect that of obese patients as a whole. Moreover, alot of time and effort was spent in evaluating these patients, explaining management plans and discussing with the patients why and how such management plans were advised, and the alternative options.

Thus, the author's advice in dealing with obese patients is first, that the anaesthetist should be aware of his or her own feelings, attitudes and prejudices concerning obese people, and should be careful to identify and suppress those which might convey to the patient an unsympathetic or condescending attitude. The patient should be evaluated in a thorough, sympathetic and non-judgemental fashion with particular emphasis on the difficulties that obesity presents to the anaesthetist. The patient should be involved in the management plan as much as possible. Time should be taken to allow the patient to detail previous adverse experiences with previous anaesthetics and operations, and any anxieties they may have with their forthcoming experience. The various potential difficulties and the specific anaesthesia plan advised to minimize or avoid such difficulties should be discussed in detail with the patient, as should the likely postoperative course.

Pharmacokinetics in the obese patient
(Abernathy & Greenblatt, 1981)

Although there is a dearth of specific data available concerning pharmacokinetics in the obese patient, some inferences on the effects of the pathophysiology of obesity upon drug disposition can be made. The smaller proportion of body water and muscle mass to total body weight, and the greater proportion of body fat in the obese patient may lead to changes in the proportion of drug distributed to various body compartments. Drug biotransformation may be altered by hepatic disease, diabetes or changes in splanchnic blood flow. Renal drug excretion may be changed owing to changes in glomerular filtration rates and biliary excretion may be affected by the increased incidence of gallstones and pancreatitis. Finally, the high incidence of hyperlipoproteinaemia may affect drug protein-binding.

In the obese patient, hydrophilic drugs have similar absolute values of volume of distribution, elimination half-life and metabolic clearance as in non-obese patients. Fat-soluble drugs, e.g. benzodiazepines (Abernathy et al., 1984; Greenblatt et al., 1984) and thiopentone (Mayersohn et al., 1981) have an increased volume of distribution, more selective distribution to fat stores and a longer elimination half-life, but similar clearance values when compared with normals. The finding of these changes in the handling of fat-soluble drugs suggests that the administration of fat-soluble anaesthetic agents may lead to prolonged elimination and therefore slow recovery from these agents. However, theoretical calculations imply that for prolonged recovery to occur, such agents would have to be administered for periods in excess of 24 h (Ladergaard-Pederson, 1981). Clinical studies of recovery from such agents following their administration to MO patients for 2–4 h have shown that prolonged recovery does not occur (Cork et al., 1981). Interestingly, fentanyl, a relatively fat-soluble drug, has a similar distribution, elimination half-life, volume of distribution and clearance in obese and non-obese patients (Bentley et al., 1981a). In patients 60% above IBW, sufentanil — also a fat-soluble drug — is distributed evenly throughout body mass, suggesting that dose regimens should be based on total body weight. Moreover, as half-life and clearance of sufentanil is similar to normals, speed of recovery should be similar to normals (Schwartz et al., 1986a). In comparison to non-obese patients, alfentanyl in the MO has a similar steady-state volume of distribution but a longer elimination half-life, as a consequence of slower clearance (Bentley et al., 1983). However, these data do not tell us a great deal about the pharmacodynamics of CNS active drugs in the obese patient, a subject that remains to be studied.

Perioperative management

Premedication

Premedication, if any, should be given orally or intravenously, as intrafat (as opposed to intramuscular) injections do not produce predictable blood concentrations of drug in the obese patient. Because the effects of CNS-depressant drugs are not predictable in the obese patient, personal bias dictates against administering any such medications until the patient reaches the operating theatre. That is the case particularly in patients with any degree of cardiovascular or respiratory compromise, as sedation and respiratory depression, with or without airway obstruction, may not be detected on the wards or on the journey to the operating theatre. Even with the patient in the operating theatre, he/she must be monitored vigilantly to detect any respiratory depression or airway obstruction.

As the risk of airway soiling is high in the obese patient, the preoperative administration of H_2-blockers, metoclopramide and antacids is probably advisable to lower the volume of gastric contents and raise gastric fluid pH (Wilson et al., 1981; Lam et al., 1986; Manchikanti et al., 1986). Anticholinergic agents may assist in speeding gastric emptying and should be given in an attempt to reduce secretions if awake tracheal intubation is anticipated, or if a particularly difficult asleep intubation is anticipated.

Operating theatre preparation, positioning and surgical retraction

It is important to ensure that such equipment as trolleys, operating tables and lithotomy stirrups are capable of bearing the unusual load of the obese patient. Large loads are imposed upon heels, buttocks and shoulders of these patients, and therefore they are prone to develop decubitus ulcers. Operating tables should be fitted therefore with suitable foam pads, or an inflatable mattress. There is an increased incidence of deep vein thrombosis in the obese patient, so the use of devices which produce intermittent leg compression should be considered.

Body fat may make the usual positions on the operating table hazardous for the obese patient, e.g. excessive posterior extension of the shoulder with the potential for brachial plexus injury when a patient with a large posterior thoracic fat pad is placed in the supine position with his or her arms abducted at 90°; or excessive cervical spine extension in a patient with a large upper posterior thoracic fat pad if the head is not supported correctly; or excessive hip extension and consequent increase in lumbar lordosis when a patient with large amounts of buttock fat is lain supine. Thus, when an obese patient is placed on the operating table, care should be taken to ensure that the various body parts are placed in positions which do not put other body parts, and in particular, neural structures, at risk. A rolled towel or inflated 1-litre intravenous bag placed in the lumbar region when the patient is supine may help to decrease the incidence of backache. Trendelenberg or lithotomy positions may increase intra-abdominal pressure with decreases in lung volume and hypoxaemia. During intra-abdominal operations, vigorous retraction and either caudad or cephalad displacement of panniculus may be necessary to afford adequate abdominal exposure. Such manoeuvres may also produce decreases in lung volume and Pao_2 (Vaughan & Wise, 1976) and cardiovascular collapse (Hodgkinson & Hussein, 1980a). Thus, when changes in position occur, the patient should be monitored particularly vigilantly.

Monitoring

Cardiovascular monitoring should include a V_5 or equivalent ECG lead. Arterial pressure monitoring by a sphygmomanometer cuff may be difficult and inaccurate. If cuff-pressure measurements are to be used, the cuff should be of appropriate size — the inflatable bladder should encompass at least 70% of the circumference of the arm — and should fit snugly. Because of the inaccuracies and difficulties with cuff measurements, it is the author's practice to use intra-arterial pressure measurement in all but the shortest of cases, particularly if frequent arterial blood gas measurements are necessary. Paradoxically, while intravenous catheter placement is often difficult in the obese patient, placement of an intra-arterial catheter is usually no more difficult than in a non-obese patient. In patients with documented cardiac disease, with evidence of raised pulmonary artery pressure, OHS or Pickwickian syndrome, and those undergoing extensive operations, placement of a pulmonary artery catheter should be considered. In the obese patient with myocardial dysfunction, transoesophageal echocardiography may be of assistance.

As perioperative hypoxia is a constant threat to MO patients, arterial oxygenation should be monitored either by pulse oximetry or by frequent arterial blood gas measurements. Measurement of end-tidal carbon dioxide is helpful in ensuring correct tracheal tube placement and in judging the adequacy of artificial ventilation.

As there are few data to guide the anaesthetist on the dose requirement of non-depolarizing neuromuscular-blocking agents in the obese patient, any neuromuscular block should be monitored with a peripheral nerve stimulator. The use of percutaneous needle electrodes should be considered, since considerable amounts of fat may separate skin electrodes from the relevant nerve.

Obese patients are as likely to lose body heat intraoperatively as non-obese patients; thus, body temperature should be monitored and maintained as for the latter. It is particularly important to avoid postoperative shivering in obese patients since this may produce further arterial desaturation in patients who may already be on the borderline in this regard.

Intraoperative management

Airway maintenance

It is suggested that, other than for the shortest of general anaesthetics (GA) in highly selected patients, tracheal intubation is used in all obese patients. This is advocated as it may be difficult or even impossible to maintain a gas-tight mask fit and a patent airway while attending also to the other manual tasks necessary during an anaesthetic. Moreover, airway protection is essential because the risk of regurgitation or vomiting of gastric contents is high and a tracheal tube is needed to provide intermittent positive-pressure ventilation (IPPV). Spontaneous ventilation by the MO under GA may result in an unacceptable increase in $Paco_2$.

Difficulties with tracheal intubation should be anticipated in all obese patients, and all possible hazards defined in the preoperative visit. Appropriate airway management equipment should be available, including tracheal tubes and laryngoscope blades of different types and sizes, tracheal tube stylets, intubation stylets and a selection of oropharyngeal and nasopharyngeal airways. If it is anticipated that chest-wall fat may obstruct the standard laryngoscope handles, a 'polio blade' laryngoscope should be available. Fibre-optic intubation stylets, or fibre-optic laryngoscopes, bronchoscopes and equipment for cricothyrotomy and transtracheal jet ventilation should also be available. The choice between an awake or an asleep tracheal intubation should be made for each case, bearing in mind the anticipated difficulties and expertise of the anaesthetist. Under GA, the reported incidence in the MO of difficult tracheal intubations is 13% in patients with a mean BMI of 46 (Buckley et al., 1983), 2.4% for weight 1.5–1.75 IBW, and 7.3% for weight 1.75–2.0 IBW (Lee et al., 1980). The latter authors performed awake tracheal intubations in 19% of patients of weight 2.0–2.5 IBW, in 50% of patients when weight was in excess of 2.5 IBW and recommend awake intubation when patient's weight is in excess of 1.75% IBW.

When confronted with intubating the trachea of an obese patient, a useful policy is to anaesthetize the oropharynx topically with local anaesthetic and then to introduce the laryngoscope into the mouth gently, attempting to visualize the epiglottis and, if possible, the larynx. If it is possible to see these structures, it is likely that asleep oral intubation can be performed. If not, awake intubation should be performed by direct visualization with a standard laryngoscope or with a fibre-optic laryngoscope or bronchoscope, following suitable topical anaesthesia and supplemental oxygen administration. Any CNS depressant administered in these circumstances should be kept to a minimum and its effects observed closely. While blind nasal intubation has been advocated strongly (Bromage, 1980), this technique should be attempted only by those skilful in the technique and who have a high success rate. Personal use of blind nasal intubation in MO patients has resulted in several brisk and voluminous epistaxes.

Patients with symptoms suggestive of an obstructive sleep apnoea syndrome, or those who are to undergo operations to alleviate such conditions, inevitably present formidable tracheal intubation difficulties. The high incidence of failure of intubation, the subsequent difficulty in mask and bag ventilation, and consequent life-threatening hypoxia when such intubations are attempted under GA dictate that intubation of the trachea should be performed in the awake patient. In these patients, as in others, the use of a pulse oximeter provides useful information on the occurrence of arterial desaturation during the course of such manoeuvres.

Asleep intubation of the trachea should be performed in a manner designed to avoid hypoxia and regurgitation–vomiting and aspiration of gastric contents. As intubation may take longer than normal or be impossible, and as MO patients have only a small intrapulmonary oxygen store (low FRC) and a high $\dot{V}o_2$, they are at particular risk of hypoxaemia during this phase of the anaesthetic (Jense et al., 1991). Thorough denitrogenation/preoxygenation either by the usual 3 min preoxygenation or by the four-breath technique (Moyer & Rein, 1986) is essential. For asleep intubations it is advisable to have two experienced anaesthetists available. In the event that intubation of the trachea is not successful and it becomes necessary to ventilate the patient's lungs with mask and bag, it may take one person to maintain both a gas-tight mask fit and the airway, the second person being available to squeeze the bag. A further experienced anaesthetist may be useful for other difficult circumstances. Cricothyroid pressure (Sellick's manoeuvre) should be applied in all cases. After induction of unconsciousness, suxamethonium 1.0–1.2 mg/kg should be administered to produce relaxation. This dose is higher than normal, as obese patients have a higher-than-normal level of pseudocholinesterase activity (Bentley et al., 1981b). Confirming correct tracheal placement by auscultation may be difficult because of the thickness of the chest wall and supplementary aids such as end-tidal carbon dioxide monitoring or fibre-optic bronchoscopy may be useful.

Choice of anaesthetic techniques

General anaesthesia

As implied above, if a GA is to be used for the obese patient, it should be delivered almost always via a tracheal tube. Under GA, obese patients hypoventilate to a greater extent than do non-obese patients when allowed to breathe spontaneously, often resulting in unacceptable hypercapnia with resultant cardiovascular disturbances, and possibly hypoxia.

The doses of induction agents used for the obese patient should be larger than for the non-obese patient. Doses of thiopentone should be of the order of 7.5 mg/kg but allowance should be made for the patient's cardiovascular fitness. Nitrous oxide is a good choice of agent as it has a swift onset of action, is fat insoluble and is subject to little biotransformation. However, even in the healthiest MO patients, an F_1o_2 in excess of 0.5 may be necessary to maintain an adequate Pao_2 (Vaughan & Wise, 1976), thus limiting the usefulness of nitrous oxide. Obese patients metabolize volatile anaesthetics to greater degrees than non-obese patients. Compared with non-obese patients, serum fluoride concentrations produced by metabolism of methoxyflurane, halothane and enflurane are greater in MO patients (Vaughan, 1982b). Serum bromide concentrations are also higher following halothane anaesthesia in MO patients than in non-obese patients and, as 'halothane hepatitis' is alleged to occur more frequently in the obese patient, halothane should probably be used with caution. However, irrespective of the choice of volatile agent, simple tests of hepatic function are similarly marginally impaired after halothane or enflurane. Isoflurane, which is metabolized to a lesser extent than halothane or enflurane (Strube et al., 1987), is the logical agent of choice.

The belief that a prolonged recovery from a volatile GA may occur in the obese patient because large stores of volatile GA may take a long time to leach out from fat deposits has been disproven elegantly in theory (Ladergaard-Pederson, 1981), and this has been confirmed by clinical studies of speed of awakening (Cork et al., 1981). Little information exists on the pharmacokinetics or pharmacodynamics of opioid agents in the obese patient (see above). Published work on inhalation anaesthetics in the obese patient describes usually a mixture of opioid (usually fentanyl) with a volatile agent.

The absolute dose of pancuronium necessary to produce a given degree of neuromuscular block in the obese patient is greater than normal but, if the dose is related to body surface area, doses are almost identical to those used for non-obese patients (Tseueda et al., 1978). When administered on a mg/kg body-weight basis, recovery from metocurine (Schwartz et al., 1986b) and vecuronium (Weinstein et al., 1986) is slower than in non-obese patients. In contrast, when atracurium is administered on a mg/kg body-weight basis, speed of recovery is similar to that in normals (Weinstein et al., 1986; Varin et al., 1990), despite the fact that at the defined point of recovery of neuromuscular block the blood levels of atracurium are higher in the obese patient than in non-obese patients (Varin et al., 1990). Atracurium would appear to be the logical choice of non-depolarizing neuromuscular-blocking drug. In the obese patient, the degree of neuromuscular block should be monitored always with a peripheral nerve stimulator to ensure correct dosage and adequate recovery/reversal.

Paramount amongst the physiological abnormalities produced by GA are respiratory abnormalities.

With the induction of GA there is a further disruption of the already altered FRC:CC relationship with ensuing $\dot{V}:\dot{Q}$ abnormalities or frank right−left shunt. All obese patients should be considered at risk of arterial hypoxaemia under GA and should not receive a F_IO_2 of less than 0.5. In those with respiratory disease, an F_IO_2 of 1.0 is indicated. The F_IO_2 may be titrated against the Sao_2 obtained from a pulse oximeter or against Pao_2 obtained from repeated arterial blood-gas measurements. Even in the healthy obese patient, the assumption of the Trendelenberg and lithotomy positions or the placement of sub-diaphragmatic packs and retractors is associated with further reductions in Pao_2 (Vaughan & Wise, 1976). However, it has been shown that MO patients may be maintained safely through transthoracic operations necessitating single-lung anaesthesia via a double-lumen tube (Brodsky et al., 1985). Spontaneous respiration under GA is relatively contra-indicated because of the hypoventilation produced by GA. IPPV is accomplished best with large tidal volumes* at a rate of 8−10 breaths/min. The application of positive end-expiratory pressure may increase Pao_2 to some extent (Eriksen et al., 1978; Salem et al., 1984). Particular attention should be paid to the patient's Pao_2 following changes in position and when the abdomen is opened during abdominal operations. Hypocapnia with a $Paco_2$ of less than 4 kPa (30 mmHg) is best avoided as this may result in an increase in shunt fraction (In-amani et al., 1985).

It deserves reiteration that the studies concerning GA and the obese patient have been performed in those who are otherwise healthy. It is likely that patients who have respiratory or cardiovascular disease have even more marked changes in respiratory variables during GA and require more careful attention.

At the conclusion of surgery, it is essential that residual neuromuscular block is antagonized completely, as judged by the response to peripheral nerve stimulation, and that the conditions for tracheal extubation are fulfilled. The trachea should not be

---

* By rearranging the BMI equation [BMI = wt (kg)/ht^2 (m) to BMI × ht^2 (m) = wt (kg)] one may calculate various body weights for the individual, e.g. true body weight (TBW), low body weight (LBW), where BMI = 30 and IBW where BMI = 25. Thus, a patient with a TBW of 139 kg and a height of 1.77 m has a BMI of 139/1.77^2 = 44.4. Thus, for this patient IBW = 25 × 1.77^2 = 78 kg and LBW = 30 × 1.77^2 = 90 kg. IPPV at a tidal volume of 12 ml/kg at LBW at a rate of 8−10 breaths/min achieves a $Paco_2$ of approximately 4 kPa (30 mmHg) (Ferguson et al., 1986).

extubated until the patient is fully awake and in control of his/her airway in order to avoid hazards of pulmonary aspiration or airway obstruction. It should be ensured, either by pulse oximetry or arterial blood-gas measurements, that hypoxia is not present prior to extubation.

Regional anaesthesia

Because of the problems encountered with GA in obese patients, regional anaesthesia (RA) would appear to be a useful alternative to GA, but it brings its own constellation of difficulties. The presence of much body fat and the indistinct nature of bony landmarks make RA techniques difficult. For peripheral nerve blocks this may be circumvented by the use of insulated needles and a peripheral nerve stimulator to ensure correct needle and drug placement.

Subarachnoid block (SAB) may be more difficult to perform in obese patients than in non-obese patients, but the difficulties are not insurmountable. The midline of the back in the lumbar region does not generally have as thick a layer of fat as do the more lateral portions, and subarachnoid puncture may be made easier by having the patient in the sitting position. Often, needles longer (15 cm or 6 in) than usual may be needed. For a given age and height, the dose requirement for SAB in the obese patient is approximately 75–80% of that of the non-obese patient (McCulloch & Littlewood, 1986; Pitkainan, 1987; Taivanen et al., 1990), and is also more variable (Taivanen et al., 1990). Evidence from case reports implies that not only is the level of block produced by an SAB not very predictable, but also that the block is of slow onset and creeps insidiously higher during the first 30 min (Catennacci et al., 1961). Anecdotal reports suggest that a high SAB tends to produce respiratory compromise, especially if patients are sedated (Catennacci et al., 1961). However, in obese patients with a block at T5, both respiratory volumes (Catennacci & Sampathakar, 1969) and arterial blood-gas values (Blass, 1979) show minimal change from baseline. If the block does extend higher in the thoracic area than T5, there is a distinct possibility of respiratory compromise, particularly in obese patients with respiratory disease. Moreover, the high extension of the block, with the variable extent of the autonomic block above the somatic block (Chamberlain & Chamberlain, 1986) may lead to cardiovascular compromise which can be precipitated also by panniculus retraction (Hodgkinson & Hussein, 1980a). Because it may be

difficult to deal with respiratory or cardiovascular emergencies in the MO, it is critical that such potential hazards are detected as early as possible by vigilant monitoring, and remedied by vigorous early intervention. Monitoring should be as intensive as for a GA, and supplementary oxygen should be used in all cases. A strong case may be made for using a continuous subarachnoid block in MO patients. This would provide all the benefits of RA and yet enable the anaesthetist to titrate the dose of drug necessary to achieve the desired extent of block, and no more.

While technically more exacting than SAB, extradural blocks have been used widely and described in obese patients (Bromage, 1980; Fox et al., 1981; Buckley et al., 1983), particularly for abdominal operations. The technique usually consists of a high-lumbar or thoracic puncture, with the introduction of a catheter and the induction of a segmental block. Catheter placement may be made easier by the use of fluoroscopic assistance (Gelman & Vitek, 1980). The technique is used usually in combination with a light GA via a tracheal tube and IPPV. Such a technique bypasses many of the problems of GA, reduces the requirement of volatile agent, eliminates the need for neuromuscular-blocking agents and permits rapid postoperative mobilization. As for SABs, the dose requirement for extradural blocks is approximately 75–80% of that of non-obese patients (Hodgkinson & Hussein, 1980b; Buckley et al., 1983). The use of extradural analgesia may confer some benefits on MO patients intraoperatively and postoperatively — lower shunt fraction, decrease in left ventricular work, $(a-v)o_2$ and lower $\dot{V}o_2$ (Gelman et al., 1980). The use of an extradural technique may be made more desirable by the fact that the catheter may be used to provide postoperative analgesia either with a local anaesthetic (LA) or opioids, which may be particularly beneficial in the MO patient (Buckley et al., 1983; Rawal et al., 1984).

The anaesthetist should not embark on a RA unless he or she is prepared to convert it to a GA, should the RA be unsatisfactory for the surgical procedure or should the patient develop respiratory difficulties. Irrespective of the RA technique used, careful monitoring, of no lesser an intensity than that for patients receiving GA, i.e. ECG, arterial pressure and arterial oxygenation, is essential. Sedation should be used sparingly, supplemental oxygen should be delivered, and respiratory function should be monitored closely.

Postoperative care

Obese patients with a previous history of respiratory disease, OHS, Pickwickian syndrome, or having had major abdominal and thoracic operations are likely to have a high incidence of respiratory complications. Thus, it may be wise to admit these patients electively to an intensive therapy unit (ITU). Management in the ITU depends on the individual patient but should include IPPV if necessary, and aggressive prophylaxis against the development of respiratory complications. Obese patients are highly immobile postoperatively, and measures should be taken to assist them in moving by the provision of an adjustable bed, overhead trapezes and the availability of sufficient nursing staff.

Respiratory function

Even in healthy obese patients, postoperative hypoxaemia is a universal hazard. Supplemental oxygen should be given during transport from operating theatre to the recovery room, and in the recovery room. Respiratory monitoring should be particularly aggressive in the recovery room and should include pulse oximetry and arterial blood-gas measurement. Before discharge, patients should be reviewed carefully by the use of any appropriate investigations. Patients should not be discharged to the ward until they have been shown not to be hypoxaemic, and it may be appropriate to use long-term oxygen therapy on the ward. Following intra-abdominal operations, arterial hypoxaemia may last for 4—6 days (Vaughan et al., 1974), and is of greater magnitude following vertical rather than horizontal incisions. Postoperative hypoxaemia can be minimized by nursing patients in the sitting position. There is some evidence that the use of RA techniques intra- and postoperatively reduces the incidence of postoperative respiratory complications (Buckley et al., 1983; Rawal et al., 1984).

Immobilization

Obese patients have a high incidence of postoperative deep vein thromboses and pulmonary emboli. The use of mini-heparin prophylaxis may be appropriate for this problem. The use of RA techniques may decrease the incidence of deep vein thrombosis and pulmonary emboli (Fox et al., 1981; Buckley et al., 1983).

Analgesia

Personal experience and published experience (Rand et al., 1985) implies that the MO may exhibit a lesser need for opioid analgesics than non-obese patients.

The routine use of fixed doses of intramuscular opioid analgesics for postoperative pain has been shown to be associated with several pharmacokinetic and pharmacodynamic liabilities in the non-obese patient (Chapter 76). There is a wide range of variability in the minimum effective analgesic concentration and the fixed doses of opioid produce highly variable blood levels of drug. In the obese patient, a further variable may be present, i.e. the unpredictability of absorption of drug from an intra-fat injection. Thus, if systemic opioids are to be used to provide analgesia they should probably be given in a manner which circumvents these problems. Patient controlled analgesia is a logical choice as it bypasses the unpredictability of injections and allows the patient to titrate the opioid to desired effect. Patient controlled analgesia has been successfully used in the MO and may be associated with superior analgesia and lesser total opioid use than intramuscular administration (Bennett et al., 1982a,b).

If patients have had an extradural catheter placed for operative anaesthesia, this may be used as the route for injecting either LA or opioid to provide analgesia postoperatively. The use of LA (Buckley et al., 1983) or opioid (Rawal et al., 1984; Brodsky et al., 1985) is associated with a greater speed of postoperative recovery and a reduced incidence of respiratory complications than the use of conventional opioid techniques. The doses of either LA (Buckley et al., 1983) or opioid (Rawal et al., 1984; Brodsky et al., 1985) necessary to provide postoperative analgesia appear to be similar to those in non-obese patients. If extradural opioid analgesia is used, it has a potential for producing delayed respiratory depression and, given the difficulty of maintaining or securing airways in the obese patient, those receiving extradural opioids should probably be nursed in a closely monitored environment, i.e. an ITU, until the potential for such a complication has passed.

References

Abernathy D.R. & Greenblatt D.S. (1981) Pharmacokinetics of drugs in obesity. *Clinical Pharmacokinetics* **7**, 108—24.
Abernathy D.R., Greenblatt D.S., Divoll M., Smith R.B. & Shader R.I. (1984) The influence of obesity on the pharmacokinetics of oral alprazolam and triazaolam. *Clinical Pharmaco-*

kinetics **9**, 177—83.

Alexander J.K. (1985) The cardiomyopathy of obesity. *Progress in Cardiovascular Disease* **28**, 325—46.

Alper M.A., Singh A. & Terry B.E. (1989) Effect of exercise on left ventricular function and reserve in morbid obesity. *American Journal of Cardiology* **63**, 1478—82.

Anderson J., Rasmusson J.P. & Eriksen J. (1977) Pulmonary function in obese patients scheduled for jejunoileostomy. *Acta Anaesthesiologica Scandinavica* **21**, 346—51.

Bennett R.L., Batenhorst R.L. & Graves D. (1982a) Patient controlled analgesia: a new concept in postoperative pain relief. *Annals of Surgery* **195**, 700—5.

Bennett R.L., Batenhorst R.L., Graves D., Foster T.S., Griffen W.O. & Wright B.D. (1982b) Postoperative pulmonary function with patient controlled analgesia. *Anesthesia and Analgesia* **61**, 171.

Bentley J.B., Borel J.D., Gillespie T.S., Vaughn R.W. & Gandolfi A.J. (1981a) Fentanyl pharmacokinetics in obese and non-obese patients. *Anesthesiology* **55**, 177A.

Bentley J.B., Bond I.D., Vaughan R.W. & Gondolfi A.J. (1981b) Weight, pseudocholinesterase activity and succinylcholine requirements. *Anesthesiology* **57**, 48—9.

Bentley J.B., Finley J.M. & Humphrey R.J. (1983) Obesity and alfentanil pharmacokinetics. *Anesthesia and Analgesia* **62**, 251.

Blass N.M. (1979) Regional anesthesia in the morbidly obese. *Regional Anesthesia* **5**, 20—2.

Brodsky J.E., Wyner J., Ehrenwerth S. & Cohn R.B. (1985) One lung anesthesia in morbidly obese patients. *Anesthesiology* **57**, 32—4.

Bromage P.R. (1980) *Epidural Analgesia*. W.E. Saunders, Philadelphia.

Buckley F.P., Robinson N.B., Simonowitz D.A. & Dellinger E.P. (1983) Anesthesia in the morbidly obese. A comparison of anesthetic and analgesic regimens for upper abdominal surgery. *Anesthesia* **38**, 840—51.

Burwell C.S., Robin E.D., Whaley R.D. & Bickelman A.G. (1956) External obesity associated with alveolar hypoventilation — a Pickwickian syndrome. *American Journal of Medicine* **25**, 815—20.

Catennacci A.J. & Sampathakar D.R. (1969) Ventilation studies in the obese patient during spinal anesthesia. *Anesthesia and Analgesia* **48**, 48—54.

Catennacci A.J., Anderson J.D. & Boersma D. (1961) Anesthetic hazards of obesity. *Journal of the American Medical Association* **175**, 657—65.

Chamberlain D.D. & Chamberlain B.D.L. (1986) Changes in skin temperature and their relationship to sympathetic blockade during spinal anesthesia. *Anesthesiology* **65**, 139—43.

Chung F. & Crags R.R. (1980) Sleep apnoea syndrome and anaesthesia. *Canadian Anaesthetists' Society Journal* **29**, 439—45.

Cork R.C., Vaughan R.W. & Bentley J.B. (1981) General anesthesia for morbidly obese patients; an examination of postoperative out-comes. *Anesthesiology* **54**, 310—14.

Corrello B.A. & Gittens L. (1987) The cardiac mechanisms and function in obese, normotensive persons with normal coronary arteries. *American Journal of Cardiology* **59**, 469—73.

Eriksen J., Andersen J., Rasmussen J.P. & Sorensen B. (1978) Effects of ventilation with large tidal volumes or positive end expiratory pressure on cardiorespiratory function in anesthetized obese patients. *Acta Anaesthesiologica Scandinavica* **22**, 241—8.

Farebrother M.J.B. (1979) Respiratory function and cardio-respiratory response to exercise in obesity. *British Journal of Diseases of the Chest* **73**, 211—39.

Ferguson L.L., Sivashankaran S. & Dauchot P.J. (1986) Ventilator settings to mitigate hypocarbia in the obese patient. *Anesthesia and Analgesia* **65**, 553.

Fisher A., Waterhouse T.D. & Adams A.P. (1975) Obesity: its relation to anaesthesia. *Anesthesia* **30**, 633—47.

Fox G.S. (1975) Anaesthesia for intestinal short circuiting in the morbidly obese with reference to the pathophysiology of gross obesity. *Canadian Anesthetists' Society Journal* **22**, 307—12.

Fox G.S., Whalley D.G. & Bevan D.R. (1981) Anesthesia for the morbidly obese. Experience with 550 patients. *British Journal of Anesthesia* **53**, 811—16.

Gelman S. & Vitek J.J. (1980) Thoracic epidural catheter placement under fluoroscopic control in morbidly obese patients. *Regional Anesthesia* **4**, 19.

Gelman S., Laws M.L., Potzick J., Strong S., Smith L. & Erdemir M. (1980) Thoracic epidural vs. balanced anesthesia in morbid obesity: an intraoperative and postoperative hemodynamic study. *Anesthesia and Analgesia* **59**, 902—8.

Greenblatt D.F., Abernathy D.R., Lorniskar D., Narmatz J.J., Limjuco R.A. & Shader R.I. (1984) Effect of age, gender and obesity on midazolam kinetics. *Anesthesiology* **61**, 27—33.

Hamm C.W. & Koehler L.S. (1979) The implication, of morbid obesity for anesthesia. *Anesthesiology Review* **4**, 29—35.

Hedenstierna G. & Santesson J. (1976) Breathing mechanics, dead space and gas exchange in the extremely obese breathing spontaneously and during anaesthesia with intermittent positive pressure ventilation. *Acta Anaesthesiologica Scandinavica* **20**, 334—42.

Hodgkinson R. & Hussein F.J. (1980a) Caesarian section associated with gross obesity. *British Journal of Anaesthesia* **52**, 919—23.

Hodgkinson R. & Hussein F.J. (1980b) Obesity and the spread of analgesic following epidural administration of bupivacaine for caesarian section. *Anesthesia and Analgesia* **59**, 89—93.

In-amani M., Kikuta Y., Nagai H. & Okada K. (1985) The increase in pulmonary venous admixture by hypocapnia is enhanced in obese patients. *Anesthesiology* **63**, 520A.

Jense H.G., Dubin S.A., Silverstein P.I. & O'Leary-Escolas U. (1991) Effect of obesity on safe duration of apnea in anesthetised humans. *Anesthesia and Analgesia* **72**, 89—93.

Ladergaard-Pederson M.J. (1981) Recovery from general anesthesia in obese patients. *Anesthesiology* **55**, 720.

Lam A.M., Grace D.M., Penny F.F. & Vesina W.C. (1986) Prophylactic IV cimetidine reduces the risk of acid aspiration in morbidly obese patients. *Anesthesiology* **65**, 684—7.

Lee J.J., Larson R.M., Buckley J.J. & Roberts A.E. (1980) Airway maintenance in the morbidly obese. *Anesthesiology Review* **7**, 33—6.

Leibel R.L. & Hirsch J. (1985) Metabolic characterization of obesity. *Annals of Internal Medicine* **103**, 1000—2.

Luce J.M. (1980) Respiratory complications of obesity. *Chest* **78**, 626—31.

Manchikanti L., Roush J.R. & Colliver J.R. (1986) Effect of

preanesthetic ranitidine and metoclopramide on gastric contents in morbidly obese patients. *Anesthesia and Analgesia* **65**, 195–9.

Mayersohn M., Calkins J.M., Perrier D.G., Jung D. & Saunders R.J. (1981) Thiopental kinetics in obese patients. *Anesthesiology* **55**, 178A.

McCulloch W.J.D. & Littlewood D.G. (1986) Influence of obesity on spinal analgesia with bupivacaine. *British Journal of Anaesthesia* **58**, 610–14.

Moyer G.A. & Rein P. (1986) Preoxygenation in the morbidly obese patient. *Anesthesia and Analgesia* **65**, 106S.

Nakajima T., Fujioka S. & Tokunaga K. (1989) Correlation of intraabdominal fat accumulation and left ventricular performance in obesity. *American Journal of Cardiology* **64**, 369–73.

Norton M.L. & Brown A.C.D. (1990) Evaluation of the patient with a difficult airway for anesthesia. *Otolaryngology Clinics of North America* **23**, 771–85.

Paul D.R., Hoyt J.L. & Boutros A.R. (1976) Cardiovascular and respiratory changes in response to change of posture in the obese. *Anesthesiology* **45**, 73–8.

Peiris A.N., Sothmann M.S. & Hoffman R.G. (1989) Adiposity, fat distribution and cardiovascular risk. *Annals of Internal Medicine* **110**, 867–72.

Pitkainan M.J. (1987) Body mass and the spread of spinal anaesthesia with bupivacaine. *British Journal of Anaesthesia* **66**, 127–33.

Rand C.S.W., Kuldau J.M. & Yost R.L. (1985) Obesity and postoperative pain. *Journal of Psychosomatic Research* **29**, 43–8.

Rawal N., Sjostrand V., Christofferson E., Dahlstrom N., Arwill A. & Rydman H. (1984) Comparison of intramuscular and epidural morphine for postoperative analgesia in the grossly obese. Influence on postoperative ambulation and pulmonary function. *Anesthesia and Analgesia* **63**, 583–92.

Reisin E. & Frolich E.D. (1981) Obesity. Cardiovascular and respiratory pathophysiological alterations. *Archives of Internal Medicine* **141**, 431–4.

Rosenbaum S., Skinner R.F., Knight A.B. & Garrow J.S. (1985) A survey of height and weight in Great Britain 1980. *Annals of Human Biology* **12**, 115–27.

Salem M.R., Joseph N., Lim R. & Rao T.K.N. (1984) Respiratory and hemodynamic response to PEEP in grossly obese patients. *Anesthesiology* **61**, 511A.

Schwartz A.E., Matteo R.S., Ornstein E., Chow F.T. & Diaz J. (1986a) Pharmacokinetics of sufentanyl in the obese. *Anesthesiology* **65**, 652A.

Schwartz A.E., Matteo R.S., Ornstein E., Chow F.T. & Diaz J.

(1986b) Pharmacokinetics and dynamics of metocurine in the obese. *Anesthesiology* **65**, 295A.

Strube P.J., Hulands G.M. & Halsey M.J. (1987) Serum fluoride levels in morbidly obese patients: enflurane compared with isoflurane. *British Journal of Anaesthesia* **42**, 685–9.

Taivanen T., Tuominen M. & Rosenberg P.M. (1990) Influence of obesity on the spread of spinal analgesia after injection of plain 0.5% bupivacaine at the L3–4 or L4–5 interspace. *British Journal of Anaesthesia* **64**, 542–6.

Thawley S.E. (1985) Surgical treatment of sleep apnea. *Medical Clinics of North America* **69**, 1337–58.

Tseueda K., Warren J.E. & McCafferty L.A. (1978) Pancuronium bromide requirement during anesthesia for the morbidly obese. *Anesthesiology* **48**, 483–539.

Van Itallie T.B. (1985) Health implications of overweight and obesity in the United States. *Annals of Internal Medicine* **103**, 983–8.

Varin F., Ducharme J. & Thoret Y. (1990) The influence of extreme obesity on the body disposition and neuromuscular blocking effect of atracurium. *Clinical Pharmacology and Therapeutics* **48**, 18–25.

Vaughan R.W. (1982a) Pulmonary and cardiovascular derangements in the obese patient. In *Anesthetics and the Obese Patient* (Ed. Brown B.R.) pp. 19–39. Contemporary Anesthesia Practice Series. F.A. Davis, Philadelphia.

Vaughan R.W. (1982b) Biochemical and biotransformation alterations in obesity. In *Anesthetics and the Obese Patient* (Ed. Brown B.R.) pp. 55–70. Contemporary Anesthesia Practice Series. F.A. Davis, Philadelphia.

Vaughan R.W. & Wise L. (1976) Intraoperative oxygenation in obese patients. *Annals of Surgery* **184**, 35–42.

Vaughan R.W., Engelhart R.C. & Wise L. (1974) Postoperative hypoxemia in obese patients. *Annals of Surgery* **180**, 872–7.

Vaughan R.W., Bauer S. & Wise L. (1975) Volume and pH of gastric juice in obese patients. *Anesthesiology* **43**, 686–9.

Wadden T.A. & Stunkard A.J. (1985) Social and psychological consequences of obesity. *Annals of Internal Medicine* **103**, 1062–7.

Weinstein J.E., Matteo R.S. & Ornstein E. (1986) Pharmacodynamics of vecuronium and atracurium in the obese surgical patient. *Anesthesia and Analgesia* **65**, 684–7.

Wilson S.L., Manaltea N.R. & Malvesa J.D. (1981) Effects of atropine, glycopyrollate and cimetidine on gastric secretions in markedly obese patients. *Anesthesia and Analgesia* **60**, 37–40.

Wittels E.M. & Thompson S. (1990) Obstructive apnoea and obesity. *Otolaryngology Clinics of North America* **23**, 751–61.

Anaesthesia for Transplantation Surgery and Management of the Organ Donor

A.M. BURNS AND G.R. PARK

Transplantation of major organs is increasingly becoming common and more successful. Anaesthetists may be involved as part of the 'transplant team', not only with the perioperative care of the recipient, but also with the intensive care of the donor and management during organ retrieval. In addition, patients who have undergone transplantation are now presenting for anaesthesia and surgery for unrelated procedures.

Organization

The transplant team

The successful outcome of a transplant operation depends on teamwork between medical, nursing, theatre, technical and administrative staff (Table 57.1). All members of the team have special areas of expertise enabling them to contribute to these complex operations.

The transplant co-ordinator

Key members of transplant teams include the transplant co-ordinators. They organize all administrative matters connected with the transplant, including communication with the donor hospital. In addition, they co-ordinate the surgical and anaesthetic teams, the operating theatres and support staff, and the intensive care unit (ICU), and are involved with the recipient and their families. The transplant co-ordinators also liaise with national (e.g. UK Transplant Service Special Authority) and international organizations (e.g. Eurotransplant), enabling organs to be matched and transferred to places where there are suitable recipients.

Table 57.1 Members of the transplant team and their responsibilities

The transplant co-ordinator:	Donor
	Recipient
The surgical team:	Organ retrieval
	Recipient
The anaesthetic team:	Recipient
	Organ retrieval
The intensive care unit staff:	Donor
	Recipient
Medical and nursing staff in the transplant surgical and medical units:	Recipient
Operating theatre nursing and technical staff:	Organ retrieval
	Recipient
Laboratory staff:	Blood transfusion and haematology
	Biochemistry
	Histopathology

Logistics

Unless properly organized, any major transplant programme disrupts the ordinary work of a hospital. Factors such as facilities to perform the recipient surgery, including the availability of intensive care beds, limit the number of transplants that can be performed. Most transplants are undertaken with some degree of urgency, but improvements in organ preservation allow many transplant operations to be performed within normal working hours. The degree of specialist knowledge and expertise needed for major transplant procedures requires the involvement of senior members of the team. Major grafting operations often take several hours to perform, and the anaesthetic team may be involved with continuing care in the ICU. Allowances need to be made for this when organizing duty rotas.

Brainstem death and organ donation

The success of organ transplantation has greatly improved and in many transplant units, the problem now lies not with recipient survival but in the supply of donors. It has been estimated that only about 1200 people of the 500 000 who die each year in Britain are potential organ donors (Gore et al., 1989). Increasing emphasis is now being placed on management of the brain-dead organ donor. This is because it is recognized that improved quality of care of the donor may increase the number of organs that are suitable for transplantation and improve their function after grafting. Careful management of one donor may benefit up to seven patients with end-stage disease.

When perfusion of organs with oxygenated blood ceases, ischaemic damage and autolytic processes start. This necessitates organ procurement from a 'beating heart' donor for most organs. Occasionally, it may be possible to perform kidney retrieval within 60 min of the heart stopping with satisfactory graft function. The cornea and heart valves survive cessation of the circulation for a considerable period, making it possible to remove them after the heart has stopped.

The ethical issues surrounding organ donation continue to arouse debate. It is clearly undesirable for the anaesthetist to be involved in the care of both the potential donor and the recipient as this may result in a conflict of interests. In addition, some doctors feel unhappy with the idea of brainstem death and the 'beating heart' donor. It is important that colleagues are available to continue the care of the donor in such a situation.

Table 57.2 Clinical criteria for the diagnosis of brainstem death in the UK

Known cause of irreversible and severe brain injury
Absence of hypothermia, electrolyte and endocrine
 abnormalities
No residual sedative, analgesic or neuromuscular blocking
 drug effects
No pupillary response to light
Absent corneal reflex
Absent caloric responses
No motor response to painful stimuli within distribution of
 cranial nerves
No gag or bronchial reflex
Apnoea in the presence of $Paco_2$ >6.65 kPa (50 mmHg)

Brainstem death

The British criteria for recognition of brainstem death were described by the Conference of the Medical Royal Colleges and their Faculties in the UK in 1976 and revised in 1979, resulting in the publication of a Code of Practice. The clinical criteria for the diagnosis of brainstem death in the UK are shown in Table 57.2. Formal tests confirming brainstem death should be performed according to the Code of Practice by two doctors who are independent of the transplant team. The time of death is when the second set of tests confirm brainstem death.

Consent to organ donation

Only the person lawfully in possession of the body may authorize the removal of organs. In a British hospital, the health authority is deemed to be lawfully in possession of a body within a hospital. The health authority delegates this responsibility to the consultant who is at the time of death principally in charge of the patient's care. Such a 'designated person' may authorize the removal of organs by a surgical transplant team.

In practice it is usual, and recommended, that permission from relatives for organ donation is obtained. If the patient carried a donor card, there is no requirement to discuss consent with the relatives, but it is still advisable to do so. At present in Britain it is usually a senior member of the medical team looking after the patient who asks for consent. The transplant co-ordinator may also be able to provide information and support for the relatives. Most relatives gain some comfort from the act of donation and this provides some relief from an otherwise tragic situation. The special problems relating to paediatric donation have been reviewed elsewhere (Hill & Park, 1990).

Organ donation is best discussed with the relatives after the first set of tests have been performed. Waiting until after the second set of tests have been completed may result in both unnecessary distress for the relatives and delay in obtaining the organs. When brain death and organ donation are being discussed with relatives, the idea of the 'beating heart' donor should be clearly explained. It is also important that multiple organ donation is discussed, as this increases organ availability.

Both good and bad publicity have surrounded the practice of organ donation. This has led to fluctuations in supply but there is still a large deficit of some donor organs. In the UK, an 'opting in' system exists, using widely available donor cards. This has not been very successful owing to low acceptance rates by the public. 'Opting out' procedures have been implemented in some countries. In these countries, individuals have to register on a central computer if they *do not* wish to donate organs. 'Required request' has been introduced as Federal Law in many States in the USA (Grenvik, 1988). This legislation requires that the physician looking after a potential organ donor discusses the possibility of organ donation with the relatives. There is no evidence that the supply of donors has increased because of this legislation. A compromise has been proposed in the form of 'required discussion' where physicians must discuss potential donors with the local transplant team who could then approach the relatives (Rudge, 1987). Collins (1989) has shown that admitting patients who have suffered a severe cerebral vascular accident to an ICU increases subsequent organ-donation rates. These patients are breathing spontaneously (and therefore are not brain dead) and if their neurological condition deteriorates further and respiratory arrest occurs, prompt action can be taken. After this, tests to diagnose brainstem death can be performed. If these confirm the diagnosis then, assuming consent has been given, organ donation can take place. There are many ethical and moral problems arising from this idea that remain to be resolved before this is accepted as common medical practice (Park *et al.*, 1993).

A British survey has shown that relatively few potential organ donors are missed (Gore *et al.*, 1991). Based on this survey, recommendations have been made to increase the number of organs donated. These include an increased awareness of the transplant programmes and education to promote consent for donation, and earlier referral to a transplant centre allowing suitability for organ donation to be assessed. In addition, greater emphasis is now being placed on optimal and aggressive management of the potential donor to improve organ function after transplantation (Soifer & Gelb, 1989; Gelb & Robertson, 1990; Ghosh *et al.*, 1990; Hill & Park, 1990).

Criteria for organ donation

Any previously healthy individual with severe and irreversible brain injury of known cause may be a potential organ donor. A few absolute contraindications apply to all potential donor organs: hepatitis B infectivity, proven infection with human immunodeficiency virus (HIV), known viral infection, a history of intravenous drug abuse, malignancy (except primary CNS tumours) and concurrent bacterial sepsis. The potential donor known or suspected to have been an active homosexual should be carefully considered; several months may elapse between latent HIV infection and seroconversion. Age, diabetes mellitus and the presence of other disease processes are relative contraindications. A history of cardiac arrest is not a contraindication to organ donation. Individual donor organs have more specific criteria (Hill & Park, 1990). Size matching for children and for heart/lung and lung transplantation is important, and the age range for heart and heart/lung donation is more strictly defined than for other organs. In all cases a potential donor should be discussed with a transplant centre. Ultimately, the surgeon responsible for the recipient operation must decide on the suitability of a potential donor.

Transmitted bacterial infection should be avoidable by careful screening of donors for clinical and laboratory signs of sepsis and the use of routine prophylactic broad-spectrum antibiotics during organ procurement. Viral and protozoal infections are more of a problem owing to their silent carriage in donor organs, and the lack of effective drugs for their treatment. In the immunosuppressed patient cytomegalovirus and *Toxoplasma gondii* may cause life-threatening infections.

Donor maintenance

After the criteria for brainstem death have been satisfied and consent for donation obtained, patient care becomes donor maintenance. The emphasis in management is now placed on donor-organ protection. Failure to ensure that the organs are in optimal condition on removal may result in graft failure. Brainstem dysfunction results in physiological disturbances that must be recognized and appropriately managed if organ function is to be preserved (Table 57.3). Ultimately, cardiac arrest occurs, but the management of the donor aims to intervene in this natural course of events, until organ retrieval is complete. The main aims of management are to maintain optimal organ perfusion and oxygenation; correct electrolyte concentrations, acid–base and fluid balance disturbances; and to prevent infection. As a simple guide these goals have been summarized by Gelb and Robertson (1990) as the 'rule of 100s' (Table 57.4).

Ideally, when the diagnosis of brainstem death is confirmed, the duration of support should be as short as possible. Advice on management of the donor may be available from the transplant centre and individual units may have published guidelines.

Table 57.3 Management problems encountered in organ donors

Cardiovascular system	*Metabolic*
Hypotension	Hyperglycaemia
Bradycardia	Diabetes insipidus
Ventricular arrhythmias	Electrolyte disturbances
Hypovolaemia	Acid–base abnormalities
Renal function	*Haematological*
Oliguria	Coagulopathy
Polyuria	
Thermal	
Hypothermia	

Table 57.4 The aims of management of the organ donor: 'the rule of 100s'. (Data from Gelb & Robertson, 1990)

Systolic blood pressure	>13 kPa (100 mmHg)
Urine output	>100 ml/h
Pao_2	>13 kPa (100 mmHg)
Haemoglobin	>100 g/litre

An experienced anaesthetist may accompany the retrieval team, particularly for heart and heart/lung donations. The aim of the following information is to provide guidelines for the care of the donor for the anaesthetist who may not have immediate access to such advice and support.

Monitoring

Most organ donors are managed in a general or neurosurgical ICU and have already undergone a period of intensive observation. If not already established, the following should be monitored: direct arterial and central venous pressures (CVP); hourly urine output; arterial blood-gas tensions; serum electrolyte concentrations; and core (rectal) and peripheral temperatures. Peripheral intravenous access with a large cannula (12–14 g) should allow rapid infusion of fluid. The left radial artery and right internal jugular or subclavian vein should be used for invasive monitoring, as the right subclavian artery and brachiocephalic vein are divided early during retrieval of the heart. In some donors a pulmonary artery catheter (PAC) may be useful.

Cardiovascular system and fluid balance

Hypotension is common in the donor because of several factors. Damage to the vasomotor centre and loss of sympathetic tone results in progressive vasodilatation. The destruction of the nucleus ambiguous in the brainstem abolishes resting vagal tone and, combined with the loss of sympathetic drive, results in bradycardia that does not respond to atropine. In addition, there is depletion of the high-energy stores in the myocardial cells and increasing anaerobic metabolism occurs (Cooper *et al.*, 1989). This predisposes to myocardial ischaemia and arrhythmias, which may exacerbate hypotension. These factors are often compounded by hypovolaemia secondary to fluid restriction and diuretics used, during life, to reduce cerebral oedema.

Correction of hypovolaemia

The first step when correcting hypotension is to expand the intravascular volume. CVP, urine output and core-to-peripheral temperature gradients are useful guides to adequate replacement. Correction of hypovolaemia may allow inotropic therapy to be reduced or even stopped. Blood losses should be replaced with whole blood or packed cells to a haematocrit of 30%. The choice of other fluids for the correction of hypovolaemia is controversial. Colloid should be given to produce a CVP of 1–1.33 kPa (8–10 mmHg). A PAC may be useful in the fluid management of some donors. Modified gelatin solutions, hetastarch and 4.5% human albumin solution have been used for this purpose. Crystalloid may be used for fluid maintenance, but care should be taken as excessive crystalloid administration may be associated with pulmonary oedema and liver congestion. The use of 0.9% saline may also exacerbate hypernatraemia. If heart/lung donation is a possibility, then particular care must be taken to avoid pulmonary oedema and cardiac distension. Minimal amounts of crystalloid should be used, and CVP or pulmonary artery occlusion pressure should be no greater than 0.66 or 1.33 kPa (5 or 8 mmHg), respectively (Ghosh *et al.*, 1990; Large & Schofield, 1991).

Management of diabetes insipidus

Lack of antidiuretic hormone, secondary to posterior pituitary failure, results in polyuria. Severe fluid depletion and hypernatraemia occur if losses are not replaced. Diabetes insipidus presents as large volumes of dilute urine (osmolality <200 mosmol/kg) with a low sodium content, and an increasing plasma osmolality and serum sodium. If urinary losses exceed $4 \, ml \cdot kg^{-1} \cdot h^{-1}$, they should be replaced with dextrose 5%, with sodium and potassium added as needed. However, the early use of hormone replacement in controlling polyuria greatly simplifies fluid management; the administration of large volumes of cold, crystalloid solutions is avoided and electrolyte disturbances are minimized. Vasopressin may be given by infusion (0.5–15 u/h). Alternatively, the synthetic form of vasopressin, DDAVP, can be given intravenously 1–4 µg once or twice daily. DDAVP is associated with less vasoconstriction and has a longer duration of action than vasopressin.

Inotropic therapy

If hypotension persists after correction of hypovolaemia, inotropic agents should be used. The initial choice of agent is currently dopamine as it causes renal and splanchnic vasodilatation at doses below $5\,\mu g \cdot kg^{-1} \cdot min^{-1}$; higher doses cause vasoconstriction and end-organ ischaemia may occur. If this dose is insufficient to maintain organ perfusion, dobutamine, $2–10\,\mu g \cdot kg^{-1} \cdot min^{-1}$, can be added. Hypotension may occur with this agent because of peripheral vasodilatation. Drugs with predominantly vasoconstrictor properties, such as phenylephrine and noradrenaline, should only rarely be required if the above steps are followed, but may be appropriate in some donors to maintain perfusion pressure without excessive fluid. The use of inotropic support should be discussed with the transplant team, especially if heart transplantation is being considered, as this may affect the suitability of organs for donation.

Arrhythmias

Ventricular arrhythmias and conduction defects are common, as are bradycardias. In addition to brainstem dysfunction and increased intracranial pressure, other causes include hypotension, myocardial ischaemia, electrolyte imbalance and the use of inotropes. Arrhythmias should be managed in a similar way to those occurring in other situations. The atropine-resistant bradycardia seen with brainstem death responds to sympathomimetic drugs, such as isoprenaline, which act directly on β-adrenergic receptors in the heart. Cardiac arrest may occur, and particularly if the donor is already in the operating theatre, a short period of resuscitation should be performed. This may allow most organs to be retrieved, although, if prolonged, it may preclude the use of the heart for transplantation.

Aims of cardiovascular support

Systemic arterial pressure should not be considered in isolation as a guide to organ perfusion; a maximally vasodilated circulation may provide good organ perfusion, despite hypotension. A PAC is useful in ensuring optimal cardiac performance, and therefore optimal oxygen transport and organ perfusion. A PAC may be of particular value in assessing the suitability of a heart for donation.

Ventilatory support

Continued artificial ventilation is necessary in the organ donor. Arterial blood-gas tensions should be measured frequently and the ventilator adjusted to give a $Paco_2$ of 5.3–5.6 kPa (40–42 mmHg). Low minute volumes or the addition of deadspace to the ventilator circuit may be necessary to maintain normocapnia as carbon dioxide production is low in brainstem death. Pao_2 should be maintained at a value greater than 10 kPa (75 mmHg). Positive end-expiratory pressure (PEEP) may impair organ perfusion and, unless specifically indicated to improve oxygenation or if lung donation is being considered, should be avoided. Regular physiotherapy and tracheal suction should be continued.

If lung donation is a possibility then careful attention to ventilatory support may improve the quality of the donated organ. Particular care should be taken to avoid pulmonary oedema, and the addition of PEEP at 5 cmH$_2$O may reduce alveolar collapse. Inspired oxygen should be kept as low as possible to reduce the risk of pulmonary oxygen toxicity. Artificial ventilation should be continued for as short a time as possible to reduce the risk of bacterial colonization of the trachea and pulmonary infection.

Renal function

Impairment of renal function may have already occurred, and is not an absolute contraindication to transplantation. However, if renal perfusion is maintained, by avoiding hypotension and hypovolaemia, then renal function should be preserved. Ideally, urine output should be maintained at a rate greater than $1\,ml \cdot kg^{-1} \cdot h^{-1}$, as urine output before nephrectomy may affect immediate graft function (Lucas et al., 1987). If this is not achieved, despite adequate volume replacement, a renal vasodilator, such as dopamine, $2\,\mu g \cdot kg^{-1} \cdot h^{-1}$, should be used. Small doses of frusemide (10–40 mg intravenously) may also promote diuresis. Immediately before organ retrieval mannitol, 0.5 g/kg over 30 min, may be given to stimulate a diuresis.

Temperature control

Brainstem death causes loss of the normal central control of body temperature. The temperature of the donor decreases to that of the environment. Hypothermia is harmful as it causes progressive vasoconstriction and cardiac instability. Body core (rectal) temperature should be monitored and steps taken to maintain temperature to as near normal as possible. Intravenous blood and fluids should be warmed, inspired gases should be heated and humidified, and the donor should be placed on a warming mattress and covered by reflective insulating blankets.

Endocrine failure

Posterior pituitary failure, manifest by diabetes insipidus, is common in brain death and is described above. The anterior pituitary may also be damaged, when brain death occurs. There is loss of diurnal cortisol variation and plasma concentrations of tri-iodothyronine, thyroxine and thyroid-stimulating hormone are reduced. Novitsky and colleagues (1987) have suggested that endocrine failure may contribute to haemodynamic instability in the brain dead. It may be that hormone replacement improves haemodynamic instability and is beneficial in the management of organ donors, but further work is needed to establish the role of such therapy.

Hypoglycaemia and hyperglycaemia should be avoided and blood glucose concentration monitored hourly. An insulin infusion should be used if blood glucose concentration is >10 mmol/litre.

Coagulopathy

Disseminated intravascular coagulation may complicate fatal head injuries. This is probably a result of release of necrotic tissue from the ischaemic brain. Coagulation abnormalities should be suspected and corrected with appropriate blood products, to minimize blood loss at organ retrieval. A severe coagulopathy may make organ retrieval difficult and deterioration in the clinical state or laboratory studies should prompt rapid transfer to theatre.

The donor operation

When death has been certified and consent obtained, arrangements are made by the transplant co-ordinator, together with the surgical teams, for organ retrieval at the donor hospital. Much of the care of the organ donor in the ICU is continued in the operating theatre. However, specific points about the intraoperative management are discussed below.

Theatre preparation, equipment and monitoring

Multiple organ retrieval is a major surgical procedure. It should not be delegated to those inexperienced in intensive care and/or anaesthesia. It may take up to 6 h to complete the surgery, during which time significant blood and fluid losses may occur. When multiple organ retrieval is planned, equipment for invasive pressure monitoring must be available, and infusion pumps may be needed for infusion of inotropes (Table 57.5). When preparations are complete, the donor is transferred to the operating theatre. The donor is placed supine on the operating table and the arms are usually placed by the sides to allow the surgeons access to the donor.

General care

The use of analgesic and anaesthetic agents to produce anaesthesia is illogical in organ donors. However, anaesthetic agents may be used to depress possibly harmful spinal reflexes, such as tachycardia and hypertension, related to surgical incision (Wetzl et al., 1985). Most anaesthetists continue to use nitrous oxide as a carrier gas to avoid the administration of 100% oxygen from anaesthetic machines without a supply of compressed air.

Stimulation, such as occurs on skin incision, may trigger intact spinal reflexes in donors. These may manifest themselves as muscle twitches through to complex limb movements. Unless these changes are anticipated and understood by attending staff, anxieties may arise on the validity of brainstem death criteria. Reflex increases in muscle tone may also limit surgical access at laparotomy. A muscle relaxant, such as pancuronium, 0.1 mg/kg, may be given before surgical incision.

Intraoperative fluid balance, haemodynamics and temperature control

Large losses of fluids from an open abdomen and chest should be anticipated during the dissection phase. Blood transfusion may be needed during the dissection phase, and blood should be cross-matched before the operation; two units are usually sufficient. Further volume replacement may be achieved with colloid solutions. Hypothermia may be a problem in

Table 57.5 Preparation of the operating theatre and donor before multiple organ retrieval

Administration:	Liaise with transplant co-ordinator
	Liaise with operating theatre staff
	Maintain contact with donor's relatives
	Check consent for organ donation
Equipment:	Appropriate ventilator and humidifier
	Infusion pumps
	Rapid infusion device (pressure bag)
	Fluid warmer
	Warming blanket
Monitor:	Oximeter
	ECG
	Direct arterial pressure
	Central venous pressure
	Capnograph
	Temperature (core and peripheral)
	Urine output
	Pulmonary artery pressure and cardiac output (optional)
Drugs:	Muscle relaxant (pancuronium)
	Inotropes and vasoconstrictors
	Vasodilators (sodium nitroprusside, isoflurane)
	Antiarrhythmic agents
	Diuretics
	Heparin
	Antibiotics
	Specific requests (methylprednisolone)
Vascular access:	Two 12–14 g peripheral venous cannulae
	Triple-lumen central venous catheter
	Radial artery cannula
	Pulmonary artery catheter (optional)
Fluids:	Two units of cross-matched blood
	Colloid
	Crystalloid
	Mannitol
Laboratory support:	Haematology
	Biochemistry
	Arterial blood-gas analysis
	Electrolytes and glucose

nitroprusside may also be used. Hypotension may occur during mobilization of the liver, because of kinking of the inferior vena cava, and during dissection of the mediastinal pleura. Prostacyclin may be used to perfuse the lungs, where it is thought to improve pulmonary perfusion and reduce cellular aggregation within the lung vasculature. This may cause systemic hypotension and the infusion rate is usually started at a low rate and gradually increased to avoid this.

For heart and heart/lung retrieval central venous lines and, if present, the PAC, must be withdrawn before the superior vena cava is divided.

Ventilatory support

Standard anaesthetic equipment is used to provide ventilatory support using the same F_IO_2 and PEEP (if used), but occasionally a more sophisticated ventilator may be required if oxygenation is a problem. Arterial blood-gas tensions should be measured hourly throughout the operation.

For heart/lung donors, full inflation of the lungs should occur with each inspiratory cycle. During tracheal dissection and mobilization ventilation may be difficult. When the lungs are perfused they should be slowly (4 breaths/min) manually inflated. Pharyngeal toilet and tracheal suction should be performed before deflating the cuff of the tracheal tube. After full inflation of the lungs the tube is withdrawn, the trachea is clamped, and ventilation stopped.

Specific drug requirements

Heparin (3 mg/kg) is given intravenously after dissection and mobilization of the intra-abdominal organs has been completed, to avoid coagulation around perfusion cannulae. Transplant teams may have specific drug administration requirements; this may include antibiotic prophylaxis and steroid administration. The anaesthetist should be advised of the exact choice of agents.

Discontinuation of donor maintenance

The point of death is defined as the time the second set of brainstem function tests have been completed. However, supportive care of the organs continues until cross-clamping of the aorta and the start of organ cooling with preservation solutions. This time should be recorded as it marks the beginning of cold ischaemia for the organs to be transplanted. At this

the operating theatre when the donor has an open chest and abdomen. Heat losses should be minimized using the methods described above.

Reflex cardiovascular responses, including tachycardia and hypertension, may occur when the donor is stimulated. Initially, any inotropes that are in use should be stopped. If hypertension continues, vasodilatation with a volatile agent, such as isoflurane, may be most convenient, but nitrates and sodium time, ventilatory support; other supportive measures and monitoring should be stopped.

Operative details

The first part of the operation is a thorough inspection of the abdomen and thorax. This may reveal unsuspected disease or injury to the organ; if so, the procedure may have to be modified or abandoned. After that, exact operative details differ between centres.

If all transplantable organs are to be removed the chest and abdomen are opened with a long midline incision from the jugular notch to the symphysis pubis. The sternum is split but the pleura and pericardium are left intact until the abdominal organs have been dissected and mobilized. When dissection is complete, heparin is given. The pleura and pericardium are opened and the heart, or heart and lungs, mobilized. Cannulae are placed in the aortic root, the main pulmonary artery, the lower abdominal aorta, the inferior vena cava and the portal vein in preparation for cold perfusion of the organs. Circulatory arrest is produced first with cold cardioplegic solution, after which the lungs are perfused. The heart or heart/lung unit is then removed. After removal, the lungs are deflated to two-thirds vital capacity, and the trachea is stapled. Dissection, cold perfusion and removal of the abdominal organs is then completed. The organs are put in sterile bags and transported, packed in ice, to the recipient hospital. Using current preservation techniques, kidneys may be stored for up to 40 h (although organ survival after 72 h has been documented), livers up to 20 h, and heart and heart/lungs up to 4 h. Even longer times may be possible in the future.

Organ preservation

Organ ischaemia results in depletion of high-energy phosphate compounds, leading to breakdown of the cell-membrane sodium pump. Sodium and water enter the cells, which become swollen. This is of particular importance in the capillary endothelium, where swelling of the cells makes perfusion of the organ difficult. Preservation therefore aims to prevent cells swelling and to minimize the acidosis and depletion of high-energy phosphate.

All preservation techniques now employ cooling to retard the cellular processes that lead to deterioration of the organ. However, cooling alone does not prevent all the harmful effects that occur, and additional measures are necessary to produce effective preservation. These include the use of drugs and chemicals that stabilize cell membranes, reduce cellular swelling, maintain colloid osmotic pressure, act as buffers, preserve the ability to synthesize high-energy phosphate, reduce the production of free radicals, and prevent blood clotting and platelets aggregating (Belzer & Southard, 1988). The organ is initially perfused with cold solution to flush out the blood, followed by simple preservation in ice at 4°C. Individual organs have differing requirements for preservation and various solutions are available. Improvements in organ preservation have resulted in improved graft function, more distant organ procurement, less wastage of organs and the opportunity to change the night-time practice of transplantation to a semielective procedure during the day.

The recipient operation

Preoperative assessment

Most patients considered for organ transplantation have end-stage disease for which medical treatment is no longer effective. The success of a transplant programme depends on careful recipient selection; although with increasing experience patients with concurrent disease may successfully receive a transplanted organ. Individual transplant units have guidelines for the selection of patients who may benefit from an organ transplant. These are based on known outcome for specific groups of patients. Before they are placed on the waiting list, most patients are admitted to hospital for a period of assessment and investigation. For liver and heart/lung transplantation this usually includes anaesthetic assessment. A record of this assessment is of great value when patients are subsequently admitted for the operation, as problems can then be readily identified by the duty anaesthetist. If the patient is accepted into the transplant programme, the assessment period may also be used to optimize the physical condition of the patient and to prepare them psychologically for organ transplantation.

Operations

There are three groups of operations that may be performed on transplant recipients:
1 The actual grafting operations.
2 Related procedures needed by these patients, such as re-exploration of the graft to deal with complications.
3 Operations unrelated to the original pathology.

Transplant procedures

Anaesthetic principles

Although patients receiving organ grafts may undergo different procedures needing refinement of anaesthetic technique, the same anaesthetic needs apply in all patients. The anaesthetic team should be familiar with the pathophysiology of the disease needing transplantation and the surgical techniques. The choice of anaesthetic technique should aim to provide optimal conditions for graft function and, wherever possible, recovery from anaesthesia should not depend on graft function. The anaesthetist may be involved in the administration of special requirements such as antibiotic prophylaxis and immunosuppressive agents. Patients for organ transplantation are often admitted at short notice and may require precautions against aspiration of stomach contents.

Renal transplant

Renal transplantation is the treatment of choice for patients with chronic renal failure (CRF). At present, at least 80% of renal grafts function for at least 1 year, and 60–70% are still working after 5 years. The complications of CRF and the choice of anaesthetic for patients with CRF are discussed in Chapter 62. Anaesthesia for renal transplantation has been reviewed by Cottam & Eason (1991): the main principles are highlighted below.

Preoperative assessment

Patients normally undergo a period of dialysis before surgery. It is essential in any patient with fluid and electrolyte abnormalities, in particular those with hyperkalaemia, acidosis and pulmonary oedema. Haemodialysis can sometimes result in hypokalaemia and reduced intravascular volume before operation. This is seldom a risk with peritoneal dialysis. Serum potassium concentration should always be measured immediately before and after surgery.

Chronic anaemia does not usually require transfusion, but it should be considered if the haemoglobin is less than 80 g/litre. Where necessary, blood should be given during a period of dialysis before operation to prevent fluid overload and an increase in serum potassium concentration.

Patients on haemodialysis usually have an arteriovenous fistula, most commonly in the forearm and this limb must not be used for blood sampling, intravenous infusions or arterial pressure measurement. The limb should be clearly identified, and kept warm and protected with gamgee.

A common cause of renal failure is diabetes mellitus. The management of the diabetic patient is described in Chapter 51. Angina, left ventricular failure and hypertension are common. The patient's normal medication should be continued in the perioperative period.

The operation

The operation consists of inserting the donor kidney into the right or left lower quadrant of the abdomen, with vascular and ureteric anastomoses. After operation, careful attention must be paid to cardiovascular observations, urine output and fluid management, and any problems dealt with promptly to preserve graft function.

Monitoring should include ECG, oximetry, non-invasive arterial pressure, capnography and urine output. A CVP catheter is useful during and after the operation for fluid management. In the critically ill patient, direct measurement of arterial pressure and invasive haemodynamic monitoring with a PAC will be required. Intravenous administration of frusemide and mannitol may be requested after the arterial anastomosis has been performed to promote a diuresis from the newly transplanted kidney.

Liver transplantation

Survival after liver transplantation is now 80–85% at 1 year, and 60–70% at 5 years. Aspects of liver transplantation have been reviewed elsewhere (Calne, 1987; Cosimi, 1991). The clinical features of liver disease and the choice of anaesthetic agents and techniques are described in Chapter 61. However, anaesthetic care of the patient receiving a liver transplant consists of more than the choice of agents; cardiovascular and metabolic changes are encountered, and massive blood transfusion may be required. Particular problems encountered during liver transplantation include the following.

Preoperative assessment

Where possible, fluid, electrolyte, acid–base, coagulation and haemodynamic disturbances should be corrected. Some patients may be critically ill before surgery and require a period of intensive care before transfer to the operating theatre. Before surgery, blood, fresh frozen plasma (FFP) and platelets should be arranged with transfusion services. At the authors' centre it is usual to cross-match 20 units of blood, 4 units of FFP and 5 units of platelets.

The operation

The operation is divided into three phases and takes at least 6 hours to perform. During the dissection phase the diseased liver is dissected free of all peritoneal attachments. The vena cava, hepatic artery and portal vein are then clamped (see below) and the liver removed. This marks the start of the anhepatic phase. The donor liver is then removed from storage and placed in the hepatic fossa. The suprahepatic inferior vena cava and portal vein anastomoses are performed. After flushing of the liver with a colloid solution, to wash out accumulated potassium and hydrogen ions, the clamps are removed and the liver revascularized. During the reperfusion phase the inferior vena cava below the liver, the hepatic artery and the biliary anastomoses are performed. The abdomen is then closed and the patient transferred to the ICU.

Monitoring

In view of the haemodynamic instability that may occur, invasive haemodynamic monitoring is essential. Facilities to measure rapidly arterial blood-gas tensions, electrolytes, ionized calcium, haemoglobin, platelets and clotting must be available. These are monitored throughout the procedure and guide replacement.

Cardiovascular effects and bypass circuits

When the inferior vena cava is clamped, venous return from the lower half of the body almost ceases and the cardiac output decreases by approximately 50%. These changes persist throughout the anhepatic period, which usually lasts between 30 min and 1 h, and reverse when the clamps are removed. Trial clamping of the inferior vena cava is usually performed before the liver is removed. If this produces a large reduction in vascular pressures, pump-assisted bypass is used to decompress the portal vein and inferior vena cava. This also returns blood to the systemic circulation, allowing a normal cardiac output to be maintained. Bypass consists of a venovenous femorosubclavian shunt in association with a magnetically operated centrifugal pump. The system is coated with heparin, and systemic administration of heparin is not required. In some centres it is routinely used in all adult patients.

Blood loss and coagulopathy

A large blood loss should be anticipated. The average loss in adults at the authors' centre is 4 litres, but it may be much greater because of a prolonged dissection phase, coagulopathy and portal hypertension. The problems of massive transfusion are discussed in Chapter 29. A rapid infusion device allows prompt replacement of losses. Increasing use of a centrifugal cell-washer, enabling up to 50% of the lost erythrocytes to be transfused, reduces the demands on the blood transfusion service. With this system plasma is not preserved and must be replaced with crystalloid and albumin solution.

Coagulopathy is a common feature of liver failure and should be corrected before operation. Further FFP and platelets are given on reperfusion of the new liver. Cryoprecipitate may be used to correct hypofibrinogenaemia and Factor VIII depletion. Use of citrated blood lowers the plasma concentration of ionized calcium, resulting in cardiac depression. This should be corrected with calcium chloride. The prophylactic use of aprotinin, a proteinase inhibitor, may reduce blood loss incurred during liver transplantation.

Electrolyte and acid–base disturbances

When the donor liver is reperfused potassium and hydrogen ions are washed into the general circulation. This may result in hypotension and ECG changes. These cardiotoxic effects are mainly a result of hyperkalaemia and may be counteracted with calcium chloride. Other substances that are vasoactive may also be released. The metabolic acidosis present before operation can deteriorate, particularly during the anhepatic phase and immediately after reperfusion. However, sodium bicarbonate is used rarely, as rapid correction occurs spontaneously. Significant hypernatraemia may occur, particularly in children because of the large sodium load. The sources of the sodium include saline solutions, used to flush the numerous cannulae, and blood products that use sodium citrate as the anticoagulant. If the patient was hyponatraemic before operation, slow correction before surgery is important to avoid central pontine myelinosis (Laureno & Karp, 1988).

Temperature

Precautions should be taken against heat loss during this long procedure. A reduction in body temperature of 1–2°C is associated with the insertion of the ice-cold donor liver, and this is exacerbated by massive blood transfusion and prolonged surgery.

Renal function

These patients often have some degree of renal impairment before operation and oliguria may occur during the operation. In addition to maintaining cardiac output and systemic arterial pressure, active measures employed to maintain urine flow include the use of mannitol infusion, $0.5\,g \cdot kg^{-1} \cdot h^{-1}$, and dopamine, $2\,\mu g \cdot kg^{-1} \cdot min^{-1}$, throughout the operation.

Postoperative care

After completion of the operation, the patient is transferred to the ICU and ventilation-supported until the patient is stable and warm. The initial period after surgery can present many problems including fluid and electrolyte balance, infection, renal failure and nutrition. Some patients may need prolonged management in the ICU.

Heart, heart/lung and lung transplantation

Heart transplantation is considered for patients with advanced cardiac disease that cannot be treated by other forms of cardiac surgery and in whom medical treatment is no longer effective (Large & Schofield, 1991). Patients with increased pulmonary vascular resistance or chronic lung disease are not suitable for heart transplantation but may be considered for heart/lung or lung transplantation (LeGal, 1990; Cooper, 1991). Survival after heart transplantation is now 90% after 1 year and 78% after 5 years. The major problems with lung transplantation are the lack of effective protection against lung ischaemia, and the breakdown of the bronchial anastomosis. Survival after heart/lung transplantation is now 62% at 2 years. Experience with lung transplantation is still being gained but survival rates after this operation continue to improve (Cooper, 1991).

Heart and heart/lung transplantation is performed using cardiopulmonary bypass. Lung transplantation is performed through a lateral thoracotomy; cardiopulmonary bypass is used only if the patient is haemodynamically unstable or oxygenation cannot be maintained with single-lung anaesthesia. The principles and choice of anaesthetic technique for patients with cardiac and respiratory disease are discussed in Chapters 59 and 60. Meticulous haemostasis, particularly at the site of pleural adhesions, is

essential. After operation, the patient is transferred to the ICU and ventilatory support given until it is certain that there is no further bleeding requiring re-exploration. Ventilatory support after single-lung transplant may be complicated by differences in compliance between the transplanted lung and the remaining diseased lung, and may need differential lung ventilation.

Multiple-organ transplantation

A recent trend is to consider patients for transplantation who are suffering from failure of more than one organ. This includes patients with simultaneous liver and kidney disease such as polycystic disease and α_1-antitrypsin deficiency. A heart, lungs and liver graft has been successfully performed (Wallwork et al., 1987). In these cases each graft procedure is treated separately, and is performed in turn in its own conventional manner.

Corneal grafting

Patients for corneal grafting may be of any age but are usually healthy in other respects. Immunosuppressant drugs are not required to prevent rejection. The operation consists of the removal of a central disc of opaque cornea and its replacement with a similar sized disc of donor tissue. This involves opening the eye and at which time there is a risk of prolapse of intraocular contents. Anaesthesia aims to facilitate the surgery by reducing intraocular pressure. A full description is given in Chapter 38.

Bone marrow transplantation

Marrow may be aspirated from a patient for subsequent reinfusion after a course of chemotherapy or radiotherapy, or from a healthy donor. Marrow aspiration is painful and general anaesthesia is usually necessary. The procedure, which involves aspiration from multiple sites, mainly from the iliac crests, may take one to two hours. The donor is prone for most of that time. Because of this, tracheal intubation and ventilatory support are usually needed, as is the use of opioid analgesic agents. A plasma volume expander may be needed to maintain intravascular volume.

General anaesthesia is not required for the infusion of bone marrow in this form of tissue grafting, but the anaesthetist may be involved in the intensive care management of these patients. Before grafting, the recipient's own marrow must be destroyed using cytotoxic agents and/or whole-body irradiation. This results in anaemia, leucopenia and thrombocytopenia. The patients are vulnerable to infection and are nursed in isolation. Supportive management includes infusions of red cells, white cells and platelets. Antibiotics and antifungal agents are given, but infections are common and septicaemia may herald multisystem organ failure. Intensive care management includes ventilatory, circulatory and renal support, but the survival rate is low.

Other organs and tissue

Pancreatic transplantation has been successfully performed (Corry, 1991), often in combination with renal transplantation in patients with diabetes mellitus and renal failure. Interest is now focusing on combined small-bowel and liver transplantation (Grant *et al.*, 1990). Adrenal and fetal tissue has been implanted in the midbrain of patients with Parkinson's disease but results are, as yet, inconclusive (Williams, 1990).

Immunosuppression

The ideal immunosuppressive regimen would produce tolerance only to the transplanted organ, while allowing the immune system to mount a normal response to infection. Unfortunately this ideal does not yet exist. Many units now use triple therapy with low doses of azathioprine, corticosteroids and cyclosporin A. The aim of this combination therapy is to prevent graft rejection while reducing the risk of dose-related side-effects. However, the toxicity of current drugs continues to be a major problem (Table 57.6). The development of malignant disease, particularly skin cancers and lymphomas, has also been reported in recipients. Antibodies directed against specific targets, such as antilymphocyte globulin and antithymocyte globulin, are now commonly used both for initial immunosuppression and in the treatment of rejection. Monoclonal antibodies, such as OKT3, have been used in the management of steroid-resistant rejection. Whole-body irradiation, in combination with cytotoxic agents, is used to suppress the reticuloendothelial system of patients undergoing bone marrow transplantation.

Individual transplant units have specific protocols for immunosuppression depending on the organ to be transplanted. Most centres start immunosuppression during surgery and further measures may be introduced after operation. Subsequent management depends on the response of the patient,

Table 57.6 Unwanted effects of immunosuppressive agents

Corticosteroids
Delayed healing
Gastrointestinal perforation
Impaired glucose tolerance
Pituitary—adrenal axis suppression
Hypertension
Osteoporosis
Cushingoid appearance
Cataracts
Avascular necrosis
Hypokalaemia

Azathioprine
Bone marrow suppression
  Anaemia
  Thrombocytopenia
  Granulocytopenia
Hepatotoxicity
Pulmonary infiltrates

Cyclosporin
Nephrotoxicity
Neurotoxicity
  Fits
  Altered consciousness
Tremor
Hepatotoxicity
Gastrointestinal upset
Hyperuricaemia
Gum hypertrophy
Skin rashes

monitoring of the plasma concentration of cyclosporin, the full blood count and the development of complications such as infection and rejection.

Complications of immunosuppression

Infection

This is the commonest and most important complication of immunosuppression. In addition to bacterial infections, opportunistic infections with agents, such as *Pneumocystis carinii*, cytomegalovirus, *Toxoplasma gondii* and *Candida albicans*, and reactivation of *Herpes zoster* or *Herpes simplex*, may occur. Before the patient is considered for transplantation septic foci (such as carious teeth) should be eliminated and viral screening performed. The risk of infection is compounded by the often extensive surgery, the use of intravascular catheters, surgical drains and urinary catheters, malnutrition, infections present in the donor, or intercurrent disease in the recipient, such as diabetes mellitus. Scrupulous attention to infection control is essential. Aseptic techniques should be used for all invasive procedures. Equipment should, whenever possible, be disposable or autoclavable. Anaesthetic machines and ventilators should be carefully cleaned before and after each use. Disposable heat and moisture exchangers combined with bacterial and viral filters should be used in the breathing circuit.

Prophylaxis against infection includes broad-spectrum antibiotic cover started at the time of operation. Selective decontamination of the digestive tract has been advocated after liver transplantation (Stoutenbeck et al., 1986). The prevention of candidiasis with nystatin is of value in the perioperative period.

Rejection

The ease with which rejection is suppressed depends on the type of response, and also its severity. Rejection mediated by cellular infiltrates responds to immunosuppressive treatment, but antibody-mediated humoral reactions are relatively resistant. Liver grafts are rejected less rapidly than kidneys, while transplanted hearts are rejected more rapidly.

Signs of rejection depend on the organ involved. For example, oliguria and deterioration in renal function may indicate renal-graft rejection, increasing concentrations of transaminase and bilirubin may suggest liver-graft rejection and ECG changes may herald heart-transplant rejection. Fever often accompanies rejection. However, these indicators are non-specific and often fail to distinguish between infection, infarction and rejection. Angiography or isotope scanning may provide further information about graft function, but a definite diagnosis usually requires biopsy. In the case of the heart, an endo-myocardial biopsy can be taken via a transvenous catheter. Lung biopsies can be obtained either bronchoscopically or by open lung biopsy.

When the diagnosis is made, and infection or ischaemia excluded, antirejection treatment may be started. Episodes are usually managed by initiating or increasing steroid treatment. Relatively large doses of methyl prednisolone are given and then gradually reduced to a new maintenance dose.

Anaesthesia and immunosuppression

Anaesthesia and surgery are believed generally to suppress immune responses (Simpson, 1988). This may be of benefit to patients having organ grafts.

From a practical point of view, the choice, dose and time of administration of immunosuppressive agents is not affected. Anaesthetists may be asked to administer immunosuppressant agents intraoperatively. Both azathioprine and methylprednisolone if injected intravenously and rapidly may cause hypotension.

Anaesthesia for related procedures

Patients who require re-exploration of the graft have similar anaesthetic requirements to those for the original procedure. If bleeding is the major problem the patient may be haemodynamically unstable, and is often more unwell than when they initially presented for transplantation.

Many other associated operations may be needed, including biopsy of the transplanted organ. When a needle biopsy is performed, it is usually obtained using local anaesthesia. General anaesthesia is required for open biopsies in adults, and usually for children undergoing needle biopsy.

Regional techniques can be used in certain situations. For example, formation of an arteriovenous fistula, or exploration of a blocked fistula, can be performed using a brachial plexus block. This may also facilitate surgery owing to vasodilatation secondary to sympathetic block.

Anaesthesia for operations unrelated to the original pathology

The anaesthetic needs depend on the procedure being performed, the organ that has been grafted and its function. In the patient who has undergone a successful transplant, the problems related to the original pathology and chronic disease should be largely resolved. The general principles of anaesthesia in this situation are outlined below. If these are applied, then most patients may be safely managed with either general or local anaesthesia.

Before surgery it is advisable to contact the appropriate medical/transplant team. Immunosuppression may require adjustment to a different dose and/or formulation in the period after surgery. Anaesthetic management should maintain graft perfusion and function. Chronic rejection may impair graft function, which may influence the choice of anaesthetic technique. The anaesthetist must be aware of the complications of immunosuppressive drugs, especially corticosteroids, and of drug interactions, for example, the concurrent use of nephrotoxic drugs such as cyclosporin, aminoglycosides and frusemide. Anaesthetic techniques that reduce liver blood flow may increase the concentration of cyclosporin, increasing the risk of toxicity. The advantages of invasive techniques and monitoring should be balanced against the risk of infection. Appropriate antibiotic cover should always be given. If the patient becomes unwell after the operation, infection and rejection must be considered.

Anaesthesia for patients after heart and heart/lung transplantation

Many patients who have undergone heart transplantation are now presenting for unrelated surgery (Shaw et al., 1991; White & Latimer, 1991). In the presence of satisfactory graft function, few difficulties should be encountered during anaesthesia for these patients. However, it is important that the anaesthetist has some understanding of the alterations in physiology that occur after heart and lung transplantation. Both the transplanted heart and lungs are denervated and have no autonomic nerve supply. Thus, the heart does not accelerate in the normal way to sympathetic stimulation. Initially, alterations in the cardiovascular response to stress result in cardiac output being increased by an increase in stroke volume (Frank–Starling mechanism), rather than by reflex tachycardia. The heart rate response in the denervated heart is a result of stimulation of β_1-adrenoceptors by circulating catecholamines, and takes several minutes to be established. As a result, hypovolaemia is poorly tolerated, and preload should be maintained. Heart rate is also a poor guide to depth of anaesthesia. Furthermore, heart rate is unresponsive to atropine but responds to direct-acting agents such as isoprenaline. Inotropic agents and vasoconstrictors should be readily available. In the first 6 months after transplantation arrhythmias are common. These decrease in frequency with time. They should be treated by conventional methods. Regional anaesthesia has been successfully used in cardiac transplant patients. Hypotensive responses may be exaggerated and adequate hydration and prophylactic use of ephedrine has been advised.

Patients after lung transplantation who, before operation, depended on the hypoxic drive to ventilation, regain the normal response to carbon dioxide over a period of months. The respiratory pattern and the pulmonary response to exercise is normal. Stimulation of the airway below the anastomosis does not elicit a cough reflex because the lung is denervated. The tracheas of patients after heart/lung transplantation should be extubated only when they are able to respond to verbal commands to cough. All lung transplant patients need physiotherapy after operation. Excessive airway pressure should be avoided in single-lung transplant patients during ventilation, and fluid overload should be avoided as the transplanted lung lacks lymphatic drainage.

Summary

A successful transplant depends on teamwork and the combining of many areas of expertise. One-year survival rates after transplantation now approach 90% for renal, liver and heart transplantation. For the recipient a successful transplant means a dramatic improvement in the quality of life, often with a full return to normal activities and employment. Cost–benefit studies have shown that transplantation is of value not only to the recipient, but also to health care resources. A major limiting factor on the transplant programme is donor organ supply and emphasis is now being placed on donor maintenance.

Acknowledgement

This chapter has been revised from that published in the first edition of Anaesthesia and written by the late John V. Farman.

References

Belzer F.O. & Southard J.H. (1988) Principles of solid-organ preservation by cold storage. Transplantation 45, 673–6.

Calne R.Y. (Ed.) (1987) Liver Transplantation 2nd edn. Grune and Stratton, London.

Collins C. (1989) Organs for transplantation. British Medical Journal 299, 1463.

Conference of Medical Royal Colleges and their Faculties in the UK (1976) Diagnosis of brain death. British Medical Journal ii, 1187–8.

Conference of Medical Royal Colleges and their Faculties in the UK (1979) Diagnosis of brain death. British Medical Journal i, 332.

Cooper D.K.C., Novitzky D. & Wicomb W.N. (1989) The pathophysiological effects of brain death on potential donor organs, with particular reference to the heart. Annals of the Royal College of Surgeons of England 71, 261–6.

Cooper J.D. (1991) Current status of lung transplantation. Transplantation Proceedings 23, 2107–14.

Corry R.J. (1991) Status report on pancreas transplantation. Transplantation Proceedings 23, 2091–4.

Cosimi A.B. (1991) Update on liver transplantation. Transplantation Proceedings 23, 2083–90.

Cottam S. & Eason J. (1991) Anaesthesia for renal transplantation. In Anaesthesia Review vol. 8. (Ed. Kaufman L.) pp. 159–78. Churchill Livingstone, Edinburgh.

Gelb A.W. & Robertson K.M. (1990) Anaesthetic management of the brain dead for organ donation. Canadian Journal of

Anaesthesia **37**, 806—12.

Ghosh S., Bethune D.W., Hardy I., Kneeshaw J., Latimer R.D. & Oduro A. (1990) Management of donors for heart and heart—lung transplantation. *Anaesthesia* **45**, 672—5.

Gore S.M., Hinds C.J. & Rutherford A.J. (1989) Organ donation from intensive care units in England. *British Medical Journal* **299**, 1193—7.

Gore S.M., Ross Taylor R.M. & Wallwork J. (1991) Availability of transplantable organs from brain stem dead donors in intensive care units. *British Medical Journal* **302**, 149—53.

Grant D., Wall W., Mimeault R., Zhong R., Ghent C., Gancia B., Stillen C. & Duff J. (1990) Successful small bowel/liver transplantation. *Lancet* **335**, 181—3.

Grenvik A. (1988) Ethical dilemmas in organ donation and transplantation. *Critical Care Medicine* **16**, 1012—18.

Hill S.A. & Park G.R. (1990) Management of multiple organ donors. *Baillière's Clinical Anaesthesiology* **4**, 587—605.

Large S.R. & Schofield P.M. (1991) Heart transplantation. *Hospital Update* **17**, 808—16.

Laureno R. & Karp B.I. (1988) Pontine and extrapontine myelinosis following rapid correction of hyponatraemia. *Lancet* **1**, 1439—41.

LeGal Y.M. (1990) Heart and heart—lung transplantation. *Annals of Thoracic Surgery* **49**, 840—4.

Lucas B.A., Baughn W.L., Spees E.K. & Sanfillipo F. (1987) Identification of donor factors predisposing to high discard rates of cadaver kidneys and increased graft loss within one year post transplantation: SEOPF 1977—1982. *Transplantation* **43**, 253—8.

Novitzky D., Cooper D.K.C. & Reichard B. (1987) Hemodynamic and metabolic responses to hormonal therapy in brain-dead potential organ donors. *Transplantation* **43**, 852—4.

Park G.R., Gunning K.E., Lindop M.J. & Roe P.G. (1993) Organ donation. *British Medical Journal* **306**, 145.

Rudge C.J. (1987) Consent for transplantation. *British Journal of Hospital Medicine* **38**, 93—4.

Shaw I.H., Kirk A.J.B. & Conacher I.D. (1991) Anaesthesia for patients with transplanted hearts and lungs undergoing non-cardiac surgery. *British Journal of Anaesthesia* **67**, 772—8.

Simpson P.J. (1988) Immunology and anaesthesia. In *Anaesthesia Review* vol. 5. (Ed. Kaufman L.) pp. 67—84. Churchill Livingstone, Edinburgh.

Soifer B.E. & Gelb A.W. (1989) The multiple organ donor: identification and management. *Annals of Internal Medicine* **110**, 814—23.

Stoutenbeck O.P., van Saene H.K.F., Miranda D.R., Zandstra D.F. & Langrehe D. (1986) Nosocomial Gram-negative pneumonia in critically ill patients. *Intensive Care Medicine* **12**, 419—23.

Wallwork J., Williams R.S. & Calne R.Y. (1987) Transplantation of liver, heart and lungs for primary biliary cirrhosis and primary pulmonary hypertension. *Lancet* **2**, 182—5.

Wetzl R.C., Setzer N., Stiff J.L. & Rogers M.C. (1985) Haemodynamic responses in brain dead organ donor patients. *Anesthesia and Analgesia* **64**, 125—8.

White D.A. & Latimer R.D. (1991) Cardiac transplantation. *Current Opinions in Anaesthesiology* **4**, 83—9.

Williams A. (1990) Cell implantation in Parkinson's disease. *British Medical Journal* **301**, 301—2.

Anaesthesia and Sedation for Induced Hypotension, Radiology and Radiotherapy

P.J. SIMPSON

Hypotension

Intraoperative bleeding may be (i) arterial, in which case it is directly related to mean arterial pressure (MAP); (ii) capillary, when it is dependent upon local flow in the capillary bed; or (iii) venous, when it is related to venous return, venous tone and therefore posturally dependent. Arterial bleeding can only be abolished by the use of a tourniquet but can be considerably reduced by agents producing a reduction in MAP or heart rate. Capillary flow is also reduced by elective hypotension and by localized vasoconstriction produced, for example, by adrenaline infiltration or metabolic factors such as acid−base imbalance. Venous tone may be completely abolished by spinal or extradural anaesthesia and by direct acting vasodilators such as sodium nitroprusside.

Physiological background

The most important factor determining the extent of intraoperative haemorrhage is the MAP. This is directly related to both cardiac output and total peripheral resistance. While cardiac output is dependent upon myocardial contractility, determining stroke volume, and heart rate, peripheral resistance is a function of vascular dilatation. Peripheral vascular tone is controlled by sympathetic activity, vasodilatation being mainly produced by interruption of sympathetic pathways rather than by any parasympathetic effect. Some cholinergic vasodilator fibres do exist, e.g. in the smooth muscle of the gut. Hypotension due to reduction in total peripheral resistance may be mediated either centrally by drugs such as volatile agents acting on the vasomotor centre or peripherally at the level of the sympathetic ganglia, postganglionic noradrenergic (alpha) terminals, or directly on the blood vessels themselves.

Effects of hypotension on pulmonary gas exchange

As pulmonary blood flow is dependent upon gravity, the head-up position produces a reduction in flow to the apical segments of the lung. However, alveolar ventilation occurs throughout most of the lung, including the upper segments, resulting in considerable ventilation : perfusion ($\dot{V} : \dot{Q}$) mismatching and an increase in physiological deadspace. This may be as great as 80% of tidal volume (Eckenhof *et al.*, 1963) and is of particular importance in spontaneously breathing patients. The reduction in alveolar ventilation and increase in physiological shunt is an additional reason for the use of intermittent positive-pressure ventilation (IPPV) during elective hypotension. Furthermore, increasing the inspired oxygen concentration during elective hypotension minimizes the effects of this ventilation : perfusion imbalance.

Pharmacological methods of vasodilatation

Volatile anaesthetic agents

Halothane and enflurane

Although halothane produces a moderate degree of vasodilatation, the overall reduction in total peripheral resistance is only of the order of 15−18%. Vasodilatation in the skin and splanchnic vascular beds is balanced by vasoconstriction in skeletal muscle, most of the hypotension produced by halothane being a direct result of myocardial depression. In addition, bradycardia induced by the stimulant effect of halothane on the vagus nerve further reduces cardiac output. Although halothane has been extensively used in the past as a sole hypotensive agent (Prys-Roberts *et al.*, 1974) these potent side-effects make it less attractive than other volatile agents such as isoflurane. Its use should now be restricted in this situation to low concentrations employed as a background to hypotensive anaesthesia. This is of particular importance in neurosurgery if the increase in intracranial pressure from vasodilatation is to be avoided.

The mechanisms and effects of hypotension induced by enflurane are similar to those of halothane. Myocardial depression and vagal stimulation are still significant factors if excessive doses of the drug are used and for this reason it should also only be employed in moderate doses as a background agent.

Isoflurane

Unlike both halothane and enflurane, isoflurane has much less effect on myocardial contractility. Its vasodilator effect is readily reversible by alterations in inspired concentration of the drug. For this reason, it is becoming increasingly used as a hypotensive agent, particularly when only moderate reduction in arterial pressure is required. It has the additional benefit that increasing doses not only produce vasodilatation and hypotension but also central nervous depression, minimizing any reflex vasoconstriction or tachycardia which may occur as a result of baroreceptor stimulation under relatively light anaesthesia. Isoflurane also appears to have less effect than either halothane or enflurane on cerebral blood flow and therefore intracranial pressure, in patients in whom normal values are present preoperatively (Murphy *et al.*, 1974).

Sympathetic ganglionic block

Trimetaphan and pentolinium

These drugs produce autonomic ganglionic block by competitive inhibition of acetylcholine. Their effects are not confined to the sympathetic system as acetylcholine transmission also occurs in parasympathetic ganglia. Interruption of sympathetic outflow produces vasodilatation, which tends to be relatively slow in onset and recovery. The duration of hypotension produced by trimetaphan is relatively short (10−15 min) and for this reason the drug is often administered by intravenous infusion (3−4 mg/min). In contrast, a single injection of 5−15 mg pentolinium produces hypotension for approximately 45 min and allows a slow return of arterial pressure to normal values.

Although several gastrointestinal and urinary symptoms may result from concomitant parasym-

pathetic block, the two of clinical importance during induced hypotension are mydriasis and tachycardia. The increase in heart rate which often accompanies hypotension produced by ganglion block may severely impair the effectiveness of these drugs in reducing bleeding. Tachyphylaxis, that is the need for increasing doses of the drug to produce the same effect, is particularly marked with trimetaphan and may make a stable level of hypotension difficult to achieve. Continuous infusion is considerably superior to intermittent bolus dose administration in this respect.

Non-depolarizing neuromuscular blocking drugs

Alcuronium and D-tubocurarine

The use of non-depolarizing neuromuscular blocking drugs such as curare to facilitate IPPV as an adjunct to elective hypotension has been advocated for some time. Both D-tubocurarine and alcuronium are associated with histamine release, which induces vasodilatation. This far outweighs any hypotensive effect due to mild sympathetic ganglionic block.

Alpha-adrenoceptor block

Phentolamine, phenoxybenzamine, chloropromazine and droperidol

Alpha-adrenoceptor-blocking agents produce vasodilatation by competitive block of postsynaptic noradrenergic receptors within the sympathetic system. While the effects of phentolamine are relatively short (20−40 min) and easily reversible, those of phenoxybenzamine may last several days, as this drug, a nitrogen mustard derivative, forms an irreversible receptor complex. Phentolamine also exerts a direct myocardial stimulant effect, increasing both oxygen consumption and heart rate. Phenoxybenzamine may produce considerable sedation. While phentolamine, 5−10 mg, is used in the rapid production of intraoperative vasodilatation, phenoxybenzamine, 0.5−2.0 mg/kg for 10 days, is more commonly employed for chronic vascular expansion before surgery to minimize the effects of circulating catecholamines, e.g. in the surgical removal of phaeochromocytoma. Both chlorpromazine and droperidol induce mild α-adrenoceptor block, which is often useful in the preoperative preparation of patients before hypotensive anaesthesia and/or hypothermia.

Beta-adrenoceptor block

Propranolol, atenolol, oxprenolol, labetalol and practolol

The main advantages of the β-adrenoceptor antagonists in induced hypotension are reduction in heart rate and cardiac output. Considerable reduction in operative bleeding can be achieved by the maintenance of a slow heart rate without additional hypotension and propranolol has often been used to produce this 'rheostatic' hypotension. Although preoperative oral therapy (40 mg t.d.s.) is probably best, 1–2 mg intravenously can be used during anaesthesia. Beta-adrenoceptor block with either propranolol or oxprenolol is also employed either preoperatively or intraoperatively to counteract the tachycardia produced as a side-effect of induced hypotension with either ganglion-blocking or direct-acting vasodilator drugs. Again, it is best to administer the drugs orally rather than intravenously as this produces a steady intraoperative blood level of the drug. Although the combined α- and β-adrenoceptor-blocking drug labetalol would seem ideal for use in induced hypotension, it is important to realize that its α-blocking effect only lasts for 30 min compared with a 90 min duration of beta block. In addition, the β-blocking effect is five to seven times as potent as the alpha block. The perioperative use of beta block with either propranolol or labetalol may have considerable benefit in the prevention of wide fluctuations in blood pressure, particularly in patients with subarachnoid haemorrhage and vasospasm or those undergoing peripheral vascular surgery.

Direct-acting vasodilators

Sodium nitroprusside

The interest in direct-acting vasodilator drugs began with the reintroduction into clinical practice of sodium nitroprusside (SNP) (Moraca et al., 1962; Jones & Cole, 1968). The main advantage of this drug is its extremely evanescent action, allowing rapid reduction in arterial pressure and equally rapid restoration to normal levels. It is the only drug capable of predictably producing 'dial-a-pressure' hypotension over relatively short periods, e.g. in the prevention of bleeding in meningiomas and major vascular surgery, or to facilitate clipping of cerebral aneurysms. As a vasodilator, SNP inevitably produces an increase in intracranial pressure and for this reason should not be used during neurosurgery before the skull is open in a patient with raised intracranial pressure. Nevertheless, autoregulation under induced hypotension with SNP is maintained at cerebral perfusion pressures considerably lower than with other drugs (Stoyka & Schutz, 1975).

Metabolism and toxicity of sodium nitroprusside (Fig. 58.1)

Shortly after the introduction of SNP into clinical practice, reports of fatalities during its use were directly attributed to cyanide poisoning (Jack, 1974; Merrifield & Blundell, 1974; Davies et al., 1975). Each molecule of SNP contains five cyanide radicals which are liberated on breakdown of the drug in either plasma or red blood cells. Several studies, however, have failed to demonstrate significant effects upon red-cell oxygen transport of cyanide liberated during routine clinical use of SNP (du Cailar et al., 1978; Vesey et al., 1980).

The normal metabolic pathway of SNP breakdown is non-enzymatic, occurring in both red cells and plasma. The intracellular reaction is catalysed by the conversion of haemoglobin to methaemoglobin. Ultimately, more than 98% of the cyanide produced from SNP is contained within the red blood cells while a small proportion is combined with either methaemoglobin or vitamin B_{12}. Most of the cyanide is metabolized in the liver by the enzyme rhodanese to thiocyanate, which is then excreted in the urine. The rate-limiting factor in cyanide metabolism appears to be the availability of sulphydryl groups and the administration of sodium thiosulphate can considerably enhance thiocyanate production and therefore reduce blood cyanide concentrations (Krapez et al., 1981). The use of thiosulphate does not appear to affect the hypotension produced by SNP. At the maximum safe doses recommended for SNP administration, 1.5 mg/kg (Vesey et al., 1975) or $10\,\mu g \cdot kg^{-1} \cdot min^{-1}$ (Tinker & Michenfelder, 1976), small increases in plasma lactate occur which are mirrored by increases in arterial base deficit. These changes are only minor, the maximum base deficit being of the order of -6 to -7 mmols/litre, and are spontaneously reversible on discontinuation of SNP therapy. The routine measurement of acid–base balance during SNP therapy provides adequate clinical information on the development of cyanide toxicity during routine clinical use.

The use of SNP in patients already anaesthetized with a background hypotensive anaesthetic technique would still appear to be the method of choice for the production of extreme hypotension for neuro-

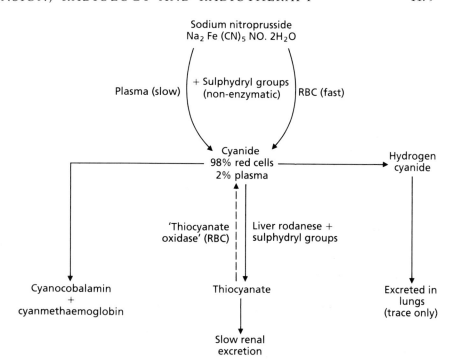

Fig. 58.1 Metabolic pathway of sodium nitroprusside. RBC, red blood cell.

surgery. No other drug at present provides the predictable and rapid hypotensive effect necessary for many aspects of intracranial surgery. For longer-term infusion and in the presence of adequate sulphydryl groups as the substrate for cyanide detoxification by rhodanese, a maximum dose rate of 8 μg/kg (Michenfelder & Tinker, 1977) has been shown to be satisfactory.

Trinitroglycerine

Intravenous trinitroglycerine (TNG) was introduced into clinical anaesthetic use as being particularly beneficial in the treatment of hypertensive crises in patients with ischaemic heart disease (Viljoen, 1968; Kaplan, 1981). Aveling and Verner (1981) subsequently investigated its potential for induced hypotension. In common with SNP, TNG metabolism has been extensively studied (Michenfelder & Tinker, 1977). Hepatic metabolism of trinitrate produces di- and mononitrate and finally glycerol. The vasodilator activity of these smaller nitrate molecules is reduced as their size decreases. TNG produces a steadier and less dramatic reduction in arterial pressure, having a greater effect on systolic than diastolic pressure and tending to maintain blood flow. Recovery from TNG-induced hypotension is also less rapid, taking between 10 and 20 min in contrast to the 2–4 min with SNP. It has been suggested that this slower effect of TNG produces less overshoot of arterial pressure either at induction of hypotension or following restoration of normal arterial pressure but as the drug appears less effective in some cases in the production of extreme hypotension, its use may not be ideal in all situations. Although TNG has been advocated as a direct acting vasodilator for neurosurgery, in one study, hypotension to 50 mmHg was not possible in three of 22 patients (Chestnut *et al.*, 1978). Unlike SNP, which dilates both resistance and capacitance vessels equally, TNG exerts its effect principally upon the venous capacitance system. As a result, diastolic arterial pressure is maintained at higher levels than with SNP and for this reason TNG maintains coronary artery perfusion more effectively than SNP. While this is probably of little importance in healthy patients, it may be of considerable advantage in patients with impaired myocardial or cerebral circulation. However, the increase in intracranial pressure produced by TNG may be even greater than with SNP.

Spinal and extradural anaesthesia

Pharmacological sympathectomy using local anaesthetic agents is a very effective way of inducing hypotension. The use of lumbar extradural anaesthesia produces arteriolar dilatation and hypotension together with a reduction in venous tone. This is enhanced by posturally dependent pooling of venous blood leading to a reduction in venous return and therefore cardiac output. If the block is extended to the mid-thoracic region, the cardiac sympathetic fibres passing in segments T1 to T4 are also blocked, preventing the compensatory tachycardia which otherwise occurs. This also limits any baroreceptor response, and prevents tachycardia occurring as a result of other pharmacological methods of induced hypotension.

Regional anaesthesia is most commonly employed in lower abdominal or pelvic surgery to minimize blood loss, particularly that occurring from the pelvic venous plexuses. The complete abolition of venous tone is extremely effective in minimizing blood loss without the need for profound arteriolar hypotension. If adrenaline is added to the local anaesthetics used, systemic absorption may partially counteract the hypotensive effect of the regional block. Adrenaline has the advantage of prolonging the effects of the local anaesthetics used, although this can be satisfactorily achieved more simply by the use of intermittent or continuous extradural injections.

Effects of posture

Posture influences intraoperative bleeding both by producing regional ischaemia if the operation site is elevated above the level of the heart, and also by augmenting the effect of agents, such as sympathetic-ganglion-blocking drugs, by pooling of venous blood. The effect of posture on regional cerebral perfusion pressure in relation to MAP at heart level is considerable. For each 2.5 cm of vertical height above the heart, arterial pressure decreases by 0.26 kPa (2 mmHg). This is of extreme importance when measuring arterial pressure in the arm while tilting the patient significantly head-up during a period of elective hypotension. Operations below heart level may equally be improved by a head-down tilt, but this is not such an effective way of reducing arterial pressure as it tends to improve venous return and therefore maintain arterial pressure. Whenever possible, posture should be used to augment pharmacological methods of induced hypotension, particularly those which depend upon venous pooling, such as trimetaphan.

Effects of intermittent positive-pressure ventilation

During normal inspiration, the negative intrathoracic pressure created enhances venous return to the heart, even against the force of gravity. With IPPV, inspiration is associated with positive intrathoracic pres-

sure, inevitably resulting in a reduction in venous return. If this effect is augmented by posture, the resultant reduction in venous return and therefore cardiac output may be considerable. However, Prys Roberts and colleagues (1967) have shown that in normotensive anaesthetized subjects, IPPV has little effect on cardiac output. This is primarily because of the reflex vasoconstriction produced in response to what is effectively a limited Valsalva manoeuvre. In addition, the baroreceptor response to hypotension induces reflex tachycardia. Two methods of inducing hypotension may be associated with a considerable reduction in cardiac output in response to IPPV, both due to temporary autonomic paralysis. Both ganglion-blocking drugs and β-adrenoceptor antagonists produce a partial or completely blocked Valsalva maneouvre (Blackburn et al., 1973), thus limiting the production of a normal compensatory response.

In general, IPPV is a useful adjunct to any hypotensive technique, largely because it augments pharmacological methods of pressure reduction, limiting the dose necessary to produce the desired effect and also the postoperative duration of hypotension. In addition, artificial ventilation allows the application of positive end-expiratory pressure to the airway, another method of limiting venous return during expiration and reducing arterial pressure.

Effects of carbon dioxide control

Carbon dioxide is a vasodilator and hyperventilation with hypocapnia induces vasoconstriction. Carbon dioxide control can be achieved either by IPPV using moderate hyperventilation or by carbon dioxide absorption in a circle system using soda lime. Care, however, must be taken during hyperventilation with patients in the head-up position as vasoconstriction may reduce cerebral blood flow to critical levels.

Monitoring during induced hypotension

Although instruments such as the cerebral function monitor are potentially available for use during hypotensive anaesthesia, their use and, indeed, their possible benefits are relatively limited (Patel, 1981). Routine monitoring involves either direct or indirect arterial pressure measurement in the knowledge that, assuming a normal intracranial pressure and with the appropriate postural adjustments, the measurement is directly related to cerebral perfusion pressure. In addition, the ECG provides an indication of the development of relative myocardial ischaemia under conditions of impaired perfusion due to excessive hypotension. The measurement of oxygen saturation and end-tidal carbon dioxide concentration has greatly improved the perioperative assessment of cardiorespiratory function.

Measurement of arterial pressure

Direct measurement

The use of an indwelling arterial cannula is the ideal method of arterial pressure measurement. The transducer must be positioned at the level at which pressure measurement is required so that if the mean arterial blood pressure at head level is desired, the transducer should be placed at this height. Although indirect methods of measurement are used during relatively mild hypotensive techniques, such as intermittent ventilation with isoflurane, extradural anaesthesia, or even in some cases, the use of ganglion-blocking drugs, direct monitoring is an essential part of the technique when rapidly acting direct vasodilators such as SNP are employed.

Indirect measurement

These methods involve modifications of the classical Riva—Rocci cuff and as such are subject to errors in observation and interpretation. Those chiefly employed are the oscillotonometer and the automated versions of this method, such as the Dinamap. Hutton and Prys-Roberts (1982) have shown that errors in interpretation of oscillotonometry have tended to err on the side of safety as what was originally thought to be systolic arterial pressure has now been demonstrated to represent more closely the mean pressure. The semiautomated versions are an improvement as they remove the observer bias and indeed display not only systolic but also mean and diastolic pressures. All these methods depend upon regular sensation of pulsation at the cuff which is rendered inaccurate by irregular cardiac rhythm such as atrial fibrillation. Moreover, as with all indirect methods of pressure measurement, they are most accurate within the normal ranges of pressure and become increasingly inaccurate at excessively low or high pressures. If one is anticipating hypotension below a systolic pressure of 9.3 kPa (70 mmHg), direct arterial monitoring should be considered essential.

Electrocardiographic monitoring

During hypotensive anaesthesia, ECG monitoring is mandatory to demonstrate two vital signs of inadequate myocardial perfusion — the development of ectopic beats and ST-segment depression. Although a single-channel ECG is incapable of demonstrating the exact site of any ischaemia, ST-segment changes do occur and are readily reversible by increasing arterial pressure. The myocardial response to relative hypoxia and hypoperfusion is a sensitive monitor of hypotension being excessively exploited.

Measurement of respiratory gas exchange

Perioperative measurement of oxygen saturation and end-tidal carbon dioxide concentration provides valuable information about oxyen uptake, availability and utilization and about the efficiency of respiratory excretion of carbon dioxide. This is of particular importance in elective hypotension where reduction in systemic arterial pressure is reflected in the pulmonary circulation, producing alterations in pulmonary gas exchange. When significant head-up tilt is used to reduce blood loss, a sudden decrease in end-tidal carbon dioxide concentration provides a reliable and important warning of air embolism.

Practical technique of induced hypotension

No single agent is capable of providing the ideal conditions for all operations, the requirements of surgery falling into three broad groups.

The first requires relatively slow onset and sustained moderate hypotension with a slow return to normal pressures, and is ideal for most plastic, maxillofacial and ENT surgery when rapid return to normal pressures may cause reactionary haemorrhage.

In the second, where massive blood loss is anticipated, moderate sustained hypotension together with a reduction in heart rate is probably all that is required.

In the third group, some operations are not only impossible without profound hypotension but also require short periods of excessively low pressures, e.g. during clipping of a cerebral aneurysm.

Further indications include resection of aortic coarctation where rapid fluctuations in arterial pressure necessitating immediate control are required. In general, there is a need for two basic methods of hypotension: elective, slow-onset slow-recovery hypotension on the one hand and 'dial-a-pressure' hypotension on the other.

In all cases, a background anaesthetic against which hypotension can be induced is essential, the principles of balanced anaesthesia dictating that it is better to employ individual agents to achieve specific effects rather than to pursue the toxic properties of a sole agent such as halothane in the production of hypotension by myocardial depression. An ideal background anaesthetic consists of omission of atropine premedication, as this induces tachycardia, but the use of generous sedation or analgesia. It is essential to avoid preoperative anxiety and the release of adrenaline, as the effects take some time to abate under anaesthesia.

Induction of anaesthesia with thiopentone, fentanyl and a long-acting, non-depolarizing muscle relaxant, either D-tubocurarine or alcuronium, is followed by topical anaesthesia of the larynx and intubation with either a new or a non-kinking tracheal tube to remove any possible risk of partial airway obstruction and carbon dioxide retention. Moderate hyperventilation with nitrous oxide and oxygen together with 0.5−1.0% isoflurane provides a suitable background technique against which hypotensive agents can be used. Under these stable conditions, specific hypotensive drugs can then be employed with the minimum of side-effects, e.g. tachycardia or excessive hypotension. During hypotension the inspired oxygen concentration may be increased to 40 or even 50% if excessively low pressures are being employed over a short period, e.g. during neurosurgery.

Postoperative management

Regular arterial pressure monitoring must be continued into the recovery period, together with meticulous airway care to avoid carbon dioxide retention and partial obstruction. The patient's position should be determined by the arterial pressure measured, and postural changes may be necessary for several hours to ensure adequate cerebral perfusion. Supplementary oxygen should be administered in all cases until the patient is adequately awake and may be required for longer where oxygenation is thought to be critical. In cases where pharmacological modification of sympathetic responses has been undertaken, such as with the use of ganglion-blocking drugs, patients should remain in bed for 12−18 h postoperatively and, if necessary, lying virtually flat until they are able to sit up without feeling dizzy.

Contraindications to induced hypotension

Although many anaesthetists are reluctant to employ induced hypotension, there are very few patients in whom it cannot be used safely. Most would refrain from utilizing the technique in patients with evidence of severe cardiovascular or cerebrovascular disease, although both these are relative contraindications if, for example, cerebral aneurysm surgery is proposed.

Myocardial ischaemia

This is made worse by an increase in the rate pressure product but, since hypotensive techniques are designed to reduce both heart rate and arterial pressure, the amount of cardiac work is normally considerably reduced. Many such patients are already receiving β-adrenoceptor block and this should be continued intraoperatively. In cases where a reduction in afterload is produced by direct acting vasodilators such as SNP, myocardial work may be further reduced.

Hypertension

Although patients with treated hypertension may be abnormally sensitive to hypotensive drugs, such techniques can still be employed with care. Untreated hypertension, however, is a relative contraindication, as arterial pressure may be extremely labile and profound hypotension may result. Volatile anaesthetic agents may enhance the hypotensive effects of drugs which the patient is already receiving for routine control. Monitoring the ECG is essential in patients with cardiovascular disease. Rollason and Hough (1960) demonstrated ST depression in hypertensive patients and Simpson and colleagues (1976) noted similar changes during anaesthesia and SNP-induced hypotension. While the importance of such changes is probably doubtful, they do demonstrate the need for care when utilizing hypotension in such patients.

Respiratory disease

Limitations to the use of hypotensive anaesthesia in patients with chronic respiratory disease are related to the disturbance in normal pulmonary physiology. The increase in physiological deadspace caused by ventilation : perfusion imbalance is more important in patients in whom preoperative gas exchange is limited. Under normal circumstances, hypoxic pulmonary vasoconstriction occurring in poorly ventilated segments of the lung prevents gross disorders of ventilation : perfusion. Vasodilatation induced by direct-acting drugs such as SNP, abolishes this response and therefore makes shunting worse.

Reversible airways obstruction and bronchospasm may be made worse by the use of either ganglion-blocking drugs or β-adrenoceptor antagonists, which are not cardiospecific and such drugs are contraindicated in asthmatics. High-inflation pressures may lead to carbon dioxide retention and severe hypotension due to impairment of venous return.

Diabetes mellitus

This relative contraindication to induced hypotension is related to the drugs used rather than to the technique employed. Ganglion-blocking drugs, by producing sympathetic block, impair stress induced gluconeogenesis mediated by adrenaline. Beta blockers may also potentiate hypoglycaemia in insulin-dependent diabetics and it is the combination of hypoglycaemia plus hypotension which may produce severe consequences, particularly on cerebral metabolism. Under normal circumstances, however, it is safe to employ volatile agents, direct-acting vasodilators or local-anaesthetic techniques without impairment of blood sugar concentrations.

Complications of induced hypotension

Failed hypotension

Although not regarded by many as a complication of hypotensive anaesthesia, failure to appreciate this may lead to the excessive use of certain agents and consequent toxic effects. Some patients, e.g. those with a sensitive renin−angiotensin system have been shown to be 'resistant' to SNP. If hypotension using one drug is not sufficient, a second agent acting at a different site in the sympathetic system should be employed. This has been put to good effect, e.g. by the combination of either ganglion-blocking drugs such as trimetaphan, or isoflurane with SNP.

Excessive hypotension

It is very unlikely that moderate hypotension, particularly when induced by vasodilatation and accompanied by additional oxygen administration in healthy patients, should lead to any permanent adverse effect. Nevertheless, situations have arisen where permanent damage has resulted from the use of more extreme levels of elective hypotension. This is related either to excessive hypotension, impaired oxygenation or inadequate arterial pressure monitoring. Lindop (1975), surveying the evidence concerning the effects of hypotension on vital organs, stressed the importance of flow rather than pressure in the development of complications. This is particularly

important as normal oxygen extraction by most organs with the exception of the heart is only about 25% of their potential.

In considering the effects of hypotension on the brain, it has been shown experimentally (Stoyka & Schutz, 1975) that the lower limit of autoregulation is better preserved with SNP-induced hypotension than with trimetaphan, flow remaining constant down to mean pressures of 5.3−6.6 kPa (40−50 mmHg). These figures need to be interpreted with some caution when extrapolated to humans because of the effects of anaesthesia and other metabolic derangements upon cerebral blood flow. More detailed studies, such as continuous EEG monitoring (Patel, 1981) and jugular venous oxygen measurements (Larson et al., 1967), have produced inconclusive results. Probably the most important rule is not to reduce the intraoperative systolic pressure to below the preoperative diastolic, and to avoid, where possible, severe head-up tilt unless arterial pressure is being measured at the head level.

The monitoring of ST-segment depression to detect myocardial ischaemia would appear to be the most reliable method of demonstrating adverse cardiac effects due to hypotension (Simpson et al., 1976). Provided myocardial work is reduced and compensatory tachycardia due to hypotension does not occur, severe problems appear to be very rare.

Although those antagonistic to hypotensive anaesthesia may always cite cases of permanent damage or even death related directly to the lowering of arterial pressure, large series, particularly that collected by Enderby (1980) do not bear this out. At East Grinstead, the mortality rate was 1 : 4128 cases of induced hypotension and Kerr (1977) in a separate series reported no mortality or morbidity in a series of 700 patients.

Sedation

Although several groups of sedative drugs, in particular the benzodiazepines, the butyrephenones and the major tranquillizers are frequently used as single doses administered for a particular procedure, their use either continuously or intermittently as part of a sedative regimen is increasing. In a similar way to balanced anaesthesia, specific drugs providing sedation, analgesia and relaxation are frequently administered to patients on IPPV. Several drugs are now available to provide a suitably balanced regimen. These fall into five main groups: (i) intravenous anaesthetic agents; (ii) benzodiazepines; (iii) opioid analgesics; (iv) non-opioid analgesics;

and (v) a miscellaneous group, which includes both the major tranquillizers and nitrous oxide.

Any ideal sedative regimen, either intermittent or continuous should fulfil the criteria summarized in Table 58.1.

Several properties assume proportionately greater significance depending upon whether single-dose or continuous therapy is used, whether the trachea is intubated and the lungs ventilated or breathing spontaneously and whether cardiovascular instability is a problem. Special circumstances may also exist, e.g. raised intracranial pressure, severe head injury, renal or hepatic failure and multiple trauma requiring considerable analgesia in addition to sedation.

Comparative pharmacology of sedative agents

Intravenous anaesthetics

Thiopentone

Thiopentone infusions have been used for continuous sedation for many years, particularly in the field of cerebral protection, associated with severe head injury. Barbiturate infusions are known to reduce cerebral metabolic oxygen consumption and provided the circulation is maintained with fluid and inotropic support, are thought to increase survival of compromised brain. As a routine sedative, however, thiopentone is exceedingly cumulative, thus failing to fulfil one of the criteria listed in Table 58.1. As a rule of thumb its sedative effects continue for as long after cessation of the infusion as therapy lasted in the first place. It is a useful anticonvulsant in status epilepticus and in the long-term sedation of head injuries but otherwise is probably of limited use.

Table 58.1 Properties of the ideal sedative drug regimen

Rapid onset of action following intravenous administration
Predictable duration of action
Uniform and narrow dose range
Wide therapeutic ratio
No adverse cardiovascular effects
No respiratory depression
No postsedation confusion
Non-cumulative
No hypersensitivity
Non-irritant, water soluble

Propofol

This is at present only officially available for intermittent use or for infusions in adults. It is an excellent agent, which is becoming exceedingly popular and is rapidly metabolized and noncumulative. Its use produces very little postsedation confusion and allows rapid awakening or by contrast, easy sedative control during short- or long-term ventilation. It is a significant respiratory depressant and, therefore, may not be suitable for patients breathing spontaneously under sedation. Propofol produces good cardiovascular stability but at the concentration currently available, its use implies that a daily infusion volume of approximately 500 ml is necessary to provide adequate sedation. As the drug is suspended in Intralipid, this produces a significant lipid load in patients receiving prolonged sedation.

Ketamine

Although ketamine is not widely used as an intravenous induction agent in the UK, it possesses many properties suitable for infusion sedation. It is a profound analgesic, without being a respiratory depressant, maintains cardiovascular stability by release of catecholamines, particularly noradrenaline and has a volume of distribution which, together with its metabolic profile, makes it suitable for use as a continuous sedative infusion. Its main disadvantage of hallucinations would appear to be minimized by concomitant use of a benzodiazepine drug and its use has been advocated in the treatment of severe bronchospasm resistant to conventional sympathomimetic therapy (Strube & Hallam, 1986).

Etomidate

In a study of etomidate sedation in intensive care, Ledingham and Watt (1983) came to the conclusion that continuous etomidate infusions combined with opioid therapy in severely ill patients were associated with a doubling of the mortality rate which they could only ascribe to a change from their previously used regimen of benzodiazepines and opioids. Subsequent work showed that etomidate infusions were associated with adrenal suppression and reduced levels of circulating corticosteroids (Fellows et al., 1983; Watt & Ledingham, 1984). As a result, etomidate is now no longer licensed for use by infusion.

Benzodiazepines

The benzodiazepines, undoubtedly, comprise the most widely used group of sedative drugs both for acute procedures and for continuous sedation. They possess many of the ideal properties listed in Table 58.1, although none of them is at present completely satisfactory for all situations. In addition, they are only sedative drugs and do not possess any analgesic qualities. For this reason, during painful procedures or in patients requiring analgesia in addition to sedation by infusion, their use must be supplemented by appropriate drugs if a satisfactory state is to be achieved. They also possess several important properties including retrograde amnesia and anxiolysis, both of which are of particular importance in intensive care.

Diazepam

This drug has been widely used for many years as a single-dose sedative given orally or intravenously. Although a moderate cardiovascular and respiratory depressant, it produces good sedation, amnesia and relaxation. Its chief disadvantage lies in its metabolism (Fig. 58.2). The active metabolite, desmethyldiazepam, has a longer half-life than the parent drug and continuous administration of diazepam results in cumulation and prolonged sedation. Another significant disadvantage is that of thrombophlebitis related to the particular solubilizing agents used such as propylene glycol, but its suspension in intralipid as Diazemuls has considerably reduced this problem.

Lorazepam

Unlike diazepam, lorazepam is mainly metabolized by conjugation in the liver and subsequently excreted in the urine, only 15% being transformed into minor metabolites. Lorazepam has a long half-life but in view of its metabolism is not cumulative (Fig. 58.2). It provides good, predictable sedation, retrograde amnesia and is suitably stable for prolonged sedation. Its long duration of action makes it unsuitable for continuous administration, but it can be satisfactorily given on a regular 6-hourly basis, allowing assessment of the patient before each dose. Lorazepam is an excellent anxiolytic and particularly advantageous when trying to wean anxious patients from ventilators.

Midazolam

Midazolam is a water-soluble benzodiazepine with a shorter half-life than diazepam. Its onset of action is relatively slow and mild venous irritation may occur, but midazolam can satisfactorily be given as a continuous infusion through a cannula. In common with other drugs in this group, it produces retrograde amnesia and has become widely used as one of the currently 'fashionable' intensive-care sedatives. Its chief disadvantage lies in the relative unpredictability of its duration of action.

There appear to be two separate groups of patients who metabolize the drug differently, so that while recovery after prolonged infusion may take only minutes in the majority of patients, in some it may take up to 48 h. This is due to an altered metabolic pathway similar, for example, to that seen with isoniazid, where patients can be slow or fast acetylators of the drug. Despite this, however, midazolam is widely used and in conjunction with opioid infusions, provides excellent sedation with good cardiovascular stability in the majority of patients.

Opioid analgesics

In patients in whom analgesia is considered

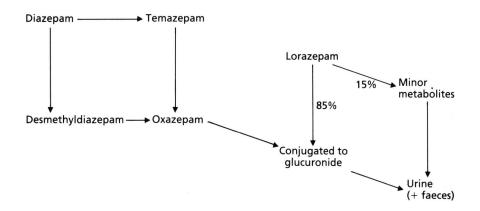

Fig. 58.2 Metabolic pathway of diazepam and lorazepam.

necessary, and in addition those in whom respiratory depression is desirable, e.g. during prolonged ventilation, opioid analgesics have many advantages. They produce profound analgesia, sedation, euphoria, cardiovascular stability and have a suitable metabolic profile. They do, however, reduce gastrointestinal motility and may impair absorption. Dependence can develop relatively rapidly, particularly when large doses are employed and their use over prolonged periods should be avoided.

Morphine and papaveretum

Both these drugs have a relatively low lipid solubility and are slow to cross the blood–brain barrier. Their elimination half-lives are of the order of 2 h, 90% being excreted following conjugation to the glucuronide in the liver. They provide good cardiovascular stability and, in general, appear to provide superior analgesia when administered as an intravenous infusion to that achieved with intermittent bolus doses (Rutter *et al.*, 1980).

Fentanyl, phenoperidine and alfentanil

The synthetic opiates are significantly more fat-soluble than the morphine group, producing considerable sedation and central nervous depression. This results in profound respiratory depression but good cardiovascular stability. While phenoperidine is customarily administered by intermittent bolus dose, the shorter-acting agents fentanyl and alfentanil are suitable for intravenous infusion. Fentanyl, however, may produce muscular rigidity and is sequestered in muscle and stomach, resulting in recirculation and further respiratory depression. High doses of fentanyl given intermittently have also been shown to diminish the stress response to surgery (Hall *et al.*, 1978) and it is possible that high-dose infusions may be disadvantageous, particularly in the multiple injured patients in whom a stress response is an essential part of normal recovery.

Non-opioid analgesics

Pentazocine, buprenorphine, nalbuphine and meptazinol

As partial agonists, these drugs antagonize opioids administered by other routes, e.g. extradurally. They produce good cardiovascular stability, mild-to-moderate respiratory depression and as they do not mask neurological signs, may be advantageous in patients with head injury or after neurological surgery. Their main disadvantage is that they are probably not sufficiently potent, either as analgesics or respiratory depressants, to be of great value as a substitute for the opioids. However, their use in patients requiring prolonged analgesia should not be underestimated and as buprenorphine, in particular, can be given sublingually, it does not require gastrointestinal absorption to be effective.

Miscellaneous sedatives

Chlormethiazole

Unlike many of the drugs already considered, chlormethiazole produces relatively uncontrolled sedation and is particularly long-acting. It is cumulative and has mainly been used to treat delirium tremens, status epilepticus and other prolonged states of agitation. It is both an anticonvulsant and an antiemetic, producing relatively mild cardiovascular and respiratory depression. Its unpredictable duration of action makes it unsuitable for acute, reversible sedation.

Phenothiazines (chlorpromazine, promethazine and trimeprazine)

These major tranquillizers produce good, though relatively unpredictable sedation. They are commonly given intermittently and in addition to sedation produce vasodilatation and hypothermia, often to considerable advantage in head-injured patients. Chlorpromazine also produces α-adrenoceptor antagonism, leading to vasodilatation and hypotension. Their chief benefits are improvement of perfusion in patients with peripheral shut-down related to shock or cold and, in combination with pethidine, profound continuous sedation by infusion as 'lytic cocktail'.

Butyrephenones (droperidol)

These drugs are potent sedatives, antagonizing central nervous transmission at dopamine, noradrenaline, serotonin and γ-aminobutyric acid sites. They are also vasodilators, producing their effect, in common with chlorpromazine, by α-adrenoceptor antagonism. They produce long-acting and uncontrolled sedation, together with hypothermia. Droperidol has a mild anticholinergic effect and is a good antiemetic, acting on the chemoreceptor trigger zone. It is often very effective in patients following maxillofacial surgery.

Nitrous oxide

Nitrous oxide/oxygen mixtures, in the form of Entonox, were used for a time in intensive care, producing excellent sedation and good analgesia. Nitrous oxide is a moderate cardiovascular depressant and may pass into other air-filled cavities such as the gastrointestinal tract, a pneumothorax or the tube of a tracheal tube cuff, increasing pressure within the cavity. Its use for prolonged sedation, however, has been discontinued because of bone marrow depression. This appears to be a dose-dependent and reversible phenomenon, although it is too serious a side-effect to allow continued use of nitrous oxide over prolonged periods.

Isoflurane

Isoflurane has been used successfully by Kong and Colleagues (1989) to produce rapidly reversible sedation with minimal cardiovascular effects in normovolaemic patients. It has little residual effect as it is almost entirely excreted unchanged and the dose required for effective sedation is confined to a narrow range of 0.1–0.4%. It is relatively cumbersome to administer through some ventilators and requires an effective extraction system to avoid environmental pollution.

Optimum sedation regimens usually include sedation in the form of a benzodiazepine, such as midazolam, together with an opioid infusion, either of morphine, fentanyl or alfentanil. This allows limitation of opioid dosage and reduces the likelihood of dependence developing to the drug. This may still be a problem if infusions are used for several days and the classical signs of withdrawal should be looked for as they are often masked in a patient recovering from severe illness and being weaned from a ventilator.

Neuroleptanalgesia (-anaesthesia)

Neuroleptanalgesia is a dissociative state similar to that induced by ketamine, in which the patients are profoundly sedated and analgesic. Unlike ketamine, however, they are still able to respond to command. It is normally achieved by the combination of a butyrephenone, such as droperidol, with an opioid such as fentanyl, in moderate dose to allow spontaneous ventilation. Suitable commercially produced combinations such as Innovar contain droperidol (2.5 mg/ml) and fentanyl (0.05 mg/ml). Although neuroleptanaesthesia is widely used in Europe, and in particular Scandinavia, its use in the UK has mainly been confined to induction of anaesthesia in patients in whom circulatory homeostasis is compromised. A droperidol/fentanyl induction maintains excellent cardiovascular stability and protects against catecholamine-induced arrhythmias. Increasing the dose of fentanyl to produce respiratory depression, together with neuromuscular block facilitates tracheal intubation and ventilation.

True neuroleptanaesthesia is employed both as an adjunct to local anaesthetic techniques in place of more conventional sedation with drugs such as benzodiazepines. It is also extremely useful in procedures where the anaesthetist is required to be remote from the patient, e.g. invasive radiological procedures, radiotherapy and other investigations. In such circumstances, patients may be sedated and unaware, but they turn over or move limbs in response to command but lie still while radiology takes place. The provision of profound analgesia prevents the procedure being unpleasant for the patient and any factual recall is absent. The dissociative state produced during neuroleptanaesthesia is very similar to that produced by ketamine anaesthesia and, as such, is an extension of the sedative techniques already described.

Radiological procedures

The need for general anaesthesia during routine radiological procedures is relatively limited, the main indications being the need for profound analgesia and keeping children or restless, uncooperative patients still. Most procedures are carried out under oral or intravenous sedation using diazepam or midazolam, supplemented where necessary by opioid premedication and/or local anaesthesia.

Most radiology departments are remote from theatres, intensive care and resuscitation equipment such as defibrillators. Many relatively ill patients including those from intensive therapy units (ICU) need to be transferred to the radiology department for investigation, not infrequently with the trachea intubated and the lungs ventilated artificially. Good anaesthetic equipment and, in particular, monitoring is essential for two reasons: first, to continue that already being used in a sick patient, and second, because the anaesthetist is remote from the patient for a large part of the procedure to avoid radiological exposure. Telemetric ECG monitoring and automatic non-invasive arterial pressure monitoring are ideal in this situation.

Anaesthetics are often given in very adverse conditions, with inadequate trained help and lack of appreciation by the radiological staff as to the anaesthetist's needs. Poor lighting, the absence of piped gases necessitating the use of cylinders and equipment disconnection or failure are frequently encountered. All these make the use of full monitoring, oxygen failure and disconnection alarms essential. General anaesthesia in some situations is preferable to heavy sedation as recovery facilities are often non-existent and rapid awakening allows early return of protective reflexes and transfer to the ward. A further advantage of general anaesthesia is that some patients suffer an acute anaphylactic response to the contrast media used and a patient who is well oxygenated with trachea intubated and the lungs ventilated, under the care of an anaesthetist is well prepared for immediate resuscitation.

Vascular radiology

Translumbar aortography and angiography

General anaesthesia is still frequently used for these procedures for several reasons. Many of the patients are relatively elderly and suffer from widespread peripheral vascular disease. Translumbar aortography and several angiographic techniques require the patient to lie prone for a considerable time and IPPV can be used to prevent inadequate ventilation, hypoxia and atelectasis. The use of IPPV also allows hyperventilation, the resultant hypocapnia inducing vasoconstriction. This slows the flow of contrast and by increasing the density of dye in the vessels, improves the quality of the X-rays. The rapid injection of contrast medium also produces severe burning pain in the legs which would necessitate profound analgesia in the absence of general anaesthesia.

Embolization

This technique is rapidly becoming the treatment of choice for devascularization of haemangiomata and other vascular tumours, either as an alternative or before surgical removal. They are frequently lengthy procedures and general anaesthesia may be far more pleasant for the patient, particularly if surgical exposure of the feeding vessels is required initially. In some cases, however, patient co-operation is necessary to monitor the development of neurological or mechanical deficit arising from inadvertent occlusion of flow to vital areas. In this case, intermittent anaesthesia with Diprivan and alfentanil or midazolam sedation are the most suitable techniques, allowing patient co-operation when required.

Endoscopy and biopsy

Most endoscopic radiological procedures are carried out using fibre-optic instruments and therefore only require sedation. These include endoscopic retrograde cannulation of the pancreas with sphincterotomy and biopsy under radiological control. Demonstration of individual gland circulation by angiography or of duct systems by retrograde cannulation and contrast injection is not usually sufficiently unpleasant or painful to require general anaesthesia. Biopsy procedures of tumours or individual glands such as the liver are performed 'closed' using a 'Tru-cut' needle, often under image intensification. Patient co-operation is necessary to stop respiration and movement both of the liver and other structures while the biopsy is taken.

Computerized tomography

Whole-body scanning is rapidly becoming widely available and the demand for anaesthesia is correspondingly increasing. As it is non-invasive and painless, the requirements are simply those of rendering children or restless, uncooperative patients immobile.

Patients undergoing mechanical ventilation in the ICU are frequently transferred for computerized tomography (CT) scanning and require full ventilatory, anaesthetic and monitoring support. Although the whole scan may take 20–30 min, each 'slice' only lasts about 20 s and at suitable points, scanning can cease to allow minor movement in an awake patient. Some, particularly children, find the whole procedure extremely daunting and general anaesthesia may be required if profound sedation is to be avoided. Care must be taken to avoid hypothermia in small infants during prolonged CT scanning in a relatively cold environment.

Magnetic resonance imaging (nuclear magnetic resonance)

Magnetic resonance imaging (MRI) involves the use of a high field strength magnet and radiofrequencies to produce an image in any plane. MRI is extremely sensitive to changes in water content of the brain, by imaging the hydrogen protons. It is particularly useful in investigating lesions of the posterior cranial fossa and spinal cord, providing far greater detail than CT scanning.

As immobility is essential during the procedure, the indications for general anaesthesia are similar to CT scanning, but there is no radiation risk. Mechanical anaesthetic problems are related to the powerful electromagnetic field, which precludes the presence of any ferromagnetic-containing objects, including pacemakers, etc. All anaesthetic equipment must either be non-ferrous or significantly remote from the patient. Telemetric monitoring is frequently used, together with plastic or rubber arterial pressure cuffs and stethoscopes. The rhythmic drum-like noise of the scanner may prevent routine auscultatory monitoring.

Suitable modifications to anaesthetic equipment and circuits include the use of plastic Jackson–Rees modifications of Ayre's T-piece or elongated Bain coaxial tubing together with plastic laryngoscopes and tracheal tubes. Intravenous anaesthesia may also be used with spontaneous respiration. Resuscitation poses a particular problem as all equipment malfunctions in the electromagnetic field. If the magnet is turned off, several hours are required before a stable field can be re-established for subsequent investigations.

Bronchography

This procedure is infrequently carried out except in specialized thoracic units. It is used to demonstrate pathology of the smaller divisions of the bronchial tree, such as bronchiectasis. Contrast (usually Dionosil) is instilled through a fibre-optic broncho-scope and the patient is then positioned to allow dissemination throughout the smaller bronchi and bronchioles. Although bronchography, particularly unilateral, can be satisfactorily carried out under topical anaesthesia, bilateral procedures, together with the associated bronchospasm, coughing and relative hypoxia make general anaesthesia desirable. Tracheal intubation and spontaneous ventilation with enflurane or isoflurane allows the gradual introduction of contrast into the main bronchi. IPPV can also be used, but this tends to disperse contrast rapidly to the distal bronchioles. Volumes of Dionosil in excess of 20 ml are required for each lung and must be aspirated at the end of the procedure before extubation.

Cardiac catheterization

As these procedures involve differential pressure and oxygen saturation measurement, any form of anaesthesia or sedation may affect the information produced. Many of the patients are relatively poor risks for general anaesthesia, with impaired myo-cardial contractility, valvular defects, ischaemic heart disease and conduction abnormalities. In children,

the main problems are those of abnormal circulations and intracardiac shunts. In most circumstances general anaesthesia is avoided, preference being given to sedative techniques which do not produce myocardial depression and allow spontaneous respir-ation on air or a minimal amount of added oxygen. General anaesthesia with spontaneous ventilation using volatile agents is unsuitable for patients with severe myocardial disease and IPPV alters pulmonary haemodynamics, therefore affecting flow and pres-sure measurement. If intubation and ventilation is considered necessary (e.g. in neonates), then a nitrous oxide/oxygen relaxant technique is most commonly used.

Anaesthesia for patients with malignant disease

Radiotherapy

Although radiotherapeutic procedures are painless, they do require the full co-operation of the patient, both in the planning stage and lying completely still during the actual procedure. In adults, this is carried out without anaesthesia and with minimum sedation in anxious patients. In children, however, general anaesthesia is frequently used, necessitating a tech-nique which allows the anaesthetist to be remote from the patient. The treatment programme involves daily radiotherapy and so multiple repeat anaes-thetics are required. Ketamine, either 10 mg/kg i.m. or 2 mg/kg i.v., preceded by diazepam premedi-cation to minimize side-effects is most frequently used as it allows spontaneous respiration with air and maintenance of laryngeal reflexes. The problems associated with alternative techniques of general anaesthesia in this situation are considerable.

Intravenous or intrathecal cytotoxic drug therapy

This is frequently required in young children suffer-ing from leukaemia which may involve the CNS. General anaesthesia is required to facilitate intra-venous cannulation or lumbar puncture before administration of large doses of frequently painful cytotoxic drugs. A straightforward inhalation tech-nique with nitrous oxide, oxygen and a volatile agent is usually all that is required to allow the patient to tolerate the procedure. As with radiotherapy, multiple repeat anaesthetics may be required and venous access may be extremely limited or non-existent, necessitating inhalation induction.

References

Aveling W. & Verner I.R. (1981) Profound hypotension with intravenous nitroglycerin. In *The International Symposium on the Clinical use of Tridil, Intravenous Nitroglycerin* (Eds Robinson B.F. & Kaplan J.A.) p. 35. The Medicine Publishing Foundation Symposium Series, Oxford.

Blackburn J.P., Conway C.M., Davies R.M., Enderby G.E.H., Eldridge A., Leigh J.M., Lindop M.J. & Strickland D.A.P. (1973) Valsalva responses, and systolic time intervals during anaesthesia and induced hypotension. *British Journal of Anaesthesia* **45**, 704–10.

Chestnut J.S., Albin M.S., Gonzales-Abola E., Newfield P. & Maroon J.C. (1978) Clinical evaluation of intravenous nitroglycerin for neurosurgery. *Journal of Neurosurgery* **48**, 704–11.

Davies D.W., Kadar D., Steward D.J. & Munroe I.R. (1975) A sudden death associated with the use of sodium nitroprusside for the induction of hypotension during anaesthesia. *Canadian Anaesthetists' Society Journal* **22**, 547–52.

du Cailar J., Mathieu-Dande J.C., Duschade J., Lamarche Y. & Castel J. (1978) Nitroprusside, its metabolites and red cell function. *Canadian Anaesthetists' Society Journal* **25**, 92–105.

Eckenhoff J.E., Enderby G.E.H., Larson A., Eldridge A. & Judevine D.E. (1963) Pulmonary gas exchange during deliberate hypotension. *British Journal of Anaesthesia* **35**, 750–8.

Enderby G.E.H. (1980) Hypotensive anaesthesia. In *General Anaesthesia* 3rd edn. (Eds Gray T.C., Nunn J.F. & Utting J.E.) pp. 1149–68. Butterworth, London.

Fellows I.W., Bastow M.D., Byrne A.J. & Allison S.P. (1983) Adrenocortical suppression in multiply injured patients: a complication of etomidate treatment. *British Medical Journal* **287**, 1835–7.

Hall G.M., Young C., Holdcroft A. & Alaghband-Zadeh J. (1978) Substrate mobilisation during surgery. *Anaesthesia* **33**, 924–30.

Hutton P. & Prys-Roberts C. (1982) The oscillotonometer in theory and practice. *British Journal of Anaesthesia* **54**, 581–93.

Jack R. (1974) The toxicity of sodium nitroprusside. *British Journal of Anaesthesia* **46**, 952.

Jones G. & Cole P.V. (1968) Sodium nitroprusside as a hypotensive agent. *British Journal of Anaesthesia* **40**, 804.

Kaplan J.A. (1981) Nitroglycerin for the treatment of hypertension during coronary artery surgery. In *The International Symposium on the Clinical use of Tridil, Intravenous Nitroglycerin* (Eds Robinson B.F. & Kaplan J.A.) p. 26. The Medicine Publishing Foundation Symposium Series, Oxford.

Kerr A. (1977) Anaesthesia with profound hypotension for middle ear surgery. *British Journal of Anaesthesia* **49**, 447–52.

Kong K.L., Willatts S.M. & Prys-Roberts C. (1989) Isoflurane compared with midazolam for sedation in the intensive care unit. *British Medical Journal* **298**, 1277–80.

Krapez J.R., Vesey C.J., Adams L. & Cole P.V. (1981) Effects of cyanide antidotes used with sodium nitroprusside infusion: sodium thiosulphate and hydroxycobalamin given prophylactically to dogs. *British Journal of Anaesthesia* **53**, 793–804.

Larson C.P. Jr., Ehrenfeld W.K., Wade J.G. & Wylie E.J. (1967) Jugular venous oxygen saturation as an index of adequacy of cerebral oxygenation. *Surgery* **62**, 31–9.

Ledingham I.McA. & Watt I. (1983) Influence of sedation on mortality in critically ill multiple trauma patients. *Lancet* **i**, 1270.

Lindop M.J. (1975) Complications and morbidity of controlled hypotension. *British Journal of Anaesthesia* **47**, 799–803.

Merrifield A. & Blundell M. (1974) Toxicity of sodium nitroprusside. *British Journal of Anaesthesia* **46**, 324.

Michenfelder J.D. & Tinker J.H. (1977) Cyanide toxicity and thiosulphate protection during chronic administration of sodium nitroprusside in the dog. *Anesthesiology* **47**, 441–8.

Moraca P.P., Bitte E.M., Hale D.E., Wasmuth C.E. & Poutasse E.F. (1962) Clinical evaluation of sodium nitroprusside as a hypotensive agent. *Anesthesiology* **23**, 193–9.

Murphy F.L. Jr., Kennell E.M., Johnstone R.E. *et al.* (1974) The effects of enflurane, isoflurane and halothane on cerebral blood flow and metabolism in man. *Abstracts of Scientific Papers, Annual Meeting of the American Society of Anesthesiologists* pp. 61–2.

Patel H. (1981) Experience with the cerebral function monitor during deliberate hypotension. *British Journal of Anaesthesia* **53**, 639–45.

Prys-Roberts C., Kelman G.R., Greenbaum R. & Robinson R.H. (1967) Circulatory influences of artificial ventilation during nitrous oxide anaesthesia in man. II. Results: the relative influence of mean intrathoracic pressure and arterial carbon dioxide tension. *British Journal of Anaesthesia* **39**, 533–48.

Prys-Roberts C., Lloyd J.W., Fisher A., Kerr J.H. & Patterson T.J.S. (1974) Deliberate profound hypotension induced with halothane. Studies of haemodynamics and pulmonary gas exchange. *British Journal of Anaesthesia* **46**, 105–16.

Rollason W.N. & Hough J.M. (1960) A study of hypotensive anaesthesia in the elderly. *British Journal of Anaesthesia* **32**, 276–85.

Rutter P.C., Murphy F. & Dudley H.A.F. (1980) Morphine: controlled trial of different methods of administration for postoperative pain relief. *British Medical Journal* **280**, 12–13.

Simpson P., Bellamy D. & Cole P. (1976) Electrocardiographic studies during hypotensive anaesthesia using sodium nitroprusside. *Anaesthesia* **31**, 1172–8.

Stoyka W.W. & Schutz H. (1975) The cerebral response to sodium nitroprusside and trimetaphan controlled hypotension. *Canadian Anaesthetists' Society Journal* **22**, 275–82.

Strube P.J. & Hallam P.L. (1986) Ketamine by continuous infusion in status asthmaticus. *Anaesthesia* **41**, 1017–20.

Tinker J.H. & Michenfelder J.D. (1976) Sodium nitroprusside; pharmacology, toxicology and therapeutics. *Anesthesiology* **45**, 340–54.

Vesey C.J., Cole P.V. & Simpson P.J. (1975) Sodium nitroprusside in anaesthesia. *British Medical Journal* **3**, 229.

Vesey C.J., Krapez J.R. & Cole P.V. (1980) The effects of sodium nitroprusside and cyanide on haemoglobin function. *Journal of Pharmacy and Pharmacology* **32**, 256–61.

Viljoen J.F. (1968) Anaesthesia for internal mammary implant surgery. *Anaesthesia* **23**, 515–20.

Watt I. & Ledingham I.McA. (1984) Mortality amongst multiple trauma patients admitted to an intensive therapy unit. *Anaesthesia* **39**, 973–82.

Anaesthesia and Respiratory Disease

I.S. GRANT

Successful anaesthetic management of the patient with severe respiratory disease depends on optimization of gas exchange preoperatively, and preservation of adequate gas exchange both intra- and postoperatively. It demands an understanding of the effects of anaesthesia and surgery on respiratory function, notably with respect to the postoperative period.

Postoperative respiratory complications which impair gas exchange such as pneumonia, lung collapse and respiratory failure are essentially the culmination of a pathophysiological process initiated by anaesthesia and surgery, and depend to a large extent on the site and severity of the surgery.

In the patient with pre-existing respiratory disease, the changes occurring are superimposed on previously deranged pulmonary function and complications are both more frequent and severe. Preoperative assessment should be made in the light of the nature of the surgery proposed, to predict perioperative problems in respect of oxygenation, adequacy of ventilation and sputum clearance. Perioperative management aims to treat pre-existing disease, to modify the pathophysiological process, and thus to avert complications. All aspects of this care should be planned and applied carefully, in the form of analgesia, physiotherapy, oxygen therapy, intravenous fluid administration and respiratory support. Monitoring over the postoperative period, clinically, radiologically and by arterial blood-gas estimation, should be meticulous, and complications detected and treated early.

Effects of anaesthesia on respiration and the pulmonary circulation

In healthy patients, oxygen consumption is reduced by approximately 15% during uncomplicated anaesthesia. However, it may be increased markedly during the immediate postoperative period, e.g. when shivering occurs following halothane anaesthesia.

Commonly used inhalation anaesthetic agents such as halothane, enflurane and isoflurane depress the Pco_2/ventilation response curve. Likewise, intravenous agents such as thiopentone, methohexitone and propofol, and opioid analgesics have similar respiratory-depressant effects. The ventilatory response to hypoxia is even more depressed (Knill & Gelb, 1978), and while this effect is relevant only when Pao_2 decreases to below 8 kPa (60 mmHg), and so should not occur during satisfactory anaesthesia, it may be important in the postoperative period in patients with obstructive lung disease when a subanaesthetic concentration of a volatile agent may depress ventilatory response to hypoxia significantly.

During anaesthesia with spontaneous ventilation, there is selective loss of the intercostal component of ventilation. Overall minute volume is governed by the respiratory-depressant effects of the anaesthetic agents balanced against the effect of surgical stimulation of ventilation.

Lung volumes

General anaesthesia, involving either spontaneous or controlled ventilation, leads to a reduction in functional residual capacity (FRC) of approximately 400 ml, which is compounded by the reduction occurring in the supine posture (Hewlett et al., 1974a,b). Thus, FRC decreases towards the volume at which significant basal airway closure occurs (closing capacity = closing volume + residual volume). Closing volume (CV) increases markedly with age, obesity, smoking and rapid infusion of crystalloid fluid (Table 59.1), and while FRC increases also in elderly people as a result of loss of elastic recoil of the lung, the reduction caused by anaesthesia and the

Table 59.1 Factors affecting functional residual capacity (FRC) and closing volume (CV)

	FRC	CV
Age	↑	↑ ↑
Supine posture	↓	—
Obesity	↓	↑
Smoking	—	↑
Crystalloid fluid infusion	↓	↑
Anaesthesia	↓	—
Upper abdominal surgery	↓	—

↑ Increase; ↓ decrease.

supine position results in airway closure during tidal ventilation, spontaneous and controlled. This results in dependent areas of lung being markedly underventilated, while still being perfused, explaining the increased alveolar–arterial (A–a) Po_2 difference observed during anaesthesia.

The cause of this reduction in FRC has not been explained fully. During anaesthesia the diaphragm appears to lie in a cephalad position, possibly because of loss of residual end-expiratory muscle tone (Hedenstierna et al., 1986). The static compliance of lungs and chest wall decreases, and since this occurs both with spontaneous ventilation and with muscle relaxation and controlled ventilation, this finding can be attributed to increased lung recoil (Westbrook et al., 1973). A further contribution to the reduction in FRC may come from a redistribution of blood from peripheral to large central vessels. The use of positive end-expiratory pressure (PEEP) restores FRC to normal, but increases Pao_2 only in those patients suffering the greatest degree of pulmonary venous admixture (Nunn et al., 1965). CV is affected little by anaesthesia, hence the decrease in the FRC–CV relationship.

Distribution of ventilation and perfusion

During anaesthesia, both with spontaneous (Rehder & Sessler, 1973) and controlled ventilation (Rehder et al., 1977), there is redistribution of ventilation away from dependent lung areas, while there is little change in the distribution of perfusion, with dependent areas preferentially perfused (Hulands et al., 1970). Thus, there are areas with a ventilation : perfusion ($\dot{V}:\dot{Q}$) ratio of zero (true shunt), or approaching zero.

Matching of perfusion to ventilation requires an intact pulmonary vascular response to hypoxia (hypoxic pulmonary vasoconstrictor reflex), hyper-

capnia and acidaemia. Chronic hypoxia causes pulmonary vasoconstriction and hypertension, and, ultimately, right heart failure. Volatile anaesthetic agents have been reported to depress the hypoxic pulmonary vasoconstrictor reflex in animals (Sykes et al., 1973) or not to affect it (Mathers et al., 1977). In man, during differential lung ventilation, one lung with oxygen and the other with nitrogen, halothane anaesthesia increases the percentage of cardiac output perfusing the hypoxic lung indicating inhibition of hypoxic pulmonary vasoconstriction (Bjertnaes et al., 1976). Recent evidence suggests that inhibition of hypoxic pulmonary vasoconstriction is minimal if pulmonary vascular pressures are normal, but may be enhanced when vascular pressures are reduced (Eisenkraft, 1987).

Overall, a calculated true shunt of 10% occurs during anaesthesia in patients with normal gas exchange preoperatively, and in view of the increased (A–a) Po_2 difference, an inspired oxygen concentration of 30% is required to guarantee a Pao_2 above the patient's normal level during uncomplicated anaesthesia. This percentage may need to be increased in patients with pre-existing gas exchange problems and during thoracic anaesthesia.

Physiological deadspace is increased markedly (by greater than 50%) as a result of ventilation of unperfused alveoli (Campbell et al., 1958). This increase is mitigated partly by a reduction in carbon dioxide production, and by the use of a tracheal tube which reduces anatomical deadspace.

Mechanics of ventilation

Airways resistance during uncomplicated anaesthesia increases to double its normal value in the conscious subject. This occurs in parallel with the reduction in lung volume, but may be compounded by secretions or bronchospasm.

Lung compliance decreases as described above in parallel with the reduction in FRC. The work of breathing thus tends to increase.

In summary, oxygenation is impaired during anaesthesia, with the increase in (A–a)Po_2 difference demanding an inspired oxygen concentration of 30–35% to maintain an arterial oxygen tension of 13.5 kPa (100 mmHg) in normal subjects. This is caused by a reduction in FRC, basal airway closure, and ventilation : perfusion ($\dot{V}:\dot{Q}$) mismatching related partly to inhibition of the hypoxic pulmonary vasoconstrictor reflex.

During spontaneous ventilation, $Paco_2$ increases as a result of respiratory-depressant effects of anaesthetic agents, and an increase in physiological deadspace.

These changes may become important in patients with pre-existing respiratory disease.

Postoperative respiratory function and development of postoperative respiratory complications

Immediate effects

The physiological changes associated with anaesthesia continue into the immediate postoperative period, usually for approximately 1–2 h after the end of anaesthesia. The arterial oxygen tension on breathing air decreases by approximately 4 kPa (30 mmHg) from the preoperative value, and is treated simply by the inhalation of 30–35% oxygen by face mask (Drummond & Milne, 1977). In addition, there is a slight transient reduction in Pao_2 caused by dilution of alveolar oxygen content by nitrous oxide diffusing out into the alveoli on return to breathing air after nitrous oxide anaesthesia (diffusion hypoxia). This may be avoided by using 100% oxygen for 5–10 min at the end of anaesthesia. By 2 h postoperatively, patients who have undergone limb or other body-surface surgery do not show deterioration in respiratory function. In these patients the presence of a respiratory disorder postoperatively implies either pre-existing lung disease or some incident such as pulmonary aspiration or thromboembolism.

Abdominal and thoracic surgery

After major abdominal or thoracic surgery, a disturbance of lung function for up to 4–5 days is inevitable, even in previously healthy individuals. This may culminate in respiratory failure, especially in obese and elderly patients, cigarette smokers and patients with pre-existing lung disease (Garibaldi et al., 1981).

The intraoperative impairment of oxygenation continues for over 48 h, the magnitude of the reduction in Pao_2 being related to the site of surgical incision (Alexander et al., 1973a). With upper midline or paramedian incisions, a reduction of 3.4 kPa (25 mmHg) occurs when breathing air (Spence & Smith, 1971).

A parallel reduction in FRC occurs which is related also to the site of surgery, being approximately 30% after open cholecystectomy and only 15% after inguinal hernia repair (Alexander et al., 1973a). With the CV not being affected by surgery, the FRC–CV difference decreases and actual airway closure and

gas trapping occurs during tidal ventilation in dependent areas of lung which are best perfused. There is a significant correlation between the reduction in Pao_2 and the reduction in FRC–CV.

By 24 h, areas of collapse of lung tissue occur in the areas of air trapping, but this is not clinically or radiologically evident until after 24 h. Retention of secretions, notably in the dependent areas, is aggravated by suppression of ciliary activity, lack of humidification, suppression of the normal occasional deep breath or sigh, and an inability to cough adequately on account of pain. Retained secretions can block off bronchi to produce lung collapse or become infected leading to development of bronchopneumonia.

Cause of reduction in functional residual capacity in relation to closing volume

1 Wound pain is the principal cause, with pain causing reflex muscle spasm, increasing abdominal pressure and assisting expiration. Loss through pain of the intermittent physiological sigh tends also to result in alveolar collapse and reduction in FRC (Caro et al., 1960).

2 Abdominal distension. Loss of bowel tone and mobility leads to distension which may be increased by absorption of nitrous oxide. Opioid analgesia may exacerbate ileus also. Pneumoperitoneum contributes also to abdominal distension; this effect can be minimized through drainage of air by suction before peritoneal closure.

3 Posture. The relationship between FRC and CV is least favourable in the supine position, in which many patients are nursed postoperatively.

4 Intrapulmonary water. Pulmonary venous congestion leads to an increase in CV in relation to FRC. Postoperative fluid retention and simultaneous excessive crystalloid infusion may thus contribute to hypoxaemia (Skillman et al., 1970; Collins et al., 1973).

Patients at risk

The following groups have been shown to be at a greater risk of postoperative respiratory complications, especially following upper abdominal surgery (Garibaldi et al., 1981):

1 Cigarette smokers. Smokers tend to have an increased CV predisposing to basal air trapping. This, compounded by hypersecretion of mucus and effects on immune function, tends to lead to postoperative atelectasis and pneumonia. The effects on immune function include decreased neutrophil activity, immunoglobulin concentrations and natural killer activity. These effects take at least 6 weeks of abstinence from smoking to return to normal.

In addition to purely respiratory problems, there is clear evidence that smokers have an overall increased perioperative risk, and that even a short (12 h) period of abstinence decreases this risk (Pearce & Jones, 1984; Jones et al., 1987). Nicotine, being a transmitter at sympathetic ganglia increases heart rate, blood pressure and systemic vascular resistance. An increased carboxyhaemoglobin level reduces available oxygen by up to 25%, resulting in a situation of increased myocardial oxygen demand with a simultaneous decrease in supply. Abstinence for even only 12 h reduces carboxyhaemoglobin concentration and improves cardiovascular reserve.

2 Obese people. The resting Pao_2 in these patients is reduced, as a result of reduced FRC and basal airway closure. Total compliance is decreased, thus increasing the work of breathing, and leading to a risk of respiratory muscle fatigue (Vaughan et al., 1975). Upper airway obstruction is likely also to be a problem in the immediate postoperative period.

3 Malnourished patients, with low serum albumin concentration.

4 Elderly patients. Evidence of an increased risk of pulmonary complications is less clear in this group, but these patients are more liable to suffer from pre-existing cardiorespiratory disease, and their CV is increased markedly, thus causing airway closure during tidal ventilation, explaining their lower resting Pao_2. They may also be more sensitive to the effects of anaesthetic agents and opioid analgesics.

5 Patients with pre-existing pulmonary disease. Patients with chronic obstructive airways disease have twice the incidence of postoperative respiratory complications compared with previously healthy patients. The overall quoted incidence of postoperative chest complications after upper abdominal surgery varies widely from 17.5% (Garibaldi et al., 1981) and 25% in patients with chronic pulmonary disease (Gracey et al., 1979) to 50–80% (Morran & McArdle, 1980). These variations presumably reflect the difficulties in defining such complications.

Surgical aspects affecting risk

1 Prolonged operations of greater than 4-h duration (Garibaldi et al., 1981). This is associated presumably with the anaesthesia-related reduction in FRC, and perhaps also the inadequate humidification of inspired gases.

2 Surgical incision. In patients with chronic obstructive airways disease, transverse incisions appear to be associated with less disturbance of pulmonary function and to reduce the incidence of bronchopneumonia in comparison with midline incisions (Becquemin et al., 1985).

3 Reduction of intra-abdominal pressure postoperatively by decompression of bowel where it is unduly distended, and by peritoneal drainage (Bevan, 1961) may improve postoperative respiratory function and reduce frequency of complications.

Careful preoperative preparation, good analgesia, physiotherapy and prompt recognition and treatment of sequelae may avert severe complications (Palmer & Sellick, 1953; Gracey et al., 1979; Morran & McArdle, 1980).

Laparoscopic abdominal surgery

Newer laparoscopic techniques of surgery such as laparoscopic cholecystectomy avoid, to a large extent, the postoperative pulmonary sequelae of abdominal surgery. The carbon dioxide insufflated into the peritoneal cavity is rapidly absorbed postoperatively, and the lack of a major incision reduces pain and muscle spasm. Little analgesia is required, and patients are able to breathe deeply and cough easily. The experience in the author's hospital of 400 laparoscopic cholecystectomies without significant pulmonary complications despite chronic lung disease in 5–10% of the patients attest to laparoscopic surgery's advantages.

Clinical assessment of the patient with respiratory disease

The aims of preoperative assessment are five-fold:
1 To detect any pre-existing respiratory disorder.
2 To define the nature of the disorder.
3 To evaluate the severity of functional impairment.
4 To detect other risk factors in relation to possible respiratory complication, e.g. obesity, skeletal abnormalities.
5 To consider the implications of the proposed surgery on pulmonary function in order to predict postoperative complications, and plan perioperative management.

Clinical history

The usual symptoms of respiratory disease should be elicited: dyspnoea, cough, sputum, haemoptysis, chest pain and wheeze.

Dyspnoea may be defined as the subjective state in

which the effort of breathing impinges on consciousness under circumstances in which a healthy person would not be aware of his or her breathing. It gives the best indication of functional impairment; specific questioning is required to define the extent to which activity is limited by dyspnoea. Dyspnoea at rest or on minor exertion (e.g. walking on the level) indicates significant disease, requiring further investigation. It does not, however, define diagnosis, since it may occur in conditions associated with high airways resistance such as asthma or chronic bronchitis, in conditions where chest-wall or lung compliance are low such as kyphoscoliosis or fibrosing alveolitis, or where hypoxaemia or hypercapnia increase respiratory drive.

Where a cough is present, the nature and volume of any sputum produced should be sought. The patient's ability to clear sputum should be evaluated with the help of the physiotherapist. Haemoptysis suggests the possibility of bronchial carcinoma, tuberculosis, bronchiectasis or pulmonary infarction, and patients with this symptom should be investigated before elective surgery.

A history of smoking or occupational exposure to dust may point to pulmonary pathology. Cardiovascular pathology co-exists often, and thus a history of ischaemic heart disease, hypertension and cardiac failure should also be pursued. Drug therapy, and past history of problems associated with anaesthesia should also be noted.

The patient with chronic lung disease is able generally to give a good overall assessment of the current activity of his or her illness.

Examination

A full physical examination is required with emphasis on detecting signs of:
1 Airways obstruction.
2 Restricted lung expansion.
3 Increased effort in breathing.
4 Sputum production and clearance.
5 Evidence of active infection.
6 Respiratory failure.
7 Right heart failure.

On initial inspection during history taking, the patient's build (obesity), skeletal abnormalities, colour (plethora, cyanosis, anaemia), respiratory rate, depth and pattern, presence of cough and finger clubbing may be noted.

Airways obstruction is suggested by hyperinflation of the chest, hyper-resonance to percussion, prolonged expiration, and expiratory rhonchi on auscultation. An audible wheeze may occur in severe obstruction, while no rhonchi may be audible during quiet respiration or where obstruction is so severe that air entry is reduced markedly. A simple forced expiratory manoeuvre reveals airways obstruction, with a forced expiratory time of greater than 4 s abnormal, and greater than 10 s indicating severe obstruction (Rigg & Jones, 1978). A clinical finding of airways obstruction suggests that pulmonary function testing, and possibly arterial blood-gas estimation is required.

By contrast, in upper airways obstruction caused, e.g. by epiglottitis, acute laryngotracheobronchitis or external compression (see Chapter 40), inspiration is prolonged typically, with inspiratory stridor.

Restricted lung expansion may be suggested by skeletal abnormalities such as kyphoscoliosis, neuromuscular weakness as in myasthenia gravis, restricted respiratory excursion, and decreased air entry noted on auscultation usually at the lung bases. An ineffective cough may indicate severe reduction in vital capacity, or else vocal-cord dysfunction.

Increased work of breathing is suggested by an increased respiratory rate and heart rate, use of accessory muscles, tracheal tug and intercostal indrawing.

Sputum production and effectiveness of clearance can be assessed by asking the patient to cough. Crepitations noted on auscultation may clear following coughing.

Active infection is suggested by pyrexia, leucocytosis, purulent sputum and localized signs on auscultation; bronchial breath sounds, increased vocal resonance, and crepitations indicating an area of pneumonic consolidation.

Agitation and confusion may indicate hypoxaemia; sweating, vasodilatation and drowsiness may be a result of hypercapnia. Chronic hypoxaemia may be indicated by signs of pulmonary hypertension such as a parasternal heave, accentuation of the pulmonary second sound and signs of right heart failure, with raised jugular venous pressure, and peripheral oedema.

Additional investigations

Radiological examination

The chest X-ray should *not* be employed as a routine investigation in all patients presenting for surgery (Fowkes, 1986). It should, however, be carried out in the following groups (Roberts, 1984):

1 Patients with acute respiratory symptoms and signs.
2 Patients with possible metastases.
3 Patients with suspected or established cardio-respiratory disease who have not had a chest X-ray in the previous 12 months.
4 Recent immigrants (who have not had a chest X-ray in the previous 12 months) from countries where tuberculosis is still endemic.

In addition, patients over 40 years of age who are undergoing major abdominal surgery, and elderly patients of 65 years or more, should have preoperative chest X-rays as a baseline measurement, since postoperative complications in these groups are common, and interpretation of subsequent X-rays is simplified greatly (Seymour *et al.*, 1982).

The chest X-ray is a poor indicator of functional impairment, but it may reveal a number of features of importance to anaesthetists. These include thoracic-cage abnormalities (Fig. 59.1), tracheal deviation or compression, localized disease of the lung and pleura not detected on clinical examination, e.g. neoplasm, collapse, consolidation, effusion, emphysematous bullae (Fig. 59.2), or pneumothorax, generalized disease underlying acute pulmonary symptoms, e.g. pulmonary fibrosis, and cardiomegaly and failure.

On a standard inspiratory posteroanterior chest X-ray, the right dome of the diaphragm lies at the level of fifth to seventh rib and is approximately 1–2 cm higher than the left dome, the shadow of the left hilum is slightly smaller and approximately 1 cm

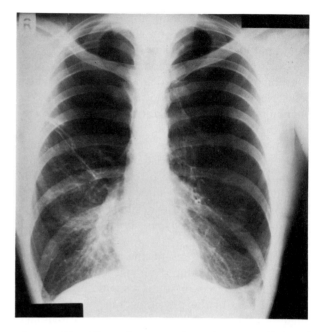

Fig. 59.2 Chest X-ray of patient with emphysema and bilateral large apical bullae.

higher than the right, the horizontal fissure cuts the sixth rib in the mid-axillary line, and the transverse diameter of the heart is less than 50% of that of the chest.

Sometimes, in particularly ill patients, only supine portable anteroposterior films can be obtained. In these, it is important to make adjustment for cardiac and mediastinal shadow, height of diaphragm, and not to miss pleural effusions which appear only as a generalized loss of lucency over the affected lung field.

Where localized lesions are present, further elucidation of the site and nature of the lesion can be obtained from lateral film, tomography and computerized tomography (CT scan). Where available, CT scan is probably now obligatory in the preoperative investigation of patients with bronchial neoplasm or mediastinal masses (Fig. 59.3).

Electrocardiogram

In the patient with severe pulmonary disease, evidence of right atrial or ventricular hypertrophy may be found. This is indicated by right axis deviation; tall, peaked P-wave (P-pulmonale) in lead II and dominant R-wave in leads V_{1-3} (Fig. 59.4). In emphysematous patients, clockwise rotation with an rS pattern across the praecordial leads is common (Fig. 59.5).

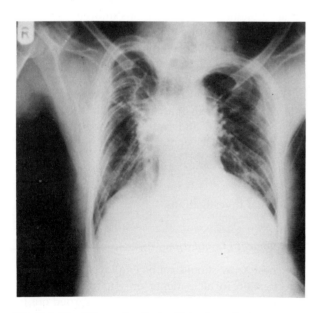

Fig. 59.1 Chest X-ray of patient with kyphoscoliosis.

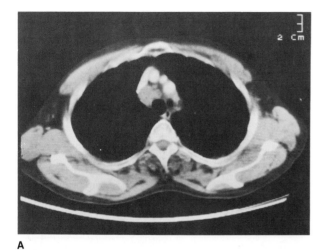

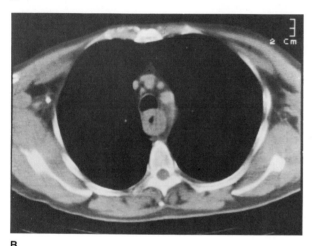

Fig. 59.3 Computerized tomography scans of mediastinum (contrast enhanced). (A) R-paratracheal lymph node mass. (B) Carcinoma of oesophagus.

Haematology

Polycythaemia may be primary or secondary to chronic hypoxaemia. To exclude the latter, arterial blood-gas analysis should be performed if a haemoglobin concentration of greater than 17 g/dl is found. Anaemia of whatever cause decreases oxygen carriage, and should be investigated and corrected to a concentration of approximately 10 g/dl before elective surgery. Leucocytosis may indicate active infection, while leucopenia may occur in immune-compromised patients suffering from fulminating infection. Eosinophilia may occur in allergic disorders, e.g. asthma, and in polyateritis nodosa.

Sputum culture

This is essential in patients with chronic lung disease or suspected acute infection, while in the investigation of the latter, blood sampling for viral antibody titres is also appropriate.

Pulmonary function tests

As successful perioperative management depends on the preservation of adequate gas exchange, it follows that measurement of the arterial partial pressures of oxygen and carbon dioxide are the best preoperative index of overall lung function in relation to metabolic requirements.

There are in addition a large number of pulmonary function tests which may be of value preoperatively both to provide a physiological diagnosis of the lung function disturbance, and as an objective measure of its severity (Cotes, 1979).

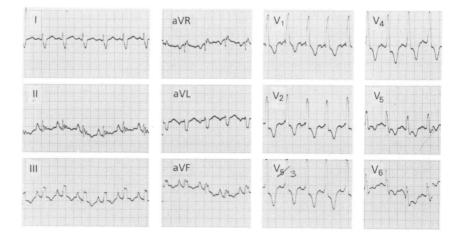

Fig. 59.4 Electrocardiogram of patient with chronic obstructive airways disease. R-axis deviation; P-pulmonale; R-ventricular hypertrophy; R-bundle branch block.

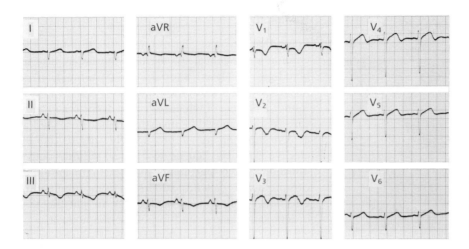

Fig. 59.5 Electrocardiogram of patient with chronic obstructive airways disease. R-axis deviation — clockwise rotation; P-pulmonale; R-ventricular 'strain'.

$FEV_{1.0}$, FVC and PEFR

In practical terms, the tests of most value are the forced expiratory volume in 1 s ($FEV_{1.0}$), forced vital capacity (FVC), and the peak expiratory flow rate over 10 ms (PEFR). These tests can be performed easily at the bedside, the first two using a dry spirometer (Vitalograph) and the latter using a Wright's peak flowmeter. All should be performed at least three times and the best results noted. The results should be compared with standard values adjusted for age, height and sex. In both obstructive airways disease and disorders where restriction of lung expansion occurs, the FVC is decreased, with the two types of disorder differentiated by the $FEV_{1.0}$:FVC ratio, and additionally by measurement of lung volumes (see below). A ratio of less than 0.70 indicates some obstruction of larger airways. Its reversibility should be assessed by repeating the test 5−10 min after inhalation of a bronchodilator aerosol, e.g. salbutamol 200 μg. In severe obstructive disease, a slow vital capacity measurement may be greater than FVC.

After major abdominal surgery, $FEV_{1.0}$ and FVC decrease by approximately 50% (Rutter *et al.*, 1980), and thus in the patient with low $FEV_{1.0}$ and FVC preoperatively, the additional reduction may lead to impairment of sputum clearance and respiratory failure postoperatively. In obstructive disease, an $FEV_{1.0}$ of less than 50% of predicted, or less than 1 litre, is associated with a marked increase in the risk of postoperative morbidity (Lockwood, 1973; Appleberg *et al.*, 1974). Such patients should be assessed further by measurement of arterial blood-gas tensions. Likewise, an FVC of less than 50% of predicted, or less than 1.5 litres should be followed up by arterial blood-gas estimation.

In the case of thoracic surgery where lobectomy or pneumonectomy is contemplated, due allowance should be made for loss of functioning lung tissue with vital capacity decreasing by approximately 35% after pneumonectomy. Removal of severely diseased tissue may, however, improve function occasionally. A preoperative $FEV_{1.0}$ of 1.5 litres is required before pneumonectomy to avoid a risk of postoperative respiratory failure.

Lung volumes

Total lung capacity (TLC), FRC and residual volume (RV) may be measured using a closed-circuit spirometer system, with the FRC being calculated first by helium dilution within the circuit, and the other values being calculated from FRC following a maximal inspiration and expiration. Table 59.2 summarizes the changes to be found in lung volumes in obstructive and restrictive disease.

The maximum expiratory flow−volume (MEFV) curve (flow measured at the mouth by a pneumotachograph during forced expiration plotted against change in lung volume) allows differentiation between obstruction in large and small airways, e.g. upper airway compression by a thyroid swelling and airways obstruction caused by asthma (Fig. 59.6).

Other, more elaborate tests of mechanical function such as measurement of dynamic compliance are made using a body plethysmograph with oesophageal balloon to measure intrapleural pressure, but are of limited value in the preoperative assessment of patients with respiratory disease.

The concept of CV and its relationship with FRC is of fundamental importance in explaining the problems of intraoperative and postoperative gas

Table 59.2 Pulmonary function test abnormalities in obstructive and restrictive disease

	Obstructive			Restrictive		
	Chronic bronchitis	Emphysema	Asthma	Fibrosing alveolitis	Sarcoidosis	Kyphoscoliosis
$FEV_{1.0}$	↓↓	↓↓↓	↓↓	↓↓	N/↓	↓
FVC	↓	↓↓	↓	↓↓	N/↓	↓
FEV/FVC	↓	↓↓	↓	N	N	N
TLC	N/↑	↑↑	N/↑	↓	N	↓
RV	↑	↑↑↑	N/↑	N/↓	N	↓
RV/TLC	↑	↑↑	↑	N/↑	N	N
T_{CO}	↓	↓↓	N/↑	↓↓	↓	N
PEFR	↓	↓	↓	↓	↓	↓

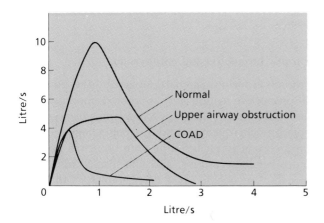

Fig. 59.6 Maximum expiratory flow—volume (MEFV) curves in upper airway obstruction and chronic obstructive airways disease.

exchange impairment, but its measurement has little place in preoperative assessment.

Assessment of gas exchange

Arterial hypoxaemia while breathing air is caused by:

1 Reduced alveolar ventilation, from either respiratory centre depression, e.g. by drugs or hypercapnia, or from airways obstruction. There is associated hypercapnia.

2 Perfusion of non-ventilated lung tissue (intrapulmonary shunting).

3 Perfusion of relatively underventilated lung tissue ($\dot{V}:\dot{Q}$ mismatch).

4 Diffusion defect across alveolar—capillary membrane from, e.g. interstitial fibrosis.

Defective gas exchange caused by defective diffusion or $\dot{V}:\dot{Q}$ mismatching such as in diffuse pulmonary fibrosis can be assessed non-invasively by measurement of the transfer factor for carbon monoxide (T_{CO}). This value is affected by lung volume and the corrected value (K_{CO}) is a better measure of gas transfer. In certain situations, usually in connection with lung surgery, it may be useful to investigate regional ventilation and perfusion, and this can be undertaken using radioisotope ventilation and perfusion scan.

Normally, in the preoperative patient with respiratory disease, gas exchange is assessed by measurement of arterial blood-gas tensions, which should be carried out with the patient breathing air (unless the patient is clinically hypoxic when measurement should be made in relation to a known inspired concentration of oxygen). Blood-gas tensions should be checked when clinical examination or pulmonary function tests indicate severe pulmonary disease. Measurements of $FEV_{1.0}$ and FVC of less than 50% of predicted, or an $FEV_{1.0}$ less than 1 litre, or an FVC less than 1.5 litres, would all be indications (Milledge & Nunn, 1975).

A decreased Pao_2 in association with increased $Paco_2$ indicates alveolar hypoventilation associated most often with chronic obstructive airways disease. The $Paco_2$ is a good predictor of the likelihood of perioperative respiratory complications. A patient with a $Paco_2$ of 6.7 kPa (50 mmHg) or more is likely to require a period of postoperative ventilation following major surgery, while a preoperative level of 6 kPa (45 mmHg) or less can be managed usually with controlled oxygen therapy and careful blood-gas monitoring (Milledge & Nunn, 1975). More recently, Nunn and colleagues (1988) have raised doubts as to the importance of an elevated $Paco_2$ level in predicting the need for postoperative ventilation. In a group of 42 patients with very severe chronic obstructive airways disease ($FEV_{1.0}$ 0.3—1.02), they found a low Pao_2 to be the best predictor of postoperative respiratory insufficiency. Nevertheless, in their series, only

12 patients overall, and only one out of 9 patients with raised Pa_{CO_2}, actually underwent upper abdominal surgery. Further checks of arterial blood-gas tensions with known $F_I_{O_2}$ of 24 or 28% may elucidate the degree of ventilatory response to oxygen and carbon dioxide, and allow the $F_I_{O_2}$ to be set for optimal blood-gas levels.

A decreased Pa_{O_2} in association with a normal or low Pa_{CO_2} is associated with a diffusion defect, intrapulmonary shunting or $\dot{V}:\dot{Q}$ mismatching. An increased $F_I_{O_2}$ raises the Pa_{O_2} where diffusion defect or $\dot{V}:\dot{Q}$ mismatch is the cause of hypoxaemia.

Drug therapy in respiratory disease

This may commonly include bronchodilator therapy, corticosteroids and treatment for co-existing cardiac failure, i.e. digoxin and diuretics.

Bronchodilator agents are of three types; β_2-adrenergic agonists such as salbutamol, which appear to act through augmentation of cyclic adenosine monophosphate (AMP) concentrations in the bronchial walls; phosphodiesterase inhibitors such as aminophylline which delay the breakdown of cyclic AMP; and anticholinergic agents such as ipratropium bromide. In general, bronchodilator therapy should be continued over the perioperative period; the β_2-agonists and ipratropium bromide, which are administered usually from metered-dose inhalers, are probably best administered via nebulizer in the postoperative period when patients may be less able to co-operate in using inhalers. The theophylline preparations, taken normally as sustained-release tablets, may be given by intravenous infusion when oral intake is not possible. Theophylline has a relatively narrow range of therapeutic plasma concentrations, and its elimination is reduced in elderly patients, those with liver disease or low cardiac output, and, conceivably, in patients in the postoperative period. Plasma concentrations should be monitored to avoid toxic drug concentrations.

Corticosteroids are administered either by inhalation (e.g. beclomethasone dipropionate, 200–800 µg/day) or systemically. Adrenal suppression does not occur by inhalation in correct dosage, and perioperative systemic supplementation is not required for this purpose, although it may be required to control the patient's asthma during the perioperative period. If the patient has been receiving systemic steroid therapy for more than 2 weeks immediately prior to surgery or for any long-term course within 1 year of surgery, cover should be supplemented over the perioperative period. Hypo-

kalaemia may occur, and requires potassium supplementation prior to surgery.

Principles of anaesthetic and postoperative management

Because chronic obstructive airways disease is by far the most common and problematical pulmonary disease in relation to anaesthesia and surgery, the principles of preoperative preparation, choice of anaesthetic technique, anaesthetic and postoperative management are considered in relation to this disease. Many of the principles outlined are applicable to other conditions, but where differences occur, they are discussed in the appropriate section for each disease.

Chronic bronchitis and emphysema

Chronic bronchitis is characterized by the presence of productive cough for at least 3 months in 2 successive years. There is excessive mucus secretion from bronchial glands, and a variable degree of airways obstruction, caused by both bronchial oedema and retained secretions, and which may initially be partially reversible by bronchodilator therapy. Repeated episodes of infection occur with eventual persistent cough and sputum production. The disease progresses variably:

1 Some patients, the bronchitic or 'blue bloater' group develop hypoxia, hypercapnia and right ventricular failure. These patients demonstrate loss of ventilatory sensitivity to carbon dioxide, depending for their ventilatory drive on a degree of hypoxia.
2 Others, the so-called 'pink puffers', develop emphysema characterized by lung overdistension, destruction of alveolar walls with loss of gas exchange surface, loss of elastic recoil, and airway obstruction. An increased $\dot{V}:\dot{Q}$ ratio or deadspace requires the patient to hyperventilate to maintain normocapnia, hence the 'pink puffer' label.

Emphysema may occur also as a primary familial disease from α_1-antitrypsin deficiency, where lung dysfunction occurs through the patient's inability to inactivate proteolytic enzymes.

In practice, many patients have a mixed picture of chronic bronchitis with emphysema.

Patients with chronic bronchitis present three particular problems in relation to anaesthesia and surgery.

1 Excess sputum which, if cleared inadequately, leads to postoperative atelectasis and bronchopneumonia.
2 Airways obstruction.

3 Loss of ventilatory response to carbon dioxide, with dependence on a hypoxic stimulus.

In addition, as with previously healthy patients, bronchitic patients are more liable to postoperative respiratory complications following upper abdominal or thoracic procedures (Tarhan *et al.*, 1973), prolonged surgery and if they are obese (Garibaldi *et al.*, 1981).

Preoperative preparation should deal with these problems, whilst choice of anaesthetic technique must be made both in relation to these problems and the nature of the surgery planned. Elective surgery should be timed for a period of remission, avoiding episodes of infective exacerbation.

Sputum clearance

Preoperative chest physiotherapy, consisting of supervised deep breathing and coughing, and postural drainage is essential in reducing postoperative morbidity (Palmer & Sellick, 1953). Sputum should be collected for culture and an appropriate antibiotic prescribed. There is evidence that prophylactic antibiotics reduce the frequency of postoperative infective complications (Morran & McArdle, 1980). The commonest organisms are *Streptococcus pneumoniae* or *Haemophilus influenzae*, for which amoxycillin or co-trimoxazole are appropriate treatment. In patients who are more ill and hospitalized, infection with β-lactamase producing coliform organisms is increasingly common, for which cefuroxime or the combination of amoxycillin with a β-lactamase inhibitor, clavulanic acid, are good choices.

Airway obstruction

Where the patient is receiving bronchodilator therapy routinely, it should be continued over the perioperative period. In those patients not receiving treatment, but in whom pulmonary function testing reveals evidence of obstruction and reversibility to dilator, a trial of salbutamol, 200 µg (2 puffs), by metered-dose inhaler, or 2.5 mg in 2.5 ml saline by nebulizer 4−6 hourly, possibly in combination with oral sustained release aminophylline, 225−450 mg, twice daily is worthwhile. Used in combination, ipratropium bromide may also occasionally be effective by inhalation, 40 µg (2 puffs) 6-hourly. Used in combination with chest physiotherapy, humidification and antibiotics, bronchodilator therapy appears to decrease the incidence of postoperative respiratory complications following upper abdominal surgery (Gracey *et al.*, 1979).

Corticosteroid therapy has rarely a place in the treatment of chronic obstructive airways disease, and should not be used electively without monitoring of pulmonary function to detect any benefit, but in the patient with intractable airways obstruction presenting for urgent surgery, especially if already receiving inhaled corticosteroid, systemic steroid therapy, prednisolone, 15−20 mg 6-hourly, or the equivalent, should be administered.

Carbon dioxide responsiveness

The relationship of a raised Pa_{CO_2} level of more than 6.7 kPa (50 mmHg) with postoperative problems after major abdominal surgery, and the need for respiratory support has been emphasized above. The inspired oxygen concentration, usually 24−28%, should be adjusted to achieve the optimal blood-gas tensions with an adequate Pa_{O_2} [8 kPa (60 mmHg)] without excessive carbon dioxide retention [Pa_{CO_2} preferably less than 7.5−8 kPa (55−60 mmHg)].

Smoking

Smoking should, of course, be discouraged in all patients presenting for surgery. To gain all possible benefits in respect of perioperative morbidity, smoking should stop at least 6 weeks before operation. Those benefits include a reduction in carboxyhaemoglobin, a reduction in coronary and systemic vascular resistance, improved neutrophil activity, improved clearance of tracheobronchial secretions, and reversal of small airway obstruction (Jones *et al.*, 1987).

Obesity

Obese patients should be encouraged to reduce weight before elective surgery, for reasons outlined previously.

Treatment of heart failure

Cor pulmonale in the 'blue bloater' should be treated with diuretics and, debatably, with digoxin; likewise, left ventricular failure which may result from concurrent ischaemic heart disease.

Premedication

In patients with severe disease, and particularly if Pa_{CO_2} is raised, opioids should be avoided. If secretions are very copious, anticholinergic agents such as atropine or hyoscine are useful; they may, however, increase viscosity, making secretions more difficult to clear. Generally, light benzodiazepine premedication with, e.g. temazepam, 10–20 mg, or diazepam is satisfactory.

Choice of anaesthetic technique

Two approaches to anaesthetic management may be taken depending on the clinical state of the patient and the nature of the surgery planned.

Minimal anaesthesia approach

This approach should be employed for minor procedures such as surgery on the limbs, lower abdomen and perineum, and other body surface areas. It involves maintenance of spontaneous ventilation, the use, where appropriate, of local or regional anaesthesia alone or in combination with light general anaesthesia, or the use of light general anaesthesia preferably without tracheal intubation. Opioid analgesia should be avoided generally, and other sedation kept to a minimum. If tracheal intubation is felt to be essential, topical local anaesthesia improves toleration of the tube by an irritable larynx and trachea.

The minimal techniques aim to avoid interference with an irritable tracheobronchial tree, to minimize respiratory depression and to avoid the difficulty of restoration of spontaneous ventilation after controlled ventilation techniques.

The disadvantages of this approach is the danger of hypoventilation if alveolar ventilatory capacity is critical. Sedation and light general anaesthesia should be avoided normally if the preoperative Pa_{CO_2} is greater than 6.7 kPa (50 mmHg). Furthermore, in emphysematous patients where Pa_{CO_2} is maintained in the normal range through hyperventilation, light volatile anaesthesia may depress ventilation markedly leading to an increased Pa_{CO_2} (Pietak *et al.*, 1975). Clearance of secretions may be a problem also. In the patient with a raised Pa_{CO_2} or very depressed $FEV_{1.0}$, this approach should be used with caution, and only for minor procedures, with close respiratory monitoring.

The almost universal availability of non-invasive respiratory monitoring in the operative theatre (pulse oximetry and end-tidal P_{CO_2}) has tended to reduce the use of intra-operative arterial blood-gas measurement. It is important not to rely on end-tidal P_{CO_2} measurement in this population, as the increased physiological deadspace leads to a considerable divergence between arterial and end-tidal P_{CO_2}

values, with the latter understating arterial measurements.

Role of local and regional anaesthesia

Nerve and plexus blocks for operations on head, neck, eyes and limbs offer freedom from respiratory side-effects and avoidance of the complications of general anaesthesia such as ciliary paralysis, tracheobronchial irritation, introduction of infection and respiratory depression. Nevertheless, the patient must be able to lie reasonably flat and refrain from coughing.

Low subarachnoid and lumbar or caudal extradural block have similar advantages for lower abdominal or pelvic surgery. Overall, however, the morbidity resulting from general anaesthesia for such operations is low, and it is only, perhaps, in the patient verging on respiratory failure that significant advantage accrues.

Combination of a local anaesthetic block with general anaesthesia allows much lighter anaesthesia to be employed with obvious benefits. Examples include ilioinguinal nerve block for inguinal herniorrhaphy, or wrist block for hand surgery.

The use of local and regional anaesthesia for procedures associated with considerable postoperative pain has obvious advantage in decreasing the need for opioid analgesia with its attendant respiratory depression.

The role of regional block in upper abdominal and thoracic surgery is considered in relation to postoperative analgesia (p. 1204).

Maximal support approach

This approach involves the use of muscle relaxation, tracheal intubation and controlled ventilation, allowing control of Pa_{O_2} and Pa_{CO_2} and clearance of secretions. It requires generally a period of postoperative respiratory support, at least until elimination of intravenous and inhalational anaesthetic agents, muscle relaxants and excess opioids has occurred, and adequate analgesia established. Thus, adequate recovery-room or intensive care facilities are necessary.

Where major abdominal and thoracic surgery is involved, and in patients with a raised Pa_{CO_2} preoperatively, this approach is advisable. Minute ventilation should be adjusted to maintain the Pa_{CO_2} at or only slightly less than usual levels, according to arterial samples. A flow-generator, volume-preset ventilator should be used, employing a low inspiratory flow rate, thus avoiding excessive airway pressure, and a prolonged expiratory time. The inspired oxygen concentration during anaesthesia should be increased to maintain a $Paco_2$ at a minimum of approximately 10 kPa (75 mmHg). PEEP, which may have application in increasing FRC during anaesthesia in patients with pulmonary restrictive disorders, has no place in chronic obstructive disease.

In emphysematous patients, the increased deadspace necessitates a high minute volume to maintain $Paco_2$ at normal levels. This should be provided with care to avoid high airway pressure and barotrauma, and to allow adequate expiratory time to avoid air trapping. In patients with large bullae, it is advisable to avoid nitrous oxide which leads to expansion of the bulla, and one must be prepared for the possibility of bullous rupture into the pleural space with tension pneumothorax resulting. Where IPPV is considered essential, consideration should be given to passage of a double-lumen tube to isolate the affected lung.

Short-term ventilatory support

Certain operations (e.g. laparoscopic cholecystectomy, certain ophthalmic or ENT procedures), do not readily allow maintenance of spontaneous ventilation intraoperatively, but are otherwise associated with minimal postoperative sequelae. The availability of a properly staffed and equipped recovery room allows short-term (up to 1–2 h) postoperative ventilation after such operations until full recovery of consciousness is achieved, with early extubation and restoration of spontaneous ventilation.

Postoperative care

Postoperative hypoxaemia is the result both of respiratory depression and the reduction in FRC with consequent airway closure, shunting and atelectasis. The complications of postoperative pneumonia and respiratory failure develop as a result of these factors, and thus attention must be directed towards minimizing respiratory depression, and the reduction in FRC.

In patients with chronic obstructive airways disease, the respiratory depression may be exacerbated by loss of the carbon dioxide ventilatory drive, and the airway closure–atelectasis problem exacerbated by failure to clear excess secretions. Such patients must be monitored very intensively with respect to ability to ventilate adequately and clear secretions. This involves pulse oximetry, monitoring of blood-gas tensions and repeated clinical and radiological examination to detect pulmonary collapse or consolidation.

Respiratory depression: analgesic considerations

This is unlikely to be a problem in patients who have undergone minor or body surface procedures under local or regional techniques. Nevertheless, if procedures are likely to lead to severe postoperative pain, such as certain orthopaedic procedures, analgesia must be provided with care, ideally with a regional technique. Examples include extradural analgesia, either with local anaesthetic (bupivacaine, 0.25–0.5% by intermittent injection or 0.125% by continuous infusion) or opioid (diamorphine, 2.5–5 mg in 5–10 ml sodium chloride, 0.9%); brachial plexus block or femoral nerve block repeated as required through indwelling cannulae. Non-opioid analgesics are increasingly used, either in combination with local analgesia or opioids, or as sole agents for less painful procedures. Some non-steroidal anti-inflammatory drugs are available for parenteral administration (diclofenac; ketorolac) or by suppository. These agents have clear advantages in view of their lack of respiratory depressant effects, but may be associated with bleeding, renal or gastric side-effects. Systemic opioids should be titrated to effect, ideally with a small intravenous bolus dose followed initially by an infusion, e.g. morphine, 1–2 mg/h. While there are indications that opioid analgesia has some beneficial effect on pulmonary function with respect to sparing the reduction in FRC occurring after major surgery (Alexander et al., 1973b), there is little doubt that the opioids may lead to episodes of apnoea and hypoxia especially during sleep (Catley et al., 1985).

Where the preoperative $Paco_2$ is greater than 6.7 kPa (50 mmHg), opioids should be avoided in the spontaneously breathing patient. Throughout the postoperative period, $Paco_2$ should be maintained in line with preoperative values, and certainly not greater than 7.5–8 kPa (55–60 mmHg). Failure to achieve this is an indication for controlled ventilation.

In those patients who have undergone major abdominal or thoracic surgery with a maximum support technique, elective postoperative ventilation allows adequate oxygenation and control of $Paco_2$, analgesia without respiratory depression, and clearance of secretions by physiotherapy, tracheal suction and fibre-optic bronchoscopy. Intermittent positive-pressure ventilation (IPPV) should be continued at least until cardiovascular status has been optimized, any fluid deficitor overload corrected and residual anaesthetic agents eliminated. The use of regional techniques, e.g. thoracic or lumbar extradural block, avoiding the use of systemic opioids, may allow an earlier return to spontaneous ventilation. In general, however, IPPV until the following day is more prudent in patients with severe disease, as close monitoring of arterial blood-gas tensions is required on return to spontaneous ventilation.

Controlled inspired oxygen therapy is required with the concentration titrated to maintain a Pao_2 of $8-9$ kPa ($60-67$ mmHg) and a $Paco_2$ below $7.5-8$ kPa ($55-60$ mmHg).

Effects on postoperative functional residual capacity

In view of the relationship between reduction in FRC and airway closure, hypoxaemia and atelectasis following upper abdominal surgery (Alexander *et al.*, 1973b), it is logical that a major aim of postoperative management should be to minimize this effect.

Analgesia

By reducing abdominal muscle spasm, analgesia should theoretically minimize the reduction in FRC and associated hypoxaemia. Thoracic extradural bupivacaine does achieve this, being associated with significantly higher Pao_2 values on the first 3 postoperative days than conventional morphine analgesia provided either by intermittent intramuscular or continuous intravenous routes (Spence & Smith, 1971; Spence & Logan, 1975; Cuschieri *et al.*, 1985). More intense administration of opioid analgesia, e.g. by infusion, does not appear to achieve a similar improvement in postoperative pulmonary function, presumably because of its inability to control the sharp pain associated with deep breathing and coughing (Cuschieri *et al.*, 1985). Lumbar extradural analgesia following lower abdominal surgery does not appear to confer a similar advantage (Drummond & Littlewood, 1977), and where there is an initial low FVC, a further reduction resulting from extradural anaesthetic may lead to a reduction in cough effectiveness and respiratory failure (Takasaki & Takahashi, 1980; Harrop-Griffiths *et al.*, 1991).

Posture

A semi-recumbent posture is associated with less reduction in FRC and basal airway closure than the supine posture (Table 59.1) and should be adopted when adequate conscious level and cardiovascular

stability are achieved postoperatively. Abdominal distension should be minimized, with very distended bowel decompressed, and peritoneal suction drainage to reduce pneumoperitoneum (Bevan, 1961).

Fluid therapy

Excessive crystalloid fluid administration increases CV and contributes to postoperative hypoxaemia. Thus, there should be a daily maximum of 2 litres, colloid being used for intravascular volume replacement (Twigley & Hillman, 1985).

Physiotherapy and respiratory therapy

Various physiotherapeutic manoeuvres may help to reduce basal airway closure. Supervised deep breathing is intended to ventilate the dependent underventilated lung regions preventing atelectasis, and encouraging the coughing of retained secretions.

Voluntary maximal inspiratory manoeuvres using an 'incentive spirometer' have been claimed to decrease atelectatic pulmonary complications (Bartlett *et al.*, 1973), but this has not been confirmed by other workers (Gale & Sanders, 1980). Intermittent positive-pressure breathing (IPPB) using a Bird or Bennett ventilator has had similar mixed results. A new method for the prophylaxis and treatment of postoperative atelectasis is the application of continuous positive airways pressure (CPAP) using a tightly fitting face mask (Paul & Downs, 1981; Dehaven *et al.*, 1985). This requires further evaluation to decide the required frequency and duration of therapy.

Doxapram infusion, $250-300$ mg, over a period ranging from 30 min to 4 h, has been subject to a number of investigations in relation to postoperative hypoxaemia and complications. It may produce only marginal benefits.

Bronchodilator therapy should be continued postoperatively by nebulizer which is used more easily by the patient suffering from abdominal pain than conventional inhalers. If carbon dioxide retention is present, nebulization should be in air or low concentration oxygen (salbutamol, 2.5 mg in 2.5 ml saline $4-6$ hourly). Aminophylline may be given by intravenous infusion ($0.5-0.8$ mg $\cdot$ kg^{-1} $\cdot$ h^{-1}).

Clearance of secretions

Sputum retention compounds the effect of FRC reduction in producing atelectasis and pneumonia. Successful clearance of secretions requires adequate analgesia, best provided by extradural analgesia.

Entonox (50% nitrous oxide in oxygen) is useful for short-term analgesia prior to physiotherapy which may be required four times per day. Humidification of inspired air aids expectoration (Gawley & Dundee, 1981).

Where the patient's vital capacity is reduced to such an extent as to render coughing ineffective (less than 1 litre), direct suction from the trachea may be necessary, involving tracheal intubation, bronchoscopy, or tracheostomy. In many cases, intubation of the trachea requires sedation, with the danger of respiratory depression and thus the need for IPPV.

A percutaneous technique of cricothyrotomy or minitracheotomy allows access to the trachea for suction without sedation and maintaining the patient's voice and cough (Matthews & Hopkinson, 1984). However, there have been reports of severe haemorrhage during the use of this technique.

Infective complications suggested by pyrexia, leucocytosis, purulent sputum, and clinical and radiological signs require appropriate antibiotic therapy after sputum culture.

Asthma

Asthma is characterized by reversible airways obstruction, and can be classified into one of two groups: 'extrinsic' and 'intrinsic'. Extrinsic asthma develops usually in childhood or young adulthood, frequently following a history of eczema in infancy, and a strong family history of allergic disorders. Hypersensitivity to one or more allergens can be demonstrated on skin testing, or a response to a specific chemical irritant. By contrast, intrinsic asthma, although characterized also by reversible obstruction, develops at a later age, and no external allergen can be demonstrated. In early asthma, airway obstruction demonstrated by a low $FEV_{1.0}:FVC$ ratio returns to normal between asthmatic attacks, while in more advanced disease, and especially in intrinsic asthma, some obstruction persists between attacks.

Preoperatively, the current activity of the disease should be assessed from history, examination and pulmonary function testing. In particular, frequency and severity of attacks, factors provoking attacks, and drug history should be noted. Examination should be directed towards evidence of obstruction (rhonchi, prolonged expiration, overdistension of chest) and infection. The ratio of $FEV_{1.0}:FVC$ should be measured before and after bronchodilator and compared with previous results if available.

Elective surgery should not be undertaken unless or until asthma is well controlled. Pre-existing bronchodilator, corticosteroid, or sodium cromoglycate therapy should be continued throughout the perioperative period, while, where asthma is controlled inadequately, therapy should be commenced or modified prior to surgery. Pulmonary infection requires treatment with an appropriate antibiotic.

Appropriate bronchodilator therapy would consist of a β_2-adrenoceptor agonist such as salbutamol, 200 µg (2 puffs), by inhaler four to six times per day, possibly in combination with aminophylline or theophylline by sustained-release tablet twice daily. This therapy should be commenced several days preoperatively. A dose of salbutamol by inhalation should be administered 15–30 min before induction of anaesthesia, whilst an oral dose of aminophylline should be given on the morning of surgery. Occasionally, patients with intrinsic asthma respond well to the anticholinergic agent, ipratropium bromide, 40 µg (2 puffs), by inhaler.

Over the perioperative period, salbutamol is best administered by nebulization and aminophylline by infusion as described previously.

Patients with severe asthma requiring maintenance topical or systemic corticosteroid therapy, those with a history of previous systemic steroid therapy or those still exhibiting significant airways obstruction despite conventional bronchodilator therapy, require systemic steroid therapy to cover the perioperative period. Oral prednisolone, 40–100 mg daily, should be given preoperatively, and hydrocortisone, 100 mg i.m., with premedication and 100 mg i.m. four times daily for the first postoperative day, decreasing thereafter. Oral prednisolone in equivalent dosage may be substituted on resumption of oral intake. Essentially, steroid dosage in this situation is titrated to the severity of the asthma.

Anaesthesia

Anaesthetic management should be aimed towards avoiding triggering of bronchospasm either through mechanical irritation by, for example, tracheal intubation, or through histamine-releasing drugs such as morphine, D-tubocurarine or atracurium.

Premedication should consist of a sedative agent such as a benzodiazepine, e.g. temazepam, with atropine to block vagal reflex-induced bronchospasm. Pethidine and promethazine are recommended also.

Halothane, being bronchodilator, is well tolerated in asthma, while ether has been recommended also in cases of severe bronchospasm. Ketamine has been used successfully by infusion to control bronchospasm in patients with status asthmaticus (Strube & Hallam,

1986), and enflurane and isoflurane appear also to have bronchodilator effects in asthmatics (Parnass et al., 1987). They have the added benefit over halothane of not sensitizing the myocardium to the arrhythmogenic effects of β_2-agonists and aminophylline.

Bronchoconstriction is provoked most commonly immediately after induction and intubation, by a combination of light anaesthesia, drug-induced histamine release and mechanical stimulation by the tracheal tube. It can be avoided best by employing an adequate depth of anaesthesia, use of agents not associated with histamine release (pethidine or fentanyl rather than morphine; vecuronium or pancuronium rather than atracurium), and spraying the vocal cords and trachea with local anaesthetic prior to tracheal intubation.

In patients with severe airways obstruction, controlled ventilation should employ a low inspiratory flow rate, low frequency and prolonged expiratory phase. A raised $Pa\text{co}_2$ may have to be accepted, to avoid excessively high airway pressure. Pneumothorax is a possible complication requiring early detection and drainage.

If severe bronchospasm occurs, aminophylline, 250 mg, by slow intravenous injection, is the first drug of choice; it should, however, be used with caution if the patient is already receiving oral phosphodiesterase inhibitor preparations. Salbutamol, 125—250 µg i.v., should be used with extreme caution in the presence of halothane. Hydrocortisone, 100—200 mg i.v., should be administered simultaneously although it has no immediate effect. Nebulized salbutamol by positive-pressure ventilation either intermittently (2.5 mg in 2.5 ml saline 2—4-hourly) or continuously from an ultrasonic nebulizer (50—100 µg/ml of water) may be effective also.

Where feasible, local or regional anaesthetic techniques are to be preferred in severe asthma.

Pulmonary eosinophilia, a mixed Type I and Type III immune reaction to the fungus *Aspergillus fumigatus*, consists of a mixed picture of airways obstruction and diffuse alveolar eosinophilic infiltrates. Polyarteritis nodosa may present with a similar picture.

Bronchiectasis

Bronchiectasis is characterized by overproduction of purulent sputum from dilated, disorganized bronchi. It may follow childhood whooping cough or measles, or from persistent pulmonary infection in cystic fibrosis. It may be localized (e.g. to a single lobe in

which case lobectomy provides a cure) or generalized throughout both lungs. There is generally some degree of airways obstruction, but bronchodilator therapy is of limited value. Later, fibrosis causes a restrictive defect. A wide range of bacterial pathogens may be involved, commonly *Staphylococcus aureus* and *Pseudomonas* species. Sputum culture is essential to determine appropriate antibiotic therapy.

Patients should be admitted approximately 1 week prior to elective surgery, and intensive physiotherapy with postural drainage instituted, together with appropriate antibiotic therapy.

Anaesthesia for minor surgery is provided best by local or regional techniques, but for major procedures, tracheal intubation for clearance of secretions and controlled ventilation is advisable. In patients with localized bronchiectasis, consideration should be given to isolating the diseased lobe using a double-lumen tube.

Prevention of postoperative complications depends on adequate clearance of secretions, for which good analgesia is essential to allow the necessary physiotherapy and coughing. Regional techniques, or Entonox used with physiotherapy are both useful. Minitracheotomy may have a place for removal of secretions.

In cystic fibrosis, chronic hypoxaemia leads eventually to pulmonary hypertension and cor pulmonale. Arterial $Pa\text{o}_2$ is decreased initially with a low or normal $Pa\text{co}_2$ early in the disease, a raised $Pa\text{co}_2$ being a sign of advanced disease. In patients with a raised $Pa\text{co}_2$ preoperatively, elective postoperative ventilation is essential (Lamberty & Rubin, 1985).

Restrictive disorders of lung and chest wall

Restricted lung expansion can result from:
1 Interstitial lung disease, e.g. sarcoidosis, fibrosing alveolitis.
2 Deformities of the thoracic cage, e.g. kyphoscoliosis, ankylosing spondylitis.
3 Pleural conditions, e.g. effusion, empyema, mesothelioma.
4 Neuromuscular disorders, e.g. Guillain—Barré syndrome, motorneurone disease, myasthenia gravis.

It is important to distinguish restriction resulting from interstitial lung disease from that produced by extrapulmonary factors. Pulmonary interstitial disorders are associated usually with impaired gas exchange (Table 59.2), while the defect in those patients with extrapulmonary restriction may be purely mechanical. In both there is a reduction in both $FEV_{1.0}$ and FVC with a normal ratio, and a decreased FRC and TLC. Ultimately, in both groups hypoxaemia occurs, as the reduction in lung volume leads to basal airway closure during tidal ventilation with consequent shunting. The reduction in vital capacity impedes the ability to cough and clear secretions. A vital capacity of less than 1 litre, i.e. twice normal tidal volume, is likely to be associated with an ineffective clearance of secretions, atelectasis and infection.

Total compliance is reduced in both groups, often more so in the extrapulmonary group, so that the work of breathing and the airway pressure required to ventilate the lungs adequately is increased.

Anaesthesia

Following anaesthesia and surgery, there is generally little further reduction in lung volume, and thus little further deterioration in gas exchange. Nevertheless, the residual effects of anaesthetic agents, analgesic drugs, ineffective coughing produced by pain and the reduction in vital capacity all contribute to a hazardous postoperative period.

Anaesthesia for minor, body surface and limb operations is achieved probably most suitably by local or regional techniques. In major abdominal and thoracic surgery, however, maximal support with controlled ventilation is advisable.

Effective analgesia must be administered to allow coughing and clearance of secretions. Regional techniques such as extradural analgesia are useful, although in severe disease where vital capacity is reduced markedly, extradural local anaesthetic block should be avoided as this reduces vital capacity further (Drummond & Littlewood, 1977). After major surgery, a short period of controlled ventilation, usually not greater than 24 h, is advisable to allow adequate analgesia, facilitate clearance of secretions, and prevent atelectasis. In patients with extremely severe restrictive lung disease, negative pressure ventilation with an iron lung has been advocated following conventional light general anaesthesia to facilitate weaning to spontaneous ventilation (Patrick et al., 1990). Oxygen may be administered in high concentrations without causing respiratory depression. Intense respiratory monitoring with frequent arterial blood-gas tension measurements is essential.

Interstitial lung disease is the term covering pulmonary diseases characterized by thickening of alveolar walls by oedema, cellular exudate, or fibrosis. Causes include:

1 Pulmonary oedema from left ventricular failure or mitral valve disease.
2 Extrinsic allergic alveolitis, such as farmers' lung.
3 Fibrosing alveolitis associated with connective tissue disorders such as systemic lupus erythematosis.
4 Idiopathic fibrosing alveolitis.
5 Sarcoidosis.

Patients with connective tissue disorders and sarcoidosis may have other systemic involvement e.g. cardiovascular or renal, and may be receiving systemic corticosteroid therapy, requiring augmentation over the perioperative period. Radiological appearance does not always reflect functional impairment.

Adult respiratory distress syndrome

The term adult respiratory distress syndrome (ARDS) is used to describe a type of acute respiratory failure associated with a predisposing, frequently septic, illness. It is characterized by hypoxaemia necessitating mechanical ventilation with high F_IO_2, bilateral diffuse infiltrates on chest X-ray, a low pulmonary compliance and absence of heart failure [pulmonary artery occlusion pressure less than 2.4 kPa (18 mmHg)]. A detailed description of ARDS is included in Chapter 84. In general anaesthetic practice, a considerable number of patients with ARDS present for operation, usually for eradication of abdominal sepsis. These patients generally come from the intensive therapy unit already ventilated and return there for intensive care, postoperatively. Meticulous care is required in the transfer of these patients, and the use of arterial, central venous pressure (CVP) and pulmonary arterial catheters to allow optimal cardiorespiratory monitoring and support is essential. Mortality in ARDS is generally associated with the development of sepsis and multiple organ failure, and maintenance of a supranormal level of oxygen delivery appears to be beneficial. Intraoperatively, the emphasis should be on the maintenance of cardiorespiratory stability as a continuation of the process of intensive care.

Pleural disease

Pleural effusion is caused most commonly by pneumonia, tuberculosis, malignant disease and pulmonary infarction.

Large effusions clearly restrict lung expansion, and should be aspirated or drained before anaesthesia. Chronic effusions may cause fibrous thickening of the visceral pleura, so that even on drainage, lung expansion is limited. This requires treatment by decortication. Empyema, caused either by suppurative pneumonia or tuberculosis, requires drainage by a wide-bore chest drain and appropriate antibiotic therapy.

Pneumothorax occurs more commonly in patients with chronic bronchitis, emphysema or asthma, with large subpleural bullae liable to rupture into the pleural space when positive-pressure ventilation is instituted. Where a large bulla is found on chest X-ray preoperatively, nitrous oxide is best avoided, as it diffuses out into the bulla; where positive-pressure ventilation is essential, consideration should be given to use of a double-lumen tube to isolate the lung containing the bulla, or of high-frequency jet ventilation.

If pneumothorax occurs in the anaesthetized patient undergoing artificial ventilation, it is liable to expand rapidly with lung collapse, mediastinal shift and cardiovascular collapse. Clinical signs include cyanosis, increased airway pressure, hypotension and raised CVP. Immediate drainage is essential, in extreme emergencies using a 14-gauge intravenous cannula before placement of an intercostal drain with underwater seal either in the fourth or fifth intercostal space in the axilla, or in the second intercostal space in the mid-clavicular line.

Failure of pneumothorax to resolve with adequate underwater seal drainage reflects either a persistent air leak (bronchopleural fistula) or failure of a non-compliant lung to re-expand. The former may seal if suction of $10-20\,cmH_2O$ is applied to the drain, expanding the lung against the chest wall around the leak, but failure to achieve this is an indication for pleurodesis or parietal pleurectomy. Re-expansion of a non-compliant lung may be achieved using CPAP or IPPV, in combination with pleural suction drainage.

Acute respiratory tract infections

Clearly, elective surgery should not be conducted where evidence of acute respiratory tract infection is present: productive cough, pyrexia, leucocytosis and clinical or radiological signs in the chest. In cases where surgery cannot be delayed, management should be directed towards monitoring of gas exchange, oxygen therapy, physiotherapy and antibiotic therapy. Whilst bacterial infection is the most common causation of pneumonia and acute bronchitis, increasingly *Mycoplasma pneumoniae*, *Legionella pneumophila* and opportunistic pathogens

such as *Pneumocystis carinii* are causative organisms. *Pneumocystis carinii* pneumonia is an increasingly common condition, both in patients with the acquired immune deficiency syndrome (AIDS) and in patients receiving immunosuppressive therapy. It is characterized by dyspnoea, hypoxaemia and bilateral infiltrates on chest X-ray, with development into ARDS. Diagnosis is made by a fluorescent antibody technique using sputum induced by breathing nebulized hypertonic saline or bronchoalveolar lavage fluid obtained by bronchoscopy. Where no clear organism is isolated early, erythromycin should be included in the antibiotic treatment to cover mycoplasma and legionella, while high-dose co-trimoxazole is required for *Pneumocystis carinii* pneumonia.

Tuberculosis

While relatively uncommon now, pulmonary tuberculosis should still be considered in patients with persistent pulmonary infection, especially if elderly or associated with weight loss and haemoptysis. Its relevance to the anaesthetist is less through its functional impairment than its potential for cross-infection through contaminated anaesthetic equipment. All equipment must therefore be sterilized after use.

Tumours of the lung and mediastinum

Most tumours of the lung are malignant, with a poor prognosis. Problems for the anaesthetist relate to the frequently coincidental chronic obstructive airways disease which is associated also with cigarette smoking, and to the nature and site of the tumour.

Assessment of fitness for anaesthesia for pneumonectomy or lobectomy is made on the basis of pulmonary function tests, arterial blood-gas tensions and an assessment of the contribution to overall function of the lung or lobe to be resected.

Centrally sited tumours may cause partial or complete obstruction of a bronchus, with distal collapse and accumulation of secretions. Peripheral tumours generally have less effect on pulmonary function. Local spread of tumour may occur to the brachial plexus or sympathetic chain from an apical (Pancoast) tumour, to the phrenic nerve causing diaphragmatic paralysis, to the recurrent laryngeal nerve, pericardium, oesophagus, trachea and pleura, causing effusion, and to the ribs. Compression of the superior vena cava by tumour causes swelling, venous engorgement and petechial haemorrhages of head, neck and upper limbs, associated often with tracheal or oesophageal compression. A head-up tilt, followed by radiotherapy to the tumour, relieves symptoms usually. Where anaesthesia is required for mediastinal biopsy, infusions established in the lower limbs, tracheal intubation and controlled ventilation are essential.

Alveolar-cell carcinoma spreads within the lung along alveolar walls, while secondary tumour may spread along pulmonary lymphatics (lymphangitis carcinomatosis). Both of these diffuse infiltrations lead to rapidly progressive dyspnoea, and typical restrictive defect.

Oat-cell carcinomas may in rare instances secrete various hormones, most commonly adrenocorticotrophic hormone (ACTH) causing Cushing's syndrome (see Chapter 52) and antidiuretic hormone (ADH), causing dilutional hyponatraemia.

A myasthenic syndrome is another manifestation of bronchial carcinoma, with muscle weakness and a sensitivity to neuromuscular-blocking drugs (see Chapter 55).

Benign tumours are rare, but bronchial adenomata may cause haemoptysis or bronchial obstruction with distal collapse and infection. They may also contain carcinoid tissue and secrete serotonin (carcinoid syndrome, see Chapter 55).

Secondary tumours tend to be multiple and bilateral, and are commonly from breast, kidney, uterus, ovary, testis, thyroid, or lung itself.

Mediastinal tumours

Mediastinal tumours may present similarly to centrally situated bronchial tumours, with compression of superior vena cava, trachea and oesophagus.

Causes include:

1 Lymph node enlargement from secondary tumour, lymphoma and sarcoidosis.
2 Thymoma.
3 Intrathoracic goitre.
4 Neurofibroma.
5 Developmental tumours/cysts.
6 Thoracic aortic aneurysm.

Anaesthesia may be required for mediastinal biopsy either by mediastinoscopy or parasternal mediastinotomy. Such patients may well have tracheal compression, sometimes close to the carina, in which case passage of a tracheal tube past the obstruction may be difficult. A careful preoperative clinical assessment with X-rays of the chest and thoracic inlet and maximum expiratory flow–volume studies should elucidate the degree of tracheal obstruction present. A range of tracheal tubes of different sizes should be available, and muscle relaxation should not be employed until successful tracheal intubation under deep inhalation anaesthesia with spontaneous ventilation.

References

Alexander J.I., Spence A.A., Parikh R.K. & Stuart B. (1973a) Role of airway closure in post-operative hypoxaemia. *British Journal of Anaesthesia* **45**, 34–40.

Alexander J.I., Parikh R.K. & Spence A.A. (1973b) Post-operative analgesia and lung function: a comparison of narcotic analgesic regimens. *British Journal of Anaesthesia* **45**, 346–52.

Appleberg M., Gordon L. & Fatti L.P. (1974) Preoperative pulmonary evaluation of surgical patients using vitalograph. *British Journal of Surgery* **16**, 57–9.

Bartlett R.H., Brennan M.L., Gazzaniga A.B. & Hanson E.L. (1973) Studies on the pathogenesis and prevention of postoperative pulmonary complications. *Surgery, Gynecology and Obstetrics* **137**, 925–33.

Becquemin J.P., Piquet J., Becquemin M.H., Melliere D. & Harf A. (1985) Pulmonary function after transverse or midline incision in patients with obstructive pulmonary disease. *Intensive Care Medicine* **11**, 247–51.

Bevan P.G. (1961) Post-operative pneumoperitoneum and pulmonary collapse. *British Medical Journal* **2**, 609–13.

Bjertnaes L.J., Hauge A., Nakken K.F. & Bredesen J.E. (1976) Hypoxic pulmonary vasoconstriction: inhibition due to anaesthesia. *Acta Physiologica Scandinavica* **96**, 283–5.

Campbell E.J.M., Nunn J.F. & Peckett B.W. (1958) A comparison of artificial ventilation and spontaneous respiration with particular reference to ventilation–blood flow relationships. *British Journal of Anaesthesia* **30**, 166–75.

Caro C.G., Butler J. & Du Bois A.B. (1960) Some effects of restriction of chest cage expansion on pulmonary function in man. *Journal of Clinical Investigation* **39**, 573–83.

Catley D.M., Thornton C., Jordan C. & Lehane J.R. (1985) Pronounced, episodic oxygen desaturation in the postoperative period: its association with ventilatory pattern and analgesic regimen. *Anesthesiology* **63**, 20–8.

Collins J.V., Cochrane G.M., Davis J., Benatar S.R. & Clark J.H. (1973) Some aspects of pulmonary function after rapid saline infusion in healthy subjects. *Clinical Science and Molecular Medicine* **45**, 407–10.

Cotes J.E. (1979) *Lung Function: Assessment and Application in Medicine* 4th edn. Blackwell Scientific Publications, Oxford.

Cuschieri R.J., Morran C.G., Howie J.C. & McArdle C.S. (1985) Postoperative pain and pulmonary complications: comparison of three analgesic regimens. *British Journal of Surgery* **72**, 495–8.

Dehaven C.B., Hurst J.M. & Branson R.D. (1985) Post-extubation hypoxaemia treated with a continuous positive airway pressure mask. *Critical Care Medicine* **13**, 46–8.

Drummond G.B. & Littlewood D.G. (1977) Respiratory effects of extradural analgesia after lower abdominal surgery. *British Journal of Anaesthesia* **49**, 999–1004.

Drummond G.B. & Milne A.C. (1977) Oxygen therapy after

thoracotomy. *British Journal of Anaesthesia* **49**, 1093−101.

Eisenkraft J.B. (1987) Hypoxia pulmonary vasoconstriction and anesthetic drugs. *Mount Sinai Journal of Medicine* **54**, 290−6.

Fowkes F.G.R. (1968) The value of routine pre-operative chest X-rays. *British Journal of Hospital Medicine* **35**, 120−3.

Gale G.D. & Sanders D.E. (1980) Incentive spirometry: its value after cardiac surgery. *Canadian Anaesthetists' Society Journal* **27**, 475−80.

Garibaldi R.A., Britt M.R., Coleman M.L., Reading J.C. & Pace N.L. (1981) Risk factors for post-operative pneumonia. *American Journal of Medicine* **70**, 677−80.

Gawley T.H. & Dundee J.W. (1981) Attempts to reduce respiratory complications following upper abdominal surgery. *British Journal of Anaesthesia* **53**, 1073−8.

Gracey D.R., Divertie M.B. & Didier E.P. (1979) Pre-operative pulmonary preparation of patients with chronic obstructive pulmonary disease. *Chest* **76**, 123−9.

Harrop-Griffiths A.W., Ravalia A., Browne D.A. & Robinson P.W. (1991) Regional anaesthesia and cough effectiveness. *Anaesthesia* **46**, 11−13.

Hedenstierna G., Tokics L., Strandberg A.A., Lundquist H. & Brismer B. (1986) Correlation of gas impairment to development of atelectasis during anaesthesia and muscle paralysis. *Acta Anaesthesiologica Scandinavica* **30**, 183−91.

Hewlett A.M., Hulands G.H., Nunn J.F. & Heath J.R. (1974a) Functional residual capacity during anaesthesia II. Spontaneous ventilation. *British Journal of Anaesthesia* **46**, 486−94.

Hewlett A.M., Hulands G.H., Nunn J.F. & Milledge J.S. (1974b) Functional residual capacity during anaesthesia III. Artificial ventilation. *British Journal of Anaesthesia* **46**, 495−503.

Hulands G.H., Greene R., Iliff L.D. & Nunn J.F. (1970) Influence of anaesthesia on the regional distribution of perfusion and ventilation in the lung. *Clinical Science* **38**, 451−60.

Jones R.M., Rosen M. & Seymour L. (1987) Smoking and anaesthesia (Editorial). *Anaesthesia* **42**, 1−2.

Knill R.L. & Gelb A.W. (1978) Ventilatory responses to hypoxia and hypercapnia during halothane sedation and anesthesia in man. *Anesthesiology* **49**, 244−51.

Lamberty J.M. & Rubin B.K. (1985) The management of anaesthesia for patients with cystic fibrosis. *Anaesthesia* **40**, 448−59.

Lockwood P. (1973) The relationship between pre-operative lung function test results and post-operative complications in carcinoma of the bronchus. *Respiration* **30**, 105−16.

Mathers J., Benumof J.L. & Wahrenbrock E.A. (1977) General anesthetics and regional hypoxic pulmonary vasoconstriction. *Anesthesiology* **46**, 111−14.

Matthews H.R. & Hopkinson R.B. (1984) Treatment of sputum retention by minitracheotomy. *British Journal of Surgery* **71**, 147−50.

Milledge J.S. & Nunn J.F. (1975) Criteria of fitness for anaesthesia in patients with obstructive lung disease. *British Medical Journal* **3**, 670−3.

Morran C.G. & McArdle C.S. (1980) The reduction of postoperative chest infection by prophylactic co-trimoxazole. *British Journal of Surgery* **67**, 464−6.

Nunn J.F., Bergman N.A. & Coleman A.J. (1965) Factors influencing the arterial oxygen tension during anaesthesia with artificial ventilation. *British Journal of Anaesthesia* **37**, 898−914.

Nunn J.F., Milledge J.S., Chan D. & Dore C. (1988) Respiratory criteria of fitness for surgery and anaesthesia. *Anaesthesia* **43**, 543−51.

Palmer K.N. & Sellick B.A. (1953) The prevention of postoperative pulmonary atelectasis. *Lancet* **i**, 164−8.

Parnass S.M., Feld J.M., Chamberlin W.H. & Segil L.J. (1987) Status epilepticus treated with isoflurane and enflurane. *Anesthesia and Analgesia* **66**, 193−5.

Patrick J.A., Meyer-Witting M., Reynolds F. & Spencer G.T. (1990) Peri-operative care in restrictive lung disease. *Anaesthesia* **45**, 390−5.

Paul W.L. & Downs J.B. (1981) Postoperative atelectasis. *Archives of Surgery* **116**, 861−3.

Pearce A.C. & Jones R.M. (1984) Smoking and anesthesia: preoperative abstinence and perioperative morbidity. *Anesthesiology* **61**, 576−84.

Pietak S., Weenig C.S., Hickey R.F. & Fairley H.B. (1975) Anesthetic effects on ventilation in patients with chronic obstructive pulmonary disease. *Anesthesiology* **42**, 160−6.

Rehder K. & Sessler D. (1973) Function of each lung in spontaneously breathing man anesthetised with thiopental−meperidine. *Anesthesiology* **38**, 320−7.

Rehder K., Sessler D. & Rodarte R. (1977) Regional intrapulmonary gas distribution in awake and anaesthetised-paralysed man. *Journal of Applied Physiology* **42**, 391−402.

Rigg J.R.A. & Jones N.L. (1978) Clinical assessment of respiratory function. *British Journal of Anaesthesia* **50**, 3−13.

Roberts C.J. (1984) The effective use of diagnostic radiology. *Journal of the Royal College of Physicians of London* **18**, 62−5.

Rutter P.C., Murphy F. & Dudley H.A.F. (1980) Morphine: controlled trial of different methods of administration for postoperative pain relief. *British Medical Journal* **280**, 12−13.

Seymour D.G., Pringle R.P. & Shaw J.W. (1982) The role of the routine pre-operative chest X-ray in the elderly general surgical patient. *Postgraduate Medical Journal* **58**, 741−5.

Skillman J.J., Parikh B.M. & Tanenbaum B.J. (1970) Pulmonary arteriovenous admixture. Improvement with albumin and diuresis. *American Journal of Surgery* **119**, 440−7.

Spence A.A. & Logan D.A. (1975) Respiratory effects of extradural nerve block in the post-operative period. *British Journal of Anaesthesia* **47**, 281−3.

Spence A.A. & Smith G. (1971) Postoperative analgesia and lung function: a comparison of morphine with extradural block. *British Journal of Anaesthesia* **43**, 144−8.

Strube P.J. & Hallam P.L. (1986) Ketamine by continuous infusion in status asthmaticus. *Anaesthesia* **41**, 1017−19.

Sykes M.K., Davies D.M., Chakrabarti M.K. & Loh L. (1973) The effects of halothane, trichloroethylene, and ether on the hypoxic pressor response and pulmonary vascular resistance in the isolated, perfused cat lung. *British Journal of Anaesthesia* **45**, 655−63.

Takasaki M. & Takahashi T. (1980) Respiratory function during cervical and thoracic extradural analgesia in patients with normal lungs. *British Journal of Anaesthesia* **52**, 1271−6.

Tarhan S., Moffitt E.A., Sessler A.D., Douglas W.W. & Taylor W.F. (1973) Risk of anesthesia and surgery in patients with chronic bronchitis and chronic obstructive pulmonary disease. *Surgery* **74**, 720−6.

Twigley A.J. & Hillman K.M. (1985) The end of the crystalloid era? A new approach to perioperative fluid administration.

Anaesthesia **40**, 860—71.

Vaughan R.W., Engelhardt R.C. & Wise L. (1975) Post-operative alveolar—arterial oxygen tension difference: its relation to the operative incision in obese patients. *Anesthesia and Analgesia* **54**, 433—7.

Westbrook P.R., Stubbs S.E., Sessler A.D., Rehder K. & Hyatt R.å. (1973) Effects of anaesthesia and muscle paralysis on respiratory mechanics in normal man. *Journal of Applied Physiology* **34**, 81—6.

60

Anaesthesia and Cardiac Disease

S. REIZ, D.T. MANGANO AND S. BENNETT

Over the next several decades, it is expected that cardiac disease, particularly ischaemic heart disease, will present continuing and challenging problems to the anaesthetist. Currently, a high prevalence of ischaemic heart disease exists, despite advances in medical diagnosis and therapy. For example, it is estimated that in the USA, approximately 10 million patients are diagnosed with ischaemic heart disease, 4 million of whom have had a previous myocardial infarction and 700 000 of whom die each year from ischaemic heart disease. The result is a significant increase in diagnostic and surgical therapeutic procedures. Thus, 1 million cardiac catheterizations and 300 000 coronary artery bypass operations are performed each year. It appears that this trend will continue over the next few decades because of our rapidly ageing population. The fastest growing segment of the population is the over-80 age group, which is also the segment with the highest prevalence of ischaemic heart disease. To anaesthetists, these statistics are important, for a large number of patients will undergo both cardiac, and more importantly, non-cardiac surgery.

Of the 25 million patients undergoing anaesthesia and surgery in the USA each year, 1 million have ischaemic heart disease, an additional 2–3 million have two or more risk factors for ischaemic heart disease, 5 million undergo major surgery and 7 million are over the age of 65. Thus, a significant portion of this population of 25 million (perhaps 20% or more) are older, at risk for ischaemic heart disease and undergo major non-cardiac surgery. Anaesthetists will be challenged with a number of important questions regarding the preoperative care of these patients: preoperative assessment of risk and optimization of therapy, intraoperative choice of monitoring, anaesthetic agents and regimens, drug therapies and postoperative disposition. Furthermore, these decisions will become more difficult for

the anaesthetist as cost-containment is an important issue. Outpatient surgery will force the anaesthetist to make preoperative decisions with less diagnostic information. In addition, there will be more pressure to discharge patients during the early postoperative course.

Given these challenges, three approaches can be taken.

1 We can improve assessment of perioperative risk to identify the highest-risk patients and either optimize their preoperative medical therapy or divert them to an alternative procedure (angioplasty or coronary artery bypass surgery).

2 We can identify mechanisms by which anaesthetic agents and regimens and the stress of surgery influence the systemic and coronary circulations and the incidence of intra-anaesthetic myocardial ischaemia.

3 We can introduce increasingly sensitive detectors of intraoperative myocardial ischaemia and treat early ischaemic changes in an effort to minimize perioperative morbidity. Examples of this new technology include multiple-lead, quantitated electrocardiography and transoesophageal echocardiography (TOE). Although these recently introduced techniques are exciting, their influence on perioperative morbidity has not been determined. In this chapter, we focus on the first two of these issues, namely, predictors of perioperative cardiac morbidity and the action of anaesthetic agents and techniques upon the systemic and coronary circulations.

Preoperative prediction of cardiac risk

Many studies have attempted to define preoperative risk factors in patients with coronary artery disease (CAD). The majority of these studies have focused on one particular factor, the occurrence of a prior myocardial infarction. From these studies, it was determined that the risk of a new perioperative infarction was increased by approximately 30-fold (from 0.2 to 6%) if the patient had suffered a myocardial infarction at any time before surgery. However, the incidence of perioperative infarction in these series ranged from 6 to 37%, depending on the time from previous myocardial infarction. Until 1976, prior myocardial infarction was the only major perioperative risk factor that was studied extensively. Goldman and colleagues (1977) used a multivariate approach to identify a number of risk factors. Although the results of this study have been questioned, it was the first to attempt to order preoperative risk factors with respect to predictive ability. Rao and colleagues (1983) rechallenged the prior myocardial infarction data and demonstrated improved statistics using a more aggressive approach to stabilizing perioperative haemodynamics. However, no study has verified these results since then.

Over the past 3 years, several studies have attempted to assess increasingly sophisticated pre-operative diagnostic techniques, including exercise stress testing, radionuclear ventriculography and dipyridamole–thallium imaging. Although each of these purports to hold potential in identifying at-risk patients, significant controversy still exists as to their usefulness. In addition, because preoperative diagnostic testing may be very costly (e.g. a dipyridamole–thallium scintigram costs around £500), and the at-risk population may be large (10 million patients per year, worldwide), recommendation of any one preoperative test has significant cost implications. Thus, identification of the most important preoperative risk factors is important from both a clinical and cost-containment viewpoint. In this section, we will review 17 of these risk factors. However, only two of these remain uncontroversial with respect to their ability to predict perioperative cardiac morbidity: previous (recent) myocardial infarction and congestive heart failure. In addition, one intraoperative factor has been identified: major vascular surgery on the aorta. Most surprisingly, a number of other preoperative and intraoperative potential predictors remain controversial, e.g. angina, hypertension, diabetes or age.

Previous myocardial infarction

Previous myocardial infarction has been identified as a risk factor for perioperative cardiac morbidity (Table 60.1). Following anaesthesia and surgery, the risk of myocardial infarction is less than 0.2% for the general population (Plumlee & Boetner, 1972; Tarhan et al., 1972). In contrast, patients with previous myocardial infarction have a reinfarction rate of between 5 and 8% (Knapp et al., 1962; Topkins & Artusio, 1964; Plumlee & Boetner, 1972; Steen et al., 1978), with an associated mortality of between 40 and 70%.

The time-period from previous myocardial infarction appears to be the most important predictor. If

Table 60.1 Previous myocardial infarction

	Studies supporting	Studies refuting
Previous myocardial infarction (recent, <6 months)	Knapp et al. (1962) Topkins and Artusio (1964) Arkins et al. (1964) Frazer et al. (1967) Tarhan et al. (1972) Hertzer (1981) Goldman et al. (1977) Steen et al. (1978) Eerola et al. (1980) von Knorring (1981) Schoeppel et al. (1983)	Wells and Kaplan (1981) Rao et al. (1983)
Previous myocardial infarction (old, undetermined)	Topkins and Artusio (1964) Sapala et al. (1975) Cooperman et al. (1978) von Knorring (1981) Schoeppel et al. (1983)	Mauney et al. (1970) Goldman et al. (1977) Carliner et al. (1985)
Location of myocardial infarction	Arkins et al. (1964)	Steen et al. (1978)

infarction occurred within 3 months, the risk of reinfarction ranges from 30 to 100% (Knapp *et al.*, 1962; Topkins & Artusio, 1964; Plumlee & Boetner, 1972; Steen *et al.*, 1978; Goldman, 1983). Infarctions occurring from 3 to 6 months before surgery are associated with a reinfarction rate of approximately 15%; and after 6 months the rate decreases to 5%.

The above data have been challenged by Rao and colleagues (1983), Wells and Kaplan (1981) and Reiz and colleagues (1982a). Wells and Kaplan (1981) studied 873 patients with ischaemic heart disease, 48 of whom had surgical procedures within 3 months of an infarction. None suffered myocardial reinfarction. The average infarction rate was 1.1%. Rao and colleagues (1983) found a reinfarction rate of 1.9% in 733 patients who had a previous myocardial infarction. When the previous infarction was less than 3 months old, perioperative reinfarction occurred in only 5.7% of patients. When the previous infarction was 4–6 months old, reinfarction occurred in 2.3% of patients. Over 80% of Rao's patients were subjected to radial and pulmonary artery catheterization. Intraoperative arterial pressure and heart rate were not allowed to fluctuate more than 20% from preinduction values. Arrhythmias were treated aggressively, and 596 of the 733 patients were monitored in an intensive therapy unit for the first 24–36 h following surgery. Reiz and colleagues (1982a) studied intraoperative ischaemia and postoperative outcome of 45 patients with infarction within 3 months of major vascular surgery. The incidence of intraoperative infarction was 6.7%. At the end of the first postoperative week, the reinfarction rate had increased to 13%. The total number of deaths from myocardial infarction as diagnosed by autopsy during the first postoperative month was 9%. The reinfarction rates reported in these studies are significantly lower than those reported previously by most investigators and warrant further study. The implications of these results are significant and demand independent verification. Preoperative optimization of the patient's status, aggressive invasive monitoring, and prompt treatment of any haemodynamic aberration may decrease perioperative morbidity and mortality. However, none of the studies addressed the effect of any of these factors on final outcome. Further controversy concerns healed or remote previous myocardial infarction as risk factors (Table 60.1).

Congestive heart failure

Clinical and radiological evidence of left ventricular failure in patients with coronary artery disease is associated with a poor prognosis (Cohn *et al.*, 1979). In patients with ejection fractions of less than 40%, determined by radioisotope imaging, the 1-year cumulative mortality is 30%. In patients with compensated left ventricular function [pulmonary capillary wedge pressure (PCWP) less than 2 kPa (15 mmHg) with normal stroke volume index], the 2-year mortality rate is 10%. Conversely, in patients with elevated filling pressure [greater than 2 kPa (15 mmHg)] and depressed stroke work (less than 20 g/metre), the 2-year mortality rate exceeds 78% (Moraski *et al.*, 1975).

Several studies (Goldman *et al.*, 1977; Cooperman *et al.*, 1978; Rao *et al.*, 1983) have identified preoperative congestive heart failure as a risk factor in the surgical population (Table 60.2). In terms of prognosis, the most valuable indicators are a third heart sound (S_3) and jugular venous distension. If these are excluded, Goldman (1978) found that other signs of congestive heart failure were not significant risk factors. A decreased preoperative ejection fraction (less than 35%), determined by radionuclide angiography, has been found to correlate with early perioperative infarction (Pasternack *et al.*, 1985).

Peripheral vascular disease and surgery

Peripheral vascular surgery is associated with high rates of perioperative myocardial infarction (up to 20%) (Young *et al.*, 1977; Hertzer, 1981, 1982, 1983). This is not surprising as vascular disease involving the carotid artery, the aorta and other peripheral circulatory beds is associated commonly with coronary artery disease (Brown *et al.*, 1981; Crawford *et al.*, 1981; Rokey *et al.*, 1984). Most studies have demonstrated that peripheral vascular disease is a risk factor (Table 60.3). However, Goldman and colleagues (1977) appear to refute this. Their study found that although aortic operations were associated with the highest risk of postoperative pulmonary oedema (11%), neither aortic nor peripheral vascular procedures carried an increased risk of postoperative infarction or cardiac death.

Table 60.2 Congestive heart failure

Studies supporting	Studies refuting
Goldman *et al.* (1977)	—
Cooperman *et al.* (1978)	—
Rao *et al.* (1983)	—

Table 60.3 Vascular surgery

Studies supporting	Studies refuting
Driscoll *et al.* (1961)	Goldman *et al.* (1977)
Jeffrey *et al.* (1983)	
Schoeppel *et al.* (1983)	
Boucher *et al.* (1985)	

Table 60.4 Angina

Studies supporting	Studies refuting
Driscoll *et al.* (1961)	Wells and Kaplan (1981)
Tarhan *et al.* (1972)	Rao *et al.* (1983)
Sapala *et al.* (1975)	
Goldman *et al.* (1977)	
Cooperman *et al.* (1978)	
Steen *et al.* (1978)	
von Knorring (1981)	
Carliner *et al.* (1985)	

Table 60.5 Diabetes mellitus

Studies supporting	Studies refuting
Driscoll *et al.* (1961)	Mauney *et al.* (1970)
Tarhan *et al.* (1972)	Goldman *et al.* (1977)
Hertzer (1981)	Steen *et al.* (1978)
	von Knorring (1981)

Angina pectoris

Classical angina is a sensitive and specific predictor for identification of patients with coronary artery disease (Diamond *et al.*, 1979). These patients are at higher risk of cardiac complications (sudden death, myocardial infarction) than the general population. Surprisingly, stable angina pectoris is not considered a perioperative cardiac risk factor (Table 60.4). For example, Goldman and colleagues (1977) found that Classes I and II angina were univariate correlates of risk for operative morbidity. However, angina was not significant from a multivariate analysis. Similarly, Rao and colleagues (1983) found that angina was significant as a risk factor only when accompanied by heart faiure. The pattern and severity of angina have not been well studied with regard to risk prediction. The aforementioned studies address only Classes I and II angina. The risk associated with more severe stable angina or unstable angina are unknown.

Diabetes mellitus

The leading cause of death in adult diabetics is ischaemic heart disease (Waller *et al.*, 1980). However, ischaemic heart disease is difficult to detect in diabetic patients because of their neuropathy, and painless myocardial infarction occurs frequently. Diabetic patients appear to be at increased risk compared with the general population, having as much as a two- to three-fold increased risk of clinical atherosclerotic disease (Kannel & McGee, 1979). In addition, infarct size is usually larger (Rennart *et al.*, 1985), and survival rate following infarction is lower than in a non-diabetic population (Beard *et al.*, 1967). Myocardial perfusion defects are common in asymptomatic diabetic males during thallium stress testing (Abenavoli *et al.*, 1981). Ambulatory monitoring studies reveal that the transient ST-depression is more frequent in diabetics than in non-diabetics with ischaemic heart disease.

Diabetes is associated also with cerebral atherosclerosis, microangiopathy, surgical and non-surgical infections and renal transplant rejections (Cruse & Foord, 1973). However, the perioperative risk in diabetic patients is controversial (Table 60.5), and the data tend to refute diabetes as a major individual risk factor (Goldman *et al.*, 1977; Steen *et al.*, 1978; von Knorring, 1981).

Hypertension

The association between hypertension and ischaemic heart disease was established by the Framingham study (Kannel & Sorlie, 1975). Both the degree of hypertension (systolic and diastolic) and the presence of other major risk factors contribute to the importance of this risk factor. Fatal and non-fatal myocardial infarction in patients with diastolic hypertension [greater than 12 kPa (90 mmHg)] are increased, especially with hypercholesterolaemia, cigarette smoking and ECG abnormalities (Pooling Project Research Group, 1978). The risk of preoperative hypertension for postoperative cardiac morbidity remains controversial (Table 60.6). For example, Goldman and colleagues (1977) found that preoperative hypertension [diastolic blood pressure between 12 and 14.6 kPa (90−110 mmHg)] was not an independent predictor of cardiac death, postoperative myocardial infarction, heart failure, or arrhythmias. In contrast, Prys-Roberts and colleagues (1971) who studied a small group of individuals with untreated hypertension [mean arterial pressure of 17.3 kPa (130 mmHg)] found that these patients had a larger decrease in perioperative arterial pressure and a

Table 60.6 Hypertension

Studies supporting	Studies refuting
Driscoll *et al.* (1961)	Goldman *et al.* (1977)
Mauney *et al.* (1970)	Cooperman *et al.* (1978)
Prys-Roberts *et al.* (1971)	Riles *et al.* (1979)
Tarhan *et al.* (1972)	Rao *et al.* (1983)
Steen *et al.* (1978)	
Schneider (1983)	
von Knorring (1981)	

higher incidence of arrhythmias and myocardial ischaemia than patients with treated hypertension.

Cigarette smoking

The Framingham study (Kannel *et al.*, 1976) demonstrated an increased risk of myocardial infarction in smokers. However, the effect of cigarette smoking on perioperative cardiac outcome has not been studied.

Acute and chronic cigarette smoking induce significant effects on the cardiovascular system. The acute effects include an increased rate–pressure product and increased myocardial oxygen consumption. Direct vasoconstrictor effects of nicotine may cause increased coronary vascular resistance, especially in patients with proximal stenosis of the left anterior descending coronary artery (Nicod *et al.*, 1984), resulting in an unfavourable myocardial oxygen supply:demand ratio. Increases in carboxyhaemoglobin concentrations with the resultant decrease in systemic oxygen transport, in addition to a decrease in plasma volume and an increase in blood viscosity, tend to aggravate the supply–demand imbalance further. Chronic cigarette smoking may produce vasoconstriction, enhance platelet aggregation and loss of endothelial integrity, leading to accelerated atherosclerosis (Klein, 1984).

The adverse cardiovascular effects, including the well-documented detrimental effects on the respiratory system (Pearce & Jones, 1984) may place the cigarette-smoking patient at greater risk for cardiac morbidity. The causes can be either direct (coronary vasoconstriction or increased rate–pressure product) or indirect (hypoxaemia from respiratory complications and carboxyhaemoglobin formation).

Hypercholesterolaemia

The perioperative risk in patients with hypercholesterolaemia is unknown generally. Patients with familial hypercholesterolaemia have a high incidence

of premature ischaemic heart disease (Jensen *et al.*, 1967; Goldstein & Brown, 1982). They are also at risk for both valvular and supravalvular aortic stenoses in addition to atherosclerosis of the carotid and femoral arteries. It is of interest that patients with familial hypercholesterolaemia have a higher than expected incidence of proximal lesions in the left main coronary artery (Forman *et al.*, 1982).

Age

In the USA, a 1.4% annual growth rate in the population over 65 is projected. However, an increase of only 0.5% is projected for those aged 16–54. It is predicted also that by the year 2055, the over-65 age group will constitute 20% of the population (Anderson, 1984). An increasing number of patients from this older age group will undergo surgery.

In the elderly population, myocardial infarction is the leading cause of postoperative death (Port *et al.*, 1980). Although resting ejection fraction, end-diastolic volume and regional wall motion are not affected by age (Port *et al.*, 1980; Fleg *et al.*, 1984), the response of the elderly heart to stresses, such as exercise and catecholamine stimulation, is depressed (Port *et al.*, 1980; Weisfeldt, 1980; Bertrand, *et al.*, 1984). In addition, elderly patients incur more surgical complications requiring more intensive and costly hospital care (Hicks *et al.*, 1975). Because there are problems in assessing age as a predictor variable independent of associated diseases (Gerstenblith *et al.*, 1976; Fleg *et al.*, 1984), it is difficult to evaluate its predictive power. Controversy still exists (Table 60.7).

Arrhythmias

Cardiac arrhythmias are associated with more serious ischaemia and ventricular dysfunction in ambulatory patients with coronary artery disease (Table 60.8). Ventricular arrhythmias or conduction disturbances detected in the late-hospital phase of an acute myo-

Table 60.7 Age

Studies supporting	Studies refuting
Driscoll *et al.* (1961)	Mauney *et al.* (1970)
Dack (1963)	Tarhan *et al.* (1972)
Arkins *et al.* (1964)	Steen *et al.* (1978)
Goldman *et al.* (1977)	von Knorring (1981)
Carliner *et al.* (1985)	Rao *et al.* (1983)

Table 60.8 Arrhythmia

Studies supporting	Studies refuting
Goldman et al. (1977)	—
Cooperman et al. (1978)	—
Goldman (1978)	—

cardial infarction are associated with a poor prognosis (Vismara et al., 1975; Schulze et al., 1976). Particularly ominous is their occurrence in association with left ventricular dysfunction (Olson et al., 1984). In patients with chronic ischaemic heart disease, frequent premature ventricular contractions increase risk.

The risk associated with preoperative arrhythmias is generally unknown. Frequent premature ventricular contractions and premature atrial contractions, in addition to rhythms other than normal-sinus or atrial fibrillation, appear to be risk factors (Goldman et al., 1977). Atrial and ventricular arrhythmias may be risk factors in patients with peripheral vascular disease undergoing major vascular surgery (Pasternack et al., 1985). However, the data are insufficient to draw definite conclusions.

Electrocardiographic abnormalities

A number of studies (Table 60.9) have suggested ECG abnormalities, other than arrhythmias, as preoperative risk factors. For example, the preoperative ECG was as strong a predictor of postoperative cardiac complications as exercise stress testing (Carliner et al., 1985). Conversely, other studies have found that ECG abnormalities, including old myocardial infarction, ST-segment or T-wave changes, or bundle branch blocks are not significant risk factors (Goldman et al., 1977). Thus, aside from changes consistent with infarction, the proper approach to the patient who has an abnormal ECG before surgery remains controversial.

Table 60.9 Electrocardiographic abnormalities

Studies supporting	Studies refuting
Driscoll et al. (1961)	Goldman et al. (1977)
Baers et al. (1965)	
Hunter et al. (1968)	
Mauney et al. (1970)	
Cooperman et al. (1978)	
von Knorring (1981)	
Carliner et al. (1985)	

Echocardiographic abnormalities

Wall motion abnormalities, detected by ventriculography, are predictive of perioperative ventricular dysfunction (Mangano, 1985). However, the predictive power of preoperative echocardiographic wall motion or other abnormalities has not been studied. The relationship between reduction or cessation of coronary blood flow and the degree of dysfunction of segmental regions of the ventricle is well known (Weyman et al., 1977; Ross, 1983). The characteristics of segmental wall motion abnormalities (number, type, degree) dictate the overall degree of ventricular dysfunction (Heger et al., 1980) and have prognostic importance for long-term morbidity and mortality (Burggraf & Parker, 1975). In nearly all patients with transmural infarction, abnormality of left ventricular wall motion can be detected (Bloch et al., 1979; Drobar, 1979; Heger et al., 1979, 1980). Regional ischaemia is associated with segmental wall-motion and wall-thickening changes, and requires multiple views to ensure specificity. Wall-thickening changes are perhaps more sensitive predictors of outcome than wall-motion abnormalities (Lieberman et al., 1981; Topol et al., 1984). Techniques that allow precise quantitation of the degree of systolic wall thickening and wall thinning using two-dimensional echocardiography are being developed currently.

Chest X-ray abnormalities

The presence of a tortuous or calcified aorta has been suggested as a significant risk factor; however, cardiomegaly has not (Table 60.10) (Goldman et al., 1977). This is surprising, as abnormalities in the chest X-ray have been shown to be predictive of ventricular function abnormalities detected by ventriculograms in patients with ischaemic heart disease (Mangano et al., 1982). The cost-effectiveness of preoperative chest X-rays in patients under 60 or those without cardiac disease has been questioned recently (Sagal et al., 1974; Rees et al., 1976; Neuhauser, 1977). In patients with ischaemic heart disease, the usefulness of the preoperative chest X-ray remains controversial.

Table 60.10 Chest X-ray

Studies supporting	Studies refuting
Mangano et al. (1982)	Goldman et al. (1977)

Valvular heart disease

In patients with valvular heart disease, associated conditions such as ventricular dysfunction, arrhythmias, pulmonary hypertension, or ischaemic heart disease confound perioperative risk assessment. Few data are available regarding the risk of valvular heart disease in patients undergoing anaesthesia and surgery. Aortic stenosis and regurgitation have been associated with increased perioperative mortality, whereas mitral stenosis and regurgitation have not (Skinner & Pearce, 1964).

Goldman and colleagues (1977) found that aortic stenosis was associated with a 14-fold greater incidence of perioperative cardiac death. Also, mitral regurgitation (Grades II/VI or greater) was associated with a higher mortality rate. However, multivariate analyses revealed that mitral regurgitation did not add to cardiac risk in the absence of other risk factors such as an S_3 gallop, jugular venous distension, or recent myocardial infarction. Although all four valvular lesions were associated with increased risk of postoperative congestive heart failure, neither aortic regurgitation nor mitral stenosis predicted increased mortality.

Previous coronary artery bypass graft surgery or coronary angioplasty

Previous coronary artery bypass grafting (CABG) appears to offer protection from perioperative myocardial infarction (Table 60.11). However, the data are incomplete, and until a larger population is studied rigorously, we can only speculate that prior bypass surgery confers significant protection. Prior coronary angioplasty might provide protection also but no data are available.

Predictors from non-routine testing

A number of preoperative invasive and non-invasive tests have been investigated for determination of perioperative risk (Table 60.12). Exercise stress testing

Table 60.11 Previous coronary artery bypass grafting

Studies supporting	Studies refuting
Mahar et al. (1978)	—
Kimbris and Segal (1981)	—
Schoeppel et al. (1983)	—
Crawford et al. (1981)	—
Wells and Kaplan (1981)	—

Table 60.12 Predictors from non-routine studies

Studies supporting	Studies refuting
Gage et al. (1977)	Carliner et al. (1985)
Cutler et al. (1979, 1981)	
Pasternack et al. (1984)	
Boucher et al. (1985)	

(Gage et al., 1977; Cutler et al., 1979, 1981), radionuclide angiography (Pasternack et al., 1984) and dipyridamole–thallium imaging (Boucher et al., 1985) have been used to identify high-risk patients with myocardial ischaemia or abnormalities of ventricular function. In isolated studies, several of these tests have been shown to be predictive of perioperative cardiac morbidity and mortality. However, other isolated studies have demonstrated no significant advantage. For example, exercise testing has been shown to have no advantage over the routine 12-lead ECG (Carliner et al., 1985). One of the major health care, cost-containment questions today is the use of highly sensitive cardiac testing for preoperative identification of perioperative risk. At present, the data are inconclusive, and the widespread use of additional preoperative diagnostic testing remains controversial.

Risk indices

The use of risk indices has been popular since the formation of the American Society of Anesthesiologists' (ASA) classification (Dripps et al., 1963). Other applied risk indices include: cardiac risk index (CRI) (Goldman et al., 1977), the New York Heart Association (NYHA) classification (Braunwald, 1984), and the Canadian Cardiovascular Society (CCS) classification of angina (Coronary Artery Surgery Study, 1978). Although these indices may be easy to calculate and applied readily, their accuracy when applied to perioperative patients is controversial (Table 60.13).

Table 60.13 Risk indices

Studies supporting	Studies refuting
Vacanti et al. (1970) (ASA)	Lewin et al. (1971) (ASA)
Goldman et al. (1977) (CRI)	Goldman et al. (1977) (ASA)
Djokovic et al. (1979) (ASA)	Jeffrey et al. (1983) (CRI)
	Carliner et al. (1985) (CRI)

For example, the ASA classification has been shown to be useful in predicting perioperative mortality by some researchers (Pasternack et al., 1984; Boucher et al., 1985) and not useful by others (Dripps et al., 1963; Goldman et al., 1977). Although CRI compares the patient's preoperative state with the incidence of life-threatening or fatal postoperative cardiovascular complications, the accuracy of this index has been challenged in the same hospital using the same criteria (Jeffrey et al., 1983). Without question, a CRI would be useful if it were applicable generally and accurate consistently. However, no such consistently accurate CRI exists.

In summary, the only preoperative predictors of perioperative cardiac morbidity that have been identified are: recent myocardial infarction, present congestive heart failure and major vascular surgery on the aorta. Others, such as angina pectoris, hypertension and diabetes are more controversial. Few rigorous outcome studies of perioperative cardiac morbidity exist. The challenge anaesthetists now face is analogous to that faced by cardiologists in the 1950s. Only where predictors of CAD were identified by studies like that in Framingham (Kannel et al., 1976) could rational approaches to prevention and treatment be devised and morbidity thereby reduced.

Recent results

We have recently published an article investigating the predictors of perioperative cardiac morbidity in at-risk patients undergoing elective non-cardiac surgery (Mangano et al., 1990). We studied 474 men with (243) or at high risk of (231) CAD, collecting historical, clinical, laboratory and physiological data during hospitalization and for 6–24 months after operation. We assessed myocardial ischaemia by continuous ECG monitoring beginning 2 days before operation and continuing for 2 days after.

Postoperative cardiac events occurred in-hospital for 83 patients (18%) and were classified as ischaemic events (cardiac death, myocardial ischaemia, or unstable angina), detected in 15 patients; congestive heart failure, detected in 30 patients; and ventricular tachycardia, detected in 38 patients (Tables 60.14, 60.15 and 60.16). Postoperative myocardial ischaemia occurred in 41% of the patients monitored and was associated with a 2.8-fold increase in the odds of all adverse cardiac outcomes (95% confidence interval, 1.6–4.9; $p < 0.004$). Multivariate analysis disclosed no other clinical, historical or perioperative variable as independently associated with ischaemic events, including CRI, history of previous myocardial

ischaemia or congestive heart failure, or the occurrence of preoperative or intraoperative ischaemia.

Our results demonstrate that postoperative myocardial ischaemia during the first 48 h after operation confers a nearly three-fold increase in the odds of having an adverse cardiac outcome and, more importantly, a nine-fold increase in the odds of having an ischaemic event. Thus, these results highlight the importance of the postoperative period, extending the work of previous investigators who have demonstrated the importance of the patient's preoperative chronic disease state and of physiological changes during operation. They also suggest greater emphasis on the postoperative period, during which early postoperative ischaemia is an important correlate of adverse cardiac outcome. Patients may warrant more intensive monitoring and intervention during this period than previously assumed. Most significantly, these results suggest that increased attention and resources focusing on the prevention of (and possibly therapy for) postoperative ischaemia may well be the key to reducing perioperative cardiac morbidity.

Effects of anaesthetic drugs and regimens on the heart

Over the last few years, a whole new body of experimental and clinical work has provided knowledge on how anaesthetic drugs, regimens and the trauma of surgery, affect cardiac function and the regulation of the delicate myocardial oxygen supply–demand balance. A close correlation between prebypass myocardial ischaemia and postoperative myocardial infarction has been documented in patients undergoing CABG (Slogoff & Keats 1985, 1986). In comparison, intraoperative myocardial ischaemia has not been documented as a risk factor for adverse cardiac outcome in male non-cardiac surgical patients with known or strongly suspected CAD (Mangano et al., 1990). These patients did, however, demonstrate a close correlation between postoperative ischaemia and cardiac complications. Most recent data support the concept that postoperative myocardial ischaemia is one of the main risk factors for adverse cardiac outcome (Mangano et al., 1992a). It therefore appears important to apply intra- and postoperative monitoring techniques with high sensitivity and specificity for myocardial ischaemia in patients with known or suspected CAD. Two examples are automated ECG ST-segment recordings and TOE. Both techniques have revealed that perioperative myocardial ischaemia is far more common than thought previously

Table 60.14 Variables associated with 83 cardiac outcomes among 474 patients undergoing non-cardiac surgery

	Odds ratio	95% confidence interval	p value	No. with outcome and variable/no. with variable
*Univariable models**				
Previous myocardial infarction	1.7	1.1–2.8	0.03	38/167
Definite coronary artery disease	1.9	1.2–3.1	0.01	54/248
History of arrhythmia	2.8	1.7–4.7	0.0001	37/123
History of congestive heart failure	2.9	1.6–5.0	0.0002	25/77
History of claudication	2.7	1.7–4.4	0.0001	42/150
Diabetes mellitus (treated with medication)	1.6	0.94–2.8	0.08	22/93
Preoperative use of nitrates	1.6	0.97–2.6	0.06	30/132
Preoperative use of digoxin for congestive heart failure	5.8	2.3–15	0.0001	10/19
Serum creatinine >0.023 µmol/litre†	2.3	1.1–5.0	0.03	11/35
ASA score ≥3	2.5	1.3–5.0	0.007	72/354
Cardiac risk index (per 10 units)	1.8	1.2–2.7	0.002	
Vascular surgery	2.4	1.5–3.9	0.0003	44/168
Narcotic anaesthesia	2.2	1.2–4.2	0.01	16/54
Preoperative Holter ischaemia‡	3.1	1.8–5.3	0.0001	28/84
Intraoperative Holter ischaemia§	2.1	1.2–3.7	0.005	27/104
Postoperative Holter ischaemia¶	3.3	1.9–5.6	0.0001	46/167
Multivariable model				
History of arrhythmia	2.2	1.3–3.9	0.006	
Preoperative use of digoxin for congestive heart failure	3.32	1.1–11	0.04	
Vascular surgery	1.8	1.1–3.2	0.03	
Postoperative Holter ischaemia	2.8	1.6–4.9	0.0002	

* All variables are binary (yes/no) unless otherwise indicated; † values in parentheses are 95% confidence intervals; ‡ based on a denominator of 429 patients; § based on a denominator of 423 patients; ¶ based on a denominator of 407 patients. ASA, American Society of Anesthesiologists.

Table 60.15 Variables associated with 15 coronary artery disease outcomes among 474 patients undergoing non-cardiac surgery

	Odds ratio	95% confidence interval	p value	No. with outcome and variable/no. with variable
*Univariable models**				
History of claudication	3.4	1.2–9.7	0.02	9/150
Activity level ≥5†	4.3	1.2–16.0	0.02	3/28
Preoperative use of nitrates	2.3	0.83–6.6	0.1	7/132
Serum creatinine ≥0.023 µmol/litre‡	5.0	1.5–17.0	0.004	4/35
Postoperative Holter ischaemia§	9.2	2.0–42.0	0.004	12/167
Multivariable model				
Postoperative Holter ischaemia	9.2	2.0–42.0	0.004	

* All variables are binary (yes/no) unless otherwise indicated; † severely limited (bed to chair) or medically restricted; ‡ equivalent to 2 mg/dl; § based on denominator of $n = 407$ patients.

Table 60.16 Results of multivariable analysis of variables associated with 30 congestive heart failure outcomes among 459 patients without coronary artery disease outcomes, and 38 ventricular tachycardia outcomes among 430 patients without coronary artery disease or congestive heart failure outcomes

	Odds ratio	95% confidence interval	p value
Variables associated with congestive heart failure*			
History of arrhythmia†	3.0	1.4−6.7	0.006
Diabetes mellitus (treated with medication)†	2.4	1.0−5.7	0.04
Duration of anaesthesia and surgery (per h)‡	1.2	1.1−1.4	0.002
or			
Vascular surgery†	3.5	1.6−7.9	0.002
Narcotic anaesthesia‡	2.5	1.0−6.5	0.05
or			
Isoflurane/opioid anaesthesia†	0.35	0.16−0.76	0.008
Variables associated with ventricular tachycardia*			
Preoperative Holter ischaemia	7.8	2.9−21.0	0.0001
Preoperative use of digoxin for congestive heart failure	12.0	2.8−50.0	0.0009

* All variables are binary (yes/no); † statistics for model containing history of arrhythmias, diabetes, vascular surgery and isoflurane/opioid anaesthesia; ‡ statistics for model containing history of arrhythmias, diabetes, duration of anaesthesia and surgery, opioid anaesthesia.

(Smith *et al.*, 1985; Knight *et al.*, 1988; London *et al.*, 1988; Häggmark *et al.*, 1989; London *et al.*, 1990; Mathew *et al.*, 1992). In addition, some studies indicate that ischaemia at this time is often the result of insufficient myocardial oxygen supply rather than increased demand (Slogoff & Keats 1985, 1986; Kleinmann *et al.*, 1986; Lowenstein & Reiz, 1987). Recent experimental and clinical studies using a variety of anaesthetic agents and techniques for ischaemia detection have also shown that careful haemodynamic control could significantly reduce the incidence of myocardial ischaemia (Nathan 1988, 1989; Leung *et al.*, 1991). Finally, it now appears established that choice of anaesthetic agent or technique has little or no influence on cardiac outcome (Slogoff & Keats 1989; Tuman *et al.*, 1989a; Forrest *et al.*, 1990; Baron *et al.*, 1991; Slogoff *et al.*, 1991). In contrast, there are indications from some recent studies that effective therapeutic interventions against risk factors for myocardial ischaemia, principally tachycardia, pain and hypoxaemia, would reduce the incidence of insufficient myocardial oxygenation. Although not yet scientifically proven, there are suggestions that these interventions might have the potential to improve cardiac outcome after non-cardiac surgery (Tuman *et al.*, 1991; Mangano *et al.*, 1992b).

This part of the chapter is not aimed at providing encyclopaedic data for the anaesthetic management of the patient with cardiac disease. We discuss, in depth, how the new experimental and clinical research data might be incorporated into clinical practice for anaesthesia to patients with cardiac disease, with emphasis on coronary artery disease and its complications.

In order to understand the effects of anaesthetic agents on the heart, we have to analyse first their intrinsic actions upon the normal and diseased myocardium and the vasculature. In the intact organism, these effects are altered by the complex cardiovascular reflex system. In patients with cardiac disease, these reflexes are often attenuated and the effects of the anaesthetic agents upon the circulation are obscured further by chronic drug therapy, premedication, blood volume, vascular volume, degree of somatic afferent stimulation, etc.

Intravenous induction agents

Barbiturates

Barbiturates depress the heart in a dose-dependent and reversible mode. Krebs and Kersting (1979) demonstrated that barbiturates, such as barbituric acid, which do not produce anaesthesia, were not cardiodepressant. In the isolated heart preparation, the degree of cardiodepression by thiobarbiturates was greater than that of the oxybarbiturates (Fig. 60.1). This difference was ascribed to the former's higher lipid solubility. Both ouabain and catecholamines antagonized effectively the cardiodepressant action of barbiturates. This indicates that myocardial calcium turnover is the primary site of action for the cardiodepression by these anaesthetic agents. Whether the interaction with myocardial calcium turnover is related mainly to the calcium influx across the cell membrane or to cellular metabolism, i.e. to the calcium content of the sarcoplasmic reticulum, has not been established yet (Price & Ohnishi, 1980).

Barbiturates in anaesthetic doses dilate arterioles and in some cases muscular venules (Altura *et al.*, 1980). In addition, they antagonize non-specifically the vasopressor response to neurohumoral substances like angiotensin II, catecholamines, serotonin, etc., and to potassium ions (Altura *et al.*, 1980). Boer and colleagues (1991) studied the influence of 4 mg/kg of thiopentone on the human systemic circulation during cardiopulmonary bypass. Since systemic blood flow is kept constant in this situation, the resultant effect on systemic blood pressure provides an estimate of the influence of the drug on systemic vascular tone. In another recent human experiment, Rouby and colleagues (1991) investigated the pulmonary and systemic circulatory effects of 5 mg/kg of thiopentone in patients awaiting cardiac

transplantation with an implanted Jarvik heart. The results of these two studies indicate that thiopentone reduces arterial and venous tone by approximately 20%. Available data suggest that vasodilatation is related to interference with calcium ion flux over the vascular cell membrane and/or to cellular calcium metabolism.

In intact animals and in humans, high clinical doses of barbiturates depress the sensitivity of the baroreflex control of heart rate (Brown & Hilton, 1956; Bristow *et al.*, 1969).

The complexity of the action of barbiturates on cardiac performance, vascular tone, barostatic reflexes and endogenous sympathetic tone in combination with pre-existing cardiac function, blood volume and preoperative cardiac and sedative medication explains the variable circulatory effects of barbiturates in patients with cardiac disease. The systemic haemodynamic effects of the short-acting barbiturates in healthy subjects are well documented (Etsten & Li, 1955). They consist of dose-dependent decreases in arterial pressure and cardiac output, and a reflex increase in heart rate. Sonntag and colleagues (1975) studied the coronary haemodynamic effects of thiopentone administered in a dose of 4 mg/kg to healthy individuals undergoing varicose vein resection. The systemic haemodynamic effects of the compound were similar to those described previously. The drug increased myocardial blood flow and decreased coronary vascular tone in proportion to the increase in myocardial oxygen demand (+55%). Glucose, lactate and pyruvate metabolism were increased also. In contrast, Reiz and colleagues (1981a), who studied a mixed group of patients with coronary artery disease during induction of anaesthesia for vascular surgery, found that 6 mg/kg of thiopentone decreased arterial pressure and cardiac output but did not alter heart rate. Hence, myocardial oxygen consumption decreased (−39%) in combination with unaltered lactate metabolism. The different heart-rate response to thiopentone in the two studies is the likely cause of the conflicting results.

Two studies have recently evaluated the influence of barbiturates on cardiac contractility using techniques which estimate left ventricular volume. Lepage and colleagues (1991) applied nuclear imaging techniques to study 22 unpremedicated urological patients with CAD, but without hypertension or other cardiovascular complications. Induction of anaesthesia was made with either methohexital or propofol, both at 2 mg/kg, followed by a continuous infusion of the respective drug at $100 \, \mu g \cdot kg^{-1} \cdot min^{-1}$. The patients were ventilated with pure oxygen and

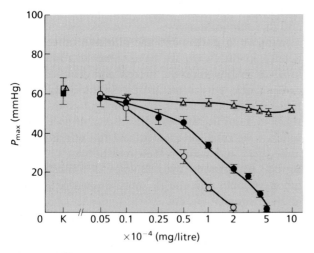

Fig. 60.1 Effects on intraventricular pressure of increasing doses of the anaesthetically effective barbiturates pentobarbital (closed circles) and thiopentone (open circles) compared with barbituric acid (triangles) which has no anaesthetic action. K indicates the control values before drug administration. (Redrawn from Krebs & Kersting, 1979.)

muscle relaxation was provided with vecuronium. Methohexital produced a 15% decrease in mean arterial pressure, a 20% reduction of cardiac output and a peak increase in heart rate of around 20%. Systemic vascular resistance thus remained unchanged. The decrease in cardiac index was associated with decreased left ventricular (LV) ejection fraction, increased end-systolic volume and evidence of unchanged preload. These findings suggest that methohexital produced its circulatory effects mainly by cardiodepression. The findings after propofol will be further discussed below. In the other study, Mulier and colleagues (1991) compared the effects of thiopentone and propofol on systemic haemodynamics and systolic function using the systolic LV short-axis diameter by TOE as an estimate of end-systolic LV volume. ASA Classes I or II patients scheduled for orthopaedic surgery were selected. The authors found that 4 mg/kg of thiopentone moderately decreased systolic blood pressure and LV end-diastolic volume without changes in heart rate, LV end-systolic volume or the slope of the end-systolic pressure–volume relationship. After 6.5 mg/kg of thiopentone, there was a more pronounced decrease of systolic blood pressure and LV end-diastolic volume. Heart rate increased by 10% while end-systolic volume remained unchanged, though the slope of the end-systolic pressure–volume relationship decreased. With the exception of the fall in systemic blood pressure, most changes were short-lived, peaking at 2–4 min after the end of thiopentone administration. The findings indicate that the 4 mg/kg dose of thiopentone reduced systemic blood pressure mainly through systemic vasodilatation, whereas the negative inotropic effect of thiopentone contributed as well after the 6.5 mg/kg dose. It should be noted that both the use of the slope of the end-systolic pressure–volume relationship derived from pressure measurements in the radial artery, and the assumption that the position of Vd (i.e the intercept of the systolic pressure–volume relationship with the volume axis) remains constant, as done by Mulier and colleagues have recently been seriously questioned (Coddens & Deloof, 1992).

Numerous studies have demonstrated that short-acting agents such as barbiturates may produce both hypotension and tachycardia when used for induction of anaesthesia. As previously discussed, it appears as if the effect of barbiturates on heart rate is attenuated in patients with cardiovascular disease. This may be particularly evident in patients on beta-blocker medication (Stone et al., 1988). Moreover, these induction agents do not offer adequate cardiac

protection from the stress of intubation (Coriat et al., 1982; Fusciardi et al., 1986; Stone et al., 1988). The haemodynamic changes observed after induction of anaesthesia with barbiturates explain many of the ischaemic episodes recorded during and after tracheal intubation. Numerous adjunct techniques have been proposed to reduce the circulatory stress response to laryngoscopy and intubation. They include volatile anaesthetic agents, opioids, intravenous lignocaine, vasodilators, beta blockers and laryngeal nerve blocks. From the most recent literature, it appears as if opioids such as fentanyl (Fusciardi et al., 1986) or alfentanil (Chraemmer-Jørgensen et al., 1992) reduce the risk for myocardial ischaemia and preserve ventricular pump function (Fig. 60.2) during the stress of intubation performed after thiopentone induction.

Propofol

Propofol belongs to the family of alkylphenols and its anaesthetic action was first described by James and Glen (1980). It was formulated primarily in aqueous Cremophor, which seems to have haemodynamic effects of its own, but is reformulated now in a soya bean emulsion (Glen & Hunter, 1984). In the isolated heart, propofol appears to be moderately more cardiodepressant than thiopentone, calculated on a molar basis (Stowe et al., 1992). Other isolated heart studies using a different technique to assess contractility have suggested thiopentone to be more cardiodepressant than propofol (Park & Lynch, 1992). Finally, it appears as if propofol markedly attenuates coronary autoregulation, i.e. produces powerful coronary vasodilatation in the isolated heart preparation (Stowe et al., 1992). In contrast, Puttick and colleagues (1992) could not find any disruption of coronary flow regulation in the intact dog administered propofol. In healthy subjects propofol decreases systemic pressure, mainly by reducing systemic vascular resistance (Prys-Roberts et al., 1983). Other studies have revealed markedly increased sensitivity to propofol in elderly patients with regard to induction dose and acute toxicity (Dundee et al., 1986). When compared with an equipotent anaesthetic dose of thiopentone, in middle-aged patients without cardiac disease, propofol produced a greater decline in arterial pressure, stroke volume and systemic vascular resistance (Grounds et al., 1985). Patients with CAD and preserved LV function had a significantly greater decrease in arterial pressure after 1.5 mg/kg of propofol than after 2 mg/kg of thiopentone (Patrick et al., 1985). Neither drug changed cardiac output. The decline in arterial pressure after propofol was

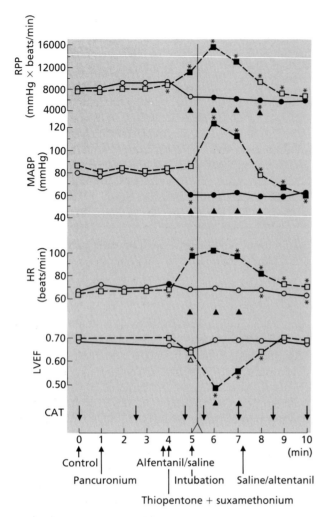

Fig. 60.2 Relationship between rate pressure product (RPP), mean arterial blood pressure (MABP), heart rate (HR) and left ventricular ejection fraction (LVEF) in patients given alfentanil (open and closed circles) or saline (open and closed squares) before tracheal intubation. Closed symbols (circles and squares) indicate statistically significant changes from control values ($p < 0.01$). Closed triangles indicate a statistically significant difference between groups ($p < 0.01$). *Indicates a statistically significant difference from the previous value ($p < 0.01$). Open triangle indicates a statistically significant difference from the previous value ($p = 0.02$). Open arrows indicate time of blood sampling for analysis of catecholamine concentrations (CAT). Median values are shown. These results were interpreted to indicate that adjunct alfentanil preserved LV pump function during orotracheal intubation following rapid sequence induction with thiopentone–suxamethonium. (Data from Chraemmer-Jorgensen *et al.*, 1992.)

caused by a fall in vascular resistance. Eight of 10 patients administered propofol were reported to have systolic pressure below 13.3 kPa (100 mmHg) and two below 9.3 kPa (70 mmHg).

In human experiments performed under cardiopul-

monary bypass Boer and colleagues (1991) demonstrated that 2 mg/kg of propofol produced a reduction of systemic vascular tone comparable to 4 mg/kg of thiopentone. In comparison, Rouby and colleagues (1991) who investigated the effects of these drugs in patients with a Jarvik heart documented that propofol at 2.5 mg/kg was a more powerful venous and arterial vasodilator than 5 mg of thiopentone. In ASA Classes I and II patients, peripheral venodilatation has been observed after 2.5 mg/kg of propofol but not after 4 mg/kg of thiopentone (Muzi *et al.*, 1992). These results in humans largely support the findings by Goodchild and Serrao (1989) in dogs with autonomous block.

The difficulty in distinguishing the influence of vasodilatation from that of cardiodepression upon systemic blood pressure in the intact human has led to some recent controversy with regards to propofol (Sebel & Lowdon, 1989; Lippmann & Mok, 1990; Merin, 1990; Van Aken & Brüssel, 1990). As with thiopentone, it is reasonable to assume that propofol will cause circulatory changes which are influenced by the pre-existing cardiovascular disease state. For instance, Fairfield and colleagues (1991) who investigated the influence of 2.5 mg/kg of propofol in ASA Class I unpremedicated patients by the use of echocardiographic and Doppler techniques found that the drug produced initial systemic vasodilatation followed by a delayed decrease in LV function. Lepage and colleagues (1988) investigated the circulatory effects of 2 mg/kg of propofol followed by a continuous infusion at $100 \, \mu g \cdot kg^{-1} \cdot min^{-1}$ vecuronium and positive-pressure ventilation with oxygen in patients with stable CAD and normal LV function. The authors could not document any cardiodepressant effect of the drug as measured by gated radionuclide imaging. Thus, the observed reduction in blood pressure was entirely due to vasodilatation. In addition, in contrast to most other investigators, they did not record any increase in heart rate. A later study from the same investigators in similar patients (Lepage *et al.*, 1991) largely supports their previous findings and concludes that 'propofol preserves LV performance despite a likely negative inotropic effect'.

Finally, Mulier and colleagues (1991) have provided TOE data which indicate that propofol reduces blood pressure mainly through its negative inotropic properties. They also suggest that the cardiodepressant effect of propofol would be more powerful than that of an equipotent dose of thiopentone. As previously discussed in this chapter, their choice of methodology and thus their conclusions have recently been seriously questioned (Coddens & Deloof, 1992).

Stephan and colleagues (1986) studied the systemic and coronary haemodynamic effects of propofol, given as a bolus dose of 2 mg/kg, followed by a continuous infusion at 200 μg · kg^{-1} · min^{-1} to patients with normal LV function subjected to coronary bypass grafting. After induction, 70% nitrous oxide in oxygen was added and fentanyl, 10 μg/kg i.v., was administered before sternotomy. Induction of anaesthesia produced a moderate decline in arterial pressure, left and right ventricular filling pressure, and cardiac output. Systemic vascular resistance remained constant and heart rate increased slightly. Myocardial blood flow decreased more than expected from the decline in perfusion pressure but in proportion to myocardial oxygen demand. Myocardial lactate production was observed in one of 12 patients. Sternotomy was followed by normalization of all systemic haemodynamic variables except cardiac output. As previously described for some other anaesthetic agents (Rydvall et al., 1984; Reiz et al., 1987), somatic afferent stimulation produced coronary vasoconstriction and myocardial lactate production was observed in one additional patient.

These data suggest that propofol administered to patients with CAD and normal LV function produces a variable and sometimes pronounced decline in arterial pressure. The relative contribution of cardiodepression and vasodilatation to the decline in blood pressure has, as yet, not been well established. Therefore, it may cause myocardial ischaemia. This might potentially produce myocardial ischaemia. In contrast to animal experimentation (Stowe et al., 1992), the drug does not appear to produce coronary vasodilatation when used clinically. When administered as a continuous infusion and combined with a low dose of fentanyl, propofol does not protect against the coronary vasoconstrictive action of surgical stimulation.

Benzodiazepines and flumazenil

In the isolated, modified Langendorf preparation, diazepam produces a dose-dependent depression of cardiac function (Reves et al., 1984). In the intact, pentobarbitone-anaesthetized dog, it lowers systemic vascular resistance (Abel et al., 1970a). In healthy subjects, diazepam induces minor reductions of arterial pressure, cardiac output and ventricular performance (Dechenne & Destrosiers, 1969; Blackburn et al., 1971; Rao et al., 1972). Similar, insignificant haemodynamic effects have been reported in patients subjected to valvular surgery or CABG (Dundee, 1969; Knapp & Dubow, 1970; Samuelson

et al., 1980). Nitrous oxide inhalation added to diazepam does not alter systemic haemodynamics in patients with CAD (McCammon et al., 1980). High-dose fentanyl does not produce significant cardio-depression (Sebel et al., 1982). Interestingly, the combination of diazepam and fentanyl may cause pronounced decline in arterial pressure, cardiac output and systemic vascular resistance (Stanley & Webster, 1978; Tomichek et al., 1983). It has been speculated that this interaction is due to peripheral vasodilatation rather than cardiodepression (Reves et al., 1984).

Midazolam has been studied extensively in healthy subjects and in patients with cardiac disease (Reves et al., 1979; Forster et al., 1980; Al-Khudhairi et al., 1982; Lebowitz et al., 1982; Schulte-Sasse et al., 1982). In healthy subjects, 0.15 mg/kg produced small reductions in diastolic pressure (10%) and moderate increases in heart rate (18%) (Forster et al., 1980). In patients with CAD, 0.3 mg/kg of midazolam produced haemodynamic changes similar to those recorded after 3−4 mg/kg of thiopentone (Al-Khudhairi et al., 1982). Schulte-Sasse and colleagues (1982) compared the cardiovascular effects of 0.2 mg/kg of midazolam administered as induction agent to flunitrazepam-premedicated patients with CAD and preserved LV function [PCWP less than 1.6 kPa (12 mmHg), ejection fraction greater than 0.5] and valvular patients with impaired LV function [PCWP greater than 2.5 kPa (19 mmHg), ejection fraction less than 0.5]. Mean arterial pressure decreased similarly in both groups. Stroke volume was maintained in the patients with depressed LV function but was reduced in the group having normal LV function. The authors suggested that pump function was maintained in the patients with valvular disease by unloading of the left ventricle. Haemodynamic changes observed after induction of anaesthesia with midazolam in patients with cardiac disease show only minor differences from those reported after diazepam or flunitrazepam (Morel et al., 1981; Samuelson et al., 1981; Kawar et al., 1985).

In one randomized study, Lepage and colleagues (1986) demonstrated marginally different effects on LV ejection fraction and systemic haemodynamics of diazepam, flunitrazepam and midazolam administered as induction agents to patients with CAD. Diazepam produces minor changes of coronary blood flow. A slight coronary vasodilating action has been proposed (Abel et al., 1970b; Cote et al., 1974). Flunitrazepam given in a dose of 15 μg/kg to patients with CAD, studied in the cardiac catheterization laboratory, produced a decrease in mean arterial and

LV end-diastolic pressures and increases in heart rate and LV maximal velocity of contraction ($\dot{V}_{max}$). Despite a fall in myocardial oxygen consumption, coronary blood flow remained unchanged and myocardial oxygen extraction declined (Nitenberg et al., 1983). Consequently, flunitrazepam produced coronary vasodilatation, unrelated to metabolic changes, i.e. the drug interferes with normal coronary autoregulation. However, none of the patients demonstrated electrocardiographic or metabolic evidence of ischaemia during the study.

The same group of investigators (Marty et al., 1986) published data obtained under comparable conditions in similar patients administered midazolam, 0.2 mg/kg i.v.; 5–15 min after this drug, coronary blood flow had decreased in proportion to the decline in myocardial oxygen consumption (24% versus 26%). There was a slight elevation of coronary venous oxygen saturation indicating some coronary vasodilatation. As in the flunitrazepam study, no ischaemia was observed following midazolam.

Recently, Marty and colleagues (1991) documented the circulatory and cardiometabolic effects of flunitrazepam given in a sleep dose to patients undergoing coronary angiography and followed by flumazenil titrated to reverse the sedation. Flunitrazepam produced circulatory changes which were similar to those previously described, i.e. a small reduction of systemic blood pressure without change in myocardial oxygen consumption or coronary sinus blood flow. The main circulatory effects of flumazenil consisted of a reversal of the changes produced by flunitrazepam. These observations agree with previous findings where no evidence of adrenergic activation has been reported in association with arousal from benzodiazepine anaesthesia/sedation (Alon et al., 1987; Sage et al., 1987; White et al., 1989).

Etomidate

Etomidate, a short-acting, non-barbiturate, intravenous anaesthetic agent held great promise as an induction agent for patients with compromised cardiac reserve due to the initial reports of minimal effects on systemic haemodynamics (Gooding et al., 1979; Criado et al., 1980). After the recognition that etomidate inhibits adrenocortical function during surgery (Wagner & White, 1984), its usage has been limited. Like most other anaesthetic agents, etomidate decreases force of contraction in the isolated heart muscle. In this preparation it was significantly less depressant than equianaesthetic doses of thiopentone (Kissin et al., 1983). In healthy patients,

0.4 mg/kg of etomidate produced haemodynamic changes similar to 4 mg/kg of thiopentone (Giese et al., 1985). Administered as a continuous infusion to patients with valvular heart disease, the circulatory effects of etomidate could not be distinguished from those of thiopentone (Karliczek et al., 1982).

The effects of etomidate on the coronary circulation in patients with cardiac disease have not been documented. In healthy subjects, 0.3 mg/kg i.v. produced an increase in myocardial blood flow and a decline in myocardial oxygen consumption (Kettler et al., 1974). These findings suggest that etomidate has a direct dilatory action on coronary blood vessels. Studies in patients on cardiopulmonary bypass have demonstrated that etomidate, similar to thiopentone and propofol, decreases systemic vascular resistance (Boer et al., 1991). Since this drug has little effect on myocardial function (De Hert et al., 1990), it appears as if systemic vasodilatation is the main mechanism behind the reduction in blood pressure observed after etomidate.

Ketamine

In the intact species, the well-documented cardiodepressant action of ketamine (Dowdy & Kaya, 1968; Goldberg et al., 1970; Valicenti et al., 1973; Berry, 1974) is masked by its centrally induced sympathetic stimulation manifested by increased concentrations of adrenaline and noradrenaline (Ivankovic et al., 1974; White et al., 1982; Zsigmond, 1974). Intravenous administration of anaesthetic doses of the drug results in increased arterial pressure, heart rate and cardiac output (White et al., 1982). In patients with limited cardiac reserve, these adverse haemodynamic effects can produce failure or myocardial ischaemia (Tweed et al., 1972; Spotoft et al., 1979). Cardiac decompensation has also been documented in critically ill patients in whom ketamine has been used for anaesthetic induction (Waxman et al., 1980). All of these findings may be explained from recent animal experimentation where ketamine has been shown to prolong isovolumic relaxation and decrease ventricular compliance evaluated by regional LV chamber stiffness (Pagel et al., 1992). The cardiovascular stimulation and the concomitant increases in plasma catecholamine concentrations may be counteracted effectively by premedication with diazepam (Kumar et al., 1978; White et al., 1982; Zsigmond, 1974) or droperidol (Bålfors et al., 1983).

The effects of ketamine on the coronary circulation have been studied in healthy subjects (Sonntag et al., 1973) and in vascular surgical patients (Bålfors et al.,

1983). In both groups, ketamine, 2 mg/kg i.v., produced changes in coronary blood flow which paralleled its effect on myocardial oxygen consumption. No changes in myocardial oxygen extraction were observed. Hence, ketamine does not interfere with normal coronary autoregulation when administered in an effective anaesthetic dose.

Droperidol

Animal and human investigations have demonstrated that droperidol by itself has no effect on cardiac function (Ostheimer et al., 1975; Stanley, 1978). In patients with CAD investigated in the cardiac catheterization laboratory, 150 µg/kg of the drug lowered systemic arterial and LV end-diastolic pressures and increased heart rate moderately consistent with dilatation of capacitance vessels and decreased venous return (Marty et al., 1982). Similar haemodynamic changes were recorded after 200 µg/kg of droperidol administered before ketamine induction of anaesthesia in vascular surgical patients (Bålfors et al., 1983). Coronary blood flow studies in the same patients did not demonstrate any direct action on the coronary vasculature by the drug. In patients studied during coronary bypass surgery, the addition of droperidol, 250 µg/kg, to high-dose fentanyl anaesthesia, 100 µg/kg, resulted in less of an increase in myocardial oxygen consumption following sternotomy (Heikkilä et al., 1985b). These results were attributable to the modification of the systemic haemodynamic effects of surgical stimulation by droperidol rather than to a direct cardiac effect of the drug.

Opioid analgesics used for anaesthesia

High-dose opioid/oxygen anaesthesia has gained tremendous popularity in cardiac surgery because of the intraoperative haemodynamic stability provided (Lowenstein et al., 1969; Arens et al., 1972; De Castro et al., 1979; Waller et al., 1981). When the cardiac-depressant properties of the different, clinically used opioids were compared, morphine and fentanyl did not depress the isolated ventricular tissue in doses used clinically (Strauer, 1972; Motomura et al., 1984; Reves et al., 1984). In contrast, pethidine was a potent cardiodepressant compound, approximately 20 times more depressant than morphine (Table 60.17). In addition, the drug is a powerful systemic vasodilator (Strauer, 1972; Freye, 1974; Motomura et al., 1984). These properties explain the often unexpected profound decline in arterial pressure and cardiac output reported in animal and human studies (King et al., 1952; Stanley & Liu, 1977). Morphine may also produce undesirable circulatory effects, such as histamine-induced hypotension, hypertension, bradycardia and severe cardiodepression when combined with nitrous oxide inhalation. These haemodynamic aberrations were common particularly in patients with preserved LV function. In addition, prolonged respiratory depression and increased peri- and postoperative fluid requirements have been described (Hasbrouk, 1970; Lowenstein, 1971; Stanley et al., 1973; Stoelting & Gibbs, 1973). With the availability of the more recent opioids, fentanyl, sufentanil and alfentanil, all of these data suggest that neither pethidine nor morphine is a suitable anaesthetic drug for patients with cardiac disease.

The haemodynamic effects of various doses of fentanyl have been described in a large number of animal and clinical studies (Bovill et al., 1984a). The drug produces remarkably small circulatory changes even in high doses (up to 100 µg/kg) administered to patients with valvular or CAD. The effects do not seem to be dose related and consist of moderate declines in heart rate and arterial pressure. Despite a minimal intrinsic cardiodepressant action, other anaesthetic drugs such as nitrous oxide inhalation or diazepam added to fentanyl in patients with cardiac disease may produce significant haemodynamic abnormalities (Stanley & Webster, 1978; Lunn et al., 1979; Tomichek et al., 1983). Studies in the isolated

Table 60.17 Relative myocardial contractile-depressant properties of equipotent doses of three opioid analgesics. (Data from Strauer, 1972)

	Dose (mg)	Relative potency	Relative myocardial contractile-depressant property
Morphine	10	1	1
Meperidine (pethidine)	70	0.1–0.2	100–200
Fentanyl	0.1–0.2	50–100	2–4

heart preparation have confirmed the clinical find-ings but have not been able to reveal by which mechanism cardiodepression occurs (Reves *et al.*, 1984). Interestingly, alfentanil has been described to have direct positive inotropic and negative chrono-tropic effects in the isolated rabbit heart (Zhang *et al.*, 1990). This is one possible explanation for the obser-vation that alfentanil added to thiopentone for rapid sequence induction in patients without cardiac dis-ease is associated with maintained LV function (Chraemmer-Jørgensen *et al.*, 1992). Milocco and col-leagues (1985) compared the effects of fentanyl/droperidol/nitrous oxide in patients with CAD and varying LV function. In patients with poor LV func-tion, the circulation was depressed markedly by the drugs (fentanyl, 15 μg/kg, and droperidol, 300 μg/kg, administered with 100% oxygen). Addition of nitrous oxide resulted in further hypotension. In patients with good LV function, the same regimen of anaesthesia produced minimal cardiodepression. Sufentanil is approximately 5—10 times as potent as fentanyl (Van de Walle *et al.*, 1976; Rolly *et al.*, 1979). In comparison, the potency of alfentanil is only 20—30% of fentanyl (Niemegeers & Janssen, 1981). Among all clinical studies published on the cardio-vascular effects of opioids, only one derives data from a double-blind investigation. Flacke and col-leagues (1985) compared the effects of equipotent doses of morphine, pethidine, fentanyl and sufentanil administered with thiopentone and nitrous oxide/oxygen on arterial pressure, heart rate and plasma catecholamine concentrations in healthy patients undergoing orthopaedic or general surgery. They found that sufentanil provided the best peri-induc-tion and intraoperative cardiovascular stability with the least demand for supplementation with inhalation agents. Most intraoperative circulatory side-effects were observed in the pethidine group, and postoper-atively, morphine-anaesthetized patients had a sig-nificantly higher incidence of respiratory depression. In open, randomized studies of patients anaes-thetized for coronary artery surgery, and hence administered higher doses of fentanyl (100 μg/kg) and sufentanil (15—20 μg/kg), other authors have failed to demonstrate major haemodynamic differ-ences between the drugs or the effects of surgical stimulation (Rosow *et al.*, 1984; Howie *et al.*, 1985). Neither drug could be shown to cause histamine release (Rosow *et al.*, 1984). More recent randomized studies in patients anaesthetized for CABG, which included the muscle relaxants pancuronium or vec-uronium added to either fentanyl or sufentanil, demonstrated similar circulatory changes as in pre-vious studies. The circulation was best maintained

with fentanyl—pancuronium as evidenced by unchanged cardiac output. Regardless of opioid, heart rate increased with the use of pancuronium and decreased with vecuronium (Gravlee *et al.*, 1988). Thus, the reduction in systemic vascular resistance, alternatively hypotension, reported after sufentanil in some patients (Sebell & Bovill, 1982) cannot be attributed to liberation of histamine.

Alfentanil has a significantly shorter action than fentanyl (De Lange & De Bruijn, 1983). In patients premedicated with lorazepam and with anaesthesia induced with etomidate for abdominal surgery, fentanyl, 30 μg/kg, or alfentanil, 120 μg/kg, were administered randomly after induction (Rucquoi & Camu, 1983). Both drugs decreased mean arterial pressure (30—33%), heart rate (25%) and cardiac index (25%) at 10 min. After 60 min, before surgical incision, the same dose of each drug was admin-istered. Only minor and clinically insignificant haemodynamic differences between the groups were recorded during the following 60-min observation period. Induction of anaesthesia with fentanyl, mean dose 110 μg/kg, or alfentanil, mean dose 1379 μg/kg, in lorazepam-premedicated patients scheduled for coronary bypass surgery was associated with clini-cally insignificant and similar haemodynamic alter-ations. Nor were the haemodynamic consequences of sternotomy different in the two groups (Hynynen *et al.*, 1986). Bovill and colleagues (1984a) assigned patients with valvular heart disease randomly to anaesthesia with fentanyl, 75 μg/kg, sufentanil, 15 μg/kg, or alfentanil, 120 μg/kg, with oxygen/air after premedication with lorazepam. Before surgery, additional fentanyl or sufentanil was given as a bolus, whereas alfentanil was administered in a continuous infusion. Mean arterial pressure decreased on average 25% after induction with sufentanil in patients with mitral valve disease. In patients with aortic valve disease, mean arterial pressure and systemic vascular resistance increased by about 10% in response to sternotomy in the fentanyl group. No other haemo-dynamic changes were observed. Transient hypo-tension following induction of anaesthesia with sufentanil in some patients in this study is consistent with previous observations in patients with CAD by the same group of investigators (Sebel & Bovill, 1982).

Over recent years, several groups have studied the coronary haemodynamic and cardiac metabolic effects of opioids, alone or in comparison with other anaesthetic agents. Blaise and colleagues (1990) docu-mented that fentanyl was devoid of effects on coron-ary vasoreactivity and myocardial metabolism in dogs. In one randomized study, Wilkinson and colleagues (1981) compared morphine, 2 mg/kg, and halothane, 0.2–1% end-tidal, in nitrous oxide/oxygen (50:50) in patients subjected to coronary artery surgery. Coronary perfusion pressure was better preserved with morphine than with halothane. Coronary blood flow decreased in proportion to the fall in myocardial oxygen consumption and the decline in coronary perfusion pressure. With sternotomy, arterial pressure increased more in morphine-anaesthetized patients. Coronary autoregulation was preserved in both groups. Myocardial lactate production was recorded in six of 14 halothane patients and was associated with hypotension before surgical incision. In patients anaesthetized with morphine, metabolic evidence of ischaemia was present in three of 12 patients and associated with hypertension and high heart rates during surgery.

Sethna and colleagues (1982) administered morphine (250 µg/kg) to conscious, secobarbitone-premedicated patients with CAD before induction of anaesthesia. The drug produced a decrease of approximately 15% in mean arterial pressure and systemic vascular resistance without changes in myocardial oxygen consumption or coronary blood flow. Coronary vascular resistance decreased and coronary sinus oxygen content increased, indicating coronary vasodilatation. No ischaemia was observed. The reasons for the conflicting results of the two studies which utilized the same thermodilution technique for coronary blood flow measurements are not clear.

Since the early 1970s, the Göttingen group headed by Sonntag has presented data on the coronary circulatory effects of various anaesthetic agents in patients with and without cardiac disease using the argon wash-in technique. Particularly alarming were their findings of a high incidence of myocardial ischaemia associated with high-dose fentanyl anaesthesia in patients with CAD (Sonntag et al., 1982). Patients were investigated after induction with 10 and 100 µg/kg in 100% oxygen. After 10 µg/kg, minimal systemic haemodynamic effects were recorded. However, both coronary vascular resistance and myocardial lactate extraction decreased. After 100 µg/kg, diastolic pressure had decreased slightly, PCWP was unaltered and heart rate had increased by an average 6 beats/min. Despite a reduction in myocardial oxygen supply, five of the nine patients studied demonstrated myocardial lactate production. With sternotomy, heart rate increased markedly (+22 beats compared with awake), whereas coronary perfusion pressure remained at awake values. Coronary vascular resistance declined. At this time, myocardial oxygen consumption was approximately 40% above the awake

value and eight of the nine patients had metabolic evidence of ischaemia.

The same group of investigators have also documented the influence of sufentanil anaesthesia and sternotomy on systemic and coronary haemodynamics (Sonntag et al., 1989). They provided anaesthesia for CABG with either sufentanil at 1 µg/kg followed by a continuous infusion at $0.015 \mu g \cdot kg^{-1} \cdot min^{-1}$ combined with 70% nitrous oxide or with sufentanil at 10 times this dose combined with oxygen. Both formats of anaesthesia resulted in identical haemodynamic changes at induction and following sternotomy. After sternotomy, 56% of patients had signs of myocardial ischaemia as evidenced by myocardial hypoxanthine production, 2 or 3 of which were unassociated with haemodynamic changes. As previously documented (Windsor et al., 1988), these data demonstrate that there is little effect on the circulation by changing the dose of sufentanil by a factor of 5 to 10. Furthermore, it appears that sufentanil, like fentanyl (Sonntag et al., 1982), does not protect the myocardium from autonomic sympathetic responses.

In similar patients anaesthetized with a similar dose of fentanyl, 75 µg/kg at induction and 25 µg/kg before surgery, Heikkilä and colleagues (1985a) found that one of 12 patients only developed ischaemia after sternotomy. In contrast to Sonntag's patients, surgical stimulation induced coronary vasoconstriction compared with the awake measurements, as shown by increased coronary vascular resistance and myocardial oxygen extraction. Administration of droperidol, 250 µg/kg, before sternotomy counteracted the coronary vasoconstrictive response to sternotomy but did not affect the incidence of ischaemia (Heikkilä et al., 1985a). The reasons for the conflicting results in the two studies can be attributed probably to the different study protocols. It is likely that the extended study period in Sonntag's study resulted in lower fentanyl plasma concentrations before surgery than in the study by Heikkilä, where part of the drug was administered immediately before surgical incision. When ischaemia develops, maximal coronary vasodilatation is likely to occur, hence the difference in coronary vascular resistance between the two studies. The high incidence of ischaemia in the study by Sonntag and colleagues (1982) illustrates the importance of maintaining heart rate close to normal values even in the face of unaltered arterial diastolic and LV filling pressures.

In patients with CAD undergoing vascular surgery and anaesthetized with the NLA II technique (fentanyl, 15 µg/kg, droperidol, 150 µ/kg, and nitrous oxide/oxygen, 75:25) coronary autoregulation was maintained well. Abdominal incision was associated with coronary vasoconstriction and a shift from myocardial release to uptake of noraderenaline. No ischaemia was observed. When NLA II anaesthesia was combined with thoracic extradural analgesia in comparable patients, the coronary vasoconstrictive response to surgical stimulation was abolished (Reiz et al., 1981b, 1982a).

More recent, randomized studies from the same group of investigators in similar patients have not confirmed the same degree of coronary vasoconstriction caused by surgical stimulation under fentanyl (10–20 μg/kg)–nitrous oxide anaesthesia (Fig. 60.3) (Hohner et al., 1993a). In contrast to the previous studies (Reiz et al., 1981b, 1982a), the patients had been given heavy morphine premedication and had less sympathetic activity as evidenced by lower catecholamine levels.

Inhaled anaesthetic agents

Effects of volatile anaesthetics on cardiac function and haemodynamics

Halogenated anaesthetics

The inhalation anaesthetics decrease a variety of indices of papillary muscle contraction, such as mean $\dot{V}_{max}$ and developed force (F_M) (Kemmotsu et al., 1973). In common with the barbiturates, halothane restricts calcium flow to the contractile proteins and/or inhibits the reaction between calcium and the contractile proteins (Price, 1974). Brown and Crout

(1971) found that contractility was depressed equally by five inhalation agents. On the basis of these observations they suggested that the cellular mechanism for cardiodepression was identical. This hypothesis was strengthened further by studies in the intact dog by Merin and Basch (1981) who found similarities between the changes in contractile function and myocardial metabolism during halothane, enflurane and isoflurane anaesthesia. In total contrast to these concepts, Lynch (1986) demonstrated recently a differential depression of the isolated guinea pig papillary muscle preparation by halothane, enflurane and isoflurane (Fig. 60.4).

The failing heart muscle preparation is more sensitive to inhalation agents than the non-failing (Kemmotsu et al., 1974). Prys-Roberts and colleagues (1976) studied dogs with myocardial infarction established by ligation of coronary arteries 7–10 days before the exposure to thiopentone/halothane/nitrous oxide anaesthesia. After 60 min, they found aortic blood flow acceleration and cardiac output to be reduced without changes in LV dP/dT, arterial pressure, or heart rate. More recently, Lowenstein

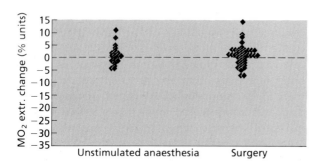

Fig. 60.3 Difference in myocardial oxygen extraction (MO₂ extr.) between awake values and values measured before and during abdominal vascular surgery under fentanyl–nitrous oxide anaesthesia. Each patient is represented by one value during unstimulated anaesthesia and two during surgery (10 and 30 min after abdominal incision). The results indicate that fentanyl does not limit coronary vasodilator reserve, i.e. has no direct effect on coronary resistance vessels. (Data from Hohner et al., 1993a.)

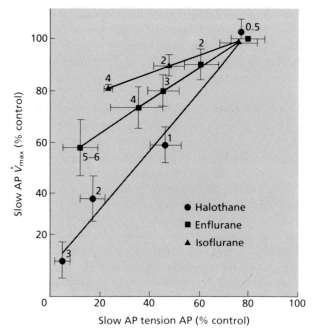

Fig. 60.4 Effects of halothane, enflurane and isoflurane on the relationship between depression of slow action potential (AP) $\dot{V}_{max}$ and the simultaneously measured depression in peak tension of guinea pig papillary muscles at 0.3 Hz. The numbers beside the points represent the anaesthetic concentration in percent bubbled through the perfusion medium. The data suggest a differential depression of myocardial contractility by the three agents. (Redrawn from Lynch, 1986.)

and colleagues (1981) demonstrated that halothane did not alter systemic haemodynamics in dogs with severe regional myocardial dysfunction induced by a critical constriction of the left anterior descending coronary artery. The inhalation agents depress baroreceptor function in animals and in humans (Bristow et al., 1969; Duke et al., 1977; Duke & Trosky, 1980; Morton et al., 1980). However, it has been suggested that barostatic reflexes are maintained better during isoflurane anaesthesia (Skovsted & Sapthavichaikul, 1977; Seagard et al., 1983; Kotrly et al., 1985).

Halothane, enflurane and isoflurane produce relaxation of vascular smooth muscle (Vatner & Smith, 1974; Östman et al., 1985). Sprague and colleagues (1974) studied the effects of halothane and isoflurane on phenylephrine-induced contraction of the rat aorta. Both drugs inhibited the vasoconstrictor response. Neither halothane nor isoflurane seems to affect α- or β-receptors (Sprague et al., 1974; Östman et al., 1986). As it was noted that cyclic AMP : ATP ratio increased with both drugs, it has been suggested that vascular relaxation was related to cyclic AMP formation (Sprague et al., 1974).

The inhalation agents affect the specific vascular beds differently. Halothane administered to primates produced vasodilatation in the renal and iliac beds whereas vasoconstriction was noted in the mesenteric bed (Vatner & Smith, 1974). Gelman and colleagues (1984) compared the effects of isoflurane and halothane on regional body flow distribution. One minimum alveolar concentration (MAC) halothane increased flow to the brain and decreased pancreatic flow. Perfusion of other vascular beds was unaffected. An equipotent concentration of isoflurane increased flow to the heart, brain and liver but decreased perfusion of the stomach, small intestine and pancreas. Halothane, enflurane and isoflurane dilate coronary blood vessels. However, their coronary vasodilating potency is markedly different (Domenech et al., 1977; Tarnow et al., 1977; Hickey et al., 1988). These differences are discussed in depth later in this chapter (pp. 1233−7).

The effects of the halogenated anaesthetics on systemic haemodynamics have been studied extensively in healthy subjects (Eger et al., 1970; Calverly et al., 1978; Eger, 1981) and in patients with cardiovascular disease (Mallow et al., 1976; Delaney et al., 1980; Eger, 1981). In healthy volunteers, cardiac output was maintained better during isoflurane than during halothane or enflurane anaesthesia. Stroke volume was decreased equally by halothane and isoflurane. Heart rate increased by about 20% with isoflurane but was not affected by halothane. Such pronounced differ-

ences could not be reproduced in the Isoflurane New Drug Application Study (1982). The systemic haemodynamic effects of the more recent inhalation anaesthetics, sevoflurane and desflurane, appear to be largely similar to those of isoflurane (Holaday et al., 1981; Lerman et al., 1990; Cahalan et al., 1991; Merin et al., 1991; Pagel et al., 1991a,b; Thompson et al., 1991; Weiskopf et al., 1991; Warltier & Pagel, 1992).

Only one investigation compares the cardiovascular effects of inhalation agents in a clinical setting and with a double-blind, randomized protocol. Hohner and colleagues (1993a) studied the circulatory effects of halothane and isoflurane in morphine-premedicated vascular surgical patients with CAD after induction with fentanyl, 3 µg/kg, and thiopentone, 2−4 mg/kg. Muscle paralysis was maintained with pancuronium and ventilation controlled at around 4.2 kPa (31.5 mmHg) with nitrous oxide/oxygen (60 : 40). Either drug was administered according to clinical needs. Haemodynamic abnormalities not responding to changes in anaesthetic dose were treated by the appropriate vasoactive drugs; phenylephrine was administered if mean arterial pressure declined to below 70% of the awake value. Nitroglycerine was administered if mean arterial pressure exceeded 120% of the awake value or if persistent elevation of PCWP by more than 30% was noted, despite increasing the inspired volatile concentration. Measurements after induction included the period after surgical preparation before incision and 10 and 30 min after abdominal incision. The mean anaesthetic doses, corrected for the difference in MAC, of the agents used at the various measurement periods were not different. Neither the use of or doses of phenylephrine nor nitroglycerine differed between the groups. As shown in Fig. 60.5, the overall systemic and coronary haemodynamic effects of the two anaesthetics and surgical stimulation were indistinguishable. It should be noted that some of the haemodynamic effects which would normally have been observed with the respective volatile agents were probably offset by the use of the intervention drugs.

One other randomized study (Smith et al., 1988) investigated the effects of 1 MAC halothane or isoflurane, used for carotid artery surgery, on systolic wall stress (SWS) and rate-corrected velocity of circumferential fibre shortening (Vcfc by TOE). Both anaesthetics produced similar and moderate changes in blood pressure and heart rate. SWS was comparable in the two groups whereas Vcfc was significantly lower in halothane patients. As Vcfc is regarded as an index of myocardial contractility independent of

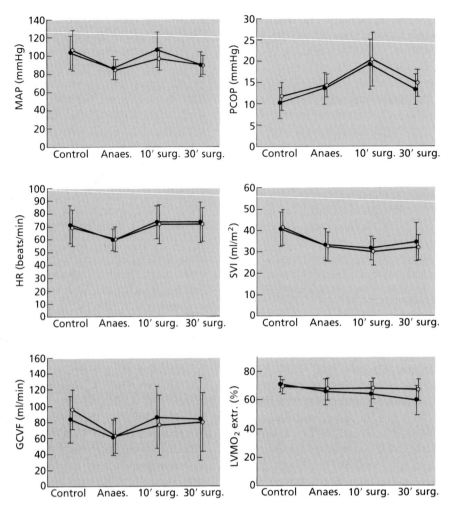

Fig. 60.5 Systemic and coronary haemodynamic changes observed during halothane (open symbols) versus isoflurane (closed symbols) nitrous oxide anaesthesia and abdominal vascular surgery. The anaesthetics were administered at identical MAC for each measurement period according to a randomized, double-blind protocol. Hypotension, hypertension, LV failure and tachycardia were treated pharmacologically according to the protocol. The number of such interventions was not different between groups. Under these circumstances, the only significant difference between groups was a greater decline of LV myocardial oxygen extraction in isoflurane patients. This finding, indicating lesser coronary vasodilator reserve with isoflurane, was due to the use of high concentrations of the anaesthetic during surgery and not an affect of prolonged exposure to the drug. MAP, mean arterial pressure; PCOP, pulmonary arteriolar occlusion pressure; HR, heart rate; SVI, stroke volume index; GCVF, great cardiac venous blood flow; LVMO$_2$ extr., myocardial oxygen extraction in the territory drained by the great cardiac vein, principally the left anterior descending coronary artery territory. (Data from Hohner *et al.*, 1993a.)

preload but variable with afterload (Colan *et al.*, 1984), these results indicate that isoflurane produces less depression of contractility than halothane. These data agree with preliminary findings by Brusset and colleagues (1986) who, in a random fashion, administered isoflurane or halothane to treat hypertension during major vascular surgery. Both these studies (Brusset *et al.*, 1986; Smith *et al.*, 1988) and that by Hohner and colleagues (1993a) derive data from vascular surgical patients, who are known to have high endogenous sympathetic tone, depressed baroreceptor function, a high incidence of systemic hypertension and concomitant use of cardiovascular

medication. It is likely that withdrawal of sympathetic tone caused by anaesthetic induction in this patient population has more influence on the circulation than the respective drug *per se*. This would explain some of the previous contradictory findings on the circulatory effects of volatile agents in vascular patients (Roizen *et al.*, 1981) as compared to other patient populations (Hess *et al.*, 1983).

Hess and colleagues (1983) and Roizen and colleagues (1981) studied the efficacy of inhalation agents upon surgically induced hypertension and raised PCWP. Hess and colleagues (1983) noted that isoflurane reduced arterial pressure and filling pressure by systemic vasodilatation, whereas arterial pressure reduction with halothane was achieved by cardio-depression. In contrast, Roizen and colleagues (1981) could not distinguish the effects of halothane and isoflurane. Both agents lowered filling pressure by reducing systemic vascular resistance. Why the conflicting results? Hess's group studied patients with good LV function undergoing coronary artery surgery. Roizen and colleagues (1981) studied a group of vascular surgical patients who have been noted to have an increased proportion of individuals with depressed LV function and raised basal sympathetic tone. In such patients, the effects on PCWP by reducing impedance to LV ejection has been shown to dominate over the cardiodepressant action of halothane (Reiz *et al.*, 1982b).

Effects of inhaled anaesthetics upon the coronary circulation and myocardial oxygenation

Halothane

In animal studies halothane has little effect upon coronary vascular tone or autoregulation (Tarnow *et al.*, 1977; Verrier *et al.*, 1980; Hickey *et al.*, 1988) (Fig. 60.6). Animals with intact or blocked autonomic function demonstrate coronary blood flow changes proportional to myocardial oxygen demand (Kenny *et al.*, 1991). Dogs with a critical coronary artery stenosis show regional dysfunction and decreased flow associated with lowered systemic pressure and therefore distal perfusion pressure in the area sup-

plied by a narrowed coronary artery, whereas regions supplied by a normal coronary artery had a decrease in coronary blood flow proportional to myocardial oxygen requirements (Francis *et al.*, 1982). The resultant ischaemia and regional dysfunction has been confirmed by Buffington (1986) to be due to decreased perfusion pressure rather than a specific effect of halothane.

In patients scheduled to undergo coronary artery surgery, randomized to receive halothane (0.2 to 1.0% end-tidal) or morphine, 2 mg/kg, ventilated with 50% nitrous oxide in oxygen, a 20% reduction in myocardial oxygen consumption was seen in both groups and was related to the decline in blood pressure. Coronary blood flow decreased less than 10% in both groups but myocardial oxygen extraction decreased to a greater extent with halothane than with morphine (Wilkinson *et al.*, 1981). Another study in a similar patient group using halothane with or without nitrous oxide found the same result (Moffitt *et al.*, 1983). This mild coronary vasodilatation agrees with earlier work by Sonntag and colleagues (1979) in subjects without coronary artery disease and has been shown in vascular surgical patients with coronary artery disease and a clinical history of impaired LV function (Reiz *et al.*, 1982b) both groups using a halothane/air/oxygen mixture. More recently in a randomized double-blind study comparing halothane and isoflurane (in nitrous oxide/oxygen) in patients with CAD undergoing abdominal aortic surgery, Hohner and colleagues (1993a) have demonstrated that halothane produced mild coronary vasodilation which was unrelated to the dose being administered (Fig. 60.7). This study shows the

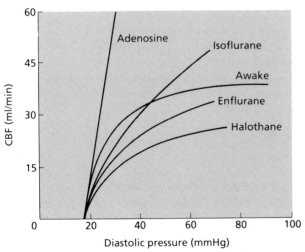

Fig. 60.6 Diastolic pressure–coronary blood flow (CBF) relationships in the awake and anaesthetized dog. The coronary vasodilating properties of the volatile agents are isoflurane >>> enflurane > halothane. None of the drugs impairs autoregulation in comparison with adenosine. (Data from Hickey *et al.*, 1988.)

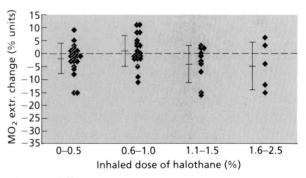

Fig. 60.7 Difference in myocardial oxygen extraction (MO₂ extr.) between awake values and values recorded during various inhaled steady-state concentrations of halothane. Halothane was not associated with a significant decrease in myocardial oxygen extraction at any dose level, hence the anaesthetic did not limit coronary vasodilator reserve. Note, however, that some patients demonstrated a marked reduction of myocardial oxygen extraction, indicating individual coronary vasodilator sensitivity to the anaesthetic. (Data from Hohner *et al.*, 1993a.)

majority of ischaemic events being related to haemo-dynamic changes such as tachycardia, hypotension and/or LV failure though a few of these events appeared to be spasm-induced, as suggested by a decreased coronary flow despite unchanged heart rate and coronary perfusion pressure.

One study in patients undergoing CABG with halothane has failed to demonstrate a decrease in myocardial oxygen extraction with halothane (Hilfiker *et al.*, 1983).

In summary, the probable mild coronary vaso-dilating action of halothane in humans with CAD appears to have negligible importance for the devel-opment of myocardial oxygen supply/demand imbal-ance compared to the effects of changes in the systemic circulation.

Enflurane

Experiments in dogs show the coronary vasodilating action of enflurane to be more powerful than that produced by halothane (Tarnow *et al.*, 1977; Hickey *et al.*, 1988) (Fig. 60.6).

Vascular patients with CAD and coronary artery bypass patients administered enflurane with or without nitrous oxide also demonstrated significant coronary vasodilatation (Moffitt *et al.*, 1984a; Rydvall *et al.*, 1984). For instance, in one study performed in patients with normal LV function, 0.5–3% inspired enflurane in oxygen decreased coronary perfusion pressure by 33%, myocardial oxygen consumption by 50% and myocardial oxygen extraction by 20% (Moffitt *et al.*, 1984a). Another study has demonstrated coronary vasodilatation following induction of anaes-thesia with enflurane 2–3% inspired concentration, in oxygen, which was no longer present at 1% inspired enflurane prior to surgical incision although coronary inflow pressure, heart rate and pulmonary artery occlusion pressure (PAOP) levels remained comparable (Moffitt *et al.*, 1986b). Even at 1% enflurane, myocardial lactate production and new V5 ECG changes failed to indicate myocardial ischaemia. All these data suggest that enflurane pro-duces coronary vasodilatation which might be dose dependent, e.g. demonstrable only at high inspired concentrations. However, myocardial oxygenation remains adequate even at markedly decreased coron-ary perfusion pressures as demonstrated by lack of metabolic or ECG signs of ischaemia in all published studies.

Isoflurane

Experiments in several animal species and in humans

with or without CAD have demonstrated that iso-flurane produces coronary vasodilatation even at nor-mal coronary inflow pressure (Tarnow *et al.*, 1977; Lundeen *et al.*, 1983; Gelman *et al.*, 1984; Buffington *et al.*, 1987; Hickey *et al.*, 1988; Sahlman *et al.*, 1988; Leclerc *et al.*, 1990; Kenny *et al.*, 1991) (Figs 60.6 and 60.8). This vasodilatation has been shown to be dose dependent both in animals and in patients with CAD (Fig. 60.9) (Cutfield *et al.*, 1988; Hohner *et al.*, 1993a). The mechanism by which this occurs is mediated by the vascular endothelium (Blaise *et al.*, 1987). The principal site of action appears to be on coronary resistance vessels (Sill *et al.*, 1987). Certainly this property is seen despite autonomic block and with normal haemodynamics (Kenny *et al.*, 1991), and is greater than that seen with enflurane or halothane but less than with adenosine and dipyridamole (Hickey *et al.*, 1988; Habazettl *et al.*, 1989).

In Hohner's study (1993a) of patients with CAD having vascular surgery, an inspired isoflurane con-centration greater than 1–1.5% (in oxygen/nitrous oxide) was required to produce significant coronary vasodilatation. An interesting observation, seen also with halothane (Fig. 60.7), was that in some patients low concentrations of isoflurane produced substantial coronary vasodilatation unaccompanied by signifi-cant systemic haemodynamic changes (Fig. 60.9), suggesting a variable individual sensitivity of coron-ary vasculature to volatile anaesthetics.

Reiz and colleagues in 1983 suggested that the coronary vasodilating property of isoflurane might contribute to the development of myocardial ischaemia in patients with CAD. Before surgery patients received 1 MAC isoflurane in an air–oxygen mixture. At steady state, coronary perfusion pressure had fallen by 35% with clinically insignificant changes of heart rate or PAOP. However, ECG and/or metabolic evidence of ischaemia was present in five of 10 patients. Next, normalization of coronary perfusion pressure and control of heart rate and filling pressure was performed. Despite this, three of the five ischaemic patients continued to demonstrate ischaemia even though there was evidence of total coronary flow being in excess of demand.

Subsequently, there have been many studies addressing the issue of isoflurane and the redistri-bution of myocardial blood flow either regionally or transmurally, and whether isoflurane is associated with more ischaemic cardiac complications than other agents. In answering these issues it is useful to consider four aspects of the current literature: (i) is it possible to produce an anatomical model in which 'steal' can be demonstrated and do such patients exist? (ii) is the coronary vasodilatation sufficient to

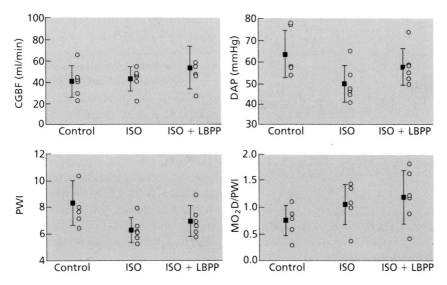

Fig. 60.8 Coronary graft blood flow (CGBF), diastolic arterial pressure (DAP), pressure work index (PWI, external myocardial work) and myocardial oxygen delivery in relation to demand (MO$_2$D/PWI) during isoflurane anaesthesia compared to sedated control. The dose of the anaesthetic was titrated so as to produce an approximate 20% decline in systemic blood pressure (ISO). After measurements, diastolic blood pressure was raised approximately to the pre-isoflurane value by the use of a G-suit [ISO + lower body positive pressure (LBPP)]. The results indicate coronary vasodilatation by isoflurane, with oxygen delivery in excess of demand. Measurements were obtained 6 h after coronary artery surgery when coronary autoregulation is normalized, using implantable micro-Doppler flow probes. Values are means ± SD (closed squares) and individual (open circles). (Redrawn from data by Leclerc *et al.*, 1990.)

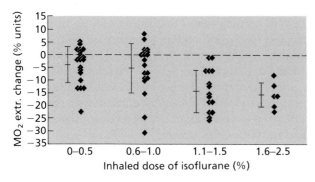

Fig. 60.9 Difference in myocardial oxygen extraction (MO$_2$ extr.) between awake values and values recorded during various inhaled steady-state concentrations of isoflurane. Isoflurane was associated with a significant, dose-dependent limitation of coronary vasodilator reserve. Little coronary vasodilatation was observed in most patients below an inhaled concentration of 1%. Note, however, that some individuals, similar to what was observed with halothane (Fig. 60.7) displayed a marked coronary vasodilator sensitivity to isoflurane even with the lowest inhaled concentrations. (Data from Hohner *et al.*, 1993a.)

cause redistribution of myocardial blood flow if one controls the wider systemic effects of isoflurane, particularly tachycardia and hypotension? (iii) if redistribution of myocardial blood flow occurs with isoflurane, does it lead to myocardial ischaemia (iv) are outcome studies sensitive enough to distinguish the possible coronary vasodilator properties of iso-

flurane from all the other contributing factors producing cardiac morbidity?

Coronary steal

In 1978 Becker described the phenomenon of *regional flow maldistribution* (coronary steal) during dipyridamole infusion using a canine model in which coronary artery occlusion accompanied by collateral development was produced over a 4-week period. Blood flows (total and transmural) were measured by the microsphere technique. Dipyridamole was administered intravenously, with maintenance of coronary inflow pressure and heart rate, this resulted in a reduced poststenotic pressure of 4 kPa (30 mmHg). Flow to normal myocardium doubled as a result of the dilatation of resistance vessels while blood flow in the collateral dependent zone decreased by half due to the reduction of collateral driving pressure (Fig. 60.10). *Transmural flow maldistribution* was demonstrated by Gallagher and colleagues (1982) in awake exercising dogs with critical stenosis of a single epicardial coronary artery (Fig. 60.11).

The incidence of 'steal-prone' anatomy as described by Becker has been reported to be 23% in patients included in the coronary artery surgery study (CASS) (Buffington *et al.*, 1988) (Fig. 60.12) and is in the order of 7% in patients with abdominal aortic aneurysm/occlusion (Coriat, 1992, personal communication).

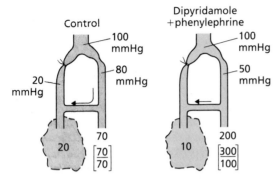

Fig. 60.10 Schematic diagram of the coronary circulation showing proposed mechanism for a vasodilator-induced coronary steal. The coronary artery divides into two branches, one completely occluded, and the other stenosed but providing collaterals to the first. In the control situation on the left, distal pressure is low in the occluded arterial bed and there is a small gradient in mean pressure across the stenosis. Flow in the ischaemic region (dotted area) is $20\,ml \cdot min^{-1} \cdot 100\,g^{-1}$ and is determined by the collateral driving pressure, or the difference between distal pressures in the bed supplying collaterals [10.6 kPa (80 mmHg)] and the ischaemic bed [2.6 kPa (20 mmHg)]. Flow in the distribution of the stenotic vessel is normal at $70\,ml \cdot min^{-1} \cdot 100\,g^{-1}$ and is evenly distributed between subendocardium (lower value in brackets) and subepicardium (upper value in brackets). During dipyridamole administration, with blood pressure maintained constant by phenylephrine, flow increases in the non-ischaemic bed to $200\,ml \cdot min^{-1} \cdot 100\,g^{-1}$, but becomes maldistributed between subendocardium and subepicardium. In addition, pressure distal to the stenosis falls to 6.6 kPa (50 mmHg), causing a reduction in collateral driving pressure. As a result, flow to the ischaemic region decreases to $10\,ml \cdot min^{-1} \cdot 100\,g^{-1}$, interpreted as a coronary steal. (Redrawn from Becker, 1978.)

The prevalence of critical coronary artery stenosis is unknown. An infinite number of combinations including stenosis severity and distensibility, haemodynamic alterations, changes in inotropy and myocardial oxygen requirements, will determine if a coronary stenosis is 'critical' at a given moment (i.e. that the hyperaemic response to a brief occlusion of this artery would be abolished).

Is isoflurane capable of producing myocardial blood-flow redistribution?

Using Becker's dog model (1978) (Fig. 60.10) some workers have demonstrated regional flow maldistribution using isoflurane (Buffington *et al.*, 1987) others have not (Cason *et al.*, 1987). Buffington and colleagues (1987) found both regional and transmural flow redistribution away from the collateral dependent zone when moderate hypotension was simulated by decreasing total coronary flow by 16–26% below the autoregulated value (Fig. 60.13). With greater or lesser flow reductions maldistribution was

not observed. During the former, coronary vasodilator reserve was probably exhausted, hence isoflurane could not produce further vasodilatation. During the latter, simulating normotension, the coronary vasodilator effect of isoflurane was most likely insufficient to produce maldistribution. It thus appears as if some degree of hypotension would be needed for isoflurane to produce flow maldistribution in this model.

One other study by Tatekawa and colleagues (1987) observed dose-dependent transmural-flow maldistribution in dogs. Unfortunately, heart rate was markedly higher during isoflurane than before. The effect on myocardial-flow distribution by the anaesthetic was therefore indistinguishable from that of tachycardia.

In summary it appears as if some of the haemodynamic changes produced by isoflurane (e.g. hypotension and/or tachycardia) have to be present for myocardial-flow maldistribution to occur in animal models with coronary artery stenosis.

Myocardial-flow maldistribution and ischaemia

Various animal experiments by Buffington and colleagues (1987) and Preibe and Foëx (1987) have documented coronary-flow maldistribution by isoflurane capable of causing regional ventricular dysfunction, thought to represent ischaemia, in the territory deprived of flow. Invariably, some degree of hypotension accompanied these observations. In contrast, less regional ventricular dysfunction was observed when halothane was given in a concentration producing the same effects as isoflurane on blood pressure, heart rate and LV dP/dT (Priebe & Foëx, 1987). These results are best explained by the different effects of the two anaesthetics on coronary vascular tone.

In comparison, Tatekawa and colleagues (1987) recorded transmural-flow maldistribution with isoflurane, unaccompanied by new mechanical dysfunction despite hypotension and/or tachycardia. No study has documented new regional contraction abnormalities without myocardial flow maldistribution. Thus, it appears as if isoflurane is unable to produce regional ventricular contraction abnormalities without simultaneous underperfusion of the territory displaying dysfunction. It is also probable that neither flow maldistribution, nor regional ventricular dysfunction can occur without some degree of adverse haemodynamic change. In addition, and in analogy with what has been previously described for nifedipine and adenosine (Gewirtz *et al.*, 1984), the negative inotropic action of isoflurane would

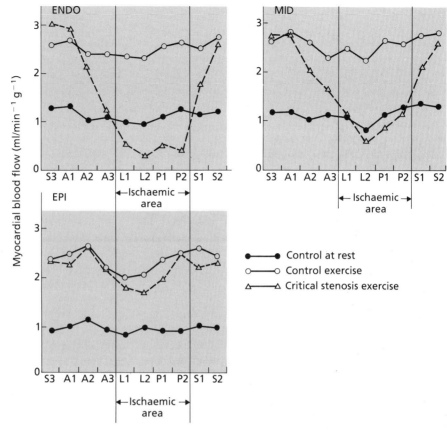

Fig. 60.11 Intramyocardial blood flow redistribution distal to a narrowed coronary artery is shown in one dog. Myocardial blood flow was measured in the absence of a stenosis at rest and during exercise, and in the presence of a stenosis during exercise. Flow to the subepicardial myocardium achieved normal levels during exercise, flow to the mid-myocardium was attenuated, and flow to the epicardium was virtually absent. Arrows indicate location of tissue samples spanned by dimension gauges. (Redrawn from Gallagher *et al.*, 1982.)

dose dependently counteract its direct coronary vaso-dilating effect and hence reduce the risk for flow maldistribution and ischaemia.

Technical problems still limit the ability to study myocardial-flow distribution in humans. In a clinical setting, Hohner and colleagues (1993a) compared the coronary haemodynamic effects of isoflurane, halothane and fentanyl (in oxygen/nitrous oxide) at comparable systemic haemodynamics. They used regional coronary flow techniques and recorded new myocardial ischaemia by 12-lead ECG, myocardial lactate and anterior LV wall function by cardiokymography as previously described by Häggmark and colleagues (1989). Although the total incidence of myocardial ischaemia was comparable in the three groups, significantly more ischaemic events unexplained by systemic haemodynamic aberrations were recorded in isoflurane patients. When ischaemia was observed in these patients, whether caused by systemic haemodynamic changes or not, and in contrast to halothane and fentanyl patients, it was almost invariably accompanied by a marked decrease in myocardial oxygen extraction. This indicates a limitation of coronary vasodilator reserve by isoflurane which could decrease the tolerance to haemodynamic aberrations.

Morbidity studies

Even in the large clinical studies of Slogoff and Keats (1985, 1986) only weak associations between intra-operative myocardial ischaemia and adverse post-operative cardiac outcomes have been shown. By tightening the definitions for haemodynamic abnormality, one still finds an approximate 25% incidence of intraoperative ischaemia unrelated to haemodynamic events (Hohner *et al.*, 1993a). Likewise, a high incidence of postoperative cardiac events after cardiac and non-cardiac surgery in patients with known or suspected CAD are unrelated to intra-operative events (Slogoff & Keats 1985; Mangano *et al.*, 1990). Attempts, therefore, to isolate isoflurane as a single factor in morbidity have proved impossible. With the exception of one study (Inoue *et al.*, 1990) all present data suggest that the choice of primary anaesthetic agent has no direct influence on the cardiac complication rate after surgery (Slogoff & Keats, 1989; Tuman *et al.*, 1989a; Forrest *et al.*, 1990; Leung *et al.*, 1991; Stühmeier *et al.*, 1992) (Table 60.18). The main reason for this lack of correlation is most likely that postoperative rather than intra-operative factors determine cardiac outcome after surgery in patients with CAD (Mangano *et al.*, 1990).

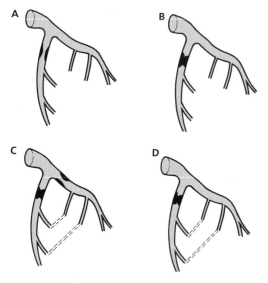

Fig. 60.12 Angiograms in the CASS Registry were sorted into these four anatomic variants. A schematic diagram of the left coronary artery is shown, but collateral connections with the right coronary artery were included in the analysis as well. (A) Fifty-one percent of the 16 249 angiograms surveyed had one or more stenoses but no occluded vessels. (B) Ten percent had a total occlusion but no collateral supply to the distal bed. Of those angiograms with a total occlusion and intercoronary collaterals (dashed lines), about 60% had a haemodynamically significant stenosis of the artery supplying the collateral vessels (C) and about 40% did not (D). (For the purposes of this study, any stenosis with a 50% or greater diameter reduction of the artery was considered 'haemodynamically significant'.) Intercoronary steal is most likely to occur in the anatomic variant at (C) because arteriolar dilatation decreases pressure distal to the stenosis and reduces flow through the high-resistance collateral network. This variant was present in 23% of 16 249 angiograms examined.

Desflurane and sevoflurane

In a dog model Pagel and colleagues (1991a,b) found that desflurane produced systemic and coronary haemodynamic changes which were indistinguishable from those induced by an equipotent dose of isoflurane. Human coronary blood flow data are lacking. Helman and colleagues (1992) studied patients undergoing coronary bypass surgery following induction of anaesthesia with thiopentone/vecuronium followed by either desflurane or sufentanil. During induction, they observed greater haemodynamic stability and less myocardial ischaemia with sufentanil. Later during surgery, the incidence of ischaemia was comparable. There was no difference in cardiac outcome following surgery between the groups. It would appear that the advantages of desflurane, e.g. rapid onset and offset, do not include

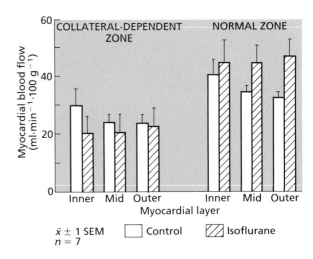

Fig. 60.13 At the mid-flow range, when total coronary flow was reduced to approximately 80% of the autoregulated value, the addition of isoflurane (0.94% end-tidal) increased blood flow to the outer layers of the normal zone of the expense of blood flow to the inner layers of the collateral-dependent zone.

any further advantages for the patients with cardiac disease. Clinical data on sevoflurane are less available than for desflurane. In a rat model Habazettl and colleagues (1991) found sevoflurane reduced coronary flow more than isoflurane whereas Bernard and colleagues (1990) found isoflurane and sevoflurane had the same effect on coronary vessels in the dog.

Nitrous oxide

Nitrous oxide stimulates the sympathetic nervous system to release noradrenaline (Smith & Corbascio, 1966). In the isolated heart preparation, the drug produces a dose-dependent depression (Price & Helrich, 1955; Price, 1976; Motomura *et al.*, 1984). Many of the confounding results of studies of the circulatory effects of nitrous oxide may be related to inappropriate study designs. Few studies have used constant anaesthetic dose and/or inspired oxygen concentration. High oxygen tensions produce vasoconstriction. Substituting nitrous oxide for oxygen therefore provides an inadequate control value for systemic vascular resistance. In the intact dog, nitrous oxide increases heart rate and lowers stroke volume (Lundborg *et al.*, 1966). In healthy volunteers, nitrous oxide is associated with minimal cardiodepression as judged by the ballistocardiographic technique (Eisele & Smith, 1972). Nitrous oxide delivered in hyperbaric conditions produces a hyperdynamic circulation, indicating massive activation of the sympathetic nervous system (Winter *et al.*, 1972). Ebert (1990) noted that nitrous oxide decreased baroreflex-

Table 60.18 Influence of choice of primary anaesthetic agent/technique on cardiac outcome after cardiac and non-cardiac surgery (randomized studies)

	Agent(s)/technique	No.	Surgery	Outcome affected
Valentin *et al.* (1986)	Spi./GA	578	Acute hip	No
Forrest *et al.* (1990)	Volatile/fentanyl	17 201	Non-cardiac	No
Reiz *et al.* (1982a)	TEA + GA/GA	45	Acute major vascular	No
Yeager *et al.* (1987)*	TEA + GA/GA	53	High-risk abdominal	Yes
Kozmary *et al.* (1990)	Isoflurane-N$_2$O/isoflurane-O$_2$	63	Carotid artery	No
Tuman *et al.* (1991)*	TEA + GA/GA	80	Vascular	Yes
Baron *et al.* (1991)	TEA + GA/GA	173	Major vascular	No
Hohner *et al.* (1993a,b)	Volatile/fentanyl	119	Major vascular	No
Stühmeier *et al.* (1992)	Isoflurane/halothane	500	Vascular	No
Slogoff and Keats (1989)	Volatile/sufentanil	1012	Coronary bypass	No
Tuman *et al.* (1989a)	Volatile/i.v.	1094	Coronary bypass	No
Inoue *et al.* (1990)	Isoflurane/enflurane	1178	Coronary bypass	Yes
Leung *et al.* (1991)	Isoflurane/sufentanil	186	Coronary bypass	No
Helman *et al.* (1992)	Desflurane/sufentanil	200	Coronary bypass	No

* Pain relief by the epidural route was extended into the postoperative period. Spi., spinal anaesthesia; GA, general light; balanced anaesthesia; TEA, thoracic extradural anaesthesia.

mediated tachycardia. Interestingly, baseline sympathetic nerve activity directed to skeletal muscle blood vessels (MSNA) increased and at the same time nitrous oxide preserved the reflex augmentation in MSNA in response to nitroprusside. Seventy percent nitrous oxide substituted for nitrogen in 30% oxygen and added to enflurane, adjusted to keep anaesthetic dose at 1 MAC in vascular surgical patients with CAD, produced evidence of mild cardiodepression (Rydvall *et al.*, 1984). Addition of nitrous oxide to an opioid anaesthetic agent may result in severe circulatory depression, the mechanism of which has still not been clarified (Bovill *et al.*, 1984b).

There are few investigations of the coronary circulatory effects of nitrous oxide. Wilkowski and colleagues (1987) published animal data on regional myocardial blood flow at different nitrous oxide concentrations. By the use of microangiographic techniques, these authors found that 60% nitrous oxide constricted epicardial coronary arteries. Philbin and colleagues (1985) studied dogs who had received high-dose fentanyl or sufentanil anaesthesia and observed postsystolic shortening in the region supplied by a narrowed coronary artery when nitrous oxide was substituted for nitrogen. Coronary perfusion pressure, heart rate, LV filling pressure and regional coronary blood flow remained unchanged. Thus, there was no indication of a direct coronary vasoconstrictive effect of nitrous oxide. The results suggest, but are not diagnostic of nitrous oxide-

induced myocardial ischaemia. In comparison, other more recent data collected in dogs administered isoflurane demonstrate that nitrous oxide produced LV segmental wall dysfunction only in the presence of decreased coronary perfusion pressure (Nathan, 1988, 1989). The magnitude of blood pressure reduction associated with new mechanical dysfunction in these studies was, however, well within limits well tolerated in clinical practice.

Preliminary results which partly agree with these animal data and with the report by Bovill and colleagues (1984b) have recently been obtained in vascular surgical patients with CAD randomized to anaesthesia with isoflurane/fentanyl with or without nitrous oxide (Hohner *et al.*, 1993b). After induction of anaesthesia but before the start of surgery there were no haemodynamic differences between the groups and the incidence of myocardial ischaemia by 12-lead ECG, myocardial lactate and/or new anterior LV wall motion abnormalities was identical. During surgical stimulation, however, the patients administered 60% nitrous oxide in oxygen demonstrated a much greater need for supplemental nitroglycerine to treat LV dysfunction and more myocardial ischaemia than those given an air/oxygen mixture. These observations were made at comparable total MAC levels in the two groups and suggest that nitrous oxide impaired LV function during the stress of surgery. The most likely explanation is that the cardiodepressant effect of nitrous oxide dominates over its sympathomimetic action in the face of increased sympathetic activity.

At first sight, these data appear to be in conflict with results from three recent studies employing TOE to document new systolic wall-motion abnormalities during anaesthesia for coronary bypass surgery in patients with normal or impaired LV function (Cahalan *et al.*, 1987; Slavik *et al.*, 1988; Mitchell *et al.*, 1989). As in the investigation by Hohner and colleagues (1993b), none of these studies documented new systolic wall-motion abnormalities during the period preceeding the start of surgery. Unfortunately, no data were collected during surgery. One other recent study has documented ECG and TOE data during carotid artery surgery (Kozmary *et al.*, 1990). The authors were unable to demonstrate any difference in the incidence of ischaemia in patients randomized to nitrous oxide/oxygen/isoflurane or oxygen/isoflurane. However, isoflurane concentrations were significantly higher in the isoflurane/oxygen group which could have influenced the results. Furthermore, the lack of specificity of systolic wall motion abnormalities for myocardial ischaemia during increased loading conditions was not respected (see monitoring section, p. 1250). The data by Hohner and colleagues, which agree with much clinical experience in major vascular surgery, therefore await further scientific confirmation.

The study by Hohner and colleagues (1993b) also examined the coronary haemodynamic effects of nitrous oxide in the presence of isoflurane and fentanyl in an effort to explain the finding of an increased incidence of myocardial ischaemia. There was, however, no evidence of any coronary haemodynamic effect induced by nitrous oxide in the setting of their study. This contrasts with data by Rydvall and colleagues (1984) who studied the influence of nitrous oxide in the presence of enflurane in comparable patients. They observed that regional coronary blood flow distribution was altered towards awake values by nitrous oxide, indicating that this agent counteracted the coronary vasodilating action of enflurane.

Extradural/subarachnoid anaesthesia

In general, the circulatory effects of spinal or extradural anaesthesia are dependent on:
1 The degree to which the block affects the regulation of vasomotor tone.
2 Whether or not the block affects the cardiac sympathetic nervous outflow to the heart.
3 Whether or not the block is combined with general anaesthesia.

4 The amount of local anaesthetic agent absorbed from the site of injection or inadvertently injected or released into the systemic circulation.
5 Whether vasoconstrictors are added to the local anaesthetic agent.
6 The relationship between vascular volume and circulating blood volume.
7 The patient's cardiac medication, in particular the use of ACE inhibitors and β-blocking drugs.

The onset of haemodynamic changes following spinal anaesthesia is more rapid and may therefore be more pronounced than those recorded in association with extradural analgesia. However, qualitatively they are similar. Extradural analgesia has been refined to a degree where the caudal, lumbar, thoracic and cervical regions may be blocked selectively. Extradural anaesthesia therefore provides the best model for the understanding of the circulatory effects of sympathetic denervation by local anaesthetic agents at different levels of the spinal cord.

Block of the lumbar sympathetic nervous outflow results in reduction of arterial and venous tone in the blocked area and reduced venous return to the heart. Recent data suggest that central hypovolaemia leading to a reduction of venous return during extradural anaesthesia may be responsible for the profound bradycardia observed in some patients (Jakobsen *et al.*, 1992). Animal experimentation has demonstrated that this protective reflex during central hypovolaemia which causes a decrease in heart rate and sympathetic activity is vagal and originates from mechanoreceptors in the left ventricle (Öberg & White, 1970). These findings agree with the observation that bradycardia during extradural anaesthesia is associated with marked decrease in LV diameter and concomitant increase in vagally mediated polypeptides (Jakobsen *et al.*, 1992). Thus, severe bradycardia during spinal/extradural anaesthesia should be treated with volume alone and possibly a vasopressor, increasing venous return, rather than with atropine. A reflex increase of vascular tone in nonblocked areas has been described in both animal experimentation models and in humans (Sjögren & Wright, 1972; Ottesen *et al.*, 1978). Hypotension can be corrected by intravenous infusion of fluids and/or by the use of vasopressors. Baron and colleagues (1987) presented data on the effects of lumbar extradural anaesthesia and volume loading on global and regional LV function of patients with stable CAD. These patients had slightly depressed EFs compared with patients without cardiac disease (mean EF 0.54 as compared with 0.64), assessed by gated bloodpool scintigraphic techniques. The authors found that a block which did not reach the level of the cardiac sympathetic nervous outflow to the heart resulted in improvement of both global and regional LV function as indicated by an improved EF and less asynergy of the left ventricle (Table 60.19).

This occurred despite a reduction in cardiac and stroke-volume indices and was combined always with a decreased arterial pressure. In contrast, normal patients who had similar systemic haemodynamic changes demonstrated an unchanged ejection fraction. Volume loading of the patients with CAD resulted in restoration of systemic haemodynamics and global and regional LV function to pre-extradural values. This study illustrates the beneficial effects on LV performance of reducing impedance to LV ejection and LV end-diastolic volume. Conflicting data have recently been presented by another French group. Saada and colleagues (1989) investigated the global and regional functional effects of lumbar extradural anaesthesia by the use of echocardiography in patients with peripheral vascular disease and CAD. The block extended over the same segments as that by Baron and colleagues (1987) and resulted in identical haemodynamic changes. Nevertheless, four of the 10 patients demonstrated impaired LV wall function at the peak of the haemodynamic changes, paralleled in a few patients by ECG changes, all suggestive of myocardial ischaemia. In the remaining patients, the unloading of the left ventricle resulted in increased systolic wall motion, similar to that which was described by Baron and colleagues (1987). The reasons for the conflicting results are most likely found in the differences in patient population. Whereas Baron and colleagues studied orthopaedic patients with stable CAD, Saada and colleagues had

selected vascular patients who are known to have a high prevalence of more severe, widespread and/or diffuse coronary disease than other patient populations (Hertzer et al., 1984). The data from these two studies also illustrate the danger of accepting absolute or derived limits for the degree of blood pressure reduction which should be accepted in patients with CAD.

The cardiac sympathetic outflow emerges from the C5 to T5 levels with the main supply to the ventricles from T1 and T2 (Randall et al., 1957). It has been suggested previously that the sympathetic block in extradural and spinal anaesthesia spreads a couple of segments rostrally to the limit of sensory block (Greene, 1958). However, recent data have demonstrated that the sympathetic block following spinal anaesthesia may spread up to 10 segments cranially to the somatic block (Chamberlain & Chamberlain, 1986). These findings may explain why pure α-agonists and fluid loading reverse hypotension only partially in some patients with sensory loss in low thoracic and lumbar regions.

Hotvedt and colleagues (1983) studied the electrophysiological effects of thoracic extradural analgesia with bupivacaine in pentobarbital-anaesthetized dogs. They found a prolongation of the cardiac action potential and force of contraction similar to that recorded after β-adrenergic block. Thoracic extradural analgesia performed after pharmacological beta block resulted in additive effects on the action potential prolongation and force of contraction (Hotvedt et al., 1984). Intravenous administration of bupivacaine to a plasma concentration similar to that recorded after extradural analgesia in the same animal model did not result in haemodynamic or electrophysiological

Table 60.19 Cardiac functional effects of lumbar extradural analgesia and volume loading in normal subjects (Group I) and patients with coronary artery disease (Group II). (Data from Baron et al., 1987)

		Control	Extradural analgesia	
			Before volume loading	After volume loading
Stroke-volume index (ml/m^2)	Group I	51 ± 4	38 ± 3	44 ± 2
	Group II	48 ± 3	39 ± 3	43 ± 3
End-diastolic volume (ml)	Group I	75 ± 4	59 ± 2	70 ± 3
	Group II	88 ± 7	69 ± 6	71 ± 7
End-systolic volume (ml)	Group I	28 ± 3	22 ± 2	26 ± 3
	Group II	43 ± 5	32 ± 5	39 ± 4
LV ejection fraction (%)	Group I	64 ± 2	65 ± 3	64 ± 3
	Group II	54 ± 2	59 ± 3	54 ± 2

changes (Hotvedt *et al.*, 1985). The results conflict partly with data by Wattwil and colleagues (1985) who investigated the circulatory effects of thoracic extradural analgesia from T1 to T5 with bupivacaine in healthy volunteers. They then compared them with those recorded after intramuscular injections of the drug to comparable plasma concentrations in the same subjects. These authors found the extradural block to produce a 33% reduction of cardiac output compared with 20% after intramuscular injection of bupivacaine. They concluded that part of the haemodynamic effects were due to systemic resorption of the local anaesthetic agent.

Reiz (1985) investigated the effects of thoracic extradural analgesia from T1 to T5 with bupivacaine on cardiac performance in vascular surgical patients with CAD. Arterial pressure, PCWP and heart rate were maintained at pre-extradural values by intravenous administration of phenylephrine and nitroglycerine and atrial pacing. In this experimental setting, the block decreased cardiac output (approximately contractility) by about 20% and myocardial oxygen consumption by 25% without signs of an altered coronary vascular tone. Earlier studies from the same group of investigators in similar patients (Reiz *et al.*, 1979) have shown that thoracic extradural anaesthesia from T1 to T12 may result in hypotension which can be reversed only partly by selective β_1-agonism, which does not alter systemic vascular resistance. These findings support the suggestions that a combination of vasodilatation and cardiodepression is responsible for the hypotension following thoracic extradural analgesia. Under conditions of impaired LV function, unloading of the impedance to ejection for the left ventricle may dominate over the cardiodepressant

effect of the block. This may result in significant improvement of cardiac output (Fig. 60.14).

Cervical extradural analgesia produces vasodilatation in areas of the body which, under resting conditions, contribute insignificantly to venous return in comparison with the splanchnic and lower-limb regions. The orthostatic reaction is largely unaffected by cervical extradural analgesia (Fig. 60.15) and exercising capacity is reduced only slightly (Ottesen, 1978). Takeshima and Dohi (1985) investigated the circulatory responses to baroreflexes, Valsava manoeuvre and sympathetic stimulation during acute cardiac sympathectomy by extradural analgesia from C4 to T7 with lignocaine in healthy volunteers. Compared with individuals who had lumbar extradural anaesthesia, they found the cardiac sympathetic block to be associated with a slightly depressed baroreceptor function following the pressor test to phenylephrine. The depressor test to nitroglycerine was not affected by the block. Partly in contrast to what was reported by Sundberg and Wattwil (1986), the authors found the responses in heart rate and arterial pressure to Valsalva manoeuvre and sympathetic stimulation to be suppressed slightly by the block. No predominant parasympathetic reactions were observed following any of the manoeuvres performed during cervical extradural analgesia. Therefore, Takeshima and Dohi (1985) concluded that the sympathetic control of heart rate serves as an inhibitor of the vagus rather than as an active cardiac accelerator.

Addition of general anaesthesia to lumbar or thoracocervical extradural analgesia may result in profound hypotension. The order of performance of the anaesthetic procedures does not seem to affect

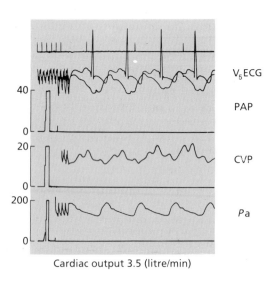

Cardiac output 3.5 (litre/min)

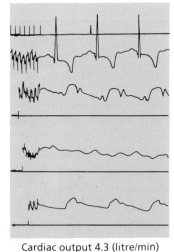

Cardiac output 4.3 (litre/min)

Fig. 60.14 Circulatory effects of adding thoracic extradural anaesthesia (right panel) to a patient with coronary artery disease during myocardial ischaemia caused by abdominal surgical stimulation (left panel). Reduction of arterial blood pressure (*Pa*) unloaded the left ventricle, resulting in reduction of pulmonary artery diastolic and central venous pressures, increase of cardiac output and lesser ST-depression.

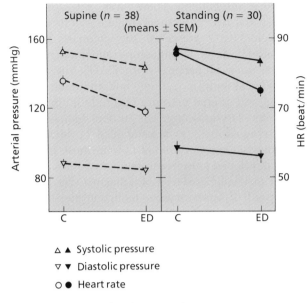

Δ ▲ Systolic pressure

▽ ▼ Diastolic pressure

○ ● Heart rate

Upper level: C4.1 ± 1.3

Lower level: T5.3 ± 1.2 (means ± SD)

Fig. 60.15 Changes in heart rate (HR) and blood pressure produced by cardiac sympathectomy with bupivacaine administered extradurally (ED) to surgical patients. Systolic blood pressure and heart rate were decreased significantly ($p < 0.001$) by the block but orthostatic function remained intact. C, control.

the magnitude of haemodynamic changes (Germann et al., 1979). The predominant mechanism for the hypotension is withdrawal of the increased vascular tone in non-blocked areas. If general anaesthetic agents which possess direct negative inotropic and vasodilating actions are utilized, these properties may contribute further to hypotension. Thoracic extradural anaesthesia combined with fentanyl/nitrous oxide anaesthesia in patients with CAD taking beta blockers, results in greater circulatory depression than recorded in similar patients without beta block (Reiz et al., 1982c).

The first report of the coronary circulation during anaesthesia studied the effects of lumbar spinal anaesthesia (Hackel et al., 1956). The block decreased coronary blood flow in proportion to the reduction of the peripheral determinants of myocardial oxygen demand, mainly afterload. Thoracic extradural anaesthesia from T1 to T12 in patients with CAD resulted in considerable reduction of coronary perfusion pressure and evidence of coronary vasodilatation disproportional to the decline in myocardial oxygen consumption (Reiz et al., 1980). The coronary vasodilatation is explained best by inadequate coronary perfusion pressure, as similar patients with control

of coronary perfusion pressure to pre-extradural values did not demonstrate a decline in coronary vascular tone (Reiz, 1985). In animal experimentation models of acute myocardial infarction, however, thoracic extradural anaesthesia including the upper thoracic segments has been demonstrated to redistribute blood from subepicardial to subendocardial areas of the myocardium (Klassen et al., 1980) and to reduce infarct size (Davis et al., 1986). The group headed by Ricksten has recently provided a large body of animal and clinical data on the effects of high extradural anaesthesia in ischaemic heart disease (Blomberg et al., 1989, 1990; Kock et al., 1990). In keeping with previous electrophysiological findings, they have demonstrated that high extradural anaesthesia decreases ventricular arrhythmias in experimental myocardial ischaemia. In addition, the neural block abolishes chest pain in patients with unstable angina pectoris and decreases the magnitude of ischaemia and improves LV function during bicycle exercise testing. The mechanism for alleviation of myocardial ischaemia has been proposed to be linked to a direct vasodilator effect in dynamic coronary artery stenoses (Blomberg et al., 1990). Since high extradural anaesthesia also reduces the two most important contributors to myocardial oxygen requirements, contractility and heart rate, it appears as if both myocardial oxygen demand and supply are shifted in a favourable direction.

All available data indicate that extradural anaesthesia might preserve LV function and reduce the incidence of myocardial ischaemia provided coronary perfusion pressure is well controlled. Several studies published over the past decade (Reiz et al., 1982a; Yeager et al., 1987; Baron et al., 1991; Tuman et al., 1991) have tried to establish if these effects could have a beneficial influence on cardiac outcome after non-cardiac surgery. The results of these studies are conflicting. At the present time it appears as if the choice of extradural anaesthesia for surgery does not influence outcome, whereas extension of neural block into the postoperative period might be associated with improved cardiac outcome. Large multicentre studies are required to finally establish if, and by which mechanisms, extradural anaesthesia could reduce cardiac morbidity after surgery.

Effects of interventions during anaesthesia

Laryngoscopy, tracheal intubation and extubation, and the stress of surgery produce circulatory changes which are often more pronounced than those elicited by anaesthetic drugs. In general, these perturbations are associated with release of noradrenaline and adrenaline, manifested by increased arterial pressure, heart rate and cardiac output. In patients with cardiac disease, cardiac failure and myocardial ischaemia frequently accompany the increase in resistance to LV ejection and the tachycardia. Until recently, the ischaemia has been regarded to be a consequence of excess demand rather than of inadequate supply of oxygen to the myocardium. Moffitt and colleagues (1985) studied patients with CAD and preserved LV function anaesthetized with halothane or morphine during laryngoscopy and intubation. Despite increases of the peripheral determinants of myocardial oxygen demand, the authors did not record any change in coronary blood flow. Oxygen demand was met by increased myocardial extraction suggesting the presence of an increased coronary vascular tone. Kleinmann and colleagues (1986) investigated the effects of tracheal intubation on myocardial perfusion assessed by thallium scintigraphy. The authors studied patients with CAD induced with thiopentone/halothane or high-dose fentanyl. Despite absence of systemic haemodynamic changes, 45% of their patients had evidence of regional hypoperfusion following intubation. There was no difference between the two anaesthetic regimens. Lowenstein and Reiz (1987) presented the coronary haemodynamic effects of laryngoscopy and intubation in vascular surgical patients with CAD. Anaesthesia was induced with thiopentone and enflurane or isoflurane, and arterial pressure was reduced by about 30% before laryngoscopy. The authors demonstrated that laryngoscopy was accompanied by immediate reductions in coronary blood flow in those patients who developed electrocardiographic, mechanical and/or metabolic evidence of ischaemia (Fig. 60.16). The speed of onset of flow reduction suggested a neurogenically mediated vasoconstriction. In contrast, patients who did not become ischaemic had no reduction of coronary blood flow despite comparable systemic haemodynamic changes. The data from these three clinical studies suggest that increased coronary vascular tone with decreased myocardial oxygen supply rather than excess oxygen demand is responsible for myocardial ischaemia during laryngoscopy and tracheal intubation. Consequently, therapeutic approaches to prevent coronary vasospasm might be an effective adjunct to interventions

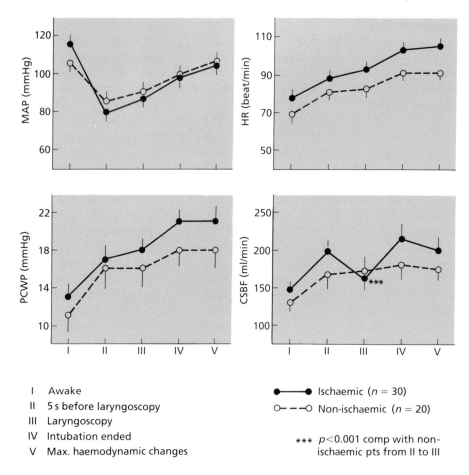

I   Awake
II   5 s before laryngoscopy
III Laryngoscopy
IV   Intubation ended
V   Max. haemodynamic changes

●——● Ischaemic (n = 30)
○– ––○ Non-ischaemic (n = 20)

*** p<0.001 comp with non-ischaemic pts from II to III

Fig. 60.16 Systemic and coronary haemodynamic changes before, during and following laryngoscopy and tracheal intubation in 30 patients who became ischaemic and 20 matched patients who did not. Coronary blood flow decreased rapidly and transiently with laryngoscopy in patients who developed ischaemia, suggesting a neurogenic mechanism. For further discussion see text. (Data from Lowenstein & Reiz, 1987.)

aimed at controlling myocardial oxygen demand in order to reduce further the incidence of myocardial ischaemia associated with laryngoscopy and tracheal intubation.

Only a few investigations report coronary vascular responses to surgery. The same lack of agreement exists between studies as previously noted in the haemodynamic effects of surgery.

Moffitt and colleagues (1984a) reported the systemic and coronary haemodynamic effects of sternotomy in patients anaesthetized with high-dose fentanyl, 75 µg/kg, followed by a continuous infusion at 10 µg · kg^{-1} · h^{-1}. Surgical stimulation did not result in any systemic or coronary circulatory changes, nor was myocardial ischaemia observed in any of the 10 patients. Sonntag and colleagues (1982) found that seven of nine patients anaesthetized for CABG with high-dose fentanyl, 100 µg/kg, given as a bolus during induction, developed myocardial lactate production in association with sternotomy. At the same measurement period, Heikkilä and colleagues (1985b), who studied similar patients under the same format and dose of anaesthesia, with the exception that 25% of the fentanyl was administered immediately before skin incision, observed lactate production in one of 12 patients only. There was a moderate and comparable increase in arterial pressure in the two studies. However, Sonntag's patients demonstrated a 22 beats/min rise in heart rate compared with an unchanged heart rate in Heikkilä's patients. The data from these three studies emphasize the importance of controlling heart rate to avoid myocardial ischaemia.

In the study by Wilkinson and colleagues (1981), sternotomy during halothane/nitrous oxide anaesthesia was associated with increases in coronary perfusion pressure, myocardial oxygen consumption and coronary blood flow. Heart rate remained unchanged. The rise in coronary blood flow was inadequate as shown by increased myocardial oxygen extraction and myocardial ischaemia was observed in nine of the 14 patients. In similar patients investigated by Hilfiker and colleagues (1983), sternotomy during halothane/nitrous oxide anaesthesia was not associated with either systemic or coronary haemodynamic changes, nor was ischaemia detected in any patient.

Moffitt and colleagues (1984b) did not observe any systemic or coronary haemodynamic effects of sternotomy during enflurane/oxygen anaesthesia. Heikkilä and colleagues (1985a) studied the effects of sternotomy during enflurane/oxygen anaesthesia, supplemented with fentanyl, 2.5 µg/kg, in similar patients. These authors found that surgical stimu-

lation produced increases by 18% of heart rate and of 43% in coronary perfusion pressure accompanied by a 47% rise in myocardial oxygen consumption and a 41% increase in coronary blood flow. Myocardial oxygen extraction remained stable and none of the 12 patients had evidence of myocardial ischaemia as detected by myocardial lactate production or ECG ST-segment changes. In comparison, patients with CAD subjected to major vascular surgical procedures during enflurane/nitrous oxide anaesthesia did not demonstrate any change in heart rate or coronary blood flow despite increases in systemic pressure and PCWP and hence myocardial oxygen requirements (Reiz et al., 1985). Myocardial oxygenation was maintained adequately as judged by unchanged ECG and myocardial lactate extraction, by a pronounced increase in oxygen extraction to awake values.

One of few randomized studies compared the systemic and coronary circulatory effects of enflurane and isoflurane/nitrous oxide anaesthesia in patients undergoing CABG (Larsen et al., 1984). Both agents produced similar systemic haemodynamic changes. There was evidence of a greater coronary vasodilating effect of isoflurane. With sternotomy, important differences became apparent. As in the study cited above (Reiz et al., 1983), myocardial oxygen extraction increased to awake values in enflurane patients. Lactate extraction remained normal in all patients. In contrast, myocardial oxygen extraction remained profoundly decreased in isoflurane patients, demonstrating persistent coronary vasodilatation during surgery. Myocardial lactate production was observed in three of the 10 isoflurane patients.

Systemic haemodynamic changes caused by abdominal incision were similar in vascular surgical patients with CAD allocated randomly to receive halothane or isoflurane/nitrous oxide anaesthesia according to a double-blind protocol (Hohner et al., 1993a). However, the coronary haemodynamic changes were markedly different. In halothane patients, coronary autoregulation was maintained and both coronary blood flow and myocardial oxygen extraction increased to meet with the increased demand for oxygen caused by surgical stimulation (Fig. 60.5). In contrast to these findings and similarly to the results by Larsen and colleagues (1984), the isoflurane patients demonstrated persistent coronary vasodilatation during surgery.

In summary, laryngoscopy, tracheal intubation and surgical stimulation have profound effects on the coronary circulation of patients with CAD. Part of the effects may be explained from the systemic haemodynamic changes induced by these perturbations.

However, coronary blood flow reduction may occur without systemic haemodynamic changes. These findings suggest that coronary vasospasm exists also in anaesthetized patients. It seems to be particularly common during laryngoscopy and tracheal intubation. Coronary autoregulation is preserved adequately during high-dose fentanyl anaesthesia and seems effective also during halothane and enflurane anaesthesia. In contrast, patients anaesthetized with isoflurane have evidence of coronary vasodilatation even with obvious signs of myocardial tissue deprivation. It appears, therefore, as if myocardial hypoperfusion and hyperfusion may coexist during isoflurane anaesthesia.

Prediction of cardiac risk from perioperative events

Most documentation available in which intra-anaesthetic cardiac events have been compared with postoperative outcome has been collected in patients subjected to coronary bypass surgery. It can be questioned if such data can be transferred to non-cardiac surgery. The dominating risk factor for postoperative cardiac morbidity (e.g. myocardial infarction) in these studies was myocardial ischaemia, as detected by new ECG ST-segment changes, noted during the period from arrival into the operating room till the patient was on bypass (Slogoff & Keats, 1985, 1986). Other, non-anaesthetic cardiac risk factors were the duration of myocardial ischaemia during aortic cross-clamping and the surgeon's estimate of the quality of the distal coronary anastomosis. The incidence of new, electrocardiographically detected, myocardial ischaemia in the two studies from the same authors was 37% and 55%, respectively. The incidence of perioperative infarction was related directly to the degree of ST-segment depression (Table 60.20). Haemodynamic aberrations, most commonly tachycardia, were associated with myocardial ischaemia in approxi-

mately 50% of instances of myocardial oxygen deprivation. Neither hypotension nor hypertension correlated with ischaemia. More interestingly, approximately 50% of the ischaemic events were unrelated to haemodynamic aberrations, suggesting non-metabolically related reduction of coronary blood flow (e.g. coronary vasospasm) as the cause of ischaemia. It indicates also that ischaemia cannot always be prevented by optimizing systemic haemodynamics (Fig. 60.17).

In non-cardiac surgery, mainly vascular, the incidence of intra-anaesthetic myocardial ischaemia, detected by the ECG, has been reported to be in the same range as for coronary bypass surgery (Roy *et al.*, 1979; Coriat *et al.*, 1982). With more sophisticated technology for diagnosis of ischaemia, vascular surgical patients with CAD have been documented to have an incidence around 70% (Häggmark *et al.*, 1989). Almost one-third of these episodes were detected before induction of anaesthesia and were not accompanied by haemodynamic changes, chest pain, or discomfort. Recent data from the SPI research group in San Francisco have demonstrated that intraoperative ischaemia correlated with postoperative myocardial ischaemia but was a poor predictor of adverse cardiac outcome in patients with documented or suspected CAD undergoing non-cardiac surgery

Table 60.20 Relationship between degree of ST-segment depression and incidence of perioperative myocardial infarction (PMI). (Data from Slogoff & Keats, 1985)

	Perioperative ST-segment depression		
	None	0.10−0.19 mV	≥0.20 mV
Number of patients	646	291	86
Incidence of PMI (%)*	2.5	6.2	9.3

* $p < 0.005$ by multiple chi-squared (χ^2).

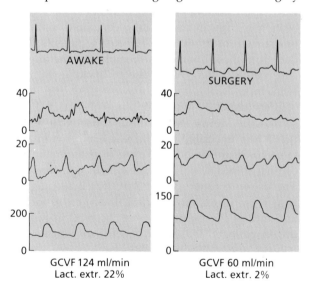

GCVF 124 ml/min
Lact. extr. 22%

GCVF 60 ml/min
Lact. extr. 2%

Fig. 60.17 The V_5 ECG, pulmonary artery, central venous and arterial pressures (top to bottom), awake (left panel) and during abdominal surgery (right panel) in a patient with coronary artery disease. ST-segment depression and metabolic changes suggestive of ischaemia developed despite comparable heart rate, pulmonary artery-occluded pressure and systemic blood pressure. The pronounced decline in blood flow through the territory perfused by the left anterior descending coronary artery (GCVF) suggests coronary vasospasm as the mechanism for ischaemia.

(Mangano *et al.*, 1990). In comparison, postoperative myocardial ischaemia correlated closely with both immediate and long-term cardiac morbidity after surgery (Browner *et al.*, 1992; Mangano *et al.*, 1992a). These findings appear logical for several reasons; (i) intraoperative myocardial ischaemia is considerably less common than postoperative ischaemia and is therefore outweighed in a multiple regression analysis; (ii) the postoperative period is more stressful than either daily life, the preinduction or the intra-operative periods. Patients with overt and covert CAD are therefore more likely to display and have their coronary disease documented at this time than at any other time. Because CAD, independent of the patient's age, is associated with decreased life expectancy, it is not surprising that patients who display myocardial ischaemic events would have worse short-, intermediate- and long-term cardiac outcome than those who do not (Mangano *et al.*, 1992a).

It has recently been documented that strict control of systemic haemodynamic variables decreases the incidence of peri-operative myocardial ischaemia (Leung *et al.*, 1991). There is, however, still no data confirming that this results in decreased cardiac morbidity. Much data also support the assumption that myocardial ischaemia may develop even with strict control of haemodynamic variables. Myocardial ischaemia caused by coronary vasodilating agents which redistribute coronary blood flow is easily avoidable by not using such agents in patients with the anatomical basis for coronary steal (e.g. an occluded territory perfused by collaterals via a stenosed coronary artery). The possibility of treating or preventing intra-anaesthetic coronary vasospasm has not been analysed yet. This field seems to be of particular interest to explore as haemodynamically related and unrelated episodes of ischaemia carry the same risk of perioperative myocardial infarction (Slogoff & Keats, 1986).

Anaesthetic management

Monitoring

Most patients with CAD require no more physiological surveillance than that which is now standard for the general population. Invasive arterial monitoring is indicated if rapid blood loss or pharmacological manipulation of circulation is anticipated.

In some populations with known or suspected CAD, in particular the vascular surgical patient, there is a need for more precise monitoring of myocardial ischaemia, volume status and LV function. It is useful to apply some non-routine preoperative tests in order to identify patients who need these additional monitoring devices. For instance, it is our practice to examine preoperative LV function by transthoracic two-dimensional echocardiography as this allows a good estimation of which patients are at risk for intra- and postoperative failure. Similar information can be obtained from nuclear ventriculography (Pasternack *et al.*, 1984; Pedersen *et al.*, 1990). There are several recent studies which have evaluated if preoperative Holter ECG ST-segment recording can identify patients at risk for perioperative myocardial ischaemia and subsequent major ischaemic complications (Pasternack *et al.*, 1989; Raby *et al.*, 1989, 1992; Fleisher *et al.*, 1991). The results of these studies show that this test has a high negative predictive value (89−99%), i.e. that patients with CAD who do not display new ischaemic ST-segment changes in daily life have little risk of having peri-operative myocardial ischaemia. Fleisher and colleagues (1991) compared the results obtained in vascular versus non-vascular patients. They demonstrated a lower negative predictive value of preoperative myocardial ischaemia in the former than in the latter group (89% versus 99%), whereas the positive predictive value was identical (38%). In comparison, the negative predictive value of a standard 12-lead resting ECG in vascular surgical patients with CAD is in the order of 90% (Reiz, 1993, personal communication). Although some studies have demonstrated a good positive predictive value of new ST-segment depression on Holter ECG (Raby *et al.*, 1992) for perioperative cardiac morbidity, most studies report it to be disappointingly low. Evidently, the positive predictive value is a function of the incidence of perioperative myocardial ischaemia and the patient population in which the technique is applied. The usefulness of the Holter ECG as we see it is thus, to denote low-risk CAD patients and to identify whether or not myocardial ischaemia in daily life is heart-rate dependent or not. In the case of the former, the anaesthetist will be alerted to the heart rate at which ischaemia might develop; in the case of the latter, the ischaemia is probably spasm related and the patient might benefit from calcium-channel block therapy prior to surgery.

The use of a pulmonary artery catheter (PAC) for the monitoring of volume status and ventricular function during non-cardiac surgery has been under intense debate ever since the notion that this device could lead to increased morbidity (Robin, 1985). This concern is not primarily related to the fairly infrequent technical complications of pulmonary artery catheterization but rather to the fact that values derived from the PAC might not represent what they are thought to represent. Therefore, it is mainly the therapy guided from these measurements that could cause morbidity. This could be one reason to explain why patients with normal or impaired LV function undergoing coronary bypass surgery with medical and volume therapy directed from a PAC did not have lower cardiovascular morbidity than those in whom the central venous pressure was used to guide therapy (Tuman et al., 1989b).

During anaesthesia hypovolaemia occurs frequently without being accompanied by tachycardia. This is mainly because anaesthetics depress baroreflexes and because the right atrial volume receptors are unloaded by the decrease in venous return. It has only recently been recognized that the PAOP poorly reflects preload when mechanical ventilation is used during and after surgery. There are several reasons why PAOP can over-estimate LV end-diastolic pressure at this time: (i) hypovolaemia leads to displacement of the PAC tip from the west zone 3 towards zone 2 or 1. Thereby, the measured pressure reflects alveolar rather than intravascular pressure; (ii) atrial contraction makes an important contribution to LV filling during hypovolaemia. This increases the LV to pulmonary arteriolar pressure gradient; (iii) if tachycardia develops, the premature closure of the mitral valve increases the left atrial to LV pressure gradient while the shortened pressure equilibration time leads to a pressure gradient between the left atrium and the pulmonary artery; (iv) hypovolaemia is often accompanied by normal or elevated PAOP in the presence of LV hypertrophy which impairs LV compliance.

Accurate estimates of preload are readily available by the use of TOE as long as the patient is under anaesthesia or sedation. LV cross-sectional end-diastolic area measured at the level of the insertion of the papillary muscles has been shown to correlate well with end-diastolic volume measured by gated nuclear ventriculography (Urbanowicz et al., 1990). The preload information derived from the TOE is particularly useful during and after major vascular surgery since over 50% of this population has chronic hypertension with LV hypertrophy (Baron et al., 1991). If TOE is not available, the variation in systolic arterial pressure is a direct reflection of preload during mechanical ventilation. The initial phase of lung inflation augments the filling of the LV by squeezing the pulmonary veins at the same time as venous return to the right ventricle is reduced. Hypovolaemia augments the resulting influence on the systolic blood pressure variation. Both experimentally

and clinically, the magnitude of systolic blood pressure variation during positive-pressure ventilation (i.e. Δ down, Fig. 60.18) has been shown to correlate closely with preload derived from the TOE. Although PAOP reliably reflected preload changes during graded haemorrhage in dogs (Perel et al., 1987), this was not the case in vascular surgical patients studied postoperatively during mechanical ventilation (Vrillon et al., 1990).

Measurements of stroke volume and PAOP by the PAC have long been used to assess LV function during and after anaesthesia. LV dysfunction could be described as systolic and/or diastolic. The former is the result of decreased inotropy and/or increased LV impedance. In most instances of systolic dysfunction, end-systolic and end-diastolic volumes increase in parallel, resulting in little change of stroke volume. Diastolic dysfunction is characterized by LV stiffness resulting in an increased PAOP. However, other mechanisms, such as volume overload or systolic dysfunction requiring completely different therapy could also cause an elevation of PAOP. The filling of the LV requires an elevated left atrial pressure when LV compliance is reduced. Therefore, even a minor fall in venous return may lead to a major reduction of LV size resulting in inadequate LV ejection. Such an event is only rarely reflected by a noticeable decrease in PAOP. All these considerations explain why construction of haemodynamic profiles or LV function curves using data derived from the PAC have serious limitations. TOE provides important additional information when estimation of LV function is needed, since the technique allows fairly precise measures of end-diastolic and end-systolic volumes (Urbanowicz et al., 1990). Hence, the mechanisms behind a low cardiac output measured by thermodilution or an elevated PAOP can be more clearly understood. As regards the diagnosis of systolic dysfunction, TOE allows on-line information. In comparison detection of diastolic dysfunction is more difficult since the Doppler flow pattern over the mitral valve is affected by the preload changes which frequently occur during anaesthesia and surgery. Nevertheless, a beat-to-beat assessment of LV filling pattern allows the anaesthetist a better understanding of the changes related to volume loading, myocardial ischaemia and vasopressor and/or intropic interventions. A summary of the accuracy of the PAC and the TOE to diagnose various circulatory aberrations is presented in Table 60.21.

There is strong experimental and clinical evidence that myocardial ischaemia leads to regional mechanical ventricular dysfunction and stunning which

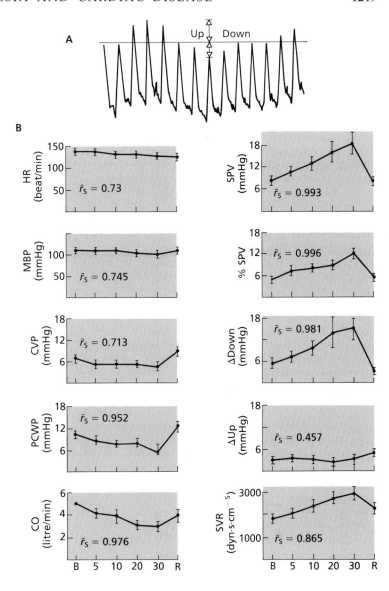

Fig. 60.18 (A) The definition of the Δ up and Δ down components of systolic pressure ventilation following positive-pressure ventilation. The horizontal reference line indicates systolic blood pressure during end-expiration. (B) Effects of graded haemorrhage and retransfusion during mechanical ventilation on: heart rate (HR), mean blood pressure (MBP), central venous pressure (CVP), pulmonary capillary wedge pressure (PCWP), cardiac output (CO), systolic pressure variation (SPV), percentage SPV (% SPV), Δ down component of SPV, Δ up component of SPV, and systemic vascular resistance (SVR). On the abscissae are the stages of the experiment: B_2 baseline after vest inflation: 5, 10, 20, and 30, the amount of blood removed as percent of blood volume; R, retransfusion of shed blood. For each parameter, the mean Spearman's rank coefficient correlation ($\bar{r}_s$) to haemorrhage is shown. (Summary of Figs 1 and 3, redrawn from Perel *et al.*, 1987.)

precede elevation of intraventricular pressure and ECG changes (Battler *et al.*, 1980; Wohlgelernter *et al.*, 1986). However, these findings do not suggest that all

Table 60.21 Ability of the pulmonary artery catheter (PAC) and transoesophageal echocardiography (TOE) to detect various states of perioperative circulatory abnormalities

	PAC	TOE
LV dysfunction	Moderate	High
Risk of acute pulmonary oedema	High	Not useful
Hypovolaemia	Poor	High
Myocardial ischaemia	Moderate	Poor
Assessment of diastolic wall stress	High	Not useful

LV, left ventricular.

new systolic wall motion abnormalities (SWMA) are of ischaemic origin. Recent experimental studies have demonstrated a lack of correlation between new SWMA and myocardial ischaemia in the presence of increased ventricular loading conditions (Buffington *et al.*, 1991; Lowenstein *et al.*, 1991). In addition, SWMAs are difficult to diagnose during tachycardia, the most common cause of myocardial ischaemia. In contrast to what has previously been generally accepted, the new SWMAs detected by TOE have recently been shown to have no better sensitivity and probably less specifity than multiple-lead ECG techniques (Table 60.22). Thus, at the present time, automated ST-segment analysis appears to be the simplest and most sensitive and specific way to monitor for myocardial ischaemia in the operating

Table 60.22 Percentage of new abnormalities regarded as indicators of myocardial ischaemia by various ischaemia monitoring techniques. Sixteen anaesthetized patients with proximal left anterior descending coronary artery stenosis were first paced to myocardial lactate production while arterial pressure was kept stable. Thereafter, while heart rate was kept constant at the control level, they had their arterial pressure increased or decreased, in a random fashion, to the same rate−pressure product (SAP × HR) and pressure rate ratio (MAP : HR), respectively, as calculated when myocardial lactate production first became evident during pacing. The results demonstrate that computerized vectorcardiography had the highest sensitivity for metabolically documented ischaemia during pacing followed by transoesophageal echocardiography (TOE). The 12-lead ECG was the least sensitive technique. During hypertension and hypotension, ischaemia by lactate production was far less common and only discovered on one occasion by the various monitoring techniques [i.e. by vector cardiography (VCG)]. Abnormalities by 12-lead ECG and TOE did not once coincide with myocardial lactate production during these two measurement periods. The reason for the low sensitivity of the 12-lead ECG compared to the VCG was probably that most ischaemia was confined to the interventricular septum (as seen by the TOE), which produces more R-wave amplitude changes than ST-segment depression during subendocardial ischaemia. (From unpublished data by Reiz and colleagues)

	End-point pacing	Max. arterial pressure	Min. arterial pressure
Myocardial lactate production	100	13	19
12-lead ECG	56	0	0
Computerized VCG	94	0	6
TOE	78	33	14

SAP, same arterial pressure; MAP, mean arterial pressure.

room and the postoperative care unit (Eisenberg *et al.*, 1992). If a three-lead system is available, the optimal leads to choose are V4, V5 and II, by which 96% of ischaemic ST-segment abnormalities detected by a standard 12-lead ECG are discovered (London *et al.*, 1988) (Fig. 60.19). Improvement in sensitivity beyond that of the 12-lead ECG can be obtained by alternative electrode positioning, possible only if the territory at risk is known, or by the use of a spatial technique such as vectorcardiography (Table 60.22).

Pre- and intraoperative management

The principles regarding patients with CAD for non-cardiac surgery and cardiac surgery are similar, i.e. the maintenance of circulatory stability at, or near, the patient's normal values, thereby reducing the risk of myocardial ischaemia.

Appropriate premedication is the key to avoiding preinduction ischaemia, which is otherwise a frequent problem (Mangano *et al.*, 1990). Bearing in mind that most preoperative ischaemia is silent (Mangano *et al.*, 1990, 1991; Muir *et al.*, 1991), i.e. not reported by the patient as chest pain but detected by the ECG, our practice is to give a single oral dose of a benzodiazepine the night before surgery followed by the same dose the next morning along with a subcutaneous injection of morphine and hyoscine. Also, the patient receives his or her regular cardiac medication with the exception of angiotensin-converting enzyme inhibitors which are stopped 24 h beore surgery to avoid exacerbating hypotension at induc-

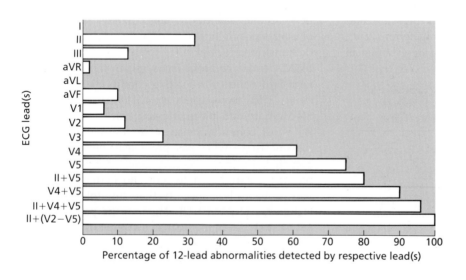

Fig. 60.19 Percentage of new ST-segment abnormalities on a 12-lead ECG detected by respective lead or lead combination. The results indicate that monitoring of lead I would not detect a single ischaemic event recorded by the 12-lead ECG, whereas the combination of II + V5 and II + V4 + V5 would pick up 80 and 96% of ischaemic events on the 12-lead ECG. Note, however, that the 12-lead ECG has poor sensitivity for ischaemia in the right ventricle, the interventricular septum and the higher parts of the posterior wall. Detection of ischaemia in these territories requires different electrode positioning or the use of spatial ECG techniques. (Data redrawn from London *et al.*, 1988.)

tion (Colson *et al.*, 1992). This approach will cause respiratory depression, thus the patient receives supplemental oxygen from the time of administration of morphine until induction. Even so, some patients exhibit low arterial oxygen saturation on arrival at the operating room but this has been shown to cause less myocardial ischaemia than tachycardia does (Entwistle *et al.*, 1992). Using this approach, our incidence of preinduction ischaemia is less than 1%.

Induction should produce minimal haemodynamic changes whilst preventing the adverse response to intubation and noxious stimuli. No single agent can achieve these aims. With the exception of ketamine, all other induction agents reduce myocardial oxygen requirements. This is by differential effects on inotrophy, heart rate, ventricular loading conditions and wall stress. The haemodynamic changes observed are principally a negative inotropic effect and depression of CNS activity, leading to decreased venous and arterial tone. In patients with LV hypertrophy, this can cause severe impairment of ventricular systolic function. High-dose opiate techniques offer haemodynamic stability but may not be suitable for non-cardiac surgery, though the efficacy of moderate doses of alfentanil have recently been demonstrated at induction (Chraemmer-Jørgensen *et al.*, 1992). The short-acting agents like thiopentone and propofol have been shown to produce hypotension and slight tachycardia, while not protecting against the stress of intubation (Martin *et al.*, 1982; Fusciardi *et al.*, 1986; Stone *et al.*, 1988). At equipotent doses, however, propofol has been shown to be less negatively inotropic than thiopentone (Park & Lynch, 1992). Hence, using a moderate dose of opiate with a small dose of benzodiazepine or thiopentone has been shown to achieve the desired effect (Fusciardi *et al.*, 1986). Non-anaesthetic adjuncts commonly used to blunt the haemodynamic changes are beta blockers (Cucchiara *et al.*, 1986; Stone *et al.*, 1988) and glyceryl trinitrate (Fusciardi *et al.*, 1986).

The choice of muscle relaxant is associated with few problems. Pancuronium has been reported to produce tachycardia and increase the risk of myocardial ischaemia but has little haemodynamic effect when administered with a combination of benzodiazepine and fentanyl (Thompson & Putnins, 1985). However, the combination of vecuronium and fentanyl has been shown to cause bradycardia (Salmenperä *et al.*, 1983). The mechanism of this is not yet fully understood.

The choice of primary maintenance agent is based on the same principle as the choice of induction agent. Having said that there has been no convincing study to show that the particular agent has any bearing on the outcome (Table 60.18). Therefore, when choosing volatile versus intravenous or general versus regional, it is logical to select a technique appropriate to the surgery. When using a volatile agent, we select isoflurane as it maintains left ventricular function better than halothane as seen on TOE (Brusset *et al.*, 1986; Smith *et al.*, 1988) and to infuse the opiate for continuous analgesia. If propofol is used to prevent awareness rather than isoflurane, it too is infused to minimize rapid haemodynamic changes. The depth of anaesthesia can be altered with either isoflurane or propofol according to the degree of surgical stimulation while allowing good recovery at the end of surgery. In choosing these drugs, the need for adjunctive hypotensive medication is reduced. The documented tachycardia associated with isoflurane does not appear to be a problem in this patient population using a balanced anaesthetic technique. In vascular surgical patients, we tend to use air rather than nitrous oxide after our work showing that nitrous oxide decreased ventricular function during surgical stimulation (Hohner *et al.*, 1993b).

For limb surgery central regional blocks are used. The extradural technique with divided doses is preferred since spinal anaesthesia often produces a rapid onset of haemodynamic changes. Experience is still limited with spinal catheters but these do seem to offer the advantage of a titratable block with low doses of local anaesthetic. For abdominal and thoracic surgery, general anaesthesia with an extradural catheter placed at the appropriate dermatome level for the anticipated pain is used. Nowadays, most frequently, extradural local anaesthetics are not administered during surgery but rather postoperatively in combination with opiates to provide pain relief, since they may cause profound hypotension when combined with general anaesthetics. Reiz and colleagues (1982a) showed that the incidence of intraoperative ischaemia was reduced when thoracic extradural anaesthesia was combined with light general anaesthesia compared to general anaesthesia alone, but that the combined technique did not improve cardiac outcome. These findings are supported by a recent study by Baron and colleagues (1991) but are in conflict with data by Yeager and colleagues (1987). It is probable that the benefit of adding extradural anaesthesia to general anaesthesia as regards the risk for major cardiac complications is entirely confined to the ability to provide good postoperative pain relief by this technique (Breslow *et al.*, 1989; Tuman *et al.*, 1991).

References

Abel R.M., Staroscik R.N. & Reis R.L. (1970a) The effects of diazepam (Valium) on left ventricular function and systemic vascular resistance. *Journal of Pharmacology and Experimental Therapeutics* **173**, 364−70.

Abel R.M., Reis R.L. & Staroscik R.N. (1970b) Coronary vasodilatation following diazepam (Valium). *British Journal of Pharmacology* **38**, 620−31.

Abenavoli T., Rubler S., Fisher V.J., Axelrod H.I. & Zuckerman K.P. (1981) Exercise testing with myocardial scintigraphy in asymptomatic diabetes males. *Circulation* **63**, 54−64.

Al-Khudhairi D., Whitwam J.G., Chakrabarti M.K., Askitopoulou H., Grundy E.M. & Powrie S. (1982) Haemodynamic effects of midazolam and thiopentone during induction of anaesthesia for coronary artery surgery. *British Journal of Anaesthesia* **54**, 831−5.

Alon E., Baitella L. & Hossli G. (1987) Double-blind study of the reversal of midazolam supplemented general anaesthesia with Ro 15−1788. *British Journal of Anaesthesia* **59**, 455−8.

Altura B.M., Altura B.T., Carella A. *et al.* (1980) Vascular smooth muscle and general anesthetics. *Federation Proceedings* **39**, 1584−91.

Anderson J.M. (1984) *The National Institute on Aging Macroeconomic Demographic Model* pp. 59−62. US Department of Health and Human Services, National Institute on Aging. Bethesda, Maryland.

Arens J.F., Bennow B.P., Ochsner J.L. & Theard R. (1972) Morphine anesthesia for aorto-coronary bypass procedures. *Anesthesia and Analgesia* **51**, 901−9.

Arkins R., Smessaert A.A. & Hicks R.G. (1964) Mortality and morbidity in surgical patients with coronary artery disease. *Journal of the American Medical Association* **190**, 485−8.

Baers S., Nakhjavan F. & Kajani M. (1965) Postoperative myocardial infarction. *Surgery, Gynecology and Obstetrics* **120**, 315−22.

Bålfors E., Häggmark S., Nyhman H. *et al.* (1983) Droperidol inhibits the effects of intravenous ketamine on central hemodynamics and myocardial oxygen consumption in patients with generalized atherosclerotic disease. *Anesthesia and Analgesia* **62**, 193−7.

Baron J.-F., Coriat P., Mundler O., Fauchet M., Bousseau D. & Vicars P. (1987) Left ventricular global and regional function during lumbar epidural anesthesia in patients with angina pectoris. Influence of volume loading. *Anesthesiology* **66**, 621−7.

Baron J.-F., Bertrand M., Barré E. *et al.* (1991) Combined epidural and general anesthesia versus general anesthesia for abdominal aortic surgery. *Anesthesiology* **75**, 611−18.

Battler A., Froelicher V.F., Gallagher K.P. *et al.* (1980) Dissociation between regional myocardial dysfunction and ECG changes during ischaemia in the conscious dog. *Circulation* **62**, 735−44.

Beard O.W., Hipp H.R., Robins M. *et al.* (1967) Survival in myocardial infarction. *American Heart Journal* **73**, 317−21.

Becker L.C. (1978) Conditions for vasodilator-induced coronary steal in experimental myocardial ischemia. *Circulation* **57**, 1103−10.

Bernard J.-M., Wouters P.F., Doursout M.-F. *et al.* (1990) Effects of sevoflurane and isoflurane on cardiac and coronary dynamics in chronically instrumented dogs. *Anesthesiology* **72**, 659−62.

Berry D.G. (1974) Effects of ketamine on the isolated chicken embryo heart. *Anesthesia and Analgesia* **53**, 919−23.

Bertrand Y.M., Boelens D., Collin L. *et al.* (1984) Preoperative assessment in geriatric patients for elective surgery. *Acta Anaesthesiologica Belgica* **35** (Suppl.), 155−65.

Blackburn J.P., Conway C.M., Leigh J.M., Lindop M.J. & Reitan J.A. (1971) The effects of anaesthetic induction agents upon myocardial contractility. *Anaesthesia* **26**, 93−4.

Blaise G., Sill J.C., Nugent M. *et al.* (1987) Isoflurane causes endothelium-dependent inhibition of contractile responses of canine coronary arteries. *Anesthesiology* **67**, 513−17.

Blaise G.A., Witzeling T.M., Sill J.C. *et al.* (1990) Fentanyl is devoid of major effects on coronary vasoreactivity and myocardial metabolism in experimental animals. *Anesthesiology* **72**, 535−41.

Bloch A., Morard J., Major C. & Perrenoud J.-J. (1979) Crosssectional echocardiography in acute myocardial infarction. *American Journal of Cardiology* **43**, 387A.

Blomberg S., Emanuelsson H., Ricksten S.-E. (1989) Thoracic epidural anesthesia and central hemodynamics in patients with unstable angina pectoris. *Anesthesia and Analgesia* **69**, 558−62.

Blomberg S., Emanuelsson H., Kvist H. *et al.* (1990) Effects of thoracic epidural anesthesia on coronary arteries and arterioles in patients with coronary artery disease. *Anesthesiology* **73**, 840−7.

Boer F., Bovill J.G., Ros P. & Van Ommen H. (1991) Effect of thiopentone, etomidate and propofol on systemic vascular resistance during cardiopulmonary bypass. *British Journal of Anaesthesia* **67**, 69−72.

Boucher C.A., Brewster D.C., Darling C.R., Okada R.D., Strauss H.W. & Pohost G.M. (1985) Determination of cardiac risk by dipyridamole−thallium imaging before peripheral vascular surgery. *New England Journal of Medicine* **312**, 389−94.

Bovill J.G., Sebel P.S. & Stanley T.H. (1984a) Opioid analgesics in anesthesia: with special reference to their use in cardiovascular anesthesia. *Anesthesiology* **61**, 731−55.

Bovill J.G., Warren P.J., Schuller J.L. *et al.* (1984b) Comparison of fentanyl, sufentanil, and alfentanil anesthesia in patients undergoing valvular heart surgery. *Anesthesia and Analgesia* **63**, 1081−6.

Braunwald E. (1984) The history. In *Heart Disease: A Textbook of Cardiovascular Medicine* (Ed. Braunwald E.) pp. 1−13. W.B. Saunders, Philadelphia.

Breslow M.J., Jordan D.A., Christopherson R. *et al.* (1989) Epidural morphine decreases postoperative hypertension by attenuating sympathetic nervous system hyperactivity. *Journal of the American Medical Association* **261**, 3577−81.

Bristow J.D., Prys-Roberts C., Fisher A., Pickering T.G. & Sleight P. (1969) Effects of anesthesia on baroreflex control of heart rate in man. *Anesthesiology* **31**, 422−8.

Brown B.R. & Crout R. (1971) A comparative study of the effects of five general anesthetics on myocardial contractility: I: Isometric conditions. *Anesthesiology* **34**, 236−45.

Brown R.V. & Hilton J.G. (1956) The effectiveness of the baroreceptors under different anesthetics. *Journal of Pharmacology and Experimental Therapeutics* **118**, 198−203.

Brown O.W., Hollier L.H., Pairolero P.C., Kazmier F.J. &

McCready R.A. (1981) Abdominal aortic aneurysm and coronary artery disease. *Archives of Surgery* **116**, 1484—8.

Browner W.S., Li J., Mangano D.T. & the SPI group (1992) In-hospital and long-term mortality in male veterans following noncardiac surgery. *Journal of the American Medical Association* **268**, 228—32.

Brusset A., Coriat P. & Pazvanska E. (1986) Isoflurane vs. halothane in control of intraoperative hypertension. Effects on left ventricular function. *Anesthesiology* **65**, 2A.

Buffington C.W. (1986) Impaired systolic thickening associated with halothane in the presence of a coronary stenosis is mediated by changes in hemodynamics. *Anesthesiology* **64**, 632—40.

Buffington C.W. & Coyle R.J. (1991) Altered load dependence of postischemic myocardium. *Anesthesiology* **75**, 464—74.

Buffington C.W., Romson J.L., Levine A. et al. (1987) Isoflurane induced coronary steal in a canine model of chronic coronary occlusion. *Anesthesiology* **66**, 280—92.

Buffington C.W., Davis K.B., Gillispie S. & Pettinger M. (1988) The prevalence of steal-prone coronary anatomy in patients with coronary artery disease: an analysis of the coronary artery surgery study registry. *Anesthesiology* **69**, 721—7.

Burggraf G.W. & Parker J.O. (1975) Prognosis in coronary disease: angiographic, hemodynamic and clinical factors. *Circulation* **51**, 146—56.

Cahalan M.K., Prakash O., Rulf E.N.R. et al. (1987) Addition of nitrous oxide to fentanyl anesthesia does not induce myocardial ischemia in patients with ischemic heart disease. *Anesthesiology* **67**, 925—9.

Cahalan M.K., Weiskopf R.B., Eger E.I. II et al. (1991) Hemodynamic effects of desflurane/nitrous oxide anesthesia in volunteers. *Anesthesia and Analgesia* **73**, 157—64.

Calverly R.K., Smith N.T., Jones C.W. et al. (1978) Cardiovascular effects of enflurane anesthesia during controlled ventilation in man. *Anesthesia and Analgesia* **57**, 619—28.

Carliner N.H., Fisher M.L., Plotnick G.D. et al. (1985) Routine preoperative exercise testing in patients undergoing major non-cardiac surgery. *American Journal of Cardiology* **56**, 51—8.

Cason B.A., Verrier E.D., London M.I. et al. (1987) Effects of isoflurane and halothane on coronary vascular resistance and collateral myocardial blood flow: their capacity to induce coronary steal. *Anesthesiology* **67**, 665—75.

Chamberlain D.P. & Chamberlain B.D.L. (1986) Changes in the skin temperature of the trunk and their relationship to sympathetic blockade during spinal anesthesia. *Anesthesiology* **65**, 139—43.

Chraemmer-Jørgensen B., Hoilund-Carlsen P.F., Bjerre-Jepsen K. et al. (1992) Does alfentanil preserve left ventricular pump function during rapid sequence induction of anaesthesia? *Acta Anaesthesiologica Scandinavica* **36**, 362—8.

Coddens J.A. & Deloof T. (1992) End-systolic pressure—volume relationship and arterial elastance: the optimal method to evaluate myocardial contractile effects of anesthetic agents? (Letter) **74**, 165.

Cohn P.F., Gorlin R., Cohn L.H. et al. (1979) Left ventricular ejection fraction as a prognostic guide in surgical treatment of coronary and valvular heart disease. *American Journal of Cardiology* **34**, 136.

Colan S.D., Borow K.M. & Neumann A. (1984) Left ventricular end-systolic wall stress-velocity of fibre shortening relation: a load-independent index of myocardial contractility. *Journal of the American College of Cardiology* **4**, 715—24.

Colson P., Saussine M., Séguin J.R. et al. (1992) Hemodynamic effects of anesthesia in patients chronically treated with angiotensin-converting enzyme inhibitors. *Anesthesia and Analgesia* **74**, 805—8.

Cooperman M., Pflug B., Martin E.W. Jr. & Evans W.E. (1978) Cardiovascular risk factors in patients with peripheral vascular disease. *Surgery* **84**, 505—9.

Coriat P., Harari A., Daloz M. & Viars P. (1982) Clinical predictors of intraoperative myocardial ischaemia in patients with coronary artery disease undergoing non-cardiac surgery. *Acta Anaesthesiologica Scandinavica* **26**, 287—90.

Coronary Artery Surgery Study (CASS) (1978) *Manual of Operations* II. Data Collection and Storage. Collaborative Studies in Coronary Artery Surgery. Washington DC, National Heart, Lung and Blood Institute, University of Washington, Seattle.

Cote P., Gueret P. & Bourassa M.G. (1974) Systemic and coronary hemodynamic effects of diazepam in patients with normal and diseased coronary arteries. *Circulation* **50**, 1210—16.

Crawford E.S., Morris G.C., Howell J.F., Flynne W.F. & Moorhead D.T. (1978) Operative risk in patients with previous coronary artery bypass. *Annals of Thoracic Surgery* **26**, 215—21.

Crawford E.S., Bomberger R.A., Glaeser D.H., Saleh S.A. & Russel W.L. (1981) Aortoiliac occlusive disease: factors influencing survival and function following reconstructive operation over a twenty-five year period. *Surgery* **90**, 1055—67.

Criado A., Maseda J., Navarro E., Escarpa A. & Avello F. (1980) Induction of anaesthesia with etomidate: heamodynamic study of 36 patients. *British Journal of Anaesthesia* **52**, 803—5.

Cruse P.J. & Foord R. (1973) A 5-year prospective study of 23 649 wounds. *Archives of Surgery* **107**, 206—10.

Cucchiara R.F., Benefield D.J., Matteo R.S. et al. (1986) Evaluation of esmolol in controlling increases in heart rate and blood pressure during endotracheal intubation in patients undergoing carotid endarterectomy. *Anesthesiology* **65**, 528—31.

Cutfield G.R., Francis C.M., Foëx P. et al. (1988) isoflurane and large coronary artery heamodynamics. A study in dogs. *British Journal of Anaesthesia* **60**, 784—90.

Cutler B.S., Wheeler H.B., Paraskos J.A. & Cardullo P.A. (1979) Assessment of operative risk with electrocardiographic exercise testing in patients with peripheral vascular disease. *American Journal of Surgery* **137**, 484—90.

Cutler B.S., Wheeler H.B., Paraskos J.A. & Cardullo P.A. (1981) Applicability and interpretation of electrocardiographic stress testing in patients with peripheral vascular disease. *American Journal of Surgery* **141**, 501—6.

Dack S. (1963) Symposium on cardiovascular—pulmonary problems before and after surgery: postoperative problems. *American Journal of Cardiology* **12**, 423—30.

Davis R.F., DeBoer L.W.V. & Maroko P.R. (1986) Thoracic epidural anesthesia reduces myocardial infarct size after coronary artery occlusion in dogs. *Anesthesia and Analgesia* **65**, 711—17.

De Castro J., Van de Walter A., Wouters L. et al. (1979) Comparative study of cardiovascular, neurological and metabolic side effects of eight narcotics in dogs. *Acta Anaesthesiologica*

Belgica **30**, 5–54.

Dechenne J.P. & Destrosiers R. (1969) Diazepam in pulmonary surgery. *Canadian Anaesthetists' Society Journal* **16**, 162–6.

De Hert S.G., Vermeyen K.M. & Adriaensen H.F. (1990) Influence of thiopental, etomidate and propofol on regional myocardial function in the normal and acute ischemic heart segment in dogs. *Anesthesia and Analgesia* **70**, 600–7.

De Lange S. & De Bruijn N.P. (1983) Alfentanil–oxygen anaesthesia: Plasma concentrations and clinical effects during variable-rate continuous infusion for coronary artery surgery. *British Journal of Anaesthesia* **55**, 183S–9S.

Delaney T.J., Kistner J.R., Lake C.L. *et al.* (1980) Myocardial function during halothane and enflurane anesthesia in patients with coronary artery disease. *Anesthesia and Analgesia* **59**, 240–4.

Diamond G.A. & Forrester J.S. (1979) Analysis of probability as an aid in the clinical diagnosis of coronary-artery disease. *New England Journal of Medicine* **300**, 1350–8.

Djokovic J.L. & Hedley-Whyte J. (1979) Prediction of outcome of surgery and anesthesia in patients over 80. *Journal of the American Medical Association* **242**, 2301–6.

Domenech R.J., Macho P., Valdes J. & Penna M. (1977) Coronary vascular resistance during halothane anesthesia. *Anesthesiology* **46**, 236–40.

Dowdy E.G. & Kaya K. (1968) Studies of the mechanism of cardiovascular response to CI-581. *Anesthesiology* **29**, 931–43.

Dripps R.D., Lamont A. & Eckenhoff J.E. (1963) New classification of physical status. *Anesthesiology* **24**, 111.

Driscoll A.C., Hobika J.H., Etsten B.E. & Proger S. (1961) Clinically unrecognized myocardial infarction following surgery. *New England Journal of Medicine* **264**, 633–9.

Drobar M. (1979) Complicated acute myocardial infarction: the importance of two-dimensional echocardiography. *American Journal of Cardiology* **43**, 387.

Duke P.C. & Trosky S. (1980) The effect of halothane with nitrous oxide on baroreflex control of heart rate in man. *Canadian Anaesthetists' Society Journal* **27**, 531–4.

Duke P.C., Townes D. & Wade J.G. (1977) Halothane depresses baroreflex control of heart rate in man. *Anesthesiology* **46**, 184–7.

Dundee J.W. (1969) Diazepam. *International Anesthesiology Clinics* **7**, 91–121.

Dundee J.W., Robinson F.P., McCollum J.S.C. & Patterson C.C. (1986) Sensitivity to propofol in the elderly. *Anaesthesia* **41**, 482–5.

Ebert T. (1990) Differential effects of nitrous oxide on baroreflex control of heart rate and peripheral sympathetic nerve activity in humans. *Anesthesiology* **72**, 16–22.

Eerola M., Eerola R., Kaukinen S. & Kaukinen L. (1980) Risk factors in surgical patients with verified preoperative myocardial infarction. *Acta Anaesthesiologica Scandinavica* **24**, 219–23.

Eisele J.H. & Smith N.T. (1972) Cardiovascular effects of 40 percent nitrous oxide in man. *Anesthesia and Analgesia* **51**, 956–63.

Eisenberg M.J., London M.J., Leung J. *et al.* (1992) Monitoring for myocardial ischemia during non-cardiac surgery. A technology assessment of transesophageal echocardiography and 12-lead electrocardiography. *Journal of the American Medical Association* **268**, 210–16.

Eger E.I. (1981) Isoflurane: a review. *Anesthesiology* **55**, 559–76.

Eger E.I., Smith N.T., Stoelting R.K. *et al.* (1970) Cardiovascular effects of halothane in man. *Anesthesiology* **32**, 396–409.

Entwistle M.D., Sommerville D. & Jones J.G. (1992) Effect of brief hypoxaemia on the resting ECG in patients with exercise-induced cardiac ischaemia. *British Journal of Anaesthesia* **69**, 536P–7P.

Etsten B. & Li T.H. (1955) Hemodynamic changes during thiopental anesthesia in humans: cardiac output, stroke volume, total peripheral resistance and intrathoracic blood volume. *Journal of Clinical Investigation* **34**, 500–10.

Fairfield J.E., Dritsas A. & Beale R.J. (1991) Haemodynamic effects of propofol: induction with 2.5 mg/kg. *British Journal of Anaesthesia* **67**, 618–20.

Flacke J.W., Bloor B.C., Kripke B.J. *et al.* (1985) Comparison of morphine, meperidine, fentanyl and sufentanil in balanced anesthesia: a double blind study. *Anesthesia and Analgesia* **64**, 897–912.

Fleg H.R., Gerstenblidth G. & Lakatta E.G. (1984) Pathophysiology of the aging in heart and circulation. In *Cardiovascular Disease in the Elderly* (Ed. Messerli F.) pp. 11–34. Martinus Nijhoff, Boston.

Fleisher L.A., Rosenbaum S.H. & Barash P.G. (1991) The predictive value of preoperative silent ischemia for postoperative ischemia cardiac events in vascular and nonvascular surgery patients. *American Heart Journal* **122**, 980–6.

Forman M.B., Kinsley R.H. & Duplessis J.P. (1982) Surgical correction of combined supravalvular and valvular aortic stenosis in homozygous familial hypercholesterolemia. *South African Medical Journal* **61**, 579–82.

Forrest J.B., Cahalan M.K., Rehder K. *et al.* (1990) Multicenter study of general anesthesia. II. Results. *Anesthesiology* **72**, 262–8.

Forster A., Gardaz J.P., Suter P.M. & Gemperle M. (1980) I.V. midazolam as an induction agent for anaesthesia: a study in volunteers. *British Journal of Anaesthesia* **52**, 907–11.

Francis C.M., Foex P., Lowenstein E. *et al.* (1982) The interaction between regional myocardial ischaemia and left ventricular performance under halothane anaesthesia. *British Journal of Anaesthesia* **34**, 965–80.

Frazer J.G., Ramachandran M.B. & Davis H.S. (1967) Anesthesia and recent myocardial infarction. *Journal of the American Medical Association* **199**, 96.

Freye E. (1974) Cardiovascular effects of high dosage of fentanyl, meperidine and naloxone in the dog. *Anesthesia and Analgesia* **53**, 40–7.

Fusciardi J., Godet G., Bernard J.M. *et al.* (1986) Roles of fentanyl and nitroglycerin in prevention of myocardial ischemia associated with laryngoscopy and tracheal intubation in patients undergoing operations of short duration. *Anesthesia and Analgesia* **65**, 617–24.

Gage A.A., Bhayana J.N., Balu V. & Hook N. (1977) Assessment of cardiac risk in surgical patients. *Archives of Surgery* **112**, 1488–92.

Gallagher K.P., Osakada G., Matsuzaki M. *et al.* (1982) Myocardial blood flow and function with critical coronary stenosis in exercising dogs. *American Journal of Physiology* **12**, H698–707.

Gelman S., Fowler K.C. & Smith L.R. (1984) Regional blood flow during isoflurane and halothane anesthesia. *Anesthesia and Analgesia* **63**, 557–65.

Germann P.A.S., Roberts J.G. & Prys-Roberts C. (1979) The combination of general anaesthesia and epidural block. I. The effects of sequence of induction on haemodynamic variables and blood gas measurements in healthy patients. *Anaesthesia and Intensive Care* **7**, 229–38.

Gerstenblith G., Lakatta E.G., Weisfeldt M.L. (1976) Age changes in myocardial function and exercise response. *Progress in Cardiovascular Disease* **19**, 1–21.

Gewirtz H., Gross S., Williams D.O. & Most A.S. (1984) Contrasting effects of nifedipine and adenosine on regional myocardial flow distribution and metabolism distal to severe coronary arterial stenosis: observations in sedated closed-chest, domestic swine. *Circulation* **69**, 1048–57.

Giese J.L., Stockham R.J., Stanley T.H., Pace N.L. & Neussen R.H. (1985) Etomidate versus thiopental for induction of anesthesia. *Anesthesia and Analgesia* **64**, 871–6.

Glen J.B. & Hunter S.C. (1984) Pharmacology of an emulsion formulation of ICI 35, 868. *British Journal of Anaesthesia* **56**, 617–26.

Goldberg A.H., Keane P.W. & Phear W.P.C. (1970) Effects of ketamine on contractile performance and excitability of isolated heart muscle. *Journal of Pharmacology Experimental Therapeutics* **175**, 388–94.

Goldman L. (1978) Supraventricular tachyarrhythmias in hospitalized adults after surgery. *Chest* **73**, 450–4.

Goldman L. (1983) Cardiac risks and complications of noncardiac surgery. *Annals of Internal Medicine* **98**, 504–13.

Goldman L., Caldera D.L., Nussbaum S.R. *et al.* (1977) Multifactorial index of cardiac risk in noncardiac surgical procedures. *New England Journal of Medicine* **297**, 845–50.

Goldstein J.L. & Brown M.S. (1982) The LDL receptor defect in familiar hypercholesterolemia: implications for pathogenesis and therapy. *Medical Clinics of North America* **66**, 335–62.

Goodchild C.S. & Serrao J.M. (1989) Cardiovascular effects of propofol in the anaesthetized dog. *British Journal of Anaesthesia* **63**, 87–92.

Gooding J.M., Weng J.-T., Smith R.A., Berninger G.T. & Kirby R.R. (1979) Cardiovascular and pulmonary responses following etomidate induction of anesthesia in patients with demonstrated cardiac disease. *Anesthesia and Analgesia* **58**, 40–1.

Gravlee G.P., Ramsey F.M., Roy R.C. *et al.* (1988) Rapid administration of a narcotic and neuromuscular blocker: a hemodynamic comparison of fentanyl, sufentanil, pancuronium and vecuronium. *Anesthesia and Analgesia* **67**, 39–47.

Greene N.M. (1958) The area of differential block during spinal anesthesia with hyperbaric tetracaine. *Anesthesiology* **19**, 45–50.

Grounds R.M., Twigley A.J., Carli F. *et al.* (1985) The haemodynamic effects of intravenous induction. Comparison of the effects of thiopentone and propofol. *Anaesthesia* **40**, 735–40.

Habazettl H., Conzen P.F., Hobbhahn J. *et al.* (1989) Left ventricular oxygen tensions in dogs during coronary vasodilation by enflurane, isoflurane and dipyridamole. *Anesthesia and Analgesia* **68**, 286–94.

Habazettl H., Conzen P.F., Vollmar B. *et al.* (1991) Effects of sevoflurane and isoflurane on regional blood flow distribution in rats. *Anesthesiology* **75**, 549A.

Hackel D.B., Sancetta S.M. & Kleinerman J. (1956) Effects of hypotension due to spinal anesthesia on coronary blood flow and myocardial metabolism in man. *Circulation* **13**, 92–7.

Häggmark S., Hohner P., Östman M. *et al.* (1989) Comparison of hemodynamic, electrocardiographic, mechanical and metabolic indicators of intraoperative myocardial ischemia in vascular surgical patients with coronary artery disease. *Anesthesiology* **70**, 19–25.

Hasbrouk J.D. (1970) Morphine anesthesia for open heart surgery. *Annals of Thoracic Surgery* **10**, 364–9.

Heger J.J., Weyman A.E., Wann L.S., Dillon J.C. & Feigenbaum H. (1979) Cross-sectional echocardiography in acute myocardial infarction: Detection and localization of regional left ventricular asynergy. *Circulation* **60**, 531–8.

Heger J.J., Weyman A.E., Wann S.L. *et al.* (1980) Cross-sectional echocardiographic analysis of the extent of left ventricular asynergy in acute myocardial infarction. *Circulation* **61**, 1113–18.

Heikkilä H., Jalonen J., Arola M. & Laaksonen V. (1985a) Surgical stimulation during high-dose fentanyl anaesthesia: effects of dehydrobenzperidol on the haemodynamics and myocardial oxygenation. *Acta Anaesthesiologica Scandinavica* **29**, 259–64.

Heikkilä H., Jalonen J., Arola M. & Laaksonen V. (1985b) Haemodynamics and myocardial oxygenation during anaesthesia for coronary artery surgery: comparison between enflurane and high-dose fentanyl anaesthesia. *Acta Anaesthesiologica Scandinavica* **29**, 457–64.

Helman J.D., Leung J.M., Bellows W.H. *et al.* (1992) The risk of myocardial ischemia in patients receiving desflurane versus sufentanil anesthesia for coronary artery bypass surgery. *Anesthesiology* **77**, 47–62.

Hertzer N.R. (1981) Fatal myocardial infarction following lower extremity revascularization: two hundred seventy-three patients followed six to eleven postoperative years. *Annals of Surgery* **193**, 492–8.

Hertzer N.R. (1982) Fatal myocardial infarction following peripheral vascular operations; a study of 951 patients followed 6 to 11 years postoperatively. *Cleveland Clinic Quarterly* **49**, 1–11.

Hertzer N.R. (1983) Myocardial ischemia. *Surgery* **93**, 97–101.

Hertzer N.R., Beven E.G., Young J.R. *et al.* (1984) Coronary artery disease in peripheral vascular patients. A classification of 1000 angiograms and results of surgical management. *Annals of Surgery* **199**, 223–33.

Hess W., Arnold B., Schulte-Sasse U. & Tarnow J. (1983) Comparison of isoflurane and halothane when used to control intraoperative hypertension in patients undergoing coronary bypass surgery. *Anesthesia and Analgesia* **62**, 15–20.

Hickey R.F., Sybert P.E., Vervier E.D. & Cason B.A. (1988) Effects of halothane, enflurane and isoflurane on coronary blood flow autoregulation and coronary vascular reserve in the canine heart. *Anesthesiology* **68**, 21–30.

Hicks G.L., Eastland M.W., DeWeese J.A., May A.G. & Rob G.G. (1975) Survival improvement following aortic aneurysm resection. *Annals of Surgery* **181**, 863–9.

Hilfiker O., Larsen R. & Sonntag H. (1983) Myocardial blood flow and oxygen consumption during halothane–nitrous oxide anaesthesia for coronary revascularization. *British Journal of Anaesthesia* **55**, 927–32.

Hohner P., Nancarrow C., Häggmark S. *et al.* (1993a) Isoflurane produces dose-dependent coronary vasodilation in vascular surgical patients with coronary artery disease. *Acta Anaesthesiologica Scandinavica* (In press).

Hohner P., Backman C., Diamond G. *et al.* (1993b) Anesthesia for abdominal aortic surgery in patients with coronary artery disease—effects of nitrous oxide on systemic and coronary hemodynamics, regional ventricular function and incidence of myocardial ischemia. *Acta Anaesthesiologica Scandinavica* (In press).

Holaday D.A. & Smith F.R. (1981) Clinical characteristics and biotransformation of sevoflurane in healthy human volunteers. *Anesthesiology* **54**, 100–6.

Hotvedt R., Refsum H. & Platou E.S. (1983) Electrophysiological effects of thoracic epidural analgesia in the dog heart *in situ*. *Cardiovascular Research* **17**, 259–66.

Hotvedt R., Refsum H. & Platou E.S. (1984) Cardiac electrophysiological and hemodynamic effects of beta-adrenoreceptor blockade and thoracic epidural analgesia in the dog. *Anesthesia and Analgesia* **63**, 817–24.

Hotvedt R., Refsum H. & Helgesen K.G. (1985) Cardiac electrophysiologic and hemodynamic effects related to plasma levels of bupivacaine in the dog. *Anesthesia and Analgesia* **64**, 388–94.

Howie M.B., McSweeney T.D., Lingam R.P. & Maschke S.P. (1985) A comparison of fentanyl–O_2 and sufentanil–O_2 for cardiac anesthesia. *Anesthesia and Analgesia* **64**, 877–87.

Hunter P.R., Endrey-Walder P., Bauer G.E. & Stephens F.D. (1968) Myocardial infarction following surgical operations. *British Medical Journal* **4**, 725–8.

Hynynen M., Takkunen O., Salmenperä M. & Haataja H. (1986) Continuous infusion of fentanyl or alfentanil for coronary artery surgery. Plasma opiate concentrations, haemodynamics and postoperative course. *British Journal of Anaesthesia* **58**, 1252–9.

Inoue K., Reichelt W., El-Banayosy A. *et al.* (1990) Does isoflurane lead to a higher incidence of myocardial infarction and perioperative death than enflurane in coronary artery surgery? A clinical study of 1178 patients. *Anesthesia and Analgesia* **71**, 469–74.

Isoflurane New Drug Application Study (1982) Clinical evaluation of isoflurane: pulse and blood pressure. *Canadian Anaesthetists' Society Journal* **29**, 15S–27S.

Ivankovic A.D., Miletich D.J., Reimann S., Albrecht R.F. & Zahel B. (1974) Cardiovascular effects of centrally administered ketamine in goats. *Anesthesia and Analgesia* **53**, 924–33.

Jakobsen J., Sofelt S., Brocks V. *et al.* (1992) Reduced left ventricular diameters at onset of bradycardia during epidural anaesthesia. *Acta Anaesthesiologica Scandinavica* **36**, 831.

James R. & Glen J.B. (1980) Synthesis, biological evaluation and preliminary structure–activity considerations of a series of alkylphenols as intravenous anaesthetic agents. *Journal of Medical Chemistry* **23**, 1350–7.

Jeffrey C.C., Kunsman J., Cullen D.J. & Brewster D.C. (1983) A prospective evaluation of cardiac risk index. *Anesthesiology* **58**, 462–4.

Jensen D., Blankenhorn D.H. & Kornerup V. (1967) Coronary disease in familial hypercholesterolemia. *Circulation* **36**, 77–82.

Kannel W.B. & McGee D.L. (1979) Diabetes and cardiovascular risk factors: the Framingham Study. *Circulation* **59**, 8–13.

Kannel W.B. & Sorlie P. (1975) Hypertension in Framingham. In *Epidemiology and Control of Hypertension* (Ed. Paul O.) pp. 553–93. Symposia Specialist, Florida.

Kannel W.B., McGee D. & Gordon T. (1976) A general cardiovascular risk profile: the Framingham Study. *American Journal of Cardiology* **38**, 46–51.

Karliczek G.F., Brenken U., Schokkenbrock R. *et al.* (1982) Etomidate—analgesic combinations for the induction of anaesthesia in cardiac patients. *Anaesthetist* **31**, 213–30.

Kawar P., Carson I.W., Clarke R.S.J., Dundee J.W. & Lyons S.M. (1985) Haemodynamic changes during induction of anaesthesia with midazolam and diazepam (Valium) in patients undergoing coronary artery bypass surgery. *Anaesthesia* **40**, 767–71.

Kemmotsu O., Hashimoto Y. & Shimosato S. (1973) Inotropic effects of isoflurane on mechanics of contraction in isolated cat papillary muscles from normal and failing hearts. *Anesthesiology* **39**, 470–7.

Kemmotsu O., Hashimoto Y. & Shimosato S. (1974) The effects of fluoxene and enflurane on contractile performance of isolated papillary muscles from failing hearts. *Anesthesiology* **40**, 252–60.

Kenny D., Proctor L.T., Schmelling W.T. *et al.* (1991) Isoflurane causes only minimal increases in coronary blood flow independent of oxygen demand. *Anesthesiology* **75**, 640–9.

Kettler D., Sonntag H., Donath U., Regensburger D. & Schenk H.D. (1974) Haemodynamik, Myokardmechanik, Sauerstoffbedarf und Sauerstoffversorgung des menschlichen Herzens unter Narkoseeinleitung mit Etomidate. *Der Anaesthetist* **23**, 116–21.

Kimbris D. & Segal B.L. (1981) Coronary disease progression in patients with and without saphenous vein bypass surgery. *American Heart Journal* **102**, 811–18.

King B.D., Elder J.D. & Dripps R.D. (1952) The effect of the intravenous administration of meperidine upon the circulation of man and the circulatory response to tilt. *Surgery, Gynecology and Obstetrics* **94**, 591–7.

Kissin I., Motomura S., Aultman D.F. & Reves J.G. (1983) Inotropic and anesthetic potencies of etomidate and thiopental in dogs. *Anesthesia and Analgesia* **62**, 961–5.

Klassen G.A., Bramwell R.S., Bromage P.R. & Zborowska-Sluis D.T. (1980) Effect of acute sympathectomy by epidural anesthesia on the canine coronary circulation. *Anesthesiology* **52**, 8–15.

Klein L.W. (1984) Cigarette smoking atherosclerosis and the coronary hemodynamic response: a unifying hypothesis. *Journal of the American College of Cardiology* **4**, 972–4.

Kleinman B., Henkin R.E., Glisson S.N. *et al.* (1986) Qualitative evaluation of coronary flow during anesthetic induction using thallium 201 perfusion scans. *Anesthesiology* **64**, 157–64.

Knapp R.B. & Dubow H. (1970) Comparison of diazepam with thiopental as an induction agent in cardiopulmonary disease. *Anesthesia and Analgesia* **49**, 722–6.

Knapp R.B., Topkins M.J. & Artusio J.F. (1962) The cerebrovascular accident and coronary occlusion in anesthesia. *Journal of the American Medical Association* **182**, 322–4.

Knight A.A., Hollenberg M., London M.J. *et al.* (1988) Perioperative myocardial ischemia: importance of the perioperative ischemic pattern. *Anesthesiology* **68**, 681−8.

Kock M., Blomberg S., Emanuelsson H. *et al.* (1990) Thoracic epidural anesthesia improves global and regional left ventricular function during stress-induced myocardial ischemia in patients with coronary artery disease. *Anesthesia and Analgesia* **71**, 625−30.

Kotrly K.J., Ebert T.J., Vucins E. *et al.* (1985) Baroreceptor reflex control of heart rate during isoflurane anesthesia in humans. *Anesthesiology* **60**, 173−9.

Kozmary S.V., Lampe G.H., Benefiel D., Cahalan M.K., Wauk L.Z., Whitendale P., Schiller N.B. & Eger E.I. II (1990) No finding of increased myocardial ischemia during or after carotid endarterectomy under anesthesia with nitrous oxide. *Anesthesia and Analgesia* **71**, 591−6.

Krebs R. & Kersting F. (1979) The effects of barbiturates on the myocardium and its reversibility. *Progress in Pharmacology* **2**, 3.

Kumar S.M., Kothary S.P. & Zsigmond E.K. (1978) Plasma-free norepinephrine and epinephrine concentrations following diazepam−ketamine induction in patients undergoing cardiac surgery. *Acta Anaesthesiologica Scandinavica* **22**, 593−600.

Larsen R., Hilfiker O., Merkel G., Sonntag H. & Drobnik L. (1984) Myocardial oxygen balance during enflurane and isoflurane anaesthesia for coronary artery surgery. *Anesthesiology* **61**, 4A.

Lebowitz P.W., Cote M.E., Daniels A.L. *et al.* (1982) Comparative cardiovascular effects of midazolam and thiopentol in healthy patients. *Anesthesia and Analgesia* **61**, 771−5.

Leclerc D., Fratacci M.D., Dupuy P. & Payen D. (1990) Coronary bypass graft flow (CGBF) vasodilation (VD) induced by isoflurane has only negligible effects on left ventricular (LV) systolic function. *Anesthesiology* **73**, 147A.

Lepage J.-Y., Blanloeil Y., Pinaud M.L. *et al.* (1986) Hemodynamic effects of diazepam, flunitrazepam and midazolam in patients with ischemic heart disease: Assessment with a radionuclide approach. *Anesthesiology* **65**, 678−83.

Lepage J.-Y., Pinaud M.L., Hélias J.H. *et al.* (1988) Left ventricular function during propofol and fentanyl anesthesia in patients with coronary artery disease: assessment with a radionuclide approach. *Anesthesia and Analgesia* **67**, 949−55.

Lepage J.-Y., Pinaud M.L., Hélias J.H. *et al.* (1991) Left ventricular performance during propofol or methohexital anesthesia: Isotopic and cardiac monitoring. *Anesthesia and Analgesia* **73**, 3−9.

Lerman J., Oyston J.P., Gallagher T.M. *et al.* (1990) The minimum alveolar concentration (MAC) and hemodynamic effects of halothane, isoflurane and sevoflurane in newborn swine. *Anesthesiology* **73**, 717−21.

Leung J.M., Goehner P., O'Kelly B.F. *et al.* (1991) Isoflurane anesthesia and myocardial ischemia: comparative risk versus sufentanil anesthesia in patients undergoing coronary artery bypass graft surgery. *Anesthesiology* **74**, 838−47.

Lewin I., Lerner A.G. & Green S.H. (1971) Physical class and physiological status in the prediction of operative mortality in the aged sick. *Annals of Surgery* **174**, 217−31.

Lieberman A.N., Weiss J.L., Jugdutt B. *et al.* (1981) Two-dimensional echocardiography and infarct size: relationship of regional wall motion and thickening to the extent of myocardial infarction in the dog. *Circulation* **63**, 739−46.

Lippman M. & Mok M.S. (1990) Propofol causes cardiovascular depression. III. *Anesthesiology* **72**, 395.

London M.J., Hollenberg M., Wong M.G. *et al.* (1988) Intraoperative myocardial ischemia: localization by 12-lead ECG. *Anesthesiology* **69**, 232−41.

London M.J., Tubau J., Wong M.G. *et al.* (1990) The 'natural history' of segmental wall motion abnormalities in patients undergoing noncardiac surgery. *Anesthesiology* **73**, 644−55.

Lowenstein E. (1971) Morphine 'anesthesia' − a perspective. *Anesthesiology* **35**, 563−5.

Lowenstein E. & Reiz S. (1987) Circulatory effects of inhalation anesthetics. In *Cardiac Anesthesia* 2nd edn. (Ed. Kaplan J.A.) pp. 3−35. Grune and Stratton, New York.

Lowenstein E., Hollowell P., Levine F.H. *et al.* (1969) Cardiovascular response to large doses of intravenous morphine in man. *New England Journal of Medicine* **281**, 1389−93.

Lowenstein E., Foëx P., Francis C.M., Davies W.L., Yusuf S. & Ryder W.A. (1981) Regional ischemic ventricular dysfunction in myocardium supplied by a narrowed coronary artery with increasing halothane concentrations in the dog. *Anesthesiology* **55**, 349−59.

Lowenstein E., Haering J.M. & Douglas P.S. (1991) Acute ventricular wall motion heterogeneity: A valuable but imperfect index of myocardial ischemia. *Anesthesiology* **75**, 385−7.

Lundborg R.O., Milde J.H. & Theye R.A. (1966) Effect of nitrous oxide on myocardial contractility of dogs. *Canadian Anaesthetists' Society Journal* **13**, 361.

Lundeen G., Manohar M. & Parks C. (1983) Systemic distribution of blood flow in swine while awake and during 1.0 and 1.5 MAC isoflurane anesthesia with or without 50% nitrous oxide. *Anesthesia and Analgesia* **63**, 499−512.

Lunn J.K., Webster L.R., Stanley T.H. & Woodward A. (1979) High dose fentanyl anesthesia for coronary artery surgery: plasma fentanyl concentrations and influence of nitrous oxide on cardiovascular responses. *Anesthesia and Analgesia* **58**, 390−5.

Lynch C. (1986) Differential depression of myocardial contractility by halothane and isoflurane *in vitro*. *Anesthesiology* **64**, 620−31.

McCammon R.L., Hilgenberg J.C. & Stoelting R.K. (1980) Hemodynamic effects of diazepam and diazepam−nitrous oxide in patients with coronary artery disease. *Anesthesia and Analgesia* **59**, 438−41.

Mahar L.J., Steen P.A., Tinker J.H. *et al.* (1978) Perioperative myocardial infarction in patients with coronary artery disease with and without aorta-coronary artery bypass grafts. *Journal of Thoracic and Cardiovascular Surgery* **76**, 533−7.

Mallow J.E., White R.D. & Cucchiara R.F. (1976) Hemodynamic effects of isoflurane and halothane in patients with coronary artery disease. *Anesthesia and Analgesia* **55**, 135−8.

Mangano D.T. (1985) Biventricular function after myocardial revascularization in humans: deterioration and recovery patterns during the first 24 hours. *Anesthesiology* **62**, 571−7.

Mangano D.T., Hedgcock M. & Wisneski J.A. (1982) Noninvasive prediction of ventricular dysfunction: Coronary artery disease. *Anesthesiology* **57**, 21A.

Mangano D.T., Browner W., Hollenberg M., London M.J., Tubau J.F., Tateo I.M., SPI Research Group (1990) Association of perioperative myocardial ischemia with cardiac morbidity and mortality in men undergoing noncardiac surgery. *New England Journal of Medicine* **323**, 1781−8.

Mangano D.T., Hollenberg M., Fegert G. *et al.* (1991) Perioperative myocardial ischemia in patients undergoing noncardiac surgery, I: incidence during the 4-day perioperative period. *Journal of the American College of Cardiology* **17**, 843—50.

Mangano D.T., Browner W., Hollenberg M. *et al.* (1992a) Long-term cardiac prognosis following noncardiac surgery. *Journal of the American Medical Association* **268**, 233—9.

Mangano D.T., Siliciano D., Hollenberg M. *et al.* (1992b) Postoperative myocardial ischemia. Therapeutic trials using intensive analgesia following surgery. *Anesthesiology* **76**, 342—53.

Martin D.E., Rosenberg H., Aukburg S.J. *et al.* (1982) Low-dose fentanyl blunts circulatory responses to tracheal intubation. *Anesthesia and Analgesia* **61**, 680—4.

Marty J., Nitenberg A., Blanchet F. *et al.* (1982) Effects of droperidol on left ventricular performance in humans. *Anesthesiology* **57**, 22—5.

Marty J., Nitenberg A., Blanchet F., Zouioueche S. & Desmonts J.-M. (1986) Effects of midazolam on the coronary circulation in patients with coronary artery disease. *Anesthesiology* **64**, 206—10.

Marty J., Nitenberg A., Philip J.P. *et al.* (1991) Coronary and left ventricular hemodynamic responses following reversing of flunitrazepam-induced sedation with flumazenil in patients with coronary artery disease. *Anesthesiology* **74**, 71—6.

Mathew J.P., Fleisher L.A., Rinehouse J.A.S. *et al.* (1992) ST segment depression during labour and delivery. *Anesthesiology* **77**, 635—41.

Mauney M.F. Jr., Ebert P.A. & Sabiston D.C. Jr. (1970) Postoperative myocardial infarction; a study of predisposing factors, diagnosis and mortality in a high risk group of surgical patients. *Annals of Surgery* **172**, 497—503.

Merin R.G. (1990) Propofol causes cardiovascular depression I. *Anesthesiology* **72**, 393.

Merin R.G. & Basch S. (1981) Are the myocardial functional and metabolic effects of isoflurane really different from those of halothane and enflurane? *Anesthesiology* **55**, 398—408.

Merin R.G., Bernard J.-M., Doursout M.-F. *et al.* (1991) Comparison of the effects of isoflurane and desflurane on cardiovascular dynamics and regional blood flow in the chronically instrumented dog. *Anesthesiology* **74**, 568—74.

Milocco I., Schlossman D., William-Olsson G. & Appelgren L.K. (1985) Fentanyl—droperidol—nitrous oxide anaesthesia in patients with ischaemic heart disease and various degrees of left ventricular functional impairment. *Acta Anaesthesiologica Scandinavica* **29**, 683—92.

Mitchell M.M., Prakash O., Rulf N.R. *et al.* (1989) Nitrous oxide does not induce myocardial ischemia in patients with ischemic heart disease and poor left ventricular function. *Anesthesiology* **71**, 526—34.

Moffitt E.A., Sethna D., Gray R. *et al.* (1983) Nitrous oxide added to halothane reduces coronary flow and myocardial oxygen consumption in patients with coronary disease. *Canadian Anaesthetists' Society Journal* **30**, 5—9.

Moffitt E.A., Scovill J.E., Barker R.A. *et al.* (1984a) Myocardial metabolism and haemodynamic responses during high-dose fentanyl anaesthesia for coronary patients. *Canadian Anaesthetists' Society Journal* **31**, 6.

Moffitt E.A., Sethna D.H., Gray R.J. *et al.* (1984b) Rate—pressure product correlates poorly with myocardial oxygen consump-tion during anesthesia in coronary patients. *Canadian Anaesthetists' Society Journal* **31**, 5—12.

Moffitt E.A., Sethna D.H., Bussell J.A. *et al.* (1985) Effects of intubation on coronary blood flow and myocardial oxygenation. *Canadian Anaesthetists' Society Journal* **32**, 105—11.

Moffitt E.A., Barker R.A., Glenn J.J., Imrie D.D., DelCampo C., Landymore R.W., Kinely C.E. & Murphy D.A. (1986a) Myocardial metabolism and hemodynamic responses with isoflurane anesthesia for coronary arterial surgery. *Anesthesia and Analgesia* **65**, 53—61.

Moffitt E.A., McIntyre A.J., Barker R.A. *et al.* (1986b) Myocardial metabolism and hemodynamic responses with fentanyl—enflurane anesthesia for coronary artery surgery. *Anesthesia and Analgesia* **65**, 46—52.

Moraski R.E., Russel R.O., Smith M. & Rackley C.E. (1975) Left ventricular function in patients with and without myocardial infarction and one, two or three vessel coronary artery disease. *American Journal of Cardiology* **35**, 1—10.

Morel D., Forster A., Gardaz J.P. *et al.* (1981) Comparative haemodynamic and respiratory effects of midazolam and flunitrazepam as induction agents in cardiac surgery. *Arzneimittel—Forschung/Drug Research* **31**, 2264—7.

Morton M., Duke P.C. & Ong B. (1980) Baroreflex control of heart rate in man awake and during enflurane and enflurane—nitrous oxide anesthesia. *Anesthesiology* **52**, 221—3.

Motomura S., Kissin I., Aultman D.F. & Reves J.G. (1984) Effects of fentanyl and nitrous oxide on contractility of blood-perfused papillary muscle of the dog. *Anesthesia and Analgesia* **63**, 47—50.

Muir A.D., Reeder M.K., Foëx P. *et al.* (1991) Preoperative silent myocardial ischaemia: incidence and predictors in a general surgical population. *British Journal of Anaesthesia* **67**, 373—7.

Mulier J.P., Wouters P.F., Van Aken H. *et al.* (1991) Cardiodynamic effects of propofol in comparison with thiopentone: assessment with the transesophageal echocardiographic approach. *Anesthesia and Analgesia* **72**, 28—35.

Muzi M., Berens R.A., Kampine J.P. & Ebert T.J. (1992) Venodilation contributes to propofol-mediated hypotension in humans. *Anesthesia and Analgesia* **74**, 877—83.

Nathan H.J. (1988) Nitrous oxide worsens myocardial ischemia in isoflurane-anesthetized dogs. *Anesthesiology* **68**, 407—15.

Nathan H.J. (1989) Control of hemodynamics prevents worsening of myocardial ischemia when nitrous oxide is administered to isoflurane-anesthetized dogs. *Anesthesiology* **71**, 686—94.

Nicod P., Rehr R., Winniford M.D. *et al.* (1984) Acute systemic and coronary hemodynamic and serologic responses to cigarette smoking in long-term smokers with atherosclerotic coronary artery disease. *Journal of the American College of Cardiology* **4**, 964—71.

Neuhauser D. (1977) Cost-effective clinical decision making. *Pediatrics* **60**, 756—9.

Niemegeers C.J.E. & Janssen P.A.J. (1981) Alfentanil, a particularly shortacting intravenous narcotic analgesic. *Drug Development and Research* **1**, 83.

Nitenberg A., Marty J., Blanchet S. *et al.* (1983) Effects of flunitrazepam on left ventricular performance, coronary haemodynamics and myocardial metabolism in patients with coronary artery disease. *British Journal of Anaesthesia* **55**, 1179—84.

Öberg B. & White S. (1970) The role of vagal nerves and arterial baroreceptors on the circulatory adjustments to hemorrhage in the cat. *Acta Physiologica Scandinavica* **80**, 395−403.

Olson H.G., Lyons K.P., Troope P. *et al.* (1984) The high-risk acute myocardial infarction patients at 1-year follow-up: Identification at hospital discharge by ambulatory electro-cardiography and radionuclide ventriculography. *American Heart Journal* **107**, 358−66.

Ostheimer G.W., Shanahan E.A., Guyton R.A., Daggett W.M. & Lowenstein E. (1975) Effects of fentanyl and droperidol on canine left ventricular performance. *Anesthesiology* **42**, 288−91.

Östman M., Biber B., Martner J. & Reiz S. (1985) Effects of isoflurane on vascular tone and circulatory autoregulation in the feline small intestine. *Acta Anaesthesiologica Scandinavica* **29**, 389−94.

Östman M., Henriksson R., Sundström S. & Reiz S. (1986) Isoflurane — a study of its adrenoreceptor interaction in the isolated rat parotid gland. *Anesthesiology* **64**, 734−8.

Ottesen S. (1978) The influence of thoracic epidural analgesia on the circulation at rest and during physical exercise in man. *Acta Anaesthesiologica Scandinavica* **22**, 537−47.

Ottesen S., Renck H. & Jynge P. (1978) Thoracic epidural analgesia — an experimental study in sheep of the effects of central circulation, regional perfusion and myocardial performance during normoxia, hypoxia and isoproterenol administration. *Acta Anaesthesiologica Scandinavica* **69**, 1.

Pagel P.S., Kampine J.P., Schmeling W.T. & Warltier D.C. (1991a) Influence of volatile anesthetics on myocardial contractility in vivo: desflurane versus isoflurane. *Anesthesiology* **74**, 900.

Pagel P.S., Kampine J.P., Schmeling W.T. & Warltier D.C. (1991b) Comparison of the systemic and coronary hemodynamic actions of desflurane, isoflurane, halothane and enflurane in the chronically instrumented dog. *Anesthesiology* **74**, 539−51.

Pagel P.S., Schmeling W.T., Kampine J.P. & Warltier D.C. (1992) Alteration of canine left ventricular diastolic function by intravenous anesthetics *in vivo*. Ketamine and propofol. *Anesthesiology* **76**, 419−25.

Park W.K. & Lynch C. III (1992) Propofol and thiopental depression of myocardial contractility. A comparative study of mechanical and electrophysiologic effects in isolated guinea pig ventricular muscle. *Anesthesia and Analgesia* **74**, 395−405.

Pasternack P.F., Imparato A.M. & Bear G. (1984) The value of radionuclide angiography as a predictor of perioperative myocardial infarction in patients undergoing abdominal aortic aneurysm resection. *Journal of Vascular Surgery* **1**, 320−5.

Pasternack P.F., Imparato A.M., Riles T.S. *et al.* (1985) The value of radionuclide angiogram in prediction of perioperative myocardial infarction in patients undergoing lower extremity revascularization procedures. *Circulation* **72** (Suppl. II), 13−17.

Pasternack P.F., Grossi E.A., Baumann F.G. *et al.* (1989) The value of silent myocardial ischemia monitoring in the prediction of perioperative myocardial infarction in patients undergoing peripheral vascular surgery. *Journal of Vascular Surgery* **10**, 617−25.

Patrick M.R., Blair I.J., Feneck R.O. & Sebel P.S. (1985) A comparison of the haemodynamic effects of propofol (Diprivan) and thiopentone in patients with coronary artery disease. *Postgraduate Medical Journal* **61** (Suppl. 3), 23−7.

Pearce A.C. & Jones R.M. (1984) Smoking and anesthesia: Preoperative abstinence and perioperative morbidity. *Anesthesiology* **61**, 576−84.

Pedersen T., Kelbaek H. & Munck O. (1990) Cardiopulmonary complications in high-risk surgical patients: the value of preoperative radionuclide cardiography. *Acta Anaesthesiologica Scandinavica* **34**, 183−9.

Perel A., Pizov W.R. & Cotev S. (1987) Systolic blood pressure variation is a sensitive indicator of hypovolemia in ventilated dogs subjected to graded hemorrhage. *Anesthesiology* **67**, 498−502.

Philbin D.M., Foëx P., Drummond G. *et al.* (1985) Postsystolic shortening of canine left ventricle supplied by a stenotic coronary artery when nitrous oxide is added in the presence of narcotics. *Anesthesiology* **62**, 166−74.

Plumlee J.E. & Boetner R.B. (1972) Myocardial infarction during and following anesthesia and operation. *Southern Medical Journal* **65**, 886−9.

Pooling Project Research Group (1978) Relationship of blood pressure, serum cholesterol, smoking habit, relative weight and ECG abnormalities to incidence of major coronary events: final report of the Pooling Project. *Journal of Chronic Diseases* **31**, 201−306.

Port S., Cobb F.R., Coleman R.E. *et al.* (1980) Effect of age on the response of the left ventricular ejection fraction of exercise. *New England Journal of Medicine* **303**, 1133−7.

Price H.L. (1974) Calcium reverses myocardial depression caused by halothane: site of action. *Anesthesiology* **41**, 576−9.

Price H.L. (1976) Myocardial depression by nitrous oxide and its reversal by Ca^{++}. *Anesthesiology* **44**, 211−15.

Price H.L. & Helrich M. (1955) Effects of cyclopropane, diethyl ether, nitrous oxide, thiopental and hydrogen ion concentration upon myocardial function of the dog heart lung preparation. *Journal of Pharmacology and Experimental Therapeutics* **115**, 206−16.

Price H.L. & Ohnishi S.T. (1980) Effects of anesthetics on the heart. *Federal Proceedings* **39**, 1575−9.

Priebe H.J. (1988) Isoflurane causes more severe myocardial dysfunction than halothane in dogs with a critical coronary artery stenosis. *Anesthesiology* **69**, 12−83.

Priebe H.-J. & Foëx P. (1987) Isoflurane causes regional myocardial dysfunction in dogs with critical coronary artery stenoses. *Anesthesiology* **66**, 293−300.

Prys-Roberts C., Meloche R. & Foëx P. (1971) Studies of anesthesia in relation to hypertension: Cardiovascular responses of treated and untreated patients. *British Journal of Anaesthesia* **43**, 122−37.

Prys-Roberts C., Roberts J.G., Foëx P. *et al.* (1976) Interaction of anaesthesia, beta-receptor blockade and blood loss in dogs with induced myocardial infarction. *Anesthesiology* **45**, 326−9.

Prys-Roberts C., Davies J.R., Calverly R.K. & Goodman N.W. (1983) Haemodynamic effects of infusion of diisopropyl phenol (ICI 35868) during nitrous oxide anaesthesia in man. *British Journal of Anaesthesia* **55**, 105−11.

Puttick R.M., Diedericks J., Sear J.W. *et al.* (1992) Effect of graded infusion rates of propofol on regional and global left ventricular function in the dog. *British Journal of Anaesthesia* **69**, 375–81.

Raby K.E., Goldman L., Creager M.A. *et al.* (1989) Correlation between preoperative ischemia and major cardiac events after peripheral vascular surgery. *New England Journal of Medicine* **321**, 1296–300.

Raby K.E., Barry J., Creager M.A. *et al.* (1992) Detection and significance of intraoperative and postoperative myocardial ischemia in peripheral vascular surgery. *Journal of the American Medical Association* **268**, 222–7.

Randall W.C., McNally H., Cowan J. *et al.* (1957) Functional analysis of the cardioaugmentor and cardioaccelerator pathways in the dog. *American Journal of Physiology* **191**, 213–17.

Rao S., Sherbaniuk R.W., Prasad K. *et al.* (1972) Cardiopulmonary effects of diazepam. *Clinical Pharmacology and Therapeutics* **14**, 182–9.

Rao T.L., Jacobs K.H. & El-Etr A.A. (1983) Reinfarction following in anesthesia in patients with myocardial infarction. *Anesthesiology* **59**, 499–505.

Rees A.M., Roberts C.J. & Bligh A.S. (1976) Routine preoperative chest radiography in non-cardio-pulmonary surgery. *British Medical Journal* **1**, 1333–5.

Reiz S. (1985) Systemic and coronary hemodynamic effects of thoracic epidural analgesia in patients with ischemic heart disease. In *Alternative Methoden der Anästhesie* (Eds Lawin P., Van Aken H. & Schneider U.) p. 57. Georg Thieme Verlag, Berlin.

Reiz S., Nath S. & Ponten E. (1979) Haemodynamic effects of prenalterol, a beta-1-adrenoreceptor agonist, in hypotension induced by high thoracic epidural block in man. *Acta Anaesthesiologica Scandinavica* **23**, 93–6.

Reiz S., Nath S. & Rais O. (1980) The effects of thoracic epidural block and prenalterol on coronary vascular resistance and myocardial metabolism in patients with coronary artery disease. *Acta Anaesthesiologica Scandinavica* **24**, 11–16.

Reiz S., Bålfors E., Friedman A., Häggmark S. & Peter T. (1981a) Effects of thiopentone on cardiac performance, coronary haemodynamics and myocardial oxygen consumption in chronic ischaemic heart disease. *Acta Anaesthesiologica Scandinavica* **25**, 103–10.

Reiz S., Bålfors E., Häggmark S. *et al.* (1981b) Myocardial oxygen consumption and coronary haemodynamics during fentanyl–droperidol–nitrous oxide anaesthesia in patients with ischaemic heart disease. *Acta Anaesthesiologica Scandinavica* **25**, 286–92.

Reiz S., Bålfors E., Bredgaard Sörensen M., Häagmark & Nyhman H. (1982a) Coronary hemodynamic effects of general anesthesia and surgery: Modification by epidural analgesia in patients with ischemic heart disease. *Regional Anesthesia* **7** (Suppl.), 8S.

Reiz S., Bålfors E., Gustavsson B. *et al.* (1982b) Effects of halothane on coronary haemodynamics and myocardial metabolism in patients with ischaemic heart disease and heart failure. *Acta Anaesthesiologica Scandinavica* **26**, 133–8.

Reiz S., Häggmark S., Rydvall A. & Östman M. (1982c) Beta-blockers and thoracic epidural analgesia. Cardioprotective and synergistic effects. *Acta Anaesthesiologica Scandinavica* **76** (Suppl.), 54.

Reiz S., Bålfors E., Sorensen M.B., Ariola S., Friedman A. &

Truedsson H. (1983) Isoflurane — a powerful coronary vasodilator in patients with coronary artery disease. *Anesthesiology* **59**, 91–7.

Reiz S., Rydvall A. & Häggmark S. (1985) Coronary haemodynamic effects of surgery during enflurane-nitrous oxide anaesthesia in patients with ischaemic heart disease. *Acta Anaesthesiologica Scandinavica* **29**, 106–12.

Reiz S., d'Ambra M.N. & Östman M. (1987) Myocardial ischemia during inhalation anesthesia in surgical patients with coronary artery disease. In *Inhalation Anesthetics — New Aspects* (Eds Peter K., Brown B.R., Martin E. & Norlander O.) Band 185, p. 187. Springer-Verlag, Berlin.

Rennart G., Saltz-Rennert H., Wanderman K. & Weitzman S. (1985) Size of acute myocardial infarcts in patients with diabetes mellitus. *American Journal of Cardiology* **55**, 1629–30.

Reves J.G., Samuelson P.N. & Lewis S. (1979) Midazolam meleate induction in patients with ischaemic heart disease: haemodynamic observations. *Canadian Anaesthetists' Society Journal* **26**, 402–9.

Reves J.G., Kissin I., Fournier S.E. & Smith L.R. (1984) Additive negative inotropic effect of a combination of diazepam and fentanyl. *Anesthesia and Analgesia* **63**, 97–100.

Riles T.S., Kopelman I. & Imparato A.M. (1979) Myocardial infarction following carotid endarterectomy: a review of 683 operations. *Surgery* **85**, 249–52.

Robin E.D. (1985) The cult of the Swan–Ganz catheter. Overuse and abuse of pulmonary flow catheters. *Annals of Internal Medicine* **103**, 445–9.

Roizen M.F., Hamilton W.K. & Sohn Y.J. (1981) Treatment of stress-induced increases in pulmonary capillary wedge pressure using volatile anesthetics. *Anesthesiology* **55**, 446–50.

Rokey R., Rolak L.A., Harati Y., Kutka N. & Verani M.S. (1984) Coronary artery disease in patients with cerebrovascular disease: a prospective study. *Annals of Neurology* **16**, 50–3.

Rolly G., Kay B. & Cocks F. (1979) A double blind comparison of high doses of fentanyl and sufentanil in man. Influences of cardiovascular, respiratory and metabolic parameters. *Acta Anaesthesiologica Belgica* **30**, 247–54.

Rosow C.E., Philbin D.M., Keegan C.R. & Moss J. (1984) Hemodynamics and histamine release during induction with sufentanil or fentanyl. *Anesthesiology* **60**, 489–91.

Ross J. (1983) Myocardial ischemia. In *Cardiac Therapy* (Eds Rosen M.R. & Hoffman B.F.) pp. 45–71. Martinus Nijhoff, Boston.

Rouby J.-J., Andreev A., Léger P. *et al.* (1991) Peripheral vascular effects of thiopental and propofol in humans with artificial hearts. *Anesthesiology* **75**, 32–42.

Roy W.L., Edelist G. & Gilbert B. (1979) Myocardial ischemia during non-cardiac surgical procedures in coronary patients. *Anesthesiology* **51**, 393–7.

Rucquoi M. & Camu F. (1983) Cardiovascular responses to large doses of alfentanil and fentanyl. *British Journal of Anaesthesia* **55**, 223S–30S.

Rydvall A., Häggmark S., Nyhman H. & Reiz S. (1984) Effects of enflurane on coronary haemodynamics in patients with ischaemic heart disease. *Acta Anaesthesiologica Scandinavica* **28**, 690–5.

Saada M., Duval A.-M., Bonnet F. *et al.* (1989) Abnormalities in myocardial segmental wall motion during lumbar epidural anesthesia. *Anesthesiology* **71**, 26–32.

Sagal S.S., Evens R.G., Forrest J.V. & Bramson R.T. (1974) Efficacy of routine screening and lateral chest radiographs in a hospital-based population. *New England Journal of Medicine* **291**, 1001–4.

Sage D.J., Close A. & Boas R.A. (1987) Reversal of midazolam sedation with anexate. *British Journal of Anaesthesia* **59**, 459–64.

Sahlman L., Henriksson B.-Å., Martner J. *et al.* (1988) Effects of halothane, enflurane and isoflurane on coronary vascular tone, myocardial performance and oxygen consumption during controlled changes in aortic and left atrial pressure. Studies on isolated working rat hearts *in vitro*. *Anesthesiology* **69**, 1–10.

Salmenperä M., Peltola K., Takkunen O. & Heinonen J. (1983) Cardiovascular effects of pancuronium and vecuronium during high-dose fentanyl anesthesia. *Anesthesia and Analgesia* **62**, 1059–64.

Samuelson P.N., Lell W.A., Kouchoukos N.T. *et al.* (1980) Hemodynamics during diazepam induction of anesthesia for coronary artery bypass grafting. *Southern Medical Journal* **73**, 332–4.

Samuelson P.N., Reves J.R., Kouchnoukos N.T. *et al.* (1981) Hemodynamic responses to anesthetic induction with midazolam or diazepam in patients with ischemic heart disease. *Anesthesia and Analgesia* **60**, 802–9.

Sapala J.A., Ponka J.L. & Duvernoy W.F. (1975) Operative and non-operative risks in the cardiac patient. *Journal of the American Geriatrics Society* **23**, 529–34.

Schneider A.J. (1983) Assessment of risk factors and surgical outcome. *Surgical Clinics of North America* **63**, 1113–26.

Schoeppel L.S., Wilkinson C., Waters J. & Meyers S.N. (1983) Effects of myocardial infarction on perioperative cardiac complications. *Anesthesia and Analgesia* **62**, 493–8.

Schulte-Sasse U., Hess W. & Tarnow J. (1982) Haemodynamic responses to induction of anaesthesia using midazolam in cardiac surgical patients. *British Journal of Anaesthesia* **54**, 1053–8.

Schulze R.A., Strauss H.W. & Pitt B. (1976) Sudden death in the year following myocardial infarction. Relation to ventricular premature contractions in the last hospital phase and left ventricular ejection fraction. *American Journal of Medicine* **62**, 192–9.

Seagard J.L., Elegbe E.O., Hopp F.A. *et al.* (1983) Effects of isoflurane on the baroreceptor reflex. *Anesthesiology* **59**, 511–20.

Sebel P.S. & Bovill J.G. (1982) Cardiovascular effects of sufentanil anesthesia. *Anesthesia and Analgesia* **61**, 115–19.

Sebel P.S. & Lowdon J.D. (1989) Propofol: a new intravenous anesthetic. *Anesthesiology* **71**, 260–77.

Sebel P.S., Bovill J.G., Boekhorst R.A.A. & Rog N. (1982) Cardiovascular effects of high-dose fentanyl anaesthesia. *Acta Anaesthesiologica Scandinavica* **26**, 308–15.

Sethna D.H., Moffitt E.A., Gray R.J. *et al.* (1982) Cardiovascular effects of morphine in patients with coronary artery disease. *Anesthesia and Analgesia* **61**, 109–14.

Sill J.C., Boye A.A., Nugent M. *et al.* (1987) Effects of isoflurane on coronary arteries and coronary arterioles in the intact dog. *Anesthesiology* **66**, 273–9.

Sjögren S. & Wright B. (1972) Circulatory changes during continuous epidural blockade. *Acta Anaesthesiologica Scandinavica* **16**, 5–25.

Skinner J.F. & Pearce M.L. (1964) Surgical risk in the cardiac patient. *Journal of Chronic Diseases* **17**, 57–72.

Skovsted P. & Sapthavichaikul S. (1977) The effects of isoflurane on arterial pressure, pulse rate, autonomic nervous activity, and barostatic reflexes. *Canadian Anaesthetists' Society Journal* **24**, 304–14.

Slavik J.R., LaMantia K.R., Kopriva C.I. *et al.* (1988) Does nitrous oxide cause regional wall motion abnormalities in patients with coronary artery disease? *Anesthesia and Analgesia* **67**, 695–700.

Slogoff S. & Keats A.S. (1985) Does perioperative myocardial ischemia lead to postoperative myocardial infarction? *Anesthesiology* **62**, 107–14.

Slogoff S. & Keats A.S. (1986) Further observations on perioperative myocardial ischemia. *Anesthesiology* **65**, 539–42.

Slogoff S. & Keats A.S. (1989) Randomized trial of primary anesthetic agents on outcome of coronary bypass operations. *Anesthesiology* **70**, 179–88.

Slogoff S., Keats A.S., Dear W.E. *et al.* (1991) Steal-prone anatomy and myocardial ischemia associated with four primary anesthetic agents in humans. *Anesthesia and Analgesia* **72**, 22–7.

Smith N.T. & Corbascio A.N. (1966) The cardiovascular effects of nitrous oxide during halothane anesthesia in the dog. *Anesthesiology* **27**, 560–6.

Smith J.S., Cahalan M.K., Benefield D.J. *et al.* (1985) Intraoperative detection of myocardial ischemia in high-risk patients: electrocardiography versus two-dimensional transesophageal echocardiography. *Circulation* **72**, 1015–21.

Smith J.S., Roizen M.F., Cahalan M.K. *et al.* (1988) Does anesthetic technique make a difference? Augmentation of systolic blood pressure during carotid endarterectomy: effect of phenylephrine versus light anesthesia and of isoflurane versus halothane on the incidence of myocardial ischemia. *Anesthesiology* **69**, 846–53.

Sonntag H., Heiss H.W., Knoll D. *et al.* (1973) Der Einfluss von Ketamin auf den myokardialen Metabolismus. *Anaesthesiologie und Wiederbelebung* **69**, 37.

Sonntag H., Hellberg K., Schnek H.-D. *et al.* (1975) Effects of thiopental (Trapanal) on coronary blood flow and myocardial metabolism in man. *Acta Anaesthesiologica Scandinavica* **19**, 69–78.

Sonntag H., Merin R.G., Donath U., Radke J. & Schenk H.D. (1979) Myocardial metabolism and oxygenation in man awake and during halothane anesthesia. *Anesthesiology* **51**, 204–10.

Sonntag H., Larsen R., Hilfiker O. *et al.* (1982) Myocardial blood flow and oxygen consumption during high-dose fentanyl anesthesia in patients with coronary artery disease. *Anesthesiology* **56**, 417–22.

Sonntag H., Stephan H., Lange H. *et al.* (1989) Sufentanil does not block sympathetic responses to surgical stimuli in patients having coronary artery revascularization surgery. *Anesthesia and Analgesia* **68**, 584–92.

Spotoft H., Korshin J.D., Sorensen M.B. & Skovsted P. (1979) The cardiovascular effects of ketamine used for induction of anaesthesia in patients with valvular heart disease. *Canadian Anaesthetists' Society Journal* **26**, 463–7.

Sprague D.H., Yang J.C. & Ngai S.H. (1974) Effects of isoflurane and halothane on contractility and the cyclic 3',5'-adenosine monophosphate system in the rat aorta. *Anesthesiology* **40**, 162—7.

Stanley T.H. (1978) Cardiovascular effects of droperidol during enflurane and enflurane-nitrous oxide anaesthesia in man. *Canadian Anaesthetists' Society Journal* **25**, 26—9.

Stanley T.H. & Liu W.S. (1977) Cardiovascular effects of nitrous oxide—meperidine anesthesia before and after pancuronium. *Anesthesia and Analgesia* **56**, 669—73.

Stanley T.H. & Webster L.R. (1978) Anesthetic requirements and cardiovascular effects of fentanyl—oxygen and fentanyl—diazepam—oxygen anesthesia in man. *Anesthesia and Analgesia* **57**, 411—16.

Stanley T.H., Gray N.H., Stanford W. & Armstrong R. (1973) The effects of high-dose morphine on fluid and blood requirements in open-heart procedures. *Anesthesiology* **38**, 536—41.

Steen P.A., Tinker J.H. & Tarhan S. (1978) Myocardial reinfarction after anesthesia and surgery. *Journal of the American Medical Association* **239**, 2566—70.

Stephan H., Sonntag H., Schenk H.D., Kettler D. & Khambuttu H.J. (1986) Effects of propofol on cardiovascular dynamics, myocardial blood flow and myocardial metabolism in patients with coronary artery disease. *British Journal of Anaesthesia* **58**, 969—75.

Stoelting R.K. & Gibbs P.S. (1973) Hemodynamic effects of morphine and morphine-nitrous oxide in valvular heart disease and coronary artery disease. *Anesthesiology* **38**, 45—52.

Stone J.G., Foëx P., Sear J.W. *et al.* (1988) Myocardial ischemia in untreated hypertensive patients: effect of a single small dose of a beta-adrenergic blocking agent. *Anesthesiology* **68**, 495—500.

Stowe D.F., Bosnjak Z.J. & Kampine J.P. (1992) Comparison of etomidate, midazolam, propofol and thiopental on function and metabolism of isolated hearts. *Anesthesia and Analgesia* **74**, 547—58.

Strauer B.E. (1972) Contractile responses to morphine, piritramide, meperidine and fentanyl: a comparative study of effects on the isolated ventricular myocardium. *Anesthesiology* **37**, 304—10.

Stühmeier K.D., Mainzer B., Sandmann W. & Tarnow J. (1992) Isoflurane does not increase the incidence of intraoperative myocardial ischaemia compared with halothane during vascular surgery. *British Journal of Anaesthesia* **69**, 602—6.

Sundberg A. & Wattwil M. (1986) Circulatory and respiratory effects of high thoracic epidural anaesthesia — with special reference to the sympathetic block and the systemic effects of the local anaesthetic. PhD thesis, Uppsala University.

Takeshima R. & Dohi S. (1985) Circulatory responses to baroreflexes, Valsalva maneuver, coughing, swallowing and nasal stimulation during acute cardiac sympathectomy by epidural blockade in awake humans. *Anesthesiology* **63**, 500—8.

Tarhan S., Moffitt E., Taylor W.F. & Ginliani (1972) Myocardial infarction after general anesthesia. *Journal of the American Medical Association* **220**, 1451—4.

Tarnow J., Eberlein H.J., Oser G. *et al.* (1977) Haemodynamik, Myokardkontraktilität, Ventrikelvolumina und Sauerstoffversorgung des Herzens unter verschiedenen Inhalationsanaesthetika. *Der Anaesthetist* **26**, 220—30.

Tatekawa S., Traber K.B., Hantler C.B. *et al.* (1987) Effects of isoflurane on myocardial blood flow and oxygen consump-tion in the presence of critical coronary stenosis in dogs. *Anesthesia and Analgesia* **66**, 1073—82.

Thompson I.R. & Putnins C.L. (1985) Adverse effects of pancuronium during high-dose fentanyl anesthesia for coronary artery bypass grafting. *Anesthesiology* **62**, 708—13.

Thompson I.R., Bowering J.B., Hudson R.J. *et al.* (1991) A comparison of desflurane and isoflurane in patients undergoing coronary artery surgery. *Anesthesiology* **75**, 776—81.

Tomichek R.C., Rosow C.E., Philbin D.M. *et al.* (1983) Diazepam—fentanyl interaction: hemodynamic and hormonal effects in coronary artery surgery. *Anesthesia and Analgesia* **62**, 881—4.

Topkins M.J. & Artusio J.F. (1964) Myocardial infarction and surgery: A five year study. *Anesthesia and Analgesia* **43**, 716—20.

Topol E.J., Weiss J.L., Guzman P.A. *et al.* (1984) Immediate improvement of dysfunctional myocardial segments after coronary revascularization: detection by intraoperative transesophageal echocardiography. *Journal of the American College of Cardiology* **4**, 1123—34.

Tuman K.J., McCarthy R.J., Spiess B.D. *et al.* (1989a) Does choice of anesthetic agent significantly affect outcome after coronary artery surgery? *Anesthesiology* **70**, 189—98.

Tuman K.J., McCarthy R.J., Spiess B.D. *et al.* (1989b) Effect of pulmonary artery catheterization on outcome in patients undergoing coronary artery surgery. *Anesthesiology* **70**, 199—206.

Tuman K.J., McCarthy R.J., March R.J. *et al.* (1991) Effects of epidural anesthesia on coagulation and outcome after major vascular surgery. *Anesthesia and Analgesia* **73**, 696—704.

Tweed W.A., Minuck M. & Mymin D. (1972) Circulatory responses to ketamine anesthesia. *Anesthesiology* **37**, 613—19.

Urbanowicz J.H., Shaaban M.N., Cohen N.G. *et al.* (1990) Comparison of transesophageal echocardiographic and scintigraphic estimates of left ventricular end-diastolic volume index and ejection fraction in patients following coronary artery bypass grafting. *Anesthesiology* **72**, 607—12.

Vacanti C.J., Van Houten R.J. & Hill R.C. (1970) A statistical analysis of the relationship of physical status to postoperative mortality in 68,388 cases. *Anesthesia and Analgesia* **49**, 564—6.

Valentin N, Lomholt B., Jensen J.S. *et al.* (1986) Spinal and general anaesthesia for surgery of the fractured hip. A prospective study in 578 patients. *British Journal of Anaesthesia* **58**, 284—91.

Valicenti J.F., Newman W.H., Bagwell E.E., Pruett K.L. & Rpboe N.W. (1973) Myocardial contractility during induction and steady-state ketamine anesthesia. *Anesthesia and Analgesia* **52**, 190—4.

Van Aken H. & Brüssel T. (1990) Propofol causes cardiovascular depression. II. *Anesthesiology* **72**, 394.

Van de Walle J., Lauwers P. & Adriaensen H. (1976) Double blind comparison of fentanyl and sufentanil in anaesthesia. *Acta Anaesthesiologica Belgica* **27**, 129—38.

Vatner S.F. & Smith N.T. (1974) Effects of halothane on left ventricular function and distribution of regional blood flow in dogs and primates. *Circulation Research* **34**, 155—67.

Verrier E.D., Edelist G., Macke C. *et al.* (1980) Greater coronary vascular reserve in dogs anesthetized with halothane. *Anesthesiology* **53**, 445—9.

Vismara L.A., Amsterdam E.A. & Mason D.T. (1975) Relation to ventricular arrhythmias in the late hospital phase of acute myocardial infarction to sudden death after hospital discharge. *American Journal of Medicine* **59**, 6–12.

von Knorring J.V. (1981) Postoperative myocardial infarction: a prospective study in a riskgroup of surgical patients. *Surgery* **90**, 55–60.

Vrillon M., Le Bret F., Vrints J. *et al.* (1990) Systolic blood pressure variation in postoperative ventilated patients. A sensitive indicator of low preload states. *Anesthesiology* **73**, 243A.

Wagner R.L. & White P.F. (1984) Etomidate inhibits adrenocortical function in surgical patients. *Anesthesiology* **61**, 647–51.

Waller B.F., Palumbo P.J., Lie J.T. & Roberts W.C. (1980) Status of the coronary arteries at necropsy in diabetes mellitus with onset after age 30 years: Analysis of 229 diabetic patients with and without clinical evidence of coronary heart disease and comparison to 183 control subjects. *American Journal of Medicine* **69**, 498–506.

Waller J.L., Hug C.C., Nagle D.N. & Craver J.M. (1981) Hemodynamic changes during fentanyl–oxygen anesthesia for aortocoronary bypass operations. *Anesthesiology* **55**, 212–17.

Warltier D.C. & Pagel P.S. (1992) Cardiovascular and respiratory actions of desflurane: is desflurane different from isoflurane? *Anesthesia and Analgesia* (Suppl. 75), 17S–29S.

Wattwil M., Sundberg A., Arvill A. & Lennquist C. (1985) Circulatory changes during high thoracic epidural anaesthesia-influence of sympathetic block and of systemic effects of the local anaesthetic. *Acta Anaesthesiologica Scandinavica* **29**, 849–55.

Waxman K., Shoemaker W.C. & Lippman M. (1980) Cardiovascular effects of anesthetic induction with ketamine. *Anesthesia and Analgesia* **59**, 355–8.

Weisfeldt M.L. (1980) Aging of the cardiovascular system. *New England Journal of Medicine* **303**, 1172–4.

Weiskopf R.B., Cahalan M.K., Ionescu P. *et al.* (1991) Cardiovascular actions of desflurane with and without nitrous oxide during spontaneous ventilation in humans. *Anesthesia and Analgesia* **73**, 165–74.

Wells P.H. & Kaplan J.A. (1981) Optimal management of patients with ischemic heart disease for noncardiac surgery by complementary anesthesiologist and cardiologist inter-

action. *American Heart Journal* **102**, 1029–37.

Weyman A.E., Franklin T.D., Egenes K.M. & Green D. (1977) Correlation between extent of abnormal regional wall motion and myocardial infarct size in chronically infarcted dogs. *Circulation* **56**, 271A.

White P.F., Way W.L. & Trevor A.J. (1982) Ketamine: its pharmacology and therapeutic uses. *Anesthesiology* **56**, 119–36.

White P.F., Shafer A., Boyle W.A. *et al.* (1989) Benzodiazepine antagonism does not provoke a stress response. *Anesthesiology* **70**, 636–9.

Wilkinson P.L., Hamilton W.K., Moyers J.R. *et al.* (1981) Halothane and morphine–nitrous oxide anesthesia in patients undergoing coronary artery bypass operation. *Journal of Thoracic and Cardiovascular Surgery* **82**, 372–82.

Wilkowski D.A.W., Sill J.C., Bonta W., Owen R. & Bove A.A. (1987) Nitrous oxide constricts epicardial coronary arteries without effect on coronary arterioles. *Anesthesiology* **66**, 659–65.

Windsor J.P.W., Sherry K., Feneck R.O. & Sebel P.S. (1988) Sufentanil and nitrous oxide anaesthesia for cardiac surgery. *British Journal of Anaesthesia* **61**, 662–8.

Winter P.M., Hornbein T.F. & Smith G. (1972) Hyperbaric nitrous oxide anesthesia in man: determination of anesthetic potency (MAC) and cardiorespiratory effects. *Abstracts of American Society of Anesthesiologists Annual Meeting.* p. 103, Boston.

Wohlgelernter D., Cleman M., Highman H.A. *et al.* (1986) Regional myocardial dysfunction during coronary angioplasty: evaluation by two-dimensional echocardiography and 12-lead electrocardiography. *Journal of the American College of Cardiology* **7**, 1245–54.

Yeager M.P., Glass D., Neff R.K., Brinck-Johnsen T. (1987) Epidural anesthesia and analgesia in high-risk surgical patients. *Anesthesiology* **66**, 729–36.

Young A.E., Sandberg G.W. & Couch N.P. (1977) The reduction of mortality of abdominal aortic aneurysm resection. *American Journal of Surgery* **134**, 585–90.

Zhang C.-C., Su J.Y. & Calkins D. (1990) Effects of alfentanil on isolated cardiac tissues of the rabbit. *Anesthesia and Analgesia* **71**, 268–74.

Zsigmond E.K. (1974) Guest discussion. *Anesthesia and Analgesia* **53**, 931–3.

Anaesthesia and Liver Disease

B.R. BROWN JR

Patients with hepatic disease are extreme risks for surgery, more so than those with cardiac disease. In this chapter, the incidence, complications, preoperative therapy and assessment, and intraoperative management of individuals with liver disease are described. Some discussion of anaesthetic recommendations for the individual with cholestatic (obstructive) jaundice is included.

Incidence of liver disease

There are numerous causes of acute and chronic liver disease. However, the most common severe hepatic lesion in Western nations is cirrhosis. Many physicians associate all cirrhosis with excess alcohol intake, but it has been estimated that 50% of cirrhosis in Europe and North America is secondary to alcoholism and 50% results from postviral hepatitis and cryptogenic causes. In a Danish study, the death rate for alcoholic and cryptogenic cirrhosis was 10 per 100 000 inhabitants per year (Malchow-Moller *et al.*, 1985). In this study, individuals with alcoholic cirrhosis had only a 62% 1-year survival rate following the diagnosis. Patients with cryptogenic cirrhosis had only a 56% 1-year survival following diagnosis. These high mortality rates are for medical patients without surgery. The incidence of cirrhosis in the USA among males is 48:100 000, whereas alcoholic hepatitis is found in approximately 20:100 000 (Garagliano *et al.*, 1979). Alcoholic liver disease is the third leading cause of death for individuals age 25–64 years in New York City, and the fifth leading cause of death in Canada in men of this same age. One of the major issues from an anaesthesia standpoint is that the incidence of cirrhosis is increasing in Western countries. For example, in the USA from 1950–74, deaths from cirrhosis increased by 72% while many other diseases, particularly cardiovascular disease, declined (Lieber & Leo, 1982). The incidence of liver disease is increasing in parallel with increasing alcohol consumption observed in Western industrialized countries. This unfortunate trend implies that more individuals with problems of liver disease will be candidates for surgery and anaesthesia.

Risk factors in the patient with liver disease

Child's classification has been used as the gold standard for risk assessment in the patient with cirrhosis for over two decades (Childs, 1963) (Table 61.1). Originally, this risk assessment in patients with parenchymal hepatic disease from cirrhosis was derived from data analysed from patients undergoing portocaval shunt surgery. However, the general principles involved have been extrapolated frequently and probably quite appropriately to all major surgical procedures in patients with cirrhotic liver disease.

Pugh and colleagues in 1973 amended Child's classification by adding the prothrombin test which was not available at the time Child's guidelines were originally formulated. Alteration of the prothrombin time is not linearly correlated with mortality. Prolongation of the prothrombin test for more than 4 s implies significant risk. Aranha and colleagues (1982) performed a retrospective study for the years 1971–9 and reported mortality and morbidity of a single major surgical procedure (e.g. cholecystectomy) in cirrhotics compared with non-cirrhotic patients (Table 61.2). The mortality rate in patients with severe cirrhosis was very high. This group employed the prothrombin test as a single measure of liver function and, in certain respects, this is probably appropriate.

More recent studies have confirmed that the patient with parenchymal hepatic disease has significant risk for surgery. Garrison and colleagues (1984)

Table 61.1 Child's classification of risks for cirrhotic patients undergoing surgery

	Group A	Group B	Group C
Serum bilirubin (μmol/litre)	<40	40−50	>50
Serum albumin (g/litre)	>35	30−35	<30
Ascites	None	Controlled	Not controlled
Neurological disorder	None	Minimal	Advanced
Nutritional status	Excellent	Good	Poor‡
Surgical risk	Good*	Moderate†	Poor‡

* <10% mortality; † approximately 30% mortality; ‡ >40% mortality.

Table 61.2 Mortality following cholecystectomy in patients with cirrhosis. (Data from Aranha *et al.*, 1982)

		Mortality rate	
	n	*n*	%
Normal liver function	314	4	1
Moderate cirrhosis: Prothrombin test <2.5 s above control	43	4	9
Severe cirrhosis: Prothrombin test >2.5 s	12	10	83

Table 61.3 Preoperative variables and mortality rates in cirrhotic patients. (Data from Garrison *et al.*, 1984)

Variable	Mortality rate if present (%)
Child's classification	
A	10
B	30
C	76
Albumin <3 g/dl	58
Antibiotics >2	82
Ascites	58
Bilirubin >50 μmol/litre	62
Cardiac failure	92
Emergency surgery	57
Hepatic failure	66
Infection	64
Prothrombin test >1.5 times control	63
Pulmonary failure	100

examined various factors before surgery which seemed to contribute to increased mortality rates in patients with cirrhosis (Table 61.3). A variety of seemingly incidental phenomena can increase mortality rates in these patients. For example, in the Garrison study, the combination of severe liver disease and pulmonary failure produced a mortality rate of 100%.

Studies of this type indicate that individuals with these problems are at high risk. However, a glimmer of light is also shed by these reports. For example, treating ascites and nutritional status in an appropriate fashion preoperatively seems to reduce mortality rate in the surgical patient. Thus, correction of the stigmata of liver disease decreases overall surgical mortality. Essentially, such information suggests that careful preparation can improve outcome.

Preoperative considerations

Cardiovascular consequences

There are several cardiovascular consequences of liver disease. For reasons that are not known, the patient with liver disease tends to develop significant numbers and different types of shunts. The well-known cutaneous spider angioma is, in reality, an arteriovenous shunt. Several types of shunts seen in liver disease are listed in Table 61.4. These shunts produce several side-effects: a common one is increased cardiac output. The author has seen an individual of 60 kg with moderate liver disease who had a resting cardiac output of 12 litres/min. Many patients of normal size with cirrhosis have cardiac outputs in the region of 7−9 litres/min. Data from individuals who had hepatic transplantation show that restoration of normal liver function (by transplantation) caused a reduction of this increased cardiac output.

In hepatic disease, there occurs also a diminution

Table 61.4 Types of shunt observed in cirrhotic patients

Cutaneous shunts ('spiders')
Intrapulmonic shunts
Portapulmonary shunts
Pleural shunts

in peripheral vascular resistance. Coupled with these changes is a general increase in plasma volume. Patients with liver disease have activation of the renin–angiotensin system which causes an increase in plasma volume and interstitial extracellular fluid volume. In contrast, alcoholics may have low cardiac output and failure secondary to alcoholic cardiomyopathy. In such patients, left ventricular stress produces a marked increase in pulmonary wedge pressure without an increase in left ventricular stroke work (Limas *et al.*, 1974). Cardiac arrhythmias, commonly ventricular extrasystoles, are observed frequently in alcoholic hepatitis. In addition, nutritional deficiencies including beriberi heart disease can cause significant decreases in cardiac reserve. Pulmonary hypertension is observed in the cirrhotic on occasion, but is not a universal feature.

One good feature of this otherwise dim outlook is that the patient with cirrhosis seems to have a less-than-usual incidence of arteriosclerosis. However, if the patient has a history of heavy smoking, this may not be so. Even with the low incidence of coronary thrombosis, congestive heart failure is a constant threat in patients with parenchymal liver disease.

The patient with liver disease should be investigated adequately for cardiac disease before surgery. Signs and symptoms of congestive failure should be sought and treatment given if necessary.

Ascites

Ascites is one of the more common manifestations of liver failure and its presence indicates severe liver disease. There is uniform opinion that the presence of ascites in a patient dictates that the individual has a graver surgical risk than the individual who does not have ascites. Ascites in liver disease is produced by three mechanisms.
1 Decreased albumin synthesis by the liver with consequent lowered plasma oncotic pressure.
2 Weeping of the liver because of increased lymphatic pressure.
3 Dilutional hyponatraemia secondary to sodium and fluid retention.

The exact role of each of these three mechanisms varies from patient to patient. There is no doubt that marked sodium retention accompanies ascites invariably. There is also no question that this sodium and water retention is at times a difficult problem. A real clinical problem entails distinguishing between water retention and true hyponatraemia. Frequently, the patient with liver disease is found to have marked serum hyponatraemia (e.g. a serum sodium of 130 mmol/litre is not unusual). In many instances, this does not indicate that the patient has a deficit of sodium stores. Instead, it indicates that water retention is greater than sodium retention, and that overall the patient may have a fairly normal body content of sodium. In this circumstance, water diuresis rather than sodium addition is appropriate therapy. This differentiation requires care by the hepatologist and anaesthetist to determine what is appropriate treatment under such circumstances.

Ideally, therapy of ascites, which reduces surgical risk, is initiated at an early stage before the proposed surgical procedure. The hepatologist should begin adequate carbohydrate and protein diet combined with a restricted sodium intake of approximately 45 mmol/day or less. Diuretics are started cautiously. It should be emphasized that inappropriate or too rapid diuretic therapy is one of the leading causes of hepatic failure in the cirrhotic patient. These individuals are extremely sensitive to hypokalaemia and great care and time should be taken with diuretic therapy. The aldosterone antagonist, spironolactone, is the usual diuretic used because of its potassium-sparing ability. After initiation of treatment with this drug, it is usual to add small amounts of a diuretic such as frusemide. The problems of diuretic therapy in these individuals include not only hypokalaemia but also hypochloraemia and hyponatraemia, all of which may aggravate metabolic alkalosis and augment the development of hepatic failure and hepatic encephalopathy.

The role of paracentesis is still debatable. In earlier eras of medicine, paracentesis was performed commonly with the abrupt removal of 5–8 litres of fluid which alleviated ascites quickly. The advent of more potent diuretics reduced the frequency of use of this technique. However, there is some indication that the technique may be undergoing a revival, and that complications are not as grave as once thought. An interesting aspect on the patient with chronic liver disease and ascites is that those individuals with distinguishable clinical peripheral oedema may have more preferential mobilization of oedema fluid and can undergo diuresis safely at a rapid rate (greater than 2 kg/day) (Pockros & Reynolds, 1986).

In certain centres, another technique used to treat intractable ascites is the LeVeen shunt. Basically, this is a peritoneovenous shunt with a one-way valve from peritoneal cavity to jugular vein. These are generally inserted under local anaesthesia. A variety of complications may occur with this treatment of ascites, although the result of diminution of ascitic fluid is generally dramatic. Complications include:

1 Disseminated intravascular coagulation (appearing in as many as 60% of these individuals).
2 Cardiac failure.
3 Infection.
4 Venous thrombosis.

If the anaesthetist encounters an individual with the LeVeen shunt, great care should be taken to study coagulation indices before and during surgery, as disseminated intravascular coagulation and other alterations of clotting factors by contamination from various peptides from the peritoneal cavity, known and unknown, may occur.

Pulmonary considerations

Table 61.5. lists some of the alterations in pulmonary status and gas exchange observed in patients with moderate to severe cirrhosis. Fifteen to 45% of patients with established cirrhosis can present with some type of pulmonary abnormality (Krowka & Cortese, 1985). True intrapulmonary shunting with low Pao_2 in patients with cirrhosis may be quite marked and can occur in the absence of other stigmata of liver disease such as significant ascites, splenomegaly, or distal clubbing (Georg et al., 1960). Shunting may amount to 70% of total cardiac output. Pleural effusions can further augment problems of pulmonary gas exchange in these patients. Pleural effusions may be present in up to 10% of cirrhotics. The hypoxaemia evoked by intrapulmonary shunting coupled with mechanical effects of pleural effusion may cause severe changes in arterial blood-gas tensions. An additional problem is the frequent presence of ventilation : perfusion mismatches ($\dot{V}:\dot{Q}$ abnormalities). Krowka and Cortese (1989) state that dilated pulmonary capillaries are a major cause of hypoxia in liver disease. These diluted capillaries do not allow oxygen from alveoli to enrich the central axial stream of blood. Thus, an outer shell of oxygenated blood mixes with a core of unoxygenated blood. Assuming a supine position lessens basilar pulmonary segment capillary dilatation and oxygenation is improved. This correlates well with the finding that many patients with liver disease suffer from platypnoea

Table 61.5 Pulmonary states and altered gas exchange observed in patients with cirrhosis

Restrictive defects due to abdominal ascites
Pleural effusions
True intrapulmonic shunts
Ventilation : perfusion mismatches ($\dot{V}:\dot{Q}$ abnormalities)
Restricted alveolar diffusion

(breathing better in the supine than in the upright position) and orthodeoxia (oxygen tension in arterial blood greater in the supine than in the upright position). Obviously, true shunts are not amenable to therapy with an increased F_Io_2, although the $\dot{V}:\dot{Q}$ mismatch is improved. Several minor abnormalities such as changes in haemoglobin P_{50} and alveolar diffusion defects have been noted, but these are not common. It must be emphasized that intrapulmonary shunting is real and common in these patients.

Many alcoholics are heavy smokers. Thus, the problems of liver disease on gas exchange may be compounded by chronic obstructive airways disease. Appropriate chest physiotherapy, bronchodilators and other forms of treatment for chronic obstructive pulmonary disease may be required in an effort to bring these patients up to the best level of gas exchange for surgery. Again it must be emphasized that without a change in the underlying hepatic disease progression, little alteration can be made in the hypoxaemia secondary to true shunts. In the author's experience, patients with cirrhosis who are non-smokers have Pao_2 in the range of 9.3 kPa (70 mmHg) because of shunts which cannot be changed by an increase in inspired oxygen concentration.

In addition to pleural effusions, mechanical restriction of ventilation occurs from ascites which causes an upward deviation of the diaphragm. This may be improved by appropriate diuretic therapy and/or paracentesis. If the patient has associated chronic obstructive airways disease, the anaesthetist should remember also that clearances of bronchodilators such as theophylline may be depressed significantly in patients with parenchymal liver disease. (Mangione et al., 1978). It may be wise to measure plasma concentrations of these drugs as a guide to therapeutic and non-toxic concentrations.

Renal, endocrine and metabolic changes in the cirrhotic

Two types of renal failure are seen in individuals with liver disease: the so-called 'hepatorenal failure' (unique to liver disease) and acute tubular necrosis. If the former diagnosis is made, the mortality approaches 100%, whereas the latter condition has a much better prognosis. In any patient with liver disease and ascites, one can make the assumption that there exists alteration of renal tubular function and there is increased absorption of sodium and water. In these individuals, renal failure can develop quite rapidly even though normal kidney function may have been present before surgery. Renal failure is a common cause of death in the patient with cirrhosis. In the postoperative period, it is manifest by oliguria, and it may be confused frequently with hypovolaemia. There are several characteristics to distinguish oliguria from hepatorenal syndrome and oliguria from tubular necrosis in these patients. Hepatorenal syndrome is characterized by negligible amounts of sodium in the urine and absence of casts. In acute tubular necrosis there is oliguria, but sodium can be detected in urine and a variety of different cellular casts are observed. Therapy is different. Management of the hepatorenal syndrome is basically expectant whereas therapy for developing acute tubular necrosis consists of various dialysis techniques. Prerenal azotaemia characterized by oliguria, sodium-containing urine and low circulating volume is generally treated with fluid administration.

Maintenance of urinary output during surgery must be a major therapeutic goal of the anaesthetist to prevent either one of these tragedies from occurring. Conduct of this therapy is discussed more fully in the section on management during anaesthesia. One issue may cause some confusion. In many low renal output syndromes, particularly those encountered in the cardiac patient, dopamine is often therapeutic. Dopamine increases glomerular filtration rate via an increase in renal blood flow produced by an increase in cardiac output. This is not a problem in patients with cirrhosis as they have normal renal blood flows and increased cardiac output. Thus, the use of dopamine is of no avail in these individuals.

Infection, particularly with Gram-negative bacteria, is ominous in the patient with cirrhosis, as those types of infections which tend to cause an increase in plasma levels of endotoxin when associated with a high bilirubin (greater than 300 μmol/litre) are particularly dangerous to the kidneys. Thus, aggressive treatment of infections preoperatively, particularly those of the Gram-negative bacterial origin, is necessary.

Fluid administration in these patients is difficult intraoperatively. It must be remembered that sodium-containing solutions are often harmful in these patients because of their avid degree of sodium retention. Although balanced salt solutions are not contraindicated absolutely, certainly the volume administered should be reduced in these individuals. Dextrose 5% solution has been advocated as a fluid of choice, again with certain restrictions, notably that one should not use a large volume of glucose solutions as hypo-osmolality and water intoxication may result. During prolonged surgery, the author usually carries out hourly intraoperative screening for sodium, potassium and serum osmolality as a guide towards administration of fluids.

Patients with cirrhosis usually have a metabolic alkalosis. The reasons for this are unknown. However, coupled with the metabolic alkalosis is an obligatory kaliuresis. The status of potassium should be noted carefully in the preoperative patient with liver disease, and correction made as necessary. It is also of some interest that the portal vein responds to alkalosis by decreases in blood flow. This may certainly be disadvantageous in certain patients with liver disease who have restricted flows already because of portal hypertension.

The endocrine responses of patients with cirrhosis are variable. In early to moderate cirrhosis, individuals have a diabetic pattern of blood glucose concentrations, i.e. they have prolonged glucose tolerance curves and mildly elevated fasting blood glucose concentrations (approximately 8 mmol/litre). They may be somewhat abnormal in their response to insulin. Although of little concern to the anaesthetist, many of the individuals have feminism associated with cirrhosis. The exact reason for this is unknown although it may be a result of impairment of degradation of female-type hormones in liver disease.

Bleeding and clotting problems

Table 61.6 lists some of the important bleeding and clotting abnormalities in patients with cirrhosis. In addition to alteration of plasma clotting factors, both from a qualitative and quantitative point of view, there are similar changes which occur in platelet numbers and platelet function. The reason for the thrombocytopenia may not be known, but it may

Table 61.6 Common causes of coagulation factor abnormalities and platelet deficiencies in hepatic disease

Decreased synthesis of coagulation factors
Isolated or single-factor reduction
Reduced vitamin K-dependent coagulation factors (Factors II, VII, IX, X)
Reduced non-vitamin K-dependent coagulation factors (Factors V, XIII, fibrinogen)

Shortening circulating half-lives of coagulation factors
Increased utilization (disseminated intravascular coagulation; hyperfibrinolysis)
Loss from variceal bleeding

Platelet abnormalities
Quantitative platelet deficiencies
Qualitative platelet deficiencies

be secondary to the hypersplenism noted in these patients. Whatever the cause, non-mechanical post-operative bleeding is an important cause of surgical mortality. The haemostatic system should be assessed most carefully before surgery and assurance made that appropriate replacement therapy will be available when required. Good co-ordination with the blood bank is mandatory for extensive surgery in patients with liver disease.

Preoperative laboratory studies

Table 61.7 lists what the author considers to be minimum preoperative investigations for these patients. In so far as renal function is concerned, creatinine, particularly creatinine clearance, is of value, but urea is not. The reason for this is that urea is synthesized in the liver before renal excretion. If liver parenchymal disease exists, urea synthesis does not occur and even in the face of renal disease such patients can have fallaciously low urea concentrations.

In patients with cryptogenic cirrhosis, every effort should be made to ascertain whether or not they are infectious to operating theatre personnel. This can be done as a routine screening test by measurement of hepatitis antigen (HBsAG). Better confirmatory serological data for infectivity of blood is the presence of HBeAG positivity. Fasting glucose concentrations help to establish the degree of glucose utilization by these individuals.

In addition to these chemical values, the anaesthetist should take a history of drug therapy. It would be unusual for one to find drugs which are potential hepatotoxins being administered to the patient with known liver disease. However, occasionally such anachronisms do exist. For example, the author has encountered patients who have liver disease and are prescribed α-methyldopa for hypertension. Alpha-

Table 61.7 Minimal preoperative laboratory studies for the patient with cirrhosis

Serum electrolytes (Na$^+$, K$^+$, Cl$^-$)
Creatinine (preferably creatinine clearance)
Glucose
Full blood count (cell counts, platelet counts, haemoglobin, haematocrit)
Prothrombin time, partial thromboplastin generation time
Albumin
HBsAG, anti-HBs; HBeAG
Bilirubin
Aminotransferases (AST, ALT)
Urinalysis
Arterial blood-gas analysis

methyldopa can have significant hepatocellular effects in addition to the fact that in certain individuals it produces a positive Coomb's reaction which makes it extremely difficult for the blood bank to type and cross-match blood transfusions for the patients.

Management of portal hypertension in the preoperative phase

Discussion has been focused on ascites already. It is important to decrease ascites as presence of this sign of liver disease indicates a patient at greater risk. Infection must be controlled with antibiotics. The patient may have been treated with a variety of drugs. Two of the more common are neomycin and lactulose. Neomycin is used to sterilize the gastrointestinal tract killing bacteria which produce ammonia. Ammonia is absorbed in the gastrointestinal tract and, in cases of portal hypertension, is shunted directly into the systemic circulation where it is thought to produce hepatic encephalopathy. Thus, the physician aims to decrease the production of this noxious substance by sterilization of the gastrointestinal tract with neomycin. Although neomycin causes few problems, some of it is absorbed and can influence the action of neuromuscular-blocking drugs, e.g. prolongation of D-tubocurarine and other competitive neuromuscular-blocking drugs. Lactulose seems to present no problems in so far as the anaesthetic is concerned. It is used to decrease ammonia production but by a different mechanism from that of neomycin. Whereas neomycin actually kills bacteria, lactulose causes an unfavorable pH in the gastrointestinal tract so that conversion of amino acids to ammonia by bacterial urease is inhibited.

Bleeding and clotting variables must be as close to normal as possible before surgery. Non-mechanical bleeding is a leading cause of death in these individuals (Table 61.8). Although vitamin K given several days before surgery has been advocated, in most cases of moderate to severe parenchymal liver disease this therapeutic procedure is not effective in combating deficiencies in clotting factors simply because the liver is incapable of synthetic reactions.

Table 61.8 Major causes of death in the surgical patient with cirrhosis (ranked in order)

Infection
Bleeding
Renal failure
Hepatic failure and encephalopathy

Usually correction of clotting factor abnormalities is provided by infusions of fresh frozen plasma preoperatively, intraoperatively and postoperatively. Fresh frozen plasma corrects all the factors deficiencies (usually Factors II, VII, V and IX) but it does not influence fibrinogen concentrations. If the fibrinogen level is abnormally low, it must be replaced with cryoprecipitate. Fresh frozen plasma and/or cryoprecipitate may be given with an end-point being normal prothrombin time and partial thromboplastin generation times.

There may be several additional therapeutic measures employed in these individuals, particularly if they have rather severe liver disease. The Sengstaken–Blakemore tube is a large-diameter triple-lumen tube used to produce mechanical compression of bleeding oesophageal varices. The disadvantage of such a tube to the anaesthetist is that a face-mask fit becomes impossible because of the tube protruding from the mouth. Of value to the anaesthetist is the fact that it is almost impossible for the patient to inhale gastric contents with a Sengstaken–Blakemore tube in the correct position. If such a tube is in place, the author frequently employs an awake, topical tracheal tube insertion technique.

Another drug used occasionally in therapy of individuals with cirrhosis is propranolol. This is given to decrease splanchnic blood flow and thereby decrease the potential for variceal haemorrhage. Obviously, propranolol can interact with some of the inhalation anaesthetics to enhance negative inotropic effects on myocardial contractility. Cimetidine is also prescribed for patients with cirrhosis. These individuals have a high incidence of gastric ulcer and they are given cimetidine prophylactically to inhibit stomach acidity and thus decrease the potential for ulcer formation. Cimetidine causes alterations in hepatic blood flow and inhibition of hepatic microsomal cytochrome P450 such that the metabolism of some drugs which are cleared rapidly by the liver (i.e. metabolized rapidly) are altered. Pharmacokinetic activity of fentanyl, for example, is prolonged following cimetidine therapy in humans.

Surgical procedures in the patient with liver disease

Obviously, the patient with liver disease may have other medical problems, e.g. colon carcinoma, appendicitis or another pathological condition which necessitates laparotomy. Regarding the liver disease *per se*, there are three primary procedures which necessitate general anaesthesia: (i) injection sclerotherapy; (ii) portasystemic shunt surgery; and (iii) transoesophageal variceal ligation.

Injection sclerotherapy is employed commonly to treat one of the major complications of portal hypertension (variceal bleeding). In essence, it consists of the introduction of a fibre-optic gastroscope through which a short bevelled needle can protrude. The hepatologist injects varices as they are seen with sclerosing substances such as sodium morrhuate (a mixture of cod liver oils). This effectively seals off the varices. Endoscopic sclerotherapy for oesophageal varices is considered now to be the treatment of choice and is certainly superseding far more major procedures of portasystemic shunts (Markuz & Schwartz, 1984). The most serious complication of this procedure is oesophageal stricture, a rather late development which, although of concern to the patient, is not an acute one for the anaesthetist. There have been various reports, however, of the sodium morrhuate transported from the site of injection into the pulmonary and cardiac circulations where it may cause a negative inotropic effect on the myocardium. No deaths have been reported from these complications. Anaesthesia for transoesophageal variceal ligation is generally rather brief. It has been demonstrated that atracurium may be an excellent neuromuscular-blocking drug for use in patients with severe liver disease. Its short duration of action (approximately 20–30 min) is appropriate for the procedure of variceal injection sclerotherapy (Bell *et al.*, 1985).

In patients who have not responded to medical therapy, occasionally transoesophageal ligation is used. In addition to the use of the Sengstaken–Blakemore tube, medical therapy includes intravenous vasopressin infusion. Vasopressin decreases splanchnic blood flow and thereby decreases variceal bleeding. Patients may be scheduled for emergency transoesophageal ligation if such medical regimens do not control bleeding effectively. Most surgeons employ a transthoracic approach for this. There may be some advantages gained by the use of a bronchial blocker, although in the face of the classic pulmonary shunts in these patients, this may cause severe hypoxia.

The incidence of portasystemic shunt surgery seems to be decreasing. Many years ago, it was employed to decrease portal hypertension for both elective and emergency cases. Many older anaesthetists may recall the midnight battles in which this extensive procedure was performed, however, too often ending with a high mortality rate. Portasystemic shunts are used in most centres only on an elective basis, primarily in Child's A and B classification patients. The most commonly employed types of shunt surgery are the portacaval shunt, particularly in Europe, and the selective distal splenorenal shunt (Warren shunt), particularly in the USA. The advantage of the Warren shunt is that it leads to less hepatic encephalopathy postoperatively, although technically it is far more difficult to perform than the classic portacaval shunt.

The anaethetist should be aware of the reason for portasystemic shunt procedures. They are not designed to improve function of the liver; they are designed to decrease bleeding from oesophageal varices by decreasing venous pressure in these vessels simply by shunting blood away from the liver back into the systemic circulation (i.e. the vena cava). A brief review of the blood supply of the liver shows that the organ is somewhat unique in that it derives oxygenated blood from two sources, one arterial and one venous. The first source is the hepatic artery which accounts for approximately 40% of the oxygen supply of the organ. The portal vein supplies some 70% of total blood flow, but 60% of total liver oxygen requirement. Thus, the liver is unique as a large organ which is more dependent upon venous than arterial oxygen sources. If the surgeon transfers the portal venous flow back into the right side of the heart with a portasystemic shunt, the liver's blood supply is reduced drastically. The reduction in blood flow decreases venous pressure in varices but the decrease in blood flow causes also an exacerbation of the underlying hepatocellular disease. Following portacaval shunts, hepatic function abnormalities are exaggerated. Bilirubin may increase, transaminases and a variety of liver functions undergo a magnification of pathology. The question is often asked: should one avoid the anaesthetics which impair hepatic blood flow for portasystemic shunt procedures? The answer is that whatever the anaesthetic does concerning reducing blood flow the result is only a temporary phenomenon whereas the surgeon reduces blood flow of the liver dramatically for the rest of the patient's life.

Altered drug disposition in liver disease

The patient with liver disease may undergo a variety of changes in drug disposition from lack of responsiveness to drugs to extreme sensitivity. Table 61.9 lists some of those areas in which drug pharmacokinetics may differ in the cirrhotic from the normal patient.

Ethanol causes certain types of cytochrome P450 to

Table 61.9 Factors which produce altered drug pharmacokinetics in patients with liver disease

---

Blood supply
Diminished portal venous blood supply with hepatic fibrosis decreases clearance of drugs from GI tract

Biotransformation enzymes
In early alcoholic liver disease, microsomal enzyme induction may predominate; advanced parenchymal disease causes destruction of biotransformation enzymes. Phase I reactions are generally more susceptible than are Phase II reactions

Drug albumin binding
Hypoalbuminaemia causes increased free plasma concentrations of drugs

Volume of distribution
Altered by ascites, increased extracellular fluid secondary to water–sodium retention

Decreased liver mass

---

be induced, and thus, an enhancement of biotransformation of certain drugs. Thus, in the early stages of alcoholic liver disease, the patient's liver may be able to metabolize drugs at a faster rate than it could before onset of the alcohol problem. In addition, it must be remembered that CNS sensitivity to drugs plays a most important role with respect to sedatives and hypnotics. Thus, an alcoholic may require a greater dose of sedatives and hypnotic drugs such as thiopentone than the non-alcoholic individual. Obviously, later in the course of liver disease, metabolism of drugs deteriorates. For example, in advanced liver disease, there is destruction of the cytochrome P450 system so that metabolism of drugs decreases. It is interesting that decreases in Phase I metabolism of drugs (e.g. oxidation) seems to be disturbed more easily by liver pathology than Phase II drug metabolic reactions (e.g. glucuronide conjugation). Thus, in late-stage liver disease, individuals are more prone to have prolonged half-lives of drugs that depend on Phase I oxidative reactions (barbiturates) than alterations in kinetics of drugs depending on Phase II glucuronide conjugation reactions (oxazepam).

As hypoalbuminaemia becomes manifest, binding of drugs decreases and the free drug produces a greater effect. Renal elimination of drugs may be altered also. But probably of more clinical significance is the fact that CNS responsiveness to the drugs employed commonly in anaesthesia (i.e. opioids, sedatives and tranquillizers) is altered. There seem to be changes in the blood–brain barrier of the patient with moderate to severe liver disease which cause amplification of drug transport into the brain. In addition, brain-receptor kinetics are altered such that there may be a more prolonged and profound effect per unit drug. Clinical observations must be weighed in the context of overall patient responsiveness. It cannot be assumed that the patients are either unduly sensitive or unduly resistant to drugs.

There is no reason to suspect that the hepatotoxicity of a drug such as halothane is increased because of liver disease. In fact, experimental studies in cirrhotic animals indicate that animals with cirrhosis are no more susceptible to halothane hepatotoxicity than are animals with normal hepatic function (Baden et al., 1985).

Anaesthetic management of the patient with parenchymal liver disease

There are no absolute guides for anaesthetic regimens available for these patients, as no outcome studies are available. Assuming major surgical procedures such as a portasystemic shunt surgery or bowel resection for colonic carcinoma are anticipated, the patient should be rendered as fit as possible medically. Aspects of this have been discussed already. There are no definite guidelines for premedication. In general, the sicker the individuals, the less tolerant they are of drugs, particularly those which require Phase I reactions for clearance. In patients with moderate to severe liver disease, lorazepam and oxazepam have been shown to be quite safe and effective. These benzodiazepines, as opposed to diazepam and midazolam, are cleared by glucuronidation reactions and have normal pharmacokinetics even in patients with fairly advanced liver disease. There are no contraindications to the anticholinergic drugs if these are deemed necessary.

On induction, it should be remembered that the patient with cirrhosis may have increased hyperacidity and increased gastric volume. Cimetidine therapy may be of benefit in these individuals, although the disadvantage is that there may be decreased hepatic clearance of certain drugs such as fentanyl and benzodiazepines. Induction with thiopentone, 3–4 mg/kg i.v., has been found to be quite satisfactory unless there is severe liver disease. The patient with moderate to severe liver disease does not respond well to sedatives and opioids. Therefore, the regimens which are recommended most commonly include an inhalation anaesthetic for maintenance. The author has employed either enflurane or isoflurane in combination with oxygen for maintenance anaesthesia with good results. There is no scientific documentation that either enflurane or isoflurane aggravates liver disease. These drugs are rapidly reversible and cleared easily from the brain of the cirrhotic, an advantage not held by opioids. Their use with oxygen causes less bowel distension which facilitates abdominal surgery.

There is no contraindication to any of the neuromuscular-locking drugs. Certain cirrhotics are quite resistant to D-tubocurarine. For years, it was thought this resulted from the elevated serum globulin seen in liver disease causing increased binding of D-tubocurarine. This has been found not to be the mechanism of resistance. What seems to be the explanation is the increased volume of distribution secondary to fluid and salt retention. Several studies have shown that the overall pharmacokinetics of drugs such as pancuronium and vecuronium are not altered greatly in patients with liver disease, although some resistance has been shown to pancuronium (Nana et al., 1972). In advanced liver disease, production of plasma cholinesterase may be diminished and there can be a certain slowness of return of neuromuscular block after suxamethonium (Strunin, 1977). However, the use of suxamethonium to facilitate insertion of a tracheal tube is certainly not contraindicated. In severe liver disease, the duration of action of suxamethonium may be delayed by several minutes. This is inconsequential if one is looking forward to several hours of surgery.

Careful assessment of the patient by monitoring assists the anaesthetist in fluid and blood management. Monitoring techniques recommended for extensive procedures are outlined in Table 61.10 (see also Chapter 35). Obviously, the longer and more complicated the surgery, the more reliance one must have upon intraoperative monitoring. Table 61.11 lists intraoperative biochemistry and other laboratory examinations which may be helpful in achieving the best management of these patients. For example, bleeding and clotting abnormalities can present a problem, and may be complicated by the administration of large volumes of blood often required in major surgery in these individuals. 'Wash-out' bleeding and disseminated intravascular coagulopathies (DIC) must be differentiated.

The author is compulsive about the use of normocapnic or slightly hypercapnic ventilation. Alkalosis favours transition of the ammonium ion to ammonia. Because ammonia is implicated as a causative agent of hepatic encephalopathy, it is possible that overventilation and respiratory alkalosis can enhance the penetration of this substance into the brain. Because encephalopathy and liver failure are constant threats in the postoperative period, production of ammonia

Table 61.10 Suggested monitoring for patients with moderate or advanced liver disease undergoing major surgery

Electrocardiogram
Arterial pressure, most commonly direct arterial measurement
    to facilitate blood-gas analysis
Precordial or oesophageal stethoscope
Pulse oximeter
End-tidal capnograph
Neuromuscular monitor
Central venous line
Urinary catheter
Pulmonary artery catheter (?)

Table 61.11 Suggested blood analysis intraoperatively for patients with moderate to severe liver disease undergoing major surgery

Hourly
Haemoglobin; haematocrit
Arterial blood-gas tensions
Sodium and potassium ions
Glucose

Measurements in face of significant blood loss and replacement
Platelet count
Prothrombin time
Euglobulin lysis time

should be avoided as much as possible. Thus, the author advocates the use of a capnograph to prevent carbon dioxide concentration from decreasing sufficiently to produce a state of respiratory alkalosis.

Another problem in patients with cryptogenic or posthepatitic cirrhosis is the fact that many are infectious to operating theatre personnel. If a patient is HBsAG-positive (positive hepatitis B antigen), he or she must be considered as infectious. If an HBeAG antigen is present, the patient is dangerously infective. Similarly, the presence of anti-HCV titres indicate potential for hepatitis C infectivity. Precautions such as wearing gowns and gloves are indicated for all anaesthesia personnel. Washing reusable anaesthesia equipment in a hypochlorite solution following anaesthesia is indicated.

For shorter, minor surgical procedures, such as injection sclerotherapy of bleeding oesophageal varices, the author often employs the following regimen: induction of anaesthesia with thiopentone, 3–4 mg/kg, or propofol, 2 mg/kg, followed by tracheal tube insertion facilitated by suxamethonium. After this, nitrous oxide in oxygen and atracurium are administered. The stimulation of fibre-optic oesophagoscopy is not great.

In those surgical procedures during which there is need to maintain optimal hepatic blood flow, the suggestions outlined in Table 61.12 may be considered.

Frequency of use of regional anaesthetic regimens depends on clinical judgement. Obviously, subarachnoid or extradural block or peripheral nerve block may be desirable in certain cases. They may not be possible because of bleeding and clotting abnormalities which are quite common with cirrhotics. However, each case must be taken individually and in certain circumstances, the use of skilfully administered regional anaesthesia may be of considerable benefit.

Careful evaluation of renal function during prolonged surgery is necessary. In adults, urinary output should be kept at 50 ml/h. This may be difficult, particularly if crystalloid solutions cannot be used because of the avid sodium retention exhibited by many of these patients. Dextrose 5% is used usually during surgery. If urinary output decreases, mannitol is indicated. If urinary output is kept at 50 ml/h or greater, the incidence of renal failure syndromes, both the hepatorenal syndrome and acute tubular necrosis, seems to be diminished. Therefore, this should be a paramount concern to the anaesthetist. Caution is urged with the use of frusemide. This potent loop diuretic causes real problems in the cirrhotic, e.g. exacerbation of hepatic failure and hypokalaemia.

Postoperative care

Adequate analgesia may be difficult in these cases as they do not respond normally to opioids. If the bleeding and clotting abnormalities are corrected

Table 61.12 Considerations for maintenance of hepatic blood flow during anaesthesia

1 *Techniques.* Apparently little difference between most general anaesthetic sequences and spinal/extradural
2 *Anaesthetic drugs.* Preferred drugs are isoflurane, desflurane, sevoflurane. Decreases in total hepatic blood flow generally parallel drugs in systemic arterial pressure. Avoid halothane as it causes greater decreases in total hepatic blood flow than other anaesthetics
3 *Ventilation.* Avoid hyperventilation and positive end-expiratory pressure (PEEP) if possible
4 *Circulatory volume.* Maintain circulatory volume and replace fluids and blood as needed
5 *Vasoactive drugs.* Beta-adrenergic blockers and nitroprusside decrease hepatic blood flow; ephedrine and adrenaline increase flow

preoperatively, the author has used an extradural catheter for administration of opioids postoperatively.

Following extensive surgery, postoperative ventilatory support may be needed. However, there may not be the freedom of ventilatory regimens in these patients as there is following surgery in other patients. For example, positive-pressure ventilation, and particularly positive end-expiratory pressures (PEEP) may diminish hepatic blood flow. Reduction in hepatic blood flow over a period of time may be harmful. Therefore, it is preferable to wean the patient from positive-pressure ventilatory support, as soon as possible. It must be emphasized also that production of respiratory alkalosis may be detrimental to these individuals, and therefore careful assessment of end-tidal carbon dioxide and/or blood-gas tensions to maintain normocapnia or slight hypercapnia should be the rule.

Adequate hydration and prevention of hepatic encephalopathy should be carried out in the intensive therapy unit, postoperatively. Antibiotics given systemically and enterally may be required. The author has had good results from use of extradural opioids for postoperative pain relief. Because systemic doses of opioids may precipitate development of hepatic encephalopathy, use of the extradural catheter with very low dosages of opioids is an advantage. Contraindications to this technique involve primarily abnormalities of bleeding and clotting.

The patient with obstructive liver disease

The patient with cholestatic jaundice (i.e. obstructive jaundice) is somewhat different from the individual with parenchymal liver disease. The patient with obstructive jaundice, most commonly a result of biliary tract stone or carcinoma, generally has fairly intact hepatocyte function. Thus, all problems associated with activation of the renin–angiotensin system, alteration of pharmacokinetics of drug metabolism, etc. do not apply. However, the patient still runs a high risk. For example, mortality rate can be as high as 10–15% (Pain et al., 1985). Renal failure is a specific cause of 30% of deaths of patients with obstructive jaundice following surgery. Obstructive jaundice is rather common in gall bladder disease, a mundane and common surgical procedure.

Risk factors in patient with cholestatic jaundice are outlined in Table 61.13. Some of these are correctable preoperatively to decrease risk, e.g. correction of anaemia and prothrombin time. As opposed to the individual with hepatic parenchymal diseases,

Table 61.13 Preoperative variables associated with poor prognosis (mortality rate exceeding 15%) in surgical patients for relief of extrahepatic cholestasis

Pitt et al. (1981)	Dixon et al. (1983)
Increased creatinine (i.e. renal failure)	Haematocrit <30%
Hypoalbuminaemia	Plasma bilirubin >180 mmol/litre
Bilirubin >150 mmol/litre	Malignant obstructing lesion
Alkaline PO$_4$ >100 IU	Age >60 years
	Alkaline PO$_4$ >100 IU

vitamin K is advocated in all cases of obstructive jaundice and is efficacious. The dose recommended is 10 mg vitamin K$_1$, t.i.d. i.m., for at least 72 h before surgery. Bleeding is third on the list of causes of death of individuals with obstructive jaundice following surgery, with renal failure and infection the first and second causes, respectively.

There are several measures that can be performed to decrease the hazard of renal failure. These include the use of appropriate antibiotics to reduce sepsis and endotoxaemia. During the course of the procedure, the anaesthetist should monitor intraoperative urinary output and maintain at least 50 ml/h output in adults. A crystalloid such as Ringer's lactate solution can enhance urinary output under these circumstances. The diuretic of choice is mannitol and it is particularly recommended if the serum bilirubin concentration increases to greater than 300 mmol/litre. The use of fluids and the diuretic mannitol should extend to the recovery period. Monitoring of central venous pressure in longer operations is of value to detect fluid overload. Many physicians give preoperative treatment with oral bile salts such as sodium taurocholate, which reduces gastrointestinal endotoxin production, to ameliorate problems of renal failure postoperatively. Table 61.14 lists some of the general principles of the perianaesthetic management of these patients. Note that albumin can be used to reduce free plasma bilirubin values. Some physicians and surgeons have urged the use of albumin intraoperatively not only to increase serum osmolality, but also to bind free bilirubin in an attempt to avoid renal complications postoperatively. The value of this has not been determined by extensive clinical trials and it is placed here merely for information.

With regard to selection of anaesthetic regimens, there is no absolute contraindication to any. The author frequently uses isoflurane or enflurane in oxygen preceded by thiopentone. There may be some alteration and excretion of the neuromuscular-block-

Table 61.14 General principles of anaesthetic management of patients with cholestatic jaundice

Preanaesthesia phase
Correct underlying anaemia
Reduce sepsis (e.g. antibiotics, sodium taurocholate)
Correct coagulopathies with vitamin K (prothrombin time
 should be <3 s over control)
Improve nutritional status

Intra-anaesthetic phase
Use albumin to reduce free plasma bilirubin
Maintain urinary output at least 50 ml/h
 Ringer's lactate or other crystalloid
 Mannitol
Fresh frozen plasma to maintain adequate coagulation profile
Intraoperative antibiotics as necessitated

Recovery phase
Maintain urinary output with adequate blood, fluid
replacement

ing agents by bile, but in general there are probably few in the way of clinical manifestations of altered pharmacokinetics. Thus, there exist no contraindications to the use of the commonly employed neuromuscular-blocking drugs.

The only problem that has arisen with anaesthetics concerns the opioids. Some opioids cause spasm of the sphincter of Oddi and increase intrabiliary pressures. McCammon and colleagues (1984) studied the effects of several opioids on human interbiliary tract dynamics. They found that fentanyl (as does morphine) caused a considerable increase in biliary tract pressures. Butorphanol produced the least effect. Thus, opioid supplementation in these cases might best be performed with butorphanol. Although an increase in biliary tract pressure *per se* is not dangerous in the anaesthesized patient, it does inhibit adequate intraoperative cholangiography which could give rise to incorrect diagnosis and prolongation of the surgical procedure.

Careful monitoring of clotting is indicated during surgery. In general, unless it is an emergency procedure, vitamin K administration preoperatively restores prothrombin time to normal. However, in cases that must proceed to surgery before the therapeutic effect of vitamin K is present (a period of at least 48 h) reliance must be placed on fresh frozen plasma to correct clotting abnormalities. Platelet counts are usually normal in these diseases.

Postoperative management of these patients dictates that urinary output should continue to be high to prevent renal complications. Infection must be treated aggressively with appropriate antibiotics to reduce endotoxaemia. In general, these patients may be given parenteral opioids in a similar way to patients with normal function. The pruritus of jaundice (before it is dissipated by the surgical therapy) may be somewhat of a problem and diphenhydramine has been used to alleviate this difficulty.

Conclusion

The patient with moderate to severe liver disease constitutes an extraordinary risk for the combination of surgery and anaesthesia. It is unfortunate that outcome studies with different anaesthesia regimens are not available. However, outcome studies with a combination of the two show that patients with liver disease of significant degree can have perisurgical mortality rates from 30−80%. The leading causes of death in a surgical patient with liver disease are: (i) infection; (ii) liver failure; (iii) renal failure; and (iv) clotting abnormalities. Thus, the anaesthetist with the rest of the surgical care team must try to prevent such complications. The selection of a specific anaesthetic regimen is perhaps less important than careful monitoring and prevention of the above problems from occurring during the perioperative phase. Certain features of liver disease can be changed in the preoperative period to produce a more favourable prognosis (e.g. ascites).

The patient with cholestatic jaundice is a frequent candidate for surgery. Recommendations for anaesthetic care have been considered, which include prevention of renal problems intraoperatively by maintenance of a relatively high urinary output. Again, selection of anaesthesia is probably at the discretion of the anaesthetist as there seems to be no contraindication to any type of anaesthesia. The use of opioids which increase intrabiliary pressure may at times be contraindicated.

References

Aranha G.V., Sontag S.O. & Greenlee H.B. (1982) Cholecystectomy in cirrhotic patients: a formidable operation. *American Journal of Surgery* **143**, 53−60.

Baden J.M., Kundomal Y.R., Luttropp M.E., Maze M. & Kazek J. (1985) Effects of volatile anaesthetics or fentanyl on hepatic function in cirrhotic rats. *Anesthesia and Analgesia* **64**, 1183−8.

Bell C.F., Hunter J.M., Jones R.S. & Utting J.E. (1985) Use of atracurium and vecuronium in patients with oesophageal varices. *British Journal of Anaesthesia* **57**, 160−8.

Childs C.G. (1963) The liver and portal hypertension. In *Major Problems in Clinical Surgery*, vol. I (Ed. Childs C.G.). W.B.

Saunders, Philadelphia.

Dixon J.M., Armstrong C.P., Duffy S.W. & Davies G.C. (1983) Factors affecting morbidity and mortality after surgery for obstructive jaundice: a review of 313 patients. *Gut* **24**, 845–52.

Garagliano S.F., Lilienfeld A.M. & Mendeloff A.I. (1979) Incidence rates of liver cirrhosis and related disease in Baltimore and selected areas of the United States. *Journal of Chronic Diseases* **32**, 543–54.

Garrison R.N., Cryer H.M. & Howard D. (1984) Clarification of risk factors for abdominal operations in patients with hepatic cirrhosis. *Annals of Surgery* **199**, 648–55.

Georg J., Mellemgaard K., Tygstrup N. & Winkler K. (1960) Venoarterial shunts in cirrhosis of the liver. *Lancet* **i**, 852–4.

Krowka M.J. & Cortese D.A. (1985) Pulmonary aspects of chronic liver disease in liver transplantation. *Mayo Clinic Proceedings* **60**, 407–18.

Krowka M.J. & Cortese D.A. (1989) Pulmonary aspects of liver disease and liver transplantation. *Clinical Chest Medicine* **10**, 539–616.

Lieber C.S. & Leo M.A. (1982) Alcohol and the liver. Medical disorders of alcoholism: pathogenesis and treatment. In *Major Problems in Internal Medicine*, vol. 22 (Ed. Lieber C.S.) p. 259. W.B. Saunders, Philadelphia.

Limas C.J., Guiha N.H., Lekagul O. & Cohn J.N. (1974) Impaired left ventricle function in alcoholic cirrhosis with ascites. *Circulation* **49**, 755–60.

Malchow-Moller A., Thomsen C., Hilden J., Matzen P., Mindeholm L. & Juhl E. The Copenhagen Computer Icterus Group (1985) Survival after jaundice: a prospective study of 1,000 consecutive cases. *Scandinavica Gastroenterologica* **20**, 155.

Mangione A., Imhoff T.E., Lee R.B., Shum L. & Jusko W.J. (1978) Pharmacokinetics of theophylline in hepatic disease. *Chest* **76**, 616.

Marzuk P.M. & Schwartz J.S. (1984) Endoscopic sclerotherapy for esophageal varices. *Annals of Internal Medicine* **100**, 608–10.

McCammon R.L., Stoelting R.K. & Madura J.A. (1984) Effects of butorphanol, nalbuphine, and fentanyl on intrabiliary tract dynamics. *Anaesthesia and Analgesia* **63**, 139–42.

Nana A., Cardan E. & Leitersdorfer T. (1972) Pancuronium and vecuronium bromide: its use in asthmatics and patients with liver disease. *Anaesthesia* **27**, 154–8.

Pain J.A., Cahill C.J. & Baley M.E. (1985) Perioperative complications of obstructive jaundice: therapeutic consideration. *British Journal of Surgery* **72**, 942–5.

Pitt H.A., Cameron J.L., Postier R.G. & Gadacz T.R. (1981) Factors affecting mortality in biliary tract surgery. *American Journal of Surgery* **141**, 66–72.

Pockros P.J. & Reynolds T.B. (1986) Rapid diuresis in patients with ascites from chronic liver disease: the importance of peripheral edema. *Gastroenterology* **90**, 1827–33.

Pugh R.N.H., Murray-Lyon I.M., Dawson J.L., Pietroni M.C. & Williams R. (1973) Transection of the esophagus for bleeding varices. *British Journal of Surgery* **60**, 646–9.

Strunin L. (1977) *The Liver and Anaesthesia*. W.B. Saunders, London.

Anaesthesia for Patients with Renal Dysfunction

J.W. SEAR AND D.E. HOLLAND

Approximately 78 patients per year per million population in the UK develop end-stage renal failure. The magnitude of the problem indicates, therefore, that many anaesthetists may be asked to anaesthetize these patients for vascular access procedures, renal transplantation, or incidental surgery.

The first cadaveric human kidney allograft was performed by Voronoy in 1936, and the first living related donor graft between identical twins by Merrill in Boston in 1954.

The progress of chronic renal disease is slow; symptoms and signs occur only when more than 60% of the total nephron mass is lost. With reduction of the nephron mass below 40%, patients develop anaemia, uraemia and nocturia associated with a decreased concentrating ability. Dialysis is required usually when less than 10% of the nephrons are functioning.

This chapter considers the pathophysiology and management of patients with chronic renal failure, and also those with urological problems.

Influence of renal disease on the use of drugs during anaesthesia

As renal function becomes impaired, there is an inability to excrete sodium and water. This results in water retention with peripheral oedema, hypertension and a hyperdynamic circulation. The latter is augmented by the effects of anaemia and reduced oxygen carriage. Accompanying the water retention are electrolyte disturbances — hyponatraemia, hyperkalaemia, hyperchloraemia, hypocalcaemia, hyperphosphataemia and hypermagnesaemia.

In addition, there are major changes in the pharmacokinetics of drugs in patients with chronic renal failure. These result from alterations in drug protein binding (plasma proteins and tissues), changes in the volumes of drug distribution, altered cellular metabolism and altered drug elimination (Reidenberg, 1972, 1985).

Plasma and tissue protein binding

The binding of basic drugs (i.e. pKa exceeding 7.4) is unaltered in renal failure, but there is a significant decrease in the binding of acidic drugs which bind mainly to albumin. As a result, acidic drugs may show an increased volume of distribution and altered clearance in renal failure, although free drug clearance usually remains unaltered. Three mechanisms may be responsible for the decrease in plasma and tissue protein binding.

Hypoalbuminaemia occurs as a result of both increased excretion (as in the nephrotic syndrome) and decreased synthesis.

Uraemia. High circulating urea concentrations cause altered conformation of plasma and tissue proteins, which show an altered binding of drug molecules at receptor sites.

Competition for binding sites. Endogenous substrates and drug metabolites accumulate in renal failure and compete with the parent drug for plasma protein binding sites (Verbeeck *et al.*, 1981a).

Hepatic drug metabolism in uraemia

Uraemia alters hepatic intermediary metabolism (Reidenberg, 1972; Kopple, 1978; Attman & Gustafson, 1979; Horl *et al.*, 1980), but its effects on liver drug metabolism are not fully understood. Mixed function oxidase activity is increased. The cause of this is uncertain, but it has been suggested that one of the naturally occurring indoles, which accumulate in renal failure, may be responsible. Although there is good evidence of impaired hepatic drug metabolism associated with uraemia in various animal models (Terner *et al.*, 1978; Ali *et al.*, 1979; Hogan *et al.*, 1979; Patterson & Cohn, 1984; Gibson, 1986), this does not appear to be so in humans. The rates of activity of the major pathways of drug metabolism (oxidation and glucuronidation) are either unaltered or increased in renal failure (Balant *et al.*, 1983). The efficiency of hydrolytic and reductive metabolic pathways may be reduced.

Altered drug elimination

Biodegradation in the liver produces water-soluble, inactive metabolites. These are normally excreted by passive filtration at the glomerulus; some compounds (e.g. penicillins) are eliminated by active tubular secretion. Passive drug reabsorption may occur in the distal convoluted tubules and collecting ducts. In renal failure, the reduction in glomerular filtration may lead to accumulation of metabolites in plasma and body tissues (e.g. pethidine, morphine, nitrofurantoin), with the development of toxic side-effects.

The accumulation of metabolites may lead to decreased protein binding of the parent drug, as well as reduced clearance and prolongation of the elimination half-life of the parent drug. This occurs both by metabolite-induced inhibition of hepatic enzymes (end-product inhibition) and by the law of mass action (Verbeeck *et al.*, 1981a). Examples include diflusanil and clofibrate.

The relationship between renal function (as expressed by serum creatinine or creatinine clearance) and elimination half-life of a drug was established by Kunin (1967). With decreasing creatinine clearance, the elimination half-life of drugs excreted by extrarenal routes is unchanged. However, for drugs that are eliminated primarily by the kidney, there is a different relationship. The half-life increases only slowly with deteriorating renal function until a critical creatinine clearance of 10–20 ml/min is reached. Below this value, the half-life increases asymptotically with further reductions in renal function. Examples of these two extremes are the antibiotics minocycline and cefazolin (Welling *et al.*, 1974, 1975) (Fig. 62.1).

In the patient with chronic renal failure, there may be prolonged action of water-soluble highly ionized compounds — these include atropine and neostigmine, digoxin, some β-adrenoreceptor-blocking drugs, ganglion-blocking drugs and the majority of the competitive neuromuscular-blocking drugs.

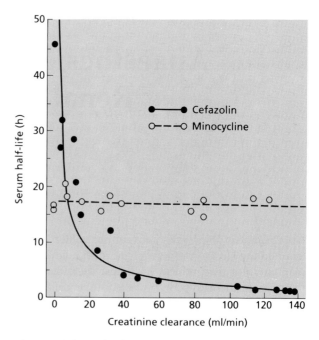

Fig. 62.1 Relationship between creatinine clearance and serum half-lives of cefazolin and minocycline. (Redrawn from Welling *et al.*, 1974, 1975.)

Influence of renal disease on pharmacokinetics of drugs used during anaesthesia

Premedicant drugs

Both atropine and glycopyrrolate are eliminated via the kidney (20–50% total dose). Thus, in patients with renal failure, accumulation may occur. In contrast, only 1% of hyoscine is recoverable from the urine. However, because of its untoward CNS effects, large doses of hyoscine should not be administered to the elderly patient.

Phenothiazine drugs are metabolized extensively in the liver, and their clearance is unchanged in renal failure. One disadvantage to their use is the additional effect of α-adrenergic block, which may accentuate the cardiovascular instability seen in response to anaesthesia in the recently dialysed, hypovolaemic patient.

Induction agents

Thiopentone is still widely used for the induction of anaesthesia — despite increased sensitivity of patients with chronic renal failure to barbiturate drugs. Dundee and Annis (1955) demonstrated that normal induction doses of thiopentone result in a prolonged loss of consciousness — the prolongation being related to the plasma urea concentration. A number of suggestions have been made as to the aetiology of this phenomenon: these include increased blood—brain barrier permeability, increased free-drug concentration from qualitative abnormalities in plasma albumin, increased non-ionized thiopentone as a result of the acidaemia, and abnormal cerebral uptake and metabolism of the barbiturate. Burch and Stanski (1982) and Christensen and colleagues (1983) all demonstrated a decrease in plasma protein binding of thiopentone in patients with renal failure — as a result of which there is an increased volume of drug distribution. There is no change in the unbound clearance of thiopentone.

The higher free-drug fraction results in higher brain concentrations of thiopentone. Assuming there is no difference in brain or cardiovascular sensitivity to thiopentone in the patient with chronic renal failure, a decreased rate of administration should be used for the induction of anaesthesia rather than a decreased drug dose (Burch & Stanski, 1982). This hypothesis is supported by the studies of Christensen and Andreasen (1978) and Christensen and colleagues (1983) who compared the dose of thiopentone (in mg/kg) required to induce anaesthesia successfully in patients suffering from renal failure and in healthy patients. No differences were found, and the arterial and venous sleep concentrations of thiopentone were similar in the two groups, indicating no alteration in brain barbiturate sensitivity.

Ketamine is best avoided for the induction of anaesthesia, as it causes an increase in both heart rate and arterial pressure which may be deleterious in the patient with coronary artery disease. Droperidol, in combination with fentanyl, causes only a small decrease in effective renal blood flow, glomerular filtration rate and urine output (Gorman & Craythorne, 1966); neuroleptanaesthesia has been recommended as a safe and suitable technique in patients with renal failure undergoing transplantation or incidental surgery (Morgan & Lumley, 1975; Lindahl-Nilsson et al., 1980).

There is little information on the disposition of other intravenous induction agents in chronic renal failure (Table 62.1), although diazepam, midazolam and etomidate all show a significant decrease in plasma protein binding in the patient with uraemia (Carlos et al., 1979; Ochs et al., 1981; Vinik et al., 1983). Disposition of propofol is unaltered in chronic renal failure (Morcos & Payne, 1985; Ickx et al., 1991; Kirvela et al., 1992).

Neuromuscular-blocking drugs and anticholinesterases

The neuromuscular-blocking drugs are amongst the most important anaesthetic drugs to be affected by renal dysfunction. Table 62.2 lists the extent that urinary excretion plays in their elimination.

Depolarizing relaxants

Wyant (1967) and Thomas and Holmes (1970) reported decreased plasma pseudocholinesterase activity in patients treated by dialysis for chronic renal failure, but this does not appear to be an important feature in patients treated by modern haemodialysis (Ryan, 1977). Prolongation of the action of suxamethonium is seen in some patients with chronic renal failure. Another problem with the depolarizing drugs is the

Table 62.1 Influence of chronic renal failure on the disposition of intravenous induction agents

	Patients with normal renal function				Patients with impaired renal function				
	$t_{\frac{1}{2}EL}$	Cl_p	V_{dss}	FF	$t_{\frac{1}{2}EL}$	Cl_p	V_{dss}	FF	Reference
Thiopentone	611	3.2	1.9	15.7	583	4.5*	3.0*	28.0*	Burch and Stanski (1982)
	588	2.7	1.4	11.0	1069	3.9	3.2*	17.8*	Christensen et al. (1983)
Etomidate	—	—	—	24.9	—	—	—	43.4*	Carlos et al. (1976)
Diazepam	5540	0.3	2.1	1.44	2196*	0.9*	2.8	6.97*	Ochs et al. (1981)
Midazolam	296	6.7	2.2	3.9	275	11.4*	3.8*	6.51*	Vinik et al. (1983)
Propofol	226	—	—	—	404	—	—	—	Morcos and Payne (1985)
	511	22.3	5.3	—	505	30.2*	9.2*	—	Ickx et al. (1991)
	1714	11.8	19.8	—	1638	12.9	22.6	—	Kirvela et al. (1992)

$t_{\frac{1}{2}EL}$, elimination half-life (min); Cl_p, plasma clearance ($ml \cdot kg^{-1} \cdot min^{-1}$); V_{dss}, volume of distribution (litre/kg); FF, free or unbound fraction of drug (%); * $p < 0.05$.

Table 62.2 Commonly used neuromuscular-blocking drugs and their dependence on renal excretion for elimination

Elimination	Drugs
>95%	Gallamine
60–90%	Pancuronium, alcuronium, pipercuronium D-methyl tubocurarine, doxacurium
25–60%	D-tubocurarine
<25%	Vecuronium, atracurium, suxamethonium, mivacurium

suxamethonium-induced increase in serum potassium concentration. Way and colleagues (1972) have shown the increase in haemodialysis patients to be the same as that seen in normal healthy surgical patients (approximately 0.5 mmol/litre). In contrast, increases as great as 5–7 mmol/litre have been reported in traumatized, burned, or neurologically injured patients. In uraemic patients where there is an already increased potassium concentration, an increase of this order is dangerous, and suxamethonium is only considered safe in the recently dialysed patient. Pretreatment with a non-depolarizing relaxant such as D-tubocurarine does not prevent this increase in potassium concentrations.

Competitive neuromuscular-blocking drugs

The influence of renal disease on the pharmacokinetics of the competitive neuromuscular-blocking drugs is shown in Table 62.3. D-tubocurarine, D-methyl tubocurarine, gallamine, alcuronium and pancuronium all undergo significant renal excretion; thus, there is a prolonged terminal half-life and reduced clearance in renal failure. In the case of pancuronium, although augmentation of biliary excretion may occur in patients with impaired renal function, the observed decreased systemic drug clearance may lead to prolonged neuromuscular block (Geha et al., 1976; McLeod et al., 1976; Somoygi et al., 1977; Buzello & Agoston, 1978).

Potentiation of neuromuscular block may occur in patients with metabolic acidosis; the acidosis also opposes the reversal by neostigmine. In the uraemic patient and the patient undergoing renal transplant surgery, other causes of potentiation include hypokalaemia, hypocalcaemia, hypermagnesaemia, some aminoglycoside antibiotics, frusemide, mannitol and methylprednisolone.

Inadequate reversal of neuromuscular block at the end of surgery may be prevented by consideration of the kinetics of the individual drugs.

D-*tubocurarine.* In healthy patients, 70% of an intra-

Table 62.3 Influence of chronic renal failure on the disposition of competitive neuromuscular-blocking drugs

	Patients with normal renal function			Patients with impaired renal function			
	$t_{\frac{1}{2}EL}$	Cl_p	V_{dss}	$t_{\frac{1}{2}EL}$	Cl_p	V_{dss}	Reference
D-tubocurarine	1.4	2.4	0.25	2.2*	1.5*	0.25	Miller et al. (1977)
Pancuronium	2.2	1.8	0.26	4.3*	0.88*	0.30	Somogyi et al. (1977)
	1.7	1.0	0.14	8.2*	0.31*	0.14	McLeod et al. (1976)
	4.2	–	–	17.5*	–	–	Buzello and Agoston (1978)
Gallamine	2.2	1.2	0.24	12.5*	0.24*	0.28	Ramzan et al. (1981)
D-methyl tubocurarine	6.0	1.2	0.57	11.4*	0.38*	0.48	Brotherton and Matteo (1981)
Vecuronium	1.32	3.0	0.19	1.62	2.5	0.24	Fahey et al. (1981)
	0.88	5.3	0.20	1.36*	3.2*	0.24	Lynam et al. (1988)
	1.95	3.2	0.51	2.48	2.6	0.47	Bencini et al. (1986)
Atracurium	0.35	6.1	0.18	0.40	6.7	0.22	Fahey et al. (1984)
	0.28	5.9	0.19	0.35	6.9	0.21	deBros et al. (1986)
	0.33	5.5	0.16	0.34	5.8	0.14	Ward et al. (1987)
Pipercuronium	2.28	2.4	0.31	4.38*	1.6*	0.44	Caldwell et al. (1989)
Doxacurium	1.65	2.7	0.22	3.68	1.2*	0.27	Cook et al. (1991)

$t_{\frac{1}{2}EL}$, elimination half-life (h); Cl_p plasma clearance (ml·kg^{-1}·min^{-1}); V_{dss} volume of distribution (litre/kg); * $p < 0.05$.

venous dose is recovered from the urine. However, in the presence of renal failure, there is a compensatory increase in biliary excretion of the drug. Thus, prolonged paralysis in the uraemic patient is seen only after administration of large or repeated doses (Gibaldi et al., 1972; Logan et al., 1974; Rouse et al., 1977). A study by Miller and colleagues (1977) has shown a decreased clearance of D-tubocurarine, and hence a slower decline in the plasma drug concentration. There is also a reduced protein binding of D-tubocurarine in patients with renal failure (Ghoneim et al., 1973).

D-methyl tubocurarine. A significant decrease in drug clearance, and prolonged half-life is observed in patients with renal failure (Brotherton & Matteo, 1981). In the healthy patient, approximately 43% of the drug is excreted unchanged in the urine within the first 24 h of administration.

Gallamine. Buzello and Agoston (1978) and Ramzan and colleagues (1981) have reported significant prolongation of the elimination half-life in renal failure. This relates closely with the high (90%) excretion of unchanged gallamine by the kidney (Feldman et al., 1969). There are several case reports of inadequate reversal and prolonged paralysis after use of gallamine in patients with renal insufficiency (Feldman & Levi 1963; Lowenstein et al., 1970). The paralysis may be reversed by haemodialysis.

Atracurium. Clinical studies by Hunter and colleagues (1982, 1984) have shown no difference in the duration of neuromuscular block following an initial dose or repeated doses of atracurium when administered to patients with normal renal function, and to anephric patients. Dynamic–kinetic studies by Fahey and colleagues (1984) and deBros and colleagues (1986) have demonstrated unaltered onset time, duration of action and recovery time in patients with renal failure. The drug may also be used by continuous infusion to maintain neuromuscular block in renal failure patients (Russo et al., 1986), with full recovery of neuromuscular function by 10 min after cessation of the infusion in 75% of patients. However, our own data (Wait et al., 1988) demonstrate considerable variability in recovery times in both healthy patients and in patients undergoing renal transplantation. These observations support the work of Nguyen and colleagues (1985), who have recorded a prolonged recovery rate and longer time to 90% recovery of initial twitch height in anephric patients.

Atracurium undergoes Hoffman degradation and ester hydrolysis. However, Fisher and colleagues (1986) have suggested that up to 50% of the clearance of atracurium cannot be accounted for by either of these mechanisms. In addition, there are higher concentrations of the metabolite laudanosine in patients with renal failure, suggesting that this metabolite is dependent partially on renal function for its elimination. Elevated blood laudanosine concentrations may result in CNS stimulation and convulsions. However, peak concentrations during general anaesthesia are of the order of 200 ng/ml compared with concentrations of 17 µg/ml which are associated with convulsions in the dog (Ward et al., 1987). In patients in the intensive therapy unit (ITU) with severe renal dysfunction, Yate and colleagues (1987) and Parker and colleagues (1988) have found the maximum laudanosine concentration following infusion of atracurium to be of the order of 5 µg/ml. Similar observations have been made during infusions of atracurium in patients undergoing renal transplantation (LePage et al., 1991).

Vecuronium. Compared with atracurium, vecuronium has a longer half-life in healthy patients (Cronnelly et al., 1984a; Fahey et al., 1984). Despite these differences, the duration of action of the drugs is similar in patients with normal excretory function.

Although Fahey and colleagues (1984) found no influence of renal failure on the duration of neuromuscular block or the kinetics of vecuronium, Lynam and colleagues (1988) have recently shown prolongation of both the elimination half-life and the drug's dynamic effect, when a single bolus dose of vecuronium, 0.1 mg/kg, was administered to renal transplant patients anaesthetized with isoflurane 1% and nitrous oxide in oxygen. Occasional resistance to vecuronium has been reported also in the very sick and acidotic patient.

In three recent studies (Bevan et al., 1984; LePage et al., 1987; Starsnic et al., 1989), there is evidence of accumulation of vecuronium in patients with renal failure. Caution should therefore be exercised to ensure complete return of neuromuscular function following prolonged surgery in anephric or transplant patients.

The altered disposition of some neuromuscular-blocking drugs in patients with renal failure obviously affects their clinical usage. If a small initial paralysing dose is given, the cessation of its effect is by distribution within the body. However, if a larger dose or multiple increments are administered, the recovery from paralysis is at a rate related to the drug's terminal half-life. Thus, the aim for *all* neuro-muscular-blocking drugs should be to avoid high plasma drug concentrations near the completion of surgery and anaesthesia.

Newer neuromuscular-blocking drugs

Mivacurium. This is a short-acting benzyl-isoquinol-inium compound, which is metabolized by plasma esterases and presumably also in the liver. In healthy subjects, deBros and colleagues (1987) demonstrated an elimination half-life of 17 min, and a clearance of $54 \, \text{ml} \cdot \text{kg}^{-1} \cdot \text{min}^{-1}$. The duration of effect is only slightly prolonged in renal failure.

Doxacurium. This is a long-acting drug, with an elimination half-life of 99 min, and clearance of $2.7 \, \text{ml} \cdot \text{kg}^{-1} \cdot \text{min}^{-1}$. It is mainly excreted unchanged by the kidney, although esterase hydrolysis may contribute in part to the termination of drug effect. Clearance is decreased in patients with renal failure, and the duration of action prolonged (Cook *et al.*, 1991).

Pipercuronium. This is eliminated mainly unchanged by the kidney and its excretion resembles that of pancuronium. Renal failure is associated with pro-longation of the elimination half-life and decreased clearance (Caldwell *et al.*, 1989).

Opioid drugs

In the healthy patient, most analgesic drugs adminis-tered during anaesthesia are metabolized to inactive metabolites which are then excreted in the urine or bile. Metabolism of pethidine, fentanyl, alfentanil and morphine in the liver is of the order of 95%, 93%, 99% and 90%, respectively. Phenoperidine differs from these opioids in that approximately 50% is eliminated normally unchanged in the urine. Thus, the action of phenoperidine is likely to be prolonged in renal failure.

In a recent study (Sloan *et al.*, 1991), regional clearances of morphine have been studied in the merino sheep. Total body clearance was 1.63 litres/min, with hepatic and renal contributions being 1.01 and 0.55 litres/min, respectively. Kidney clearance of morphine was greater than the 0.21 litres/min calcu-lated from the product of systemic clearance and urinary recovery of unmetabolized morphine, indi-cating that renal metabolism of morphine occurs. Whether this is also found in humans is unknown at present.

However, prolonged or pronounced clinical effects following intravenous doses of morphine to patients with chronic renal failure have been reported by Mostert and colleagues (1971) and Don and colleagues (1975). Despite observations suggesting that clearance of morphine was decreased in renal failure (Moore *et al.*, 1984; Sear *et al.*, 1985), it now appears that these results may have occurred because of cross-reactivity of the radioimmunoassay antibody with the pharma-cologically active metabolite morphine-6-glucuro-nide. Studies by Aitkenhead and colleagues (1984), Woolner and colleagues (1986), Chauvin and col-leagues (1987a), Sawe and Odar-Cederlof (1987) and Sear and colleagues (1989) have all indicated little effect of renal insufficiency on morphine elimination (Table 62.4). However, the accumulation of the active morphine-6-glucuronide may lead to prolonged clinical sequelae — Osborne and colleagues (1986) have indicated that its half-life in patients with renal failure is 38–103 h. In patients undergoing renal transplantation, we have found terminal half-lives of morphine-3-glucuronide and morphine-6-glucuronide to vary between 200 and 900 min (Sear

Table 62.4 Influence of chronic renal failure on the disposition of morphine in the awake and anaesthetized patient

	Patients with normal renal function					Patients with impaired renal function					Reference
	$t_{\frac{1}{2}\text{EL}}$	Cl_p	V_{dss}	$t_{\frac{1}{2}}\text{M3G}$	$t_{\frac{1}{2}}\text{M6G}$	$t_{\frac{1}{2}\text{EL}}$	Cl_p	V_{dss}	$t_{\frac{1}{2}}\text{M3G}$	$t_{\frac{1}{2}}\text{M6G}$	
Awake	210	11.5	2.8	—	—	191	10.3	1.8*	—	—	Aitkenhead *et al.* (1984)
	130	21.4	4.0	—	—	73*	28.0	3.0	—	—	Woolner *et al.* (1986)
	102	28.0	4.0	240	—	144	21.1	4.4	2976*	—	Sawe and Odar-Cederlof (1987)
Anaesthetized	186	21.3	3.7	—	—	185	17.1	2.8*	—	—	Chauvin *et al.* (1987b)
	307	11.4	3.8	258	116	302	9.6	2.4*	533*	433*	Sear *et al.* (1989)

$t_{\frac{1}{2}\text{EL}}$, elimination half-life (min); Cl_p, plasma clearance ($\text{ml} \cdot \text{kg}^{-1} \cdot \text{min}^{-1}$); V_{dss}, volume of distribution (litres/kg); M3G and M6G, morphine-3- and morphine-6-glucuronides; * $p < 0.05$.

et al., 1989). There has also been a recent report of an increase in myoclonic activity in the presence of elevated concentrations of another morphine metabolite (normorphine) (Glare et al., 1990). Similar alterations in the disposition of codeine, propoxyphene and dihydrocodeine are also observed in patients with renal failure (Gibson et al., 1980; Barnes et al., 1985; Guay et al., 1988).

Although Bion and colleagues (1986) have suggested that haemodialysis may aid the clearance of morphine in the patient with chronic renal failure who becomes overdosed, this has been contested by a recent study by Turner and colleagues (1990).

Szeto and colleagues (1977) studied the kinetics of pethidine when given chronically to patients with impaired renal function. They demonstrated accumulation of the N-demethylated metabolite, norpethidine. This metabolite is less analgesic, but has a greater convulsant activity than the parent compound. Szeto has reported two patients in renal failure where the plasma ratio of norpethidine to pethidine was increased markedly with the occurrence of excitatory side-effects. Thus, pethidine should be used with caution in the uraemic patient.

Studies of fentanyl and its congeners in renal failure indicate little change in the major pharmacokinetic variables (Table 62.5).

Early reports on the pharmacokinetics of fentanyl in renal failure suggested an increased apparent volume of distribution and an increased systemic clearance (Corall et al., 1980). Bower (1982) has demonstrated no alteration in fentanyl binding to plasma proteins in patients with renal failure. There is, however, an increase in the free fraction of alfentanil in

the uraemic patient (Chauvin et al., 1987b; Bower & Sear, 1989), together with an increased volume of distribution at steady state.

Recent data show no effect of uraemia plasma protein binding or the disposition of sufentanil (Fyman et al., 1987; Davis et al., 1988; Sear, 1989), although there are case reports of prolonged narcosis following administration of this opioid to patients with chronic renal failure (Wiggum et al., 1985; Fyman et al., 1987).

Anticholinesterases

All of these drugs are excreted by glomerular filtration and renal tubular secretion. Cronnelly and Morris (1982) have reported the pharmacokinetics of neostigmine, pyridostigmine and edrophonium in patients with renal failure (Table 62.6). A significant decrease in the clearance of the anticholinesterases is seen in the anephric patient, but there is reversion of the pharmacokinetics to those seen in the healthy individual within 1 h of a living related donor renal allograft. The elimination half-life of both pyridostigmine and edrophonium is prolonged, and exceeds the half-life of pancuronium and D-tubocurarine. Thus, it is unlikely that residual neuromuscular block or recurarization in the anephric patient results from the muscle relaxant outlasting the antagonist.

Benzodiazepines

The disposition kinetics of several drugs of this group are altered in patients with acute or chronic renal failure. Kangas and colleagues (1976) found a

Table 62.5 Influence of chronic renal failure on the plasma protein binding and disposition of opioids of the phenyl–piperidine series

	Patients with normal renal function				Patients with impaired renal function				
	$t_{\frac{1}{2}EL}$	Cl_p	V_{dss}	FF	$t_{\frac{1}{2}EL}$	Cl_p	V_{dss}	FF	Reference
Fentanyl	450	14.8	7.7	—	594*	11.8	9.5	—	Duthie (1986)
	—	—	—	—	308	10.7	3.5	—	Gulden et al. (1984)
	—	—	—	20.8	285	6.0	1.9	22.4	Sear (1987); Bower (1982)
Alfentanil	90	3.1	0.3	11.0	107	3.1	0.4*	19.0*	Chauvin et al. (1987b)
	120	3.2	0.4	10.3	142	5.3*	0.6	12.4*	Bower and Sear (1989)
	83	6.5	0.5	—	58*	5.3	0.3*	—	van Peer et al. (1986)
Sufentanil					176	11.5*	0.85*		Fyman et al. (1987)
	76	12.8	1.3	—	90	16.4	1.7	—	Davis et al. (1988)
	195	18.2	3.6	7.8	188	19.2	3.8	8.6	Sear (1989)

$t_{\frac{1}{2}EL}$, elimination half-life (min); Cl_p, plasma clearance ($ml \cdot kg^{-1} \cdot min^{-1}$); V_{dss}, volume of distribution (litres/kg); FF, free or unbound drug fraction (%); * $p < 0.05$.

Table 62.6 Influence of chronic renal disease on the pharmacokinetics of the anticholinesterases. (Data from Cronnelly & Morris, 1982)

	Patients with normal renal function			Anephric patients			Living related donor renal transplants		
	$t_{\frac{1}{2}EL}$	V_{dss}	Cl_p	$t_{\frac{1}{2}EL}$	V_{dss}	Cl_p	$t_{\frac{1}{2}EL}$	V_{dss}	Cl_p
Neostigmine	80	0.7	9.0	183*	0.8	3.4*	104	1.0	9.4
Edrophonium	110	1.1	9.6	206*	0.7	2.7*	87	0.9	9.9
Pyridostigmine	112	1.1	8.6	379*	1.0	2.1*	83	1.0	10.8

$t_{\frac{1}{2}EL}$, elimination half-life (min); V_{dss}, volume of distribution (litres/kg); Cl_p, plasma clearance (ml$\cdot$kg$^{-1}\cdot$min^{-1}); * $p < 0.05$.

decrease in the plasma protein binding of diazepam in patients with chronic renal failure, while Andreasen (1974) showed no correlation between the serum albumin concentration and diazepam binding in patients with acute renal failure. In a later investigation of the disposition of diazepam in chronic renal failure, Ochs and colleagues (1981) found an increased volume of distribution and increased systemic clearance related to an increase in the free, unbound drug fraction (from 1.4% to 7.9%). Unbound drug pharmacokinetics showed no difference in the uraemic patient with respect to systemic clearance, but there was a smaller volume of distribution in the patient with renal failure.

The pharmacokinetics of the water-soluble benzo-diazepine, midazolam, have been studied in patients with chronic renal failure (Vinik et al., 1983). There were significantly greater values for total drug clearance and the steady-state volume of distribution in the chronic renal failure patients when compared with healthy controls. These changes were secondary to an increased free fraction (6.5% compared with 3.9%). There were no differences for the unbound pharmacokinetic variables, and the elimination half-life was similar in both groups (4.6–4.9h).

There was no correlation between induction time and free-drug fraction in the renal failure patients, probably because of inherent alterations in drug sensitivity in the uraemic patient. Because the increased free fraction of unbound drug may be distributed rapidly to the vessel-rich tissues after an intravenous dose, it is probably best to slow the rate of administration of midazolam during induction of anaesthesia in the uraemic patient in order to minimize the effects of any relative overdosage of free drug to the heart, kidneys, liver and brain.

Of the other benzodiazepines, single-dose studies with lorazepam (Verbeeck et al., 1976) indicated no alteration in the elimination half-life in renal failure, although the same authors have recently shown impaired clearance of the drug following chronic administration to two patients with uraemia (Verbeeck et al., 1981b).

Inhalation agents

All general anaesthetic agents cause myocardial depression; it is not surprising therefore that halothane, enflurane and isoflurane all cause a dose-related decrease in renal blood flow, glomerular filtration rate and urine flow (Groves et al., 1990). These decreases occurred in the absence of any change in cardiac output.

Renal concentrating ability appears unaltered by isoflurane and halothane. This control is lost, however, in the presence of increased serum concentrations of the inorganic fluoride ion, as might occur if methoxyflurane or enflurane were administered for long periods to patients with impaired renal function. The excretion of inorganic fluoride is dependent on the glomerular filtration rate (GFR). Normal excretion is unlikely at rates of less than 16 ml/min. In humans, the toxic threshold concentration for serum fluoride appears to be in excess of 50 µmol/litre (Cousins et al., 1974). In healthy patients, there is little likelihood of enflurane producing fluoride concentrations of this order of magnitude. However, Wickstrom (1981) has reported the administration of enflurane (mean concentration 2.4 MAC-h) to patients undergoing renal transplantation. The mean peak fluoride concentration was 21 µmol/litre; but in one of the 10 patients studied, a peak concentration of 40 µmol/litre was achieved. Hence, enflurane should not be used routinely as the sole anaesthetic agent in the patient with impaired renal function.

Patients with impaired renal function may develop cardiac arrhythmias as a result of alterations of plasma electrolyte concentrations. There is also the additional risk during transplantation of acute haemodynamic changes associated with the release of catecholamines and renin (Freilich *et al.*, 1984). Under these circumstances, isoflurane may be more advantageous than the other two volatile agents.

There are few studies on the renal effects of volatile agents in patients with abnormal kidney function, but Mazze and colleagues (1984) demonstrated no deterioration in renal function in chronic renal failure patients anaesthetized with halothane or enflurane.

Comparison of halothane, enflurane and isoflurane as volatile supplementation in patients undergoing living related donor transplantation has shown no influence of anaesthesia on immediate postoperative renal function (Cronnelly *et al.*, 1984b).

Anaesthesia for urological surgery

Many patients for urological procedures are elderly and therefore likely to suffer from multiple diseases, related especially to the cardiovascular system, hypertension, respiratory disease and renal impairment. Renal cell mass and renal function decline with age. The 30–40% decrease in cardiac output over the age range 25–65 years is accompanied by a similar change in renal blood flow (RBF). As a result, the GFR at the age of 70 years is only 50% of that measured in the 20-year old. Creatinine clearance declines linearly after the fourth decade.

Urinary concentrating ability (a tubular function) decreases similarly with age, and with it a decrease in water-conserving capacity. This is important under circumstances of reduced fluid intake where elevation of the serum sodium concentration may occur, with symptomatic hypernatraemia.

Transurethral resection of prostate and bladder tumours

Problems related to the lithotomy position

The lithotomy position results in impairment of ventilation as a result of restriction of diaphragmatic movement by the intra-abdominal contents. The Trendelenberg posture leads also to a *decrease* in cerebral blood flow through an increase in the intracranial venous pressure. Air embolism through sectioned pelvic veins may occur also. A final problem created by patient positioning is the tendency to gastric regurgitation. These effects are exaggerated in the obese patient and in those with chronic lung disease. The longer the duration of surgery, and the more extreme the degree of leg flexion, the greater the postoperative atelectasis and hypoxia. Elevation of the legs causes increased venous return, and has

been reported to lead to acute left ventricular failure. Conversely, removal of the legs from the lithotomy position at the end of surgery should be completed slowly to avoid severe hypotension. Positional effects on arterial pressure may be exaggerated by the loss of vascular tone during regional anaesthesia.

Other problems associated with the lithotomy position include pressure necrosis to the shoulders, buttocks and lower legs, and peripheral nerve injuries.

Anaesthetic techniques

For the short procedure (e.g. cystoscopy), an inhalation agent by mask is common practice. The bronchodilator properties of halothane may be useful in those patients with chronic lung disease, but has largely been superseded by enflurane and isoflurane.

Alternative regimens include the use of subarachnoid anaesthesia, or lumbar or sacral extradural block with lignocaine or bupivacaine.

Use of local techniques for urological procedures

The bladder, lower ends of the ureters, and prostate are innervated from the inferior hypogastric plexus. The sympathetic fibres originate from roots and ganglia of T12 to L3; and the parasympathetic fibres from S2 to S4. Sympathetic stimulation causes bladder neck contraction and inhibition of detrusor muscle tone, while the parasympathetic fibres are motor to the detrusor muscle and inhibitory to the internal vesical sphincter. The external bladder sphincter is innervated by the internal pudendal nerve (S2, 3, 4).

Thus extradural or subarachnoid analgesia must be provided up to the level of T10. Suitable drugs for extradural anaesthesia are 10–20 ml of lignocaine 1.5% or bupivacaine 0.5%, and for subarachnoid anaesthesia, heavy bupivacaine 0.5%, 3–4 ml.

For cystoscopy, topical analgesia (1–2% lignocaine gel) is often satisfactory, but a 'low' subarachnoid technique, conducted with the patient in the sitting position, and using 1.5–2 ml of heavy bupivacaine, may be employed.

Whatever anaesthetic method is used, care must be taken to avoid increases in central venous pressure (CVP) which in turn causes increased haemorrhage. Factors increasing CVP include straining, vascular overload from the irrigating fluid, overtransfusion, and use of pressor drugs. Tracheal intubation and controlled ventilation may be indicated in patients undergoing prolonged surgery, or where the positioning of the patient is extreme.

Complications of transurethral resection

Surgical complications of transurethral resection (TUR) of importance to the anaesthetist are described below.

Underestimation of blood loss

Average blood loss is approximately 500 ml, but losses in excess of 2 litres may occur. Visual assessment of blood loss estimation in the patient undergoing transurethral resection of the prostate (TURP) is difficult because of dilution by the irrigation fluid. In addition, absorption of the irrigating fluid may prevent the development of the usual clinical signs of hypotension and tachycardia.

Bleeding may occur from both open prostatic arterial vessels and venous sinuses, and may be exacerbated by activation of the fibrinolytic system. Patients undergoing prostatic surgery have a higher incidence of fibrinolysis than do other surgical patients (Lombardo, 1957). This may result from release of the plasminogen activator, prostatic urokinase. The prophylactic administration of ε-aminocaproic acid (EACA) has been recommended, but use of this drug has been associated with the development of a generalized thrombotic tendency, cardiac and hepatic necrosis, and subendocardial haemorrhage and ischaemia.

Bladder perforation

The classical signs of perforation — nausea, abdominal distension, and pain — may be masked by general anaesthesia. Prompt diagnosis and treatment depend on maintenance of an accurate record of the irrigating fluid balance.

Absorption of irrigating fluid (transurethral resection syndrome)

Excessive absorption of the irrigating fluid (1.5% glycine; osmolality 220 mosmol/litre) may lead to hypervolaemia (with the potential development of left ventricular failure and pulmonary oedema), hyponatraemia, haemolysis (secondary to the hypoosmolality of the irrigating fluid), bacteraemia leading to septic shock and patient cooling.

Overhydration occurs in approximately 2–4% of all patients undergoing TUR, with an associated body weight increase of between 300 and 2000 g. Hyponatraemia is manifest by the development of hypertension, elevated jugular venous pressure, tachypnoea

and hypoxia. If uncorrected, it leads to cerebral irritation and convulsions, with an altered level of consciousness, coma and cerebral oedema (Henderson & Middleton, 1980; Allen et al., 1981). This complication may be treated readily by fluid restriction, diuretics, and (in exceptional circumstances) the cautious use of hypertonic (3%) sodium chloride by intravenous infusion. Irrigation with large amounts of glycine (an α-amino acid) may lead to elevated plasma glycine and ammonia concentrations in both experimental animals and humans. Toxicity from glycine and ammonia may produce temporary visual disturbance (Ovassapian et al., 1982; Roesch et al., 1983; Ryder et al., 1984).

For further discusson, the reader should refer to Hatch (1987) and Hahn (1991).

There is some recent epidemiological evidence suggesting an increased mortality following TURP when compared with open prostatectomy (Roos et al., 1989). The main factor appeared to be an increased risk of acute myocardial infarction in the TURP group. The cause remains unclear but it may relate to the type and duration of anaesthesia, the irrigation fluid and, possibly, activation of coagulation factors and platelets. Although Mebust and colleagues (1970) reported that cardiac output fell during TURP by an average of 17%, this is not supported by our recent observations (Lawson et al., 1993). Decreases in cardiac output were seen in those patients receiving general anaesthesia but were not observed in patients receiving spinal anaesthesia in the presence of fluid loading with crystalloid. In the absence of major intraoperative blood losses, no further fall in cardiac output occurred during prostatic resection (Fig. 62.2).

Septicaemia. Gram-negative septicaemia is common following instrumentation of the urinary tract. Prophylactic antibiotics should be given before surgery if there is evidence of urinary tract infection or an indwelling urinary catheter.

Other endoscopic or non-invasive urological procedures

Percutaneous lithotripsy

This method for the removal of renal stones has the advantages, in comparison with open pyelolithotomy, of minimal blood loss and shorter recovery periods. Percutaneous lithotripsy (PCLT) may be conducted under general or regional anaesthesia; the latter needs to extend from T8 to L3.

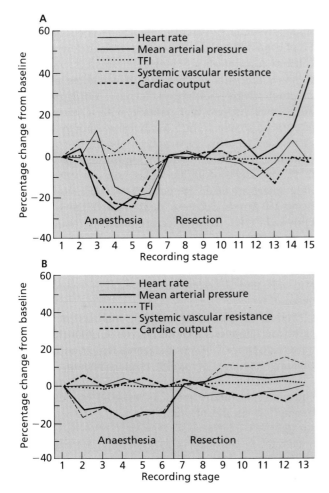

Fig. 62.2 Haemodynamic parameters at various recording stages in patients receiving general (A) or spinal (B) anaesthesia. Parameters shown as the mean percentage change from the baseline value for each recording period. TFI, thoracic fluid index. (Redrawn from Lawson *et al.*, 1993.)

A number of complications of relevance to the anaesthetist have been described.

Fluid intoxication following accidental rupture of the renal pelvis. Water overload is best avoided by use of normal saline as the irrigating fluid.

Hypothermia through use of excessive volumes of non-warmed irrigating fluids.

Pneumothorax, especially on the left side, following accidental percutaneous puncture of the pleura.

Autonomic hyperreflexia occurs in patients with previous spinal cord transections. Distension of the renal pelvis and ureter with fluid may cause hypertension and bradycardia, or cardiac arrest (Bennett *et al.*, 1984).

Bacteraemia and fever following instrumentation in the presence of renal sepsis. Organisms likely to be found are *Escherichia coli*, *Pseudomonas*, *Proteus* and *Aerobacter aerogenes*. Supportive therapy and antibiotics are required.

Posture. Prolonged periods in the lateral position require careful positioning of the patient to prevent nerve damage, and protection of the eyes.

Extracorporeal shock-wave lithotripsy

Extracorporeal shock-wave lithotripsy (ESWL) is a non-invasive method for fragmentation of renal calculi and presents a number of problems also for the anaesthetist (Abbott *et al.*, 1985). With older machines, an electrical discharge of approximately 20 kV is directed via an underwater electrode to produce an instantaneous spark, which vaporizes the water within the electrode gap, and produces shock-waves that are focused onto the calculus. The discharge is triggered by the R-wave of the ECG.

Patients are immersed in water at 36°C and anaesthesia may be provided by general or regional anaesthesia. Fluid immersion results in peripheral venous compression with a central shift of the blood volume, reflected as an increase in CVP and pulmonary capillary wedge pressure (PCWP). In addition, the warm immersion fluid may cause cutaneous vasodilatation, leading to exacerbation of postural hypotension. Patients undergoing ESWL under regional anaesthesia may suffer other cardiovascular changes (severe hypotension and bradycardia). If the nerve block extends above T4–6 levels, it may result in obtunding of the compensatory mechanisms that prevent a decrease in cardiac output associated with the head-up position.

Specific hazards of ESWL include arrhythmias if the shock-wave discharge is not timed with the R-wave of the ECG; excessive heat loss if bath temperatures decrease below 36°C; prolonged shivering during the recovery period unless the room temperature is elevated. The anaesthetist must consider also the remoteness of the patient (especially during X-ray screening), when setting up effective haemodynamic and respiratory monitoring.

In newer machines, shock waves are focused from a generator below the supine patient. Problems that arise in these patients relate to:

1 Prolonged anaesthesia.
2 The need for the anaesthetist to be remote from the patient for radiation protection.
3 The difficulty of observing the anaesthetic machine and monitoring equipment at a distance from the patient.
4 Frequent absence of piped gas supplies and scavenging/venting systems in the X-ray department.

Transvesical and retropubic prostatectomy

These operations require abdominal muscle relaxation, and may be accompanied by considerable blood loss. Anaesthesia may be achieved by extradural or subarachnoid anaesthesia, or it may involve tracheal intubation and muscle paralysis. Deliberate hypotension, either by ganglion-blocking drugs, vasodilators, or extradural block, may aid surgery, but careful replacement of blood in response to measured loss is essential.

Nephrectomy and other surgical procedures involving the lateral decubitus position

Use of this position tends to cause marked ventilation : perfusion ($\dot{V}:\dot{Q}$) imbalance, with blood supply favouring the lower lung, and positive-pressure ventilation going to the upper lung.

These cardiorespiratory effects are complicated further by use of excessive table flexion which results in direct caval compression and a decrease in venous return. Rarely, the pleura is damaged during radical kidney operations but this results in collapse of the uppermost lung, and further $\dot{V}:\dot{Q}$ inequality. An underwater seal drain may be required in the early postoperative period to aid re-expansion. Anaesthesia for nephrectomy may be achieved by regional anaesthetic techniques, but analgesia must extend to at least T8.

Other surgical procedures (e.g. cystectomy, ileal conduit formation, anterior exenteration)

These operations are conducted best under combined general and regional anaesthesia.

Clinical problems of anaesthesia in patients with renal insufficiency

Acid—base status and electrolyte imbalance

The patient with chronic renal failure is unable to excrete acid metabolites. This results in metabolic acidosis, low plasma bicarbonate concentration, hyponatraemia, hyperchloraemia and hyperkalaemia. Hyperphosphataemia is associated with low serum calcium concentrations. However, there is evidence to show that uraemic patients may tolerate mild to moderate degrees of hyperkalaemia. Although most authorities suggest that patients with a serum potassium of greater than 5.5 mmol/litre should not be anaesthetized, this is supported by little scientific evidence. It is probably safe to administer anaesthesia in the presence of higher potassium concentrations *unless* there are ECG changes of hyperkalaemia (high-peaked T-waves, decreased amplitude of the R-wave, widened QRS complex, progressive diminution in the amplitude of the P-wave). Factors which may increase further the plasma potassium concentration, e.g. spontaneous ventilation, hypoventilation and repeated doses of suxamethonium, should be avoided.

Methods available for reducing high serum potassium concentrations include glucose—insulin therapy, administration of bicarbonate and hyperventilation, calcium resonium enema (30—60 g), or haemodialysis.

Most of the electrolyte and acid—base changes in chronic renal failure may be reversed by adequate haemodialysis and ultrafiltration.

Anaemia

Anaemia was one of the major problems in the anaesthetic management of patients with chronic renal failure. Patients on haemodialysis often showed a haemoglobin of <6 g/dl, with a haematocrit of 20—25%. The picture is that of a normochromic, normocytic anaemia of complex aetiology. Causes include decreased red blood cell production from reduced erythropoietin synthesis and release, bone-marrow depression by uraemia, decreased red cell lifespan, repeated blood loss during haemodialysis and aluminium toxicity.

Other factors in the aetiology of the anaemia include deficiency of iron, folate and vitamins B_6 and B_{12}.

These problems have now been reduced by the administration of biosynthetic erythropoietin (EPO) which increases haemoglobin concentrations towards normal (Winearls et al., 1986). However, significant side-effects have been observed if the haematocrit is raised above 35% — these include hypertension, cerebrovascular accidents, thrombosis of fistulae and epileptiform activity (Eschbach et al., 1987; Winearls, 1992). There is also reduction in the need for repeated top-up blood transfusions (Eschbach et al., 1989). In the absence of a correction of the anaemia, there is compensation for the reduction in oxygen-carrying capacity by an increase in cardiac output, and an increase in red cell 2,3-diphosphoglycerate (2,3-DPG). The latter shifts the oxyhaemoglobin dissociation curve to the right, thereby improving tissue oxygenation. The shift appears to be greater in the uraemic patient on haemodialysis, in comparison with the uraemic patient not on dialysis. This may result from a secondary effect related to the influence of acidosis on the position of the oxygen dissociation curve. Severe anaemia causes also a 15—25% decrease in the blood : gas partition coefficients for the inhalation anaesthetic agents, with a predictable increase in the rates of anaesthetic onset and recovery.

Because of the need to maintain adequate tissue oxygenation during the surgical period, anaesthesia should be accomplished without increases in blood pH, and avoiding decreases in cardiac output.

Hypertension and ischaemic heart disease

These are some of the commonest presenting complications in patients with chronic renal failure; Morgan and Lumley (1975), Marsland and Bradley (1983) and Heino and colleagues (1986) have reported incidences of preoperative hypertension of 68—94% in three series of patients undergoing transplantation. The incidence of ischaemic heart disease will vary with age of the recipient; from about 5% in patients aged up to 55 years, and higher in the elderly recipients.

The aetiology of the hypertension in chronic renal failure is often the consequence of volume expansion secondary to salt and water retention (Brown et al., 1971). In other patients, where hypertension cannot be controlled by dialysis, it is suggested that an abnormal relationship exists between plasma renin activity, fluid volume and blood pressure. There may also be an inappropriate level of sympathetic nervous system activity. Improvements in dialysis technology have resulted in a significant reduction in the numbers of patients receiving antihypertensive therapy. Those needing treatment are often refractory to single agents, and require large doses of combinations of anti-hypertensive drugs (e.g. β-adrenoceptor-blocking drugs, calcium-channel blockers, vasodilators and angiotensin-converting enzyme inhibitors) which may all contribute to produce significant drug interactions with volatile and intravenous anaesthetic agents (Foëx, 1984; Jones, 1984; Prys-Roberts, 1984; Jenkins & Scoates, 1985; Gorven et al., 1986; Sear et al., 1990; Durand et al., 1991).

In the post-transplant patient where there is correction of the uraemia and fluid imbalance, persistence of hypertension may indicate either acute and/or chronic rejection of the allograft, the presence of native diseased kidneys, or transplant artery stenosis.

Cyclosporine A (CYA) therapy may also produce hypertension; this is often accompanied by renal dysfunction. It appears to be a direct vasoconstrictor response and to be an action of CYA on intracellular calcium homeostasis. CYA also reduces renal tubular sensitivity to aldosterone. Other contributory factors include the presence of CYA-induced hypomagnesaemia and the renal production of thromboxane A_2.

Patients with renal failure, especially those on dialysis, are prone to develop accelerated atherosclerosis. Uraemic cardiomyopathy and pericarditis are associated also with chronic renal disease, and result in further decreases in contractility and ejection fraction.

Coagulation

Uraemic patients may develop bleeding problems as a reflection of platelet dysfunction with decreased platelet Factor III resulting in decreased platelet adhesiveness. There is also a decrease in vitro in aggregation in response to the addition of adenosine diphosphate. In addition to thromboasthenia, thrombocytopenia may be present also. Laboratory investigations show no alterations in the prothrombin time or partial thromoboplastin time, but bleeding time is prolonged.

The decrease in platelet Factor III availability occurs because of accumulation of endogenous waste products, including guadininosuccinate, phenol and phenolic acid. These products are eliminated by adequate dialysis, with a return to normal platelet function. It has been suggested by Stewart and Castaldi (1967) that peritoneal dialysis is more effective than haemodialysis in correcting this abnormality.

Other methods of treating the uraemic bleeding diathesis include: platelet transfusion, cryoprecipitate (10 units over 30 min has an effect for 1—12 h), and the infusion of desamino-8-D-AVP (DDAVP) (Mannucci et al., 1983). The latter acts to increase the activity of factors VIII, XII, von Willebrand's Factor and high molecular weight kininogen (Mannucci, 1988).

Central nervous system

The CNS features of uraemia are manifest initially as malaise, fatigue and reduced mental ability, but may proceed to myoclonus, fitting, and on to coma and death. Patients complain of pruritus, which is particularly severe at night and at rest, and appears to be relieved by movement. Peripheral neuropathies are seen commonly in the lower limbs, and may involve the autonomic nervous system, leading to postural hypotension.

Respiratory system

Uraemic lung is the radiological entity of perihilar pulmonary venous congestion secondary to fluid retention. Excessive fluid administration may therefore result in the development of right heart failure.

Immunosuppressed patients are susceptible to pulmonary infections, with pre-existing disease often exacerbated by airway instrumentation and general anaesthesia.

Endocrine system

Uraemic osteodystrophy encompasses a number of separate skeletal problems including osteomalacia, osteosclerosis and osteitis fibrosa cystica — the latter developing as a result of secondary hyperparathyroidism. As renal function decreases, phosphate excretion falls and the resulting hyperphosphataemia leads to a reduced absorption of calcium and hyperactivity of the parathyroid glands on an attempt to maintain the serum calcium concentration. The sequel to this is bone demineralization, rendering the patients liable to spontaneous fracturing of the long bones and vertebrae.

Gastrointestinal tract

Common gastrointestinal symptoms in patients with uraemia are anorexia, nausea and vomiting, gastrointestinal bleeding, diarrhoea and hiccups, the latter being relieved best by phenothiazines (e.g. chlorpromazine). Renal failure patients have delayed gastric emptying in addition to an increase in acidity and gastric volume. Hence, patients will benefit from administration of an H_2-receptor antagonist as part of the premedication.

Immune system

The uraemic patient has a natural impairment of his or her immune system, which may be exaggerated by the use of corticosteroids and immunosuppressant drugs in the treatment of conditions such as the nephrotic syndrome. As a result, sepsis remains a major cause of morbidity and mortality. Particular attention should be paid to a strict aseptic technique when inserting a urinary catheter, invasive monitoring devices and peripheral infusions.

Abnormalities caused by haemodialysis

The main sequelae are excessive or persistent heparinization after dialysis, abnormal fluid shifts and hepatitis virus and human immunodeficiency virus (HIV). Residual heparinization presents as a bleeding diathesis occurring up to 10 h after haemodialysis. It is corrected readily by protamine sulphate (initial dose: 10 mg). If fluid and electrolyte shifts occur too rapidly during haemodialysis, a 'disequilibrium' syndrome may develop. This is characterized by dehydration, weakness, nausea and vomiting, hypotension, and occasionally by convulsions and coma. Treatment should be symptomatic and aggressive.

Hepatitis is endemic in the dialysis population of many countries, and anaesthetists should wear gloves to minimize the risk of transmission of hepatitis A and B virus. Adequate screening and immunization should be conducted for medical and nursing personnel responsible for patients with chronic renal failure.

The impact of HIV in the dialysis population is not of major consideration at present, but this should be paramount in the careful screening of further dialysis and transplant recipients.

Protection of veins, shunts and fistulae

Functioning shunts or fistulae must be protected carefully during anaesthesia and surgery, with the sphygmomanometer cuff placed on the contralateral arm. There is little indication for routine invasive arterial monitoring, and all arterial sites should be spared from cannulation as several may be needed for vascular access formation. Venous access should be restricted to peripheral veins on the dorsum of the hand — with preservation of forearm and antecubital fossa veins. Central venous cannulation (see below) is achieved best using the subclavian or internal jugular approaches.

Other preoperative complications in patients with chronic renal failure

The introduction of regular haemodialysis has improved greatly the condition of surgical patients with coincidental chronic renal failure. However, the preoperative examination should exclude evidence of congestive cardiac failure, pleural or pericardial effusions and ECG abnormalities from myocardial ischaemia.

Anaesthesia for patients with chronic renal failure

Anaesthesia for vascular and peritoneal access for dialysis

Regional anaesthesia may be a useful alternative to general anaesthesia in patients with chronic renal failure needing access for dialysis. However, the duration of both brachial plexus block (Bromage & Gertel, 1972), and subarachnoid anaesthesia (Orko et al., 1986) are reduced significantly in uraemic patients when compared with a healthy, normal population. The cause for this may be a faster tissue wash-out of the local anaesthetic agents. This may result from increased cardiac output in the uraemic patient as a result of both anaemia and the presence of shunts or fistulae. Any increase in hepatic blood flow increases the clearance of these high extraction-ratio drugs.

In addition, there is accelerated onset of sensory analgesia in patients with renal failure, through the combined effects of the acidosis increasing ionization of the local anaesthetic drugs, and a reduced intrathecal space secondary to distension of extradural and spinal veins by the hyperdynamic circulation.

However, two recent papers have failed to support these earlier data (Beauregard et al., 1987; McEllistrem et al., 1989). In addition, there is no evidence of altered bupivacaine disposition after supraclavicular plexus block in uraemic patients (Rice et al., 1991).

The use of extradural or subarachnoid anaesthesia may result in sympathetic block with a significant decrease in arterial pressure. This can be avoided by careful preoperative fluid loading.

Both extradural and subarachnoid anaesthesia and the institution of regional nerve blocks may result in haematomata at the injection site. However, this has not been considered of sufficient severity to preclude consideration of local techniques for both dialysis access and renal transplantation (Linke & Merin,

Table 62.7 Maximum safe doses of local anaesthetic agents (mg) (in a 70-kg healthy man)

	Plain solution	+ Adrenaline (1/200 000)	Relative duration of sensory block
Lignocaine	300	500	1.5
Bupivacaine	175	250	8
Mepivacaine	300	500	1.5
Etidocaine	300	400	8
Prilocaine	400	600	1.5
Chloroprocaine	600	650	0.75
Procaine	500	600	1

These doses should be decreased by 25% in the acidotic patient to avoid signs of CNS toxicity (e.g. light-headedness, dizziness, disorientation, euphoria, dysarthria, slurring of speech; progressing to twitching and generalized convulsions).

1976), and the institution of adequate dialysis brings about reversal of the primary platelet dysfunction.

Bupivacaine is the agent of choice, although a recent report has described cardiotoxic effects following its use in normal doses in a patient with renal failure (Gould & Aldrete, 1983). As a general rule, the normal maximum doses of bupivacaine and other local anaesthetic agents should be decreased by 25%, as acidosis also has an effect in reducing the CNS threshold to the toxic effects of these drugs (Table 62.7).

Regional anaesthesia is contraindicated generally in the patient with a uraemic neuropathy. Addition of vasoconstrictors to prolong the action of local anaesthetic agents is best avoided because of the risk of cardiac arrhythmias following systemic absorption in the acidotic, hyperkalaemic patient.

Anaesthesia for general surgery including renal transplantation

Patients with renal dysfunction require careful organization of their planned surgery with respect to preoperative dialysis. Uraemia may lead to unusual drug responses as a result of several different factors. These include reduced plasma protein−drug binding and low concentrations of plasma pseudocholinesterase. Electrolyte imbalance may lead to problems with reversal of the competitive neuromuscular-blocking drugs.

Premedication is of great importance, as many patients (especially at the time of transplantation) are understandably anxious. Suitable attenuation of this anxiety may be achieved with an orally administered benzodiazepine. Intramuscular premedication is best avoided because of bleeding diatheses found in uraemic patients. Vagolytic drugs may be given intravenously at the induction of anaesthesia to overcome pronounced bradycardia associated with the use of suxamethonium and combinations of opioids and the newer generation of competitive neuromuscular blocking drugs with little chronotropic effect. Chronic β-adrenoreceptor block, calcium-channel inhibitors and other cardioactive drugs should be maintained up to the morning of surgery.

With respect to the intravascular volume, it is generally wise to aim for mild overhydration. Tasker and colleagues (1974) have demonstrated that the prophylactic administration of saline preoperatively to the renal failure patient was effective in preventing further deterioration of renal function.

The routine prophylactic administration of antacids is advocated in patients with symptoms of peptic reflux. A single dose of sodium citrate (30 ml) is usual. H_2-receptor antagonists given 4 h preoperatively have been used also to reduce the gastric hyperacidity. Care should be exercised with administration of antiemetic drugs (e.g. phenothiazines), as they may result in prolonged sedation and extrapyramidal side-effects in patients with renal failure.

Anaesthesia may be induced with any of the standard induction agents given cautiously and preceded by a loading dose of a suitable opioid (fentanyl, 1–5 μg/kg; or alfentanil, 20–30 μg/kg). With such a regimen, it is possible to control the haemodynamic responses to induction of anaesthesia, laryngoscopy and tracheal intubation.

There are few studies investigating the haemodynamic effects of anaesthesia in renal patients. In a prospective study, Pouttu (1989) reported the cardiovascular responses to induction of anaesthesia, intubation and revascularization in three groups of patients (normotensive patients; hypertensive patients receiving β-adrenoceptor-blocking drugs; and hypertensive patients receiving a combination of β-adrenoceptor-blocking drugs and vasodilators) undergoing cadaveric transplantation. In all patients, anaesthesia was induced with 1 μg/kg fentanyl and a sleep dose of thiopentone to loss of eyelash reflex. Compared with the other two groups, arterial pressures were lower in the normotensive patients before and during induction of anaesthesia, and after intubation. However, the magnitude of the blood pressure and heart rate responses was comparable in all three groups, as was the incidence of intraoperative hypotension. Similar haemodynamic changes have been measured when propofol or the combination

propofol–fentanyl are used (Morcos & Payne, 1985; Nguyen et al., 1985; Kirvela et al., 1992).

Neuromuscular block is achieved with atracurium or vecuronium in doses of 0.6 and 0.1 mg/kg, respectively. Increments of these drugs should be given when clinically indicated and by monitoring neuromuscular transmission with a peripheral nerve stimulator. As an alternative, an infusion may be used — although caution must be exercised with vecuronium (see earlier). For the patient in whom there is the added problem of an inadequate period of starvation before surgery, suxamethonium may be used to facilitate intubation. An additional point of importance is that uraemia per se has the effect of prolonging gastric emptying.

All techniques for the maintenance of anaesthesia have been employed successfully. The inhalation agents have the advantages of non-renal elimination (although fluoride ion accumulation may occur with enflurane), and may be given with high inspired oxygen concentrations in the severely anaemic patient. However, all these commonly used agents cause myocardial depression. Normocapnia or mild hypocapnia should be maintained. Short periods of hypoventilation can lead to desaturation of haemoglobin, while excess hyperventilation with low carbon dioxide tensions causes a shift of the oxyhaemoglobin dissociation curve to the left.

In patients undergoing abdominal or other body cavity surgery, and in whom there is history of a recent myocardial infarction or a poor left ventricular ejection fraction, moderate- to high-dose fentanyl, 30–50 μg/kg, or sufentanil, 10–20 μg/kg, have been recommended as the main anaesthetic drugs.

At the end of anaesthesia and surgery, residual neuromuscular block may be reversed with neostigmine given with atropine or glycopyrrolate. The latter should be used in patients with associated ischaemic heart disease so as to avoid unnecessary tachycardia. All patients should receive oxygen for 12–24 h, postoperatively.

Water deprivation before surgery results in a greater volume contraction in patients with renal failure than in the healthy individual. This is because of the continued excretion of solutes, electrolytes and water in the absence of fluid intake as a result of loss of normal renal concentrating mechanisms. Dextrose 5% infused at approximately 100 ml/h overnight may alleviate the hypovolaemia.

Intraoperative fluid replacement should be undertaken to avoid volume depletion, aiming for a urine flow rate of 1 ml/min. Salt-containing solutions (but not those containing potassium) should be given to replace obligatory losses, in addition to insensible losses, surgical losses and third-space effects. There is no contraindication to the infusion of blood (see below) although excessive volume may lead to fluid overload and acute congestive cardiac failure. Failure to replace blood with blood results in a compromised circulation in the patient who is already severely anaemic. The levels of 2,3-DPG, which are low in stored blood, increase during the 24-h period after transfusion. Great care must be taken with fluid intake in patients who are anuric or anephric.

Monitoring and fluid requirements during anaesthesia

In addition to continuous measurement of heart rate and arterial pressure, the ECG should be monitored using leads in the CM5 configuration to allow early detection of myocardial ischaemia, and its treatment by control of heart rate or arterial pressure.

Measurement of CVP is as important as the arterial pressure in patients undergoing renal transplantation. Although many previous reviews have stressed the problems of overhydration and electrolyte imbalance, this has always been in poorly prepared or non-dialysed patients. Accordingly, fluid intakes of the order of $10 \, \text{ml} \cdot \text{kg}^{-1} \cdot 24 \, \text{h}^{-1}$ were advocated. By careful use of CVP, both intraoperative and postoperative fluid management can be gauged to avoid hypovolaemia and hypotension.

Recent studies by Carlier and colleagues (1982, 1986) in Brussels have demonstrated that maximal hydration during anaesthesia (up to 100 ml/kg normal saline), with an associated increase in pulmonary arterial pressure, is associated with improved early function of cadaveric renal allografts. This has been our impression also in Oxford, where the aim is to hydrate the patient with equal volumes of crystalloid (normal saline) and colloid (blood, plasma, or haemaccel) to raise the CVP by $7-10 \, \text{cmH}_2\text{O}$ at the time of renal revascularization. Fluid loads of this magnitude may precipitate pulmonary oedema in patients with poor myocardial function, and in such cases, positioning of a pulmonary artery catheter before surgery is indicated.

Postoperative fluid requirements depend on early renal function, but should aim to maintain the CVP at its intraoperative value. In practice, this equates to an initial regimen of urine output plus 50-100 ml/h. In those patients showing a prompt and profound diuresis, CVP maintenance and the avoidance of arterial hypotension should be primarily by infusion of crystalloid solutions supplemented by colloid.

Persistent hypotension in the presence of an adequate CVP normally responds to dobutamine, $1-20 \, \mu\text{g} \cdot \text{kg}^{-1} \cdot \text{min}^{-1}$. Many units routinely infuse dopamine, $2-3 \, \mu\text{g} \cdot \text{kg}^{-1} \cdot \text{min}^{-1}$, from the time of renal revascularization to promote renal arteriolar vasodilatation.

In those patients with renal failure not undergoing transplantation, fluid replacement in the anephric individual should be limited to insensible losses plus drainage, while in the patient with chronic renal insufficiency who is polyuric and unable to concentrate urine, volumes of 3-4 litres/day ($\pm$ a diuretic) may be needed.

Although it is not our practice to monitor perioperatively the plasma electrolyte (and particularly potassium) concentrations routinely, there have been reports of sudden increases in plasma potassium concentrations leading to arrhythmias and cardiac arrest (Hirshman & Edelstein, 1979). Several factors may be responsible, including administration of mannitol (Moreno et al., 1969) and stored blood, severe metabolic acidosis and hyperkalaemia associated with hyperglycaemia (Goldfarb et al., 1976). The aetiology of the last mechanism is unknown, and the prevention of this complication assumes greater significance in the diabetic patient undergoing renal transplantation.

Additional non-anaesthetic drugs given during renal transplantation

Immunosuppressive therapy

The initiation of immunosuppressive therapy (hydrocortisone, prednisolone, azathioprine, cyclosporin, antilymphocytic globulin, monoclonal antibodies) varies with respect to timing and doses between units, but often one or more of these agents is given at the time of renal revascularization. Recent work by Cirella and colleagues (1987) has shown chronic CYA therapy to prolong the duration of pentobarbitone anaesthesia in mice, and also potentiate the efficacy of analgesia induced by fentanyl. Augustine and Zemaitis (1986) have confirmed these observations to be the result of decreased levels of cytochrome P450 in animals receiving long-term cyclosporin treatment, and hence a decrease in the rate of microsomal mixed function oxidase drug metabolism. Another interaction between CYA and muscle relaxants has been reported by Sidi and colleagues (1990) who observed a greater incidence of postoperative respiratory failure in transplant patients receiving CYA as the immunosuppressant drug. Administration of intravenous cyclosporin — formulated in Cremophor

EL — should be conducted with caution, as a case of anaphylaxis has been reported (Magalini *et al.*, 1986). Drug interactions have also been reported with azathioprine (Gramstad, 1987).

Promotion of diuresis

Other drugs given by the anaesthetist are those used to promote diuresis from the grafted kidney. Carlier and colleagues (1986) have demonstrated that the incidence of delayed graft function (as a result of acute tubular necrosis) may be reduced by the techniques of maximal hydration of the recipient, the use of mannitol (Weimer *et al.*, 1983) and *in situ* perfusion of the donor organs. Mannitol has been demonstrated also to improve renal blood flow by a greater percentage than can be accounted for by vascular volume expansion alone (Johnston *et al.*, 1979).

Mannitol is the reduced form of the six-carbon sugar mannose, and its use to promote a graft diuresis has been criticized by some authorities (Salaman *et al.*, 1969). It is a small molecule that equilibrates slowly within the extracellular fluid spaces. It is filtered freely by the renal glomerulus, and is not reabsorbed in the distal renal tubules. Through its osmotic properties, water and sodium are excreted also. If, however, there is failure of adequate perfusion of the graft kidney, and hence failure of glomerular filtration, the presence of mannitol in the extracellular space may lead to intracellular dehydration with increased intravascular volume and congestive cardiac failure.

Moote and Manninen (1987) have examined the influence of mannitol on serum electrolytes in patients undergoing renal transplantation. Fifty grams of mannitol increased the CVP, and reduced serum concentrations of sodium, chloride and bicarbonate. The rise in potassium was small, but this may assume clinical importance in patients also receiving a blood transfusion.

Frusemide, in doses of 40–80 mg i.v., to stimulate diuresis, is not open to the same criticism. Its use should be coupled with preloading of the recipient with isotonic (0.154 M) saline. The administration of a fluid load acts also as a physiological stimulus to urine production. This stimulus is important, as nearly all the available analgesic and inhalation drugs given during anaesthesia cause an increase in circulating antidiuretic hormone concentrations, which influence both the *in vitro* and denervated allograft. There are data to suggest that potent diuretics should not be given to patients receiving cyclosporin, as the combination may lead to acute tubular necrosis (Whiting *et al.*, 1984).

Failure of the adequately perfused graft to respond to these diuretic stimuli may be treated by an infusion of dopamine, $3-5\,\mu g \cdot kg^{-1} \cdot min^{-1}$.

Blood transfusion

Previously, blood transfusion for potential renal transplant patients or during transplantation was avoided, to minimize sensitization to the major histocompatibility antigens. However, Opelz, Terasaki and others have confirmed a higher degree of renal graft survivals in patients transfused before surgery (Morris, 1978; Opelz & Terasaki, 1978). The optimum number of transfusions is probably between 4 and 10 units of blood, but no consensus view exists as to the optimal interval between the last transfusion and transplantation. However, the efficacy of transfusion can be seen by an increased graft survival (from 47% to 57% at 5 years). If cadaveric graft survival is compared at 1 year for patients undergoing deliberate transfusion and those transfused for medical reasons only, the respective figures are 89% and 60%.

Blood products may take the form of whole blood, packed red cells, or washed red cells; frozen–thawed blood has been found to be ineffective in increasing actuarial survival.

There is now less evidence to support the beneficial influence of blood transfusion on graft survival, because of the immunosuppressive potential of CYA (Lundgren *et al.*, 1986; Opelz, 1987; Editorial, 1988). However, donor-specific transfusions may be useful in some patients undergoing living-related donor allografting.

Postoperative care and complications of the renal transplant patient

Because of the multiple pathology exhibited by renal transplant patients, they should be nursed postoperatively in an intensive therapy unit where controlled oxygen therapy, comprehensive monitoring and, if necessary, assisted ventilation can be carried out. Systemic arterial pressure should be recorded non-invasively avoiding the arm containing the shunt or fistula. Strict monitoring of fluid input and output is essential, the intake being related to CVP, and composed of both crystalloids and colloids. Some authorities suggest that routine use of H_2-receptor antagonists to reduce the risk of stress ulceration, but this is best reserved for patients with a proven previous history of peptic ulceration.

The major postoperative anaesthetic complications are vomiting and aspiration, cardiac arrhythmias (some leading to cardiac arrest), hypoxia, hypotension and hypertension, pulmonary oedema, and delayed respiratory distress.

Analgesia in the postoperative transplant patient or the patient with chronic renal failure undergoing coincidental surgery is important if chest complications are to be avoided. Opiate drugs provide the mainstay of treatment, but possible cumulation of active metabolites may occur in the patient with a non-functioning kidney. Matzke and colleagues (1986) reported codeine-induced narcosis in uraemic patients receiving standard doses of codeine; the altered disposition of codeine and its metabolites in end-stage renal failure are well described by Guay and colleagues (1988). Excessive opioid medication may lead to delayed respiratory depression, sedation and convulsions (all relatable to both parent drug and active metabolite accumulation). The recent widespread awareness of the techniques of patient-controlled analgesia may aid the more efficient and safe titration of dosage to desired effect in the uraemic patient.

Although only a small percentage of non-steroidal anti-inflammatory drugs (NSAIDs) are eliminated unchanged via the kidney, there is evidence of reduced clearance of ketoprofen, fenoprofen, naproxen and carprofen in renal failure due to probable deconjugation of acyl glucuronide metabolites. NSAIDs may also cause reversible kidney damage — with reduction of renal blood flow and the GFR; and oedema, interstitial nephritis and papillary necrosis in the kidney. These effects are probably caused by the action of the NSAIDs on prostaglandin synthesis — the latter being integral for renal blood flow and GFR autoregulation. Hence, these drugs are best avoided in *all* patients with renal impairment.

Conclusion

In one of the first series of patients undergoing renal transplantation, Strunin (1966) reported an immediate perioperative mortality of 16%. More recent series (Lindahl-Nilsson et al., 1980; Marsland & Bradley, 1983; Heino et al., 1986) have recorded perioperative mortalities of less than 0.6%, while similar figures have been reported for the overall surgical management of the patient with chronic renal failure (Morgan & Lumley, 1975).

There is no single correct method for the anaesthetic management of the patient with end-stage renal disease. Effective and safe anaesthesia depends on an understanding of the pathophysiology and biochemistry of the uraemic patient, and their effects on the disposition and metabolism of the drugs given.

References

Abbott M.A., Samuel J.R. & Webb D.R. (1985) Anaesthesia for extracorporeal shock wave lithotripsy. *Anaesthesia* **40**, 1065–72.

Aitkenhead A.R., Vater M., Achola K., Cooper C.M.S. & Smith G. (1984) Pharmacokinetics of single-dose i.v. morphine in normal volunteers and patients with end-stage renal failure. *British Journal of Anaesthesia* **56**, 813–18.

Ali M., Nicholls P.J. & Yoosef A. (1979) The influence of old age and of renal failure on hepatic glucuronidation in the rat. *British Journal of Pharmacology* **66**, 498–9.

Allen P.R., Hughes R.G., Goldie D.J. & Kennedy R.H. (1981) Fluid absorption during transurethral resection. *British Medical Journal* **282**, 740.

Andreasen F. (1974) The effect of dialysis on the protein binding of drugs in the plasma of patients with acute renal failure. *Acta Pharmacologica et Toxicologica* **34**, 284–94.

Attman P.-O. & Gustafson A. (1979) Lipid and carbohydrate metabolism in uraemia. *European Journal of Clinical Investigation* **9**, 285–91.

Augustine J.A. & Zemaitis M.A. (1986) The effects of cyclosporine (CsA) on hepatic microsomal drug metabolism in the rat. *Drug Metabolism and Disposition* **14**, 73–8.

Balant L.P., Dayer P. & Fabre J. (1983) Consequences of renal insufficiency on the hepatic clearance of some drugs. *International Journal of Clinical Pharmacological Research* **3**, 459–74.

Barnes J.N., Williams A.J., Tomson M.J.F., Toseland P.A. & Goodwin F.J. (1985) Dihydrocodeine in renal failure: further evidence for an important role of the kidney in the handling of opioid drugs. *British Medical Journal* **290**, 740–2.

Beauregard L., Martin R. & Tetrault J.P. (1987) Brachial plexus block and chronic renal failure. *Canadian Journal of Anaesthesia* **34**, 118S.

Bencini A.F., Scaf A.H.J., Sohn Y.J., Meistelman C., Lienhart A., Kersten U.W., Schwarz S. & Agoston S. (1986) Disposition and urinary excretion of vecuronium bromide in anesthetized patients with normal renal function or renal failure. *Anesthesia and Analgesia* **65**, 245–51.

Bennett M.J., Smith R.W. & Fuchs E. (1984) Sudden cardiac arrest during percutaneous ultrasonic nephrostolithotomy. *Anesthesiology* **60**, 254–6.

Bevan D.R., Donati F., Gyasi H. & Williams A. (1984) Vecuronium in renal failure. *Canadian Anaesthetists' Society Journal* **31**, 491–6.

Bion J.F., Logan B.K., Newman P.M., Brodie M.J., Oliver J.S., Aitchison T.C. & Ledingham I.McA. (1986) Sedation in intensive care: morphine and renal function. *Intensive Care Medicine* **12**, 359–65.

Bower S. (1982) Plasma protein binding of fentanyl: the effect of hyperlipidaemia and chronic renal failure. *Journal of Pharmacy and Pharmacology* **34**, 102–6.

Bower S. & Sear J.W. (1989) Disposition of alfentanil in patients receiving a renal transplant. *Journal of Pharmacy and Pharmacology* **41**, 654–7.

Bromage P.R. & Gertel M. (1972) Brachial plexus anesthesia in chronic renal failure. *Anesthesiology* **36**, 488–93.

Brotherton W.D. & Matteo R.S. (1981) Pharmacokinetics and pharmacodynamics of metocurine in humans with and without renal failure. *Anesthesiology* **55**, 273–6.

Brown J.J., Duesterdieck G., Fraser R., Lever A.F., Robertson J.I.S., Tree M. & Weir R.J. (1971) Hypertension and chronic renal failure. *British Medical Bulletin* **27**, 128–35.

Burch P.G. & Stanski D.R. (1982) Decreased protein binding and thiopental kinetics. *Clinical Pharmacology and Therapeutics* **32**, 212–17.

Buzello W. & Agoston S. (1978) Pharmacokinetics of pancuronium in patients with normal and impaired renal function. *Der Anaesthesist* **27**, 291–7.

Caldwell J.E., Canfell P.C., Castagnoli K.P., Lynam D.P., Fahey M.R., Fisher D.M. & Miller R.D. (1989) The influence of renal failure on the pharmacokinetics and duration of action of pipercuronium bromide in patients anesthetized with halothane and nitrous oxide. *Anesthesiology* **70**, 7–12.

Carlier M., Squifflet J.P., Pirson Y., Gribomont B. & Alexandre G.P.J. (1982) Maximal hydration during anesthesia increases pulmonary arterial pressures and improves early function in human renal transplants. *Transplantation* **34**, 201–4.

Carlier M., Squifflet J.P., Pirson Y., Alexandre G.P.J., de Temmermann P. & Gribomont B.F. (1986) Anesthetic protocol in human renal transplantation: twenty two years of experience. *Acta Anaesthesiologica Belgica* **37**, 89–94.

Carlos R., Calvo R. & Erill S. (1976) Plasma protein binding of etomidate in patients with renal failure or hepatic cirrhosis. *Clinical Pharmacokinetics* **4**, 144–8.

Chauvin M., Lebrault C., Levron J.C. & Duvaldestin P. (1987a) Pharmacokinetics of alfentanil in chronic renal failure. *Anesthesia and Analgesia* **66**, 53–6.

Chauvin M., Sandouk P., Scherrmann J.M., Farinotti R., Strumza P. & Duvaldestin P. (1987b) Morphine pharmacokinetics in renal failure. *Anesthesiology* **66**, 327–31.

Christensen J.H. & Andreasen F. (1978) Individual variation in response to thiopental. *Acta Anaesthesiologica Scandinavica* **22**, 303–13.

Christensen J.H., Andreasen F. & Jansen J. (1983) Pharmacokinetics and pharmacodynamics of thiopental in patients undergoing renal transplantation. *Acta Anaesthesiologica Scandinavica* **27**, 513–18.

Cirella V.N., Pantuck C.B., Lee Y.J. & Pantuck E.J. (1987) Effects of cyclosporine on anesthetic action. *Anesthesia and Analgesia* **66**, 703–6.

Cook D.R., Freeman J.A., Lai A.A., Robertson K.A., Kang Y., Stiller R.L., Aggarwal S., Abou-Donia M.M. & Welch R.M. (1991) Pharmacokinetics and pharmacodynamics of doxacurium in normal patients and in those with hepatic or renal failure. *Anesthesia and Analgesia* **72**, 145–50.

Corall I.M., Moore A.R. & Strunin L. (1980) Plasma concentrations of fentanyl in normal surgical patients and those with severe renal and hepatic disease. *British Journal of Anaesthesia* **52**, 101A.

Cronnelly R. & Morris R.B. (1982) Antagonism of neuromuscular blockade. *British Journal of Anaesthesia* **54**, 183–94.

Cronnelly R., Fisher D.M., Miller R.D., Gencarelli P., Nguyen-Gruenke L. & Castagnoli N. (1984a) Pharmacokinetics and pharmacodynamics of vecuronium (Org NC 45) in anesthetised humans. *Anesthesiology* **58**, 405–8.

Cronnelly R., Salvatierra O. & Feduska N. (1984b) Renal allograft function following halothane, enflurane or isoflurane anesthesia. *Anesthesia and Analgesia* **63**, 202A.

Cousins M.J., Mazze R.I., Losek J.C., Hitt B.A. & Love F.V. (1974) The etiology of methoxyflurane nephrotoxicity. *Journal of Pharmacology and Experimental Therapeutics* **190**, 530–41.

Davis R.J., Stiller R.L., Cook D.R., Brandom B.W. & Davin-Robinson K.A. (1988) Pharmacokinetics of sufentanil in adolescent patients with chronic renal failure. *Anesthesia and Analgesia* **67**, 268–71.

deBros F.M., Lai A., Scott R., deBros J., Baston A.G., Goudsouzian N., Ali H.H., Cosimi A.B. & Saverese J.J. (1986) Pharmacokinetics and pharmacodynamics of atracurium during isoflurane anesthesia in normal and anephric patients. *Anesthesia and Analgesia* **65**, 743–6.

deBros F., Basta S.J., Ali H.H., Wargin W. & Welch R. (1987) Pharmacokinetics and pharmacodynamics of BW B1090U in healthy surgical patients receiving N_2O/O_2 isoflurane anesthesia. *Anesthesiology* **67**, 609A.

Don H.F., Dieppa R.A. & Taylor P. (1975) Narcotic analgesics in anuric patients. *Anesthesiology* **42**, 745–7.

Dundee J.W. & Annis D. (1955) Barbiturate narcosis in uraemia. *British Journal of Anaesthesia* **27**, 114–23.

Durand P.G., Lehot J.J. & Foëx P. (1991) Calcium-channel blockers and anaesthesia. *Canadian Journal of Anaesthesia* **38**, 75–89.

Duthie D.J.R. (1986) Renal failure, surgery and fentanyl pharmacokinetics. Abstracts of VII European Congress of Anaesthesiology, vol. I. *Beitrage zur Anaesthesiologie und Intensivmedizin* **16**, 187.

Editorial (1988) Time to abandon pre-transplant blood transfusion. *Lancet* **1**, 567.

Eschbach J.W., Egrie J.C., Downing M.R., Browne J.K. & Adamson J.W. (1987) Correction of the anemia of end-stage renal disease with recombinant human erythropoietin. Results of a combined Phase I and II Clinical Trial. *New England Journal of Medicine* **316**, 73–8.

Eschbach J.W., Abdulladi M.H., Browne J.K., Delano B.G., Downing M.R., Egrie J.C. *et al.* (1989) Recombinant human erythropoietin (rHuEpo) in anemic patients with end-stage renal disease: Results of a Phase III multicenter trial. *Annals of Internal Medicine* **111**, 992–1000.

Fahey M.R., Morris R.B., Miller R.D., Nguyen T.L. & Upton R.A. (1981) Pharmacokinetics of ORG NC45 (Norcuron) in patients with and without renal failure. *British Journal of Anaesthesia* **53**, 1049–53.

Fahey M.R., Rupp S.M., Fisher D.M., Miller R.D., Sharma M., Canfell C., Castagnoli K. & Hennis P.J. (1984) The pharmacokinetics and pharmacodynamics of atracurium in patients with and without renal failure. *Anesthesiology* **61**, 699–702.

Feldman S.A. & Levi J.A. (1963) Prolonged paresis following gallamine. A case report. *British Journal of Anaesthesia* **35**, 804–6.

Feldman S.A., Cohen E.N. & Golling R.C. (1969) The excretion of gallamine in the dog. *Anesthesiology* **30**, 593–8.

Fisher D.M., Canfell C., Fahey M.R., Rosen J.I., Rupp S.M., Sheiner L.B. & Miller R.D. (1986) Elimination of atracurium in humans: contribution of Hofmann elimination and ester hydrolysis versus organ-bound elimination. *Anesthesiology* **65**, 6–12.

Foëx P. (1984) Alpha and beta-adrenoceptor antagonists. *British Journal of Anaesthesia* **56**, 751–65.

Freilich J.D., Waterman P.M. & Rosenthal J.T. (1984) Acute hemodynamic changes during renal transplantation.

Anesthesia and Analgesia **63**, 158–60.

Fyman P., Avitable M., Moser F., Reynolds J., Casthley P., Butt K. & Kopman A. (1987) Sufentanil pharmacokinetics in patients undergoing renal transplantation. *Anesthesia and Analgesia* **66**, 62S.

Geha D.G., Blitt C.D. & Moon B.J. (1976) Prolonged neuro-muscular blockade with pancuronium in the presence of acute renal failure: a case report. *Anesthesia and Analgesia* **55**, 343–5.

Ghoneim M.M., Kramer E., Bannow R., Pandya M.S. & Routh J.L. (1973) Binding of D-tubocurarine to plasma proteins in normal man and in patients with hepatic or renal failure. *Anesthesiology* **39**, 410–15.

Gibaldi M., Levy G. & Hayton E.L. (1972) Tubocurarine and renal failure. *British Journal of Anaesthesia* **44**, 163–5.

Gibson F.P. (1986) Renal disease and drug metabolism: an overview. *American Journal of Kidney Diseases* **8**, 7–17.

Gibson T.P., Giacomini K.M., Briggs W.A., Whitman W. & Levy G. (1980) Propoxyphene and norpropoxyphene plasma concentrations in the anephric patient. *Clinical Pharmacology and Therapeutics* **27**, 665–70.

Glare P.A., Walsh T.D. & Pippenger C.E. (1990) Normorphine, a neurotoxic metabolite? *Lancet* **335**, 725–6.

Goldfarb S., Cox M., Singer I. & Goldberg M. (1976) Acute hyperkalemia induced by hyperglycemia: hormonal mechan-isms. *Annals of Internal Medicine* **84**, 426–32.

Gorman H.M. & Craythorne N.W.B. (1966) The effect of a new neuroleptic analgesic agent (Innovar) on renal function in man. *Acta Anaesthesiologica Scandinavica* **24** (Suppl.), 111.

Gorven A.M., Cooper G.M. & Prys-Roberts C. (1986) Haemo-dynamic disturbances during anaesthesia in a patient receiv-ing calcium channel blockers. *British Journal of Anaesthesia* **58**, 357–60.

Gould D.B. & Aldrete J.A. (1983) Bupivacaine cardiotoxicity in a patient with renal failure. *Acta Anaesthesiologica Scandinavica* **27**, 18–21.

Gramstad L. (1987) Atracurium, vecuronium and pancuronium in endstage renal failure. Dose-response properties and inter-actions with azathioprine. *British Journal of Anaesthesia* **59**, 995–1003.

Groves N.D., Leach K.G. & Rosen M. (1990) Effects of halothane, enflurane and isoflurane anaesthesia on renal plasma flow. *British Journal of Anaesthesia* **65**, 796–800.

Guay D.R.P., Awni W.M., Findlay J.W.A., Halstenson C.E., Abraham P.A., Opsahl J.A., Jones E.C. & Matzke G.R. (1988) Pharmacokinetics and pharmacodynamics of codeine in end-stage renal disease. *Clinical Pharmacology and Therapeutics* **43**, 63–71.

Gulden D., Koehntop D., Rodman J., Brundage D. & Hegland M. (1984) Fentanyl pharmacokinetics during renal trans-plantation. *Anesthesiology* **61**, 243A.

Hahn R.G. (1991) The transurethral resection syndrome. *Acta Anaesthesiologica Scandinavica* **35**, 557–67.

Hatch P.D. (1987) Surgical and anaesthetic considerations in transurethral resection of the prostate. *Anaesthesia and Intensive Care* **15**, 203–11.

Heino A., Orko R. & Rosenberg P.H. (1986) Anaesthesiological complications in renal transplantation: a retrospective study of 500 transplantations. *Acta Anaesthesiologica Scandinavica* **30**, 574–80.

Henderson D.J. & Middleton R.G. (1980) Coma from hypo-natremia following transurethral resection of prostate. *Urology* **15**, 267–71.

Hirshman C.A. & Edelstein G. (1979) Intraoperative hyper-kalemia and cardiac arrest during renal transplantation in an insulin dependent diabetic patient. *Anesthesiology* **51**, 161–2.

Hogan E.M., Nicholls P.J. & Yoosuf A. (1979) Hepatic micro-somal oxidative N-demethylation in rats in renal failure. *British Journal of Pharmacology* **66**, 74–5.

Horl W.H., Stepinski J. & Heidland A. (1980) Carbohydrate metabolism and uraemia — mechanisms for glycogenolysis and gluconeogenesis. *Klinische Wochenschrift* **58**, 1051–64.

Hunter J.M., Jones R.S. & Utting J.E. (1982) Use of atracurium in patients with no renal function. *British Journal of Anaesthesia* **54**, 1251–8.

Hunter J.M., Jones R.S. & Utting J.E. (1984) Comparison of vecuronium, atracurium and tubocurarine in normal patients and in patients with no renal function. *British Journal of Anaesthesia* **56**, 941–51.

Ickx B., Barvais L., Cockshott I.D., Douglas E.J., Vandesteene A. & d'Hollander A. (1991) Pharmacokinetics of propofol in patients with end-stage renal disease. A preliminary report. In *Focus on Infusion — Intravenous Anaesthesia* (Ed. Prys-Roberts C.) pp. 196–8. Current Medical Literature Ltd, London.

Jenkins L.C. & Scoates P.J. (1985) Anaesthetic implications of calcium channel blockers. *Canadian Anaesthetists' Society Journal* **32**, 436–47.

Johnston P.A., Bernard D.B., Donohoe J.F., Perrin N.S. & Levinsky N.G. (1979) Effect of volume expansion on hemo-dynamics of the hypoperfused rat kidney. *Journal of Clinical Investigation* **64**, 550–8.

Jones R.M. (1984) Calcium antagonists. *Anaesthesia* **39**, 747–9.

Kangas L., Kanto J., Forsstrom J. & Ilisalo E. (1976) The protein binding of diazepam and N-demethyldiazepam in patients with poor renal function. *Clinical Nephrology* **5**, 114–18.

Kirvela M., Olkkola, K.T., Rosenberg P.H., Yli-Hamkala A., Salmela K. & Lindgren L. (1992) Pharmacokinetics of propofol and haemodynamic changes during induction of anaesthesia in uraemic patients. *British Journal of Anaesthesia* **68**, 178–82.

Kopple J.D. (1978) Abnormal aminoacid and protein metab-olism in uremia. *Kidney International* **14**, 340–8.

Kunin C.M. (1967) A guide to use of antibiotics in patients with renal disease. *Annals of Internal Medicine* **67**, 151–8.

Lawson R.A., Turner W.H., Reeder M.K., Sear J.W. & Smith J.C. (1993) Haemodynamic effects of transurethral prostatectomy (TURP). *British Journal of Urology* **72**, 74–9.

LePage J.Y., Malinge M., Cozian A., Pinaud M., Blanloeil Y. & Souron R. (1987) Vecuronium and atracurium in patients with endstage renal failure. *British Journal of Anaesthesia* **59**, 1004–10.

LePage J.Y., Athouel A., Vecherini M.F., Malinovsky J.M. & Cozian A. (1991) Evaluation of proconvulsant effect of laudanosine in renal transplant recipient. *Anesthesiology* **75**, 780A.

Lindahl-Nilsson C., Lundh R. & Groth C.-G. (1980) Neurolept anaesthesia for the renal transplant operation. *Acta Anaesthesiologica Scandinavica* **24**, 451–7.

Linke C.L. & Merin R.G. (1976) A regional anesthetic approach for renal transplantation. *Anesthesia and Analgesia* **55**, 69–73.

Logan D.A., Howie H.B. & Crawford J. (1974) Anaesthesia and renal transplantation: an analysis of fifty six cases. *British Journal of Anaesthesia* **46**, 69–72.

Lombardo L.N. (1957) Fibrinolysis following prostatic surgery. *Journal of Urology* **77**, 289–96.

Lowenstein E., Goldfine C. & Flacke W.E. (1970) Administration of gallamine in the presence of renal failure — reversal of neuromuscular blockade by peritoneal dialysis. *Anesthesiology* **33**, 556–8.

Lundgren G., Groth C.-G., Albretchson D., Brynger H., Flatmark A., Frodin L., Gabel H., Husberg B., Klintmalm G., Maurer W., Persson H. & Thorsby E. (1986) HLA-matching and pretransplant blood transfusions in cadaveric renal transplantation — a changing picture with cyclosporin. *Lancet* **ii**, 66–9.

Lynam D.P., Cronnelly R., Castagnoli K.P., Canfell P.C., Caldwell J., Arden J. & Miller R.D. (1988) The pharmacodynamics and pharmacokinetics of vecuronium in patients anesthetized with isoflurane with normal renal function or with renal failure. *Anesthesiology* **69**, 227–31.

Magalini S.C., Nanni G., Agnes S., Citterio F. & Castagneto M. (1986) Anaphylactic reaction to first exposure to cyclosporine. *Transplantation* **42**, 443–4.

Mannucci P.M. (1988) Desmopressin: a nontransfusional form of treatment for congenital and acquired bleeding disorders. *Blood* **72**, 1449–55.

Mannucci P.M., Remuzzi C. & Pusineri F. (1983) Deamino-8-D-arginine vasopressin shortens the bleeding time in uremia. *New England Journal of Medicine* **308**, 8–12.

Marsland A.R. & Bradley J.P. (1983) Anaesthesia for renal transplantation — 5 years' experience. *Anaesthesia and Intensive Care* **11**, 337–44.

Matzke G.R., Chan G.L.C. & Abraham P.A. (1986) Codein dosage in renal failure. *Clinical Pharmacy* **5**, 15–16.

Mazze R.I., Sievenpiper T.S. & Stevenson J. (1984) Renal effects of enflurane and halothane in patients with abnormal renal function. *Anesthesiology* **60**, 161–3.

McEllistrem R.F., Schell J., O'Malley K., O'Toole D. & Cunningham A.J. (1989) Interscalene brachial plexus blockade with lidocaine in chronic renal failure — a pharmacokinetic study. *Canadian Journal of Anaesthesia* **36**, 59–63.

McLeod K., Watson M.J. & Rawlins M.D. (1976) Pharmacokinetics of pancuronium in patients with normal and impaired renal function. *British Journal of Anaesthesia* **48**, 341–5.

Mebust W.K., Brady T.W. & Valk W.L. (1970) Observations on cardiac output, blood volume, central venous pressure, fluid and electrolyte changes in patients undergoing transurethral prostatectomy. *Journal of Urology* **103**, 632–7.

Miller R.D., Matteo R.S., Benet L.Z. & Sohn T.I. (1977) The pharmacokinetics of D-tubocurarine in man with and without renal failure. *Journal of Pharmacology and Experimental Therapeutics* **202**, 1–7.

Moore A., Sear J., Baldwin D., Allen M., Hunniset A., Bullingham R. & McQuay H. (1984) Morphine kinetics during and after renal transplantation. *Clinical Pharmacology and Therapeutics* **35**, 641–5.

Moote C.A. & Manninen P.H. (1987) Mannitol administered during renal transplantation produces profound changes in fluid and electrolyte balance. *Canadian Journal of Anaesthesia*

35, 120S. (Abstr.)

Morcos W.E. & Payne J.P. (1985) The induction of anaesthesia with propofol (Diprivan) compared in normal and renal failure patients. *Postgraduate Medical Journal* **61** (Suppl. 3), 62–3.

Moreno M., Murphy C. & Goldsmith C. (1969) Increase in serum potassium resulting from the administration of hypertonic mannitol and other solutions. *Journal of Laboratory and Clinical Medicine* **73**, 291–8.

Morgan M. & Lumley J. (1975) Anaesthetic considerations in chronic renal failure. *Anaesthesia and Intensive Care* **3**, 218–26.

Morris P.J. (1978) Blood transfusion and transplantation. *Transplantation* **26**, 276.

Mostert J.W., Evers J.L., Hobika G.H., Moore R.H. & Ambrus J.L. (1971) Cardiorespiratory effects of anaesthesia with morphine or fentanyl in chronic renal failure and cerebral toxicity after morphine. *British Journal of Anaesthesia* **43**, 1053–9.

Nguyen H.D., Kaplan R., Nagashima H., Dunclaf D. & Foldes F.F. (1985) The neuromuscular effect of atracurium in anephric patients. *Anesthesiology* **63**, 335A.

Ochs H.R., Greenblatt D.J., Kaschel H.J., Klehr W., Divoll M. & Abernethy D.R. (1981) Diazepam kinetics in patients with renal insufficiency or hyperthyroidism. *British Journal of Clinical Pharmacology* **12**, 829–32.

Opelz G. (1987) Improved kidney graft survival in nontransfused recipients. *Transplantation Proceedings* **XIX**, 149–52.

Opelz G. & Terasaki P.I. (1978) Improvement in kidney-graft survival with increased number of blood transfusions. *New England Journal of Medicine* **299**, 799–803.

Orko R., Pitkanen M. & Rosenberg P.H. (1986) Subarachnoid anaesthesia with 0.75% bupivacaine in patients with chronic renal failure. *British Journal of Anaesthesia* **58**, 605–9.

Osborne R.J., Joel S.P. & Slevin M.L. (1986) Morphine intoxication in renal failure: the role of morphine-6-glucuronide. *British Medical Journal* **292**, 1548–9.

Ovassapian A., Joshi C.W. & Brunner E.A. (1982) Visual disturbance: an unusual symptom of transurethral prostatic resection. *Anesthesiology* **57**, 332–4.

Parker C.J.R., Jones J.E. & Hunter J.M. (1988) Disposition of infusions of atracurium and its metabolite laudanosine in patients with renal and respiratory failure in an ITU. *British Journal of Anaesthesia* **61**, 531–40.

Patterson S.E. & Cohn V.H. (1984) Hepatic drug metabolism in rats with experimental chronic renal failure. *Biochemical Pharmacology* **33**, 711–16.

Pouttu J. (1989) Haemodynamic responses during general anaesthesia for renal transplantation in patients with and without hypertensive disease. *Acta Anaesthesiologica Scandinavica* **33**, 245–9.

Prys-Roberts C. (1984) Anaesthesia and hypertension. *British Journal of Anaesthesia* **56**, 711–24.

Ramzan M.I., Shanks C.A. & Triggs E.J. (1981) Gallamine disposition in surgical patients with chronic renal failure. *British Journal of Clinical Pharmacology* **12**, 141–7.

Reidenberg M.M. (1972) Drug metabolism in uraemia. *Clinical Nephrology* **4**, 83–5.

Reidenberg M.M. (1985) Kidney function and drug action

(editorial). *New England Journal of Medicine* **313**, 816–18.

Reiter V., Fay R., Pire J.C., Lamiable D. & Rendoing J. (1989) Propofol a debit continu au cours des transplantations renales chez l'adulte. *Cahiers d'Anesthesiologie* **37**, 23–31.

Rice A.S.C., Pither C.E. & Tucker G.T. (1991) Plasma concentrations of bupivacaine after supraclavicular brachial plexus blockade in patients with chronic renal failure. *Anaesthesia* **46**, 354–7.

Roesch R.P., Stoelting R.K., Lingeman J.E., Kahnowski R.J., Backes D.J. & Gephardt S.A. (1983) Ammonia toxicity resulting from glycine absorption during transurethral resection of the prostate. *Anesthesiology* **58**, 577–9.

Roos N.P., Wennberg J.E., Malenka D.J., Fisher E.S., McPherson K., Andersen T.V., Cohen M.M. & Ramsey E. (1989) Mortality and reoperation after open and transurethral resection of the prostate for benign prostatic hyperplasia. *New England Journal of Medicine* **320**, 1120–4.

Rouse J.M., Galley R.L.A. & Bevan D.R. (1977) Prolonged curarisation following renal transplantation. A retrospective study. *Anaesthesia* **32**, 247–51.

Russo R., Ravagnan R., Buzzetti V. & Favini P. (1986) Atracurium in patients with chronic renal failure. *British Journal of Anaesthesia* **58** (Suppl. 1), 63S.

Ryan D.W. (1977) Preoperative serum cholinesterase concentration in chronic renal failure. *British Journal of Anaesthesia* **49**, 945–9.

Ryder K.W., Olson J.P., Kahnoski R.J., Karn R.C. & Oei T.O. (1984) Hyperammonemia after transurethral resection of the prostate: a report of 2 cases. *Journal of Urology* **132**, 995–7.

Salaman J.R., Calne R.Y., Pera J., Sells R.A., White H.J.O. & Yoffa D. (1969) Surgical aspects of clinical renal transplantation. *British Journal of Surgery* **56**, 413–17.

Sawe J. & Odar-Cederlof I. (1987) Kinetics of morphine in patients with renal failure. *European Journal of Clinical Pharmacology* **32**, 337–42.

Sear J.W. (1987) Disposition of fentanyl and alfentanil in patients undergoing renal transplantation. Proceedings of VII European Congress of Anaesthesiology, vol I. *Beitrage zur Anaesthesiologie und Intensivmedizin* **19**, 53–8.

Sear J.W. (1989) Sufentanil disposition in patients undergoing renal transplantation: influence of choice of kinetic model. *British Journal of Anaesthesia* **63**, 60–7.

Sear J., Moore A., Hunnisett A., Baldwin D., Allen M., Hand C., McQuay H. & Morris P. (1985) Morphine kinetics and kidney transplantation: morphine removal is influenced by renal ischemia. *Anesthesia and Analgesia* **64**, 1065–70.

Sear J.W., Hand C.W., Moore R.A. & McQuay H.J. (1989) Studies on morphine disposition: influence of renal failure on the kinetics of morphine and its metabolites. *British Journal of Anaesthesia* **62**, 28–32.

Sear J.W., Jewkes C., Sanders D.J. & Foëx P. (1990) Does the choice of antihypertensive therapy matter? *European Journal of Anaesthesiology* **8**, 414–15.

Sidi A., Kaplan R.F. & Davis R.F. (1990) Prolonged neuromuscular blockade and ventilatory failure after renal transplantation and cyclosporine. *Canadian Journal of Anaesthesia* **37**, 543–8.

Sloan P.A., Mather L.E., McLean C.F., Rutten A.J., Nation R.L., Milne R.W., Runciman W.B. & Somogyi A.A. (1991) Physiological disposition of i.v. morphine in sheep. *British Journal of Anaesthesia* **67**, 378–86.

Somogyi A.A., Shanks C.A. & Triggs E.J. (1977) The effect of renal failure on the disposition and neuromuscular blocking action of pancuronium bromide. *European Journal of Clinical Pharmacology* **12**, 23–9.

Starsnic M.A., Goldberg M.E., Ritter D.E., Marr A.T., Sosis M. & Larijani G.E. (1989) Does vecuronium accumulate in the renal transplant patient? *Canadian Journal of Anaesthesia* **36**, 35–9.

Stewart J.H. & Castaldi P.A. (1967) Uraemic bleeding: a reversible platelet defect corrected by dialysis. *Quarterly Journal of Medicine* (New Series) **XXXVI**, 409–23.

Strunin L. (1966) Some aspects of anaesthesia for renal homotransplantation. *British Journal of Anaesthesia* **38**, 812–22.

Szeto H.H., Inturrisi C.E., Houde R., Saal S., Cheigh J. & Reidenberg M. (1977) Accumulation of normeperidine, an active metabolite of meperidine in patients with renal failure or cancer. *Annals of Internal Medicine* **86**, 738–41.

Tasker P.R.W., MacGregor G.A. & de Wardener H.E. (1974) Prophylactic dose of intravenous saline in patients with chronic renal failure undergoing major surgery. *Lancet* **ii**, 911–12.

Terner U.K., Wiebe L.I., Noujain A.A., Dossetor J.B. & Sanders E.J. (1978) The effects of acute and chronic uremia in rats on their hepatic microsomal enzyme activity. *Clinical Biochemistry* **11**, 156–8.

Thomas J.L. & Holmes J.H. (1970) Effect of hemodialysis on plasma cholinesterase. *Anesthesia and Analgesia; Current Researches* **49**, 323–5.

Turner S.A., Denson D.D., Sollo D. & Katz J. (1990) Extraction of narcotics by hemodialysis. *Regional Anesthesia* **15** (Suppl. 15), 14 (Abstr.)

van Peer A., Vercauteren M., Noorduin H., Woestenborghs R. & Heykants J. (1986) Alfentanil kinetics in renal insufficiency. *European Journal of Clinical Pharmacology* **30**, 245–7.

Verbeeck R., Tjandramanga T.B., Verberckmoes R. & de Schepper P.J. (1976) Biotransformation and excretion of lorazepam in patients with chronic renal failure. *British Journal of Clinical Pharmacology* **3**, 1033–9.

Verbeeck R.K., Branch R.A. & Wilkinson G.R. (1981a) Drug metabolites in renal failure: pharmacokinetic and clinical implications. *Clinical Pharmacokinetics* **6**, 329–45.

Verbeeck R.V., Tjandramanga T.B., Verberckmoes R. & de Schepper P.J. (1981b) Impaired elimination of lorazepam following subchronic administration in two patients with renal failure. *British Journal of Clinical Pharmacology* **12**, 749–51.

Vinik H.R., Reves J.G., Greenblatt D.J., Abernethy D.R. & Smith L.R. (1983) The pharmacokinetics of midazolam in chronic renal failure patients. *Anesthesiology* **59**, 390–4.

Wait C.M., Goat V.A., Sear J.W. & Blogg C.E. (1988) Atracurium in chronic renal failure: closed-loop control of infusion. *Abstracts* vol. II. 9th World Congress of Anaesthesiologists, Washington, June 1988.

Ward S., Boheimer N., Weatherley B.C., Simmonds R.J. & Dopson T.A. (1987) Pharmacokinetics of atracurium and its metabolites in patients with normal renal function, and in patients in renal failure. *British Journal of Anaesthesia* **59**, 697–706.

Way W.L., Miller R.D., Hamilton W.K. & Layzer R.B. (1972) Succinylcholine-induced hyperkalemia in patients with renal failure? *Anesthesiology* **36**, 138–41.

Weimer W., Geerlings S.W., Bijnen A.B., Obertop H., van Urk H., Lameijer L.D., Wolff H.D. & Jeekel J. (1983) A controlled study on the effect of mannitol on immediate renal function after cadaver donor kidney transplantation. *Transplantation* **35**, 99–101.

Welling P.G., Craig W.A., Amidon G.L. & Kunin C.M. (1974) Pharmacokinetics of cefazolin in normal and uremic subjects. *Clinical Pharmacology and Therapeutics* **15**, 344–53.

Welling P.G., Shaw W.R., Uman S.J., Tse F.C.S. & Craig W.A. (1975) Pharmacokinetics of minocycline in renal failure. *Antimicrobial Agents and Chemotherapy* **8**, 532–7.

Whiting P.H., Cunningham C., Thompson A.W. & Simpson J.G. (1984) Enhancement of high dose cyclosporin A toxicity by frusemide. *Biochemical Pharmacology* **33**, 1075–9.

Wickstrom I. (1981) Enflurane anaesthesia in living donor renal transplantation. *Acta Anaesthesiologica Scandinavica* **25**, 263–9.

Wiggum D.C., Cork R.C., Weldon S.T., Gandolfi A.J. & Perry D.S. (1985) Postoperative respiratory depression and elevated sufentanil levels in a patient with chronic renal failure. *Anesthesiology* **63**, 708–10.

Winearls C.G. (1992) Erythropoietin. Proceedings of the Royal College of Physicians of Edinburgh **22**, 426–38.

Winearls C.G., Oliver D.O., Pippard M.J., Reid C., Downing M.R. & Cotes P.M. (1986) Effect of human erythropoietin derived from recombitant DNA on the anaemia of patients maintained by chronic haemodialysis. *Lancet* **ii**, 1175–8.

Woolner D.F., Winter D., Frendin T.J., Begg E.J., Lynn K.L. & Wright G.J. (1986) Renal failure does not impair the metabolism of morphine. *British Journal of Clinical Pharmacology* **22**, 55–9.

Wyant G.M. (1967) The anaesthetist looks at tissue transplantation: three years' experience with kidney transplants. *Canadian Anaesthetists' Society Journal* **14**, 255–75.

Yate P.M., Flynn P.J. & Arnold R.W. (1987) Clinical experience and plasma laudanosine concentrations during the infusion of atracurium in the intensive therapy unit. *British Journal of Anaesthesia* **59**, 211–17.

Anaesthesia and the Elderly Patient

S.W. KRECHEL

Because of advances in health care and growing social awareness of the importance of health maintenance, elderly people comprise an increasing percentage of the population in developing countries. More elderly people are presenting for a wide variety of surgical procedures and the anaesthetist is faced with the task of evaluating a patient and administering an anaesthetic to one who is often frail and fragile.

Precisely when an individual becomes classed as elderly is not clear, as one can obviously be old before one's time or young beyond one's years. For the purposes of discussion, however, we shall consider the age of 65 years and beyond as being the appropriate group designated elderly.

Altered physiology

The ageing process is one of inexorable decline from birth to death. Table 63.1 delineates some of these changes.

Nervous system

Brain weight decreases by approximately 18% by the age of 80 (Lytle & Altar, 1979). There appears to be an age-related decrease in neurone density with the most conspicuous loss in the cerebral and cerebellar cortices. Cerebral blood flow and cerebral oxygen consumption decline with progressing age (Kety, 1956).

Of additional importance is the fact that ageing is associated with a decrease in the rate of synthesis and an increase in the rate of destruction of various neurotransmitter substances. Two catecholamine synthetic enzymes, tyrosine hydroxylase and dopa decarboxylase show decreased brain activity with ageing. In addition, there is a concomitant increase in catabolic enzymes including monoamine oxidase and catecholmethyltransferase. Choline acetyltransferase activity is also decreased significantly with ageing. These changes in neurotransmitter substances help to explain disease processes associated with ageing such as Parkinsonism and Alzheimer's disease.

Cognitive, sensory, motor and autonomic functions are altered with ageing. For example, perceptual speed, short-term memory, arithmetic manipulations, visual and auditory reaction times decline directly with age after the second and third decades. However, many intellectual functions, including information storage, verbal skills, comprehension, mental personality and long-term memory are well preserved in the healthy elderly individual (Katzman & Terry, 1983; Goodnick & Gershon, 1984). Visually evoked responses show an increased latency period, apparently secondary to reduced nerve conduction velocity in the optic nerve, optic pathways, or both (Celesia & Daly, 1977). Conduction velocity within sensory nerves slows with ageing, possibly secondary to axonal degeneration, reduced number of nerve fibres and increased presence of connective tissue within the peripheral nerve pathways (Dorfman & Bosley, 1979). Significant hearing deficits are usually present by the age of 70 years. In addition, there is a degeneration of the organ of Corti and reduction of cochlear neurones.

Approximately 10% of persons over the age of 65 years suffer from dementia. This prevalence increases to approximately 22% for those over the age of 80 years. Dementia is not necessarily an inescapable consequence of the ageing process but instead may result from many correctable causes. Among these are drug-induced side-effects and interactions, metabolic disorders, emotional disorders, nutritional deficiencies, tumour or trauma, sensory deprivation or arteriosclerotic changes. As any of these factors may become manifest in the perioperative period, it

Table 63.1 Selected anatomical, physiological and functional changes associated with ageing (75–80 years of age compared with 30 years). (Data from Meakins & McLaren, 1986)

	Percentage of decrease	Reference
Brain weight	18	Lytle and Altar (1979)
Brain blood flow	25	Kety (1956)
Nerve conduction velocity	10	Kohn (1963)
Neurone density	48	Devaney and Johnson (1980)
Muscle strength	15–35	Robinson (1964)
Cardiac output (resting)	30	
Glomerular filtration rate	31	
Renal plasma flow	50	
Vital capacity	44	Kohn (1963)
Maximum breathing capacity	57	
Basal metabolic rate	16	
Body water content	18	

is important for the anaesthetist to be familiar with these causes.

The ageing process leads to progressive impairment of autonomic homeostasis. Elderly people have impaired autonomic response to:

1 Lower body negative pressure or impaired venous return.

2 Impaired ability to maintain arterial pressure following assumption of the upright position.

3 Attenuated carotid sinus baroreceptor responsiveness.

4 Impaired responses to thermal stress.

5 Impaired cardiac responses to hypoxia and hypercapnia (Collins *et al.*, 1980; Halter & Pieffier, 1982).

Plasma noradrenaline concentrations are increased in elderly people in both the awake and the asleep state. There is an exaggerated increase in release of noradrenaline in response to orthostatic stress especially in patients with systolic hypertension at rest (Halter & Pfeifer, 1982). Plasma noradrenaline concentrations double between the ages of 20 and 80 years in healthy volunteers at rest after an overnight fast. The positive correlation between increased plasma noradrenaline and systolic arterial pressure may be related to increased sympathetic nervous system activity.

Aberrations in sleep patterns associated with the normal ageing process include shortened total sleep time, more frequent arousals and early morning awakenings. Similarly, these changes have been associated with the increases in plasma noradrenaline (Prinz *et al.*, 1984).

Adrenaline concentrations are not increased with age although there is evidence that the clearance of adrenaline is enhanced in elderly people, suggesting that adrenal medullary release of adrenaline is increased. Elderly people also exhibit a decreased responsiveness to β-adrenergic stimulation.

Cardiovascular system

The physiological changes associated with ageing are less clear with respect to the cardiovascular system than in any other sphere. Most of the studies before 1980 were not successful in controlling for the presence of cardiovascular disease, and therefore, the physiological changes observed resulted from both the natural process of ageing and also the disease processes present in the ageing population. Studies since 1980 have been more successful in this endeavour although not totally without flaws. We encounter disease-free elderly patients infrequently. Most commonly, we treat elderly patients who have both an aged and a diseased cardiovascular system. Hence, it is important that we discuss both these subgroups. Table 63.2 summarizes the important physiological changes in the cardiovascular system associated with age.

It is important to note that while otherwise healthy elderly people increase their cardiac output with exercise, they do so in a way which is different from their younger counterparts. Elderly people maintain or increase their cardiac output by increasing stroke volume. With the increased impedance to ejection,

Table 63.2 Changes in the cardiovascular system associated with age

Decreased	Reference	Increased	Reference
Resting cardiac output Ejection volume Heart rate	Brandfonbrener et al. (1955)	Rigidity in aorta and major vessels Plasma noradrenaline concentrations	
Rate response to exercise	Coath (1984)	Systolic arterial pressure	Kannel and Gordon (1978)
Diastolic arterial pressure	—	Systemic vascular resistance	Bender (1965)
Number of pacemaker cells in sinoauricular node	Davies and Pomerance (1972)	Diastolic arterial pressure (increases to age 60 years then returns to baseline)	
		Exercise cardiac output	Becklake et al. (1965)
Response to β-adrenergic stimulation	Kuramoto et al. (1979)		
Beta-receptor affinity for agonists	Feldman et al. (1984)		

higher filling pressures are required during stress. As ventricular compliance decreases, there is a fine division between providing sufficient fluid to maintain filling pressures and exceeding this to cause congestive heart failure.

In addition, it is suggested that the more frequent development of ventricular arrhythmias in elderly people is secondary to the deterioration in sinus pacemaker activity (Roberts & Goldberg, 1979).

Evidence suggests that elderly people are at an increased risk for silent myocardial ischaemia as a direct result of a decreased ability to perceive such pain (Miller, 1990).

Respiratory system

A longitudinal study of the respiratory system with age has not been performed, but instead, coexisting populations of different ages are compared. Another problem which renders study difficult is that the changes which occur with ageing do not affect normal function but instead exclusively affect reserve capacity. Hence, the aged respiratory system is at risk only with stress. Ventilatory reserve is more than 100 litres/min, 12 times the resting ventilatory requirement at the age of 20 years; by 90 years, it has decreased to 30 litres/min, seven times the resting requirement.

Four basic changes occur which affect lung function in elderly people:
1 Decrease in motor power (this may be a detraining effect).

2 Decrease in elastic recoil of the lung (implies increased compliance).
3 Stiffening of the chest wall. (This explains why the lungs of elderly patients are more difficult to ventilate in spite of increased compliance.)
4 Decrease in the size of intervertebral spaces (when adjusted for height, total lung capacity remains relatively constant with age).

As a direct result of these factors, both residual volume and functional residual capacity increase with age while vital capacity is reduced by 20 ml/year (Campbell & Lefrak, 1984).

The primary function of the lung, i.e. gas exchange, is affected by the ageing process. As a direct result of the decrease in elastic recoil associated with ageing, airways in the dependent portion of the lung have a greater tendency to close. Air flow and distribution of alveolar gas exchange is impaired. This impairment is the major cause of the decreased arterial oxygen tension seen with advancing age. The arterial partial pressure of oxygen (Pao_2) declines progressively with age, approximately 0.5 kPa (4 mmHg) per decade beyond the age of 20 years. Assuming a normal Pao_2 at the age of 20 years of 12.8 kPa (95 mmHg), we should predict a normal Pao_2 by the age of 80 years of approximately 8.7 kPa (65 mmHg) (Sorbini et al., 1968). A second result of mismatch of ventilation and perfusion seen in elderly people is the increase of physiological deadspace. As the arterial tension of carbon dioxide does not increase, minute ventilation must increase to compensate for the wasted ventilation (Tenney & Miller, 1956).

The ageing process is associated with declining ability to adapt to abnormal situations. The elderly individual's response to hypoxia is approximately 25% of that seen in young individuals. The response to hypercapnia is also diminished markedly (Kronenberg & Drage, 1973).

Perhaps more difficult to understand is that the ventilatory response to exercise is greater in elderly people than in younger ones. This increase in ventilation during exercise seems to compensate for the increased inefficiency of gas exchange. Exercise in elderly people as in young people remains essentially isocapnic (Brischetto et al., 1984).

The diffusing capacity of the lung also decreases with age, as measured by the transfer of carbon monoxide across the alveolar membrane (Donevan et al., 1959). Of additional interest to the anaesthetist is the progressive loss of protective airway reflexes associated with advancing age (Pontoppidan & Beecher, 1960). Silent tracheal aspiration is a relatively common occurrence in older individuals. Fortunately, elderly people possess the lowest gastric volumes and the highest gastric pH of all age groups and are theoretically at a decreased risk of morbidity associated with aspiration (Manchikanti et al., 1985).

Finally, elderly people are subjects of intensive studies of sleep apnoea. It has been demonstrated that while elderly people display a lowered ventilatory response to carbon dioxide in the awake state, their ventilatory response to carbon dioxide is unaffected by sleep, whereas in younger individuals, carbon dioxide responsiveness is decreased during sleep (Martinez et al., 1984). On the other hand, elderly people experience repetitive periods of apnoea lasting greater than 10s. These are both central (cessation of respiratory efforts) and obstructive (pharyngeal obstruction to air flow with continuing respiratory effort). The anaesthetist must be particularly aware of these factors when prescribing premedication and postoperative pain relief.

Endocrine system

Very little work has been performed on changes in the endocrine systems associated with ageing. Several studies indicate that hypothyroidism is more common in elderly people (Lloyd & Goldberg, 1961; Jefferys et al., 1972; Bahemuka & Hodkinson, 1975; Sawin et al., 1985). Changes in thyroid function may have some relationship to cognitive and cardiovascular function in elderly people.

As an individual ages, a glucose load is less well tolerated for several reasons.

1 Poor diet.
2 Physical inactivity.
3 Decreased lean body mass with increase in total body fat (obesity).
4 Decreased insulin secretion.
5 Insulin antagonism.

In a review of the literature, Davidson (1979) suggests that most of the evidence indicates normal or increased release of insulin during the ageing process in conjunction with insulin antagonism, leading to relative glucose intolerance and non-insulin-dependent diabetes mellitus in elderly people. Perhaps of the most clinical significance is the finding that the percentage of haemoglobin in the glycosylated form increases with age (Graf et al., 1978). Glycosylated haemoglobin is a reflection of glucose concentrations during the previous 1–3 weeks. This implies that elderly people are chronically hyperglycaemic. In conjunction with evidence indicating an increased predisposition to wound infection and decreased tensile strength of wound-healing in patients who are hyperglycaemic (Rayfield et al., 1982), this suggests caution in administering glucose to elderly patients. One hundred to 200 ml of a 5% glucose-containing solution administered every hour alternating with a non-glucose-containing solution should be sufficient to prevent hypoglycaemia while avoiding hyperglycaemia. Frequent checks of glucose concentrations aid in achieving this goal.

Hepatic and renal systems

Studies of changes in hepatic physiology associated with ageing are of cross-sectional design, as opposed to the longitudinal (prohibitively time-consuming) variety. In addition, the majority of the studies of drug metabolism have been undertaken in aged animals and the information obtained may or may not be applicable to elderly humans. Furthermore, it is difficult to separate environmental factors, e.g. smoking, nutrition, infections, etc. from factors of ageing alone.

Liver blood flow is reduced approximately 40% in elderly people, leading to decreased clearance of high-clearance drugs such as propranolol and lignocaine (Gerber, 1982).

While several animal studies suggest that hepatic metabolism is altered with ageing (Schmucker & Wang, 1980; Rikans & Notley, 1982; Vlasuk & Walz, 1982), it appears that there is no clear evidence that microsomal cytochrome P450 content and enzyme activity decrease with age in humans. Although there is some evidence to suggest a reduction in capacity may result from a decrease in liver size associated with increasing age (Marchesini *et al.*, 1988; Wynne *et al.*, 1989).

Table 63.3 represents a summary of the anatomical and physiological changes in the renal system associated with age. The decline in function of the renal system is striking. In the otherwise healthy individual, this decline in function does not lead to any clinically apparent sequelae. However, it does imply that the elderly patient does not respond well to stress, particularly of the iatrogenic variety, e.g. intravenous fluid infusion, nephrotoxic drug administration, diuretic administration, etc. When treating elderly patients, the anaesthetist should keep these changes continually in mind and have a high index of suspicion for both hypernatraemia and hyponatraemia, in addition to adjusting drug dosages of those drugs cleared by renal mechanisms.

Altered pharmacology

Before reviewing the available information on specific drugs used in anaesthesia and the effect of the ageing process on the pharmacology of these drugs, it is important to discuss drug therapy in elderly people in general terms.

Drug absorption may be altered by physiological

Table 63.3 Changes in renal anatomy and physiology associated with age

Anatomy
↓ Total renal mass
↓ Cortical mass
↓ Number of glomeruli
↓ Surface area of glomeruli
↓ Length and volume of proximal tubules (Epstein, 1986)

Physiology
↓ Renal plasma flow (Goldring *et al.*, 1940)
↓ Mean blood flow per unit mass (most profound in cortex with sparing of deeper regions) (Hollenberg *et al.*, 1974)
↑ Filtration fraction (glomerular filtration rate/renal plasma flow) (Epstein, 1986)
↓ Glomerular filtration rate (Rowe *et al.*, 1976)
↓ Capacity to conserve sodium (Epstein & Hollenberg, 1976)
↓ Renin–aldosterone responsiveness to acute stimuli (Weidmann *et al.*, 1975)
↓ Concentrating ability (Epstein, 1979)
↑ Sensitivity to arginine vasopressin response to hyperosmolarity (Helderman *et al.*, 1978) (compensating mechanism?)
↑ Serum antidiuretic hormone (Rondeau *et al.*, 1982) (compensating mechanism?)

changes occurring in the gastrointestinal tract. These include:
1 Increased gastric pH (from decreased acid output).
2 Decreased gastrointestinal motility.
3 Decreased gastrointestinal blood flow.
4 Decreased mucosal cell absorbing area.
In the case of many drugs, these changes appear to have no effect on absorption.

Whilst drug absorption may be changed little in elderly patients, drug distribution and elimination are changed markedly. A decrease in lean body mass and concomitant decrease in total body water lead to a decrease in the volume of distribution of water-soluble drugs. The concomitant increase in total body fat leads to an increase in the volume of distribution of fat-soluble drugs.

Also of critical importance in understanding the pharmacology of elderly patients is the concept of initial volume of distribution. This is defined as the amount of drug in the body following injection and instantaneous mixing, divided by the initial blood concentration. The initial distribution volume of a drug depends on several factors, some of which are age dependent, e.g. vascular volume, cardiac output, distribution of blood flow to various organs, solubility and protein binding. The decline in cardiac output, cerebral blood flow, hepatic blood flow and renal blood flow would all be expected to contribute to a decrease in initial distribution volume in elderly patients. The importance of a decreased initial volume of distribution has been shown effectively for thiopentone (Homer & Stanski, 1985), etomidate (Arden *et al.*, 1986) and morphine (Berkowitz *et al.*, 1975).

A 15–20% decrease in plasma albumin concentration leads to decreased binding and therefore increased bioavailability of drugs which are albumin bound. Such drugs important to the anaesthetist include barbiturates and benzodiazepines. In general, the acidic drugs tend to be albumin bound.

Alpha-l-acid glycoprotein is an acute-phase reactive protein which is unchanged in healthy elderly people (Veering *et al.*, 1990), but increased in many disease states such as inflammation or malignancy. Many basic drugs bind primarily to this protein. These drugs include the opioids, local anaesthetics, propranolol, quinidine and chlorpromazine. Some of these drugs bind to both proteins; as the two proteins tend to change their concentrations in opposite directions, this may explain the overall lack of change in plasma protein binding which may be observed.

When changes in protein binding do occur, the overall effect may be marked. For example, if a drug is 50% albumin bound and the amount of binding is reduced by 10% this leads to a 20% increase in circulating free drug. On the other hand, if the drug is 98% protein bound and there is a decrease of 10% in binding, this leads to a 500% increase in free drug. It is easy to see why dosing an elderly patient according to information obtained in a young person may lead to an overdosage.

An additional factor which leads to an unexpected increase in free-drug availability in elderly patients is that they are frequently receiving a number of different medications. Often there is competition for drug binding sites on the various protein fractions. It has been shown that the incidence of adverse drug reactions increases in a linear fashion with the number of drugs that a patient is taking and reaches 100% when the patient is taking 10 or more different drugs (Vestal *et al.*, 1985).

Another factor related to drug distribution is the decrease in membrane integrity which may be seen in elderly patients, leading to increased penetration of drugs through such membranes. There is some speculation that this may be the mechanism responsible for increased drug sensitivity, particularly of the opioids, in elderly patients.

Hepatic metabolism tends to be decreased in elderly people by virtue of a decreased hepatic mass and decreased number of functional cells, rather than by decreased microsomal enzyme activity. Decreased clearance is mainly a result of decreased hepatic blood flow (Kitani, 1985).

Decreased renal blood flow, glomerular filtration rate and active tubular excretion lead to decreased excretion of drugs and metabolites. Hence, elimination half-times of many drugs tend to be increased substantially in elderly patients.

Inhalation agents

Minimal alveolar concentration (MAC) decreases with age. This decline in MAC parallels changes in cerebral oxygen consumption, cerebral blood flow and neuronal density (Kety, 1956) (Figs 63.1 and 63.2).

As might be anticipated, EEG studies of patients anaesthetized with isoflurane demonstrate an age-related difference in CNS sensitivity to this inhalation agent. Elderly patients have a greater proportion of total time in analytical silence and significantly more isoelectric periods (Schwartz *et al.*, 1989).

It has been shown that there is a difference in blood : gas partition coefficients of volatile anaesthetics in blood associated with age (Lerman *et al.*, 1984). The blood : gas partition coefficients of isoflurane,

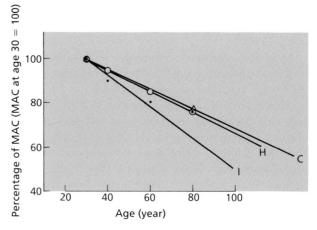

Fig. 63.1 MAC as a function of age. I, isoflurane (data from Stevens *et al.*, 1975); H, halothane (data from Gregory *et al.*, 1969); C, cyclopropane (data from Munson *et al.*, 1984).

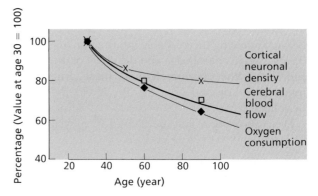

Fig. 63.2 Changes in cerebral blood flow, oxygen consumption and cortical neuronal density as a function of age. (Redrawn from Kety, 1956.)

enflurane, halothane and methoxyflurane are significantly higher in adults (mean age 30 years), than both children (mean age 5 years) and elderly adults (mean age 80 years). On the other hand, there was no difference between the solubility found in children and elderly adults. The changes in partition coefficient appear to be associated with changes in albumin, triglyceride, cholesterol and globulin concentrations. This change in blood-gas solubility may help to explain why elderly patients tend to exhibit a more rapid inhalation induction of anaesthesia.

Solubility is one factor which may alter uptake and distribution of inhalation agents. The physiological changes in both the respiratory and cardiovascular systems are additional factors. Briefly, the increase in ventilation seen in elderly patients tends to increase uptake; counterbalancing this effect is the decrease in cerebral blood flow. The increased intrapulmonary shunt seen in elderly patients tends to have the effect of decreasing uptake with the moderately soluble, volatile anaesthetics, e.g. halothane, enflurane and isoflurane, but little or no effect on highly soluble agents, e.g. diethyl ether and methoxyflurane. Perhaps the most important physiological change associated with ageing which affects uptake and distribution of the inhalation agents is the decrease in cardiac output, leading to an overall increase in uptake.

Although clinically, it is well known that elderly patients do appear to undergo a more rapid inhalation induction (Eger, 1974), only recently has an attempt been made to study the differences in rate of inhalation anaesthetic uptake between young and elderly patients (Dwyer et al., 1990). Measuring end-tidal fractional concentrations (F_E) : inspired fraction (F_I), after 15 min, the F_E : F_I ratios for isoflurane were significantly lower in elderly patients than in young patients, predicting a slower induction of anaesthesia in elderly patients.

Recovery from anaesthesia, proceeds more slowly in elderly patients. Strum and colleagues, 1991 noted delayed anaesthetic elimination and increased apparent volume of distribution at steady state. These observations may be explained by decreased tissue perfusion and increased ratio of fat to lean body mass.

The cardiovascular response of elderly patients to potent inhalation agents is different from that of younger patients. For example, isoflurane produces less increase in heart rate in elderly patients compared with young patients (2–5% versus 20%) (Linde et al., 1975). This may result from diminished autonomic nervous system responses seen in elderly patients, causing attenuation of the intrinsic sympathomimetic activity of isoflurane. All three potent inhalation agents are associated with a dose-related decrease in systemic arterial pressure in both young and old people. However, our own observations indicate a difference in the magnitude of change. There is a greater decline in systolic arterial pressures associated with enflurane and halothane as opposed to isoflurane (Krechel, 1984). This is similar to the findings of Linde and colleagues (1975).

In Linde's study, a 25% decrease in cardiac output was noted for both halothane and isoflurane in the elderly patient. This decline in cardiac output is considerably greater than that shown by Graves and colleagues (1974) in younger patients and may result from the decreased heart rate response to the administration of isoflurane seen in elderly patients. In contrast with Linde, Tarnow and colleagues (1976) found no significant decline in cardiac output associated with isoflurane anaesthesia in geriatric patients.

Most recently, the cardiovascular effects of halothane have been examined in elderly patients by Tokics and colleagues (1985). In this study, halothane caused a reduction in cardiac index, mean arterial pressure and oxygen uptake. However, no increase in either right atrial or pulmonary capillary venous pressure occurred and the arterial–venous oxygen content difference decreased. This is in contrast with studies performed in younger subjects (Eger et al., 1970; Sonntag et al., 1978). The Tokics study demonstrated also a dose-dependent decrease in systemic vascular resistance in this elderly population and they concluded that the depressant action of halothane on the myocardium was masked by peripheral vasodilatation.

There is little work on regional blood flow changes during inhalation anaesthesia in old versus young people. One study in animals (Hoffman et al., 1982) observed significant regional haemodynamic differences in young rats compared with aged rats in both anaesthetized and unanaesthetized conditions.

Intravenous anaesthetics and adjuvants

Barbiturates

The pharmacology of thiopentone has been studied extensively in elderly patients, but the results are conflicting.

Christensen and colleagues (1981) found a 30% reduction in dose requirements in elderly versus young patients. Volumes of distribution were larger in elderly patients and the terminal elimination half-lives were increased with age, as was clearance. Sear (1983) observed that the recovery time following thiopentone in elderly patients was nearly twice that seen in younger patients. Muravchick (1984) found a 44% decrease in the thiopentone dose requirement in elderly versus younger patients. In as much as thiopentone is 80% albumin bound, and albumin is decreased significantly in elderly people, one would expect that high levels of free unbound drug might explain this increased sensitivity to thiopentone. However, data from Burch and Stanski (1983) do not confirm this. In this study, a concentration-dependent decrease of thiopentone protein binding could not be demonstrated. In a subsequent study from the same laboratory (Homer & Stanski, 1985) the authors were not able to demonstrate the progressive increase in the steady-state volume of distribution of thiopentone with age, contrary to Christensen and colleagues (1981) and Jung and colleagues (1982). Homer and Stanski (1985) also found no change in brain sensitivity to thiopentone with age. EEG spectral-edge analysis confirms a lack of pharmacodynamic alteration associated with age (Stanski & Maitre, 1990). Although Stanski's group did observe a decrease in the initial volume of distribution with a resultant higher initial serum level after a given dose and concluded that this alone accounted for the increased sensitivity, they have now refuted this in favour of a decreased rapid intracompartmental clearance as the pharmacokinetic variable responsible for this increased sensitivity.

Benzodiazepines

Studies on a variety of benzodiazepines have indicated that elderly patients are more sensitive to the CNS-depressant effects of these drugs than young patients (Castelden et al., 1977; Korttilla et al., 1978; Reidenberg et al., 1978).

It is well established that elderly patients are more sensitive to the CNS-depressant effects of diazepam (Reidenberg et al., 1978). The elimination half-life of diazepam is increased markedly in elderly patients (Klotz et al., 1975; Divoll et al., 1983). Protein binding appears to be a significant factor with respect to the pharmacodynamics of diazepam. Diazepam is greater than 95% protein bound, and binding correlates with plasma albumin concentration, both decreasing with age (Davis et al., 1985).

Midazolam has also been investigated in elderly patients (Greenblatt et al., 1977a; Dundee et al., 1985; Kanto et al., 1986). Little if any change is found in the pharmacokinetics of midazolam in the elderly versus the young population. On the other hand, elderly patients are more sensitive to the CNS effects of this drug. The dose required in elderly patients is approximately half that required in younger patients (Kanto et al., 1986; Wong et al., 1991). The CNS in elderly patients appears to be intrinsically more sensitive to the effects of this drug than does that of younger individuals.

Ketamine

Ketamine may be a useful drug for elderly patients (Vaughan & Stephen, 1974; Stefansson et al., 1982). Although hallucinations occurred in approximately 7.5% of the elderly patients in Vaughan's and Stephen's studies (1974), this incidence would be expected to be attenuated by a combination of midazolam and ketamine (White, 1982).

The physiological changes noted in the cardiovascular and autonomic nervous systems lead to differences in the pharmacological effects on the cardiovascular system in elderly compared with young patients. Increases in heart rate and arterial pressure and cardiac output tend to be relatively small in elderly patients. In the absence of its sympathomimetic effects, ketamine may be a potent myocardial depressant and cause both a reduction in cardiac output and systemic arterial pressure.

Etomidate

Etomidate is an intravenous hypnotic agent of the imidazole type which is potentially very useful in elderly patients because of the haemodynamic stability seen with this drug (Colvin et al., 1979). As with thiopentone, Stanski's group demonstrated no alteration in brain sensitivity with etomidate (Arden et al., 1986). The dose required in elderly patients was approximately 50% that required in younger patients.

The steady-state volume of distribution is unchanged in elderly patients relative to young patients. Clearance decreases with advancing age, but the elimination half-life is not age related, probably secondary to the variability in the steady-state volume of distribution. The initial volume of distribution decreased by 42% between the ages of 20 and 80 years and this change alone is thought to be responsible for the increased sensitivity seen in the elderly patient.

Propofol

The newest intravenous anaesthetic — propofol — although not extensively studied in elderly patients has been used successfully in these patients under a wide variety of conditions (Dundee et al., 1986; Larsen et al., 1988; Lepage et al., 1988; Steib et al., 1988; Russell et al., 1989; Lepage et al., 1991).

As is the case with most intravenous anaesthetic and adjuvant drugs, elderly patients require approximately half the induction dose of propofol required by the younger patient (Dundee et al., 1986).

Concerns regarding the safety of this drug in elderly patients have been raised. The cardiovascular effects of propofol include a decrease in mean arterial pressure due primarily to a decrease in diastolic pressure, raising special concerns relative to coronary perfusion. Studies to date suggest this is more a theoretical concern than a practical one. Propofol has compared favourably with thiopentone (Steib et al., 1988), etomidate (Larsen et al., 1988) and with methohexitone in patients with known coronary artery disease (Lepage *et al.*, 1991). Similarly, it has been used successfully in conjunction with fentanyl for anaesthesia in patients undergoing coronary artery bypass surgery and cardiopulmonary bypass (Russell *et al.*, 1989). There is ample suggestion in the literature that propofol is a myocardial depressant and studies to date in patients with coronary artery disease have been restricted to those with good left ventricular function (Lepage *et al.*, 1991).

Opioids

As with other drugs, elderly patients seem to be more sensitive than young patients to the effect of opioids.

Bellville and colleagues (1971) observed that older patients experience or report less pain and receive more benefit from opioid analgesics. There is good evidence that this is true regardless of the route of administration, i.e. not only intramuscular and intravenous but also extradural (Moore *et al.*, 1990). Many studies have examined various opioids in an attempt to explain this phenomenon. The results remain conflicting and confusing. Berkowitz and colleagues (1975) found no difference in total distribution or elimination of morphine following intravenous administration in elderly patients compared with young patients. However, they did observe that early serum concentrations of morphine in their elderly patients were approximately 70% higher than in younger patients, indicating that the initial distribution volume was considerably less in elderly patients. On the other hand, Stanski and colleagues (1978) observed an increase in the terminal elimination half-life of morphine in addition to an increase in the volume of distribution in elderly patients versus young volunteers. However, Stanski's patients were undergoing resection of aortic aneurysm, and more recent evidence suggests that aortic cross-clamping may alter the pharmacokinetics of opioid analgesics (Hudson *et al.*, 1986).

For pethidine, Chan and colleagues (1975) reported a smaller volume of distribution and higher plasma concentrations in elderly patients. Other investigators have been unable to demonstrate any changes in pharmacokinetics of this drug in elderly patients (Mather *et al.*, 1975; Herman *et al.*, 1985). Other workers have found no change in volume of distribution, but an increase in elimination half-life and plasma clearance in elderly patients (Holmberg *et al.*, 1982). Clinically, this would imply that it may not be necessary to reduce the initial dose of pethidine in an elderly patient but it would be advisable to limit the total dose and increase the dose intervals. However, the use of pethidine in elderly patients may be questionable as it is a direct myocardial depressant and is associated with tachycardia and an increased systemic vascular resistance, especially in higher doses. Such circulatory effects may be detrimental in a geriatric patient who may already have a compromised circulatory status.

Bentley and colleagues (1982) have suggested that fentanyl has a markedly prolonged elimination half-life in elderly patients compared with younger patients. They noted a terminal elimination half-life which was approximately three times greater in elderly patients than in young ones. They found no difference in the volume of distribution of the drug but clearance was prolonged markedly.

These results have been challenged (Hudson *et al.*, 1986). It is likely that the pharmacokinetics of fentanyl are similar to sufentanil. Matteo and colleagues (1986a,b) noted a decreased plasma clearance and a decreased initial volume of distribution in elderly patients compared with younger patients. The elimination half-life was not prolonged in elderly patients and would appear to be a reflection of the fact that although the clearance rate is decreased, the total volume to be cleared is similarly depressed. It is important to note again that the smaller initial volume of distribution of fentanyl in elderly patients allows more of the drug to cross the blood–brain barrier and bind to receptors early in the course of an anaesthetic, explaining the observed increase in sensitivity.

While age has been shown to have no effect on the pharmacodynamics of alfentanil (Lemmens *et al.*, 1988a), both reduced clearance and prolonged terminal elimination half-life have been demonstrated in elderly patients compared with young patients for alfentanil (Helmers *et al.*, 1985). While the average clearance is definitely lower among elderly patients, in this study a moderate degree of variability was present in all age groups. Lemmens and colleagues (1988b) also found the drug unpredictable in elderly patients. Consequently, it would be difficult to predict how one should alter the dose or infusion rate for an elderly individual. In practice, for low doses and short infusion times, the opioid effect would be expected to be terminated through redistribution, making dose adjustments unnecessary.

Muscle relaxants

Of the competitive neuromuscular-blocking drugs, suxamethonium is the only drug used with any frequency at the present time. Elderly men show reduced levels of plasma cholinesterase and lower rates of hydrolysis of suxamethonium than their younger counterparts (Shanor et al., 1961). Such findings do not appear in elderly women.

The pharmacokinetics of pancuronium are altered in elderly patients, in that prolonged elimination half-life and decreased plasma clearance are seen relative to younger patients. Age appears to have no influence on the distribution phase or the total apparent volume of distribution for this drug (McLeod et al., 1979; Duvaldestein et al., 1982).

D-tubocurarine and metocurine behave similarly in elderly patients; both exhibit decreased plasma clearance, decreased initial volume of distribution, decreased volume of distribution, and prolonged elimination half-life (Matteo et al., 1985).

There is some conflict in the literature regarding vecuronium. D'Hollander and colleagues (1982) observed a significant decrease in dose requirement and rate of recovery from block after administration of vecuronium in elderly patients. In contrast, in a study a year later, the same group noted that the maximum effect of a standard dose of vecuronium was not altered by age, but there was a delay in the establishment of paralysis which increased with increasing age (D'Hollander et al., 1983a). Others have found no difference between young and old patients with respect to dose–response relationships for vecuronium (Lowry et al., 1985; O'Hara et al., 1985). The conflict has continued into the 1990s with reports such as that of Lien and colleagues (1991) suggesting a significantly prolonged recovery time and elimination half-life in elderly patients.

Similarly, atracurium has been shown to display no age-related changes in pharmacokinetics (D'Hollander et al., 1983b). However, the work of Kitts and colleagues (1990) has demonstrated that while total clearance of atracurium was similar in both elderly and young patients, organ clearance (liver and kidney) was lower in elderly patients at the same time that clearance by Hoffmann elimination and ester hydrolysis was higher. In this same study, contrary to expected, the volume of distribution at steady state was larger in elderly patients. In addition, the elimination half-life was slightly increased with age.

The long-acting neuromuscular-blocking drug, pipecuronium is being studied in elderly patients. Early work indicates no substantial dose–response difference between young and old with respect to this drug (Azad et al., 1989).

Many elderly patients are receiving a wide variety of drugs which may influence the pharmacodynamics of neuromuscular-blocking drugs, e.g. the anti-arrhythmic drugs such a lignocaine, quinidine and verapamil. It is wise to consider drug interactions in elderly patients and to monitor carefully the neuro-muscular junction during the administration of neuromuscular-blocking drugs.

Age-related differences are seen also in the effects of anticholinesterase drugs used for antagonism of neuromuscular block. For example, the onset time of endrophonium is slower in elderly patients (Cronnelly & Miller, 1984). However, the dose requirement is unaffected.

Increased elimination half-life and decreased clearance have been demonstrated also in the elderly patients compared with young patients (Silverberg et al., 1986). The onset time and maximum response after neostigmine is comparable for young patients and elderly patients. However, the duration of action is prolonged markedly in elderly patients (Young et al., 1984).

Matteo and colleagues (1990) have demonstrated no increased duration of action for edrophonium in elderly patients compared with young subjects and suggest, therefore, that neostigmine or pyridostig-mine are the preferred anticholinesterases for use in elderly patients since their prolonged duration of action more closely matches that of the long-acting muscle relaxants.

Prolonged muscarinic side-effects may also be important. The incidence of arrhythmias in the post-operative period has been shown to be greater in elderly patients who have received the combination of neostigmine and atropine compared with neo-stigmine and the longer-acting glycopyrronium. The latter combination would appear to be more appropriate for use in elderly patients (Owens et al., 1978; Muravchick et al., 1979).

Local anaesthetics

Several investigators have noted that elderly patients are more prone to the adverse effects of lignocaine (Lie et al., 1974; Pfeifer et al., 1976).

Nation and colleagues (1977) observed that the elimination half-life of lignocaine was prolonged markedly in elderly individuals compared with young patients. Clearance, however, was similar.

Drayer and colleagues (1983) reported a negative correlation between lignocaine clearance and age. Abernethy and Greenblatt (1983) found an increased elimination half-life and decreased total clearance for lignocaine in elderly men but no difference in these variables between young and old women, suggesting that sex in addition to age was an important variable in the pharmacokinetics of lignocaine. Others have suggested that the presence of congestive heart failure is another important variable (Cusson *et al.*, 1985).

There is no evidence to suggest that the loading dose of lignocaine is different in elderly patients, but it would appear that a lower infusion rate and close monitoring of blood concentrations would be most appropriate in elderly patients, especially in men and those patients with congestive heart failure.

Veering and colleagues (1987a, 1987b, 1988) have repeatedly observed decreased clearance of bupivacaine in elderly patients and have attributed this finding to a decrease in hepatic enzyme activity either via a direct decline in activity or a capacity reduction related to the reduced size of the liver (Marchesini *et al.*, 1988; Wynne *et al.*, 1989). This decreased clearance implies some increased risk of toxicity from bupivacaine when repeated doses are used or infusions employed in the elderly patient.

The risks of anaesthesia in elderly patients

The mortality associated with anaesthesia and surgery increases with age. This is demonstrated in data from a review by Marx and colleagues (1973) (Fig. 63.3). Obviously, age is not the only important variable with respect to mortality associated with anaesthesia and surgery. Overall physical status is known to be exceedingly important and the American Society of Anesthesiologists' physical status classification has been shown to be a good predictor of risk of death after surgery in patients aged 80 years old and over (Djokovic & Hedley-Whyte, 1979).

A clear and precise definition of the risk of anaesthesia and surgery is elusive, especially in elderly patients. Over the years, many studies have attempted to examine this question (Table 63.4). Several conclusions may be reached from these studies:

1 The overall mortality of geriatric surgical patients has decreased over the decades from the 1950s through to the 1980s, but appears to have stabilized

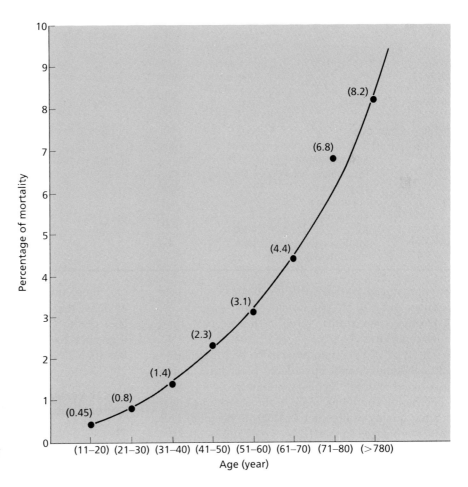

Fig. 63.3 Mortality as a function of age. (Data from Marx *et al.*, 1973.)

Table 63.4 Age-related mortality since 1946

Years	Type of procedure	Age group	Mortality Elective	Overall	Emergent	Reference
1946–55	All	>70		8.0		Parsons *et al.* (1956)
1947–49	All	>70		16.1		Bosch *et al.* (1952)
1948–52	All	>60		5.1		Cole (1953)
1950–51	Gastrointestinal	>60	5.7	9.0	21.9	Haug and Dale (1952)
1951–60	Inguinal hernia	60	1.8		12.5	Williams and Hale (1966)
1955	All	>60			8.5	Klug and McPherson (1959)
1955–60	All	80		24.3		Wilder and Fishbein (1961)
1959–64	All	≥80	25.0		37.0	Marshall and Fahey (1964)
1960–63	All	>75	5.8	7.8	24.4	Bonus and Dorsey (1965)
1960–64	Gastrointestinal	65	17.8	20.6	23.2	Cogbill (1967)
1962–71	All	≥80	11.8		20.7	Kohn *et al.* (1973)
1965–69		60–70		4.4		Marx *et al.* (1973)
		70–80		6.8		Marx *et al.* (1973)
		>80		8.2		
1967–68		≥70	9.0		66.0	Stevens and Aldrete (1969)
1969–75	Abdominal	>75			31.7	Blake and Lynn (1976)
1970–75	All	>90		12		Miller *et al.* (1977)
1970–73	All	>70		4.9		Santos and Gelperin (1975)
		>90	7.0			
1971–80	Hernias	≥65	1.3		7.5	Nehme (1983)
1972–79	Gastrointestinal	>70	6.7		2.0	Greenburg *et al.* (1981)
1974–75	All	≥65		4.88		Commission on Professional and Hospital Activities (1977)
1975–77		>80	6.2			Djokovic and Hedey-Whyte (1979)
1975–80	Hernias	≥70	0.0	6.4	22.0	Tingwald and Cooperman (1982)
1978–79	All	<65		0.75		Stephen (1984)
		>70	5.8			
	Intra-abdominal			11.3		
	Extra-abdominal			2.4		
	Open heart		15.4			
	Intrathoracic		5.4			
	Emergency				10.8	
1979–83	All	≥100		0.0		Katlic (1985)
1986–1987	Major surgery, non-thoracic	>80	5.6		10.3	Pedersen *et al.* (1990)

at approximately a 5.5% risk for major elective procedures and a 10.5% risk for emergency procedures.
2 Elective procedures carry a lower risk than emergency ones.
3 The type of operation appears to be important — intra-abdominal and open-heart procedures being associated with the highest mortalities.

Perhaps of more relevance to the elderly patient is his/her quality of life after leaving the hospital. This topic has been addressed (Palmer *et al.*, 1989). Looking specifically at major abdominal procedures in the over 80s compared with patients aged 40–65 years

old, these investigators reported very disconcerting evidence that by 6 months postoperatively more than 50% of the elderly patients were less independent than they had been preoperatively, compared with less than 20% of their younger counterparts.

Local versus regional versus general anaesthesia

There is little evidence to suggest a distinct superiority of one type of anaesthesia over another. It has been suggested that with respect to the elderly surgical patient, the choice of anaesthesia is relatively unimportant compared with the skill with which it is administered (Bosch et al., 1952; Cole, 1953).

Intuition suggests that the less the physiological trespass, the lower will be the extent of morbidity and mortality. An example of this may be the observation that the myocardial reinfarction rate after local anaesthesia for ophthalmic procedures is zero, whilst that for patients having general or major regional anaesthesia for non-ophthalmic surgery is 6.1% (Steen et al., 1978; Backer et al., 1980). This does not imply necessarily that local anaesthesia is safer than general anaesthesia, but does suggest that the physiological trespass in this type of procedure is less compared with that in non-ophthalmic surgery.

Proponents of regional anaesthesia suggest that the greater lability of heart rate and arterial pressure in the perioperative period associated with general anaesthesia is more likely to be associated with morbidity and mortality.

Proponents of general anaesthesia use a similar argument to support the opposite position.

A preliminary report from the Johns Hopkins Group indicates that myocardial ischaemia may be more common with regional anaesthesia in high-risk patients than with general anaesthesia in a similar group (Beattie et al., 1986).

Although it is often stated that transurethral resection of the prostate is safer under regional anaesthesia because the patient remains awake and alert allowing a change in sensorium to indicate early problems with excessive absorption of irrigant solution, a large study of 2000 patients revealed that anaesthesia was not a significant factor in the morbidity and mortality associated with this procedure (Melchior et al., 1974). It has, however, been shown that blood loss during spinal anaesthesia for this procedure is significantly less than under general anaesthesia (Smart, 1984).

The advantages and disadvantages of general and regional anaesthesia have been investigated extensively in the elderly patient having hip surgery for fractures (Hole et al., 1980; Wickstrom et al., 1982; Lundh et al., 1983; Modig et al., 1983a; McKenzie et al., 1984; Bigler et al., 1985). The evidence is in favour of regional anaesthesia for total hip replacement surgery. Decreased blood transfusion requirements and a decreased incidence of thromboembolism associated with extradural anaesthesia compared with general anaesthesia was noted by Modig and colleagues (1983b). In another study, extradural anaesthesia was associated with less deterioration of cerebral and pulmonary function postoperatively than was general anaesthesia (Hole et al., 1980). In support of this,

Lundh and colleagues (1983) were able to show that extradural anaesthesia did not influence the relationship between functional residual capacity and closing capacity (unlike general anaesthesia). Ventilation–perfusion relationships during extradural anaesthesia in this study showed no significant changes compared with control values, indicating a preservation of pulmonary gas exchange. Early mortality, i.e. 1 month, appears to be lower in those patients receiving spinal anaesthesia (McLaren et al., 1978; Davis & Laurenson, 1981). However, long-term studies of morbidity and mortality (2 months to 1 year), show little difference between regional and general anaesthesia (McKenzie et al., 1984). (See also Chapter 48.)

There are some special considerations for regional anaesthesia in elderly patients. Several studies indicate that advancing age influences the spread of local anaesthetic solution in the extradural space (Bromage, 1969; Grundy et al., 1978; Park et al., 1980; Veering et al., 1987b). For the most part, advancing age appears to decrease the dose and volume of local anaesthetic necessary to block a given number of spinal segments. Similar findings have been noted with spinal anaesthesia (Pitkanen et al., 1984; Veering et al., 1988). On the other hand, no correlation was found between age and the extent of sensory spread of local anaesthetics injected in the caudal space (Freund et al., 1984).

The stress factor

Cold stress

Thermal regulation is impaired in elderly people, as are many other homeostatic mechanisms (Collins et al., 1977). Vasomotor responses to temperature changes are notably impaired. Deep anaesthesia renders a patient poikilothermic whilst light planes of anaesthesia narrow the environmental range over which patients can maintain their temperature (Flacke & Flacke, 1983). In addition, regional anaesthesia has been shown to be associated with even greater heat loss than general anaesthesia (Jenkins et al., 1983). Elderly patients are noted to leave operating rooms with lower temperatures than their younger counterparts (Vaughan et al., 1981).

The most important factor relative to body temperature in the perioperative period is operating-room temperature (Morris & Wilkey, 1970; Morris 1971a; Roizen et al., 1980). The administration of fluids at room temperature and the administration of high-flow dry anaesthetic gases contribute also. Whilst one may argue that hypothermia may be beneficial because of the associated decreased metabolic rate and oxygen consumption, the disadvantages of hypothermia outweigh any advantage that this may represent. Oxygen delivery may suffer as a result of a leftward shift of the oxyhaemoglobin dissociation curve resulting from both decreased temperature and respiratory alkalosis (secondary to a decreased carbon dioxide production without compensatory ventilatory changes). Vasoconstriction occurs to some degree and filling pressures may be misleading. The associated increase in systemic vascular resistance may impose increased demands on the heart. Blood flow to the extremities may become compromised. In addition, Lunn (1969) has reported an increased incidence of postoperative deep vein thrombosis and pulmonary embolism in countries where operations are performed under cold ambient temperatures compared with the virtual lack of such complications in warm subtropical locations.

Hypothermia has profound effects on the pharmacology of anaesthetic and adjuvant drugs. The MAC of inhalation agents decreases with a falling temperature. The elimination half-life of several intravenously administered drugs may be increased secondary to decreased metabolism and decreased organ blood flow. In combination, this may lead to relative anaesthetic overdose and delayed awakening.

Perhaps the most serious consequence of inadvertent hypothermia in the perioperative period is the occurrence of shivering. A recent study has indicated that the occurrence of postanaesthetic shivering remains relatively consistent throughout life (Murphy et al., 1986). The metabolic cost of shivering is an increase in oxygen consumption from 300 to 800% (Horvath et al., 1956; Benzinger, 1969). In order to meet this increased demand for oxygen at the tissue level, the normal patient increases oxygen supply by increasing cardiac output and minute ventilation (Bay et al., 1968). The elderly patient may not be able to meet this increased demand, resulting in hypoxaemia.

It is of interest that the catabolic response to major surgical trauma may be attenuated in elderly patients who remain normothermic during and after surgery (Carli & Itiaba, 1986).

Among the most effective ways of maintaining body heat in elderly patients is maintenance of ambient temperature in the range of 21.1–23.9°C (Morris, 1971b). Also effective are the use of warming blankets (controversial), the use of a heat and humidity exchanger, the use of low fresh-gas flows and the use of a heated humidifier in the anaesthetic breathing system (Morris & Wilkey, 1970; Roizen

et al., 1980; Linko et al., 1984; Tollofsrud et al., 1984). In addition, it has been suggested that the poikilothermic state be reintroduced on the postoperative period to attenuate the metabolic stress of shivering, through the use of morphine and/or other drugs such as the phenothiazines (Rodriguez et al., 1983).

Neuroendocrine stress

There is little information on the neuroendocrine response to stress in elderly patients. The work of Arnetz suggests that there is an age-related decrease in the neuroendocrine response to surgical stress, at least with respect to the use of prolactin as a marker (Arnetz et al., 1984; Arnetz, 1985). The age-related differences in serum prolactin response were attenuated significantly by spinal anaesthesia (Arnetz, 1985). It is interesting to note from these studies that under basal conditions serum concentrations of neuroendocrine hormones were identical in young and old, suggesting a diminished reserve capacity in elderly patients. In other studies, the stress response in elderly patients was associated with an increase in plasma cortisol and glucose concentrations under general anaesthesia, attenuated by extradural anaesthesia (Hole et al., 1982; Riis et al., 1983; Hjortso et al., 1985).

A link exists between the neuroendocrine and the immune systems. A significant decrease in both number and function of lymphocytes and function of monocytes has been noted under general anaesthesia in elderly patients (Hole et al., 1982; Whelan & Morris, 1982). It is not known if this is qualitatively or quantitatively different in younger patients. Most investigators have concluded that peri- and postoperative immunosuppression is associated with the stress response elicited by surgical trauma, as opposed to some inherent mechanism associated with general anaesthesia. It is important to note, however, that both the altered immune function and the hormonal response to surgical stress appear to be blocked by spinal and extradural anaesthesia (Hole et al., 1982; Whelan & Morris, 1982). This may be an important consideration in an elderly patient undergoing major cancer surgery.

Psychological factors

From a psychiatric standpoint, elderly people have little reserve capacity. Thus, sudden changes in environment and other conditions are liable to produce acute disturbances in the form of confusional states, affective disorders or dementia (Roth, 1976).

The reason for this phenomenon is not known, but it helps to explain the common observation that elderly patients may decline rapidly from a functional standpoint when stressed with only 'minor' illnesses. There are three important points for the anaesthetist to note:

1 A simple change of environment may induce a confusional state in a patient who was otherwise functioning well in an independent fashion within his/her own structured environment.

2 Delirium may be caused by a wide variety of factors including many medical conditions and medications (Liston, 1982). This is frequently overlooked and the patient is assumed to be suffering from senile dementia (Portnoi, 1981).

3 Elderly patients, particularly men, have an increased risk of suffering major depression associated with perioperative events (LaRue & Schaeffer, 1986). This particular group is most likely to attempt and succeed at suicide.

References

Abernethy D.R. & Greenblatt D.J. (1983) Impairment of lidocaine clearance in elderly male subjects. *Journal of Cardiovascular Pharmacology* **5**, 1093−6.

Arden J.R., Holley F.O. & Stanski D.R. (1986) Increased sensitivity to etomidate in elderly: initial distribution versus altered brain response. *Anesthesiology* **56**, 19−27.

Arnetz B.B. (1985) Endocrine reactions during standardized surgical stress: the effects of age and methods of anesthesia. *Age and Aging* **14**, 96−101.

Arnetz B.B., Lahnborg G., Eneroth P. & Thunell S. (1984) Age related differences in the serum prolactin response during standardized surgery. *Life Science* **35**, 2675−80.

Azad S.S., Larijani G.E., Goldberg M.E., Beach C.A., Marr A.T. & Seltzer J.L. (1989) A dose response evaluation of pipercuronium bromide in elderly patients under balanced anesthesia. *Journal of Clinical Pharmacology* **29**, 657−9.

Backer C.L., Tinker J.H., Robertson D.M. & Vlietsra R.E. (1980) Myocardial reinfarction following local anesthesia for ophthalmic surgery. *Anesthesia and Analgesia* **59**, 257−62.

Bahemuka M. & Hodkinson H.M. (1975) Screening for hypothyroidism in elderly patients. *British Medical Journal* **2**, 601−3.

Bay J., Nunn J.F. & Prys-Roberts C. (1968) Factors influencing arterial P_{O_2} during recovery from anaesthesia. *British Journal of Anaesthesia* **40**, 398−406.

Beattie C., Christopherson R., Manolio T. & Pearson T. (1986) Myocardial ischemia may be more common with regional than general anesthesia in high risk patients. *Anesthesiology* **65**, 518A.

Becklake M.R., Frank H., Dagenais G.R., Stiguy G.L. & Guzman C.A. (1965) Influence of age and sex on exercise cardiac output. *Journal of Applied Physiology* **20**, 938−47.

Bellville J.W., Forrest W.H., Miller E. & Brown B.W. (1971) Influence of age on pain relief from analgesics; a study of postoperative patients. *Journal of the American Medical Association* **217**, 1835−41.

Bender A.D. (1965) The effect of increasing age on the distribution of peripheral blood flow in man. *Journal of the American Geriatrics Society* **13**, 192−8.

Bentley J.B., Borel J.D., Nenad R.E. & Gillespie T.J. (1982) Age and fentanyl pharmacokinetics. *Anesthesia and Analgesia* **61**, 968−71.

Benzinger T.H. (1969) Heat regulation: homeostasis of central temperature in man. *Physiology Reviews* **49**, 671−759.

Berkowitz B.A., Ngai S.H., Yang J.C., Hempstead J. & Spector S. (1975) The disposition of morphine in surgical patients. *Clinical Pharmacology and Therapeutics* **17**, 629−35.

Bigler D., Adelhoj B., Petring O.U., Pederson N.O., Busch P. & Kalhke P. (1985) Mental function and morbidity after acute hip surgery during spinal and general anaesthesia. *Anaesthesia* **40**, 672−6.

Blake R. & Lynn J. (1976) Emergency abdominal surgery in the aged. *British Journal of Surgery* **63**, 956−60.

Bonus R.L. & Dorsey J.M. (1965) Major surgery in the aged patient. *Archives of Surgery* **90**, 95−7.

Bosch D.T., Islami A., Tan C.T.C. & Beling C.A. (1952) The elderly surgical patient. *Archives of Surgery* **64**, 269−77.

Brandfonbrener M., Landowne M. & Shock N.W. (1955) Changes in cardiac output with age. *Circulation* **12**, 557−66.

Brischetto M.J., Millman R.P., Peterson D.D., Silage D.A. & Pack A.I. (1984) Effect of aging on ventilatory response to exercise and CO_2. *Journal of Applied Physiology* **56**, 1143−50.

Bromage P.R. (1969) Aging and epidural dose requirements. *British Journal of Anaesthesia* **41**, 10−16.

Burch P.G. & Stanski D.R. (1983) The role of metabolism and protein binding in thiopental anesthesia. *Anesthesiology* **58**, 146−52.

Campbell E.J. & Lefrak S.S. (1984) Physiologic process of aging in the respiratory system. In *Anesthesia and the Geriatric Patient* (Ed. Krechel S.W.) pp. 23−43. Grune and Stratton, Orlando.

Carli F. & Itiaba K. (1986) Effect of heat conservation during and after major abdominal surgery on muscle protein breakdown in elderly patients. *British Journal of Anaesthesia* **58**, 502−7.

Castelden C.M., George C.F., Marcer D. & Hallett C. (1977) Increased sensitivity to nitrozepam in old age. *British Medical Journal* **1**, 10−12.

Celesia G.G. & Daly R.F. (1977) Effects of aging on visual evoked responsives. *Archives of Neurology* **35**, 403−7.

Chan K., Kendall M.J., Mitchard M. & Wells W.D. (1975) The effect of aging on plasma pethidine concentration. *British Journal of Clinical Pharmacology* **2**, 297−302.

Christensen J.H., Andreasen F. & Jansen J.A. (1981) Influence of age and sex on the pharmacokinetics of thiopentone. *British Journal of Anaesthesia* **53**, 1189−95.

Coath A. (1984) Physiologic process of aging in the cardiovascular system. In *Anesthesia and the Geriatric Patient* (Ed. Krechel S.W.) pp. 11−21. Grune and Stratton, Orlando.

Cogbill C.L. (1967) Operation in the aged. *Archives of Surgery* **94**, 202−5.

Cole W.H. (1953) Operability in the young and the aged. *Annals of Surgery* **138**, 145−57.

Collins K.J., Dore C., Exton-Smith A.N., Fox R.H., Weaver

E.J.M., Waters A.F., Brookes J.M. & Inniss R. (1977) Accidental hypothermia and impaired temperature homeostasis in the elderly. *British Medical Journal* **1**, 353–6.

Collins A.J., Exton-Smith A.N. & James M.H. (1980) Functional changes in autonomic nervous responses with aging. *Age and Aging* **9**, 17–24.

Colvin M.P., Savege T.M., Newland P.E., Weaver E.J., Waters A.F., Brookes J.M. & Inniss R. (1979) Cardiorespiratory changes following induction of anaesthesia with etomidate in patients with cardiac disease. *British Journal of Anaesthesia* **51**, 551–6.

Commission on Professional and Hospital Activities (1977) *Hospital Mortality: PAS Hospitals. Limited States 1974–1975,* p. 150. University of Michigan Press, Michigan.

Cronnelly R. & Miller R.D. (1984) Edrophonium: dose response onset and duration of antagonism in elderly patients. *Anesthesiology* **61**, 303A.

Cusson J., Nattel S., Matthews C., Talajic M. & Lawand S. (1985) Aged dependent lidocaine disposition in patients with acute myocardial infarction. *Clinical Pharmacology and Therapeutics* **37**, 381–6.

Davidson M.B. (1979) The effect of aging on carbohydrate metabolism: a review of the English literature and a practical approach to the diagnosis of diabetes mellitus in the elderly. *Metabolism* **28**, 688–705.

Davies M.J. & Pomerance A. (1972) A quantitative study of aging in human sino-atrial nodes and internodal tracts. *British Heart Journal* **34**, 150–2.

Davis F.M. & Laurenson V.G. (1981) Spinal anaesthesia or general anaesthesia for emergency hip surgery in elderly patients. *Anaesthesia and Intensive Care* **9**, 352–8.

Davis D., Grossman S.H., Kitchell B.B., Shand G. & Routledge P.A. (1985) The effects of age and smoking on the plasma protein binding of lignocaine and diazepam. *British Journal of Clinical Pharmacology* **19**, 261–5.

Devaney K.O. & Johnson H.A. (1980) Neuron loss in the aging visual cortex of man. *Journal of Gerontology* **35**, 836–41.

D'Hollander A., Massaux F., Nevelsteen M. & Agoston S. (1982) Age dependent dose response relationship of ORG-NC 45 in anaesthetized patients. *British Journal of Anaesthesia* **54**, 653–7.

D'Hollander A.A., Nevelsteen M., Barvais L. & Baurain M. (1983a) Effective age on the establishment of muscle paralysis induced in anaesthetized adult subjects by ORG-NG 45, *Acta Anaesthesiologica Scandinavica* **27**, 108–10.

D'Hollander A.A., Luyckx C., Barvais L. & De Ville K. (1983b) Clinical evaluation of atracurium besylate requirement for a stable muscle relaxation during surgery: lack of age related effects. *Anesthesiology* **59**, 237–40.

Divoll M., Greenblatt D.J., Ochs H.R. & Shaden R.I. (1983) Absolute bioavailability of oral and intramuscular diazepam: effects of age and sex. *Anesthesia and Analgesia* **62**, 1–8.

Djokovic J.L. & Heldley-Whyte J. (1979) Prediction of outcome of surgery and anesthesia in patients over 80. *Journal of the American Medical Association* **242**, 2301–6.

Donevan R.E., Palmer W.H., Varvis C.J. & Bates D.V. (1959) Influence of age on pulmonary diffusing capacity. *Journal of Applied Physiology* **14**, 483–92.

Dorfman I.J. & Bosley T.M. (1979) Age related changes in peripheral and central nerve conduction in man. *Neurology* **29**, 38–44.

Drayer E.D., Lorenzo B., Werns S. & Reidenberg U.M. (1983) Plasma levels, protein binding and elimination data of lidocaine and active metabolites in cardiac patients of various ages. *Clinical Pharmacology and Therapeutics* **34**, 14–22.

Dundee J.W., Halliday N.J., Loughran P.G. & Harper K.W. (1985) The influence of age on the onset of anaesthesia with midazolam. *Anaesthesia* **40**, 441–3.

Dundee J.W., Robinson F.P., McCollum J.S.C. & Patterson C.C. (1986) Sensitivity to propofol in the elderly. *Anaesthesia* **41**, 482–5.

Duvaldestein P., Saada J., Berger J.L., D'Hollander A. & Mesmonts J.M. (1982) Pharmacokinetics, pharmacodynamics, and dose response relationships of pancuronium in control and elderly subjects. *Anesthesiology* **56**, 36–40.

Dwyer R., Fee J.P.H. & Clark R.S.J. (1990) End tidal concentrations of halothane and isoflurane during induction of anesthesia in young and elderly patients. *British Journal of Anaesthesia* **64**, 36–41.

Eger E.I.II (1974) *Anesthetic Uptake and Action.* Williams and Wilkins Publishing Company, Baltimore.

Eger E.I.II, Smith N.T., Stoelting R.K., Cullen D., Kadis L.D. & Witchen C.E. (1970) Cardiovascular effect of halothane in man. *Anesthesiology* **32**, 396–409.

Epstein M. (1979) Effects of aging on the kidney. *Federation Proceedings* **38**, 168–72.

Epstein M. (1986) Aging and the kidney. In *Geriatric Anesthesia, Principles and Practice* (Eds Stephen C.R. & Assaf R.A.E.). Butterworth, Boston.

Epstein M. & Hollenberg N.K. (1976) Age as a determinant of renal sodium conservation in normal man. *Journal of Laboratory and Clinical Medicine* **87**, 411–17.

Feldman R.D., Limbird L.E., Nodeau J., Robertson D. & Wood J.J. (1984) Alterations in leukocyte β-receptor affinity with aging. *New England Journal of Medicine* **310**, 815–19.

Flacke J.W. & Flacke W.E. (1983) Inadvertent hypothermia: frequent, insidious, and often serious. *Seminars in Anesthesia* **2**, 183–96.

Freund P.R., Bowdle T.A., Slattery J.T. & Bell L.E. (1984) Caudal anesthesia with lidocaine or bupivacaine, plasma local anesthetic concentration and extent of sensory spread in old and young patients. *Anesthesia and Analgesia* **63**, 1017–20.

Gerber J.G. (1982) Drug usage in the elderly. In *Clinical Internal Medicine in the Aged* (Ed. Schrier R.W.) p. 55. W.B. Saunders and Co., Philadelphia.

Goldring W., Chasis H., Ranges H.A. & Smith H.W. (1940) Relations of effective renal blood flow and glomerular filtration to tubular excretory mass in normal man. *Journal of Clinical Investigation* **19**, 739–50.

Goodnick P. & Gershon S. (1984) Chemotherapy of cognitive disorders in geriatric subjects. *Journal of Clinical Psychology* **45**, 196–209.

Graf R.J., Halter J.B. & Porte D. (1978) Glycosylated hemoglobin in normal subjects and subjects with maturity onset diabetic evidence for a saturable system in men. *Diabetes* **27**, 834–9.

Graves C.L., McDermott R.W. & Bidwaia A. (1974) Cardiovascular effects of isoflurane in surgical patients. *Anesthesiology* **41**, 486–9.

Greenblatt D.J., Abernethy D.R., Locniskar A., Harmantz J.S., Limsuco R.A. & Shader R.I. (1977a) Effect of age, gender, and obesity on midazolam kinetics. *Anesthesiology* **61**, 27–35.

Greenburg A.G., Saik R.P., Coyle J.J. & Peskin G.W. (1981) Mortality and gastrointestinal surgery in the aged, elective vs emergency procedures. *Archives of Surgery* **116**, 788–91.

Gregory G.G., Eger E.I. & Munson E.S. (1969) The relationship between age and halothane requirement in man. *Anesthesiology* **30**, 488–91.

Grundy E.M., Ramamurthy S., Patel K.P., Mani M. & Winnie A.P. (1978) Extradural analgesia revisited; a statistical study. *British Journal of Anaesthesia* **50**, 805–9.

Halter J.B. & Pieffier M.A. (1982) Aging and autonomic nervous systems function in man in biologic markers of aging. *NIH Publication*, number 82–2221, pp. 168–76.

Haug C.A. & Dale W.A. (1952) Major surgery in old people. *Archives of Surgery* **64**, 421–37.

Helderman J.H., Vestal R.E., Rowe J.W., Sobin J.D., Ardies R. & Robertson G.L. (1978) The response of arginine vasopressin to intravenous ethanol and hypertonic saline in man: the impact of aging. *Journal of Gerontology* **33**, 39–47.

Helmers J.H., Norrduin H. & vanLeeuwen L. (1985) Alfentanil used in the aged: a clinical comparison with its use in young patients. *European Journal of Anaesthesia* **2**, 347–52.

Herman R.J., McAllister C.B., Branch R.A. & Wilkinson G.R. (1985) Effects of age on meperidine disposition. *Clinical Pharmacology and Therapeutics* **37**, 19–24.

Hjortso N.C., Christensen N.J., Andersen T. & Kehlet H. (1985) Effects of the extradural administration of local anesthetic agents and morphine on the urinary excretion of cortisol: catecholamines and nitrogen following abdominal surgery. *British Journal of Anaesthesia* **57**, 400–6.

Hoffman W.E., Miletich D.J.U. & Albrecht R.F. (1982) Cardiovascular and regional blood flow changes during halothane anaesthesia in the aged rat. *Anesthesiology* **56**, 444–8.

Hole A., Terjesen T. & Breivik H. (1980) Epidural versus general anesthesia for total hip arthoplasty in elderly patients. *Acta Anaesthesiologica Scandinavica* **24**, 279–87.

Hole A., Unsgaard G. & Breivik H. (1982) Monocyte functions are depressed during and after surgery under general anesthesia but not under epidural anesthesia. *Acta Anaesthesiologica Scandinavica* **26**, 301–7.

Hollenberg N.K., Adams D.F., Soloman H.S., Rashid A., Abrams H.L. & Merril J.B. (1974) Senescence and the renal vasculature in normal man. *Circulation Research* **34**, 309–16.

Holmberg L., Odar-Cederlof I., Nilsson J.I.G., Ehrnebo M. & Boreus L.O. (1982) Pethidine binding to blood cells and plasma proteins in old and young subjects. *European Journal of Clinical Pharmacology* **23**, 457–61.

Homer T.D. & Stanski D.R. (1985) The effect of increasing age on thiopental disposition and anesthetic requirement. *Anesthesiology* **62**, 714–24.

Horvath S.M., Spurr G.B., Hutt B.K. & Hamilton L.H. (1956) Metabolic cost of shivering. *Journal of Applied Physiology* **8**, 595–602.

Hudson R.J., Thompson I.R., Cannon J.E., Frieson R.M. & Meatherall R.C. (1986) Pharmacokinetics of fentanyl in patients undergoing abdominal aortic surgery. *Anesthesiology* **64**, 334–8.

Jefferys P.M., Farrian H.E., Hoffenberg R., Fraser P.M. & Hodkinson H.M. (1972) Thyroid function tests in the elderly. *Lancet* **i**, 924–7.

Jenkins J., Fox J. & Sharwood-Smith G. (1983) Changes in body heat during transvesical prostatectomy. *Anaesthesia* **38**, 748–53.

Jung D., Mayersohn M., Perrier D., Calkins J. & Saunders R. (1982) Thiopental disposition as a function of age in female patients undergoing surgery. *Anesthesiology* **56**, 263–8.

Kannel W.B. & Gordon T. (1978) Evaluation of cardiovascular risk in the elderly; the Framingham Study Bull. *New York Academy of Medicine* **54**, 573–91.

Kanto J., Aaltonen L., Himberg J.J. & Hovi-Viander M. (1986) Midazolam as an intravenous induction agent in the elderly; a clinical and pharmacokinetic study. *Anesthesia and Analgesia* **65**, 15–20.

Katlic M.R. (1985) Surgery in centenarians. *Journal of the American Medical Association* **253**, 3139–41.

Katzman R. & Terry R.D. (1983) Normal ageing of the central nervous system. In *The Neurology of Ageing* (Ed. Katzman R. & Terry R.D.) pp. 15–50. Davis, F.A. Philadelphia.

Kety S.S. (1956) Human cerebral blood flow and oxygen consumption as related to aging. *Journal of Chronic Diseases* **3**, 478–86.

Kitani K. (1985) The role of the liver in pharmacokinetic and pharmacodynamic alterations in the elderly. In *Therapeutics in the Elderly* (Eds O'Malley K. & Waddington J.L.). Elsevier, Amsterdam.

Kitts J.B., Fisher P.M., Canfell P.C., Spellman M.J., Caldwell J.E., Heier T., Fahey M.R. & Miller R.D. (1990) Pharmacokinetics and pharmacodynamics of atracurium in the elderly. *Anesthesiology* **72**, 272–5.

Klotz V., Avant G.R., Hoyumpa A., Schenker S. & Wilkinson G.R. (1975) The effects of age and liver disease on the disposition and elimination of diazepam in adult man. *Journal of Clinical Investigation* **55**, 347–59.

Klug T.J. & McPherson R.D. (1959) Postoperative complications in the elderly surgical patient. *American Journal of Surgery* **97**, 713–17.

Kohn R.R. (1963) Human aging and disease. *Journal of Clinical Disease* **16**, 5–21.

Kohn P., Zekert F., Vormittage E. & Grabner H. (1973) Risks of operation in patients over 80. *Geriatrics* **28**, 100–5.

Korttila K., Saarnivaara L., Tarkkanen J., Himberg J.J. & Hytonen M. (1978) Effect of age on amnesia and sedation induced by flunitrazepam during local anesthesia for bronchoscopy. *British Journal of Anaesthesia* **50**, 1211–18.

Krechel S.W. (1984) Inhalation agents in the aged. In *Anesthesia and the Geriatric Patient* (Ed. Krechel S.W.) pp. 99–114. Grune & Stratton, Orlando.

Kronenberg R.S. & Drage C.W. (1973) Attenuation of the ventilatory and heart rate responses to hypoxia and hypercapnea with aging in normal men. *Journal of Clinical Investigation* **52**, 1812–19.

Kuramoto K., Matsushita S., Kuwajima I., Iwasoki T. & Murakami M. (1979) Comparison of hemodynamic effects of exercise and isoproterenol infusion in normal young and old men. *Japanese Circulation Journal* **43**, 71–6.

Larsen R., Rathgeber J., Bagdolin A., Lange H. & Rieke H. (1988) Effects with propofol on cardiovascular dynamics and coronary blood flow in geriatric patients, a comparison with etomidate. *Anaesthesia* **43**, 25–31.

LaRue A. & Schaeffer J. (1986) Psychologic reactions of elderly patients to illness and surgery. *Seminars in Anesthesia* **5**, 36–43.

Lemmens H.J.M., Bovill J.G., Hennis P.J. & Burm A.G.L. (1988a) Age has no effect on the pharmacodynamics of alfentanil. *Anesthesia and Analgesia* **67**, 956–60.

Lemmens H.J.M., Bovill J.G., Burm A.G.L. & Hennis P.J. (1988b) Alfentanil infusion in the elderly: prolonged computer-assisted infusion of alfentanil in the elderly surgical patient. *Anaesthesia* **43**, 850–6.

Lepage J.Y.M., Pinaud M.L, Hélias J.H., Juge C.M., Cozian A.Y., Farinotti R. & Souron R.J. (1988) Left ventricular function during propofol and fentanyl anesthesia in patients with coronary artery disease: assessment with a radionucleide approach. *Anesthesia and Analgesia* **67**, 949–55.

Lepage J.Y.M., Pinaud M.L., Hélias J.H., Cozian A.Y., Normand Y.L. & Souron R.J. (1991) Left ventricular performance during propofol or methohexitol anesthesia: isotopic and invasive cardiac monitoring. *Anesthesia and Analgesia* **73**, 3–9.

Lerman J., Gregory G.A., Willis M.M. & Eger E.I. (1984) Age and solubility of volatile anesthetics in blood. *Anesthesiology* **61**, 139–43.

Lie K.I., Wellens H.J., VanCapelle F.J. & Durrer D. (1974) Lidocaine in the prevention of primary ventricular fibrillation. *New England Journal of Medicine* **291**, 1324–6.

Lien C.A., Matteo R.S., Ornstein E., Schwartz A.E. & Diaz J. (1991) Distribution, elimination and action of vercuronium in the elderly. *Anesthesia and Analgesia* **73**, 39–42.

Linde H.W., Oh S.O., Homi J. & Josai C. (1975) Cardiovascular effects of isoflurane and halothane during controlled ventilation in older patients. *Anesthesia and Analgesia* **54**, 701–4.

Linko K., Honkavaara P. & Nieminen M.T. (1984) Heated humidification in major abdominal surgery. *European Journal of Anaesthesia* **1**, 285–91.

Liston E.H. (1982) Delirium in the aged. *Psychiatric Clinics of North America* **5**, 49–66.

Lloyd W.H. & Goldberg I.J.L. (1961) Incidence of hyperthyroidism in the elderly. *British Medical Journal* **2**, 1256–9.

Lowry K.G., Mirakhur R.K., Lavery G.G. & Clarke R.S.T. (1985) Vecuronium and atracurium in the elderly; a clinical comparison to pancuronium. *Acta Anaesthesiologica Scandinavica* **29**, 405–8.

Lundh R., Hedenstierna G. & Johansson H. (1983) Ventilation perfusion relationships during epidural analgesia. *Acta Anaesthesiologica Scandinavica* **27**, 410–16.

Lunn H.F. (1969) Observations on heat gain and loss in surgery. *Guy's Hospital REP* **118**, 117–27.

Lytle L.D. & Altar A. (1979) Diet, central nervous system and aging. *Federation Proceedings* **38**, 1922–6.

Manchikanti L., Colliver J.A., Marrero T.C. & Rousch J.R. (1985) Assessment of age related acid aspiration risk factors in pediatric, adult and geriatric patients. *Anesthesia and Analgesia* **64**, 11–17.

Marchesini G., Bua V., Brunori A., Bianchi G., Pisi P., Fabri A., Zoli M. & Pisi E. (1988) Galactose elimination capacity and liver volume in aging man. *Hepatology* **8**, 1079–83.

Marshall W.H. & Fahey P.J. (1964) Operative complications and mortality in patients over 80 years of age. *Archives of Surgery* **88**, 896–904.

Martinez D., Zamel N., Bradley D. & Phillipson E.A. (1984) Effect of aging on the peripheral chemo reflex during sleep in

healthy men. *American Review of Respiratory Disease* **129**, 244–50A.

Marx G.F., Mateo C.V. & Orkin L.R. (1973) Computer analysis of postanesthetic deaths. *Anesthesiology* **39**, 54–9.

Mather L.E., Tucker G.T., Pflug A.E., Lindop M.J. & Wilkerson C. (1975) Meperidine kinetics in man; intravenous injection in surgical patients and volunteers. *Clinical Pharmacology and Therapeutics* **17**, 21–30.

Matteo R.S., Backus W.W., McDaniel D.D., Brotherton W.P., Abraham R.A. & Diaz J. (1985) Pharmacokinetics and pharmacodynamics of D-tubocurarine and metocurarine in the elderly. *Anesthesia and Analgesia* **64**, 23–9.

Matteo R.S., Ornstein E., Schwartz A.E., Young W.L. & Chow F.T. (1986a) Effects of low dose of sufentanil on the EEG; elderly versus young. *Anesthesiology* **65**, 553A.

Matteo R.S., Ornstein E., Young W.L., Schwartz A.E., Port M. & Chang W.J. (1986b) Pharmacokinetics of sufentanil in the elderly. *Anesthesia and Analgesia* **65**, 94S.

Matteo R.S., Young W.L., Ornstein E., Schwartz A.E., Silverberg P.A. & Diaz J. (1990) Pharmacokinetics and pharmacodynamics of edrophonium in elderly surgical patients. *Anesthesia and Analgesia* **71**, 334–9.

McKenzie P.J., Wishart H.Y. & Smith G. (1984) Long term outcome after repair of fractured neck of femur; comparison of subarachnoid and general anaesthesia. *British Journal of Anaesthesia* **56**, 581–5.

McLaren A.D., Stockwell M.L. & Reid V.T. (1978) Anaesthesia techniques for surgical correction of fractured neck of femur. *Anaesthesia* **33**, 10–14.

McLeod K., Hull C.J. & Watson M.J. (1979) Effects of aging on the pharmacokinetics of pancuronium. *British Journal of Anaesthesia* **51**, 435–8.

Meakins J.L. & McLaren A.D. (1986) *Surgical Care of the Elderly.* Yearbook Medical Publishers, Chicago.

Melchior J., Valk W.L., Foret J.D. & Mebust W.K. (1974) Transurethral prostatectomy; computerized analysis of 2,223 consecutive cases. *Journal of Urology* **112**, 634–42.

Miller P.F. (1990) Ageing and pain perception in ischemic heart disease. *American Heart Journal* **120**, 22–30.

Miller R., Malar K. & Silvay G. (1977) Anesthesia for patients aged over ninety years. *New York State Journal of Medicine* **77**, 1421–5.

Modig J., Borg T., Bagge L. & Saldeen I.T. (1983a) Role of extradural and of general anaesthesia in fibrinolysis and coagulation after total hip replacement. *British Journal of Anaesthesia* **55**, 625–9.

Modig J., Borg T., Karlstrom G., Maripuu E. & Sahlstedt B. (1983b) Thromboembolism after total hip replacement, role of epidural and general anesthesia. *Anesthesia and Analgesia* **62**, 174–80.

Moore A.K., Bilderman S., Lubenskyi W., McCans J. & Fox G.S. (1990) Differences in epidural morphine requirements between elderly and young patients after abdominal surgery. *Anesthesia and Analgesia* **70**, 316–20.

Morris R.H. (1971a) Operating room temperature in anesthetized paralyzed patients. *Archives of Surgery* **102**, 95–7.

Morris R.H. (1971b) Influence of ambient temperature on patient temperature during intra-abdominal surgery. *Annals of Surgery* **173**, 230–3.

Morris R.H. & Wilkey B.R. (1970) The effects of ambient temperature on patient temperature during surgery not involving body cavities. *Anesthesiology* **32**, 102–7.

Munson E.S., Hoffman J.C. & Eger E.I. (1984) Use of cyclopropane to test generality of anesthetic requirement in the elderly. *Anesthesia and Analgesia* **63**, 998–1000.

Muravchick S. (1984) Effect of age and premedication on thiopental sleep dose. *Anesthesiology* **61**, 333–6.

Muravchick S., Owens W.D. & Felts J.A. (1979) Glycopyrolate and cardiac dysrhythmias in geriatric patients after reversal of neuromuscular blockade. *Canadian Anaesthetists' Society Journal* **26**, 22–5.

Murphy M.T., Lipton J.M. & Giesecke A.H. (1986) Postanesthetic shivering; incidence and implications in the elderly patient. *Anesthesia and Analgesia* **65**, 108S.

Nation R.L., Triggs E.J. & Selig M. (1977) Lignocaine kinetics in cardiac patients and aged subjects. *British Journal of Clinical Pharmacology* **4**, 439–48.

Nehme A.E. (1983) Groin hernias in elderly patients; management and prognosis. *American Journal of Surgery* **146**, 257–60.

O'Hara D.A., Fragen R.J. & Shanks C.A. (1985) The effects of age on dose response curves for vecuronium in adults. *Anesthesiology* **63**, 542–4.

Owens W.D., Waldbaum L.S. & Stephen C.R. (1978) Cardiac dysrhythmias following reversal of neuromuscular blocking agents in geriatric patients. *Anesthesia and Analgesia* **57**, 186–90.

Palmer C.A., Reece-Smith H. & Taylor I. (1989) Major abdominal surgery in the over-eighties. *Journal of the Royal Society of Medicine* **82**, 391–3.

Park W.Y., Massengale M., Kim S.I., Poon K.C. & MacNamara T.E. (1980) Age and the spread of local anaesthetic solutions in the epidural space. *Anesthesia and Analgesia* **59**, 768–71.

Parsons W.H., Whitaker H.T. & Hinton J.K. (1956) Major surgery in patients 70 years of age and over. *Annals of Surgery* **143**, 845–54.

Pederson T., Eliasen K. & Henriksen E. (1990) A prospective study of mortality associated with anesthesia and surgery: risk indicators of mortality in hospital. *Acta Anaesthesiologica Scandinavica* **34**, 176–82.

Pfeifer H.J., Greenblatt D.J. & Koch-Weiser J. (1976) Clinical use and toxicity of intravenous lidocaine. *American Heart Journal* **92**, 168–73.

Pitkanen M., Haapaiemi L., Tuominen M. & Rosenberg P.H. (1984) Influence of age on spinal anaesthesia and isobaric 0.5% bupivacaine. *British Journal of Anaesthesia* **56**, 279–84.

Pontoppidan H. & Beecher H.K. (1960) Progressive loss of protective reflexes in the airway with the advance of age. *Journal of the American Medical Association* **174**, 2209–13.

Portnoi V.A. (1981) Diagnostic dilemma of the aged. *Archives of Internal Medicine* **141**, 734–7.

Prinz P.N., Vitiello M.V., Smallwood R.G., Schoene R.B. & Halter J.B. (1984) Plasma norepinephrine in normal young and aged men: relationship with sleep. *Journal of Gerontology* **39**, 561–7.

Rayfield E.J., Ault M.J., Kuesch G.T., Brothers M.J., Nechemias C. & Smith H. (1982) Infection in diabetics; the case for glucose control. *American Journal of Medicine* **72**, 439–50.

Reidenberg M.M., Levy N., Warner H., Coutinho C.B., Schwartz M.A., Yu G. & Cheripko J. (1978) Relationship between diazepam dose, plasma level, age, and central nervous system depression. *Clinical Pharmacology and Therapeutics* **23**, 371–4.

Riis J., Lomholt B., Hatholdt O., Kehlet N., Valentin N., Danielsen V. & Joyrberg V. (1983) Immediate and long term mental recovery from general versus epidural anesthesia in elderly patients. *Acta Anaesthesiologica Scandinavica* **27**, 44–9.

Rikans L.E. & Notley B.A. (1982) Differential effects of aging on hepatic microsomal mono oxygenase induction by phenobarbital and beta-naphthoflavone. *Biochemical Pharmacology* **31**, 2339–43.

Roberts J. & Goldberg P. (1979) Changes in responsiveness to the heart with drugs during aging. *Federation Proceedings* **38**, 1927–32.

Robinson S. (1964) Physical fitness in relation to age. In *Aging of the Lung Perspectives* (Eds Cander L. & Moyer J.H.) pp. 287–301. Grune and Stratton, New York.

Rodriguez J.L., Weissman C., Damask M.C., Askanazi J., Hyman A.I. & Kinney J.M. (1983) Morphine and postoperative rewarming in critically ill patients. *Circulation* **68**, 1238–46.

Roizen M.F., Sohn Y.J., L'Hommedieu C.S., Wylie E.J. & Ota M.K. (1980) Operating room temperatures prior to surgical draping, effect on patient temperature in the recovery room. *Anesthesia and Analgesia* **59**, 852–5.

Rondeau E., DeLima J., Caillens H. & Ardaillou R. (1982) High plasma antidiuretic hormone in patients with cardiac failure; influence of age. *Mineral and Electrolyte Metabolism* **8**, 267–74.

Roth M. (1976) The psychiatric disorders of later life. *Psychiatric Annals* **6**, 57–101.

Rowe J.W., Andres R., Tobin J.D., Norris A.H. & Shock N.W. (1976) The effect of age on creatinine clearance in man; a cross sectional and longitudinal study. *Journal of Gerontology* **31**, 155–63.

Russell G.N., Wright E.L., Fox M.A., Douglas E.J. & Cockshott I.D. (1989) Propofol–fentanyl anesthesia for coronary artery surgery and cardiopulmonary bypass. *Anaesthesia* **44**, 205–8.

Santos A.L. & Gelperin A. (1975) Surgical mortality in the elderly. *Journal of the American Geriatrics Society* **23**, 42–6.

Sawin C.T., Castelli W.P., Hershman J.M., MacNamara P. & Bucharach P. (1985) The aging thyroid; thyroid deficiency in the Framingham study. *Archives of Internal Medicine* **145**, 1386–8.

Schmucker D.L. & Wang R.K. (1980) Effect of animal age and phenobarbital on rat liver glucose-6-phosphatase activity. *Experimental Gerontology* **15**, 7–13.

Schwartz A.E., Tuttle R.H. & Poppers P.J. (1989) Electroencephalographic burst suppression in elderly and young patients anesthetized with isoflurane. *Anesthesia and Analgesia* **68**, 9–12.

Sear J.W. (1983) The effect of age on recovery; a comparison of the kinetics of thiopentone and althesin. *Anaesthesia* **38**, 1158–61.

Shanor S.P., Van Hees G.R., Baart N., Frdos E.G. & Foldes F.F. (1961) The influence of age and sex on human plasma and red cell cholinesterase. *American Journal of Medical Sciences* **242**, 357–61.

Silverberg P.A., Matteo R.S. & Ornstein E. (1986) Pharmacokinetics and pharmacodynamics of edrophonium in the elderly. *Anesthesia and Analgesia* **65**, 142S.

Smart R.F. (1984) Endoscopic injection of the vasoconstrictor ornithine-8-vasopressin transurethral resection. *British Journal of Urology* **56**, 191−7.

Sonntag H., Donath U., Hillebrand W., Merin R.G. & Raoke J. (1978) Left ventricular function in conscious man during halothane anesthesia. *Anesthesiology* **48**, 320−4.

Sorbini C.A., Grassi V., Solinas E. & Muiesan G. (1968) Arterial oxygen tension in relation to age in healthy subjects. *Respiration* **25**, 3−13.

Stanski D.R. & Maitre P.O. (1990) Population pharmacokinetics and pharmacodynamics of thiopental: the effects of age revisited. *Anesthesiology* **72**, 412−22.

Stanski D.R., Greenblatt D.J. & Lowenstein E. (1978) Kinetics of intravenous and intramuscular morphine. *Clinical Pharmacology and Therapeutics* **24**, 52−9.

Steen P.A., Tinker J.H. & Tarhan S. (1978) Myocardial reinfarction after anesthesia and surgery. *Journal of the American Medical Association* **239**, 2566−70.

Stefansson T., Wickstrom I. & Haljamae H. (1982) Haemodynamic and metabolic effects of ketamine anaesthesia in the geriatric patient. *Acta Anaesthesiologica Scandinavica* **26**, 371−7.

Steib A., Freys G., Beller J.P. & Curzola U. (1988) Propofol in elderly high risk patients. A comparison of hemodynamic effects with thiopentone during induction of anesthesia. *Anaesthesia* **43**, 1111−14.

Stephen C.R. (1984) The risk of anesthesia and surgery in the geriatric patient. In *Anesthesia and the Geriatric Patient* (Ed. Krechel S.W.) pp. 231−46. Grune and Stratton, Orlando.

Stevens K.M. & Aldrete J.A. (1969) Anesthesia factors affecting surgical morbidity and mortality in the elderly male. *Journal of the American Geriatrics Society* **17**, 659−67.

Stevens W., Dolan W.M., Gibbons R.T., White A., Eger E.I., Miller R.D., De Jong R.H. & Elashoff R.M. (1975) Minimum alveolar concentration (MAC) of isoflurane with and without nitrous oxide in patients of various ages. *Anesthesiology* **42**, 197−200.

Strum D.P., Eger E.I., Unadkat J.D., Johnson B.H. & Carpenter R.L. (1991) Age effects the pharmacokinetics of inhaled anesthetics in humans. *Anesthesia and Analgesia* **73**, 310−18.

Tarnow J., Bruckner J.B., Eberlein H.J., Hess E.W. & Patschke D. (1976) Haemodynamics and myocardial oxygen consumption during isoflurane (forane) anesthesia in geriatric patients. *British Journal of Anaesthesia* **48**, 669−75.

Tenney S.M. & Miller R.M. (1956) Dead space ventilation in old age. *Journal of Applied Physiology* **9**, 321−7.

Tingwald G.R. & Cooperman M. (1982) Inguinal and femoral hernia repair in geriatric patients. *Surgery, Gynecology and Obstetrics* **154**, 704−6.

Tokics L., Brismar B. & Hedenstierna G. (1985) Halothane relaxant anaesthesia in elderly patients. *Acta Anaesthesiologica Scandinavica* **29**, 303−8.

Tollofsrud S.G., Gundersen Y. & Andersen R. (1984) Perioperative hypothermia. *Acta Anaesthesiologica Scandinavica* **28**, 511−15.

Vaughan R.W. & Stephen C.R. (1974) Abdominal and thoracic surgery in adults with ketamine, nitrous oxide and D-tubocurarine. *Anesthesia and Analgesia* **53**, 271−80.

Vaughan M.S., Vaughan R.W. & Cork R.C. (1981) Postoperative hypothermia in adults; relationship of age, anesthesia and shivering to rewarming. *Anesthesia and Analgesia* **60**, 746−51.

Veering B.T.H., Burm A.G.L., van Kleef J.W., Hennis P.J. & Spierdijk J. (1987a) Spinal anesthesia with glucose-free bupivacaine: effects of age on neuronal blockade and pharmacokinetics. *Anesthesia and Analgesia* **66**, 967−70.

Veering B.T.H., Burm A.G.L., van Kleef J.W., Hennis P.J. & Spierdijk J. (1987b) Epidural anesthesia with bupivacaine-effects of age on neural blockade and pharmacokinetics. *Anesthesia and Analgesia* **66**, 589−93.

Veering B.T.H., Burm A.G.L. & Spierdijk J. (1988) Spinal anesthesia with hyperbaric bupivacaine effects of age on neural blockade and pharmacokinetics. *British Journal of Anaesthesia* **60**, 187−94.

Veering B.T.H., Burm A.G.L., Souverijn J.H.M., Serre J.M.P. & Spierdijk J. (1990) The effect of age on the serum concentration of albumin and alpha-1-acid glycoprotein. *British Journal of Clinical Pharmacology* **29**, 201−6.

Vestal R.E., Jue S.G. & Cusack B.J. (1985) Increased risk of adverse drug reactions in the elderly; fact or myth? In *Therapeutics in the Elderly* (Eds O'Malley K. & Waddington J.L.) pp. 97−104. Elsevier Publishers, Amsterdam.

Vlasuk G.P. & Walz F.G. (1982) Liver microsomal polypeptides from fisher-344 rats affected by age, sex and zenobiotic induction. *Archives of Biochemistry and Biophysics* **214**, 248−59.

Weidmann P., Demyttenaere-Bursztein S., Maxwell M.H. & De Lima J. (1975) Effect of aging on plasma renin and aldosterone in normal man. *Kidney International* **8**, 325−33.

Whelan P. & Morris P.J. (1982) Immunological responsiveness after transurethral resection of the prostate; general versus spinal anesthetic. *Clinical and Experimental Immunology* **48**, 611−18.

White P.F. (1982) Comparative evaluation of intravenous agents for rapid sequence induction − thiopental, ketamine and midazolam. *Anesthesiology* **57**, 279−84.

Wickstrom I., Holmberg I. & Stephensson T. (1982) Survival of female geriatric patients after hip fracture surgery; a comparison of five anaesthetic methods. *Acta Anaesthesiologica Scandinavica* **26**, 607−14.

Wilder R.J. & Fishbein R.H. (1961) Operative experiences with patients over 80 years of age. *Surgery, Gynecology and Obstetrics* **113**, 205−12.

Williams J.S. & Hale H.W. (1966) The advisability of inguinal herniorrhaphy in the elderly. *Surgery, Gynecology and Obstetrics* **122**, 100−4.

Wong H.Y., Fragen R.J. & Dunn K. (1991) Dose-finding study of intramuscular midazolam preanesthetic medication in the elderly. *Anesthesiology* **74**, 675−9.

Wynne H.A., Cope L.H., Mutch E., Rawlins M.D. & James O.F.W. (1989) The effect of age upon liver volume and apparent liver blood flow in healthy man. *Hepatology* **9**, 297−301.

Young W.L., Backus W., Matteo R.S., Ornstein E. & Diaz J. (1984) Pharmacokinetics and pharmacodynamics of neostigmine in the elderly. *Anesthesiology* **61**, 300A.

Cardiopulmonary Resuscitation

P.J.F.BASKETT

In the majority of hospitals, the anaesthetist is a key member of the resuscitation team and is therefore expected to be conversant with the management of all aspects of acute cardiorespiratory arrest from any cause and regardless of whether the event occurs in the operating room, the coronary or intensive therapy unit, the accident and emergency or radiology department or in the general ward.

Pathophysiology of cardiorespiratory arrest

Primary cardiac cause — 'sudden cardiac death'

A substantial proportion of cases of cardiac arrest result from factors which are primarily cardiac in origin and these are associated frequently with an encouragingly high survival rate given prompt and appropriate resuscitation. The causes include atherosclerosis, coronary artery spasm and, rarely, embolism, valvular heart disease (principally aortic stenosis and mitral regurgitation), cardiomyopathy, myocarditis, bacterial endocarditis, conduction defects such as the Wolff—Parkinson—White syndrome and prolonged atrioventricular block, cardiac tumours and aortic dissection (Eisenberg, 1984).

Of patients presenting with sudden cardiac death, 75% have some degree of coronary artery atherosclerosis, usually with some significant previous history such as an earlier myocardial infarction, heart failure, or angina (Cobb & Werner, 1982). However, sudden cardiac death is by no means associated always with acute myocardial infarction, even in patients with pre-existing coronary artery disease. The commonest presenting rhythm in sudden cardiac death is ventricular fibrillation, and it has been shown in a series of 305 patients presenting with this rhythm that less than 20% had evidence of acute myocardial infarction, only 50% had ST-segment changes and approximately 25% had no ECG changes in the days following resuscitation (Cobb *et al.*, 1980).

The cause of ventricular fibrillation is, therefore, not determinable in every case. Clearly, in the majority, it is associated with localized myocardial ischaemia from atheroma with or without acute infarction but in others such an explanation is not tenable and different factors such as local electrolyte imbalance, platelet abnormalities, psychological stress, or abnormal secretion of neurochemical transmitter substances must be present.

On rare occasions, cardiac arrest results from acute valvular failure associated with cusp prolapse, disintegration of an artificial prosthesis, or cardiac rupture.

Primarily non-cardiac causes

A substantial number of cardiac arrests are primarily a result of non-cardiac causes whereby healthy, or relatively healthy hearts stop because they are starved of vital metabolic requirements or because of a radical disturbance of the metabolic or acid—base environment.

Respiratory failure

Myocardial failure occurs as a result of oxygen deprivation associated with unrespirable atmospheres, obstructed airways, depression or paralysis of mechanical respiratory activity, and pulmonary alveolar and capillary dysfunction. The associated carbon dioxide build-up and depression of pH levels compounds the muscle fibres' distress.

Hypovolaemia

Hypovolaemia causes hypotension and reduced tissue perfusion. The coronary arteries fill during diastole and it is this filling pressure which is crucial to myocardial nutrition and performance. Hypovolaemia may arise as a result of major blood or plasma loss or may be a result of extrusion of fluid from the vascular compartment to the extra- or intracellular spaces.

Metabolic and electrolytic disturbances

In common with all tissues, the heart depends on a particular *milieu intrèrieur* for its satisfactory function. Electrolyte (particularly potassium, calcium and sodium ions) and blood sugar concentrations must remain within relatively narrow limits and in normal balance across the cell membrane. Similarly, pH values are restricted as are the concentrations of sympathetic and parasympathetic hormones and other naturally occurring cardio- and vasoactive substances in blood and tissues.

Temperature

Cardiac rate and force of contraction are reduced by a reduction in temperature. Frequently, ventricular fibrillation (VF) occurs at a core temperature of 28–30°C, but in some patients (particularly children), slow, spontaneous, weak but organized contractions continue until very low temperatures (15–20°C) have been reached. This phenomenon, in conjunction with the cerebral protection conferred by hypothermia, accounts for the reports of survivors of near-drowning incidents who have been known to have been submerged in cold water for periods of up to 40 min.

Drugs and poisons

Cardiorespiratory function is depressed, either directly or indirectly, by a wide variety of drugs and poisons. Some agents act principally on the respiratory system and inflict damage on the myocardium through asphyxia; others act principally on the myocardium, but most anaesthetic, sedative or hypnotic agents exert a combined effect on both systems. Most drugs used in local anaesthesia are profound myocardial depressants attaching themselves to receptors in the cells, thereby impeding normal metabolic function.

Mechanical disruption of cardiac action

From time to time, cardiac arrest occurs as a result of extracardiac mechanical forces which prevent cardiac filling or ejection. These include tension pneumothorax or pneumopericardium, ruptured diaphragm or haemorrhagic cardiac tamponade and massive pulmonary thrombo- or air embolism.

Rhythms associated with cardiac arrest

Ventricular fibrillation

In VF, contraction of the myocardial fibres is no longer co-ordinated to produce forward propulsion of the ventricular contents. Instead, the fibres are activated at random and the ventricle quivers rather than contracts. Contraction of the individual fibres is at first strong (coarse VF) but weakens gradually as ischaemia supervenes (Fig. 64.1). Eventually all contractions cease, producing asystole.

VF occurs most commonly in cardiac arrest associated with pre-existing heart disease and derangement of body core temperature but can also occur with outbursts of sympathetic activity, particularly in the presence of sensitizing agents such as halothane and electric shock. In a significant number of cases, however, the cause remains unproven.

VF is rare in children.

Asystole

Asystole is characterized by complete standstill of the myocardial fibres. All untreated cases of VF end in asystole. Asystole occurs also in a number of patients without being preceded by VF. This may be confused with artifacts (disconnected ECG leads) or very fine VF (Fig. 64.2).

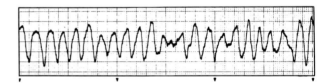

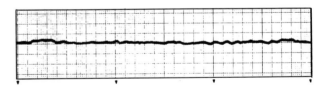

Fig. 64.1 Electrocardiogram showing ventricular fibrillation.

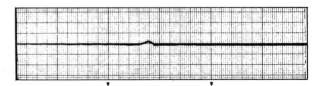

Fig. 64.2 Electrocardiogram showing asystole.

Asystole is associated with massive myocardial ischaemia or selective ischaemia involving the conducting tissues. It occurs in many of arrests from non-cardiac causes, e.g. asphyxia and hypovolaemia. It may be associated also with hyperkalaemia, hypocalcaemia, and extremes of acidosis and alkalosis. It may be provoked more easily during β-adrenergic block, especially if strong parasympathetic activity depresses the function of the sinus or atrioventricular nodes.

Asystole occurs as the primary arrhythmia in approximately 25% of cases of cardiac arrest (Eisenberg, 1984; Camm, 1986). Unlike VF, it carries a grim prognosis and is frequently a terminal unresuscitable event.

Asystole is the most common form of cardiac arrest in children.

Electromechanical dissociation

Electromechanical dissociation (EMD) is a condition of extreme pump failure, producing no cardiac output in the presence of ECG activity which is usually bizarre, but which may appear to be near normal (Fig. 64.3).

Electromechanical dissociation is a relatively rare mode of cardiac arrest and its presence should lead to a suspicion of mechanical embarrassment of the heart from tamponade, pneumothorax, pulmonary or air embolism, or exsanguination. It may occur secondarily to inappropriate drug therapy (e.g. local anaesthetics) or be associated with hypocalcaemia or extremes of pH. From time to time, fine VF degenerates into EMD before terminating in asystole.

Unless a cause can be elucidated rapidly and treated (e.g. tension pneumothorax, postoperative cardiac tamponade), the prognosis for patients with EMD is poor.

Ventricular tachycardia

Ventricular tachycardia may or may not be associated with a cardiac output sufficient to maintain cerebral function. The rhythm is composed of a sequence of bizarre rapid runs of premature ventricular contractions. Cardiac output depends on the rate. Fast rates (over 200/min) do not permit adequate time for ventricular filling. The adequacy of cardiac output can be assessed approximately by whether or not the patient remains conscious. The pulse is notoriously difficult to palpate, particularly at higher rates. Untreated ventricular tachycardia degenerates usually into VF within a few minutes, therefore treatment must be immediate.

Life-support techniques

Resuscitative life-support techniques have been designed to maintain an oxygenated circulation to the vital tissues by artificial means pending restoration of a spontaneous heartbeat and ventilation.

The techniques have been classified under two headings: *'Basic life support'* and *'Advanced life support'*. The concept of the *'Chain of survival'* outlines the sequence needed for successful outcome after cardiorespiratory arrest (Cummins *et al.*, 1991). The chain consists of assessment of the situation by the first bystander who alerts the emergency response system and applies basic life support (BLS) methods. Further links in the chain consist of early defibrillation and advanced life support techniques of airway and ventilation management, venous access and drug therapy. Various flow charts in the appendices at the end of this chapter give guidelines on the sequence of basic and advanced life-support actions.

Basic life support

BLS includes resuscitation techniques which do not rely on any equipment but depend solely on the rescuer's skills and willingness to perform. These techniques are applicable particularly for emergencies occurring outside hospital, but should certainly not be forgotten in hospital practice where they have equal priorities during the early phase of management. Recently, there have been many reports deploring the poor standard of BLS amongst doctors

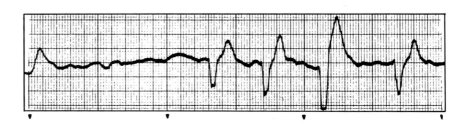

Fig. 64.3 Electrocardiogram showing electromechanical dissociation.

and medical students (Lowenstein *et al.*, 1981; Casey, 1984; Baskett, 1985; Paton, 1985; Skinner *et al.*, 1985).

Advanced life support

Advanced life support (ALS) requires equipment and particular skills. It is designed to provide airway security, sophisticated artificial ventilation and circulatory support whilst restoring a spontaneous heartbeat and respiration.

For convenience, in this chapter BLS and ALS relating to airway management, artificial ventilation and circulatory support are considered together and restoration of spontaneous activity is considered as a separate aspect of ALS.

BLS, as taught to both professionals and laymen, consists of *Assessment*, *Airway* control by manual methods, artificial *Breathing* by the mouth-to-mouth or mouth-to-nose technique, and support of the *Circulation* using external (or closed) chest compressions (ECC). The techniques may be remembered easily by the layman as A, B and C, indicating airway, breathing and circulation.

Assessment

In the emergency outside hospital or in the unmonitored hospital patient, only three requirements need to be satisfied for some form of resuscitation to be initiated.

1 Is the environment safe? (falling masonry, respirable atmosphere, electricity, traffic, etc.).
2 Has the patient suddenly become unrousable?
3 Does the patient look ghastly, i.e. very blue, very pale, or very grey?

Time should not be wasted on further assessment such as pupil size, cardiac auscultation for silence, etc. Help should be called and BLS started immediately.

Airway control

Basic measures

If contamination of the airway is suspected, the mouth should be searched for foreign material using finger sweeps and the head then placed, preferably with the occiput on a small pillow, in the 'sniffing the morning air' position with moderate cervical flexion and extension at the atlanto-occipital joint. If necessary, the tongue can be lifted further forward by chin-lift and jaw-thrust (Fig. 64.4).

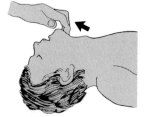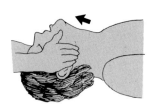

Fig. 64.4 Position for basic airway control.

Special care must clearly be taken with patients with suspected cervical spine injuries to avoid excessive movement, particularly cervical flexion. Nevertheless, the airway is paramount for the patient will surely die without its patency. Jaw thrust is the safest method.

Foreign body airway obstruction can be overcome generally by back blows to the chest with the patient in the recumbent or 'sitting forward' position. If this should fail, subdiaphragmatic abdominal thrusts (the Heimlich manoeuvre) augmented by intermittent finger sweeps may clear the expelled debris. The rescuer should stand behind the victim and place his or her clasped hands below the patient's xiphoid process and above the umbilicus in the midline. Incorrectly performed, the Heimlich manoeuvre may be associated with damage to the thoracic or abdominal viscera.

Once airway patency is assured, the rescuer must look, listen and feel for spontaneous breathing (Fig. 64.5).

If spontaneous breathing occurs, the patient should be 'log-rolled' on his/her side and placed in a stable position by flexing the upper arm and leg. If spontaneous breathing does not occur, artificial ventilation is required immediately.

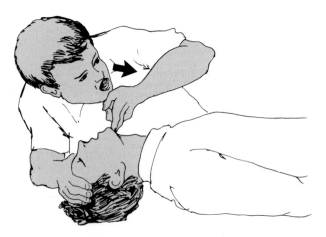

Fig. 64.5 Checking for spontaneous breathing.

Advanced measures

Clearly, the unprotected airway is a great hazard during cardiopulmonary resuscitation (CPR) and the sooner it is secured the better. The airway adjuvants are particularly familiar to the anaesthetist and include such routine items as the oro- and nasopharyngeal airways, the tracheal tube and cricothyrotomy equipment. There is no doubt that the tracheal tube provides the best possible secure airway and tracheal intubation should be accomplished as early and as competently as possible. Tracheal intubation is rarely difficult for the anaesthetist unless there are particular anatomical deformities or maxillofacial injury, but special care is required in patients with potential cervical spinal injuries.

However, tracheal intubation is a skill which takes time to learn and requires regular (though not very frequent) experience to maintain.

As a result, several efforts have been made to produce alternative equipment or techniques which are more simple to teach and acquire. These include the oesophageal obturator airway (OOA), the oesophageal gastric tube airway (OGTA), the laryngeal mask, and the use of a lighted stilete, modified oropharyngeal guide, or manual tactile methods to obviate the problem of user deficiency in manipulating a laryngoscope. Both the OOA and OGTA found initial favour in paramedic practice in certain parts of the USA but have now fallen from vogue, partly because of problems of getting a good mask—face fit, of undiagnosed incorrect placement of the tube in the trachea, oesophageal damage and rupture, and gastric regurgitation and aspiration occurring during insertion or removal. The laryngeal mask is probably the best substitute for tracheal intubation, which is currently available. While not providing an absolute guarantee of protection from aspiration of foreign material in its present form, it is far superior to the alternatives in common practice such as the oro- or nasopharyngeal airways. In addition to offering good airway patency and reasonable security, ventilation can be provided by direct attachment of the bag valve to the mask tube without the need for an airtight fit between the face and a mask (Fig. 64.6).

Artificial ventilation

Basic measures

This may be carried out using the mouth-to-mouth or mouth-to-nose method because manual methods do not work (Norley & Baskett, 1986). Certain

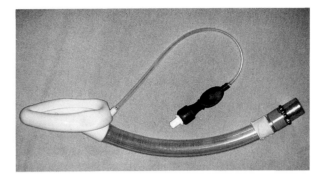

Fig. 64.6 The laryngeal mask airway.

countries have a preference for teaching one method or the other (often depending on cultural beliefs). In the UK and the USA, the mouth-to-mouth method is preferred generally and taught to the lay public. The mouth-to-nose method may give rise to problems in patients with obstructed nasal airways, particularly during expiration, unless the mouth is actively opened during this phase.

One of the commonest complications occurring during resuscitation is gastric regurgitation (Elam et al., 1960; Bjork et al., 1982) and pulmonary aspiration. This is most likely to occur if the airway control is less than perfect and if high inflation pressures are used. The American Heart Association (AHA) standards prior to 1985 demanded that, during two-person CPR, a breath of 800–1200 ml be interposed between every fifth chest compression. Since the rate of chest compressions was deemed to be 60/min, this allowed less than 1 s for the breath of approximately 1 litre and necessitated high inflation pressures to generate such flow rates. Ruben and colleagues (1961) reported that the oesophageal opening pressure was 20–25 cmH$_2$O in curarized adults. Considerably higher pressures than these were generated usually in CPR performed correctly to the old AHA standards (Melker, 1985).

Consequently, teaching has now been modified so that 1.5 s is allowed for each artificial inspiration of approximately 800 ml. For similar reasons, the initial four 'staircase' breath technique, which was recommended formerly, has now been abandoned in favour of two slow initial breaths with the aim of reducing inflation pressures (AHA, 1986). Cricoid pressure performed by professional rescuers reduces also the incidence of gastric reflux (Sellick, 1961).

Advanced measures

Mouth-to-mouth and mouth-to-nose techniques, while having many advantages, have four major disadvantages which should be overcome as quickly as possible in the sequence of events. These include:
1 Low F_1O_2 for the patient.
2 Possibility of cross-infection between the patient and the rescuer.
3 Aesthetic problems for the rescuer.
4 Fatigue for the rescuer.
   Various devices are available to overcome some or all of these disadvantages.

Mouth-to-mask and mouth-to-oropharyngeal airway devices

These devices give reasonable protection against direct physical contact. Some, with built-in oropharyngeal tubes, may help additionally with airway support and others have an additional valve arrangement to divert the patient's exhaled air away from the rescuer. Most unskilled and semi-skilled individuals find them relatively easy to use and certainly more effective than a self-inflating bag—valve—mask arrangement, because two hands can be used to achieve a seal with the face and support the airway. For this reason, they should be available in all patient areas and the technique taught to basic nurses and ancillary hospital staff. The devices have been compared and contrasted in a recent report (Hamer *et al.*, 1986). The author's personal preference is for the mask type, e.g. Laerdal pocket mask (Fig. 64.7), rather than the tube flank type, e.g. Brook airway, because it is easier to obtain a seal.

Self-inflating bag—valve—mask devices (Fig. 64.8)

These are customarily available in first-aid stations, ambulances and in all hospital patient areas. There is no doubt that, used correctly, they provide excellent, temporary, artificial ventilation. However, the skill of achieving an airtight seal and supporting the airway with one hand is not acquired readily by all, and in many cases better ventilation would be given using

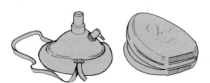

Fig. 64.7 Laerdal pocket mask.

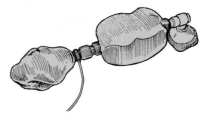

Fig. 64.8 Self-inflating bag—valve—mask devices with oxygen reservoir.

mouth-to-mouth or mouth-to-mask methods. This fact should be emphasized in all teaching programmes. The skill can be acquired reliably only by direct experience with patients in the anaesthetic room and the numbers who require training may create logistic problems. Many self-inflating bag—valve—mask devices are available and there are several excellent models to choose from. Points to look for in selection include:
1 Robust valve construction.
2 Non-perishable bag material with good 'feel'.
3 Standard fittings for face-mask and tracheal tube connectors.
4 Easy disassembly of valve for cleaning.
5 Incorrect reassembly of valve impossible.
6 Oxygen reservoir bag or tube available.
7 Positive end-expiratory pressure (PEEP) valve available.
8 Variable blow-off valve available.
9 Expense.

Automatic resuscitators

Automatic resuscitators have several advantages over manual methods:
1 In the patient without tracheal intubation, two hands are available to maintain the airway and establish a good mask—patient seal.
2 In the patient with tracheal intubation, once the resuscitation pattern is set, ventilation progresses automatically and this frees the anaesthetist for other tasks.
3 A high F_1O_2 is possible.
4 Ventilatory patterns can be consistent and PEEP and blow-off valves can be incorporated.
5 They can operate in contaminated atmospheres.
   However, they have also a number of disadvantages:
1 In the patient without a tracheal tube, the oesophagus is inflated unless the airway is controlled perfectly.

2 They are dependent on a power source, usually compressed gas.

3 Certain types are unsuitable for use during CPR.

Points to look for in selection of the most appropriate model include:

1 Robust construction with reliable valve mechanism.

2 Portability.

3 Appropriate power source availability.

4 Disassembly of parts in contact with patient expirations possible for cleaning with easy foolproof reassembly.

5 Standard fittings.

6 Blow-off and PEEP valves available.

7 Cycling arrangement unaffected by chest compressions — pressure-cycled machines are of no value as they are triggered immediately by chest compressions.

8 Appropriate flow rates — the very high flow rates associated with some manual time-cycled devices lead to a high incidence of gastric inflation and regurgitation.

On the other hand, the flow/pressure characteristics must be sufficiently flexible to ensure adequate ventilation of patients with poor chest compliance and high airway resistance.

Portable automatic resuscitators vary in complexity and versatility. Basic resuscitators are simple straightforward devices suitable for use by nurses and ambulancemen in the early stages of CPR. Transport ventilators allow sophisticated and variable respiratory patterns. The attributes and performance of both groups have been evaluated (Nolan & Baskett, 1992).

Jet ventilation

The concept of providing jet ventilation through a cricothyroid needle has a number of potential advantages when tracheal intubation is difficult, or impossible. The airway can be established rapidly and simply by needle puncture through the cricothyroid membrane and the ventilation system attached easily. Inaccurate needle placement can of course be disastrous, as can obstruction of the airway preventing expiration at or above laryngeal level.

Circulation

Once the airway has been cleared and two breaths delivered, the pulse in the carotid or femoral artery should be checked by gentle palpation over a period of 5–10 s. If the pulse is present, artificial ventilation should continue at a rate of 12/min until respiration

is re-established. If there is no pulse, ECCs should commence without delay and help sought. ECCs consist of rhythmical applications of pressure using the heel of one hand placed over the junction of the upper two-thirds and lower third of the sternum. The other hand is placed on top of the first and the fingers are kept away from the chest wall to minimize damage to the rib cage.

Pressure is applied by the rescuer keeping the elbows locked and the shoulders directly over the hands. The sternum is depressed 4–5 cm in an average adult and proportionately less in children (Fig. 64.9).

Both compression and release should occupy 50% of the cycle and the hands should not be lifted from the chest at any time. The rate should be 80–100/min. Correctly applied, chest compression can produce systemic arterial pressures of 10.6–13.0 kPa (80–100 mmHg), but the diastolic pressure (which determines coronary artery flow) is unlikely to exceed 5.3 kPa (40 mmHg) (AHA, 1986) and blood flow may not match up to optimistic pressure values. Therefore, only very minimal interruptions in chest compressions are acceptable for pulse checking, assessment after defibrillation, etc.

CAB versus ABC

It has been suggested that, in patients with primary cardiac arrest, the sequence of resuscitative efforts should be changed to begin with ECCs and follow with airway clearance and artificial ventilation a minute or so later (Crul et al., 1983). It is argued that the majority of cardiac arrests occur as a result of a primary cardiac cause and that chest compressions are a priority because the blood in the circulation is oxygenated right up to the time of arrest. This is certainly true in the witnessed arrest where the rescuer can be virtually sure of the cause and therefore can be recommended in certain situations attended

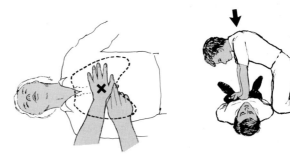

Fig. 64.9 External chest compressions.

by experienced doctors, nurses or paramedic ambulance staff. However, it is not considered appropriate for public education schemes because of the problem of precise diagnosis and is certainly not appropriate for the unwitnessed arrest because oxygen levels have fallen by the time resuscitation is commenced.

The precordial thump

The value of the precordial thump is still a matter for debate. Its use has been associated with reversion to a spontaneous heartbeat in some patients with primary heart disease and VF but in others the rhythm has deteriorated. It is recommended only in witnessed arrests and is not recommended for use by members of the lay public because of the need for precise diagnosis.

Blood flow during cardiopulmonary resuscitation

The technique of ECCs was thought originally to generate a cardiac output by direct compression of the heart between the back of the sternum and the front of the spine and it was assumed the mitral and tricuspid valves closed during the compression phase. This cardiac pump effect is supported by recent studies which have shown higher stroke volumes and better coronary blood flow during ECCs at high rates with intermittent ventilations (Maier *et al.*, 1984).

In a quest for better cardiac output during resuscitation, a group of workers in Baltimore investigated the effects of ventilation on the circulation during resuscitation (Chandra *et al.*, 1980; Rudikoff *et al.*, 1980). They suspected that high intrathoracic pressures might augment blood flow during CPR.

Animals with cardiac arrest (with the trachea intubated) were resuscitated using an automatic ventilator generating high airway pressures [9.3–13.3 kPa (70–100 mmHg)] and a mechanical device to achieve chest compression. These automatic devices were synchronized through a computer system to trigger simultaneously at a rate of 10–40/min with compression and inspiration both lasting for 60% of the cycle. The technique was termed 'new CPR' or 'simultaneous ventilation and compression' (SVC) CPR. New CPR achieved substantially higher blood flow in the common carotid vessels and modest improvements in systemic arterial pressure when compared with conventional CPR using chest compressions (60/min) and interspersed ventilations [10/min at airway pressure of 5.3 kPa (40 mmHg)].

Clearly, intrathoracic pressure had a considerable influence over common carotid blood flow during resuscitation and the question of the mechanism of forward flow during CPR was investigated further. Rudikoff and colleagues (1980) showed that right atrial, pulmonary artery, left ventricular and aortic pressures were almost identical during CPR, suggesting that the heart was acting as a simple conduit rather than a pump. The intrathoracic pressure changes were reflected within the thick-walled common carotid arteries, but much less so in the internal jugular veins. This suggested that venous collapse occurred at the thoracic inlet during peaks of intrathoracic pressure, so allowing forward flow. Rosborough and colleagues (1980), using angiography, demonstrated bicuspid valves at the thoracic inlet veins which closed during rapid rises in intrathoracic pressure but which remained open during more gradual increases in venous pressure (e.g. congestive heart failure). Niemann's group (Niemann *et al.*, 1979) confirmed also a passive role for the heart during new CPR with forward flow being generated by lung inflations. They also demonstrated similar differences between extrathoracic and intrathoracic venous system pressure during periods of high intrathoracic pressure, although there was some reflux through the inferior vena cava.

Rudikoff and colleagues also (1980) also demonstrated the value of abdominal binding in dogs, suggesting that reducing the movement of the diaphragm and the peripheral venous capacity of the lower half of the body enhanced blood flow to the upper half. Confirmation of the value of abdominal binding has also been reported in human subjects (Chandra *et al.*, 1981). Further support for the thoracic pump effect has come from studies of 'Cough CPR' by Criley and colleagues (1976), who showed that rhythmical coughing was able to sustain consciousness in patients in cardiac arrest for 1–2 min.

However, the authors of these papers relating to new CPR responsibly pointed out that their results could not necessarily be translated into human clinical practice. Most of the work has been performed on dogs which have a very different chest configuration to humans. ECCs are known to be relatively ineffective in dogs, but these animals may respond better to high inflation pressures than humans during CPR. On the other hand, the human barrel-shaped chest may be more conducive to effective ECCs. High intrathoracic pressures clearly reduce aortic diastolic pressure upon which coronary flow depends.

While better common carotid flows have been demonstrated during new CPR, there has not been confirmation that this is matched by a similar improvement in cerebral blood flow. There has been no sizeable study in humans which can demonstrate an improvement in survival using the new methods.

Finally, there are serious practical difficulties of introducing some of the laboratory techniques into routine clinical practice. Simultaneous ventilation and compressions cannot be practised using manual chest compressions in the patient without tracheal intubation. Abdominal binding, using pneumatic counterpressure suits [medical antishock trousers (MAST)] may be helpful (Bircher et al., 1980), but this has not yet been proven in human clinical practice.

During the decompression phase of standard CPR, the elasticity of the chest contributes very little to improving blood flow. Prompted by an unusual case report describing a successful cardiac resuscitation using a toilet plunger applied to the chest wall (Lurie et al., 1990), a group at San Francisco General Hospital have developed a simple CPR method which uses a hand-held suction device to actively compress and expand the chest. The active compression–decompression (ACD) device is applied to the mid-sternum. Preliminary studies in animals and humans have shown that in comparison with standard CPR, ACD resuscitation produces a significant improvement in cardiac output and ventilation (Cohen et al., 1992).

The ACD device comprises a rubber suction head, bellows and handle. The handle is a circular disc with a cushioned upper surface for compression and an undercut grip for decompression. The handle is designed to prevent tilting during compression. The ACD device has a built in monitoring system to ensure a 1.5–2 in depth of compression. Differences in chest hair or contour, and excessive sweating do not significantly affect the ability of the ACD device to generate adequate suction.

ACD resuscitation has been compared to standard methods of CPR in 10 humans during cardiac arrest (Cohen et al., 1992). Use of the ACD resuscitator resulted in significant increases in end-tidal carbon dioxide ($ETCO_2$), systolic arterial pressure, and diastolic filling times and a significant reduction in reverse flow within the heart during compression. The authors speculated that during active decompression with the ACD device, marked negative intrathoracic pressures are produced, resulting in an increase in venous return. Furthermore, in intubated patients, physiological levels of ventilation were achieved (80 ml/compression).

The increase in cardiac output produced by ACD CPR should result in improved cerebral perfusion and therefore, better long-term survival. Large studies will be necessary in order to prove a significant improvement in long-term outcome.

Open-chest cardiac compression has been recommended also as being haemodynamically superior to closed-chest methods (Bircher et al., 1980), but outcome studies in patients with cardiac arrest from non-traumatic causes have not demonstrated significant improvement in survival (Geehr & Lewis, 1986). Bearing in mind the enormous practical difficulties associated with the method, it is reasonable to reserve it for those with specific indications, such as cardiac tamponade, etc. (Robertson, 1991).

Current recommendations

Therefore, the guidelines by such organizations as the European Resuscitation Council, the AHA, the World Federation of Societies of Anaesthesiologists, the European Academy of Anaesthesiology, the Australian Resuscitation Council and the Resuscitation Council (UK) continue to recommend conventional CPR techniques using external chest compressions at a rate of 80/min, with a compression phase of at least 50% of the cycle combined with a ventilation interposed after every fifth compression in two-person CPR. They emphasize that care should be taken not to increase inflation pressures in the patient without tracheal intubation for fear of causing gastric regurgitation but, in patients with tracheal intubation, high intrathoracic pressures, even intermittently, may be valuable in boosting blood flow.

Restoration of spontaneous heartbeat

The aim of CPR is of course to re-establish a spontaneous heartbeat as soon as possible. This almost always involves advanced skills and sophisticated equipment. Hopes of survival generally fade unless a spontaneous cardiac output can be restored in 15–30 min, except in cases of hypothermia and poisoning by sedative, hypnotic, or opioid agents.

Defibrillation

The big life-saving factors in CPR are undoubtedly prompt BLS and early defibrillation. Once VF has deteriorated into asystole, the outlook is generally abysmal. To achieve really good results, defibrillation should be attempted within 2–4 min of the arrest. Good BLS has been estimated to 'buy' a further 4–5 min (Ritter et al., 1985), making a total of 6–9 min before survival figures decline exponentially (Weaver et al., 1986). The sooner defibrillation can be applied after the diagnosis of VF the better the outcome. It is therefore reasonable to work towards the day that every frontline ambulance should carry a defibrillator with someone who is capable of interpreting an ECG trace and operating the apparatus. Similarly, every nurse who is deemed fit to be placed in charge of a ward or department should be able to defibrillate in the correct circumstances. A survey has shown clearly that in hospital the majority of patients who survive cardiac arrest do so as a result of prompt BLS and defibrillation by nurses acting before the doctors arrive (Sowden et al., 1984).

Defibrillation acts by delivering a substantial electrical impulse (measured in Joules) to the heart, through paddles or large adhesive electrodes applied to the chest wall, causing simultaneous depolarization of all myocardial cells that are capable of it. After a short time the normal cardiac impulse reappears through the conducting pathways and coordinated myocardial contraction is re-established.

Manual defibrillators

Modern defibrillators are generally powered by rechargeable batteries, but some work directly from mains electricity. The rechargeable type is flexible in that it can operate in any environment but is dependent on responsible personnel ensuring that the batteries are kept fully charged. Those designed to work from mains electricity are clearly dependent on the adjacent availability of a power point, but may be eminently suitable for such sites as the operating room and critical care areas. Some defibrillators are capable of operating from either mains or battery. Modern technology has ensured that defibrillators have become relatively miniaturized so that now all are readily portable.

The controls of the modern defibrillator are simple but each model varies somewhat in the siting of these controls and it is therefore vital to be familiar with the operation of any individual machine before being called upon to use it in an emergency.

The controls consist of:

1 An on/off switch.

2 A Joules setting control which determines the amount of energy to be delivered. Calibration points indicate delivered energy and settings are generally marked at 80 J, 160 J and 320 J or 360 J.

3 A 'charge' button which may be situated on the defibrillator or on one of the paddles or may be duplicated on both. Operating this button places the apparatus in readiness to deliver the shock.

4 Discharge buttons are situated generally on each of the paddle electrodes and are pressed simultaneously to deliver the shock. The paddles should be designed to protect the operator from electric shock. Defibrillators designed solely for internal use (e.g. in cardiac surgery) have the discharge button incorporated in the machine, rather than the paddles.

The majority of defibrillators designed for prehospital and general hospital use (as opposed to operating room) have an ECG oscilloscope incorporated. The patient's ECG can be transmitted to the oscilloscope from the defibrillator paddle electrodes. Most ECG defibrillators have also a facility for monitoring the ECG trace through a conventional three-lead system after spontaneous activity has returned. In some machines there is a switch to select if the paddle route or conventional lead system is operative. In others, insertion of the conventional leads into the apparatus overrides input from the paddle electrodes automatically. It is vital that the operator should be aware of which system is 'live'; otherwise he or she may diagnose asystole inaccurately if applying paddles when the system is switched to 'leads'.

The oscilloscope may take 10 s to 'recover' after delivery of a defibrillatory shock, thus, no interpretation is possible during this period, and chest compressions should be continued until the trace is interpretable again.

Some ECG–defibrillators have a paper-recording facility which can be operated manually or may be triggered automatically by the energy-select control.

To defibrillate patients with rhythms such as refractory atrial fibrillation and preferably (but not essentially) to convert ventricular tachycardia and supraventricular tachyarrhythmias, the energy should be delivered precisely at the top of the R-wave of the ECG. Clearly, this is impossible using manual control so many ECG–defibrillators have a 'synchronize' facility which delays the application of the shock until the next R-wave arrives, regardless of when the operator presses the discharge buttons. The operator, when using the defibrillator to convert VF, must ensure that machines with this facility are in the 'manual', rather than the 'synchronize', position, otherwise the delivery of the shock is delayed awaiting the arrival of a non-existent R-wave.

Paddle placement

For defibrillation, one electrode should be placed below the right clavicle and the other just outside the cardiac apex (V_4/V_5 position) (Fig. 64.10).

The polarity of the paddles is not important for defibrillation and therefore they are interchangeable.

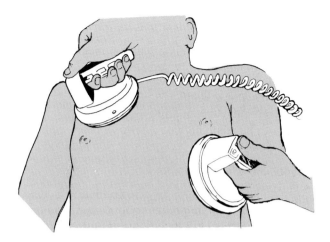

Fig. 64.10 Placing of electrodes for defibrillation.

The paddles should be placed firmly [11.25 kg (25 lb) pressure] on the chest using conductive gel pads or electrode jelly. The latter is less satisfactory as it tends to be spread across the chest wall during resuscitative efforts. If this happens, the delivered shock then arcs across the chest wall, often inflicting a surface burn, and failing to reach the heart. If conventional paddle positions are unsuccessful, anterior–posterior positions may be tried.

Defibrillators are now available, which are becoming increasingly sophisticated. Some offer a computerized facility, which provides for an initial self-check on batteries and satisfactory operation and will record also time, date, Joules delivered and transthoracic impedance through an automatic recording system.

Automated external defibrillators are now available and have brought defibrillation into the role of ambulancemen and nurses on a widespread basis. In these machines, the ECG trace is monitored and analysed through large (10 cm) adhesive electrodes. Should VF occur, the defibrillator is automatically charged to preset energy levels using a built-in algorithm system. In the semi-automatic type, the information is given on a visual display and the final delivery of the shock is carried out manually. In the fully automatic system, the operator is given an audible warning through a voice synthesizer and defibrillation occurs automatically after 15 s unless the system is overridden manually.

These systems have great potential appeal for use by personnel who may not be fully trained in ECG interpretation, e.g. basic ambulance staff, airline and railway personnel, marshalls in sports arenas, managers of large shopping complexes and intelligent relatives of patients particularly at risk. They have proved reliable in that they do not make 'errors of commission', i.e. they do not defibrillate except in patients with VF. However, they may make errors of 'omission' in patients with very fine VF, which may be mistaken for asystole.

The transoesophageal route for defibrillation has been described for patients at risk in critical care units (Aadgey *et al.*, 1991). The probe is left *in situ* in the oesophagus at cardiac level. Defibrillation can be accomplished swiftly in the monitored patient using considerably less electrical energy.

Implantable defibrillators are available now and, after being assessed in a few centres, are being used in individuals specially at risk (Mirowski *et al.*, 1980). The tiny defibrillator (approximately the same size as an implanted pacemaker) is implanted into the thoracic cavity. The cardiac electrodes sense both VF and ventricular tachycardia and deliver a shock of 10–20 J automatically. The process is said to be painless and some patients have been unaware that the device has operated.

Despite such sophistication borne of modern technology, there is now more than ever a place for the small, simple and inexpensive apparatus. It is apparent now that early defibrillation in VF has enormous potential in treating sudden cardiac death. The only way that such potential can be realized is by a much more widespread availability of defibrillators in ambulances, places of work, and even in certain homes. They must be relatively cheap and therefore may not have an ECG facility. Because asystole and EMD carry such a dismal prognosis, there is a good case for blind defibrillation of all patients with clinical cardiac arrest if an ECG trace is not available immediately. Defibrillation does not alter apparently the gloomy prognosis of asystole and EMD but increases survival rates substantially in patients with VF.

Defibrillation energy requirements

Although there have been advocates pressing industry to make defibrillators with higher-energy outputs than 360 J (delivered), clinical evidence does not support the use of much higher energy levels. A decade ago, the AHA recommended 6.0 J/kg (4.8 J/kg delivered) (Parker, 1975) and if this recommendation were followed, most machines would be inadequate for all patients over 70 kg. However, others from Belfast and Virginia have disputed the need for such high-energy levels and produced evidence from prospective series (Pantridge *et al.*, 1975; Gascho *et al.*, 1979) to show clearly that energy levels between 60 and 300 J (delivered) defibrillated 95—99% of those who were convertible. Furthermore, several patients weighing over 100 kg were defibrillated with modest energy outputs. Therefore, it would seem that apparatus currently available is offering energy in the correct range. Higher-energy application may well be counterproductive by causing myocardial damage (Crompton, 1980). It must be remembered that not all patients in VF will defibrillate and the cause is more likely to be from hypoxia, electrolyte or pH disturbance, etc. than a need for higher-energy shocks.

The European Resuscitation Council, the Resuscitation Council (UK) and the AHA have issued guidelines for energy settings to be used in defibrillation and these are in broad agreement.

Details of the sequence to be followed are included in the ALS algorithm in Appendix 2 at the end of this chapter.

Cardiac pacing

Cardiac pacing has very limited application in the management of patients with cardiac arrest. It can be effective when applied immediately to patients with asystole from sudden predominant failure of the sinus—node discharge or atrioventricular block, but is not likely to be successful in patients with extensive myocardial or systemic derangement (Camm, 1986).

The transvenous route takes time to establish and interferes with other resuscitative efforts and so recently attention has been turned to the use of rapid, less invasive methods using transoesophageal and large cutaneous adhesive transthoracic electrodes.

The transoesophageal route has met with some success but capture is dependent on the electrode position and these tend to move easily. The transthoracic route has some appeal also but may be painful and results have not yet been very encouraging, particularly within the prehospital situation (Paris et al., 1985).

Drug therapy

Drug therapy plays a major part in the management of many cardiorespiratory arrests. In this section discussion is confined to drugs used in the immediate resuscitation period. For a summary of the indications and doses for each agent the reader is referred to the end of this section.

Pharmacological considerations

The drugs used during resuscitation include:
1 Sympathomimetic vasopressors.
2 Vagolytic agents.
3 Antiarrhythmic agents.
4 Calcium and calcium antagonists.
5 Sodium bicarbonate.

Sympathomimetic vasopressors

Sympathomimetic agents are used primarily as vasopressor agents to improve cerebral and coronary perfusion, particularly by increasing aortic diastolic pressure. Adrenaline is acknowledged generally as the agent of choice at the present time, principally by virtue of its powerful α-agonistic action. Other α-adrenergic agonists such as phenylephrine, methoxamine and metaraminol produce good results also (Redding & Pearson, 1963). However, adrenaline has also β-adrenergic agonist activity which might be thought valuable in improving cardiac excitation and contractility. Against this potential benefit must be balanced the increased oxygen demand of β-agonist activity and pure beta agonists such as isoprenaline have fallen from popularity for this reason.

At the time of cardiac arrest, the principal requirement is for vasopressor activity with a degree of stimulation of the heart's action and adrenaline would appear still to be the drug of choice for patients with asystole and fading fine VF. Recently, it has been shown that the doses of adrenaline previously advocated should be revised upwards (Lindner, 1991). If the initial 1 mg fails to be effective, then further increments of 1 mg should be given. Once the heart has restarted, beta stimulation should be minimized to reduce myocardial oxygen demands, and dopamine in modest dosage has replaced the more powerful isoprenaline, which should be retained for cases with refractory heart block. Dopamine in high dosage, 40 mg i.v., has a strong α-adrenergic agonistic action and may be useful during initial resuscitation. Therefore, this drug potentially could be used during resuscitation and the postresuscitation period (Yakaitis, 1983). For the present, however, the recommendation must be adrenaline for the resuscitation period and dopamine for support afterwards.

Vagolytic agents

Atropine has been recommended as a first-line treatment for cardiac asystole. The basis for this suggestion is that excessive parasympathetic outburst can cause sinus arrest and clearly, atropine is the first drug of choice under such conditions. Parasympathetic hyperexcitation can occur during cardiac catheterization, carotid sinus stimulation, and ocular muscle stretching, and is associated also with certain drugs used commonly in anaesthesia, such as neostigmine, suxamethonium, etc. It has been argued that those patients who survive asystole do so because the cause was excessive parasympathetic activity and therefore atropine should be administered first. However, it is likely that the majority of patients develop asystole without significant parasympathetic influence and they should therefore be given the vasopressor benefits of adrenaline as soon as possible without waiting for the results of atropine therapy. It has been pointed out that there has been no significant study of the effects of atropine given alone during resuscitation (Yakaitis, 1983). Atropine is indicated for the treatment of severe bradycardia accompanied by serious hypotension because it improves sinoatrial excitation and atrioventricular conduction. The drug should be given cautiously in boluses of 0.5 mg until a satisfactory cardiac output is achieved. Excessive dosage causes tachycardia and increased myocardial work and oxygen consumption and may give rise to arrhythmias.

Antiarrhythmic agents

Lignocaine is the first choice agent in the control of multifocal premature ventricular contractions and ventricular tachycardia. It suppresses re-entrant arrhythmias. The drug appears to work satisfactorily in the presence of a low pH and hyperkalaemia and therefore is particularly suitable for use in cardiac infarction and arrest. Lignocaine is more effective in preventing VF than in enhancing the chances of defibrillation. It should be given to all patients with multifocal premature ventricular contractions and ventricular tachycardias. In established VF which has proved refractory to the initial series of 12 defibrillatory shocks, lignocaine should be given if VF is still brisk or has recurred after temporary conversion. Once conversion occurs, a continuous infusion may be required to suppress superfluous ventricular activity.

Alternative antiarrhythmic agents include procainamide, diphenylhydantoin, disopyramide, mexilitine, tocainamide, amiodarone and britylium tosylate. Apart from procainamide, most have been used to suppress multifocal premature ventricular ectopics and ventricular tachycardia, rather than to aid conversion of established VF.

The agent which is emerging with promising results is bretylium tosylate. In addition to increasing the ventricular fibrillation threshold (VFT), it reduces also the ventricular defibrillation threshold (VDT) and therefore may prove in time to be a more satisfactory drug than lignocaine for the treatment of refractory VF (Nowak et al., 1981; Yakaitis, 1983; Chamberlain, 1991). Amiodarone may also be helpful when other antiarrhythmic drugs have failed to produce successful defibrillation and its lack of cardiac depression makes it a relatively safe alternative (Waller, 1991).

Calcium and calcium antagonists

Calcium enhances myocardial contractility and excitability, and was used frequently in asystole. It has, however, no vasopressor action. It is clear (Yakaitis, 1983) that neither experimental evidence nor clinical experience supports the routine use of calcium during cardiac arrest. Calcium may be of value if there is a clear indication, e.g. hypocalcaemia following massive blood transfusion, hyperkalaemia, or calcium-channel blocker toxicity, but should be reserved for such specific occasions, and possibly for EMD. It is clear that inappropriate calcium administration can be positively harmful to the ailing heart by increasing coronary artery spasm at the same time as raising myocardial oxygen demand, hence extending any area of infarction.

The diminished use of calcium has been underlined by the positive value derived from calcium antagonists which improve coronary artery blood flow and reduce the VFT in patients with myocardial ischaemia. The use of such agents as verapamil and, to a lesser extent, nifedipine and diltiazem in cardiac arrest awaits evaluation but it is likely that their main role is in prevention or in the immediate postarrest phase.

Sodium bicarbonate

The hypoxia and reduced tissue perfusion occurring during cardiac arrest induces metabolic acidosis which in turn creates a hostile environment for attempts to restart the heart. Traditionally, sodium bicarbonate has been given early during resuscitation in an attempt to counter this vicious circle. However, it is clear that enthusiastic administration of bicarbonate is fraught with problems and that great caution should be used in its prescription (Weil *et al.*, 1985). In large doses, bicarbonate may cause hyperosmolality, hypernatraemia and hypercapnia, adding further to the problems of a disturbed *milieu intérieur*. In addition, it may reduce the activity of simultaneously administered catecholamines. The benefits of early administration of bicarbonate are certainly not proven and it is now generally agreed that good ventilation is initially a safer way of correcting the decrease in pH (Chamberlain, 1986). Bicarbonate should be withheld until 15−20 min have elapsed after the onset of cardiac arrest and then given in a dose of only 0.75 mmol/kg (50 ml of 8.4% for a 70-kg adult). Further administration should be guided by the results of arterial blood gas and pH analysis.

It should always be remembered that sodium bicarbonate is a highly irritant drug which causes serious tissue necrosis if injected extravascularly and phlebitis if injected into any but large central veins. Therefore, this agent should always be given through an indwelling cannula or catheter placed in a large vein. The drug should be given from a preloaded syringe and not as an infusion from a large-volume container as inadvertent overdosage can occur easily in the hive of activity which accompanies a resuscitation attempt.

Routes of administration for drugs used during resuscitation

Drugs may be administered by three routes during resuscitation:
1 Intravenous.
2 Intratracheal.
3 Intracardiac.

The intravenous route

This is generally the preferred route of most clinicians but it should be emphasized that central intravenous access is required. Drugs injected into an indwelling cannula on the back of the hand do not find their way rapidly into the circulation during resuscitation. Ideally, the internal or external jugular veins or the femoral vein should be cannulated. This may present technical difficulties, especially if hypovolaemia is present. Chest compressions and ventilation should not be interrupted for more than a few seconds to gain intravenous access. A large vein in the antecubital fossa is acceptable. If possible, a long catheter should be introduced from this point towards the great veins so that drugs can be flushed in reliably to their site of action with 50−100 ml of dextrose 5%.

The intratracheal route

Redding and colleagues (1967) drew attention initially to the intratracheal route for the administration of adrenaline during resuscitation. In the past decade, there has been a resurgence of interest in this route, and a number of other drugs including lignocaine, atropine, phenylephrine and naloxone have been administered by the bronchial and alveolar mucous membranes. Clearly, the intratracheal route, if effective, would be a valuable alternative to the intravenous route when cannulation of a suitable vein proves technically difficult. Drugs given intratracheally should be diluted to a volume of 10 ml in water for injection to increase uptake. Generally speaking, the doses recommended for clinical practice are twice those advocated for intravenous administration. Drugs given intratracheally may have an extended action by continual absorption from the lungs, and this should be remembered when considering further doses. Noradrenaline, sodium bicarbonate and calcium salts should not be given intratracheally because of their damaging effect on the respiratory mucous membrane. The intratracheal route is unsatisfactory in the presence of severe pulmonary oedema.

The tracheal route has been advocated for lignocaine and atropine but unfortunately this route has not proved reliable for the administration of adrenaline (Quinton *et al.*, 1987; Orlowski *et al.*, 1990). This may be due to local pulmonary vasoconstriction impeding absorption or to pulmonary congestion after prolonged resuscitation (Aitkenhead, 1991a). It is to be emphasized that the drug must be injected in a volume of 10 ml through a catheter or nebulizer tube extending below the end of the tracheal tube.

The intracardiac route

This is the least preferred route as there is clearly a significant risk of cardiac or lung damage. There seem to be no advantages of the intracardiac route over the other two available methods and therefore it should be used only as the last resort if intravenous or intratracheal access cannot be achieved.

Summary of the indications and doses of drugs used during resuscitation

Adrenaline

Indications.
1 Asystole.

2 Persistant VF.
Dosage. Intravenously, 1 mg (10 ml of 1/10 000), repeated three times and then consider a 5 mg further dose.

Dopamine

Indications. Postarrest circulatory support.
Dosage. $2-10\,\mu g \cdot kg^{-1} \cdot min^{-1}$ i.v. infusion.

Isoprenaline

Indications. Pre- or postarrest heart block or bradycardia unresponsive to atropine.
Dosage. $100\,\mu g$ i.v. and by infusion containing 2 mg in 50 ml dextrose 5% at a rate to maintain effect.

Atropine

Indications.
1 Asystole thought to be caused by parasympathetic activity.
2 Other cases of asystole after adrenaline has been given.
3 Sinus bradycardia with hypotension and circulatory compromise.
Dosage. 1 mg i.v.

Lignocaine

Indications.
1 Multifocal premature ventricular contractions.
2 Ventricular tachycardia.
3 Lively VF persisting after 12 shocks.
Dosage. 50–100 mg i.v. slow bolus or by infusion of 500 mg in 50 ml dextrose 5% at a rate to maintain effect.

Bretylium tosylate

Indications. As for lignocaine (reserved usually for occasions when lignocaine has failed but may be used as an alternative).
Dosage. 500 mg i.v.

Calcium chloride

Indications.
1 Asystole known to result from hyperkalaemia or hypocalcaemia.
2 EMD if adrenaline fails.
Dosage. 2–5 ml i.v. of 10% solution.

Sodium bicarbonate

Indications. Only after 15–20 min of refractory cardiac arrest.
Dosage. 50 ml i.v. 8.4% solution; 25 ml may be repeated after a further 15-min interval, but it is preferable to measure arterial pH to assess precise requirements.

Postresuscitation care

Although several patients recover quickly with minimal or no sequelae after cardiorespiratory arrest, a significant number have temporary or permanent complications requiring sophisticated intensive therapy. It is outside the scope of this contribution to go into the detailed treatment of single and multiorgan failure which is described in Section V of this book. The aim of this section is merely to provide outline guidance of the management to be followed after careful assessment of the patient who has been resuscitated successfully.

The potential problems

After cardiorespiratory arrest, damage may occur in the brain and other neural tissues and vital organs such as the myocardium, liver, kidney and intestine. This damage may arise as a result of ischaemia, reperfusion injury, or interorgan failure.

Ischaemia

Ischaemia causes an increase in capillary permeability resulting in oedema formation which hampers blood flow further. Poor blood flow encourages microthrombus formation and sludging in small blood vessels. Adenosine triphosphate (ATP) levels decrease dramatically and tissue glucose, especially in the brain, becomes exhausted rapidly. Tissue death follows rapidly.

Reperfusion injury

Damage may occur when oxygen is reintroduced into the ischaemic tissues if cardiopulmonary resuscitation has been successful after a period of circulatory arrest. The injury arises as a result of initial reactive hyperaemia causing oedema, acidosis and release of oxygen-derived free radicals and other toxic agents possibly associated with disturbed calcium homeostasis (Van Reempts, 1985).

Interorgan failure

Failure of one vital organ system is associated almost invariably with an adverse effect on the others. Hypotension, hypoxia, hypercapnia and hyperthermia are particularly damaging.

Immediate postresuscitation care

The following management principles should be followed (Willatts, 1988; Aitkenhead, 1991b).

Support of pulmonary gas exchange with a sufficiently high F_IO_2 to ensure adequate oxygenation using hyperventilation to achieve moderate hypocapnia [$Paco_2$ 4 kPa (30 mmHg)] for 6–8 h using myoneural-blocking agents and sedative infusions. Postresuscitation gastric dilatation, pneumothorax and pericardial tamponade should be sought using chest X-rays and treated immediately.

Cardiovascular support to ensure an adequate cardiac output and appropriate distribution to the vital organs. Normotension should be the aim, achieved by blood volume restoration and inotropic support or vasodilator drugs as required, minimizing myocardial oxygen demands as far as possible.

Cerebral protection. Intracranial pressure increase may be minimized by hyperventilation, hypothermia (35°C) and control of fits (seizures). Most authorities would support the administration of dexamethasone, 12 mg, in the initial period and mannitol may assist also in the reduction of cerebral oedema. After initial hopes (Bleyaert *et al.*, 1978), barbiturate therapy given after the arrest has not been shown to improve outcome by the Brain Resuscitation Clinical Trial I Group (Abramson, 1986). However, it is possible that certain calcium antagonists, such as nimodipine or lidoflazine, may offer some hope of improving brain recovery in the future.

Metabolic control. Acidosis should be avoided — as much by suitable perfusion and ventilation and renal function as possible. Enthusiastic administration of sodium bicarbonate may be fraught with problems and may not lead to the improvement in acidosis expected of it. Other more suitable buffers are being sought. Hyperglycaemia should be controlled by insulin to bring blood glucose concentrations to within normal limits. Variations in serum potassium concentrations can affect cardiac performance

adversely and extremes either way should be corrected, especially if the patient has been digitalized.

Renal support. Oliguria following hypoperfusion may be treated with mannitol, 50 g, and frusemide, 40–120 mg, and, if these fail, by a dopamine infusion up to 5 $\mu g \cdot kg^{-1} \cdot min^{-1}$. Nephrotoxic drugs should be monitored carefully by their blood concentrations. Dialysis should be considered early if the patient's general prognosis warrants it. Clearly, a decision to provide cardiopulmonary resuscitation implies a commitment to provide sophisticated postresuscitation care in an intensive therapy unit (Redmond, 1986).

Risk of infection during resuscitation attempts

With the recent spread of the acquired immune deficiency syndrome (AIDS) and the enormous associated publicity, it is reasonable for would-be rescuers to consider the risk to themselves of performing mouth-to-mouth ventilation for their patients. Although it is impossible to state categorically that cross-infection with the AIDS virus is absolutely impossible, it is possible to state that the likelihood is remote and no documented case has yet been reported. Furthermore, 600 family members of known victims infected with the AIDS virus have been followed up and none developed any serological evidence of infection, despite such intimacies as kissing on the mouth and sharing of cups, eating utensils, razors, towels, facecloths and toothbrushes (Levine, 1986). These numbers exclude sexual partners who, of course, are at risk.

A greater potential risk of infection occurs with the hepatitis B and the herpes viruses and with bacterial contaminants. Guidelines for minimizing risk have been issued by the Department of Health in the UK and the Centre for Disease Control in the USA and it would seem prudent to follow these carefully when dealing with at-risk patients. In resuscitation, this means using mechanical aids for artificial ventilation and taking precautions to avoid contamination with the patient's blood. Since resuscitation is commonplace in hospital, and mouth-to-mouth ventilation is displeasing to most health-care professionals (Wynne, 1986), it would be best to ensure that all in hospitals are taught the use of the mouth-to-mask (or similar) method and that the appropriate equipment should be universally available. However, this should not deter anyone, health-care professional or not, from attempting to resuscitate outside hospital using the mouth-to-mouth method. A life is at stake and the risk is infinitesimal in this environment.

Outcome after resuscitation attempts

Resuscitation is a multidisciplinary activity attracting a variety of specialties. As a result terminology is often confused and there is no uniform pattern or set of definitions which is universally accepted for reporting exerience and outcome. Consequently, it is often difficult to compare presented results.

Representatives from the European Resuscitation Council, the AHA, the Heart and Stroke Foundation of Canada, and the Australian Resuscitation Council have met and produced a glossary of uniform terms and definitions for out-of-hospital resuscitation (Task Force of Representatives, 1991).

Survival rates after resuscitation attempts vary with a number of factors:
1 Interval to BLS.
2 Interval to ALS.
3 Training of responders.
4 Presenting rhythm.
5 Underlying disease process.
6 Age and sex.

Only some of these factors, such as response intervals and training to suitable levels of expertise, are directly within the rescuer's control. Nevertheless, they make a significant difference to outcome. Given excellent training and fast-response intervals, discharge recovery rates exceeding 50% may be expected from patients developing VF in a coronary care unit (Mackintosh et al., 1979). Scott (1981) found recovery to discharge rates significantly less in patients suffering cardiac arrest outside intensive and coronary care units and emergency areas but recorded nevertheless a 28-day survival rate of 24% in patients with VF and 11.5% in patients with asystole. It is interesting to note that resuscitation survival rates were significantly higher in the middle of the day than the night. Sowden and colleagues (1984) reported VF survival rates of 45.7% but results from asystole of 2.3% in patients with myocardial infarction.

Published results seem to indicate that an overall survival rate from cardiac arrest from causes in all hospital environments seems to average 15–20%. These figures could be improved by better training and response intervals and allocation of at-risk patients to areas of high expertise and readily available ALS equipment, together with careful preselection of patients not for resuscitation. Nevertheless,

resuscitation seems to offer reasonable value for money, especially when compared with the cost of other forms of treatment in hospital, and considering that many of the patients who develop VF and recover are relatively young men who frequently live useful lives for many productive years.

Ethical aspects of resuscitation

The possibility of resuscitating someone who has died places a heavy responsibility on the medical profession to select those who should be offered such an opportunity. We must, as far as we are able, try to ensure that the opportunity that we offer is one that the patient and his/her relatives would wish, given that resuscitation attempts do not always have a happy, pain-free and untroubled aftermath.

Resuscitation attempts in the mortally ill do not enhance the dignity and serenity that we all hope for when we die. Death is inevitable for all of us at some time and it is not the role of the medical profession to postpone it for a further spell of misery by virtually prolonging the process of dying. Sadly, all too often resuscitation is begun in patients destined for a few weeks' unhappy existence as cardiac or respiratory cripples or in the terminal, painful throes of untreatable cancer. Ideally, therefore, resuscitation should be reserved for those who have a reasonable prospect of regaining a comfortable and contented existence. Clearly, we are a long way from achieving this ideal with published series revealing discharge survival rates averaging 15–20%.

In most of the series, 40–60% did not respond to initial resuscitation attempts. Although in many, no doubt, the attempts were well and truly justified, in a large proportion the resuscitative efforts were probably inappropriate with hindsight. Sowden and colleagues (1984) reported an incidence of 25% of cases where resuscitation was clearly inappropriate.

The decision not to resuscitate

Three principle problems present when trying to improve selection of cases.

The immediacy of the problem

The emergency resuscitation team has no time to go into details of the patient's history and prognosis. The junior ward nurse, unless specifically instructed not to do so, is obliged to call the team to any patient with cardiorespiratory arrest. He/she is not qualified to certify death. Therefore, the team arrives, rushes into action, and asks questions afterwards (Baskett, 1986).

Failure to predict outcome

There are still large gaps in our expertise at predicting outcome in a large number of individual patients (Older, 1985). Greater accuracy is needed to help selection of cases and it may be that some form of scoring arrangement akin to the acute physiology and chronic health evaluation (APACHE) system (Wagner *et al.*, 1983) would aid in prediction.

Doctor failure

It must be accepted that a number of clinicians fail in their duty to identify clearly those patients unsuitable for resuscitation. Often it is an unwillingness to shoulder such a weighty responsibility and sometimes, regrettably, it is a matter of medical pride in refusing to admit that the patient has reached end-stage disease. There are also those who fear medicolegal recriminations. There is a reluctance to label a mentally alert patient who is nevertheless terminally ill 'not for resuscitation'.

Several factors must influence the decision not to resuscitate, which include:

1 The patient's own wishes.

2 The opinion of the relatives, who may be reporting their own feelings, or the known feelings of a patient who cannot communicate.

3 The patient's prognosis and his/her ability to cope with disablement in one form or another.

4 The patient's social environment.

Generally speaking, clear decisions are made in the atmosphere of close individual clinical supervision of critical care units. In the general wards, however, the potential event may not be discussed in the context of every patient and inappropriate resuscitation may occur.

In the UK, the decision not to resuscitate is generally an informal one made by the clinician in charge of the patient, perhaps consulting one or two of his/her colleagues. The decision may be made at the instigation of others, such as relatives or the nursing staff.

Formal 'do not resuscitate' policies have been introduced in Canada (McPhail *et al.*, 1981) and in the USA (Lo & Steinbrook, 1983). These policies require strict protocols to be followed with formal consul-

tation with patients and/or his/her relatives and the requirement of a second opinion, on request. Correctly, the policy must be reviewed at regular intervals. The concept has the support of the General Council of the Canadian Medical Association (Canadian Medical Association, 1974).

Both formal and informal systems are capable of working and it may be that each country will adopt the most suitable arrangement to its own style of practice, its own doctor−patient relationship and its own medicolegal arrangements.

Organization of a hospital resuscitation service

Each hospital or hospital group should set up a small panel of individuals to consider and review the special resuscitation requirements of their own environment. The panel should consist of senior and junior hospital doctors (usually anaesthetists, cardiologists and emergency physicians), a nurse and a pharmacist, and an administrator, when required. The panel should determine the composition of a resuscitation team and the call-out system, the provision of equipment and its location and arrange for facilities for training of all staff to appropriate levels of competence and audit of results.

Resuscitation teams

All telephones in the hospital should have a priority number to ring in case of emergency. The hospital should arrange to have a resuscitation team capable of attending such an emergency anywhere in the complex at a moment's notice. The team consists normally of an anaesthetist and a physician, a nurse/operating department assistant (ODA), and a porter to bring equipment, as required.

It has been found convenient to use the anaesthetist on duty in the intensive therapy unit (ITU) as the team member. Each member of the team should carry a 'talking' bleep to advise them of the site of the emergency. The message relayed by the hospital switchboard should be repeated at least twice. Members of the team may find it useful to carry their own portable equipment for intravenous infusion, intubation and artificial ventilation in a small emergency case.

Equipment

All patient areas

All patient areas (wards, radiodiagnosis, outpatients, physiotherapy, occupational therapy, etc.) should hold equipment for resuscitation which should include:
1 Pocket masks and self-inflating bag—valve—masks.
2 Tracheal intubation kit.
3 Suction apparatus.
4 Intravenous cannulation and infusion kit.
5 Cardiac arrest drug pack of preloaded syringes.
6 Oxygen therapy facilities.

Ideally, this equipment should be on a trolley which can be brought to any location within the area it serves.

As many departments as possible should have a portable ECG—defibrillator. It is vital not to have to negotiate elevators or stairs to bring an ECG—defibrillator to the scene in view of the urgent need for the apparatus in patients with VF.

Other areas

A spare trolley containing all the above equipment should be available for other areas such as kitchens, administration, etc.

Training

Each hospital should have a resuscitation training room set aside for teaching staff of all grades appropriate resuscitative skills (Baskett *et al.*, 1976, Baskett, 1981). The room should be equipped with audiovisual aids, training manikins, drug packs, ECG simulator and defibrillator. A resuscitation training officer should be appointed specifically to supervise training of staff (Evans, 1986; Wynne, 1986).

The following standards of training need to be achieved:
1 All non-medical and non-nursing staff: BLS and use of the mouth-to-mask method.
2 All nursing and medical staff (including students): BLS and use of the mouth-to-mask method.
3 All medical staff and senior medical students: BLS; use of bag—valve—mask; defibrillation; laryngeal mask airway.
4 All nursing staff in charge of patient departments: BLS; use of bag—valve—mask; defibrillation, laryngeal mask airway.
5 All medical staff working in acute areas, e.g. coronary and intensive care, emergency and operating departments: full ALS.
6 All nursing staff working in acute areas, as above: BLS; use of bag—valve—mask; defibrillation; laryngeal mask airway; intravenous cannulation, and limited drug administration, e.g. adrenaline and atropine.

Acknowledgements

The algorithms (pp. 1340—3) in Appendices 64.3, 64.5 and 64.6 are based broadly on the guidelines produced by the European Resuscitation Council in 1992.

The algorithms in Appendix 64.7 are based on guidelines produced by my colleagues, Dr Jennifer Eaton and Dr Michael Wilson.

Appendices — resuscitation algorithms

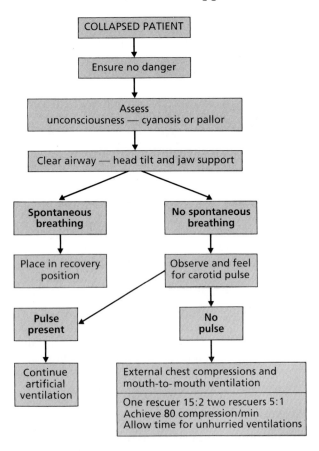

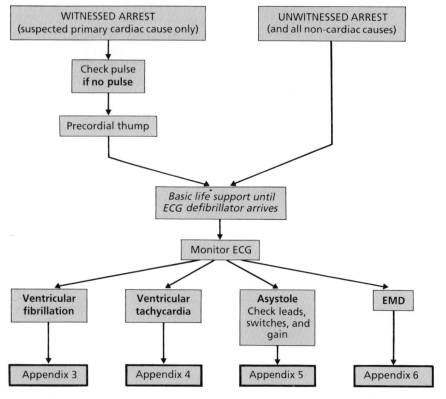

Appendix 64.1 Basic life support.

Appendix 64.2 Advanced life support.

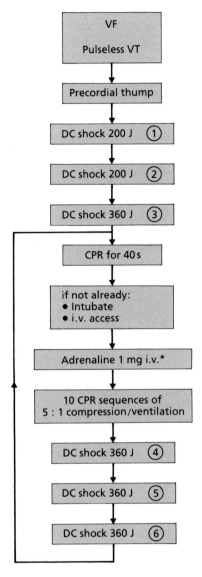

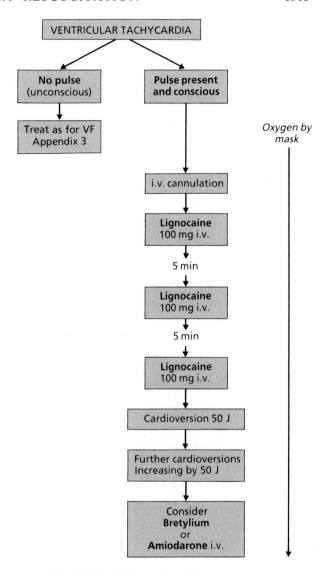

Appendix 64.4 Ventricular tachycardia.

Notes:
I The interval between shocks 3 and 4 should not be >2 min
II Adrenaline given during loop approx. every 2–3 min
III Continue loops for as long as defibrillation is indicated
IV After 3 loops consider:
● Alkalizing agents
● Antiarrhythmic agents

* If an i.v. line cannot be established, consider
giving double or triple doses of adrenaline or
atropine via a tracheal tube

Appendix 64.3 Ventricular fibrillation (VF), pulseless
ventricular tachycardia (VT). [Reproduced with permission of
the European Resuscitation Council (1992) ALS Guidelines.]

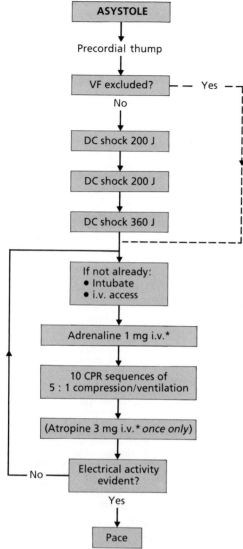

Note:
If no response after 3 cycles, consider high dose adrenaline 5 mg i.v.

* If an i.v. line cannot be established, consider giving double or triple doses of adrenaline or atropine via a tracheal tube

Appendix 64.5 Asystole. [Reproduced with permission of the European Resuscitation Council (1992) ALS Guidelines.]

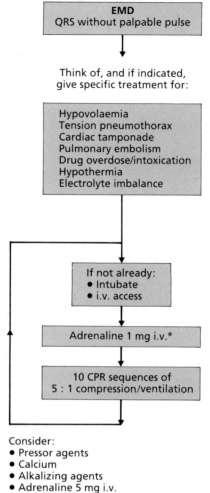

Consider:
• Pressor agents
• Calcium
• Alkalizing agents
• Adrenaline 5 mg i.v.

* If an i.v. line cannot be established, consider giving double or triple doses of adrenaline or atropine via a tracheal tube

Appendix 64.6 Electromechanical dissociation. [Reproduced with permission of the European Resuscitation Council (1992) ALS Guidelines.]

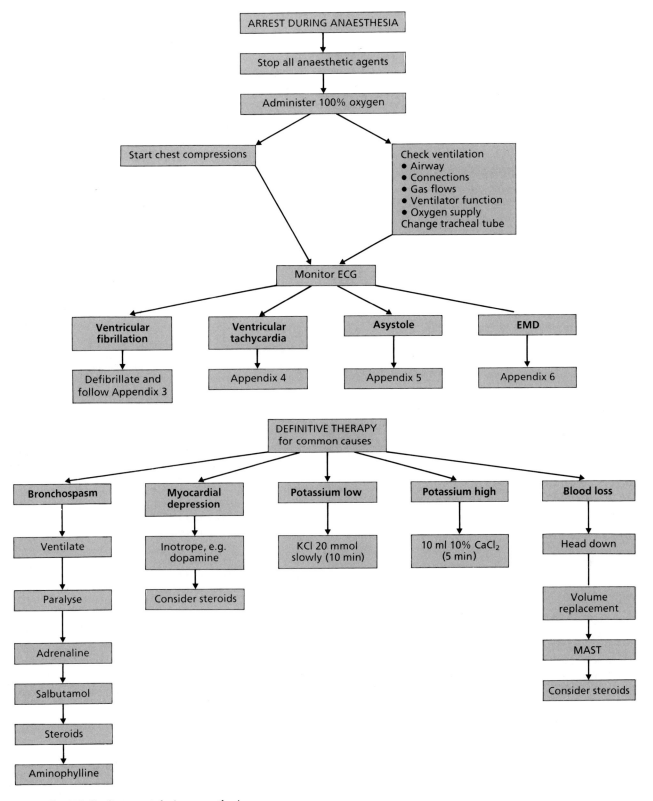

Appendix 64.7 Cardiac arrest during anaesthesia.

References

Aadgey A.A.J., Mckeown P.P. & Anderson J.McC. (1991) Cardioversion and defibrillation: the esophageal approach. In *Update in Intensive Care and Emergency Medicine* (Ed. Vincent J.L.) pp. 34–43. Springer Verlag, Berlin; Heidelberg; New York.

Abramson N.S. (1986) Randomised clinical study of thiopentol loading in comatose survivors of cardiac arrest – Brain Resuscitation Clinical Trial I. *New England Journal of Medicine* **314**, 397–403.

Aitkenhead A.R. (1991a) Drug Administration during CPR: What route? *Resuscitation* **22**, 191–6.

Aitkenhead A.R. (1991b) Cerebral protection after cardiac arrest. *Resuscitation* **22**, 197–202.

American Heart Association (1986) National Conference on Standards and Guidelines for Cardiopulmonary Resuscitation & Emergency Cardiac Care. Standards and Guidelines for Cardiopulmonary Resuscitation & Emergency Cardiac Care 1986. *Journal of the American Medical Association* **255**, 2843–989.

Baskett P.J.F. (1981) The way we teach resuscitation. *Medical Teacher* **3**, 14–19.

Baskett P.J.F. (1985) Resuscitation needed for the curriculum? *British Medical Journal* **290**, 1531–2.

Baskett P.J.F. (1986) The ABC of resuscitation – ethics of resuscitation. *British Medical Journal* **293**, 189–90.

Baskett P.J.F., Lawler P.G.P., Hudson R.B.S., Makepeace A.P. & Cooper C. (1976) Resuscitation teaching room in a district general hospital: concept and practice. *British Medical Journal* **1**, 568–71.

Bircher N., Safar P. & Stewart R. (1980) A comparison of standard, MAST augmented and open chest CPR in dogs. *Critical Care Medicine* **8**, 147–52.

Bjork R.J., Snyder B.D., Champion B.C. & Lorwenson R.B. (1982) Medical complications of cardiopulmonary arrest. *Archives of Internal Medicine* **142**, 500–3.

Bleyaert A.L., Nemoto E.M., Safar P., Stezoski W., Mickell J.J., Moossy S.J. & Rao G.R. (1978) Thiopental amelioration of brain damage after global ischaemia in monkeys. *Anesthesiology* **49**, 390–8.

Camm A.J. (1986) The ABC of resuscitation – asystole and electromechanical dissociation. *British Medical Journal* **292**, 9–10.

Canadian Medical Association (1974) *Proceedings of the Annual Meeting Including the Transactions of the General Council.* Canadian Medical Association, Ottawa.

Casey W.F. (1984) Cardiopulmonary resuscitation – a survey of standards among junior hospital doctors. *Journal of the Royal Society of Medicine* **77**, 921–4.

Chamberlain D. (1986) The ABC of resuscitation–ventricular fibrillation. *British Medical Journal* **292**, 1068–9.

Chamberlain D.A. (1991) Lignocaine and bretylium as adjunct to electrical defibrillation. *Resuscitation* **22**, 153–8.

Chandra N., Rudikoff M. & Weisfeldt M.L. (1980) Simultaneous chest compression and ventilation at high airway pressure during cardiopulmonary resuscitation in man. *Lancet* **1**(8161), 175–8.

Chandra N., Snyder L. & Weisfeldt M.L. (1981) Abdominal binding during CPR in man. *JAMA* **246**(4), 351–3.

Cobb L.A. & Werner J.A. (1982) Predictors and prevention of sudden cardiac death. In *The Heart* (Ed. Hurst J.W.). McGraw, New York.

Cobb L.A., Werner J. & Trobough G. (1980) Sudden cardiac death – a decade's experience with out of hospital resuscitation. *Modern Concepts of Cardiovascular Disease* **49**, 31–6.

Cohen T.J., Tucker K.J. & Lurie K.G. (1992) Active compression decompression resuscitation. A new method of cardiopulmonary resuscitation. *JAMA* **267**, 2916–23.

Criley J.M., Blaufuss A.H. & Kissel G.L. (1976) Cough induced cardiac compression. *Journal of the American Medical Association* **236**, 1246–50.

Crompton R. (1980) Accepted controversial and speculative aspects of ventricular defibrillation. *Progress in Cardiovascular Disease* **23**, 167–86.

Crul J.F., Meursing B.T.J. & Zimmerman A.H.E. (1983) The ABC sequence of cardiopulmonary resuscitation. *Disaster Medicine* **1**, 230–9.

Cummins R.O., Ornato J.P., Thies W.H. & Pepe P.E. (1991) Improving survival from sudden cardiac arrest: the chain of survival concept. *Circulation* **83**, 1832–47.

Eisenberg M.S. (1984) The problem of sudden cardiac death. In *Sudden Cardiac Death in the Community* (Eds Eisenberg M.S., Bergner L. & Hallstrom A.P.) pp. 1–15. Praeger Publications, New York.

Elam J.O., Greene D.G., Schneider M.A., Ruben H.M., Gordon A.S., Horstead R.F., Benson D.W. & Clements J.A. (1960) Head-tilt method of oral resuscitation. *Journal of the American Medical Association* **172**, 812–5.

Evans T.R. (1986) The ABC of resuscitation – resuscitation in hospital. *British Medical Journal* **292**, 1377–9.

Gascho J.A., Crompton R.S. & Sipes J.N. (1979) Energy levels and patient weight in ventricular defibrillation. *Journal of the American Medical Association* **242**, 1380–4.

Geehr E.C. & Lewis F.R. (1986) Failure of open-heart massage to improve survival after pre-hospital non-traumatic cardiac arrest. *New England Journal of Medicine* **314**, 1189–90.

Hamer M., Howells T.H. & Watson R. (1986) A survey of resuscitation ventilatory aids. *Journal of the British Association of Immediate Care* **9**, 31–3.

Levine P.H. (1986) The dilemma of cardiopulmonary resuscitation in patients with HTLV III/LAV infection. *National Faculty Newsletter of the American Heart Association* **9**, 1–2.

Lindner K. (1991) Vasopressor therapy in cardiopulmonary resuscitation. In *Update in Intensive Care and Emergency Medicine* (Ed. Vincent J.-L.) pp. 18–24. Springer Verlag, Berlin; Heidelberg; New York.

Lo B. & Steinbrook R.L. (1983) Deciding whether to resuscitate. *Archives of Internal Medicine* **143**, 1561–3.

Lowenstein S.R., Hansbrough J.F., Libby L.S., Hill D.M., Mountain R.D. & Scroggin C.H. (1981) Cardiopulmonary resuscitation by medical and surgical house officers. *Lancet* **ii**, 679–81.

Lurie K.G., Lindo C. & Chin J. (1990) CPR: the P stands for plumber's helper. *Journal of the American Medical Association* **264**, 1661.

Mackintosh A.F., Crabb M.E., Brennan H., Williams J.H. & Chamberlain D.A. (1979) Hospital resuscitation from ventricular fibrillation in Brighton. *British Medical Journal* **1**, 511–13.

Maier G.W., Tyson G.S. & Olsen C.O. (1984) The physiology of external cardiac massage: high impulse cardiopulmonary resuscitation. *Circulation* **70**, 86–101.

McPhail A., Moore S., O'Connor J. & Woodward C. (1981) One hospital's experience with a 'Do not Resuscitate Policy'. *Canadian Medical Association Journal* **125**, 830–6.

Melker R. (1985) Recommendations for ventilation during cardiopulmonary resuscitation. Time for change? *Critical Care Medicine* **13**, 882–3.

Mirowski M., Reid P.R. & Mower N.M. (1980) Termination of malignant ventricular arrhythmias with an implanted automatic defibrillator in human beings. *New England Journal of Medicine* **303**, 322–4.

Niemann J.T., Garner D., Rosborough J. & Criley J.M. (1979) The mechanism of blood flow in closed chest cardiopulmonary resuscitation (Abstract). *Circulation* **60** (Suppl. 2), 74.

Nolan J.P. & Baskett P.J.F. (1992) Gas powered resuscitators and portable ventilators. *Prehospital and Disaster Medicine* **7**(1), 25–34.

Norley I. & Baskett P.J.F. (1986) Manual methods of artificial respiration — how effective are they? *Journal of the British Association for Immediate Care* **9**, 27–30.

Nowak R.M., Bodmar T.I., Dronan S., Gentzkow G. & Tomlanovich, M.C. (1981) Bretylium tosylate and lidocaine as initial treatment for cardiopulmonary arrest; randomised comparison with placebo. *Annals of Emergency Medicine* **10**, 404–7.

Older P. (1985) Cardiopulmonary resuscitation in hospital. *Medical Journal of Australia* **143**, 432–3.

Orlowski J.P., Gallagher J.M. & Porenibka D.T. (1990) Endotracheal epinephrine is unreliable. *Resuscitation* **2**, 103–13.

Pantridge J.F., Adgey A.A.J., Webb S.W. & Geddes J.S. (1975) Electrical requirements for ventricular defibrillation. *British Medical Journal* **2**, 313–15.

Paris P.M., Stewart R.D., Kaplan R.M. & Whipkery R. (1985) Transcutaneous pacing for bradyasystolic cardiac arrests in prehospital care. *Annals of Emergency Medicine* **14**, 320–3.

Parker M.R. (1975) Defibrillation and synchronised conversion. In *Advanced Cardiac Life Support*. American Heart Association, Dallas.

Paton A. (1985) Resuscitation in hospital: again. *British Medical Journal* **291**, 1445–6.

Quinton D.N., O'Byrne G. & Aitkenhead A.R. (1987) Comparison of endotracheal and peripheral intravenous adrenaline in cardiac arrest. Is the endotracheal route reliable? *Lancet* **1**, 828–9.

Redding J.S. & Pearson J.W. (1963) Evaluation of drugs for cardiac resuscitation. *Anesthesiology* **24**, 203–7.

Redding J.S., Asuncion J.S. & Pearson J.W. (1967) Effective routes of drug administration during cardiac arrest. *Anesthesia and Analgesia* **46**, 253–8.

Redmond A.D. (1986) Post-resuscitation care. *British Medical Journal* **292**, 1447–8.

Ritter G., Wolfe R.A., Goldstern S., Landiz J.R., Vash C.M., Acheson A., Leighton R. & Medendrop S.V. (1985) The effect of bystander CPR on survival out of hospital cardiac arrest victims. *American Heart Journal* **110**, 932–7.

Robertson C. (1991) The value of open chest CPR for non-traumatic cardiac arrest. *Resuscitation* **22**, 203–8.

Ruben H., Knudsen E.J. & Carugati G. (1961) Gastric inflation in relation to airway pressure. *Acta Anaesthesiologica Scandinavica* **5**, 107.

Rudikoff M.T., Maughan W.L., Effron M., Freund P. & Weisfeldt M.L. (1980) Mechanisms of blood flow during cardiopulmonary resuscitation. *Circulation* **61**, 345–52.

Sellick B.A. (1961) Cricoid pressure to control regurgitation of stomach contents during induction of anaesthesia. *Lancet* **ii**, 404–6.

Scott R.P.F. (1981) Cardiac resuscitation in a teaching hospital — a survey of cardiac arrests occurring outside intensive care units and emergency rooms. *Anaesthesia* **36**, 526–30.

Skinner D.V., Camm A.J. & Miles S. (1985) Cardiopulmonary resuscitation. Skills of pre-registration house officers. *British Medical Journal* **290**, 1549–50.

Sowden G.R., Baskett P.J.F. & Robins D.W. (1984) Factors associated with survival and eventual cerebral status following cardiac arrest. *Anaesthesia* **39**, 39–43.

Task Force of Representatives from the European Resuscitation Council, American Heart Association, Heart and Stroke Foundation of Canada, Australian Resuscitation Council (1991) Recommended guidelines for uniform reporting of data from out of hospital cardiac arrest: the 'Utstein' style. *Circulation* **84**, 960–75.

Van Reempts J. (1985) Ischaemic brain injury and cell calcium: morphologic and therapeutic aspects. *American Journal of Emergency Medicine* **14**, 736–42.

Wagner D., Knaus W. & Draper E. (1983) Statistical validation of a severity of illness measure. *American Journal of Public Health* **73**, 878–84.

Waller D.G. (1991). Treatment and prevention of ventricular fibrillation: are there better agents? *Resuscitation* **22**, 159–68.

Weaver W.D., Cobb L.A., Hallstrom A.P., Fahrenbusch C., Copass M. & Ray R. (1986) Factors influencing survival after out of hospital cardiac arrest. *Journal of the American College of Cardiology* **7**, 752–7.

Weil M.H., Trevino R.P. & Racknow E.C. (1985) Sodium bicarbonate during CPR. *Chest* **88**, 487–8.

Willatts S.M. (1989) Post-resuscitation care. In *Cardiopulmonary Resuscitation*. Anaesthesia Monograph Series (Ed. Baskett P.J.F.) pp. 115–33. Elsevier, Amsterdam.

Wynne G. (1986) The ABC of resuscitation — training and retention of skills. *British Medical Journal* **293**, 30–2.

Yakaitis R.W. (1983) *The Pharmacology of Cardiopulmonary Resuscitation in Resuscitation* (Ed. Jackson S.) pp. 69–81. Churchill Livingstone, New York.

Human Immunodeficiency and Hepatitis Viruses

J.F. SEARLE

AIDS

The first reports of the acquired immune deficiency syndrome (AIDS) came from the USA during the summer of 1981 (Gottlieb *et al.*, 1981; Hymes *et al.*, 1981). Young homosexual men presented with Kaposi's sarcoma and pneumonia produced by infection with *Pneumocystis carinii*. Since then, the disease has become an escalating epidemic — 215 000 cases have been reported worldwide in the first 10 years, 126 000 of which have been in the USA. However, the total number of cases is many times more than this. By the end of the century, the World Health Organization estimates that there will be half to three-quarters of a million new cases a year in sub-Saharan Africa and more than a quarter of a million cases in Asia.

The number of reported cases in the UK continues to increase. By September 1991, 5065 cases of AIDS had been reported, of whom 3156 have died. About three new cases are being reported every day. While the epidemic continues to be associated with sexual intercourse between men and intravenous drug abuse, the virus is now endemic in the heterosexual population. Although this has always been the case in Africa, 19% of reported cases in the UK are now occurring in heterosexual adults. There are 69 known cases of children with AIDS in Britain, almost half of whom have died (Communicable Disease Report, 1991a).

The actual number of individuals infected with the AIDS virus is not known, but in the UK it probably exceeds 50 000. During the 10 years from the summer of 1981, 15 712 reports of infected individuals had been made. In 1489 of these, the virus had probably been transmitted through heterosexual intercourse (AIDS Update, 1991).

AIDS is caused by infection with the human immunodeficiency virus (HIV). This was discovered by Barre-Sinoussi and colleagues (1983) at the Institut Pasteur in Paris. HIV is a retrovirus. The genomes of retroviruses encode the enzyme reverse transcriptase, which enables DNA to be transcribed from RNA. HIV can therefore make copies of itself as DNA in host cells, the viral DNA becoming an integrated part of the cell genome. This is the basis of chronic infection and makes the development of an effective and safe antiviral agent extremely difficult. The main target of HIV is the T-helper lymphocyte, thereby rendering the patient profoundly immunologically incompetent.

Clinical features (Adler, 1991)

Infection with HIV causes many different symptoms and signs which may occur to varying degrees over many years.

The seroconversion illness. Infection following exposure to the virus may be asymptomatic. Non-specific symptoms such as sore throat, fever, fatigue, muscle and joint pains and lymphadenopathy may occur. Neurological features have been reported also, caused by an acute, reversible encephalitis, meningitis, myelopathy and neuropathy. The number of people so infected who will eventually develop AIDS is unknown. A majority will probably do so, even though this may not happen for several years.

Persistent generalized lymphadenopathy (PGL). The definition of PGL is enlarged nodes at least 1 cm in diameter, in more than one extrainguinal site that persist for at least 3 months in the absence of any current medication or illness known to cause enlarged nodes. The nodes are symmetrical.

Progression. There are two major clinical features of AIDS — Kaposi's sarcoma and opportunistic infections. Other tumours have been described, namely non-Hodgkin's lymphoma and squamous carcinoma of the mouth, rectum and anus. HIV infection declares itself in many ways. The Centres for Disease Control have classified this range of infections into four groups (Table 65.1). The opportunistic infections which occur are summarized in Table 65.2.

AIDS presents four problems to anaesthetists:

1 The use of zidovudine (AZT) in the treatment of AIDS.
2 AIDS patients who develop respiratory failure.
3 The possibility of anaesthetists and other health care workers being infected with HIV during the course of their work.
4 The anaesthetist with HIV infection and AIDS.

Zidovudine and anaesthesia (Phillips & Spence, 1987)

AZT (3'-azido-3"-deoxythymidine) is used in the treatment of AIDS and acts as a false transmitter for reverse transcriptase thereby preventing HIV incorporating its own DNA copy into the host cell. AZT inhibits host cell DNA polymerase to some degree. It also inhibits the enzyme thymidylate kinase thereby depleting cells of thymidine triphosphate and other pyrimidine bases.

Table 65.1 Summary of classification system for human immunodeficiency virus

Group I	Acute infection
Group II	Asymptomatic
Group III	Persistent generalized lymphadenopathy
Group IV	Other diseases
Subgroup A	Constitutional disease (fever > 1 month, weight loss > 10% baseline, diarrhoea > 1 month)
Subgroup B	Neurological disease (dementia, myelopathy, peripheral neuropathy)
Subgroup C	Secondary infectious diseases C1 Those specified in the surveillance definition of the Centres for Disease Control C2 Others — oral hair leucoplakia, multidermatomal, *Herpes zoster*, recurrent *Salmonella* bacteraemia, nocardiosis, tuberculosis, oral *Candida*
Subgroup D	Secondary cancers (Kaposi's sarcoma, non-Hodgkin's lymphoma, primary cerebral lymphoma)
Subgroup E	Others conditions

Table 65.2 Opportunistic infections in AIDS. (Data from Adler, 1991)

Syndrome	Features	Common organisms			
		Protozoa	Viruses	Bacteria	Fungi
Lung	Cough, shortness of breath, fever, hypoxia, chest X-ray infiltrates	*P. carinii* pneumonia	Cytomegalovirus *Herpes simplex* virus	Mycobacteria Gram-positive *Streptococcus pneumoniae* *Haemophilus influenza* *B. catarrhalis* Group B *Streptococcus*	*Cryptococcus*
Central nervous system	Meningitis/encephalitis or focal signs	Toxoplasma	Cytomegalovirus *Herpes simplex* virus Progressive multifocal leucoencephalopathy	Mycobacteria	*Aspergillus* *Cryptococcus* *Candida*
Gut	Dysphagia High-volume diarrhoea Bloody diarrhoea/colitis	*Cryptosporidium* *Isopora belli* *Microsporidia*	Cytomegalovirus *Herpes simplex* virus	*Myobacterium avium intracellulare* *M. tuberculosis* *Salmonella*	*Candida*
Pyrexia of undetermined origin	Fever, weight loss +/−lymphadenopathy	Consider all pathogens and focal or disseminated infection			

The side-effects of AZT, therefore, are mainly neurological and haematological. The extent of these should be documented fully before embarking upon anaesthesia. The inhibition of DNA polymerase in the bone marrow leads to a neutropenia and a megaloblastic anaemia. This anaemia is more severe if there is B_{12} or folate deficiency. Thus, there is the possibility of an interaction between AZT and nitrous oxide, particularly if nitrous oxide is used for many hours. As yet there is no clinical evidence that this is a significant problem.

The plasma half-life of AZT is approximately 30 min. Thirty-five percent is protein bound. It is metabolized in the liver and excreted actively in the renal tubules. Therefore, AZT may interact with other drugs which are excreted in this way, e.g. morphine, with which it may compete for glucuronic acid conjugation. Zidovudine has no serious cardiovascular side-effects.

Respirature failure in AIDS

Pulmonary disease is part of AIDS as a result of opportunistic infections. In over 80% of cases, the infecting organism is *Pneumocystis carinii*. Kaposi's sarcoma can also involve the lung. An adult respiratory distress syndrome-(ARDS)-type picture has been described, although without the appearance of hyaline membranes and haemorrhages. Multiple pathological processes may be present in the lung.

Some patients with AIDS inevitably develop respiratory failure. Most of these patients are in early or middle adult life and might reasonably expect to receive full intensive care support, including mechanical ventilation. However, they also have a fatal disease. Thus the question of whether or not to subject them to tracheal intubation and mechanical ventilation demands careful consideration.

In the early years of the epidemic, the outcome of mechanical ventilation was universally poor. In its comprehensive report on the pulmonary complications of the disease, the National Heart, Lung and Blood Institute Workshop on AIDS of the USA investigated 102 patients who required tracheal intubation and mechanical ventilation (Murray *et al.*, 1984). Almost all had advanced pneumocystis pneumonia. Eighty-six percent died in hospital, almost all in the intensive therapy unit (ITU). In another study (Stover *et al.*, 1985), 61 patients developed respiratory complications, 22 of whom were treated with mechanical ventilation; all died. In another North American study (Schein *et al.*, 1986), over a period of 18 months, 31 patients had artificial ventilation. Twenty-three of these had parenchymal lung infection (in 20 the

organism was *Pneumocystis carinii*); 21 died in hospital. Of the two survivors, one was weaned from mechanical ventilation 48 h after an open-lung biopsy and one with pneumocystis needed ventilation for only 48 h. Eight patients did not have respiratory failure. Five received ventilation after brain biopsy, one of whom died. Three patients had circulatory failure; two died.

However, more recent reports have shown a considerably better outcome. Survival rates following mechanical ventilation of 54% (Efferen *et al.*, 1989), and 36% (Friedman *et al.*, 1989) can now be achieved. Nevertheless, in both these series the median long-term survival after leaving hospital was less than 1 year. Thus, it may well be that when the matter is discussed with a patient, aggressive intensive therapy should be embarked on. However, the prognosis is very poor if the patient has had respiratory symptoms for more than 4 weeks or the episode of *Pneumocystis carinii* pneumonia is recurrent (Miller & Roberts, 1991).

Acute physiology and chronic health evaluation (APACHE) II underestimates the outcome of patients requiring intensive care for AIDS (Smith *et al.*, 1989). This is probably because of the lack of a specific diagnostic category coefficient for AIDS which accurately reflects the severity of the disease.

Prevention of infection of anaesthetists and other health care workers

The rate at which the 'AIDS epidemic' has increased in the Western World has been slower than was originally predicted, but the number of cases of HIV infection continues to increase. Furthermore, the disease can no longer be thought of as being almost entirely confined to men who have sex with other men and to intravenous drug abusers. The virus is in the heterosexual community. It is inevitable therefore that an increasing number of patients will be anaesthetized who are HIV positive. At the present time the routine testing of patients for HIV antibody without consent is not supported by the World Health Organization, the Department of Health and the General Medical Council. Thus, the HIV status of a vast majority of patients is unknown to hospital staff.

Mode of transmission

HIV has been isolated from many body fluids — saliva, urine, cerebrospinal fluid (CSF), breast milk, tears, amniotic fluid, synovial fluid, blood, semen and vaginal secretions. However, transmission is by blood, sexual contact and transplacentally from the mother to the fetus. The amount of virus in saliva is small and transmission by this route has not been reported.

Unlike the hepatitis B virus, the infectivity of HIV is low. Nevertheless, reported cases worldwide of occupational transmission have risen from five in 1988 to 60 by November 1991 (Communicable Disease Surveillance Centre, 1991b). These 60 cases may be categorized as follows:

1 Cases with documented seroconversion following specific exposure   32
2 Presumptive infection without other exposure   24
3 Other occupational/home care transmission   4

Transmission of the virus most commonly follows a needle-stick injury with a hollow needle. The risk of seroconversion following occupational exposure is 0.3%.

Precautions against occupational transmission

Precautions against occupational transmission have been set out in several publications (Arden, 1986; Gerberding 1986; UK Health Departments 1990; Association of Anaesthetists of Great Britain and Ireland, 1992). As the HIV status of any given patient is unlikely to be known, precautions should be a *routine part of anaesthetic practice*. The extent of these precautions can be categorized according to the risk of exposure to blood. Thus, in major operative procedures, a full range of protective clothing should be worn, i.e. gloves, water-repellant gowns and aprons, head and eye protection and protective footwear and masks. Where the likelihood of contact with blood or blood stained fluids is low, as when giving an intra-muscular injection, only gloves need be worn.

Anaesthesia involves an intermediate level of risk and the following precautions should be a routine part of anaesthetic practice in operating suites, intensive care units, accident departments, wards and during cardiopulmonary resuscitation.

1 Needles must *not* be resheathed. Needles, syringes with needles attached and other 'sharps' should not be handed from one person to another. They should be placed in a tray and then picked up.
2 All needles and sharps should be disposed of in an appropriately tough disposal bin. Cardboard bins are not sufficiently tough to prevent piercing of the wall of the bin.
3 Should a needle-stick injury occur, or a cut or abrasion become contaminated with blood, bleeding should be encouraged and the skin washed thoroughly with soap and water.
4 Whilst intact skin is impermeable to the virus, cuts and abrasions on the anaesthetist's skin which might become contaminated by a patient's blood or body fluid must be covered with a waterproof dressing. Where there are extensive lesions on the hands, e.g. from eczema, chapping or several scratches, gloves should be worn all the time. Particular care should be taken to prevent contamination of such skin with large amounts of blood or blood-stained fluids.
5 Gloves must be worn for performing venepuncture, setting up an intravenous infusion and inserting and removing airways and tracheal tubes. Where substantial spillage of blood may occur as, for example, in setting up an intra-arterial line, a plastic apron, a mask, and eye protection should be worn also.
6 As HIV infection is not airborne, those parts of the breathing system outside the patient do not constitute a risk either to the anaesthetist and his/her assistants or other patients unless they become contamined with blood.
7 Where possible, contaminated equipment should be autoclaved. Where this is not possible, it should be decontaminated with freshly prepared glutaraldehyde, washed thoroughly with soap and water and then left in glutaraldehyde for a further 3 h. Contaminated floors and surfaces should be washed with a 1% solution of freshly prepared sodium hypochlorite.
8 During cardiopulmonary resuscitation, expired air ventilation should be performed through an artificial airway. Ventilation via a tracheal tube should be established at the earliest possible moment.

The anaesthetist with HIV infection and AIDS

Transmission of HIV from an infected anaesthetist to patients

To date (June 1993), there is only one report of transmission of HIV from a health care worker to patients. Five patients in Florida became HIV positive after being treated by a dental surgeon with AIDS (Communicable Disease Report, 1990, 1991a, 1991b). Four studies have been published of patients who have been treated by HIV-positive staff (three surgeons and one dental student). Of the 996 patients, none had seroconverted. The numbers are, however, small (Armstrong et al., 1987; Mishu et al., 1990; Porter et al., 1990; Comer et al., 1991). Clearly, there is a risk of transmission, albeit small, should blood-to-blood contact occur.

There is considerable public anxiety about the possibility of patients being infected by health care workers. The precautions outlined above to prevent patients infecting anaesthetists will also normally prevent transmission in the other direction. However, certain procedures may place patients at risk.

These procedures have been defined as 'surgical entry into tissues, cavities or organs, or repair of major traumatic injuries, cardiac catheterization and angiography, vaginal and Caesarean deliveries and other obstetric procedures during which bleeding may occur; the manipulation, cutting or removal of any oral or perioral tissues including tooth structures during which bleeding may occur' (UK Health Departments, 1993). Thus, an anaesthetist who is HIV positive should not carry out any procedure which involves opening skin or tissues and carries with it the risk of the anaesthetist's blood contaminating the patient's blood.

HIV encephalopathy

Concern has been expressed about the competence of an anaesthetist who is developing an HIV encephalopathy (Association of Anaesthetists of Great Britain and Ireland, 1988). However, the vast majority of HIV encephalopathy presents well into the course of the disease when the patient is too ill to work. An infected anaesthetist should already be under regular medical care during the course of which impairment of mental function will have already been detected.

Patient safety, both from infection by an anaesthetist and errors due to mental impairment depend upon the anaesthetist being under regular medical care. If he/she has any reason to believe that he/she may be infected, appropriate diagnostic testing and advice must be sought (General Medical Council, 1988). A national panel of experts, which includes an anaesthetist, is available to provide infected health care workers with advice about their work and practice.

Hepatitis viruses

The term 'viral hepatitis' refers to disease caused by several different viruses. There are five main types:

Hepatitis A. This is spread by the faecal–oral route. Outbreaks occur following contamination of food and drink. Prevention is therefore a matter of public health and hygiene.

Hepatitis B. Hepatitis B is a major, worldwide health problem. There are more than 200 million carriers throughout the world. In the UK, approximately 2000 cases of hepatitis B infection are notified each year. However, the total number of cases is substantially more than this, as there is considerable underreporting. The longer-term consequences of infection include cirrhosis, chronic active hepatitis, chronic persistent hepatitis and primary liver cancer. More immediately, infection results in an acute illness and/or the carrier state. The carrier state is defined as 'persistence of hepatitis B surface antigen in the circulation for more than 6 months'. It develops in 5–10% of infected adults.

There is widespread global variation in the carrier state. The incidence in the adult population of the UK is about 1:500 (Table 65.3). Individuals who are hepatitis B surface antigen-(HBs Ag)-positive pose a serious risk to health care workers. A patient who is in the early prodromal or acute phase of hepatitis B is also a high risk from the point of view of occupational transmission of the virus. The virus is highly infectious. Although it is found in almost all body fluids, excretions and secretions, transmission is by blood-to-blood and sexual contact. Innoculation can occur

Table 65.3 Incidence of hepatitis B carrier

Area	Hepatitis B	Neonatal infection	Childhood infection
Northern, western and central Europe North America Australia	0.1–0.5%	Rare	Rare
Eastern Europe Former USSR SW Asia Central and southern America	2–7%	Frequent	Frequent
SE Asia China Tropical Africa	8–20%	Very frequent	Very frequent

through minute amounts of blood. The risk of transmission is about 20% following an innoculation accident with HBs Ag-positive blood (Seeff *et al.*, 1978; Werner & Grady, 1982). The virus is not transmitted by inhalation of droplets or by faecal–oral contamination.

Hepatitis C. This is also blood borne and is a cause of post-transfusion hepatitis. Fifty percent of patients infected with the virus develop chronic liver disease. As with hepatitis B, it may be transmitted by blood-to-blood contact during invasive procedures.

Non-A non-B hepatitis. This is currently diagnosed by excluding other causes of hepatitis.

Delta hepatitis. This is caused by a defective transmissible agent. It requires the presence of multiplying hepatitis B virus in order to replicate. Modes of transmission are similar to that of hepatitis B. Infection is found in intravenous drug abusers.

Prevention of occupational transmission of hepatitis B

As transmission occurs through blood-to-blood contact, all the precautions set out under HIV occupational transmission should be strictly adhered to in dealing with a patient in the prodromal or acute phase or who is a 'carrier'.

Immunization

Hepatitis B is a preventable disease. Safe vaccines are available. All anaesthetists (and other health care workers at risk from occupational exposure to the virus) should be actively immunized. The vaccine is 90% effective. A small proportion of the population do not mount an antibody response. Thus, postvaccination screening should be performed 2–4 months after a course of vaccine injections. Non-responders should be given a booster, but even then the response will probably be poor. These individuals need hepatitis B immunoglobulin should they be exposed to the virus.

The duration of protection conferred by modern vaccines is of the order of 3–5 years. It is absolutely essential that all anaesthetists know their state of

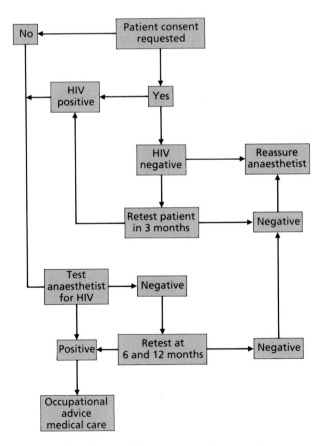

Fig. 65.1 Procedure to follow after possible occupational exposure to HIV.

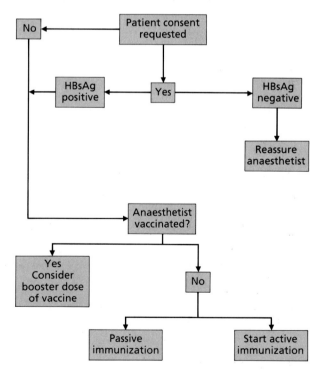

Fig. 65.2 Procedure to follow after possible occupational exposure to hepatitis B.

immunity against hepatitis B and ensure that they are protected in this way against infection.

Management of occupational exposure to HIV and hepatitis B
(UK Health Departments, 1990)

Following possible exposure, the source patient should be identified and interviewed. If there are no risk factors, the anaesthetist can be reassured. However, if the absence of risk factors cannot be established, consent should be sought from the same patient to testing for HIV and HBsAg. The procedures shown in the flow charts should then be followed (Figs 65.1 and 65.2).

The use of prophylactic zidovudine following occupational exposure has been recommended but remains controversial (Brown et al., 1991; Jeffries, 1991).

References

Adler M.W. (Ed.) (1991) Range and natural history of infection. In *ABC of AIDS* pp. 12–13. British Medical Association, London.

AIDS Update (1991) *British Medical Journal* **303**, 208.

Arden J. (1986) Anaesthetic management of patients with AIDS. *Anaesthesiology* **64**, 660–1.

Armstrong F.P., Milner J.C. & Wolfe W.H. (1987) Investigation of a health care worker with symptomatic immunodeficiency virus infection: an epidemiologic approach. *Military Medicine* **152**, 414–18.

Association of Anaesthetists of Great Britain and Ireland (1988) AIDS and Hepatitis B. *Guidelines for Anaesthetists.*

Association of Anaesthetists of Great Britain and Ireland (1992) HIV and other blood-borne viruses. *Guidelines for Anaesthetists.*

Barre-Sinoussi F., Cherman J.C., Rey F. et al. (1983) Isolation of T lymphotropic retrovirus from a patient at risk for acquired immune deficiency syndrome (AIDS). *Science* **220**, 868–71.

Brown E.M., Caul E.O., Roome A.P. et al. (1991) Zidovudine after occupational exposure to HIV. *British Medical Journal* **303**, 990.

Communicable Disease Report (1990) Possible transmission of human immunodeficiency virus to a patient during an invasive dental procedure. *Morbidity and Mortality Weekly Reports* **39**, 489–93.

Communicable Disease Report (1991a) Update: transmission of HIV infection during an invasive dental procedure — Florida. *Morbidity and Mortality Weekly Reports* **40**, 21–7.

Communicable Disease Report (1991b) Update: transmission of HIV during invasive dental procedures — Florida. *Morbidity and Mortality Weekly Reports* **40**, 377–81.

Comer R.W., Myers D.R., Steadman C.D. et al. (1991) Management considerations for an HIV positive dental student. *Journal of Dental Education* **55**, 187–91.

Communicable Disease Surveillance Centre. Public Health Laboratory Service (1991a) Communicable Disease Report. AIDS and HIV-1 infection in the United Kingdom. *Monthly Report* **41**, 185–8.

Communicable Disease Surveillance Centre. Public Health Laboratory Service (1991b) Occupational transmission of HIV. *Summary of Published Reports.* September.

Efferen L.S., Nadarajah D. & Palat D.S. (1989) Survival following mechanical ventilation for *Pneumocystis carinii* pneumonia in patients with the acquired immunodeficiency syndrome. A different perspective. *American Journal of Medicine* **87**, 401–4.

Friedman Y., Franklin C., Rackcow E.C. et al. (1989) Improved survival in patients with AIDS, *Pneumocystis carinii* pneumonia and severe respiratory failure. *Chest* **96**, 862–6.

General Medical Council (1988) HIV infection and AIDS: the ethical considerations.

Gerberding J.L. (1986) Recommended infection control policies for patients with human immunodeficiency virus infection. *New England Journal of Medicine* **315**, 1562–4.

Gottlieb M.S., Schanker H.M., Fan P.T. et al. (1981) Pneumocystis pneumonia — Los Angeles. *Morbidity and Mortality Weekly Report* **30**, 250–2.

Hymes K.B., Greene J.B., Marcus A. et al. (1981) Kaposi's sarcoma in homosexual men — a report of eight cases. *Lancet* **ii**, 598–600.

Jeffries D.J. (1991) Zidovudine after occupational exposure to HIV. *British Medical Journal* **302**, 1349–50.

Miller R.F. & Roberts C.M. (1991) Intensive care management of HIV positive patients and patients with AIDS. *Clinical Intensive Care* **2**, 17–25.

Mishu B., Schaffner W., Horan J.M. et al. (1990) A surgeon with AIDS; lack of evidence of transmission to patients. *Journal of the American Medical Association* **264**, 467–70.

Murray J.F., Felton C.P., Garay S.M. et al. (1984) Pulmonary immunodeficiency syndrome. *New England Journal of Medicine* **310**, 1682–8.

Phillips A.J. & Spence A.A. (1987) Zidovudine and the anaesthetist. *Anaesthesia* **42**, 799–800.

Porter J.D., Cruikshank J.G., Gentle P.H. et al. (1990) Management of patients treated by a surgeon with HIV infection. *Lancet* **335**, 113–14.

Schein R.M.H., Fische M.A., Pitchenik A.E. et al. (1986) ICU survival of patients with the acquired immunodeficiency syndrome. *Critical Care Medicine* **14**, 1026–7.

Seeff L.B., Wright M.P.H., Zimmerman H.J. et al. (1978) Type B hepatitis after needlestick exposure: prevention with hepatitis B immune globulin. *Annals of Internal Medicine* **88**, 285–93.

Smith R.L., Levine S.M. & Lewis M.L. (1989) Prognosis of patients with AIDS requiring intensive care. *Chest* **96**, 857–61.

Stover P.E., White D.A., Romano P.A. et al. (1985) Spectrum of pulmonary diseases associated with the acquired immune deficiency syndrome. *American Journal of Medicine* **78**, 429–37.

UK Health Department (1990) *Guidelines for Clinical Health Care Workers: Protection Against Infection with HIV and Hepatitis Viruses.* HMSO, London.

UK Health Departments (1993) *AIDS-HIV Infected Health Care Workers. Occupational Advice for Health Care Workers, Their Physicians and Employers.*

Werner B.G. & Grady G.F. (1982) Accidental hepatitis B — surface antigen positive innoculations. *Annals of Internal Medicine* **97**, 367–9.

SECTION III
LOCAL ANAESTHESIA

Local Anaesthetic Drugs: Mode of Action and Pharmacokinetics

G.T. TUCKER

Local anaesthetics cause reversible block of the conduction of impulses in the peripheral nervous system. An understanding of the principles involved in the movement of these compounds to and from their sites of action in nerves, their interaction with the axonal membrane, and the factors controlling their eventual removal from the body is essential to the practice of effective and safe regional anaesthesia. This chapter will consider the interrelationships between the chemical structure and physicochemical properties of these drugs and their mechanism of action and pharmacokinetic characteristics.

Chemical structure

A variety of chemicals are capable of blocking nerve conduction. Most of the clinically useful local anaesthetics conform to a structural sequence consisting of an aromatic ring linked by a carbonyl-containing moiety through a carbon chain to a substituted amino group (Table 66.1). The total length of the molecules is about 1.5 nm, and they are amphipathic in nature, i.e. partly lipophilic and partly hydrophilic.

For the purpose of classifying the different agents, the most important feature is the nature of the carbonyl-containing linkage group. Thus, the ester-type agents include cocaine, benzocaine, procaine, 2-chloroprocaine and amethocaine, whilst the amides include lignocaine, prilocaine, mepivacaine, bupivacaine and etidocaine. Cinchocaine is also an amide but with the group inserted the other way round, as a carbamoyl linkage. Unlike the amides, the esters are hydrolysed readily, especially on repeated autoclaving and under alkaline conditions. Rapid enzymatic hydrolysis takes place also once they are in the bloodstream. This is promoted by the addition to procaine of a chlorine atom at the 2 position (chloroprocaine), whereas the addition of a butyl group to

the aromatic nitrogen (amethocaine) has the opposite effect.

In procaine and its analogues, the aromatic moiety is incorporated into a para-aminobenzoic acid nucleus, whereas in lignocaine and its analogues the aromatic system is typically 2,6-xylidine. Prilocaine differs in being based upon o-toluidine, thereby lacking one of the aromatic methyl groups shielding the amide link.

The carbon chain consists of either one or two methylene groups as in lignocaine and procaine, respectively; it may also be branched as in prilocaine and etidocaine or incorporated into a heterocyclic ring as in mepivacaine and bupivacaine. The latter two arrangements allow for the presence of an asymmetric carbon atom. This gives rise to stereoisomeric forms with different anaesthetic, vasoactive and toxic properties. However, only the racemates of prilocaine, mepivacaine, bupivacaine and etidocaine are used clinically. Ropivacaine, a new addition to the amide series undergoing evaluation in humans has been developed as a single enantiomer.

The terminal subunit is typically a tertiary amine group. Exceptions are found in prilocaine, which has a secondary amino group, and benzocaine, which has no amino group at all. Thus, benzocaine apart, all of the clinically used local anaesthetics are weak bases, existing in solution as both non-ionized (freebase) and ionized (cation) forms.

Differences in the chemical structure of the various compounds are expressed in their physicochemical properties which in turn relate to anaesthetic and kinetic properties.

Physicochemical properties

Some physicochemical properties of the esters and the amides are shown in Table 66.2.

Table 66.1 Chemical structures of clinically important local anaesthetic agents. (Redrawn from Tucker, 1983)

	Aromatic ring	Linkage group	Carbon chain	Amino group
Esters Cocaine		COO		N.CH₃ / CH.CO.OCH₃
Benzocaine	H₂N—	COO	—CH₂.CH₃	
Procaine (novocaine)	H₂N—	COO	—CH₂.CH₂—N	C₂H₅ / C₂H₅
2 — Chloroprocaine (Nesacaine)	H₂N— (Cl)	COO	—CH₂.CH₂—N	C₂H₅ / C₂H₅
Amethocaine (tetracaine, Pontocaine, decicaine)	H₉C₄HN— (OC₄H₉)	COO	—CH₂.CH₂—N	CH₃ / CH₃
Amides Cinchocaine (dibucaine, Nupercainal)	N	CO.NH	—CH₂.CH₂—N	C₂H₅ / C₂H₅
Prilocaine (Citanest)	(CH₃)	NH.CO	—CH (CH₃)	N—H / C₃H₇
Lignocaine (lidocaine, Xylocaine)	(CH₃ / CH₃)	NH.CO—	—CH₂—	N—C₂H₅ / C₂H₅
Mepivacaine (Carbocaine)			N (CH₃)	
Bupivacaine (Marcaine)			N—C₄H₉	
Etidocaine (Duranest)			—CH (C₂H₅)	N—C₂H₅ / C₃H₇

* Indicates an asymmetric carbon atom and, therefore, the existence of stereoisomers. Ropivacaine, the *n*-propyl homologue of mepivacaine and bupivacaine, is currently under development as a single S(−)-enantiomer.

Molecular weight

Molecular weights of the agents span a relatively small range from 220 to 288. This indicates that differences in their aqueous diffusion coefficients will also be small as these values are related to the inverse of the square root of the molecular weight.

Dural permeability is claimed to be more dependent on molecular weight than lipophilicity (Moore *et al.*, 1982; Bernards & Hill, 1991). Molecular weight

Table 66.2 Physicochemical properties of local anaesthetics. (Data from Tucker & Mather, 1980; Strichartz *et al.*, 1990)

Agent	Mol.wt	pKa (25°C)	Distribution coefficient*	Protein binding (%)	Aqueous solubility† (mg HCl/ml; pH 7.37, 37°C)	Rank lipid diffusion index‡
Esters						
Procaine	236	9.0	1.7	5.8**	—	8
Chloroprocaine	271	9.3	9.0	—	—	—
Amethocaine	264	8.6	221	76**	1.4	5
Amides						
Prilocaine	220	8.0	25	55††	—	6
Lignocaine	234	7.8	43	64††	24	4
Mepivacaine	246	7.9	21	77††	15	7
Ropivacaine	274	8.2	115	90	—	3
Bupivacaine	288	8.2	346	95††	0.83	2
Etidocaine	276	7.9	800	94††	—	1

* *n*-octanol; pH 7.4; 25°C; † Dudziak and Uihlein (1978); ‡ estimated from the product of the fraction non-ionized × fraction unbound to protein × the partition coefficient of the non-ionized base (Hull, 1985) (Rank 1 = highest); ** nerve homogenate binding; †† plasma protein binding, 2 μg/ml.

might also be relevant to the movement of local anaesthetics in the sodium channel of the nerve membrane (see below).

Lipid solubility

Octanol:buffer distribution coefficients reflect the relative lipid solubility of local anaesthetics (Table 66.2), showing good rank−order correlation with *in vitro* partition into rat sciatic nerve and human extradural and subcutaneous fat (Rosenberg *et al.*, 1986).

Increases in lipid solubility are achieved by modifications at either end of the molecules. In the ester series, the lipophilicity of procaine is enhanced by addition of a chlorine atom to the aromatic ring to give 2-chloroprocaine and by butyl substitution on the aromatic amine group as in amethocaine. In the amide series, a similar effect is achieved mainly by alkyl substitution on the terminal aliphatic amine group. For example, replacement of the methyl group in mepivacaine by a butyl group gives bupivacaine, a much more lipid-soluble agent. Net lipid solubility is independent of ester or amide grouping. Thus, amethocaine is highly lipophilic, as are bupivacaine and etidocaine.

A high lipid solubility would be expected to promote diffusion through membranes, thereby speeding the onset of action, and to enhance interaction with hydrophobic components of axonal receptor sites, thereby increasing potency and duration

of effect (see below). Increased sequestration by non-specific tissue components and fat near the site of action exert also a modulating effect on the anaesthetic profile.

Ionization

The esters have higher pKa values (8.6−9.3) than the amides (7.8−8.2) and will, therefore, be more ionized at physiological pH. The effect on pKa values of differences in structure within the two main types of agents is complex, involving steric factors as well as the inductive effects of alkyl substituents on the amine nitrogen. For example, the greater pKa of bupivacaine compared with mepivacaine is explained by the effect of greater alkyl substitution making the nitrogen atom more negative. In contrast, the lower pKa of etidocaine seems to reflect the effect of bulkier substituents in decreasing cation stabilization by hydration.

By promoting ionization, a higher pKa would be expected to delay diffusion, thereby prolonging onset of action. This may account also, in part, for the relatively poor penetrance of the esters compared with the amides. The influence of pKa on onset of action is considered in more detail in the section on the dynamics of nerve block.

Ionization is relevant also to the stability, solubility, and activity of local anaesthetics and their equilibrium distribution in various body compartments.

To ensure the stability of the ester-type agents,

they must be dispensed in quite acidic solutions such that they exist predominantly in the more stable and soluble ionized form. Hence the pH of plain solutions of the esters may be as low as 2.8 compared with 4.4–6.4 for those of the amides. In turn, the lower pH of ester solutions means that less (non-ionized) drug will be available initially to diffuse to sites of action, thereby contributing to delay in blocking the nerve. Since instability is not a problem with the amides, further decreasing their ionization by alkalinization of the injected solution would be expected to shorten the latency of block (see below).

Protein binding

Besides being more lipid soluble, the more potent and longer-acting local anaesthetics are bound also more extensively to plasma and tissue proteins (Table 66.2). This suggests that the forces attracting these compounds to non-specific sites and to axonal receptors have a large hydrophobic component. Binding to non-specific proteins near the site of action may delay onset of action by lowering the concentration gradient of diffusible drug (see below).

Aqueous solubility

The aqueous solubility of a local anaesthetic is related directly to its extent of ionization (and therefore decreases as pH is raised) and related inversely to its lipid solubility (Table 66.2).

Benzocaine, which lacks an amino group attached to the carbon chain, is almost insoluble in water. For this reason, its use is confined to topical anaesthesia, although it has been injected for prolonged intercostal nerve block after solubilization with dextran.

A low aqueous solubility may be a limiting factor when selecting an agent for subarachnoid block. Thus, there has been concern over the possible neurotoxicity of 1% solutions of bupivacaine HCl as they become opalescent on mixing with cerebrospinal fluid (CSF) *in vitro* (Dudziak & Uihlein, 1978). However, whether or not precipitation of the compound occurs *in vivo* is debatable (Meyer & Nolte, 1978; Starke & Nolte, 1978; Dennhardt & Ammon, 1980), and animal studies indicate that morphological effects on the spinal cord of the less water-soluble agents are apparent only after intrathecal injection of concentrations greater than 2% (Adams *et al.*, 1974, 1977).

Mechanism of action

Covino (1980, 1987) and, more recently, Butterworth

and Strichartz (1990) provide seminal reviews of the electrophysiological and molecular mechanisms of local anaesthesia.

Electrophysiological effects

The transmission of an electrical impulse down a nerve can be likened to knocking over a sequence of dominoes. Removal of one of the dominoes in the chain is analogous to the application of a local anaesthetic. The primary electrophysiological effect of these compounds is to cause a local decrease in the rate and degree of depolarization of the nerve membrane such that the threshold potential for transmission is not achieved and the electrical impulse is not propagated down the nerve (Fig. 66.1). There is no effect on the resting or threshold potentials, but prolongation of the repolarization phase and refractory period may also play a role in anaesthetic action (Covino, 1980).

Effect on ionic fluxes

Evidence from studies in which sodium ion concentration was varied and others in which its flux was measured directly have shown that the primary effect of local anaesthetics on depolarization and repolarization of the nerve membrane is mediated by their ability to impair membrane permeability of sodium

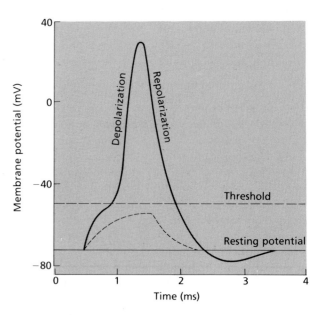

Fig. 66.1 The action potential of a peripheral nerve. On exposure to a local anaesthetic the rate and degree of depolarization are decreased (dashed line), such that the threshold potential is not attained and the impulse is not propagated down the nerve.

ions. Metabolic inhibition of the sodium pump may be discounted (Covino, 1980).

Although some anaesthetics, particularly procaine and cocaine, impair potassium ion flux also, the effect is much less than that on sodium transport and is probably not involved in conduction block (Covino, 1980). Nevertheless, this has prompted investigations into the possibility of using potassium chloride to lower resting membrane potential, thereby potentiating the effects of local anaesthetics. Earlier clinical studies did show some advantage of the combination, albeit using potentially toxic doses of potassium (Bromage & Burfoot, 1966; Aldrete *et al.*, 1969). More recent studies using lower doses found no effect on intravenous regional anaesthesia and brachial plexus block with prilocaine but faster onset of sensory block with bupivacaine injected into the brachial plexus (McKeown & Scott, 1984; Parris & Chambers, 1986).

Raising and lowering calcium ion concentration around a nerve antagonizes and enhances local anaesthetic block, respectively, and it has been suggested that local anaesthetics compete with membrane-bound calcium. Whether this action relates directly to the opening and closing of sodium channels and therefore conduction block remains controversial (Covino, 1980; Saito *et al.*, 1984).

Marked circadian variation in the duration of action of local anaesthetics when used for dental surgery may reflect circadian variation in the membrane permeability of ions (Pollmann, 1981).

Site of action of local anaesthetics

Three distinct sites have been proposed where local anaesthetics might exert their effect on sodium conductance across the nerve membrane (Ritchie, 1975). These are:

1 On the membrane surface, involving alteration of the fixed negative charge and hence transmembrane potential, without change in resting intracellular potential.
2 Within the membrane matrix, involving its lateral expansion, thereby causing distortion of the sodium channel.
3 Specific receptors within the sodium channel.

Although these possibilities are not mutually exclusive in that different agents may act at different sites, only the specific receptor theory is compatible with all of the following experimental observations (Covino, 1980):

1 Completely non-ionized drugs, such as benzocaine, are active.

2 Ionized forms act on the internal surface of the axonal membrane (evidence based upon internal and external perfusion of the giant squid axon with solutions of tertiary amine and quaternary analogues of lignocaine).
3 Optical isomers of some local anaesthetics show differential activity.
4 Local anaesthesia can be modulated by varying the frequency of nerve stimulation.

Thus, Hille (1977) has developed a model for a single receptor in the sodium channel that accommodates the actions of all clinically used local anaesthetics but which proposes different routes of access for ionized and non-ionized species. Three different conformational states of the sodium channel are postulated (Fig. 66.2).

1 A resting state (R), in which sodium activation and inactivation gates (m and h, respectively) are closed and which predominates before nerve stimulation.
2 An open state (O), in which both gates are open, allowing passage of sodium ions during stimulation. This state is present during depolarization of the membrane.
3 An inactive state (I), in which the m-gate remains open but the h-gate is closed immediately following stimulation. This state is associated with the initial phase of repolarization and the refractory period. The rest of the repolarization phase is associated with an increase in potassium ion conductance and efflux from the internal side of the membrane.

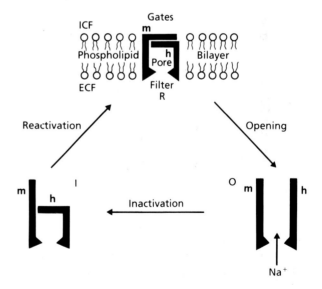

Fig. 66.2 The functional components and possible conformational states of a sodium channel. R, resting state; O, open state, allowing sodium influx; I, inactive state; ICF, intracellular fluid; ECF, extracellular fluid. (Redrawn from Wildsmith, 1986.)

Local anaesthetics bind to the receptor in all three channel states and prevent electrical conduction during the O-state. Furthermore, closure of the h-gate enhances drug–receptor interaction and promotes channel inactivation. Movement of non-ionized, lipophilic species to and from the receptor is possible in all three states via diffusion through the membrane matrix, whereas movement of ionized, hydrophilic species is only possible through the open h-gate when the channel is in the O-state (Fig. 66.3).

Although the single-site theory has aesthetic appeal, Mrose and Ritchie (1978) and Huang and Ehrenstein (1981) have presented experimental data more compatible with a two-site model which discriminates between ionized and non-ionized agents.

The effect of pH

It is clear that both ionized and non-ionized molecules can produce conduction block. However, the question as to which species contributes most to the action of partially ionized agents has not been resolved satisfactorily.

Earlier studies showed that, whereas a high external pH potentiated the effect of local anaesthetics on nerves with intact sheaths, the drugs were more effective in neutral or acidic solution when desheathed

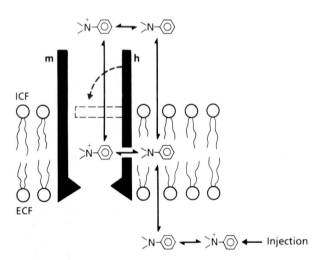

Fig. 66.3 The paths of access of local anaesthetic to the 'local anaesthetic receptor' in the neuronal sodium channel. Non-ionized and ionized forms can reach the binding site from the intracellular fluid (ICF) if activation (m) and inactivation (h) gates are both open. The non-ionized form can also reach the receptor through the membrane phase. The binding site has an important hydrophobic component and closure of the h-gate enhances the hydrophobic interaction. (Redrawn from Wildsmith, 1986.)

nerves were used (Ritchie *et al.*, 1965; Strobel & Bianchi, 1970). This has been rationalized by assuming that equilibrium block was not achieved with the sheathed preparations and that alkalinization promoted diffusion of free base to the receptor. Diffusional delays being minimal in the desheathed preparations, a greater drug potency in acidic solution signified that the cation is the active species (Covino, 1986). However, although more recent data obtained using sheathed rabbit vagus support this interpretation (Gissen *et al.*, 1986), other data obtained using sheathed and unsheathed frog sciatic nerve do not (Bokesch *et al.*, 1987a). Thus, the first of these groups showed that the rate of block with bupivacaine occurs slowly and is potentiated by alkalinization. On the other hand, Bokesch and colleagues (1987a) concluded that acidification (with hydrochloric acid) lowers the potency of lignocaine irrespective of whether the perineurium is present or not, and state that diffusional delays are insufficient to explain potentiation of block under alkaline conditions.

There is agreement that acidification with carbon dioxide increases local anaesthetic potency (Catchlove, 1972; Gissen *et al.*, 1985; Bokesch *et al.*, 1987a) and that this may be mediated by its rapid diffusion across the membrane to cause a lowering of intracellular pH. This effect would be consistent with the cationic forms of local anaesthetics being the dominant active species. In addition, whereas Bokesch and colleagues (1987a) do not exclude a direct action of carbon dioxide itself on the membrane but do discount any effect on extracellular pH, Gissen and colleagues (1985) conclude that carbonation is without effect on membrane sensitivity but does increase extracellular pH.

The effects of age and pregnancy

Increased sensitivity to local anaesthetic-induced conduction block in isolated nerves from young and old rabbits is consistent with smaller dosage requirements in paediatric and geriatric patients (Benzon *et al.*, 1988). Pregnancy is also associated with a decrease in dose requirements and increased susceptibility to nerve block (Butterworth *et al.*, 1990a). The mechanism of this change is unknown, but does not seem to be related to a direct effect of progesterone on the axonal membrane (Bader *et al.*, 1990).

Frequency-dependent block

An increase in the frequency of nerve stimulation has been shown to enhance the effect of local anaesthetics on sodium conductance and action potential (Strichartz, 1973; Courtney, 1975).

Thus, if an *in vitro* nerve preparation is stimulated at a very low frequency and exposed to a low concentration of a local anaesthetic, a constant decrease in impulse transmission develops (tonic or 'resting' block). Increasing the stimulus frequency with the same concentration of anaesthetic will increase the degree of block until a new steady state is reached (phasic, 'use-', or 'frequency-dependent' block). After a period of rest, the original level of conduction will return.

This phenomenon may be explained on the basis of Hille's 'modulated receptor' (Hille, 1977). As shown in Fig. 66.4, the drug binds to sodium channels in the O- and I-states but has a very low affinity for channels in the R-state. After a long rest, all channels are in a relative drug-free state, but binding to open and inactivated channels develops during the action potential. If dissociation from these sites is fast relative to the frequency of stimulus, there is no accumulation of block beyond the first stimulus (Fig. 66.4A). However, more rapid stimulation allows the h- and m-gates to remain open for longer periods of time, thereby maximizing access of drug to the receptor. The drug binds more tightly, dissociation is incomplete before the next stimulus is applied, and the block deepens (Fig. 66.4B). The conditions of membrane potential that favour the open-channel state enhance also the rates at which block develops and reverses.

The relevance of frequency-dependent block to clinical anaesthesia has not been established. However, somatic motor fibres have no frequency threshold whereas sensory fibres do with respect to the transmission of nociceptive stimuli. Therefore, variability in the ability of different agents to produce frequency-dependent and differential block may be related (Scurlock *et al.*, 1978). In the treatment of chronic pain, it has been suggested that onset and depth of anaesthesia might be augmented by combining the use of local anaesthetics and nerve stimulators (Covino, 1980). As repolarization of the nerve membrane depends upon the efflux of potassium ions, block of potassium channels enhances frequency-dependent block by prolonging the O-state (Drachman & Strichartz, 1991). Thus, the combination of local anaesthetics with specific potassium ion channel blockers might have clinical advantages.

Although the implications of frequency dependence for clinical nerve block are unclear, there is good reason to believe that this phenomenon contributes to the relative cardiotoxicity of some local

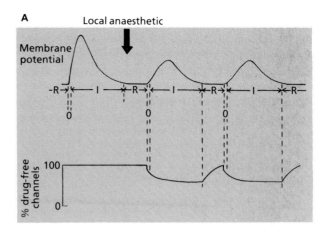

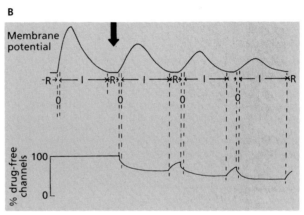

Fig. 66.4 Changes in sodium channel states and block of sodium channels associated with the nerve action potential in the presence of a local anaesthetic. (A) The effect of infrequent stimulation, leading to a tonic block. (B) The effect of frequent stimulation, leading to a phasic or 'frequency-dependent' block. The drug binds to sodium channels in open (O) and inactivated (I) states but has a very low affinity in the rested (R) state. Drug dissociation is time dependent and becomes incomplete during frequent stimulation, resulting in an accumulation of drug-associated (blocked) channels with successive impulses. (Redrawn from Clarkson & Hondeghem, 1985.)

anaesthetics. Thus, the antiarrhythmic effect of lignocaine and the greater risk of cardiac depression and arrhythmogenesis with bupivacaine are accounted for by observations suggesting that whereas lignocaine blocks sodium channels in the myocardium in a 'fast-in, fast-out' manner, bupivacaine is fast-in and slow-out (Clarkson & Hondeghem, 1985). The R(+)-isomer of bupivacaine produces a more pronounced frequency-dependent block than the S(−)-isomer (Vanhoutte *et al.*, 1991). This could contribute to differences in the lethal doses of the isomers observed in animals (Aberg, 1972; Luduena *et al.*,

1972), and to the lower cardiotoxicity of ropivacaine, which is a single S(−)-isomer, relative to that of racemic bupivacaine (Reiz *et al.*, 1989; Moller & Covino, 1990).

Structure−activity relationships

Studies of the relationships between structure and local anaesthetic activity are complicated by the need to distinguish between the relative potencies of cationic and free-base forms and between tonic and phasic block.

With regard to tonic block there is general agreement that potency increases with lipid solubility (Courtney, 1980; Wildsmith *et al.*, 1987) of both neutral and protonated species (Bokesch *et al.*, 1986). However, block does not depend uniquely on hydrophobicity as predicted if lipid partitioning alone determines potency, i.e. simple Meyer−Overton theory does not apply — equal block is not produced by equal membrane concentrations of either base or cation in a series of compounds. Similarly, neither molecular size nor the concentration of the ionized species in solution explain the experimental observations for tonic block. Therefore, specific structural features as well as physicochemical properties seem to contribute to anaesthetic potency (Bokesch *et al.*, 1986). Suggestions that esters are more potent than amides at similar lipid solubility depend on correlations using the partition coefficient of non-ionized base (Courtney, 1980; Wildsmith *et al.*, 1987). However, the esters have higher pKa values and if distribution coefficients (which are based on measurements of the sum of neutral and charged species in the aqueous phase) are used the differences are smaller. Using partition coefficient as the index of lipid solubility, within the amide series of agents it appears that incorporation of the amino nitrogen into a piperidine ring, as in mepivacaine, ropivacaine and bupivacaine, is associated with enhanced potency relative to acyclic analogues of similar lipid solubility (Wildsmith *et al.*, 1989).

According to Hille's 'modulated receptor theory', the extent and rate of frequency-dependent block are predicted to correlate inversely with lipid-solubility. Thus, ionized hydrophilic species, which can only come and go through the open gates, should exhibit greater phasic block than non-ionized, lipophilic species whose movement through the membrane is independent of gate opening. This was supported by experiments with completely ionized (quaternary) and completely non-ionized agents (Hille, 1977). It was an anomaly, therefore, that very lipid-soluble agents such as bupivacaine were found to produce marked frequency dependence at low rates of channel activation (Courtney *et al.*, 1978). Subsequent studies suggested that molecular size is important, rapid receptor-binding and unbinding of molecules like bupivacaine being impeded by their bulk (Courtney, 1980). However, further investigations with lignocaine homologues have indicated that the ability to produce frequency-dependent block is neither a simple function of molecular weight nor of partition coefficient or pKa (Bokesch *et al.*, 1986). These findings emphasized also that the molecular features for optimal tonic and phasic block are not the same, suggesting that perhaps two distinct binding sites are involved (Strichartz, 1985).

Whatever the finer details of the topography of the interaction between local anaesthetics and their axonal 'receptor(s)' eventually turn out to be, the clinical potency of these drugs is related broadly to their lipid solubility. Thus, etidocaine, bupivacaine and amethocaine are effective in lower doses than lignocaine, prilocaine and mepivacaine, while chloroprocaine and procaine are even less potent. To some extent, this order is determined also by vasoactive properties and non-specific tissue sequestration. For example, a greater intrinsic potency of lignocaine compared with prilocaine appears to be offset by its greater vasodilating effect resulting in faster systemic uptake from the site of injection. A lower potency of etidocaine with respect to bupivacaine for sensory block after extradural injection may reflect its greater solubility in adipose tissue within the extradural space.

The dynamics of nerve block

Factors affecting the onset and spread of neural block include dispersion by bulk flow of the injected solution and diffusion of the local anaesthetic agent. Duration of effect is determined by the rate of diffusion of drug away from the nerve as well as by its vascular uptake. The latter process will be considered later in the context of systemic absorption. Neural and perineural breakdown of local anaesthetics appears to be negligible and does not influence the time course of anaesthesia (Tucker & Mather, 1980).

Bulk flow

This can be assessed using marker dyes or radio-contrast media. Spread of analgesia is only partially dependent on bulk flow of the injected solution.

Subarachnoid block

Hydrodynamic considerations are more important following subarachnoid injection than any other regional anaesthetic procedure. The outcome depends on a complex interplay of baricity, posture and volume and has been reviewed in detail by Greene (1985), Wildsmith and Rocco (1985) and by Stienstra and Greene (1991).

Extradural block

Studies using radiopaque markers have shown that increasing the volume of injectate causes a disproportionately small increase in cephalad spread (Burn et al., 1973). This may reflect greater spillage into the paravertebral spaces with larger volumes and is consistent with spread of analgesia relationships (Grundy et al., 1978). Below a limiting volume (constant dose), the spread and intensity of block become independent of volume, indicating that factors other than bulk flow are more important for the ultimate dispersion of the local anaesthetic.

In general, altering the speed of injection has been found to have little influence on spread of either solution or analgesia, although confounding factors include the drug used, the age of the patient and the direction of the needle bevel (Erdemir et al., 1966; Husemeyer & White, 1980; Rosenberg et al., 1981; Cohen et al., 1984). Extremely rapid injection of bupivacaine (over 5 s) was shown to hasten onset of block and to enhance perineal anaesthesia (Griffiths et al., 1987).

Changes in posture have a minimal effect on the dynamics of extradural block (Park, 1988), although a decrease in cephalad spread of analgesia in the sitting position has been observed in obese patients (Hodgkinson & Husain, 1981).

Increases in the longitudinal spread and duration of extradural anaesthesia with increasing age have been assigned to reduced lateral leakage of solution, owing to progressive sclerotic closure of the paravertebral foramina (Bromage, 1975). Partial support for this comes from studies with radioactive markers (Nishimura et al., 1959; Burn et al., 1973). However, more recent work indicates that the relationship between decline in dose requirement and age is more complex than proposed originally (Grundy et al., 1978; Sharrock, 1978; Park et al., 1980; Park, 1988).

Intercostal block

There has been considerable debate as to the extent of spread of solutions injected into the intercostal groove. Using cadavers, radiopaque dyes, or computed tomography, some groups have concluded that the solution spreads via an extrapleural route into intercostal spaces adjacent to the one injected (Nunn & Slavin, 1980; Crossley & Hosie, 1987), whereas others found no such spread (Moore, 1981; Johansson et al., 1985). The clinical significance of this relates to the practice of multiple or continuous administration of local anaesthetics into one intercostal space to provide prolonged analgesia over an extensive field (O'Kelly & Garry, 1981; Murphy, 1983).

Brachial plexus block

Winnie and colleagues (1979) used a mixture of bupivacaine and radiopaque dye to document the spread of solution following injection into the brachial plexus sheath, and have made recommendations designed to improve the flow in the desired direction. These were based on the concept of a continuous, single fascial compartment surrounding the brachial plexus. Thompson and Rorie (1983) have challenged this view, however, with evidence from dissections and computed tomography for the presence of individual fascial compartments around each of the major branches of the plexus. They concluded that connective tissue septa interfere with circumferential spread of local anaesthetic, explaining the occasional occurrence of incomplete sensory block. Subsequently, Vester-Andersen and colleagues (1986), using gelatine injections, found no evidence for septa. Lack of contact between some of the nerves and the gelatine was accounted for by obstruction of circumferential spread of solution owing to the position of the arm during injection. More recently, Partridge and colleagues (1987) confirmed the presence of septa, but found them to be functionally incomplete and easily deranged by an appropriate single-injection technique.

Interpleural block

Studies in dogs using evoked potential technology (Riegler et al., 1989) and in humans using computed tomography (Strømskag et al., 1990) have mapped the flow of injected solution. Most of the solution collects at the lowest point of the pleural cavity, varying with body position, and distributes to the roots of the intercostal and splanchnic nerves and the sympathetic chain.

Diffusion

Once the local anaesthetic has been deposited and spread physically in the extraneural fluids it diffuses to the nerve membrane.

Subarachnoid block

After subarachnoid injection, the relatively high lipid solubility of local anaesthetics promotes local cord uptake rather than extensive cephalad spread via CSF flow. Thus, drug concentrations in the CSF decline in both directions from the point of injection and exponentially at the site of injection as uptake proceeds (Koster *et al.*, 1936; Meyer & Nolte, 1978; Post *et al.*, 1985). Direct diffusion along the concentration gradient from CSF through the pia mater directly into the cord delivers drug to superficial parts of the structure. Access to deeper areas is effected by diffusion in the CSF contained in the spaces of Virchow–Robin which connect with perineural clefts surrounding the bodies of nerve cells within the cord (Greene, 1983). Further penetration of drug into the cord may occur also through uptake into spinal radicular arteries (Fig. 66.5).

The pattern of drug distribution within the cord is a complex function of accessibility by diffusion from the CSF, the relative myelin (lipid) content of various tracts, and the rate of drug removal by local perfusion. Studies in animals using radiolabelled local anaesthetics have shown their accumulation along the posterior and lateral aspects of the cord as well as in the spinal nerve roots, with less in the dorsal root ganglion and the centre of the cord. Uptake of drug was higher in the grey matter than in the white matter and posterior nerve roots had higher concentrations than anterior roots (Howarth, 1949; Bromage *et al.*, 1963; Cohen, 1968; Post *et al.*, 1985).

Extradural block

Local anaesthetics appear rapidly in the CSF after extradural injection (Wilkinson & Lund, 1970) in sufficient concentrations to block spinal nerve roots. By 30 min, high drug concentrations are achieved also in the peripheral cord and in the spinal nerves in the paravertebral space (Bromage *et al.*, 1963).

Apart from direct diffusion of drug across the dura, access to the cord, particularly the dorsal horn region, may be mediated by diffusion and bulk flow through the arachnoid villi at the dural root sleeves [although this is contested by studies using *ex vivo* dura (Bernards & Hill, 1991)], by uptake into the posterior branch of spinal segmental arteries and by centripetal subneural and subpial spread from the remote paravertebral nerve trunks (Fig. 66.5) (Bromage, 1967, 1975). These suggestions are consistent with clinical observations of the distribution of analgesia during induction and regression of block.

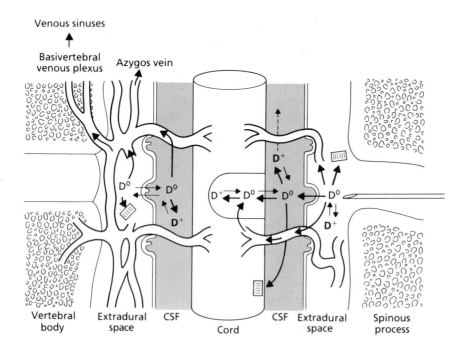

Fig. 66.5 The pathways of local distribution and systemic uptake of a local anaesthetic in the extradural and subarachnoid spaces. A needle is shown delivering drug into the extradural space, followed by attachment to non-specific lipid binding sites (shaded squares) and transfer across the dura. In the spinal cord, interaction with spinal receptors as well as non-specific lipid sites is shown. Deeper penetration of the cord is indicated via uptake into spinal arteries. Extradural veins, in close proximity to arachnoid granulations, are depicted as the major route of vascular clearance after both extradural and spinal injection. Two alternative routes of drainage, via the azygos veins or the basivertebral venous plexus, are shown. (Redrawn from Cousins & Mather, 1984.)

Venous sinuses

Basivertebral venous plexus   Azygos vein

D^0 D^0 D^+ D^0 D^0 D^0
D^+ D^+
D^+

Vertebral body   Extradural space   CSF   Cord   CSF   Extradural space   Spinous process

A segmental pattern of analgesia during onset may relate to the initial diffusion into spinal nerves and roots, with subsequent non-segmental regression resulting from ultimate diffusion to structures within the cord (Urban, 1973).

Studies with implanted electrodes in monkeys indicate that the depth of penetration of the cord increases with the concentration and lipid solubility of the local anaesthetic (Cusick et al., 1980, 1982). A marked effect of etidocaine on lower limb reflexes after thoracic extradurals in humans is consistent with block of relatively deep motor tracts within the cord (Bromage, 1974).

Much of an extradural dose of local anaesthetic may be sequestered temporarily in extraneural tissues at the site of injection. Prolonged storage in extradural fat, particularly of more lipid-soluble agents, has been shown in sheep (Tucker & Mather, 1980).

Brachial plexus block

Progression of block from upper arm to hand and then to fingers is explained by more rapid diffusion of local anaesthetic into mantle fibres that innervate more proximal regions than do core fibres (DeJong, 1977). To explain why the onset of motor block often precedes that of sensory loss, Winnie and colleagues (1977a) have suggested that this is due to the more peripheral location of motor fibres in the median nerve. According to the classical view, the sequence of recovery should be the same as that of onset: arm first, then hand and fingers (DeJong, 1977). This follows if the concentration gradient within the nerve now becomes reversed, decreasing from core to mantle. However, this has been challenged by Winnie and colleagues (1977b) who observed the reverse order of recovery with significant motor block that outlasted analgesia. To account for this, it was proposed that a more rapid vascular uptake occurs near the more distally innervating sensory fibres located in the core of the nerve. As intraneural blood vessels pass from mantle to core they become increasingly branched, thereby offering a larger surface area for drug absorption.

Differential block

As discussed with reference to extradural and brachial plexus block, the anatomical location of nerve fibres and their accessibility by diffusion may influence their susceptibility to local anaesthetic effect. In addition, there are intrinsic differences in the ability to block various types of nerve fibre subserving dif-

ferent functional modalities. Thus, the sequence of clinical observations after injection of a local anaesthetic for major nerve block is generally:

1 Elevation of skin temperature (B-block).
2 Loss of pain-temperature sensation (Aδ- and C-block).
3 Loss of proprioception (Aγ-block).
4 Loss of touch and pressure sensation (Aβ-block).
5 Loss of motor function (Aα-block).

Classically, this order is explained by increases in fibre diameter and extent of myelinization raising the intrinsic margin of safety for conduction (the anomalous position of unmyelinated C-fibres with respect to the larger B-fibres may reflect their grouping in Remak bundles). If a critical number of nodes of Ranvier must be blocked to ensure complete inhibition of impulse propagation, a lower concentration of drug should be necessary to block smaller fibres since the number of nodes is inversely proportional to fibre size. Contrary to this view, however, re-evaluation of the differential sensitivity of mammalian nerve fibres indicates that the facility of equilibrium block decreases in the order A-, B- and C-fibres (Gissen et al., 1980, 1982a,b). The apparent disparity between these in vitro findings and the sequence of clinical block was explained by the absence of equilibrium under the latter conditions. Thus, less drug reaches the larger fibres owing to the delaying effect of their diffusion barriers and attrition by vascular uptake. Some support for Gissen's conclusion is provided by other electrophysiological studies (Palmer et al., 1983; Rosenberg & Heinonen, 1983; Ford et al., 1984), but Fink and Cairns (1984) discount diffusion within a nerve as a contributory factor to differential block. They argue also that differential block is probably unrelated to fibre-size differences in susceptibility. Subsequent commentaries point to a greater importance of the length of the exposed nerve segment and the number of nodes that it contains, rather than its diameter (Fink, 1989; Raymond et al., 1989). Thus, Fink (1989) explains the persistence of differential block after extradural injection as follows. After injection of a weak solution of, for example, bupivacaine, the local anaesthetic bathes only a few millimetres of segmental nerve in the intervertebral foramina owing to a diffusion constraint beyond the extradural fat. Therefore, critical three-node block is rare in long internode (motor) fibres but likely in short internode (sensory) fibres. Fink's explanation for the differential segmental pattern of blocked physiological functions (vasoconstriction, skin temperature discrimination, pinprick pain sensibility and skeletal muscle activity) after subarachnoid injection is as follows: the cephalad decrease in root length increases the security of conduction in anaesthetic-bathed long-internode fibres more than in short-internode fibres, because the latter have more nodes available for consecutive three-node or decremental conduction block. The practical spin-offs of these arguments remain to be seen. Use of weak solutions of local anaesthetics in the interest of neurological safety may be compensated by infiltrating greater lengths of nerve, and better ways of exploiting differential block may be developed.

Drug-related factors

Concentration

An increase in local anaesthetic concentration or dose will shorten the latency of block and increase its duration. However, the gains are disproportionate, as a simple diffusion model and some experimental data indicate that duration and the reciprocal of onset time are related logarithmically to dose (Tucker & Mather, 1980).

Physicochemical properties

It has been suggested that the onset of conduction block in isolated nerves is determined primarily by the pKa of the individual agents (Covino, 1986). However, diffusion is determined not only by the fraction of non-ionized drug but also by the lipid solubility of this form. Additionally, *in vivo* non-specific binding or solubility in tissue along the diffusion pathway will modulate the rate at which local anaesthetic molecules reach their receptor sites on the nerve membrane. Therefore, a more rigorous predictor of onset of anaesthesia should be the lipid diffusion index, the product of non-ionized fraction, the partition coefficient of the free base and the fraction unbound to protein (Hull, 1985). Relative estimates of this index are given in Table 66.2. Procaine is predicted to have a slow onset followed by mepivacaine, prilocaine, then amethocaine and lignocaine, with bupivacaine and particularly etidocaine having very fast onset. Clinically, this order is modified by the dosage used. Thus, bupivacaine is relatively slow in onset when used as a 0.25% solution but latency decreases significantly on going to 0.75%. 2-chloroprocaine would be expected to have a low diffusion potential and onset, but this is overcome by its use in high concentration (3%).

Differences in diffusion index seem also to account

for differences in differential block between agents. For example, on this basis Gissen and colleagues (1982b) have explained the clinical observation that, whereas in low doses bupivacaine produces good sensory analgesia with minimum motor loss, etidocaine produces profound motor block. Thus, differences in the relative rates of onset of C(pain)- and A(motor)-fibre block for the two drugs were reproduced in an *in vitro* preparation (Fig. 66.6).

Duration of anaesthesia, like potency, is related to the lipid solubility and binding affinity of local anaesthetics and is influenced also by their intrinsic vasoactivity.

Effects of pH

If diffusion of local anaesthetics to the axonal membrane is rate limiting and rapid tissue buffering does not occur, increasing the pH of the injected solution should shorten the latency of action. This is borne out by some clinical studies showing faster onset and longer duration after adding sodium bicarbonate to bupivacaine solutions immediately before extradural (e.g. DiFazio *et al.*, 1986; McMorland *et al.*, 1986; Tackley & Coe, 1988), brachial plexus (e.g. Hilgier, 1985) and sciatic/femoral nerve injection (Coventry & Todd, 1989), and intravenous regional anaesthesia (e.g. Armstrong *et al.*, 1990a,b). However, other investigators found no useful effect of alkalinization on extradural (e.g. Benhamou *et al.*, 1989; Verborgh *et al.*, 1991) or peripheral nerve blocks (e.g. Smith *et al.*, 1986; Bedder *et al.*, 1987).

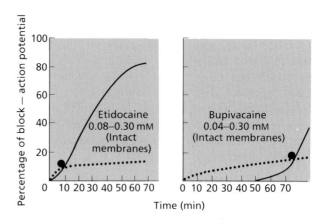

Fig. 66.6 Effects of etidocaine and bupivacaine on the onset of block of the compound action potential of the sheathed rabbit vagus nerve at 22°C. Dashed line, C-fibre response; solid line, A-fibre response. The cross-over points (closed circles), when A-block exceeds C-block, is much later with bupivacaine. (Redrawn from Gissen *et al.*, 1982b.)

The use of carbonated (CO_2) solutions of local anaesthetics might be expected to have a similar effect on latency as those to which bicarbonate is added. However, the results of controlled clinical studies are again equivocal (Brown et al., 1980; McClure & Scott, 1981; Martin et al., 1981; Morison, 1981; Nickel et al., 1986). Dissipation of the effect of carbon dioxide on intracellular pH may be too rapid in vivo, and its vasodilating effect might promote systemic absorption of local anaesthetic.

Cohen and colleagues (1968) have suggested that tachyphylaxis on repeated injection of local anaesthetics could be explained by the pH-lowering effect of their usually acidic solutions. A progressive lowering of CSF pH has been noted after subarachnoid injections (Cohen et al., 1968; Tucker & Mather, 1980) but rapid buffering seems to occur in the extradural space (Wurst & Stanton-Hicks, 1983). More peripheral injections cause sustained lowering of tissue pH, especially when adrenaline is added to the solution, but this acidosis does not appear to influence duration of block (Wennberg et al., 1982; Buckley et al., 1985). Tachyphylaxis is not explained adequately by pH effects alone (Mather, 1986).

Effects of temperature

The conduction blocking effect of local anaesthetics on isolated nerves is potentiated by low temperature (Rosenberg & Heavner, 1980). However, the use of cold solutions did not improve intravenous regional anaesthesia (Heavner et al., 1989) and produced marginal enhancement of median sensory nerve block (Butterworth et al., 1990b). In contrast, warming solutions of bupivacaine to 37°C appears to shorten the latency of subarachnoid block (Callesen et al., 1991) and to improve the quality of sensory block after extradural injection (Mehta et al., 1987).

Systemic absorption

A knowledge of the rates of systemic absorption of local anaesthetics helps to set confidence limits on the likelihood of systemic toxic reactions after the various block procedures. Indirectly, these rates suggest also the relationship between block and the amount of drug remaining at the site of injection.

In humans, measurement of drug concentration—time profiles in the peripheral circulation has been used widely to assess systemic uptake of the different agents. Because these profiles are the net result of both systemic absorption and disposition, they are of value mainly to determine relative changes in drug uptake. Variables affecting absorption are assumed usually not to influence disposition. To assess safety margins, vascular drug concentrations after perineural injection are compared with estimates of threshold values associated with the onset of significant CNS toxicity. These range from 5 to 10 µg/ml for lignocaine and from 2 to 4 µg/ml for bupivacaine and etidocaine. Although these values are useful guidelines, they refer to the mythical 'average subject' and must be interpreted in the light of a number of considerations. These include whether measurements are made of plasma or blood, total or unbound drug, ionized or non-ionized species, optical isomers, and active drug metabolites. The site of bood sampling (artery or vein) may be critical also when drug concentrations are changing rapidly (Tucker, 1986).

If blood drug concentration—time profiles are available also after intravenous administration, it becomes possible to calculate drug absorption rates using more sophisticated techniques of pharmacokinetic analysis such as deconvolution (Tucker, 1986).

Because local anaesthetics are relatively lipid-soluble compounds, their diffusion across the capillary epithelium is not likely to be rate limiting. Hence their absorption rates will primarily be related directly to blood flow and inversely to local tissue binding.

Important determinants of systemic absorption include the physicochemical and vasoactive properties of the agent, the site of injection, dosage factors, the presence of additives such as vasoconstrictors, factors related to nerve block, and pathophysiological features of the patient.

Agent

The extensive data on peak blood and plasma concentrations of the amide local anaesthetics and the times of their occurrence after various routes of injection have been tabulated elsewhere (Tucker & Mather, 1979, 1980, 1988). For example, after extradural injection of plain solutions, the increment in peak whole-blood drug concentration per 100 mg of dose is about 0.9–1.0 µg/ml for lignocaine and mepivacaine, slightly less for prilocaine, and approximately 50% as much for bupivacaine and etidocaine. Although differences in disposition kinetics contribute to this order (see below), it appears that, despite similar peak times, net absorption of the long-acting, more lipid-soluble agents is slower. This is consistent with data on residual concentrations of the agents in extradural fat after injection into sheep (Tucker & Mather, 1980) and is confirmed by pharmacokinetic calculations of the time-course of drug absorption in humans (Tucker & Mather, 1979; Burm *et al.*, 1987). The latter show that systemic uptake after extradural injection is a biphasic process, the contribution of the initial rapid phase being greater for lignocaine than for the long-acting analogues (Table 66.3; Fig. 66.7). This slower net absorption of the latter adds to their systemic safety margin after accurate injection.

Differences in the absorption rates of the various agents have implications for their accumulation during repeated and continuous administration. Whereas systemic accumulation is most marked with the short-acting amides, extensive local accumulation is predicted for bupivacaine and etidocaine, despite their longer dosage intervals (Tucker & Mather, 1975; Tucker *et al.*, 1977; Inoue *et al.*, 1985). For all agents the slow absorption-phase rate limits systemic elimination after central nerve block, and will determine the terminal plasma half-life and hence the rate of systemic accumulation.

Observations of relatively low blood concentrations of prilocaine with respect to the toxic threshold, particularly after brachial plexus block (Fig. 66.8) and intravenous regional anaesthesia, support the claim that this compound should be the agent of choice for

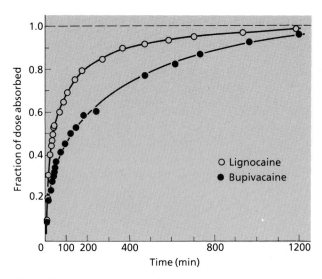

Fig. 66.7 Fraction of local anaesthetic dose absorbed into the general circulation as a function of time after extradural injection. The data points represent values determined by deconvolution of the measured plasma drug concentrations in representative subjects against the intravenous unit impulse curve in each subject. The curves represent biexponential functions fitted to the data points by non-linear regression. (Redrawn from Tucker, 1986.)

Table 66.3 Mean dose fractions (*F*) and half-lives characterizing the absorption of lignocaine and bupivacaine after subarachnoid and extradural injection in humans (Burm *et al.*, 1987, 1988). The data were obtained after deconvolution of plasma drug concentration–time profiles measured after simultaneous intravenous injection of deuterated drug and spinal/extradural injection of non-labelled drug. The time course of unabsorbed bupivacaine was described by a biexponential function after both subarachnoid and extradural injection, whereas that of lignocaine was monoexponential after subarachnoid and biexponential after extradural injection

	Lignocaine		Bupivacaine	
	Subarachnoid	Extradural	Subarachnoid	Extradural
F_1	—	0.38	0.35	0.29
$t_{\frac{1}{2}}, \text{abs}_1$ (min)	—	9.3	50	8
F_2	—	0.58	0.61	0.64
$t_{\frac{1}{2}}, \text{abs}_2$ (min)	71	82	408	371
F	1.03	0.96	0.96	0.91

F, total systemic availability compared with the intravenous injection.

such single-dose procedures (Wildsmith *et al.*, 1977). In this case, however, a high systemic clearance, rather than slow absorption, is mainly responsible for the low blood drug concentrations.

Although the rate of systemic absorption of local anaesthetics is controlled largely by the extent of local binding, their intrinsic vasoactive properties could also modulate local perfusion and hence uptake (Blair, 1975; Aps & Reynolds, 1976, 1978; Fairley & Reynolds, 1981; Jones *et al.*, 1985). However, the effects are a complex function of drug, dose, type and tone of blood vessel, and their relevance to the relative absorption of drugs after peripheral and central nerve blocks is difficult to evaluate (Burm, 1989). Nevertheless, it has been suggested, for example, that an increase in extradural blood flow (whether mediated locally or by change in cardiac output or both), with assumed increase in the systemic absorption rate of bupivacaine, is an important factor leading to regression of analgesia during continuous extradural infusion of bupivacaine (Mogensen *et al.*, 1988). Furthermore, the vasodilatory effect of racemic bupivacaine on both cutaneous and extradural blood flow contrasts strikingly with the vasoconstrictor effect of S(−)-ropivacaine, a difference which may contribute to their relative anaesthetic profiles (Kopacz *et al.*, 1989; Dahl *et al.*, 1990).

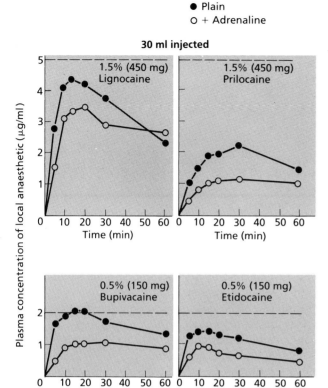

Fig. 66.8 Mean plasma concentrations of amide-type local anaesthetics after interscalene brachial plexus block. Thirty ml of agent, with (open circles) or without (closed circles) adrenaline, were injected. The broken lines indicate the putative toxic thresholds. (Redrawn from Tucker, 1986.)

Site of injection

Vascularity and the presence of tissue and fat that can bind local anaesthetics are primary influences on their rate of removal from specific sites of injection. In general, and independent of the agent used, absorption rate decreases in the order: intercostal block > caudal block > extradural block > brachial plexus block > sciatic and femoral nerve block (Tucker & Mather, 1980, 1988).

Intercostal block

Maximum circulating concentrations of the agents after intercostal blocks using plain solutions may exceed the toxic threshold, but effects are obtunded presumably by light general anaesthesia and premedication. Since sustained high plasma drug concentrations are achieved during continuous intercostal infusions, supplementary bolus injections are likely to be dangerous (Safran *et al.*, 1990).

Extradural block

The role of fat deposits within the extradural space in delaying the absorption of local anaesthetics has been discussed already. Vascular uptake will take place into the extradural veins and thence to the azygos vein. In the presence of raised intrathoracic pressure, however, absorbed drug could be redirected also up the internal vertebral venous system to cerebral sinuses (Fig. 66.5).

Vascular absorption of local anaesthetic from different regions of the extradural space (cervical, lumbar, thoracic) appears to be similar (Mayumi *et al.*, 1983). Mogensen and colleagues (1989) concluded that changes in drug absorption from the extradural space during continuous dosage do not account for tachyphylaxis since they found no time-dependent changes in the extradural distribution of radiocontrast medium nor in the rate of rise of plasma lignocaine after each injection. Unfortunately, the latter measurements are not valid indices of systemic drug absorption rate.

Brachial plexus block

The various techniques for blocking the brachial plexus are not associated with significant differences in local anaesthetic absorption rate (Vester-Andersen *et al.*, 1981; Maclean *et al.*, 1988).

Subarachnoid block

Systemic uptake after subarachnoid injection is believed to occur predominantly after passage of drug across the dura into the more vascular extradural space (Cohen, 1968), as well as from blood vessels within the spinal space, in the pia mater, and the cord itself (Fig. 66.5). Extensive diffusion into the extradural space would be expected to result in sequestration in fat, thereby retarding the absorption of the longer-acting agents to a greater extent than the short-acting ones. Pharmacokinetic analysis shows that there are differences in the pattern of systemic absorption after subarachnoid and extradural injection, and confirms that there is a slower net absorption of bupivacaine compared to lignocaine (Table 66.3). The slower initial uptake from the subarachnoid space may reflect dural diffusion. The similarity of the slower uptake phase for subarachnoid bupivacaine and the overall monoexponential uptake of subarachnoid lignocaine with the corresponding slow phases of uptake after extradural injection suggest a common rate-limiting removal from extradural fat.

Intravenous regional anaesthesia

A pharmacokinetic analysis of plasma lignocaine concentrations measured after intravenous regional anaesthesia has shown that, if the cuff is inflated correctly for at least 10 min after injection, only about 20—30% of the dose enters the systemic circulation during the first minute after cuff release. The rest emerges rather slowly, with approximately 50% of the dose still in the arm after 30 min (Tucker & Boas, 1971). Direct experimental support for this comes from observations of sustained high concentrations of local anaesthetic in the venous drainage from the blocked arm (Evans et al., 1974). Longer application of the cuff delays wash-out of drug from the arm (Tucker & Boas, 1971). Intermittent deflation of the cuff for 10—30s followed by reinflation appears to have little effect on the ultimate maximum plasma drug concentration but does prolong the time to maximum concentration (Sukhani et al., 1989).

Tracheal administration

Doses of lignocaine up to 400 mg produce peak plasma drug concentrations usually within 10—15 min and well below the toxic threshold (Tucker & Mather, 1980, 1988). The concentrations are significantly lower in spontaneously breathing patients than in paralysed patients since the former are more likely to swallow some of the dose, which then undergoes first-pass hepatic metabolism following absorption from the gut (Scott et al., 1976). Application only to areas below the vocal cords may result in excessive plasma drug concentrations because of less transfer to the gut (Curran et al., 1975). Plasma concentrations of lignocaine were found to be significantly lower when using an ultrasonic nebulizer compared to a conventional topical spray (Labedzki et al., 1990).

Interpleural block

High-dosage requirements and exposure of drug to a relatively large surface area of tissue, resulting in rapid systemic drug absorption, emphasize the small safety margin of this technique. Maximum plasma concentrations of bupivacaine are higher but occur later than when the same dose is injected for intercostal block (van Kleef et al., 1990). Mean steady-state plasma concentrations of bupivacaine during continuous interpleural infusion are consistent with those predicted from single-dose data (Kastrissios et al., 1991).

Dosage factors

Differences in absorption rates as a function of concentration and volume of injectate (constant dose) (Tucker & Mather, 1980, 1988; Denson et al., 1983) and speed of injection (Scott et al., 1972; Rosenberg et al., 1981; Vester-Andersen et al., 1984) are small. There is some evidence for a disproportionate increase in peak plasma drug concentration with increasing dose (Bridenbaugh et al., 1974; Lund et al., 1975), but again the changes are probably not of clinical significance.

Adrenaline

The degree to which adrenaline decreases the systemic absorption rate of local anaesthetic is a complex function of the type, dose and concentration of local anaesthetic and of the characteristics of the injection site (Tucker & Mather, 1980, 1988).

Although the peak plasma concentrations of local anaesthetics after most of the common regional blocks are lowered by adrenaline, it does not always prolong the time to peak (Tucker & Mather, 1979, 1980, 1988). In general, the greatest effects are seen after intercostal blocks and with short-acting rather than long-acting agents. This suggests that the greater local binding of the latter and their vasodilatory effects tend to offset the vasoconstriction caused by adrenaline. Differences in the effect of adrenaline on the systemic uptake of different local anaesthetics are reflected broadly in its effect on duration of block (Covino, 1986).

Physical and pathophysiological factors

Weight

In adults, plasma concentrations of local anaesthetics after extradural and other nerve blocks are correlated poorly with weight (Scott et al., 1972; Tucker et al., 1972; Moore et al., 1976a,b; Pihlajamäki, 1991).

Age

Using stable isotope technology to delineate absorption and disposition, Veering and colleagues (1991a; 1992) showed that the rate of the late phase of bupivacaine absorption after subarachnoid block increases with age (22—81 years), whereas no change in absorption occurs after extradural block. These findings reinforce the view that a decreased duration of analgesia in elderly patients has a pharmacodynamic rather than a pharmacokinetic basis.

Limited data are available in children which indicate somewhat faster absorption than in adults (Eyres et al., 1978, 1983; Ecoffey et al., 1984; Takasaki, 1984; Rothstein et al., 1986).

Pregnancy

Although engorgement of vertebral veins and a hyperkinetic circulation might be expected to enhance absorption of local anaesthetics after extradural block, plasma drug concentration—time profiles appear to be similar in pregnant and non-pregnant women (Morgan et al., 1977; Pihlajamäki et al., 1990).

Disease and surgery

Changes in local perfusion associated with altered haemodynamics as a result of disease or surgery may modify absorption of local anaesthetics and hence duration of anaesthesia. For example, acute hypovolaemia slows lignocaine absorption after extradural injection in dogs (Morikawa et al., 1974) and prolongs anaesthesia in patients undergoing thoracotomy with regional block (Quimby, 1965). Conversely, a decreased duration of brachial plexus block in patients with chronic renal failure was suggested to reflect a hyperkinetic circulation and enhanced systemic uptake of local anaesthetic (Bromage & Gertel, 1972). However, this hypothesis is not supported by the results of recent studies (e.g. Rice et al., 1991).

Systemic disposition

After systemic absorption local anaesthetics are distributed by the bloodstream to the organs and tissues of the body and cleared, mostly by metabolism and to a small extent by renal excretion. In pregnant women a proportion of the dose also crosses the placenta into the baby.

The role of the lung

The first capillary bed to be exposed to local anaesthetic once it has entered the systemic circulation is that in the lung. This structure acts as a capacitor, sequestering temporarily a large quantity of drug because of a high lung:blood partition coefficient. Hence, after rapid intravenous input, the arterial blood drug concentration which hits the target organs for toxicity, the brain and the heart (via the coronary circulation), is attenuated considerably compared with the drug concentration in the pulmonary artery

(Tucker & Boas, 1971; Lofstrom, 1978; Jorfeldt et al., 1979).

Arthur (1981) has shown that lung uptake of prilocaine in humans exceeds that of lignocaine and contributes to its greater systemic safety margin. The rank order of uptake in rat lung slices was found to be bupivacaine > etidocaine > lignocaine (Post et al., 1979). The extravascular pH of the lung is low relative to plasma pH and this encourages ion-trapping of local anaesthetic (Post & Eriksdotter-Behm, 1982). Conversely, a relative decrease in plasma pH impairs uptake (Palazzo et al., 1991). Other basic drugs, e.g. propranolol, may compete with local anaesthetics for pulmonary binding sites, thereby decreasing their first-pass extraction (Rothstein et al., 1987). On the other hand, general anaesthesia and severe respiratory deficiency do not appear to have a marked effect (Jorfeldt et al., 1983).

Local anaesthetic drugs injected into patients with intracardiac right—left shunts (Bokesch et al., 1987b) or injected inadvertently into the carotid or vertebral artery during attempted stellate ganglion block, bypass the lung, resulting in a high probability of CNS toxicity. Furthermore, Aldrete and colleagues (1977, 1978) have shown that the introduction of local anaesthetics, under pressure, into the lingual, brachial or femoral artery of baboons and the facial artery of dogs can produce a retrograde flow facilitating direct access of high concentrations of drug to the cerebral circulation.

Blood binding

The long-acting amides are bound in plasma to a greater extent than the short-acting ones (Table 66.4). There are two classes of binding sites: a high-affinity, low-capacity site on α_1-acid glycoprotein and a quantitatively less important low-affinity high-capacity site on albumin (Tucker et al., 1970a; Mather et al., 1971; Mather & Thomas, 1978; Piafsky & Knoppert, 1979; Routledge et al., 1980; Denson et al., 1984; Kraus et al., 1986).

The extent of binding varies with the plasma concentration of α_1-acid glycoprotein, and both are elevated considerably in patients with cancer (Jackson et al., 1982), chronic pain (Fukui et al., 1984), trauma (Edwards et al., 1982), inflammatory disease (Bruguerolle et al., 1985) and uraemia (Grossman et al., 1982), and in postoperative (Hasselstrom et al., 1985) and postmyocardial infarction patients (Barchowsky et al., 1981). Low plasma concentrations of α_1-acid glycoprotein in neonates are associated with much lower binding of local anaesthetics compared with

Table 66.4 Pharmacokinetic parameters describing the disposition kinetics of amide-type local anaesthetics in adult males. (Data from Tucker, 1986)

	Prilocaine	Lignocaine	Mepivacaine	Ropivacaine	Bupivacaine	Etidocaine
$K_{B/P}$	1.1	0.8	0.9	0.7	0.6	0.6
F_U	0.45	0.30	0.20	0.06	0.05	0.05
V_{SS}* (litre)	191	91	84	61	73	134
V_{USS}* (litre)	320	253	382	742	1028	1478
Cl* (litres/min)	2.37	0.95	0.78	0.73	0.58	1.11
E_H	?	0.65	0.52	0.49	0.38	0.74
$t_{\frac{1}{2},z}$ (h)	1.6	1.6	1.9	1.9	2.7	2.7
MBRT (h)	1.3	1.6	1.8	1.4	2.1	2.0

* Specified with respect to arterial blood drug concentration, with the exception of prilocaine and ropivacaine data, which are specified with respect to peripheral venous blood drug concentration. Note, with the exception of lignocaine and ropivacaine, all data refer to racemic drug. $K_{B/P}$, blood/plasma drug concentration ratio; V_{SS}, volume of distribution at steady state based on total blood drug concentration; V_{USS}, volume of distribution at steady state based on unbound drug concentration in plasma water; Cl, systemic clearance; F_U, fraction unbound in plasma (at 2 μg/ml total concentration); E_H, estimated hepatic extraction ratio; $t_{\frac{1}{2},z}$, terminal elimination half-life; MBRT, mean body residence time.

that in adult plasma (Tucker *et al.*, 1970b; Petersen *et al.*, 1981; Wood & Wood, 1981; Piafsky & Woolner, 1982). Binding decreases as pH decreases (Burney *et al.*, 1978; McNamara *et al.*, 1981; Coyle *et al.*, 1984).

Attachment of the agents to binding sites in or on erythrocytes is of similar order to plasma binding (Tucker *et al.*, 1970a). However, in the presence of plasma proteins, plasma binding competes with binding to the red cells. Hence, blood : plasma drug concentration ratios are related inversely to plasma binding (Table 66.4).

The role of plasma binding in the toxicity of local anaesthetics has been discussed by Tucker (1986, 1988).

Thus, it is important to allow for this phenomenon when interpreting measurements of plasma drug concentrations. For example, marked accumulation of total plasma drug concentrations postoperatively may not signify a risk of toxicity (Ross *et al.*, 1980; Richter *et al.*, 1984). This change reflects the postoperative increase in α_1-acid glycoprotein and therefore plasma drug binding. Unbound (active) drug concentrations, which are likely to be a better index of effect, are similar before and after surgery (Fig. 66.9). When systemic drug input is gradual, as after perineural injection, distribution of the dose is spread over time and a large extravascular distribution space and extensive tissue binding (see below) ensures that only a small percentage remains in the blood at any time. Under these conditions, any changes in plasma binding are buffered effectively by a high volume of distribution. Also, for drugs like bupivacaine, with relatively low hepatic extraction ratios,

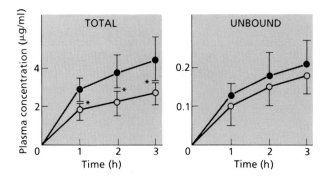

Fig. 66.9 Mean total and free plasma concentrations of bupivacaine during intravenous infusions of bupivacaine HCl 2 mg/min in seven cholecystectomy patients studied 3 h before surgery (open circles) and 72 h after operation (closed circles). * Statistically significant difference. (Redrawn from Tucker, 1986.)

any increase in freedrug concentration will be compensated by a faster elimination.

Theoretically plasma binding could limit the first-pass uptake of local anaesthetics into the brain and myocardium following rapid, inadvertent, intravenous injection, thereby modulating toxicity. However, it is probable that a toxic dose would produce sufficiently high blood drug concentrations to overwhelm the blood binding capacity on first-pass through the brain and heart. Furthermore, studies of the initial brain uptake of local anaesthetics in rats indicate that there is an enhanced dissociation from plasma binding sites in the microcirculation (Terasaki *et al.*, 1986) (Fig. 66.10). The latter observation contrasts with findings in the dog, showing that at a few minutes often rapid intravenous injection of ligno-

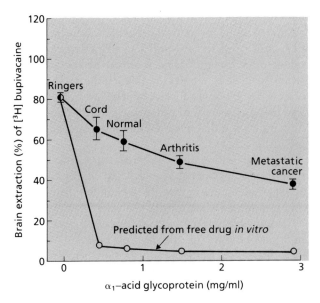

Fig. 66.10 Effect of the binding of bupivacaine to human serum on its first-pass brain uptake in rats. The closed circles represent the brain extraction of bupivacaine after carotid injection of drug (1 µg/ml) mixed in Ringer's solution or in umbilical cord, normal, arthritis or metastatic cancer human serum. Each point represents the mean ± SE for five to six experiments. The open circles represent the theoretical extraction predicted using free percentages measured *in vitro*. (Redrawn from Terasaki *et al.*, 1986.)

caine, the extent of drug distribution into brain tissue and CSF was entirely governed by the equilibrium free concentration of drug in plasma (Marathe *et al.*, 1991). Therefore, it appears important to distinguish events after even a few recirculations from those during first-pass through an organ. In either case it should not be assumed that plasma binding modulates tissue drug uptake, thereby 'protecting' against toxicity.

Tissue distribution

In the amide series of local anaesthetics, a greater extent of plasma binding is accompanied by a parallel increase in affinity for tissue components. Thus, steady-state volumes of distribution based on unbound drug (V_{USS}), which reflect net tissue binding, vary over a five-fold range, being greatest for the more lipid-soluble agents (Table 66.4). Distribution volumes based on total drug concentration in blood vary only two-fold, reflecting the balance between blood and tissue binding.

The toxicity of local anaesthetic is increased significantly by acidosis and hypercapnia (Englesson, 1974; Englesson & Grevsten, 1974). In theory, an increased

brain and myocardial concentration of free ionized drug could account for this through haemodynamic changes and ion trapping. However, the latter possibility seems unlikely, as animal studies have shown that the partition coefficients of local anaesthetics between whole brain or myocardium and blood are similar (Simon *et al.*, 1984) or reduced (Nancarrow *et al.*, 1987) during metabolic acidosis of the type associated with convulsions. This is because the lowering of blood pH is similar to, or greater than, the lowering of tissue pH. On the other hand, Simon and colleagues (1984) have hypothesized that treatment of convulsions by paralysis and artificial ventilation will tend to exacerbate entry of local anaesthetic into the brain, because prevention of the systemic acidosis, but not the cerebral acidosis, promotes ion trapping of drug in the organ (Fig. 66.11). This does not imply that ventilation with oxygen is deleterious, but it may require the use of anticonvulsants for continuation of ventilation until the drug is cleared from the brain.

Excretion

Renal excretion of unchanged local anaesthetics is a minor route of elimination, accounting for less than 1–6% of the dose under normal conditions (Tucker & Mather, 1979). Depending on the agent, acidification of the urine increases this proportion to 5–20%, which is consistent with less tubular reabsorption as a result of greater ionization. However, this increase is insufficient to warrant the use of a forced acid diuresis in treating toxicity.

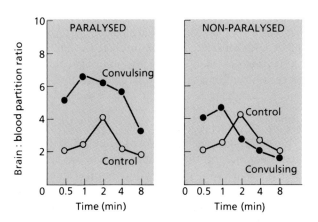

Fig. 66.11 Brain : blood partition ratios of lignocaine after intravenous injection into convulsing (closed circles) and non-convulsing (open circles) rats. The left-hand panel shows data for rats paralysed with gallamine and ventilated with nitrous oxide/oxygen; the right-hand panel shows data for non-paralysed animals. (Redrawn from Simon *et al.*, 1984.)

Metabolism

Esters

These are cleared in both the blood and the liver. *In vitro* half-lives in plasma reflect the action of pseudocholinesterase and in normal adults they vary from 10—20 s for chloroprocaine (O'Brien *et al.*, 1979; Kuhnert *et al.*, 1986), 40 s for procaine (Reidenberg *et al.*, 1972; DuSouich & Erill, 1977), to several minutes for amethocaine (Foldes *et al.*, 1965). Red cell esterases contribute also to blood clearance (Calvo *et al.*, 1980).

In vitro half-lives are longer than those measured *in vivo*, e.g. that of chloroprocaine after extradural injection is about 3 min (Kuhnert *et al.*, 1986). However, this value probably reflects rate-limiting absorption rather than metabolic clearance. After high intravenous doses of procaine, clearances of 0.04—0.08 litres·min^{-1}·kg^{-1} and elimination half-lives of 7—8 min have been observed, probably reflecting some saturation of the enzyme systems (Seifen *et al.*, 1979).

The clinical implication of the rapid clearance of the esters is that if a toxic concentration is attained after inadvertent intravenous injection, the ensuing reaction should be relatively short-lived. *In vitro* plasma half-lives are prolonged by about two to four times in patients with renal and liver disease (Reidenberg *et al.*, 1972; DuSouich & Erill, 1977). However, normal esterase activity is preserved in their erythrocytes, suggesting that they may not be significantly more susceptible to toxicity (Calvo *et al.*, 1980).

The hydrolysis products of procaine and chloroprocaine have been measured in human plasma but appear to be inactive pharmacologically (Brodie *et al.*, 1948; O'Brien *et al.*, 1979; Kuhnert *et al.*, 1980; Krogh & Jellum, 1981), although the aminobenzoic acids may contribute to the rare allergic reaction.

Amides

The amide linkage is stable in blood, and most of the clearance of these agents occurs in the liver. Mean values vary in the order: bupivacaine < ropivacaine < mepivacaine (reflecting the size of the *N*-methyl substituent in this homologous series) < lignocaine < etidocaine < prilocaine (Table 66.4). Over the whole series, there is no relationship to anaesthetic potency or to lipid solubility—protein binding. Etidocaine clearance is dependent mostly on liver perfusion, whereas that of bupivacaine should be more sensitive to changes in intrinsic

hepatic enzyme function (Tucker, 1986). Although clearance of the former is double that of the latter and they are intrinsically equitoxic, any advantage this might offer for etidocaine is offset by the fact that twice the dose is needed to establish the same quality of sensory block as that produced by bupivacaine. The blood clearance of prilocaine exceeds liver blood flow indicating that some extrahepatic metabolism of this drug occurs.

Terminal elimination half-lives and mean body residence times are between 1.5 and 3 h for all of the agents, reflecting a balance between their distribution and clearance characteristics (Table 66.4).

The evaluation of any stereoselectivity in the pharmacokinetics of the optical isomers of chiral local anaesthetics after administration as racemates is now possible with the availability of chiral h.p.l.c. columns. In humans, the plasma clearance of $R(+)$-bupivacaine, the more toxic form, is about 20% greater than that of the $S(-)$-isomer (Lee *et al.*, 1987), while the systemic clearances of $S(+)$- and $R(-)$-prilocaine are similar (Tucker *et al.*, 1990). Since the isomers of prilocaine have similar anaesthetic activity and acute toxicity in animals, a higher margin for systemic CNS toxicity is not likely to be achieved by substituting racemic prilocaine with one of its isomers.

Identification of the biotransformation products of the amides in human urine indicates three major sites of metabolic attack, namely aromatic hydroxylation, *N*-dealkylation and amide hydrolysis (Tucker & Mather, 1980, 1988; Rosenberg *et al.*, 1991; Pere *et al.*, 1991). Monoethylglycinexylidide, glycinexylidide and the 4-hydroxy products formed from lignocaine and bupivacaine, pipecolylxylidide from mepivacaine and bupivacaine, and the monodealkylated derivatives of etidocaine have all been measured in human plasma. It is likely that the first of these contributes significantly to the effects of the parent drug. On continuous infusion, unbound plasma concentrations of monoethylglycinexylidide are 70% of those of lignocaine (Drayer *et al.*, 1983), and studies in rodents indicate that it is about 70% as toxic (Blumer *et al.*, 1973). Metabolism of prilocaine to *o*-toluidine and subsequent hydroxylation of this product is responsible for methaemoglobinaemia at doses above 600 mg (Hjelm & Holmdahl, 1965). Other amides are hydrolysed to 2,6-xylidine which does not produce this problem (McLean *et al.*, 1969).

Accumulation

With the increasing use of techniques involving the

prolonged administration of local anaesthetics, it is important to assess the rate and extent of drug accumulation. Thus, toxicity could develop insidiously with time, or more suddenly if inappropriate bolus doses are superimposed on a continuous infusion. If kinetics are dose- and time-independent, it is possible to predict the extent of accumulation and to adjust dosage rate accordingly. For short-term intermittent extradural injections of lignocaine and etidocaine given over 5–10 h, increases in plasma drug concentration were consistent with single-dose data (Tucker et al., 1977). As discussed previously, following more prolonged administration in postoperative patients, a time-dependent decrease in clearance (based upon measurement of total-bound plus free-plasma drug concentration) is expected as levels of α_1-acid glycoprotein and plasma-binding increase. In addition, however, there is evidence, mostly from animal studies, for a progressive decrease in the intrinsic ability of hepatic enzymes to clear lignocaine (Lennard et al., 1983), mepivacaine and bupivacaine (Mazoit et al., 1988a; Mather, 1991), presumed to be due to product-inhibition. Recent observation that the plasma concentrations of bupivacaine during 72 h interpleural infusion were predictable from single-dose data are not consistent with either time-dependent increase in plasma binding or decrease in intrinsic hepatic clearance (Kastrissios et al., 1991).

Effects of patient variables and other drugs

Most of the information on likely effects of patient variables and other drug therapy on the disposition kinetics of local anaesthetics has been obtained from studies with intravenous lignocaine, and it may not be possible always to extrapolate the findings to patients receiving regional anaesthesia. This is a problem especially when haemodynamic factors are involved, since the cardiovascular effects of sympathetic nerve block may complicate the issue, and changes in drug elimination may be offset by opposite changes in drug absorption (Tucker, 1984). For example, although hypovolaemia decreases lignocaine clearance (Benowitz et al., 1974), plasma drug concentrations are lower following extradural block in the presence of blood loss as a result of an impaired absorption rate (Morikawa et al., 1974).

A summary of variables which have been studied with respect to the disposition kinetics of the amide local anaesthetics is given in Table 66.5. Of these, the evidence suggests that old age (uncomplicated by disease), weight, sex, race, pregnancy and renal disease have relatively minor impact, whereas cardiovascular disease and liver cirrhosis are associated with clinically more significant alterations in kinetics. Elimination half-lives are prolonged two- to threefold in neonates, reflecting increased volumes of distribution or decreased clearance or both. Along with

Table 66.5 The influence of some patient variables and other drugs on the disposition of local anaesthetic agents

Variable	Agent	Route	Change	Reference
Age				
Elderly	L	Exd	$\downarrow Cl$	Bowdle et al. (1986)
	B	Exd	$\downarrow Cl$	Veering et al. (1987, 1992)
	B	S	$\downarrow Cl$	Veering et al. (1991a)
	B	—	$\leftrightarrow F_U$	Veering et al. (1991b)
	L	i.v.	$\downarrow Cl, \leftrightarrow V, \uparrow t_{\frac{1}{2}} (\sigma)$ $\leftrightarrow Cl, V, t_{\frac{1}{2}} (\c{Q})$	Abernethy and Greenblatt (1984a)
	L	i.v.	$\leftrightarrow Cl, \uparrow V, \uparrow t_{\frac{1}{2}}$	Nation et al. (1977)
	L	i.v.	$\leftrightarrow Cl, \leftrightarrow V, \uparrow t_{\frac{1}{2}}, \downarrow F_U$	Cusack et al. (1985)
	L	i.v.	$\uparrow Cl$	Cusson et al. (1985)
Children	B	IC	$\uparrow Cl^*$	Rothstein et al. (1986)
	L	i.v.	$\leftrightarrow Cl,^* V,^* t_{\frac{1}{2}}$	Finholt et al. (1986)
	L	Caud	$\leftrightarrow Cl^*$	Ecoffey et al. (1984)
	B	Caud	$\uparrow Cl^*$	Ecoffey et al. (1985)
	B	Caud	$\uparrow Cl,^* \uparrow F_U$	Mazoit et al. (1988b)
Neonates	L	s.c.	$\leftrightarrow Cl,^* \uparrow V,^* \uparrow t_{\frac{1}{2}}$	Mihaly et al. (1978)
	M	s.c.	$\downarrow Cl,^* \uparrow V,^* \uparrow t_{\frac{1}{2}}$	Moore et al. (1978)
	B	Exd (mother)	$\uparrow t_{\frac{1}{2}}$	Magno et al. (1976); Caldwell et al. (1977)
	E	Exd (mother)	$\uparrow t_{\frac{1}{2}}$	Morgan et al. (1978)

Continued on p. 1376

Table 66.5 *Continued*

Variable	Agent	Route	Change	Reference
Weight	L, M, B	Exd, Caud, IC, Periph.	$\leftrightarrow C-T$	Scott *et al.* (1972); Tucker *et al.* (1972); Moore *et al.* (1976a,b)
	L	i.v.	$\leftrightarrow Cl,\ \uparrow V,\ \uparrow t_{\frac{1}{2}}$ (obesity)	Abernethy and Greenblatt (1984b)
	L	i.v.	$\downarrow Cl$	Cusson *et al.* (1985)
Sex	L	i.v.	$\leftrightarrow Cl,\ \uparrow V\ (♀)$	Abernethy and Greenblatt (1984a)
	L	i.v.	$\leftrightarrow Cl,\ \uparrow V,\ \uparrow t_{\frac{1}{2}},\ \leftrightarrow F_U\ (♀)$	Wing *et al.* (1984)
Race	L	i.v.	$\leftrightarrow Cl,\ V,\ t_{\frac{1}{2}},\ F_U$ (Caucasian, Oriental, Black)	Goldberg *et al.* (1982)
Pregnancy	E	Exd	$\leftrightarrow C-T$	Morgan *et al.* (1977)
	L	Exd	$\downarrow Cl,\ \leftrightarrow F_U$ (pre-eclampsia vs. normal)	Ramanathan *et al.* (1986); Bottorff *et al.* (1987)
	L	i.v.	$\leftrightarrow Cl,*\ \uparrow V,*\ \uparrow t_{\frac{1}{2}}$ (sheep)	Bloedow *et al.* (1980)
	L	i.v.	$\uparrow Cl,*\ \leftrightarrow V,*\ \leftrightarrow t_{\frac{1}{2}}$ (sheep)	Arthur *et al.* (1985)
	L	i.v.	$\uparrow Cl,\ \uparrow V,\ \leftrightarrow t_{\frac{1}{2}}$ (sheep)	Santos *et al.* (1988)
	R	i.v.	$\downarrow Cl,\ \updownarrow V,\ \leftrightarrow t_{\frac{1}{2}}$ (sheep)	Santos *et al.* (1990)
	B	—	$\uparrow F_U$	Wulf *et al.* (1991)
Disease				
Heart failure	L	i.v.	$\downarrow Cl,\ \downarrow V,\ \leftrightarrow t_{\frac{1}{2}}$	Thomson *et al.* (1973)
Orthostatic hypotension	L	i.v.	$\downarrow Cl,\ \downarrow V,\ \leftrightarrow t_{\frac{1}{2}},\ \leftrightarrow F_U$ (sitting vs. supine)	Feely *et al.* (1982a)
Cardiopulmonary resuscitation	L	i.v.	$\downarrow Cl,\ \downarrow V,\ \leftrightarrow t_{\frac{1}{2}}$	Chow *et al.* (1981, 1983)
Cirrhosis	L	i.v.	$\downarrow Cl,\ \uparrow V,\ \uparrow t_{\frac{1}{2}}$	Thomson *et al.* (1973); Huet and Villeneuve (1983)
	L	—	$\uparrow F_U$	Barry *et al.* (1990)
Chronic hepatitis	L	i.v.	$\uparrow Cl,\ \uparrow V$	Huet and LeLorier (1980)
Acute viral hepatitis	L	i.v.	$\updownarrow Cl,\ \updownarrow V,\ \updownarrow t_{\frac{1}{2}}$	Williams *et al.* (1976)
Renal failure	L	i.v.	$\leftrightarrow Cl,\ V,\ t_{\frac{1}{2}}$ ($\uparrow$ GX)	Thomson *et al.* (1973) Collinsworth *et al.* (1975)
Other drugs				
Halothane	L	i.v.	$\downarrow Cl,\ \updownarrow V,\ \updownarrow t_{\frac{1}{2}}$	Bentley *et al.* (1983)
	L	i.v.	$\downarrow Cl$ (sheep)	Mather *et al.* (1986)
Diazepam	B, E	Exd	$\updownarrow C_{max}?$	Giasi *et al.* (1980)
	B	i.v., Exd	$\leftrightarrow Cl,\ V,\ t_{\frac{1}{2}}$ $\leftrightarrow C-T$ (monkey)	Thompson *et al.* (1986)
	B	Caud	$\downarrow Cl$	Giaufre *et al.* (1988)
	L	Caud	$\leftrightarrow Cl$	Giaufre *et al.* (1988)
Midazolam	B	Caud	$\leftrightarrow Cl$	Giaufre *et al.* (1990)
	L	Caud	$\uparrow Cl$	Giaufre *et al.* (1990)

Continued

Table 66.5 *Continued*

Variable	Agent	Route	Change	Reference
Noradrenaline	L	i.v.	$\downarrow Cl$, $\downarrow V$, $\uparrow t_{\frac{1}{2}}$ (monkey)	Benowitz et al. (1974)
Isoprenaline	L	i.v.	$\uparrow Cl$, $\uparrow V$, $\downarrow t_{\frac{1}{2}}$ (monkey)	Benowitz et al. (1974)
Ephedrine	L	i.v.	$\uparrow Cl$	Wiklund et al. (1977)
Propranolol	L	i.v., p.o.	$\downarrow Cl$, $\leftrightarrow F_U$	Tucker et al. (1984); Bax et al. (1985)
	B	i.v.	$\downarrow Cl$, $\leftrightarrow V$, $\uparrow t_{\frac{1}{2}}$	Bowdle et al. (1987)
Verapamil	L	i.v.	$\leftrightarrow Cl$, V, $t_{\frac{1}{2}}$ (dog)	Chelly et al. (1987)
Cimetidine	L	i.v.	$\downarrow Cl$, $\downarrow V$, $\leftrightarrow t_{\frac{1}{2}}$, $\uparrow F_U$	Feely et al. (1982b)
	L	i.v.	$\downarrow Cl$, $\downarrow V$, $\leftrightarrow t_{\frac{1}{2}}$, $\leftrightarrow F_U$	Wing et al. (1984)
	L	i.v.	$\downarrow Cl$, $\leftrightarrow V$, $\uparrow t_{\frac{1}{2}}$	Bauer et al. (1984)
	L	i.v.	$\downarrow Cl$, $\downarrow V$, $\leftrightarrow t_{\frac{1}{2}}$	Jackson et al. (1985)
	B	i.v.	$\downarrow Cl$	Noble et al. (1987)
	L	Exd	$\leftrightarrow Cl$	Flynn et al. (1989a)
	L	Exd	$\downarrow Cl$	Kishikawa et al. (1990)
	B	Exd	$\leftrightarrow Cl$	Flynn et al. (1989b)
	B	Exd	$\leftrightarrow Cl$	O'Sullivan et al. (1988)
	B	Exd	$\leftrightarrow Cl$	Kuhnert et al. (1987)
Ranitidine	L	i.v.	$\leftrightarrow Cl$, V, $t_{\frac{1}{2}}$, F_U	Feely and Guy (1983)
	L	i.v.	$\downarrow Cl$, $\downarrow V$, $\leftrightarrow t_{\frac{1}{2}}$	Robson et al. (1985)
	L	i.v.	$\leftrightarrow Cl$, V, $t_{\frac{1}{2}}$	Jackson et al. (1985)
	B	i.v.	$\leftrightarrow Cl$	Noble et al. (1987)
	L	Exd	$\leftrightarrow Cl$	Flynn et al. (1989a)
	B	Exd	$\leftrightarrow Cl$	Flynn et al. (1989b)
	B	Exd	$\leftrightarrow Cl$, $\leftrightarrow F_U$	Brashear et al. (1991)
	B	Exd	$\leftrightarrow Cl$	O'Sullivan et al. (1988)
Phenytoin	L	i.v.	$\uparrow Cl$, $\leftrightarrow V$, $\leftrightarrow t_{\frac{1}{2}}$, $\downarrow F_U$	Perucca and Richens (1979); Routledge et al. (1981)

B, bupivacaine; E, etidocaine; L, lignocaine; M, mepivacaine; R, ropivacaine; Caud, caudal; Exd, extradural; IC, intercostal; Periph., peripheral nerve block; S, subarachnoid; Cl, clearance; V, volume of distribution (mostly derived for steady state); $t_{\frac{1}{2}}$, terminal elimination half-life; C_{max}, maximum plasma drug concentration; $C-T$, plasma drug concentration–time profile; F_U, free fraction in plasma; GX, plasma glycinexylidide; * standardized to body weight; $\uparrow$ $\downarrow$ trend only.

suggestions that absorption is faster in children than in adults, their unbound clearance (corrected for body weight) appears to be similar (lignocaine) or greater (bupivacaine). Corresponding volumes of distribution seem to be similar or higher, such that half-lives are comparable with those in adults.

A number of drugs (notably halothane, cimetidine and propranolol) have been shown to lower the clearance of local anaesthetics, mainly by direct inhibition of mixed function oxidase activity, with a smaller contribution from decreased hepatic blood flow (Table 66.5). Several *in vitro* studies showing decreased plasma binding of local anaesthetic drugs in the presence of other drugs have been described.

However, the clinical significance of these observations is questionable in view of the high concentrations used and because altered free fractions do not necessarily imply significant increases in free-drug concentrations *in vivo*.

Many studies of the potential effect of H_2-antagonists on the pharmacokinetics of local anaesthetics have been reported, with various permutations of agents, dosage, route of administration and duration of pretreatment. In isolation they all suffer from the problem of small numbers of subjects. However, in general, it seems that in single doses for premedication ranitidine has no effect and cimetidine has little or no effect on the kinetics of either extradural lignocaine or bupivacaine. On continuous dosage, cimetidine lowers the clearance of lignocaine significantly but ranitidine has little or no effect. The effects of multiple dosage of cimetidine and ranitidine on bupivacaine clearance have not been determined.

Placental transfer

Esters

After maternal injection, 2-chloroprocaine appears in both maternal and cord plasma in very low concentrations (Kuhnert et al., 1980; Abboud et al., 1983, 1984). Thus, even though elimination half-lives of chloroprocaine and procaine are twice as long in cord plasma as in maternal plasma and pregnancy is associated with a decrease in pseudocholinesterase activity (Reidenberg et al., 1972; O'Brien et al., 1979; Kuhnert et al., 1980), the absolute rate of hydrolysis in the mother remains fast and helps to reduce placental transfer and the risk of fetal intoxication.

Amides

At delivery, mean values of cord : maternal plasma concentration ratios of the amides decrease in the order: prilocaine (1.0−1.1), lignocaine (0.5−0.7), mepivacaine (0.7), bupivacaine (0.2−0.4) and etidocaine (0.2−0.3) (Tucker & Mather, 1979). These differences reflect differential maternal and fetal plasma binding of the drugs owing to relatively low fetal concentrations of α_1-acid glycoprotein. Equilibrium ratios of the agents are predicted in humans and sheep from plasma-binding data, with allowance for ion trapping due to fetal acidosis (Tucker et al., 1970b; Thomas et al., 1976; Kennedy et al., 1986, 1990). As such, therefore, these ratios are not direct predictors of relative fetal toxicity, as corresponding ratios of unbound (active) drug across the placenta are probably close to unity irrespective of the drug. (Negative followed by positive deviations from unity are expected with time as the transplacental concentration gradient reverses during the rise and fall of maternal drug concentrations.) Nevertheless, a high maternal : fetal binding ratio should delay equilibration of drug in fetal tissues, despite rapid equilibration across the placenta (Dawes, 1973; Hamshaw-Thomas et al., 1985). On the other hand, similar umbilical artery : umbilical vein concentration ratios observed for the various agents argue against large differences in their equilibration rates in the fetus (Tucker et al., 1970b).

Finster and Pedersen (1979) and Kuhnert and colleagues (1981) have suggested that relatively low cord : maternal ratios of bupivacaine, based on total plasma drug concentrations, are due to more extensive uptake of this drug by the fetal tissues. Such an explanation is kinetically unsound and certainly cannot explain low umbilical venous : maternal ratios (Carson & Reynolds, 1988).

In the event of inadvertent maternal intravascular injection of local anaesthetic, it is advisable either to effect the delivery immediately before maximum fetal uptake occurs or, providing that maternal and fetal circulations remain adequate, to delay until significant back-transfer of drug to and clearance by the mother has taken place (Gupta et al., 1986). An intermediate window will exist in which the body burden to the newborn, whose capacity to eliminate the drug may be impaired, is relatively high.

References

Abboud T.K., Kim K.C., Nouehed R., Kuhnert B.R., DerMardirossian N., Moumdjian J., Sarkis F. & Nagappala S. (1983) Epidural bupivacaine, chloroprocaine, or lidocaine for Cesarian section — maternal and neonatal effects. Anesthesia and Analgesia 62, 914−19.

Abboud T.K., Afrasiabi A., Sarkis F., Daftarian A., Nagappala S., Noueihed R., Kuhnert B.R. & Miller F. (1984) Continuous infusion epidural analgesia in parturients receiving bupivacaine, chloroprocaine or lidocaine — maternal, fetal and neonatal effects. Anesthesia and Analgesia 63, 421−8.

Aberg G. (1972) Toxicological and local anaesthetic effects of optically active isomers of two local anaesthetic compounds. Acta Pharmacologica et Toxicologica 31, 273−86.

Abernethy D.R. & Greenblatt D.J. (1984a) Impairment of lidocaine clearance in elderly male subjects. Journal of Cardiovascular Pharmacology 5, 1093−6.

Abernethy D.R. & Greenblatt D.J. (1984b) Lidocaine disposition in obesity. American Journal of Cardiology 53, 1183−6.

Adams H.J., Mastri A.R., Eicholzer A.W. & Kilpatrick G. (1974) Morphological effects of intrathecal etidocaine and tetracaine on the rabbit spinal cord. Anesthesiology 53, 904−8.

Adams H.J., Mastri A.R. & Doherty J. (1977) Bupivacaine: morphological effects on spinal cords of cats and durations of spinal anesthesia in sheep. Pharmacology Research Communications 9, 847−55.

Aldrete J.A., Barnes D.R. & Sigon M.A. (1969) Studies on effects of addition of potassium chloride to lidocaine. Anesthesia and Analgesia 48, 269−76.

Aldrete J.A., Nicholson J., Sada T., Davidson W. & Garastasu G. (1977) Cephalic kinetics of intra-arterially injected lidocaine. Oral Surgery 44, 167−72.

Aldrete J.A., Romo-Salas F., Arora S., Wilson R. & Rutherford R. (1978) Reverse arterial blood flow as a pathway for central nervous system toxic response following injection of local anesthetics. Anesthesia and Analgesia 57, 428−33.

Aps C. & Reynolds F. (1976) The effect of concentration on vasoactivity of bupivacaine and lignocaine. British Journal of Anaesthesia 48, 1171−4.

Aps C. & Reynolds F. (1978) An intradermal study of the local anaesthetic and vascular effects of the isomers of bupivacaine. *British Journal of Clinical Pharmacology* **6**, 63–8.

Armstrong P., Brockway M. & Wildsmith J.A.W. (1990a) Alkalinisation of prilocaine for intravenous regional anaesthesia. *Anaesthesia* **45**, 11–13.

Armstrong P., Watters J. & Whitfield A. (1990b) Alkalinisation of prilocaine for intravenous regional anaesthesia. Suitability for clinical use. *Anaesthesia* **45**, 935–7.

Arthur G.R. (1981) Distribution and Elimination of Local Anaesthetic Agents: The Role of Lung, Liver and Kidney. PhD Thesis, University of Edinburgh.

Arthur G.R., Morishima H.O., Finster M., Pedersen H. & Covino B.G. (1985) Effect of pregnancy on lidocaine pharmacokinetics in sheep. *Anesthesiology* **63**, 229A.

Barchowsky A., Stargel W.W., Shand D.G. & Routledge P.A. (1981) On the role of alpha$_1$-acid glycoprotein in lignocaine accumulation following myocardial infarction. *British Journal of Clinical Pharmacology* **13**, 411–15.

Bader A.M., Datta S., Moller R.A. & Covino B.G. (1990) Acute progesterone treatment has no effect on bupivacaine-induced conduction blockade in the isolated rabbit vagus nerve. *Anesthesia and Analgesia* **71**, 545–8.

Barry M., Keeling P.W.N., Weir D. & Feely J. (1990) Severity of cirrhosis and the relationship of α_1-acid glycoprotein concentration to plasma protein binding of lidocaine. *Clinical Pharmacology Therapy* **47**, 366–70.

Bauer L.A., Edwards W.A.D., Randolph F.P. & Blouin R.A. (1984) Cimetidine-induced decrease in lidocaine metabolism. *American Heart Journal* **108**, 413–15.

Bax N.D.S., Tucker G.T., Lennard M.S. & Woods H.F. (1985) The impairment of lignocaine clearance by propranolol — major contribution from enzyme inhibition. *British Journal of Clinical Pharmacology* **19**, 597–603.

Bedder M.D., Kozody R. & Craig D.B. (1987) A comparison of bupivacaine and alkalinized bupivacaine in brachial plexus anesthesia. *Anesthesia and Analgesia* **66**, 9S.

Benhamou D., Labaille T., Bonhomme L. & Perrachon N. (1989) Alkalinization of epidural 0.5% bupivacaine for Cesarian Section. *Regional Anesthesia* **14**, 240–3.

Benowitz N., Forsyth R.P., Melmon K.L. & Rowland M. (1974) Lidocaine disposition kinetics in monkey and man. II. effects of hemorrhage and sympathomimetic drug administration. *Clinical Pharmacology and Therapeutics* **16**, 99–109.

Bentley J.B., Glass S. & Gandolfi A.J. (1983) The influence of halothane on lidocaine pharmacokinetics in man. *Anesthesiology* **59**, 246A.

Benzon H.T., Strichartz G.R., Gissen A.J., Shanks C.A., Covino B.G. & Datta S. (1988) Developmental neurophysiology of mammalian peripheral nerves and age-related differential sensitivity to local anaesthetic. *British Journal of Anaesthesia* **61**, 754–60.

Bernards C.M. & Hill H.F. (1991) The spinal nerve root sleeve is not a preferred route for redistribution of drugs from the epidural space to the spinal cord. *Anesthesiology* **75**, 827–32.

Blair M.R. (1975) Cardiovascular pharmacology of local anaesthetics. *British Journal of Anaesthesia* **47**, 247–52.

Bloedow D.C., Ralston D.H. & Hargrove J.C. (1980) Lidocaine pharmacokinetics in pregnant and non-pregnant sheep. *Journal of Pharmaceutical Science* **69**, 32–7.

Blumer J., Strong J.M. & Atkinson A.J. (1973) The convulsant potency of lidocaine and its N-dealkylated metabolites. *Journal of Pharmacology and Experimental Therapeutics* **186**, 31–6.

Bokesch P.M., Post C. & Strichartz G. (1986) Structure–activity relationship of lidocaine homologs producing tonic and frequency-dependent impulse blockade in nerve. *Journal of Pharmacology and Experimental Therapeutics* **237**, 773–81.

Bokesch P.M., Raymond S.A. & Strichartz G. (1987a) Dependence of lidocaine potency on pH and Pco$_2$. *Anesthesia and Analgesia* **66**, 9–17.

Bokesch P.M., Castaneda A.R., Ziemer G. & Wilson J.M. (1987b) The influence of right-to-left cardiac shunt on lidocaine pharmacokinetics. *Anesthesiology* **67**, 739–44.

Bottorff M.B., Pieper J.A., Boucher B.A., Hoon T.J., Ramanathan J. & Sibai B.M. (1987) Lidocaine protein binding in pre-eclampsia. *European Journal of Clinical Pharmacology* **31**, 719–22.

Bowdle T.A., Freund P.R. & Slattery J.T. (1986) Age-dependent lidocaine pharmacokinetics during lumbar peridural anesthesia with lidocaine hydrocarbonate and lidocaine hydrochloride. *Regional Anesthesia* **11**, 123–7.

Bowdle T.A., Freund P.R. & Slattery J.T. (1987) Propranolol reduces bupivacaine clearance. *Anesthesiology* **66**, 36–8.

Brashear W.T., Zuspan K.J., Lazebnik N., Kuhnert B.R. & Mann L.I. (1991) Effect of ranitidine on bupivacaine disposition. *Anesthesia and Analgesia* **72**, 369–76.

Bridenbaugh P.O., Tucker G.T., Moore D.C., Bridenbaugh L.D. & Thompson G.E. (1974) Preliminary clinical evaluation of etidocaine (Duranest): a new long-acting local anesthetic agent. *Acta Anaesthesiologica Scandinavica* **18**, 165–71.

Brodie B.B., Lief P.A. & Poet R. (1948) The fate of procaine in man following its intravenous administration and methods for the estimation of procaine and diethylaminoethanol. *Journal of Pharmacology and Experimental Therapeutics* **94**, 359–95.

Bromage P.R. (1967) Physiology and pharmacology of epidural analgesia. *Anesthesiology* **28**, 592–622.

Bromage P.R. (1974) Lower limb reflex changes in segmental epidural analgesia. *British Journal of Anaesthesia* **46**, 504–8.

Bromage P.R. (1975) Mechanisms of action of extradural analgesia. *British Journal of Anaesthesia* **47**, 199–211.

Bromage P.R. & Burfoot M.F. (1966) Quality of epidural blockade. II. Influence of physicochemical factors, hyaluronidase and potassium. *British Journal of Anaesthesia* **38**, 857–65.

Bromage P.R. & Gertel M. (1972) Brachial plexus anesthesia in chronic renal failure. *Anesthesiology* **36**, 488–93.

Bromage P.R., Joyal A.C. & Binney J.C. (1963) Local anesthetic drugs: penetration from the spinal extradural space into the neuraxis. *Science* **140**, 392–3.

Brown D.T., Morison D.H., Covino B.G. & Scott D.B. (1980) Comparison of carbonated bupivacaine and bupivacaine hydrochloride for extradural anaesthesia. *British Journal of Anaesthesia* **52**, 419–22.

Bruguerolle B., Philip-Joet F., Arnaud C. & Arnaud A. (1985) Consequences of inflammatory processes on lignocaine protein binding during anaesthesia in fibreoptic bronchoscopy. *British Journal of Clinical Pharmacology* **20**, 180–1.

Buckley P., Neto G.D. & Fink B.R. (1985) Acid and alkaline solutions of local anesthetics: duration of nerve block and tissue pH. *Anesthesia and Analgesia* **64**, 477–82.

Burm A.G.L. (1989) Clinical pharmacokinetics of epidural and spinal anaesthesia. *Clinical Pharmacokinetics* **16**, 283–311.

Burm A.G.L., Vermeulen N.P.E., Van Kleef J.W., De Boer A.G., Spierdijk J. & Breimer D.D. (1987) Pharmacokinetics of lidocaine and bupivacaine in surgical patients following epidural administration. Simultaneous investigation of absorption and disposition kinetics using stable isotopes. *Clinical Pharmacokinetics* **13**, 191–203.

Burm A.G.L., Van Kleef J.W., Vermeulen N.P.E., Olthof G., Breimer D.D. & Spierdijk T. (1988) Pharmacokinetics of lidocaine and bupivacaine following subarachnoid administration in surgical patients: simultaneous investigation of absorption and disposition kinetics using stable isotopes. *Anesthesiology* **69**, 584–92.

Burn J.M., Guyer P.B. & Langdon L. (1973) The spread of solutions into the epidural space. A study using epidurograms in patients with the lumbosciatic syndrome. *British Journal of Anaesthesia* **45**, 338–44.

Burney R.G., Difazio C.A. & Foster J.H. (1978) Effects of pH on protein binding of lidocaine. *Anesthesia and Analgesia* **57**, 478–80.

Butterworth J.F. & Strichartz G.R. (1990) Molecular mechanisms of local anesthesia: a review. *Anesthesiology* **72**, 711–34.

Butterworth J.F., Walker F.O. & Lysak S.Z. (1990a) Pregnancy increases median nerve susceptibility to lidocaine. *Anesthesiology* **72**, 962–5.

Butterworth J.F., Walker F.O. & Neal J.M. (1990b) Cooling potentiates lidocaine inhibition of median nerve sensory fibers. *Anesthesia and Analgesia* **70**, 507–11.

Caldwell J., Moffatt J.R., Smith R.L., Lieberman A.B., Beard R.W., Sneddon W. & Wilson B.W. (1977) Determination of bupivacaine in human fetal and neonatal blood samples by gas liquid chromatography mass spectrometry. *Biomedical Mass Spectrometry* **4**, 322–5.

Callesen T., Jarnvig I., Thage B., Krantz T. & Christiansen C. (1991) Influence of temperature of bupivacaine on spread of analgesia. *Anaesthesia* **46**, 17–19.

Calvo R., Carlos R. & Erill S. (1980) Effects of disease and acetazolamide on procaine hydrolysis by red cell enzymes. *Clinical Pharmacology and Therapeutics* **27**, 175–83.

Carson R.J. & Reynolds F. (1988) Maternal–fetal distribution of bupivacaine in the rabbit. *British Journal of Anaesthesia* **61**, 332–7.

Catchlove R.F.H. (1972) The influence of CO_2 and pH on local anesthetic action. *Journal of Pharmacology and Experimental Therapeutics* **181**, 298–309.

Chelly J.E., Hill D.C., Abernethy D.R., Dlewati A., Doursout M.-F. & Merin R.G. (1987) Pharmacodynamic and pharmacokinetic interactions between lidocaine and verapamil. *Journal of Pharmacology and Experimental Therapeutics* **243**, 211–16.

Chow M.S.S., Ronfeld R.A., Ruffett D. & Fieldman A. (1981) Lidocaine pharmacokinetics during cardiac arrest and external cardiopulmonary resuscitation. *American Heart Journal* **102**, 799–801.

Chow M.S.S., Ronfeld R.A., Hamilton R.A., Helmink R. & Fieldman A. (1983) Effect of external cardiopulmonary resuscitation on lidocaine pharmacokinetics in dogs. *Journal of Pharmacology and Experimental Therapeutics* **224**, 531–7.

Clarkson C.W. & Hondeghem L.M. (1985) Mechanism for bupivacaine depression of cardiac conduction: fast block of sodium channels during the action potential with slow recovery from block during diastole. *Anesthesiology* **62**, 396–405.

Cohen E.N. (1968) Distribution of local anesthetic agents in the neuraxis of the dog. *Anesthesiology* **29**, 1002–5.

Cohen E.N., Levine D.A., Colliss J.E. & Gunther R.E. (1968) The role of pH in the development of tachyphylaxis to local anesthetic agents. *Anesthesiology* **29**, 994–1001.

Cohen S., Luykx W.M. & Marx G.F. (1984) High versus low flow rates during lumbar epidural block. *Regional Anesthesia* **9**, 8–11.

Collinsworth K.A., Strong J.M., Atkinson A.J., Winkle R.A., Periroth F. & Harrison D.C. (1975) Pharmacokinetics and metabolism of lidocaine in patients with renal failure. *Clinical Pharmacology and Therapeutics* **18**, 59–64.

Courtney K.R. (1975) Mechanism of frequency-dependent inhibition of sodium currents in frog myelinated nerve by the lidocaine derivative GEA 968. *Journal of Pharmacology and Experimental Therapeutics* **195**, 225–36.

Courtney K.R. (1980) Structure–activity relations for frequency-dependent sodium channel block in nerve by local anesthetics. *Journal of Pharmacology and Experimental Therapeutics* **213**, 114–19.

Courtney K.R., Kendig J.J. & Cohen E.N. (1978) The rates of interaction of local anaesthetics with sodium channels in nerve. *Journal of Pharmacology and Experimental Therapeutics* **207**, 594–604.

Cousins M.J. & Mather L.E. (1984) Intrathecal and epidural administration of opioids. *Anesthesiology* **61**, 276–310.

Coventry D.M. & Todd J.G. (1989) Alkalinisation of bupivacaine for sciatic nerve block. *Anaesthesia* **44**, 467–70.

Covino B.G. (1980) The mechanism of local anaesthesia. In *Topical Reviews in Anaesthesia*, vol. I (Eds Norman J. & Whitwam J.) pp. 85–134. J. Wright & Sons, Bristol.

Covino B.G. (1986) Pharmacology of local anesthetic agents. *British Journal of Anaesthesia* **58**, 701–16.

Covino B.G. (1987) Local anaesthetics. In *Drugs in Anaesthesia: Mechanism of Action* (Eds Feldman S.A., Scurr C.F. & Paton W.) pp. 261–91. Edward Arnold, London.

Coyle D.E., Denson D.D., Thompson G.A., Myers G.A., Arthur G.R. & Bridenbaugh P.O. (1984) The influence of lactic acid on the serum protein binding of bupivacaine: species differences. *Anesthesiology* **61**, 127–33.

Crossley A.W.A. & Hosie H.E. (1987) Radiographic study of intercostal nerve blockade in healthy volunteers. *British Journal of Anaesthesia* **59**, 149–54.

Curran J., Hamilton C. & Taylor T. (1975) Topical analgesia before tracheal intubation. *Anaesthesia* **30**, 765–8.

Cusack B., O'Malley K., Lavan J., Noel J. & Kelly J.G. (1985) Protein binding and disposition of lignocaine in the elderly. *European Journal of Clinical Pharmacology* **29**, 323–9.

Cusick J.F., Myklebust J.B. & Abram S.E. (1980) Differential neural effects of epidural anesthetics. *Anesthesiology* **53**, 299–306.

Cusick J.F., Myklebust J.B., Abram S.E. & Davidson A. (1982) Altered neural conduction with epidural bupivacaine. *Anesthesiology* **57**, 31–6.

Cusson J., Nattel S., Matthews C., Talajic M. & Lawand S. (1985) Age-dependent lidocaine disposition in patients with acute myocardial infarction. *Clinical Pharmacology and Therapeutics*

37, 381–6.

Dahl J.B., Simonsen L., Mogensen T., Henriksen J.H. & Kehlet H. (1990) The effect of 0.5% ropivacaine on epidural blood flow. *Acta Anaesthesiologica Scandinavica* **34**, 308–10.

Dawes G.S. (1973) A theoretical analysis of fetal drug equilibration. In *Fetal Pharmacology* (Ed. Boreus L.) pp. 381–99. Raven Press, New York.

DeJong R.H. (1977) *Local Anesthetics* 2nd edn. pp. 63–83. Charles Thomas, Springfield.

Dennhardt R. & Ammon K. (1980) Untersuchungen zur Loslichkeit von Bupivacain im Liquor cerebrospinalis. *Der Anaesthesist* **29**, 10–13.

Denson D.D., Bridenbaugh P.O., Turner P.A. & Phero J.C. (1983) Comparison of neural blockade and pharmacokinetics after subarachnoid lidocaine in the rhesus monkey. II: effects of volume, osmolality, and baricity. *Anesthesia and Analgesia* **62**, 995–1001.

Denson D.D., Coyle D.E., Thompson G.A. & Myers J.A. (1984) Alpha$_1$-acid glycoprotein and albumin in human serum bupivacaine binding. *Clinical Pharmacology and Therapeutics* **35**, 409–15.

DiFazio C.A., Carron H., Grosslight K.R., Moscicki J.C., Bolding W.R. & Johns R.A. (1986) Comparison of pH-adjusted lidocaine solutions for epidural anesthesia. *Anesthesia and Analgesia* **65**, 760–4.

Drachman D. & Strichartz G. (1991) Potassium channel blockers potentiate impulse inhibition by local anesthetics. *Anesthesiology* **75**, 1051–61.

Drayer D.E., Lorenzo B., Werns S. & Reidenberg M.M. (1983) Plasma levels, protein binding, and elimination data of lidocaine and active metabolites in cardiac patients of various ages. *Clinical Pharmacology and Therapeutics* **34**, 14–22.

Dudziak R. & Uihlein M. (1978) Loslichkeit von Lokalanaesthetika im Liquor cerebrospinalis und ihre Abhangigkeit von der Wasserstoffionenkonzentration. *Der Anaesthesist* **27**, 32–7.

DuSouich P. & Erill S. (1977) Altered metabolism of procainamide and procaine in patients with pulmonary and cardiac diseases. *Clinical Pharmacology and Therapeutics* **21**, 101–2.

Ecoffey C., Desparmet J., Berdeaux A., Maury M., Guidicelli J.F. & Saint-Maurice C. (1984) Pharmacokinetics of lignocaine in children following caudal anaesthesia. *British Journal of Anaesthesia* **56**, 1399–401.

Ecoffey C., Desparmet J., Maury M., Berdeaux A., Giudicelli J.F. & Saint-Maurice C. (1985) Bupivacaine in children: pharmacokinetics following caudal anesthesia. *Anesthesiology* **63**, 447–8.

Edwards D.J., Lalka D., Cerra F. & Slaughter R.L. (1982) Alpha$_1$-acid glycoprotein concentration and protein binding in trauma. *Clinical Pharmacology and Therapeutics* **31**, 62–7.

Englesson S. (1974) The influence of acid–base changes on central nervous system toxicity of local anaesthetic agents. I. *Acta Anaesthesiologica Scandinavica* **18**, 79–87.

Englesson S. & Grevsten S. (1974) The influence of acid–base changes on central nervous system toxicity of local anaesthetic agents. II. *Acta Anaesthesiologica Scandinavica* **18**, 88–103.

Erdemir H.A., Soper L.E. & Sweet R.E. (1966) Studies of factors affecting peridural anesthesia. *Anesthesia and Analgesia* **44**, 400–4.

Evans C.J., Dewar J.A., Boyes R.N. & Scott D.B. (1974) Residual nerve block following intravenous regional anaesthesia. *British Journal of Anaesthesia* **46**, 668–70.

Eyres R.L., Kidd J., Oppenheim R.C. & Brown T.C.K. (1978) Local anaesthetic plasma levels in children. *Anaesthesia and Intensive Care* **6**, 243–7.

Eyres R.L., Bishop W., Oppenheim R.C. & Brown T.C.K. (1983) Plasma bupivacaine concentrations in children during caudal epidural analgesia. *Anaesthesia and Intensive Care* **II**, 20–2.

Fairley J.W. & Reynolds F. (1981) An intradermal study of the local anaesthetic and vascular effects of the isomers of mepivacaine. *British Journal of Anaesthesia* **53**, 1211–16.

Feely J. & Guy E. (1983) Lack of effect of ranitidine on the disposition of lignocaine. *British Journal of Clinical Pharmacology* **15**, 378–9.

Feely J., Wade D., McAllister C.B., Wilkinson G.R. & Robertson D. (1982a) Effect of hypotension on liver blood flow and lidocaine disposition. *New England Journal of Medicine* **307**, 866–9.

Feely J., Wilkinson G.R., McAllister C.B. & Wood A.J.J. (1982b) Increased toxicity and reduced clearance of lidocaine by cimetidine. *Annals of Internal Medicine* **96**, 592–4.

Finholt D.A., Stirt J.A., DiFazio C.A. & Moscicki J.C. (1986) Lidocaine pharmacokinetics in children. *Anesthesia and Analgesia* **65**, 279–82.

Fink B.R. (1989) Mechanisms of differential axial blockade in epidural and subarachnoid anesthesia. *Anesthesiology* **70**, 851–8.

Fink B.R. & Cairns A.M. (1984) Diffusional delay in local anesthetic block *in vitro*. *Anesthesiology* **61**, 555–7.

Finster M. & Pedersen H. (1979) Placental transfer and fetal uptake of drugs. *British Journal of Anaesthesia* **51**, 25S–8S.

Flynn R.J., Moore J., Collier P.S. & Howard P.J. (1989a) Single dose oral H$_2$-antagonists do not affect plasma lidocaine levels. *Acta Anaesthesiologica Scandinavica* **33**, 93S–6S.

Flynn R.J., Moore J., Collier P.S. & McClean E. (1989b) Does pretreatment with cimetidine and ranitidine affect the disposition of bupivacaine? *British Journal of Anaesthesia* **62**, 87–91.

Foldes F.F., Davidson G.N., Duncalf D. & Kuwabarra S. (1965) The intravenous toxicity of local anesthetic agents in man. *Clinical Pharmacology and Therapeutics* **6**, 328–35.

Ford D.J., Prithvi Raj P., Singh P., Regan K.M. & Ohlweiler D. (1984) Differential peripheral nerve block by local anesthetics in the cat. *Anesthesiology* **60**, 28–33.

Fukui T., Hameroff S.R. & Gandolfi A.J. (1984) Alpha$_1$-acid glycoprotein and beta-endorphin alterations in chronic pain patients. *Anesthesiology* **60**, 494–6.

Giasi R.M., D'Agostino E. & Covino B.G. (1980) Interaction of diazepam and epidurally administered local anesthetic agents. *Regional Anesthesia* **3**, 8–11.

Giaufre E., Bruguerolle B., Morrison-Lacombe G. & Rousset-Rouviere B. (1988) The influence of diazepam on the plasma concentrations of bupivacaine and lignocaine after caudal injection of a mixture of the local anaesthetics in children. *British Journal of Clinical Pharmacology* **26**, 116–18.

Giaufre E., Bruguerolle B., Morrison-Lacombe G. & Rousset-Rouviere B. (1990) The influence of midazolam on the plasma concentrations of bupivacaine and lidocaine after caudal injection of a mixture of the local anesthetics in children. *Acta Anaesthesiologica Scandinavica* **34**, 44–6.

Gissen A.J., Covino B.G. & Gregus J. (1980) Differential sensitivities of mammalian nerve fibers to local anesthetic agents. *Anesthesiology* **53**, 467–74.

Gissen A.J., Covino B.G. & Gregus J. (1982a) Differential sensitivity of fast and slow fibers in mammalian nerve. II. Margin of safety for nerve transmission. *Anesthesia and Analgesia* **61**, 561–9.

Gissen A.J., Covino B.G. & Gregus J. (1982b) Differential sensitivity of fast and slow fibers in mammalian nerve. III. Effect of etidocaine and bupivacaine on fast/slow fibers. *Anesthesia and Analgesia* **61**, 570–5.

Gissen A.J., Covino B.G. & Gregus J. (1985) Differential sensitivity of fast and slow fibers in mammalian nerve. IV. Effect of carbonation of local anesthetics. *Regional Anesthesia* **10**, 68–75.

Gissen A.J., Covino B.G. & Gregus J. (1986) Differential sensitivity of fast and slow fibers in mammalian nerve. VI. Effect of pH on blocking action of local anesthetics. *Regional Anesthesia* **11**, 132–8.

Goldberg M.J., Spector R. & Johnson G.F. (1982) Racial background and lidocaine pharmacokinetics. *Journal of Clinical Pharmacology* **22**, 391–4.

Greene N.M. (1983) Uptake and elimination of local anesthetics during spinal anesthesia. *Anesthesia and Analgesia* **62**, 1013–24.

Greene N.M. (1985) Distribution of local anesthetic solutions within the subarachnoid space. *Anesthesia and Analgesia* **64**, 715–30.

Griffiths R.B., Horton W.A., Jones I.G. & Blake D. (1987) Speed of injection and spread of bupivacaine in the epidural space. *Anaesthesia* **42**, 160–3.

Grossman S.H., Davis D., Kitchell B.B., Shand D.G. & Routledge P.A. (1982) Diazepam and lidocaine plasma protein binding in renal disease. *Clinical Pharmacology and Therapeutics* **31**, 350–7.

Grundy E.M., Ramamurthy S., Patel K.P., Mani M. & Winnie A.P. (1978) Extradural analgesia revisited. *British Journal of Anaesthesia* **50**, 805–9.

Gupta N., Kennedy R.L., Vicinie A., Seifert R., Edelmann C., Mandel M., Tyler I.L., Kupke K., Miller R.P. & de Sousa H. (1986) Fetal uptake of bupivacaine following bolus intravenous injection. *Anesthesiology* **65**, 382A.

Hamshaw-Thomas A., Rogerson N. & Reynolds F. (1985) Transfer of bupivacaine, lignocaine and pethidine across the rabbit placenta: influence of maternal protein binding and fetal flow. *Placenta* **5**, 61–70.

Hasselstrom L., Nortved-Sorensen J., Kehlet H., Juel-Christiansen N., Brynjolff I., Munck O. & Tucker G.T. (1985) The influence of systemically administered bupivacaine on cardiovascular function in cholecystectomised patients. *Acta Anaesthesiologica Scandinavica* **29**, 76A.

Heavner J.E., Leinonen L., Haasio J., Kytta J. & Rosenberg P.H. (1989) Interaction of lidocaine and hypothermia in Bier Blocks in volunteers. *Anesthesia and Analgesia* **69**, 53–9.

Hilgier M. (1985) Alkalinization of bupivacaine for brachial plexus block. *Regional Anesthesia* **8**, 59–61.

Hille B. (1977) Local anesthetics: hydrophilic and hydrophobic pathways for the drug–receptor reaction. *Journal of General Physiology* **69**, 497–515.

Hjelm M. & Holmdahl M.H. (1965) Biochemical effects of aromatic amines. II. Cyanosis, methaemoglobinaemia and Heinz-body formation induced by a local anaesthetic agent (prilocaine). *Acta Anaesthesiologica Scandinavica* **9**, 99–120.

Hodgkinson R. & Husain F.J. (1981) Obesity, gravity and spread of epidural anesthesia. *Anesthesia and Analgesia* **60**, 421–4.

Howarth F. (1949) Studies with a radioactive spinal anaesthetic. *British Journal of Pharmacology* **4**, 333–47.

Huang L.-Y.M. & Ehrenstein G. (1981) Local anesthetic QX-572 and benzocaine act at separate sites on the batrachotoxin-activated sodium channel. *Journal of General Physiology* **77**, 137–53.

Huet P.-M. & LeLorier J. (1980) Effects of smoking and chronic hepatitis B on lidocaine and indocyanine green kinetics. *Clinical Pharmacology and Therapeutics* **28**, 208–14.

Huet P.-M. & Villeneuve J.-P. (1983) Determinants of drug disposition in patients with cirrhosis. *Hepatology* **3**, 913–18.

Hull C.J. (1985) The pharmacokinetics of opioid analgesics, with special reference to patient-controlled administration. In *Patient-Controlled Analgesia* (Eds Hamer M., Rosen M. & Vickers M.D.) pp. 7–17. Blackwell Scientific Publications, Oxford.

Husemeyer R.P. & White D.C. (1980) Lumbar extradural injection pressures in pregnant women. An investigation of relationships between rate of injection, injection pressures and extent of analgesia. *British Journal of Anaesthesia* **52**, 55–60.

Inoue R., Suganuma T., Echizen H., Ishizaki T., Kushida K. & Tomono Y. (1985) Plasma concentrations of lidocaine and its principal metabolites during intermittent epidural anesthesia. *Anesthesiology* **63**, 304–10.

Jackson P.R., Tucker G.T. & Woods H.F. (1982) Altered plasma binding in cancer: role of alpha$_1$-acid glycoprotein and albumin. *Clinical Pharmacology and Therapeutics* **32**, 295–302.

Jackson J.E., Bentley J.B., Glass S.J., Fukui T., Gandolfi A.J. & Plachetka J.R. (1985) Effects of histamine-2 receptor blockade on lidocaine kinetics. *Clinical Pharmacology and Therapeutics* **37**, 544–8.

Johansson A., Renck H., Aspelin P. & Jacobsen H. (1985) Multiple intercostal blocks by a single injection? A clinical and radiological investigation. *Acta Anaesthesiologica Scandinavica* **29**, 524–8.

Jones R.A., DiFazio C.A. & Longnecker D.E. (1985) Lidocaine constricts or dilates rat arterioles in a dose-dependent manner. *Anesthesiology* **62**, 141–4.

Jorfeldt L., Lewis D.H., Lofstrom B. & Post C. (1979) Lung uptake of lidocaine in healthy volunteers. *Acta Anaesthesiologica Scandinavica* **23**, 567–74.

Jorfeldt L., Lewis D.H., Lofstrom B. & Post C. (1983) Lung uptake of lidocaine in man as influenced by anaesthesia, mepivacaine infusion or lung insufficiency. *Acta Anaesthesiologica Scandinavica* **27**, 5–9.

Kastrissios H., Triggs E.J., Mogg G.A.G. & Higbie J.W. (1991) The disposition of bupivacaine following a 72 h interpleural infusion in cholecystectomy patients. *British Journal of Clinical Pharmacology* **32**, 251–4.

Kennedy R.L., Miller R.P., Bell J.U., Doshi D., de Sousa H., Kennedy M., Heald D.L. & David Y. (1986) Uptake and distribution of bupivacaine in fetal lambs. *Anesthesiology* **65**, 247–53.

Kennedy R.L., Bell J.U., Miller R.P., Doshi D., de Sousa H.,

Kennedy M.J., Heald D.L., Bettinger R. & David Y. (1990) Uptake and distribution of lidocaine in fetal lambs. *Anesthesiology* **72**, 483—9.

Kishikawa K., Namiki I., Miyashita K. & Saitoh K. (1990) Effects of famotidine and cimetidine on plasma levels of epidurally administered lignocaine. *Anaesthesia* **45**, 719—21.

Kopacz D.J., Carpenter R.L. & Mackey D.C. (1989) Effect of ropivacaine on cutaneous capillary blood flow in pigs. *Anesthesiology* **71**, 69—74.

Koster H., Shapiro A. & Leikensohn A. (1936) Procaine concentration changes at the site of injection in subarachnoid anesthesia. *American Journal of Surgery* **33**, 245—8.

Kraus E., Polnaszek C.F., Scheeler D.A., Halsall H.B., Eckfeldt J.H. & Holtzman J.L. (1986) Interaction between human serum albumin and alpha$_1$-acid glycoprotein in the binding of lidocaine to purified protein fractions and sera. *Journal of Pharmacology and Experimental Therapeutics* **239**, 754—9.

Krogh K. & Jellum E. (1981) Urinary metabolites of chloroprocaine studied by combined gas chromatography—mass spectrometry. *Anesthesiology* **54**, 329—32.

Kuhnert B.R., Kuhnert P.M., Prochaska A.L. & Gross T.L. (1980) Plasma levels of 2-chloroprocaine in obstetric patients and their neonates after epidural anesthesia. *Anesthesiology* **53**, 21—5.

Kuhnert P.M., Kuhnert B.R., Stitts J.M. & Gross T.L. (1981) The use of a selected ion monitoring technique to study the disposition of bupivacaine in mother, fetus and neonate following epidural anesthesia for Cesarian section. *Anesthesiology* **55**, 611—17.

Kuhnert B.R., Kuhnert P.M., Philipson E.H., Syracuse C.D., Kaine C.J. & Chang-hyon Y. (1986) The half-life of 2-chloroprocaine. *Anesthesia and Analgesia* **65**, 273—8.

Kuhnert B.R., Zuspan K.J., Kuhnert P.M., Syracuse C.D., Brashear W.T. & Brown D.E. (1987) Lack of influence of cimetidine on bupivacaine levels during parturition. *Anesthesia and Analgesia* **66**, 986—90.

Labedzki L., Scavone J.M., Ochs H.R. & Greenblatt D.J. (1990) Reduced systemic absorption of intrabronchial lidocaine by high-frequency nebulization. *Journal of Clinical Pharmacology* **30**, 795—7.

Lee E.J.D., Ang S.B. & Lee T.L. (1987) Stereoselective high-performance liquid chromatographic assay for bupivacaine enantiomers. *Journal of Chromatography* **420**, 203—6.

Lennard M.S., Tucker G.T. & Words H.F. (1983) Time-dependent kinetics of lignocaine in the isolated perfused rat liver. *Journal of Pharmacokinetics and Biopharmaceutics* **11**, 165—82.

Lofstrom B. (1978) Tissue distribution of local anesthetics with special reference to the lung. *International Anesthesiology Clinics* **16**, 53—72.

Luduena F.P., Bogado E.F. & Tullar B.F. (1972) Optical isomers of mepivacaine and bupivacaine. *Archives of International Pharmacodynamie* **200**, 359—69.

Lund P.C., Bush D.F. & Covino B.G. (1975) Determinants of etidocaine concentrations in the blood. *Anesthesiology* **42**, 497—503.

Maclean D., Chambers W.A., Tucker G.T. & Wildsmith J.A.W. (1988) Plasma prilocaine concentrations after three techniques of brachial plexus blockade. *British Journal of Anaesthesia* **60**, 136—9.

Magno R., Berlin A., Karlsson K. & Kjellmer I. (1976) Anesthesia for Cesarian section. IV: Placental transfer and neonatal elimination of bupivacaine following epidural analgesia for elective Cesarian section. *Acta Anaesthesiologica Scandinavica* **20**, 141—6.

Marathe P.H., Shen D.D., Artru A.A. & Bowdle A. (1991) Effect of serum protein binding on the entry of lidocaine into brain and cerebrospinal fluid in dogs. *Anesthesiology* **75**, 804—12.

Martin R., Lamarche Y. & Tetreault L. (1981) Comparison of the clinical effectiveness of lidocaine hydrocarbonate and lidocaine hydrochloride with and without epinephrine in epidural anaesthesia. *Canadian Anaesthetists' Society Journal* **28**, 217—23.

Mather L.E. (1986) Tachyphylaxis in regional anaesthesia: can we reconcile clinical observation and laboratory measurements? In *New Aspects in Regional Anaesthesia*, number 4 (Eds Wust H.J. & Stanton-Hicks M.) pp. 3—8. Springer, Heidelberg.

Mather L.E. (1991) Disposition of mepivacaine and bupivacaine evantiomers in sheep. *British Journal of Anaesthesia* **67**, 239—46.

Mather L.E. & Thomas J. (1978) Bupivacaine binding to plasma protein fractions. *Journal of Pharmacy and Pharmacology* **30**, 653—4.

Mather L.E., Long G.J. & Thomas J. (1971) The binding of bupivacaine to maternal and foetal plasma proteins. *Journal of Pharmacy and Pharmacology* **23**, 359—65.

Mather L.E., Runciman W.B., Carapetis R.J., Ilsley A.H. & Upton R.N. (1986) Hepatic and renal clearances of lidocaine in conscious and anesthetised sheep. *Anesthesia and Analgesia* **65**, 943—9.

Mayumi T., Dohi S. & Takahashi T. (1983) Plasma concentrations of lidocaine associated with cervical, thoracic, and lumbar epidural anesthesia. *Anesthesia and Analgesia* **62**, 578—80.

Mazoit J.X., Lambert C., Berdeaux A., Gerard J.-L. & Froideveaux R. (1988a) Pharmacokinetics of bupivacaine after short and prolonged infusions in conscious dogs. *Anesthesia and Analgesia* **67**, 961—6.

Mazoit J.X., Denson D.D. & Samii K. (1988b) Pharmacokinetics of bupivacaine following caudal anesthesia in infants. *Anesthesiology* **68**, 387—91.

McClure J.H. & Scott D.B. (1981) Comparison of bupivacaine hydrochloride and carbonated bupivacaine in brachial plexus block interscalene technique. *British Journal of Anaesthesia* **53**, 523—6.

McKeown D.W. & Scott D.B. (1984) Influence of the addition of potassium to 0.5% prilocaine solution during i.v. regional anaesthesia. *British Journal of Anaesthesia* **56**, 1167—70.

McLean S., Starmer G.A. & Thomas J. (1969) Methaemoglobin formation by aromatic amines. *Journal of Pharmacy and Pharmacology* **21**, 441—50.

McMorland G.H., Douglas M.J., Jeffery W.K., Ross P.L.E., Axelson J.E., Kim J.H.K., Gambling D.R. & Robertson K. (1986) Effect of pH-adjustment of bupivacaine on onset and duration of epidural analgesia in parturients. *Canadian Anaesthetists' Society Journal* **33**, 537—41.

McNamara P.J., Slaughter R.L., Pieper J.A., Wyman M.G. & Lalka D. (1981) Factors influencing serum protein binding of lidocaine in humans. *Anesthesia and Analgesia* **60**, 395—400.

Mehta P.M., Theriot E., Mehrotra D., Patel K. & Kimball B.G.

(1987) Simple technique to make bupivacaine a rapid-acting epidural anesthetic. *Regional Anesthesia* **12**, 135–8.

Meyer J. & Nolte H. (1978) Liquorkonzentration von Bupivacain nach subduraler Applikation. *Regional Anaesthesie* **1**, 38–40.

Mihaly G.W., Moore R.G., Thomas J., Triggs E.J., Thomas D. & Shanks C.H. (1978) The pharmacokinetics of the anilide local anaesthetics in neonates. I: Lignocaine. *European Journal of Clinical Pharmacology* **13**, 143–52.

Mogensen T., Højgaard L., Scott N.B., Henriksen J.H. & Kehlet H. (1988) Epidural blood flow and regression of sensory analgesia during continuous postoperative epidural infusion of bupivacaine. *Anesthesia and Analgesia* **67**, 809–13.

Mogensen T., Simonsen L., Scott N.B., Henriksen J.H. & Kehlet H. (1989) Tachyphylaxis associated with repeated epidural injections of lidocaine is not related to changes in distribution or the rate of elimination from the epidural space. *Anesthesia and Analgesia* **69**, 180–4.

Moller R. & Covino B.G. (1990) Cardiac electrophysiologic properties of bupivacaine and lidocaine compared with those of ropivacaine, a new amide local anesthetic. *Anesthesiology* **72**, 322–9.

Moore D.C. (1981) Intercostal nerve block: spread of india ink injected to the rib's costal groove. *British Journal of Anaesthesia* **53**, 325–9.

Moore D.C., Mather L.E., Bridenbaugh P.O., Balfour R.I., Lysons D.F. & Horton W.G. (1976a) Arterial and venous plasma levels of bupivacaine following peripheral nerve blocks. *Anesthesia and Analgesia* **55**, 763–8.

Moore D.C., Mather L.E., Bridenbaugh L.D., Balfour R.I., Lysons D.F. & Horton W.G. (1976b) Arterial and venous plasma levels of bupivacaine (Marcaine) following epidural and intercostal nerve blocks. *Anesthesiology* **45**, 39–45.

Moore R.G., Thomas J., Triggs E.J., Thomas B.D., Burnard E.D. & Shanks C.H. (1978) The pharmacokinetics and metabolism of the anilide local anaesthetics in neonates. III: Mepivacaine. *European Journal of Clinical Pharmacology* **14**, 203–12.

Moore R.A., Bullingham R.E.S., McQuay H.J., Hand C.W., Aspel J.B., Allen M.C. & Thomas D. (1982) Dural permeability to narcotics: *in vitro* determination and application to extra-dural administration. *British Journal of Anaesthesia* **54**, 1117–28.

Morgan D.H., Cousins M.J., McQuillan D. & Thomas J. (1977) Disposition and placental transfer of etidocaine in pregnancy. *European Journal of Clinical Pharmacology* **12**, 359–65.

Morgan D.H., McQuillan D. & Thomas J. (1978) Pharmaco-kinetics and metabolism of the anilide local anaesthetics in neonates. II: Etidocaine. *European Journal of Clinical Pharmacology* **13**, 365–71.

Morikawa K.I., Bonica J.J., Tucker G.T. & Murphy T.M. (1974) Effects of acute hypovolaemia on lignocaine absorption and cardiovascular response following epidural block in dogs. *British Journal of Anaesthesia* **46**, 631–5.

Morison D.H. (1981) A double-blind comparison of carbonated lidocaine and lidocaine hydrochloride in epidural anaes-thesia. *Canadian Anaesthetists' Society Journal* **28**, 387–9.

Mrose H.E. & Ritchie J.M. (1978) Local anesthetics: do benzo-caine and lidocaine act at the same single site? *Journal of General Physiology* **71**, 223–5.

Murphy D.F. (1983) Continuous intercostal nerve blockade for pain relief after cholecystectomy. *British Journal of Anaesthesia* **55**, 521–4.

Nancarrow C., Runciman W.B., Mather L.E., Upton R.N. & Plummer J.L. (1987) The influence of acidosis on the dis-tribution of lidocaine and bupivacaine into the myocardium and brain of the sheep. *Anesthesia and Analgesia* **66**, 925–35.

Nation R.L., Triggs E.J. & Selig M. (1977) Lignocaine kinetics in cardiac patients and aged subjects. *British Journal of Clinical Pharmacology* **4**, 439–48.

Nickel P.M., Bromage P.R. & Sherrill D.L. (1986) Comparison of hydrochloride and carbonated salts of lidocaine for epidural analgesia. *Regional Anesthesia* **11**, 62–7.

Nishimura N., Kitahara T. & Kusakabo T. (1959) The spread of lidocaine and I-131 solution in the epidural space. *Anes-thesiology* **20**, 785–8.

Noble D.W., Smith K.J. & Dundas C.R. (1987) The effects of H_2 antagonists on the elimination of bupivacaine. *British Journal of Anaesthesia* **59**, 735–7.

Nunn J.E. & Slavin G. (1980) Posterior intercostal nerve block for pain relief after cholecystectomy. *British Journal of Anaes-thesia* **52**, 253–9.

O'Brien J.E., Abbey V., Hinsvark O., Perel J. & Finster M. (1979) Metabolism and measurement of chloroprocaine, an ester-type local anesthetic. *Journal of Pharmaceutical Sciences* **68**, 75–8.

O'Kelly E. & Garry B. (1981) Continuous pain relief for multiple fractured ribs. *British Journal of Anaesthesia* **53**, 989–91.

O'Sullivan G.M., Smith M., Morgan B., Brighouse D. & Reynolds F. (1988) H_2 antagonists and bupivacaine clearance. *Anaesthesia* **43**, 93–5.

Palazzo M.G.A., Kalso E.A., Argiras E., Madgwick R. & Sear J.W. (1991) First pass lung uptake of bupivacaine: effect of acidosis in an intact rabbit lung model. *British Journal of Anaesthesia* **67**, 759–63.

Palmer S.K., Bosnjak Z.J., Hopp F., von Colditz J.H. & Kampine J.P. (1983) Lidocaine and bupivacaine differential nerve blockade of isolated canine nerves. *Anesthesia and Analgesia* **62**, 754–7.

Park W.Y. (1988) Factors influencing distribution of local anes-thetics in the epidural space. *Regional Anesthesia* **13**, 49–57.

Park W.Y., Massengale M., Kin S.-I., Poon K.C. & MacNamara T.E. (1980) Age and the spread of local anesthetic solutions in the epidural space. *Anesthesia and Analgesia* **59**, 768–71.

Parris M.R. & Chambers W.A. (1986) Effects of the addition of potassium to prilocaine or bupivacaine. Studies on brachial plexus blockade. *British Journal of Anaesthesia* **58**, 297–300.

Partridge B.L., Katz J. & Benirschke K. (1987) Functional anatomy of the brachial plexus sheath: implications for anes-thesia. *Anesthesiology* **66**, 743–7.

Pere P., Tuominen M. & Rosenberg P.H. (1991) Cumulation of bupivacaine, desbutylbupivacaine and 4-hydroxybupiva-caine during and after continuous interscalene brachial plexus block. *Acta Anaesthesiologica Scandinavica* **35**, 647–50.

Perucca E. & Richens A. (1979) Reduction of oral bioavailability of lignocaine by induction of first-pass metabolism in epi-leptic patients. *British Journal of Clinical Pharmacology* **8**, 21–31.

Petersen M.C., Moore R.G., Nation R.L. & McMeniman W. (1981) Relationship between the transplacental gradients of bupivacaine and alpha$_1$-acid glycoprotein. *British Journal of Clinical Pharmacology* **12**, 859–62.

Piafsky K.M. & Knoppert D. (1979) Binding of local anesthetics to alpha$_1$-acid glycoprotein. *Clinical Research* **26**, 836A.

Piafsky K.M. & Woolner E.A. (1982) The binding of basic drugs to alpha$_1$-acid glycoprotein in cord serum. *Journal of Pediatrics* **5**, 820−2.

Pihlajamäki K.K. (1991) Inverse correlation between the peak venous serum concentration of bupivacaine and the weight of the patient during interscalene brachial plexus block. *British Journal of Anaesthesia* **67**, 621−2.

Pihlajamäki K., Kanto J., Lindberg R., Karanko M. & Kiilholma P. (1990) Extradural administration of bupivacaine: pharmacokinetics and metabolism in pregnant and non-pregnant women. *British Journal of Anaesthesia* **64**, 556−62.

Pollmann L. (1981) Circadian changes in the duration of local anaesthesia. *Journal of Interdisciplinary Cycle Research* **12**, 187−92.

Post C. & Eriksdotter-Behm K. (1982) Dependence of lung uptake of lidocaine *in vivo* on blood pH. *Acta Pharmacologica et Toxicologica* **51**, 136−40.

Post C., Andersson R.G.G., Ryrfeldt A. & Nilsson E. (1979) Physicochemical modification of lidocaine uptake in rat lung tissue. *Acta Pharmacologica et Toxicologica* **44**, 103−9.

Post C., Freedman J., Ramsay C.-H. & Bonnevier A. (1985) Redistribution of lidocaine and bupivacaine after intrathecal injection in mice. *Anesthesiology* **63**, 410−17.

Quimby C.W. (1965) Influence of blood loss on the duration of regional anesthesia. *Anesthesia and Analgesia* **44**, 387−90.

Ramanathan J., Bottorff M., Jeter J.N., Khalil M. & Sibai B.M. (1986) The pharmacokinetics and maternal and neonatal effects of epidural lidocaine in preeclampsia. *Anesthesia and Analgesia* **65**, 120−6.

Raymond S.A., Steffensen S.C., Gugino L.D. & Strichartz G.R. (1989) The role of length of nerve exposed to local anesthetic in impulse blocking action. *Anesthesia and Analgesia* **68**, 563−70.

Reidenberg M.M., James M. & Dring L.G. (1972) The rate of procaine hydrolysis in serum of normal subjects and diseased patients. *Clinical Pharmacology and Therapeutics* **13**, 279−84.

Reiz S., Häggmark S., Johansson G. & Nath S. (1989) Cardiotoxicity of ropivacaine − a new amide local anaesthetic agent. *Acta Anaesthesiologica Scandinavica* **33**, 93−8.

Rice A.S.C., Pither C.E. & Tucker G.T. (1991) Plasma concentrations of bupivacaine after supraclavicular brachial plexus blockade in patients with chronic renal failure. *Anaesthesia* **46**, 354−7.

Richter O., Klein K., Abel J., Ohnesorge F.K., Wust H.J. & Thiessen F.M.M. (1984) The kinetics of bupivacaine (Carbostesin) plasma concentrations during epidural anesthesia following intraoperative bolus injection and subsequent continuous infusion. *International Journal of Clinical Pharmacology, Therapy, and Toxicology* **22**, 611−17.

Riegler F.X., VadeBoncouer T.R. & Pelligrino D.A. (1989) Interpleural anesthetics in the dog: differential somatic neural blockade. *Anesthesiology* **71**, 744−50.

Ritchie J.M. (1975) Mechanism of action of local anaesthetic agents and biotoxins. *British Journal of Anaesthesia* **47**, 191−8.

Ritchie J.M., Ritchie B. & Greengard P. (1965) The active structure of local anesthetics. *Journal of Pharmacology and Experimental Therapeutics* **150**, 152−9.

Robson R.A., Wing L.M.H., Miners J.O., Lillywhite K.J. & Birkett D.J. (1985) The effect of ranitidine on the disposition of lignocaine. *British Journal of Clinical Pharmacology* **20**, 170−3.

Rosenberg P.H. & Heavner J.E. (1980) Temperature-dependent nerve-blocking action of lidocaine and halothane. *Acta Anaesthesiologica Scandinavica* **24**, 314−20.

Rosenberg P.H. & Heinonen E. (1983) Differential sensitivity of A and C nerve fibres to long-acting amide local anaesthetics. *British Journal of Anaesthesia* **55**, 163−7.

Rosenberg P.H., Saramies L. & Alila A. (1981) Lumbar epidural anaesthesia with bupivacaine in old patients: effect of speed and direction of injection. *Acta Anaesthesiologica Scandinavica* **25**, 270−4.

Rosenberg P.H., Kytta J. & Alila A. (1986) Absorption of bupivacaine, etidocaine, lignocaine and ropivacaine into *n*-heptane, rat sciatic nerve, and human extradural and subcutaneous fat. *British Journal of Anaesthesia* **58**, 310−14.

Rosenberg P.H., Pere P., Hekali R. & Tuominen M. (1991) Plasma concentrations of bupivacaine and two of its metabolites during continuous interscalene brachial plexus block. *British Journal of Anaesthesia* **66**, 25−30.

Ross R.A., Clarke J.E. & Armitage E.N. (1980) Postoperative pain prevention by continuous epidural infusion. *Anaesthesia* **35**, 663−8.

Rothstein P., Arthur G.R., Feldman H., Kopf G. & Covino B.G. (1986) Bupivacaine for intercostal nerve blocks in children: blood concentrations and pharmacokinetics. *Anesthesia and Analgesia* **65**, 625−32.

Rothstein P., Cole J.S. & Pitt B.R. (1987) Pulmonary extraction of (3H) bupivacaine: modification by dose, propranolol and interaction with (14C) 5-hydroxytryptamine. *Journal of Pharmacology and Experimental Therapeutics* **240**, 410−14.

Routledge P.A., Barchowsky A., Bjornsson T.D., Kitchell B.B. & Shand D.G. (1980) Lidocaine plasma protein binding. *Clinical Pharmacology and Therapeutics* **27**, 347−51.

Routledge P.A., Stargel W.W., Finn A.L., Barchowsky A. & Shand D.G. (1981) Lignocaine disposition in blood in epilepsy. *British Journal of Clinical Pharmacology* **12**, 663−6.

Safran D., Kuhlman G., Orhant E.E., Castelain M.H. & Journois D. (1990) Continuous intercostal blockade with lidocaine after thoracic surgery. Clinical and pharmacokinetic study. *Anesthesia and Analgesia* **70**, 345−9.

Saito H., Akutagawa T., Kitahata L.M., Stagg D., Collins J.G. & Scurlock J.E. (1984) Interactions of lidocaine and calcium in blocking the compound action potential of frog sciatic nerve. *Anesthesiology* **60**, 205−8.

Santos A.C., Pedersen H., Morishima H.O., Finster M., Arthur G.R. & Covino B.G. (1988) Pharmacokinetics of lidocaine in nonpregnant and pregnant ewes. *Anesthesia and Analgesia* **67**, 1154−8.

Santos A.C., Pedersen H., Sallusto J.A., Johnson V., Morishima H., Finster M., Arthur G.R. & Covino B.G. (1990) Pharmacokinetics of ropivacaine in nonpregnant and pregnant ewes. *Anesthesia and Analgesia* **70**, 262−6.

Scott D.B., Jebsen P.J.R., Braid D.P., Ortengren B. & Frisch P. (1972) Factors affecting plasma levels of lignocaine and prilocaine. *British Journal of Anaesthesia* **44**, 1040−8.

Scott D.B., Littlewood D.G., Covino B.G. & Drummond G.B. (1976) Plasma lignocaine concentrations following endotracheal spraying with an aerosol. *British Journal of Anaesthesia* **48**, 899−901.

Scurlock J.E., Meymaris E. & Gregus J. (1978) The clinical character of local anesthetics: a function of frequency-dependent conduction block. *Acta Anaesthesiologica Scan-*

dinavica **22**, 601–8.

Seifen A.B., Ferrari A.A., Seifen A.A., Thompson D.S. & Chapman J. (1979) Pharmacokinetics of intravenous procaine infusion in humans. *Anesthesia and Analgesia* **58**, 382–6.

Sharrock N.E. (1978) Epidural anesthetic dose response in patients 20 to 80 years old. *Anesthesiology* **47**, 307–8.

Simon P., Benowitz N.L. & Culala S. (1984) Motor paralysis increases brain uptake of lidocaine during status epilepticus. *Neurology* **34**, 384–7.

Smith S., Ramamurthy S. & Walsh N. (1986) Effect of sodium bicarbonate on the onset of blockade by bupivacaine. *Regional Anesthesia* **11**, 48.

Starke P. & Nolte H. (1978) pH des Liquor spinalis wahrend subduraler Blockade. *Der Anaesthesist* **27**, 41–3.

Stienstra R. & Greene N.M. (1991) Factors affecting the subarachnoid spread of local anesthetic solutions. *Regional Anesthesia* **16**, 1–6.

Strichartz G.R. (1973) The inhibition of sodium currents in myelinated nerve by quaternary derivatives of lidocaine. *Journal of General Physiology* **62**, 37–57.

Strichartz G.R. (1985) Interactions of local anesthetics with neuronal sodium channels. In *Effects of Anesthesia* (Eds Covino B.G., Fozzard H.A., Rehder K. & Strichartz G.R.) pp. 39–52. American Physiological Society, Bethesda.

Strichartz G.R., Sanchez V., Arthur G.R., Chafetz R. & Martin D. (1990) Fundamental properties of local anesthetics. II. Measured octanol: buffer partition coefficients and pKa values of clinically used drugs. *Anesthesia and Analgesia* **71**, 158–70.

Strobel G.F. & Bianchi C.P. (1970) The effect of pH gradients on the action of procaine and lidocaine in intact and desheathed sciatic nerves. *Journal of Pharmacology and Experimental Therapeutics* **172**, 1–17.

Strømskag K.E., Hauge O. & Steen P.A. (1990) Distribution of local anesthetics injected into the interpleural space studied by computerized tomography. *Acta Anaesthesiologica Scandinavica* **34**, 323–6.

Sukhani R., Garcia C.J., Munhall R.J., Winnie A.P. & Rodvold K.A. (1989) Lidocaine disposition following intravenous regional anesthesia with different tourniquet deflation technics. *Anesthesia and Analgesia* **68**, 633–7.

Tackley R.M. & Coe A.J. (1988) Alkalinised bupivacaine and adrenaline for epidural Caesarian section. *Anaesthesia* **43**, 1019–21.

Takasaki M. (1984) Blood concentrations of lidocaine, mepivacaine and bupivacaine during caudal analgesia in children. *Acta Anaesthesiologica Scandinavica* **28**, 211–14.

Terasaki T., Pardridge W.M. & Denson D.D. (1986) Differential effect of plasma protein binding of bupivacaine on its *in vivo* transfer into the brain and salivary gland of rats. *Journal of Pharmacology and Experimental Therapeutics* **239**, 724–9.

Thomas J., Long G., Moore G. & Morgan D. (1976) Plasma protein binding and placental transfer of bupivacaine. *Clinical Pharmacology and Therapeutics* **19**, 426–34.

Thompson G.E. & Rorie D.H. (1983) Functional anatomy of the brachial plexus sheaths. *Anesthesiology* **59**, 117–19.

Thompson G.A., Turner P.A., Bridenbaugh P.O., Stuebing R.C. & Denson D.D. (1986) The influence of diazepam on the pharmacokinetics of intravenous and epidural bupivacaine in the rhesus monkey. *Anesthesia and Analgesia* **65**, 151–5.

Thomson P.D., Melmon K.L., Richardson J.A., Cohn K., Steinbrunn W., Cudihee R. & Rowland M. (1973) Lidocaine pharmacokinetics in advanced heart failure, liver disease and renal disease in humans. *Annals of Internal Medicine* **78**, 499–508.

Tucker G.T. (1983) Chemistry and pharmacology of local anaesthetic drugs. In *Practical Regional Anaesthesia* (Eds Henderson J.J. & Nimmo W.S.) pp. 1–21. Blackwell Scientific Publications, Oxford.

Tucker G.T. (1984) Absorption and disposition of local anaesthetics in relation to regional blood flow changes. In *Current Concepts in Regional Anaesthesia* (Eds Van Kleek J.W., Burm A.G.L. & Spierdijk J.) pp. 192–202. Martinus Nijhoff, Boston and The Hague.

Tucker G.T. (1986) Pharmacokinetics of local anaesthetics. *British Journal of Anaesthesia* **58**, 717–31.

Tucker G.T. (1988) Is plasma binding of local anaesthetics important? *Acta Anaesthesiologica Belgica* **39**, 147–50.

Tucker G.T. & Boas R.A. (1971) Pharmacokinetic aspects of intravenous regional anesthesia. *Anesthesiology* **34**, 538–49.

Tucker G.T. & Mather L.E. (1975) Pharmacokinetics of local anaesthetic agents. *British Journal of Anaesthesia* **47**, 213–24.

Tucker G.T. & Mather L.E. (1979) Clinical pharmacokinetics of local anaesthetic agents. *Clinical Pharmacokinetics* **4**, 241–78.

Tucker G.T. & Mather L.E. (1980) Absorption and disposition of local anesthetics: pharmacokinetics. In *Neural Blockade in Clinical Anesthesia and Management of Pain* (Eds Cousins M.J. & Bridenbaugh P.O.) pp. 45–85. Lippincott, Philadelphia.

Tucker G.T. & Mather L.E. (1988) Physicochemical properties, absorption and disposition of local anesthetic agents. In *Neural Blockade in Clinical Anesthesia and Management of Pain* 2nd edn. (Eds Cousins M.J. & Bridenbaugh P.O.) pp. 47–110. Lippincott, Philadelphia.

Tucker G.T., Boyes R.N., Bridenbaugh P.O. & Moore D.C. (1970a) Binding of anilide-type local anesthetics in human plasma. I: Relationships between binding, physicochemical properties and anesthetic activity. *Anesthesiology* **33**, 287–303.

Tucker G.T., Boyes R.N., Bridenbaugh P.O. & Moore D.C. (1970b) Binding of anilide-type local anesthetics in human plasma. II: Implications *in vivo* with special reference to transplacental disposition. *Anesthesiology* **33**, 304–14.

Tucker G.T., Moore D.C., Bridenbaugh P.O., Bridenbaugh L.D. & Thompson G.E. (1972) Systemic absorption of mepivacaine in commonly used regional block procedures. *Anesthesiology* **37**, 277–87.

Tucker G.T., Cooper S., Littlewood D., Buckley S.P., Covino B.G. & Scott D.B. (1977) Observed and predicted accumulation of local anaesthetic agents during continuous extradural analgesia. *British Journal of Anaesthesia* **49**, 237–42.

Tucker G.T., Bax N.D.S., Lennard M.S., Al-Asady S., Bharaj H.S. & Woods H.F. (1984) Effects of beta-adrenoreceptor antagonists on the pharmacokinetics of lignocaine. *British Journal of Clinical Pharmacology* **17**, 21S–8S.

Tucker G.T., Mather L.E., Lennard M.S. & Gregory A. (1990) Plasma concentrations of the stereoisomers of prilocaine after administration of the racemate: implications for toxicity? *British Journal of Anaesthesia* **65**, 333–6.

Urban B.J. (1973) Clinical observations suggesting a changing site of action during induction and recession of spinal and epidural anesthesia. *Anesthesiology* **39**, 496—503.

Vanhoutte F., Vereecke J., Verbeke N. & Carmeliet E. (1991) Stereoselective effects of the enantiomers of bupivacaine on the electrophysiological properties of the guinea-pig papillary muscle. *British Journal of Pharmacology* **103**, 1275—81.

van Kleef J.W., Burm A.G.L. & Vletter A.A. (1990) Single-dose interpleural versus intercostal blockade: nerve block characteristics and plasma concentration profiles after administration of 0.5% bupivacaine with epinephrine. *Anesthesia and Analgesia* **70**, 484—8.

Veering B.T., Burm A.G.L., van Kleef J.W., Hennis P.J. & Spierdijk J. (1987) Epidural anesthesia with bupivacaine. Effects of age on neural blockade and pharmacokinetics. *Anesthesia and Analgesia* **66**, 589—93.

Veering B.T., Burm A.G.L., Vletter A.A., van den Hoeven R.A.M. & Spierdijk J. (1991a) The effect of age on systemic absorption and systemic disposition of bupivacaine after subarachnoid administration *Anesthesiology* **74**, 250—7.

Veering B.T., Burm A.G.L., Gladines M.P.R.R. & Spierdijk J. (1991b) Age does not influence the serum protein binding of bupivacaine. *British Journal of Clinical Pharmacology* **32**, 501—3.

Veering B.T., Burm A.G.L., Vletter A.A., van den Heuvel R.P.M., Oukenhout W. & Spierdijk J. (1992) The effect of age on the systemic absorption, disposition and pharmacodynamics of bupivacaine after epidural administration. *Clinical Pharmacokinetics* **22**, 75—84.

Verborgh C., Claeys M.-A. & Camu F. (1991) Onset of epidural blockade after plain or alkalinized 0.5% bupivacaine. *Anesthesia and Analgesia* **73**, 401—4.

Vester-Andersen T., Christiansen C., Hansen A., Sorensen M. & Meisler C. (1981) Interscalene brachial plexus block: area of analgesia, complications and blood concentrations of local anesthetics. *Acta Anaesthesiologica Scandinavica* **25**, 81—4.

Vester-Andersen T., Husum B., Lindeburg T., Borrits L. & Gothgen I. (1984) Perivascular axillary block. V: blockade following 60 ml of mepivacaine 1% injected as a bolus or as 30 + 30 ml with a 20-min interval. *Acta Anaesthesiologica Scandinavica* **28**, 612—16.

Vester-Andersen T., Broby-Johansen U. & Bro-Rasmussen F. (1986) Perivascular axillary block. VI: The distribution of gelatine solution injected into the axillary neurovascular sheath of cadavers. *Acta Anaesthesiologica Scandinavica* **30**, 18—22.

Wennberg E., Haljamae H., Edwall G. & Dhuner K.-G. (1982) Effects of commercial (pH 3.5) and freshly prepared (pH 6.5) lidocaine—adrenaline solutions on tissue pH. *Acta Anaesthesiologica Scandinavica* **26**, 524—7.

Wiklund L., Tucker G.T. & Engberg G. (1977) Influence of intravenously administered ephedrine on splanchnic haemo-

dynamics and clearance of lidocaine. *Acta Anaesthesiologica Scandinavica* **21**, 275—81.

Wildsmith J.A.W. (1986) Peripheral nerve and local anaesthetic drugs. *British Journal of Anaesthesia* **58**, 692—700.

Wildsmith J.A.W. & Rocco A.G. (1985) Current concepts in spinal anesthesia. *Regional Anesthesia* **10**, 119—24.

Wildsmith J.A.W., Tucker G.T., Cooper S., Scott D.B. & Covino B.G. (1977) Plasma concentrations of local anaesthetics after interscalene brachial plexus block. *British Journal of Anaesthesia* **49**, 461—6.

Wildsmith J.A.W., Gissen A.J., Takman B. & Covino B.G. (1987) Differential nerve blockade: esters vs amides and the influence of pKa. *British Journal of Anaesthesia* **59**, 379—84.

Wildsmith J.A.W., Brown D.T., Paul D. & Johnson S. (1989) Structure—activity relationships in differential nerve block at high and low frequency stimulation. *British Journal of Anaesthesia* **63**, 444—52.

Wilkinson G.R. & Lund P.C. (1970) Bupivacaine levels in plasma and cerebrospinal fluid following peridural administration. *Anesthesiology* **33**, 482—6.

Williams R.L., Blaschke T.F., Meffin P.L., Melmon K.L. & Rowland M. (1976) Influence of viral hepatitis on the disposition of two compounds with high hepatic clearance: lidocaine and indocyanine green. *Clinical Pharmacology and Therapeutics* **20**, 290—9.

Wing L.M.H., Miners J.O., Birkett D.J., Foenander T., Lillywhite K. & Wanwimolruk S. (1984) Lidocaine disposition — sex differences and effects of cimetidine. *Clinical Pharmacology and Therapeutics* **35**, 695—701.

Winnie A.P., La Vallee D.A., Sosa B.P. & Masud K.Z. (1977a) Clinical pharmacokinetics of local anesthetics. *Canadian Anaesthetists' Society Journal* **24**, 252—62.

Winnie A.P., Tay C.-H., Patel K.P., Ramamurthy S. & Durrani Z. (1977b) Pharmacokinetics of local anesthetics during plexus blocks. *Anesthesia and Analgesia* **56**, 852—61.

Winnie A.P., Radonjic R., Akkineni S.R. & Durrani Z. (1979) Factors influencing distribution of local anesthetic injected into the brachial plexus sheath. *Anesthesia and Analgesia* **58**, 225—34.

Wood M. & Wood A.J.J. (1981) Changes in plasma drug binding and alpha₁-acid glycoprotein in mother and newborn infant. *Clinical Pharmacology and Therapeutics* **29**, 522—6.

Wulf H., Münstedt P. & Maier C. (1991) Plasma protein binding of bupivacaine in pregnant women at term. *Acta Anaesthesiologica Scandinavica* **35**, 129—33.

Wurst H.J. & Stanton-Hicks M.d'A. (1983) Changes of pH in epidural and spinal space and plasma levels of bupivacaine during acute and chronic epidurals in dogs. *Regional Anesthesia* **8**, 35—9.

General Considerations, Toxicity and Complications of Local Anaesthesia

B.G. COVINO† AND J.A.W. WILDSMITH

Chemical compounds that demonstrate local anaesthetic activity possess usually an aromatic and an amine group separated by an intermediate chain (Table 67.1). The clinically useful local anaesthetic agents fall essentially into one of two chemically distinct groups. Those agents which possess an ester link between the aromatic portion and the intermediate chain are referred to as amino esters and include procaine, chloroprocaine and amethocaine (tetracaine — USP). Local anaesthetics with an amide link between the aromatic end and the intermediate chain are referred to as amino amides and include lignocaine (lidocaine — USP), mepivacaine, prilocaine, bupivacaine and etidocaine. The ester and amide compounds differ in terms of their chemical stability, metabolic site and allergic potential. Amides are extremely stable agents whilst esters are relatively unstable in solution. The amino esters are hydrolysed in plasma by the enzyme cholinesterase, whereas the amide compounds undergo enzymatic degradation in the liver. Para-aminobenzoic acid is one of the metabolites of ester-type compounds and it can induce allergic-type reactions in a small percentage of patients. The amino amides are not metabolized to para-aminobenzoic acid and allergic reactions to these agents are extremely rare, but do occur (Brown *et al.*, 1981).

General considerations

The properties of the various local anaesthetic agents which are clinically important include potency, speed of onset, duration of anaesthetic activity and differential sensory/motor block. The clinical profile of the individual agents is determined essentially by the physicochemical characteristics of the various compounds, which in turn are dependent on their chemi-

cal structure. The physicochemical properties which influence anaesthetic activity are lipid solubility, protein binding and pKa. Minor changes in molecular structure have dramatic effects on these properties (Table 67.1).

Anaesthetic potency

Lipid solubility appears to be the primary determinant of intrinsic anaesthetic potency. The nerve membrane is basically a lipoprotein matrix, consisting of 90% lipids and 10% proteins. As a result, chemical compounds which are highly lipophilic tend to penetrate the nerve membrane more easily and they are also more potent. *In vitro* studies on isolated nerves show a correlation between the partition coefficient of local anaesthetics and the minimum concentration (C_{min}) required for conduction block (Gissen *et al.*, 1980; Wildsmith *et al.*, 1985). For example, among the amino amides, mepivacaine and prilocaine are the least lipid-soluble and weakest amide agents, while etidocaine is the most lipophilic and the most potent local anaesthetic (Fig. 67.1). A similar relationship between lipid solubility and potency exists among the ester-type drugs. Procaine is the least lipid soluble and the weakest agent, whilst amethocaine is the most lipophilic and the most potent ester-type drug.

Factors other than lipid solubility may influence anaesthetic potency also. A comparison of the partition coefficient values of the base form of ester and amide agents and their relative anaesthetic potencies indicates that the potency of the amino esters is greater than that of amino amides at similar coefficient values. It has been suggested that the amino esters may interact with a greater number of local anaesthetic receptor sites, which may explain their inherently greater potency (Wildsmith *et al.*, 1987).

In vivo studies in humans indicate that the correlation between lipid solubility and anaesthetic

† Deceased.

Table 67.1 Chemical structure, physicochemical properties and pharmacological properties of local anaesthetic agents

Agent	Chemical configuration			Physicochemical properties				Pharmacological properties		
	Aromatic lipophilic	Intermediate chain	Amine hydrophilic	Molecular weight (base)	pKa (25°C)	Partition coefficient	Percentage protein binding	Onset	Relative potency	Duration
Esters										
Procaine				236	8.9	0.02	6	Slow	1	Short
Amethocaine				264	8.5	4.1	76	Slow	8	Long
Chloroprocaine				271	8.7	0.14	—	Fast	1	Short
Amides										
Prilocaine				220	7.9	0.9	55	Fast	2	Moderate
Lignocaine				234	7.9	2.9	64	Fast	2	Moderate
Mepivacaine				246	7.6	0.8	78	Fast	2	Moderate
Bupivacaine				288	8.1	27.5	96	Moderate	8	Long
Etidocaine				276	7.7	141	94	Fast	6	Long

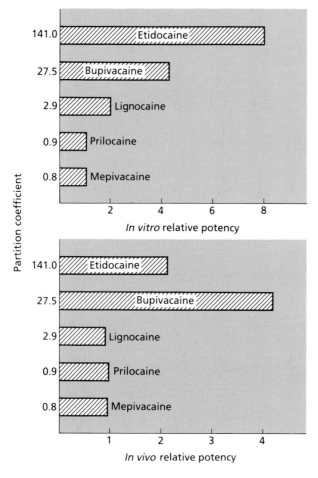

Fig. 67.1 Relationship of lipid solubility (partition coefficient) to *in vitro* and *in vivo* anaesthetic potency.

potency is not as precise as in an isolated nerve (Fig. 67.1). Lignocaine is approximately twice as potent as prilocaine and mepivacaine in an isolated preparation, but in humans, little difference in anaesthetic potency is apparent between these three agents. Similarly, etidocaine is more potent than bupivacaine in an isolated nerve while etidocaine is actually less active clinically than bupivacaine. The difference between *in vitro* and *in vivo* results is believed to be related to the vasodilator or tissue redistribution properties of the various local anaesthetics. For example, lignocaine causes a greater degree of vasodilatation than either mepivacaine or prilocaine, resulting in a more rapid vascular absorption of lignocaine such that fewer lignocaine molecules are available for neural block *in vivo*. The extremely high lipid solubility of etidocaine results in a greater uptake of this agent by adipose tissue such as in the extradural space, which again results in fewer etidocaine molecules available for neural block compared with bupivacaine.

Duration of action

The duration of anaesthesia is related primarily to the degree of protein binding of the various local anaesthetics. Local anaesthetics are believed to combine with a protein receptor located within the sodium channel of the nerve membrane. Chemical compounds which possess a greater affinity for and bind more firmly to the receptor site remain within the channel for a longer period of time, resulting in a prolonged duration of conduction block. Most of the information regarding the protein binding of local anaesthetics has been obtained from studies involving the binding of these agents to plasma proteins. It is assumed that a relationship exists between the plasma protein binding of local anaesthetics and the degree of binding to membrane proteins.

In vitro studies have demonstrated that agents such as procaine, which are poorly protein bound, are washed out rapidly from isolated nerves, whereas drugs such as amethocaine, bupivacaine and etidocaine are removed at an extremely slow rate. *In vivo* studies, including clinical investigations in humans, have confirmed the relationship between protein binding of local anaesthetics and their duration of action (Covino, 1986a). For example, procaine produces a duration of brachial plexus block of 30–60 min, while approximately 10 h of anaesthesia have been reported following the use of bupivacaine or etidocaine for brachial plexus block (Fig. 67.2).

In humans, the duration of anaesthesia is influenced markedly by the peripheral vascular effects of the local anaesthetic agents. All local anaesthetics except cocaine tend to have a biphasic effect on vascular smooth muscle. At low concentrations, these agents tend to cause vasoconstriction, whereas at clinically employed concentrations, local anaesthetics

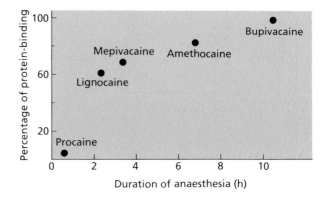

Fig. 67.2 Relationship of protein binding of various local anaesthetics to the duration of brachial plexus block.

cause vasodilatation (Johns *et al.*, 1985, 1986). However, differences exist in the degree of vasodilator activity produced by the various drugs. For example, lignocaine is a more potent vasodilator than mepivacaine or prilocaine. Although little difference in the duration of conduction block is apparent between these agents in an isolated nerve, *in vivo*, the duration of anaesthesia produced by lignocaine is shorter than that of mepivacaine or prilocaine. Addition of a vasoconstrictor drug to these three local anaesthetics results in a similar duration of action.

Onset of action

The onset of conduction block in isolated nerves is determined primarily by the pKa of the individual agents. The pKa of a chemical compound is the pH at which the ionized and non-ionized forms are present in equal amounts. The uncharged form of the local anaesthetic agent is primarily responsible for diffusion across the nerve sheath and nerve membrane and therefore the onset of action is related directly to the amount of drug which exists in the base form (Fig. 67.3). The percentage of a specific local anaesthetic drug, which is present in the base form when injected into tissue at pH 7.4, is inversely proportional to the pKa of that agent. For example, mepivacaine, lignocaine, prilocaine and etidocaine possess a pKa of approximately 7.7. When these agents are injected into tissue at a pH of 7.4, approximately 65% of these drugs exists in the ionized form and 35% in the non-ionized base form. On the other hand, amethocaine possesses a pKa of 8.6 and only 5% is present in the non-ionized form at a tissue pH of 7.4, while 95% exists in the charged cationic form. The pKa of bupivacaine is 8.1, which indicates that 15% of this agent is present in the non-ionized form at a tissue pH of 7.4, and 85% exists in the charged cationic form. Therefore, lignocaine, mepivacaine, prilocaine and etidocaine show a rapid onset of action, whereas procaine and amethocaine, with a high pKa, have a slow onset time (Fig. 67.3). Bupivacaine occupies an intermediate position in terms of pKa and latency of block.

The onset of conduction block *in vivo* is dependent in part on other miscellaneous considerations. The onset of action may be altered by the rate of diffusion through non-nervous tissue. For example, lignocaine and prilocaine possess a similar pKa and similar onset of action in an isolated nerve. However, *in vivo* prilocaine may be somewhat slower in onset than lignocaine. This difference may be related to an enhanced ability of lignocaine to diffuse through non-nervous tissue. More important, however, is the

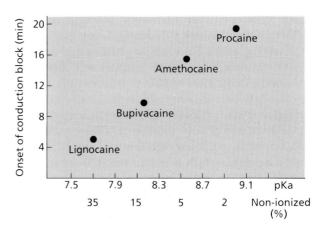

Fig. 67.3 Relationship of onset of anaesthesia of various local anaesthetic agents to their pKa and percentage of drug in non-ionized form.

concentration of local anaesthetic agent employed. For example, bupivacaine 0.25% possesses a rather slow onset of action. However, increasing the concentration to 0.75% results in a significant decrease in the latency of anaesthetic activity. The rapid onset time of chloroprocaine *in vivo* may be related in part to improved diffusion through non-nervous tissue, but also to the use of a 3% concentration of this agent. The pKa of chloroprocaine is approximately 9 and its onset of action in isolated nerves is relatively slow (Rosenberg *et al.*, 1980). However, the low systemic toxicity of this agent allows the use of high concentrations. Therefore, the rapid onset time *in vivo* of chloroprocaine may be related simply to the large number of molecules placed in the vicinity of peripheral nerves.

Differential sensory/motor block

One other important clinical consideration is the ability of local anaesthetic agents to cause a differential block of sensory and motor fibres. The intrathecal administration of varying concentrations of procaine has been employed to provide a differential block of sensory, sympathetic and motor fibres. However, it has been extremely difficult to produce sensory anaesthesia sufficient for surgery without a significant impairment of motor function. Bupivacaine was the first agent which showed a relative specificity for sensory fibres such that adequate sensory analgesia without profound inhibition of motor fibres could be achieved for surgical, obstetrical and acute and chronic pain therapy regardless of the regional anaesthetic technique employed. Bupivacaine and etidocaine provide an interesting contrast in terms of their differential sensory/motor blocking activity, although they are both potent long-acting anaesthetic agents (Fig. 67.4). For example, bupivacaine is used widely extradurally for both surgical and obstetrical procedures and relief of pain postoperatively due to its ability to provide adequate sensory analgesia with minimal block of motor fibres, particularly when used as an 0.25 or 0.5% solution. Thus, the patient in labour can be rendered pain-free and still be able to move her legs, which is one of the primary reasons why this agent has enjoyed popularity for continuous extradural block during labour. Increasing the concentration of bupivacaine to 0.75% increases the depth of both sensory and motor block while shortening also latency and producing a more prolonged duration of anaesthesia (Scott *et al.*, 1980). Etidocaine, on the other hand, shows little separation between sensory and motor block. In order to achieve adequate extradural sensory anaesthesia, 1.5% concentrations of etidocaine are required usually. At these concentrations, etidocaine has an extremely rapid onset of action and a prolonged duration of anaesthesia. However, sensory anaesthesia is associated with a profound degree of motor block. Thus, etidocaine is a valuable agent, particularly for extradural block in surgical situations where optimum muscle relaxation is desirable, as it combines a rapid onset, prolonged duration and satisfactory quality of anaesthesia combined with profound motor block. However, this marked effect on motor function renders etidocaine of limited value for obstetric analgesia and postoperative pain relief.

The factors responsible for the differential sensory/motor separation associated with bupivacaine are not known precisely. Studies on isolated nerves have shown that at low concentrations, bupivacaine blocks initially unmyelinated C-fibres followed at a later time by a block of myelinated A-fibres (Gissen *et al.*, 1982). On the other hand, etidocaine blocks both A- and C-fibres at approximately the same rate. The slow block of A-fibres by bupivacaine is believed to be a result of the relatively high pKa of this agent such that fewer uncharged molecules are available to penetrate the diffusion barriers surrounding large A-fibres. *In vivo*, the combination of the slow diffusion of bupivacaine and its absorption by the vasculature in the region of drug administration may result in a situation in which the number of bupivacaine molecules which penetrate ultimately the membrane of the large, motor A-fibres is insufficient to cause conduction block. The lack of diffusion barriers around the small sensory C-fibres allows a sufficient number of bupivacaine molecules to reach the receptor sites in the C-fibre membrane to cause sensory anaesthesia. Thus, bupivacaine may possess the optimal pKa and lipid-solubility characteristics required for differential sensory/motor block.

In summary, the pharmacological activity of local anaesthetic agents is related primarily to their physicochemical properties. However, the activity of these agents *in vivo* may be altered by other actions which are unrelated essentially to their physicochemical properties. On the basis of anaesthetic activity in humans, the various agents may be classified as follows:

1 Agents of low anaesthetic potency and short duration of action: procaine and chloroprocaine.
2 Agents of intermediate anaesthetic potency and duration of action: lignocaine, mepivacaine and prilocaine.
3 Agents of high anaesthetic potency and prolonged duration of action: amethocaine, bupivacaine and etidocaine.

In terms of latency, chloroprocaine, lignocaine, mepivacaine, prilocaine and etidocaine possess a relatively rapid onset of action. Bupivacaine is intermediate in terms of onset of anaesthesia, whilst procaine and amethocaine demonstrate a long latency period.

Factors influencing anaesthetic activity

Although the inherent pharmacological properties of the various local anaesthetic agents determine basically their anaesthetic profile, other factors may influ-

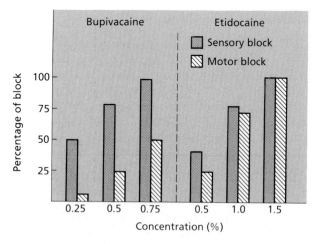

Fig. 67.4 Comparative sensory/motor block of bupivacaine and etidocaine following extradural administration.

ence the quality of regional anaesthesia also. These include:

1 Dosage of local anaesthetic administered.
2 Addition of a vasoconstrictor to the local anaesthetic solution.
3 Site of administration.
4 Carbonation or pH adjustment of local anaesthetic solutions.
5 Additives.
6 Mixtures of local anaesthetics.
7 Pregnancy.

Dosage of local anaesthetic solutions

The mass of drug administered influences the onset, depth and duration of anaesthesia (Fig. 67.5). As the dose of local anaesthetic is increased, the frequency of satisfactory anaesthesia and the duration of anaesthesia increase and the speed of onset of anaesthesia decreases. In general, the dosage of local anaesthetic administered can be increased by either administering a larger volume or a more concentrated solution. However, in clinical practice, an increase in dosage is achieved usually by employing a more concentrated solution of the specific agent. For example, increasing the concentration of extradurally administered bupivacaine from 0.125 to 0.5% whilst maintaining the same volume of injectate (10 ml) resulted in a decreased latency, improved incidence of satisfactory analgesia and an increased duration of sensory analgesia. Similarly, an increase in the concentration of extradural bupivacaine in surgical patients from 0.5% to 0.75% with a concomitant increase in dosage from approximately 100–150 mg

produced a more rapid onset and prolonged duration of sensory anaesthesia, a greater frequency of satisfactory sensory anaesthesia and an enhanced depth of motor block (Scott et al., 1980). Prilocaine, 600 mg, administered extradurally either as 30 ml of a 2% solution or 20 ml of a 3% solution showed no difference in onset, adequacy or duration of anaesthesia and onset, depth and duration of motor block, which indicates that dosage rather than volume or concentration of anaesthetic solution is the primary determinant of anaesthetic activity. The volume of anaesthetic solution may influence the spread of anaesthesia to a much lesser degree. For example, 30 ml of lignocaine 1% administered into the extradural space produced a level of anaesthesia which was 4.3 dermatomes higher than that achieved when 10 ml of lignocaine 3% was employed. With less extreme differences, variations in volume (at a constant dose) have little influence on extent of block (Duggan et al., 1988). Thus, the primary qualities of regional anaesthesia, namely, onset, depth and duration of block, are related to the mass of drug injected, i.e. the product of volume and concentration. Spread is only marginally influenced by volume.

Addition of a vasoconstrictor to local anaesthetic solutions

Vasoconstrictors, particularly adrenaline (epinephrine — USP), are added to local anaesthetic solutions frequently to decrease the rate of vascular absorption which allows more anaesthetic molecules to reach the nerve membrane and thereby improve the depth and duration of anaesthesia. Local anaesthetic solutions

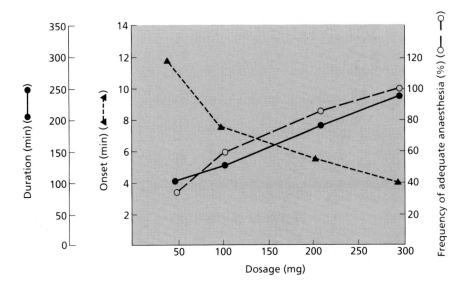

Fig. 67.5 Effect of dose of extradural etidocaine on onset, frequency and duration of anaesthesia.

contain usually a 1/200 000 (5 μg/ml) concentration of adrenaline. This concentration of adrenaline has been reported to provide an optimal degree of vasoconstriction when employed with lignocaine for extradural or intercostal use. Other vasoconstrictor agents such as noradrenaline (norepinephrine — USP) and phenylephrine have been added also to solutions of local anaesthetics. Equipotent concentrations of adrenaline and phenylephrine appear to prolong the duration of spinal anaesthesia produced by amethocaine to a similar extent (Concepcion *et al.*, 1984) (Fig. 67.6).

The effect of adrenaline on prolonging the duration of anaesthesia varies depending on the local anaesthetic employed and the site of injection. For example, the duration of action of all agents is prolonged by the addition of adrenaline when used for infiltration anaesthesia and peripheral nerve blocks. Adrenaline increases also the duration of extradural anaesthesia when added to procaine, mepivacaine and lignocaine but does not alter markedly the duration of action of extradurally administered prilocaine, bupivacaine or etidocaine. The decreased vasodilator action of prilocaine compared with lignocaine is believed responsible for the reduced effect of added adrenaline to solutions of prilocaine. The high lipid solubility of bupivacaine and etidocaine may be responsible for the diminished effect of adrenaline. These agents are taken up substantially by extradural fat and then released slowly, and this contributes to their prolonged duration of action. However, the interaction of adrenaline and the long-acting agents such as bupivacaine is dependent on the concentration of drug employed. For example, in

extradural block for labour, the frequency and duration of adequate analgesia was improved when adrenaline, 1/200 000, was added to bupivacaine 0.125% and 0.25%. However, the addition of adrenaline to 0.5% and 0.75% bupivacaine did not improve the adequacy or prolong the initial regression of extradural sensory anaesthesia in obstetrical or surgical patients. The profoundness but not the duration of motor block is enhanced following the extradural administration of adrenaline containing solutions of bupivacaine and etidocaine.

In the subarachnoid space, adrenaline extends significantly the duration of action of amethocaine (Concepcion *et al.*, 1984). Two or four segment regression of anaesthesia is not enhanced markedly when solutions of lignocaine or bupivacaine with adrenaline are administered intrathecally, although anaesthesia in the lower thoracic and lumbosacral areas is prolonged. Thus, adrenaline added to spinal solutions of lignocaine and bupivacaine may not prolong significantly the duration of effective surgical anaesthesia in the abdominal area but provides an extended duration of anaesthesia in the lower limbs. A more generalized extension of duration may be obtained by increasing the dose injected (Brown *et al.*, 1980a).

Site of injection

Although local anaesthetics are classified frequently as agents of short, moderate or long duration with a slow or rapid onset of action, these general properties are influenced by the type of anaesthetic procedure performed. In general, the most rapid onset but the shortest duration of action occurs following the intrathecal or subcutaneous administration of local anaesthetics, whilst the slowest onset times and the longest durations are observed during the performance of brachial plexus blocks. For example, an agent such as bupivacaine demonstrates an onset time of approximately 5 min and a duration of action of approximately 3—4 h when administered into the subarachnoid space. However, when bupivacaine is administered for brachial plexus block, the onset time is approximately 20—30 min, whilst the duration of anaesthesia averages 10 h. Differences in the onset and duration of anaesthesia depending on the site of injection result in part from the particular anatomy of the area of injection, the variation in the rate of vascular absorption, and the amount of drug employed for various types of regional anaesthesia. In the case of spinal anaesthesia, the lack of a nerve sheath around the spinal cord and deposition of the

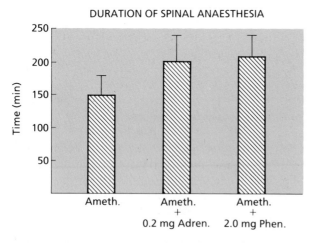

Fig. 67.6 Effect of adrenaline (Adren.) and phenylephrine (Phen.) on the duration of spinal anaesthesia produced by amethocaine (Ameth.).

local anaesthetic solution in the immediate vicinity of the spinal cord is responsible for the rapid onset of action. On the other hand, the relatively small amount of drug employed for spinal anaesthesia accounts probably for the relatively short duration of action associated with this particular technique. In the case of brachial plexus block, the onset of anaesthesia is slow because the anaesthetic agent is deposited usually at some distance from the nerve roots, and the drug must diffuse through various tissue barriers before reaching the nerve membrane. The long duration of brachial plexus block is related probably to the decreased rate of vascular absorption from that site, and also the larger doses of drug employed commonly for this regional anaesthetic technique.

Carbonation and pH adjustment of local anaesthetics

In isolated nerve preparations, carbon dioxide enhances the diffusion of local anaesthetics through nerve sheaths resulting in a more rapid onset (Fig. 67.7) and a decrease in the minimum concentration (C_{min}) of local anaesthetic required for conduction block (Gissen & Covino, 1985). The enhanced onset and depth of conduction block is believed to result from the diffusion of carbon dioxide through the nerve membrane and a decrease in the axoplasmic pH. The lower pH increases the intracellular concentration of the active cationic form of the local anaes-

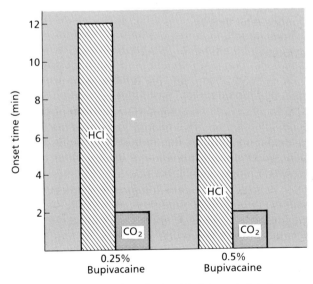

Fig. 67.7 Onset time of conduction block in an isolated nerve following exposure to bupivacaine–HCl and bupivacaine–CO_2.

thetic which binds to a receptor in the sodium channel. In addition, the local anaesthetic cation does not diffuse readily through membranes such that the drug remains entrapped within the axoplasm, a situation referred to as ion trapping. Several investigations in humans have demonstrated that lignocaine carbonate solutions produce a more rapid onset of brachial plexus and extradural block compared with the use of lignocaine hydrochloride solutions (Bromage, 1965, 1970). However, other studies have failed to demonstrate a significantly more rapid onset of action when lignocaine carbonate was compared with lignocaine hydrochloride for extradural block (Morrison, 1981). Similarly, it has been reported that bupivacaine–CO_2 is associated with a more rapid onset of action in humans. However, double-blind studies in which bupivacaine carbonate was compared with bupivacaine hydrochloride for brachial plexus or extradural block, have failed to confirm these earlier reports of a significantly shorter onset of action of the carbonated solution (Brown et al., 1980b; McClure & Scott, 1981). It is not certain if carbonation of local anaesthetic solutions decreases consistently the latency of conduction block in a clinical situation. However, it does appear that carbonated solutions do improve the profoundness of sensory anaesthesia and motor block when administered into the extradural space. The major advantage of these solutions may be in brachial plexus blocks where a more complete inhibition of conduction in the radial, median and ulnar nerves has been demonstrated.

Alkalinization of local anaesthetic solutions has also been employed in order to decrease the onset of conduction block. The addition of sodium bicarbonate increases the pH of the local anaesthetic solution which in turn increases the amount of drug in the uncharged base form. Thus, the rate of diffusion across the nerve sheath and nerve membrane should be enhanced, resulting in a more rapid onset of anaesthesia. Several clinical studies have been carried out in which the addition of sodium bicarbonate to solutions of bupivacaine or lignocaine did appear to produce a significant decrease in the latency of brachial plexus and extradural block. In addition, it has been reported also that the duration of brachial plexus block was prolonged by increasing the pH of bupivacaine (Hilgier, 1985).

Additives

Various attempts have been made to prolong the duration of anaesthesia by incorporating substances such as dextran into local anaesthetic solutions

(Loder, 1960). Discrepancies exist with regard to the effectiveness of dextran, in prolonging the duration of regional anaesthesia. In one controlled clinical study, prolonged durations of anaesthesia were observed in some individual patients but the mean duration of intercostal nerve block was not altered significantly when solutions of bupivacaine with and without dextran were compared (Bridenbaugh, 1978).

It has been suggested that the difference in results obtained by various investigators may be related to the pH of the dextran solution employed. Dextran solutions with a pH of 8.0 prolonged significantly the duration of bupivacaine-induced coccygeal nerve blocks in rats, whereas the duration of block was not altered when dextran with a pH of 4.5−5.5 was added to bupivacaine. These results indicate that alkalinization of the anaesthetic solution may be responsible for prolonged conduction block rather than the dextran itself.

Mixtures of local anaesthetics

The use of mixtures of local anaesthetics for regional anaesthesia has become relatively popular in recent years. The basis for this practice is to compensate for the short duration of action of certain agents such as chloroprocaine or lignocaine and the long latency of other agents such as amethocaine and bupivacaine.

Theoretically, mixtures of chloroprocaine and bupivacaine should offer significant clinical advantages from the rapid onset and low systemic toxicity of chloroprocaine and the long duration of action of bupivacaine. It was reported originally that a mixture of chloroprocaine and bupivacaine did result in a short latency and prolonged duration of brachial plexus blockade. However, subsequent studies indicated that the duration of extradural anaesthesia produced by a mixture of chloroprocaine and bupivacaine was significantly shorter than that obtained with solutions of bupivacaine alone. Data from isolated nerve studies suggest that a metabolite of chloroprocaine may inhibit the binding of bupivacaine to membrane receptor sites (Corke et al., 1984). At present there do not appear to be any clinically significant advantages to the use of mixtures of local anaesthetic agents. Etidocaine and bupivacaine provide clinically acceptable onsets of action and prolonged durations of anaesthesia. In addition, the use of catheter techniques for extradural anaesthesia and also for brachial plexus block makes it possible to administer repeated injection of the rapidly acting agents such as chloroprocaine or lignocaine which provide an anaesthetic duration of indefinite length.

Pregnancy

It is well known that the spread of extradural or spinal anaesthesia is greater in pregnant patients compared with non-pregnant subjects. This exaggerated spread has been attributed to mechanical factors associated with pregnancy, i.e. dilated extradural veins tend to decrease the diameter of the extradural and subarachnoid space which results in a more extensive longitudinal spread of local anaesthetic solution. Recent studies have suggested that physiological alterations associated with pregnancy may play a role also in the apparent increase in local anaesthetic sensitivity during pregnancy. For example, the spread of extradural anaesthesia is similar in patients during the first trimester of pregnancy and in term patients which indicates that mechanical factors alone cannot explain the enhanced spread of anaesthesia in parturients (Fagraeus et al., 1983). Isolated nerve studies have shown a more rapid onset and an increased sensitivity to local anaesthetic-induced conduction block in vagus nerves obtained from pregnant rabbits (Datta et al., 1983). These results suggest that hormonal changes associated with pregnancy may alter the basic responsiveness of the nerve membrane to local anaesthetics. Thus, the drug dosage for any regional anaesthetic procedure probably should be reduced in patients during all stages of pregnancy.

Specific local anaesthetic agents
(Table 67.2)

Amino ester agents

Cocaine

This compound, which was isolated from leaves of the *Erythroxylon coca* bush, was the first agent employed successfully for the production of clinical local anaesthesia. The relatively high potential for systemic toxicity and the addiction liabilities associated with its use resulted in the abandonment of this agent for most regional anaesthetic techniques. However, cocaine is an excellent topical anaesthetic agent and is the only local anaesthetic that produces vasoconstriction at clinically useful concentrations. As a result, it is still employed to anaesthetize and constrict the nasal mucosa prior to nasotracheal intubation. It is also employed frequently by otolaryngologists during nasal surgery because of its topical anaesthetic and vasoconstrictor properties.

Table 67.2 Clinical use of local anaesthetic agents

Agents	Primary clinical uses	Comments
Amino esters		
Cocaine	Topical	Limited use due to addictive potential
Procaine	Infiltration Spinal	Limited use due to: Slow onset Short duration Allergic potential
Chloroprocaine	Peripheral nerve blocks Obstetrical extradural blocks	Fast onset Short duration Low systemic toxicity
Amethocaine	Spinal anaesthesia	Limited use except for spinal anaesthesia due to: Slow onset High systemic toxicity
Amino amides		
Lignocaine	Infiltration Intravenous regional anaesthesia Peripheral nerve block Surgical and obstetrical extradural blocks Spinal anaesthesia Topical	Most versatile agent
Mepivacaine	Infiltration Peripheral nerve blocks Surgical extradural blocks	Similar to lignocaine
Prilocaine	Infiltration Intravenous regional anaesthesia Peripheral nerve blocks Surgical extradural blocks	Methaemoglobinaemia at high doses Least systemic toxicity of amide agents
Bupivacaine	Infiltration Peripheral nerve blocks Obstetrical and surgical extradural blocks Spinal anaesthesia	Sensory/motor separation
Etidocaine	Infiltration Peripheral nerve blocks Surgical extradural blocks	Profound motor block
Miscellaneous		
Nupercaine	Spinal anaesthesia	Use limited to spinal and topical anaesthesia
Benzocaine	Topical	Use limited to topical anaesthesia

Procaine

This was the first synthetic local anaesthetic agent introduced into clinical practice. Procaine is a relatively weak local anaesthetic with a slow onset and short duration of action. The relatively low potency and rapid plasma hydrolysis of this agent are responsible for the low systemic toxicity of procaine.

However, procaine is hydrolysed to para-amino-benzoic acid, which is responsible for the allergic reactions associated with the repeated use of this drug. At present, procaine is used primarily for infiltration anaesthesia, diagnostic differential spinal blocks in certain pain states and obstetrical spinal anaesthesia.

Chloroprocaine

This agent is characterized by a rapid onset of action, a short duration and low systemic toxicity. Chloroprocaine is employed primarily for extradural analgesia and anaesthesia in obstetrics because of its rapid onset and low systemic toxicity in mother and fetus. However, frequent injections are required in order to provide adequate pain relief during labour. Often extradural analgesia is established in the pregnant patient with chloroprocaine followed by the use of a longer-acting agent such as bupivacaine. Chloroprocaine has also proven of value for various regional anaesthetic procedures performed in ambulatory surgical patients in whom the duration of surgery is not expected to exceed 30−60 min. Some concern exists regarding the potential neurotoxicity of chloroprocaine solutions following reports of prolonged sensory/motor deficits after the accidental intrathecal injection of large doses. These local irritant effects are believed to be related to the low pH and presence of sodium bisulphite in chloroprocaine solutions.

Amethocaine

This agent is used primarily for spinal anaesthesia. Amethocaine may be employed as an isobaric, hypobaric or hyperbaric solution for spinal block, although hyperbaric solutions of amethocaine are probably employed most commonly. Amethocaine provides a relatively rapid onset of spinal anaesthesia, excellent qualities of sensory anaesthesia and a profound block of motor function. Plain solutions of amethocaine provide an average duration of spinal anaesthesia of 2−3 h while the addition of adrenaline can extend the total duration of anaesthesia to 4−6 h.

Amethocaine is used rarely for other forms of regional anaesthesia because of its extremely slow onset of action and the potential for systemic toxic reactions when larger doses are employed. Amethocaine possesses also excellent topical anaesthetic properties, and solutions of this agent have been employed for tracheal surface anaesthesia. The absorption of amethocaine from the tracheobronchial area is extremely rapid, and several fatalities have been reported following the use of a tracheal aerosol of this drug.

Amino amide agents

Lignocaine

Lignocaine was the first drug of the amino amide type to be introduced into clinical practice. This agent remains the most versatile and most commonly used local anaesthetic because of its inherent potency, rapid onset, moderate duration of action and topical anaesthetic activity. Solutions of lignocaine are available for infiltration, peripheral nerve blocks and extradural anaesthesia. In addition, hyperbaric lignocaine 5% is useful for spinal anaesthesia of 30−60 min duration. Lignocaine is used also in ointment, jelly, viscous and aerosol preparations for a variety of topical anaesthetic procedures.

Intravenous lignocaine has also proven of value for certain non-anaesthetic indications. This agent has gained wide acceptance as an intravenous drug for the treatment of ventricular arrhythmias. In addition, lignocaine has been employed intravenously as an antiepileptic agent, as an analgesic for certain chronic pain states and as a supplement to general anaesthesia.

Mepivacaine

This agent is similar to lignocaine in its anaesthetic profile. Mepivacaine can produce a profound depth of anaesthesia with a relatively rapid onset and a moderate duration of action. This agent may be used for infiltration, peripheral nerve blocks and extradural anaesthesia, and in some countries, 4% hyperbaric solutions of mepivacaine are available also for spinal anaesthesia.

Mepivacaine is not effective as a topical anaesthetic agent and so is less versatile than lignocaine. In addition, the metabolism of mepivacaine is prolonged markedly in the fetus and newborn such that this agent is not employed usually for obstetrical anaesthesia. However, in adults, mepivacaine appears to be somewhat less toxic than lignocaine. In addition, the vasodilator activity of mepivacaine is less than that of lignocaine. Thus, mepivacaine provides a somewhat longer duration of anaesthesia than lignocaine when the two agents are used without adrenaline.

Prilocaine

The clinical profile of prilocaine is also similar to that of lignocaine. Prilocaine has a relatively rapid onset of action, whilst providing a moderate duration of anaesthesia and a profound depth of conduction block. This agent causes significantly less vasodilatation than lignocaine and so can be used without adrenaline. In general, the duration of prilocaine without adrenaline is similar to that of lignocaine with adrenaline. Thus, prilocaine is particularly useful in patients in whom adrenaline may be contraindicated. Prilocaine is useful for infiltration, peripheral nerve block and extradural anaesthesia.

Prilocaine is the least toxic of the amino amide local anaesthetics. Thus, this agent is particularly useful for intravenous regional anaesthesia as CNS toxic effects are seen rarely following tourniquet deflation even when early accidental release of the tourniquet may occur.

Methaemoglobinaemia may occur following the use of relatively large doses of prilocaine. This unusual side-effect has essentially eliminated the use of this drug in obstetrics, although prilocaine has not been reported to cause any significant adverse effects in mother, fetus or newborn. However, the cyanotic appearance of newborns delivered to mothers who have received prilocaine for extradural anaesthesia during labour results in sufficient confusion concerning the aetiology of the cyanosis such that the obstetrical use of this potentially valuable drug has been virtually abandoned.

Bupivacaine

Bupivacaine was the first local anaesthetic that combined the properties of an acceptable onset, long duration of action, profound conduction block and significant separation of sensory anaesthesia and motor block. This agent is used for various regional anaesthetic procedures, including infiltration, peripheral nerve blocks, extradural and spinal anaesthesia. The average duration of surgical anaesthesia of bupivacaine varies from approximately 3 to 10 h. Its longest duration of action occurs when major peripheral nerve blocks, such as brachial plexus block, are performed.

The major advantage of bupivacaine appears to be in the area of extradural obstetrical analgesia for labour where satisfactory pain relief of 2–3 h duration is achieved which decreases the need for repeated injections in the pregnant patient. Moreover, adequate analgesia is achieved usually without significant motor block such that the patient in labour is able to move her legs. This differential block of sensory and motor fibres is also the basis for the widespread use of bupivacaine for postoperative extradural analgesia and for certain chronic pain states.

Etidocaine

This agent is characterized by very rapid onset, prolonged duration of action, and profound sensory and motor block. Etidocaine may be used for infiltration, peripheral nerve block and extradural anaesthesia. Etidocaine has a significantly more rapid onset of action than bupivacaine. Concentrations of etidocaine which are required for adequate sensory anaesthesia produce profound motor block. As a result, etidocaine is useful primarily as an anaesthetic for surgical procedures in which muscle relaxation is required. Thus, this agent is of limited use for obstetrical extradural analgesia and for postoperative pain relief because it does not provide a differential block of sensory and motor fibres.

Miscellaneous

Nupercaine (dibucaine — USP)

This agent is used for spinal and topical anaesthesia. It is more potent than amethocaine and, whilst the onset of action of the two agents is similar, the duration of spinal anaesthesia is slightly longer with nupercaine. The degree of hypotension and the profoundness of motor block appear to be less in patients receiving intrathecal nupercaine compared with subjects in whom amethocaine was administered into the subarachnoid space, although the spread of sensory anaesthesia was similar in the two groups.

Benzocaine

This local anaesthetic is used exclusively for topical anaesthesia. It is available in a variety of proprietary and non-proprietary preparations. The most common forms used in an operating room setting are as aerosol solutions for tracheal administration and an ointment for lubrication of tracheal tubes.

Toxicity of local anaesthetic agents

Local anaesthetic agents are relatively free from side-effects if they are administered in an appropriate dosage and in the appropriate anatomical location. However, systemic and localized toxic reactions may occur, usually from the accidental intravascular or intrathecal injection or the administration of an excessive dose of local anaesthetic agent. In addition, specific adverse effects are associated with the use of certain agents such as allergic reactions to the amino ester or procaine-like drugs, and methaemoglobin-aemia following the use of prilocaine.

Systemic toxicity

Systemic reactions to local anaesthetics involve primarily the CNS and the cardiovascular system. In general, the CNS is more susceptible to the systemic actions of local anaesthetic agents than the cardiovascular system. The dose and blood concentration of local anaesthetic required to produce CNS toxicity is usually lower than that which results in circulatory collapse. Although local anaesthetic-induced cardiovascular depression occurs less frequently than CNS reactions, adverse effects involving the cardiovascular system tend to be more serious and more difficult to manage.

Central nervous system toxicity

The initial symptoms of local anaesthetic-induced CNS toxicity involve feelings of light-headedness and dizziness followed frequently by visual and auditory disturbances such as difficulty in focusing and tinnitus. Other subjective CNS symptoms include disorientation and occasional feelings of drowsiness. Objective signs of CNS toxicity are usually excitatory in nature and include shivering, muscular twitching and tremors involving initially muscles of the face and distal parts of the extremities. Ultimately, generalized convulsions of a tonic–clonic nature occur. If a sufficiently large dose or a rapid intravenous injection of a local anaesthetic agent is administered, the initial signs of CNS excitation are followed rapidly by a state of generalized CNS depression. Seizure activity ceases and respiratory depression and ultimately respiratory arrest may occur. In some patients, CNS depression without a preceding excitatory phase is seen, particularly if other CNS-depressant drugs have been administered.

CNS excitation is believed to be the result of an initial block of inhibitory pathways in the cerebral cortex by local anaesthetic drugs (DeJong, 1977). The block of inhibitory pathways allows facilitatory neurones to function in an unopposed fashion which results in an increase in excitatory activity leading to convulsions. An increase in the dose of local anaesthetic administered leads to an inhibition of conduction in both inhibitory and facilitatory pathways resulting in a generalized state of CNS depression.

In general, a correlation exists between anaesthetic potency and intravenous CNS toxicity of various agents (Englesson, 1974). For example, in cats, the dose of procaine required to cause convulsions is approximately seven times greater than the convulsive dose of bupivacaine. However, bupivacaine is also approximately eight times more potent than procaine as a local anaesthetic agent. A similar study in dogs indicated that the relative CNS toxicity of bupivacaine etidocaine and lignocaine is $4:2:1$, which is similar to the relative potency of these agents for the production of regional anaesthesia in humans (Liu et al., 1983). Intravenous infusion studies in human volunteers have demonstrated also a relationship between the intrinsic anaesthetic potency of various agents and the dosage required to induce CNS toxicity.

The rate of injection and rapidity with which a particular blood concentration is achieved alters the intravenous toxicity of local anaesthetic agents. For example, in human volunteers an average dose of 236 mg of etidocaine and a venous blood concentration of 3.0 µg/ml were required before the onset of CNS symptoms occurred when an infusion rate of 10 mg/min was employed (Scott, 1981). When the infusion rate was increased to 20 mg/min, an average dose of 161 mg of etidocaine, which produced a venous plasma concentration of approximately 2 µg/ml, resulted in symptoms of CNS toxicity.

The acid–base status of animals and patients can affect markedly the CNS activity of local anaesthetic agents. In cats, the convulsive threshold of various local anaesthetics was related inversely to the arterial $P\text{co}_2$ level (Fig. 67.8). For example, when the $P\text{co}_2$ was elevated from 3.3–5.3 kPa (25–40 mmHg) to 8.7–10.8 kPa (65–81 mmHg) the convulsive threshold of procaine, mepivacaine, prilocaine, lignocaine and bupivacaine was decreased by approximately 50%. A decrease in arterial pH decreases also the convulsive threshold of these agents. In fact, pH exerts probably a greater influence on CNS toxicity of local anaesthetics than does $P\text{co}_2$. Respiratory acidosis with a resultant increase in $P\text{co}_2$ and a decrease in arterial pH decrease consistently the convulsant threshold of local anaesthetic agents. However, an increase in $P\text{co}_2$ in response to an elevated arterial pH (as may occur during metabolic alkalosis) exerts less of a potentiating effect on the CNS activity of local anaesthetic agents.

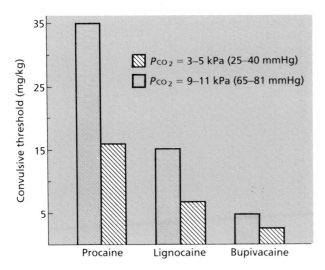

Fig. 67.8 Effect of hypercapnia on the convulsive threshold of procaine, lignocaine and bupivacaine.

This potentiating effect of acidosis and/or hypercapnia may be a result of several factors. An elevation of Pco_2 enhances cerebral blood flow so that more anaesthetic agent is delivered to the brain. In addition, in the presence of hypercapnia, diffusion of carbon dioxide across the nerve membrane may result in a reduction in intracellular pH. Intracellular acidosis augments the conversion of the base form of local anaesthetic agents to the cationic form, resulting in an increase in the intraneuronal concentration of the active form of the local anaesthetic agent. The cationic form does not diffuse well across the nerve membrane so that ionic trapping occurs, which increases also the apparent CNS toxicity of local anaesthetic agents.

Hypercapnia and/or acidosis decrease also the plasma protein binding of local anaesthetic agents. Therefore, an elevation in Pco_2 or decrease in pH increases the proportion of free drug available for diffusion into the brain. On the other hand, acidosis increases the cationic form of the local anaesthetic which should decrease the rate of diffusion.

In summary, local anaesthetic agents can exert marked effects on the CNS. In general, signs of CNS excitation leading to frank convulsions are the most common manifestation of systemic anaesthetic toxicity. Excessive doses or rapid intravenous administration of these drugs may lead also to CNS depression and respiratory arrest. In general, the potential CNS toxicity of local anaesthetics is correlated with the inherent anaesthetic potency of the various agents but the toxicity of these agents can be altered by factors such as rate of injection, hypercapnia and acidosis.

Cardiovascular system toxicity

Local anaesthetic agents can exert a direct action both on the heart and peripheral blood vessels.

Direct cardiac effects

The primary cardiac electrophysiological effect of local anaesthetics is a decrease in the maximum rate of depolarization in Purkinje fibres and ventricular muscle. This reduction in the maximum rate of depolarization is believed to result from a decrease in sodium conductance in the fast sodium channels in cardiac membranes.

Action potential duration and the effective refractory period are decreased also by local anaesthetics. However, the ratio of effective refractory period to action potential duration is increased both in Purkinje fibres and in ventricular muscle.

Qualitative differences may exist between the electrophysiological effects of various agents. Bupivacaine depresses the rapid phase of depolarization (V_{max}) in Purkinje fibres and ventricular muscle to a greater extent than lignocaine (Clarkson & Hohdeghem, 1985). In addition, the rate of recovery from a steady-state block is slower in bupivacaine-treated papillary muscles as compared with lignocaine. This slow rate of recovery results in an incomplete restoration of V_{max} between action potentials particularly at high heart rates. In contrast, recovery from lignocaine is complete, even at rapid heart rates. These differential effects of lignocaine and bupivacaine may explain the antiarrhythmic properties of lignocaine and the arrhythmogenic potential of bupivacaine.

Electrophysiological studies in intact dogs and in humans reflect essentially the findings observed in isolated cardiac tissue. As the dose and blood concentrations of lignocaine increase, a prolongation of conduction time through various parts of the heart occurs. These are reflected in the ECG as an increase in the PR interval and QRS duration. Extremely high concentrations of local anaesthetics depress spontaneous pacemaker activity in the sinus node resulting in sinus bradycardia and sinus arrest.

Local anaesthetic agents also exert profound effects on the mechanical activity of cardiac muscle. All local anaesthetics exert a dose-dependent, negative inotropic action on isolated cardiac tissue. This depression of cardiac contractility is proportional to the conduction-blocking potency of the various agents in isolated nerves (Block & Covino, 1982). Thus, the more potent local anaesthetics depress cardiac contractility at lower concentrations than the less potent drugs (Table 67.3). In general, local anaesthetics can be allocated into three groups in terms of their myocardial-depressant effect. The more potent agents, bupivacaine, amethocaine and etidocaine, depress cardiac contractility at the lowest concentrations. The agents of moderate anaesthetic potency, i.e. lignocaine, mepivacaine, prilocaine, chloroprocaine form an intermediate group of compounds in terms of myocardial depression. Finally, procaine and chloroprocaine, which are the least potent of local anaesthetics, require the highest concentration to decrease cardiac contractility.

Studies in intact dogs in which a strain-gauge arch was sutured to the right ventricle, revealed that all local anaesthetic agents evaluated exerted a negative inotropic action (Stewart *et al.*, 1963). As in the isolated cardiac tissue studies, a relationship existed between the local anaesthetic potency of various agents and their relative myocardial depressant effect (Fig. 67.9). For example, amethocaine, which is approximately 8–10 times more potent than procaine as a local anaesthetic, was approximately eight times more potent as a depressant of myocardial contractility than procaine. Haemodynamic studies in closed-chest, anaesthetized dogs have shown that amethocaine, etidocaine and bupivacaine caused a 50% decrease in cardiac output at doses of 10–20 mg/kg, whilst 30–40 mg/kg of lignocaine, mepivacaine, prilocaine and chloroprocaine were required for a similar decrease in cardiac output. A dose of 100 mg/kg of procaine was needed to reduce cardiac output by 50%.

The mechanism by which local anaesthetics depress myocardial contractility is not known precisely but may involve an interaction with calcium. Both procaine and amethocaine can increase the

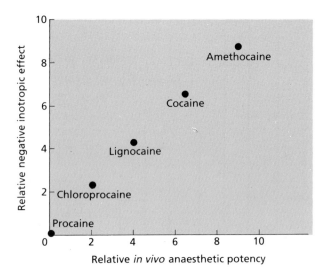

Fig. 67.9 Relationship between myocardial depressant effect and relative anaesthetic potency of various local anaesthetics.

release of calcium from isolated skeletal muscle preparations. The relative potency of amethocaine and procaine in terms of their ability to increase the rate of calcium efflux from sartorius muscle was proportional to their local anaesthetic activity. A similar displacement of calcium from cardiac muscle should result in a decrease in myocardial contractility. However, studies in the isolated guinea pig heart indicated that an increase in the extracellular concentration of calcium failed to reverse the negative inotropic action of bupivacaine or lignocaine.

Direct peripheral vascular effects

Local anaesthetic agents appear to exert a biphasic effect on peripheral vascular smooth muscle. Direct measurements of the arteriolar diameter in the cre-

Table 67.3 Comparative effect of various local anaesthetic agents on cardiac contractility and cardiac output

Agent	Relative anaesthetic potency	Contractility of isolated guinea pig heart (50% ↓) μg/ml	Cardiac output in dogs (50% ↓) mg/kg
Procaine	1	277	100
Chloroprocaine	1	102	30
Cocaine	2	56	—
Lignocaine	2	67	30
Prilocaine	2	42	40
Mepivacaine	2	55	40
Etidocaine	6	—	20
Bupivacaine	8	6	10
Amethocaine	8	6	20

master muscle of rats revealed that concentrations of lignocaine varying from 10^0 to 10^3 μg/ml produced a dose-related state of vasoconstriction varying from 88 to 60% of the control vascular diameter (Johns et al., 1985). An increase in the concentration of lignocaine to 10^4 μg/ml produced approximately a 27% increase in arteriolar diameter, indicative of a significant degree of vasodilatation. Isolated rat portal vein studies have demonstrated also that local anaesthetic drugs stimulate spontaneous myogenic contractions and augment basal tone at low concentrations but inhibit myogenic activity at higher concentrations.

In vivo studies have also confirmed the biphasic effect of local anaesthetics on the peripheral vasculature. Blood flow investigations in animals and humans have demonstrated that lower doses of local anaesthetics may decrease peripheral arterial flow without any change in systemic arterial pressure, which is indicative of an increase in peripheral vascular resistance. Higher doses of local anaesthetics result in an increased blood flow in peripheral arteries indicating a state of vasodilatation. Cocaine is the only local anaesthetic that causes vasoconstriction consistently because of its ability to inhibit the uptake of noradrenaline by storage granules. The excess concentration of free circulating noradrenaline is responsible for the vasoconstriction associated with the use of cocaine. A comparison of the peripheral vascular effects of various local anaesthetic agents has failed to demonstrate a good correlation between the relative anaesthetic potency of these agents and their ability to cause peripheral vasodilatation. However, a correlation does appear to exist between the duration of action of these agents as local anaesthetics and the duration of vasodilatation. Thus, lignocaine, mepivacaine and prilocaine cause a duration of peripheral vasodilatation of approximately 5 min following intra-arterial injection into the femoral artery of dogs. On the other hand, agents such as bupivacaine, etidocaine and amethocaine, which are long-acting local anaesthetics, produce a prolonged period of vasodilatation.

The pulmonary vasculature appears to be particularly sensitive to the stimulatory effects of local anaesthetics. Procaine increased pulmonary vascular resistance markedly in a Starling heart—lung preparation. Studies in intact anaesthetized dogs employing pulmonary artery catheters also showed that both the ester and amide agents can cause marked increases in pulmonary artery pressure and pulmonary vascular resistance. Relatively large intravenous doses of procaine, chloroprocaine and amethocaine caused increases in pulmonary vascular resistance of approximately 300%. Increases of 100—200% in pulmonary vascular resistance were observed after the administration of 3 mg/kg of bupivacaine and etidocaine. The administration of 10 mg/kg doses of mepivacaine, lignocaine and procaine resulted in increases in pulmonary vascular resistance of approximately 50—100%. At doses of local anaesthetics which approached lethal levels, decreases in pulmonary artery pressure and pulmonary vascular resistance were seen with both the ester- and amide-type local anaesthetic agents.

The biphasic peripheral vascular effect of local anaesthetic agents may be related to changes in smooth muscle concentrations of calcium. A competitive antagonism exists between local anaesthetic drugs and calcium ions in smooth muscle. Local anaesthetic compounds may displace calcium from membrane binding sites, resulting in diffusion of this ion into the smooth muscle cytoplasm. Such an increase in cytoplasmic calcium concentration should stimulate the interaction between contractile proteins leading to an increase in myogenic tone which would produce a state of vasoconstriction. However, as the concentration of local anaesthetic agent at the smooth muscle membrane is increased, the displacement of calcium by these agents decreases ultimately both the cytoplasmic calcium concentration and the interaction between the contractile protein elements of smooth muscle, which then results in a state of muscle relaxation leading to vasodilatation.

Comparative cardiovascular toxicity of local anaesthetics

In general, a direct relationship exists between the anaesthetic potency and cardiovascular depressant potential of the various agents. In recent years, the more potent drugs, i.e. bupivacaine and etidocaine, have been reported to cause rapid and profound cardiovascular depression in some patients following an accidental intravascular injection. Severe cardiac arrhythmias were observed and the cardiac depression appeared resistant to various therapeutic modalities. Thus, it has been suggested that the more potent and highly lipid-soluble drugs such as bupivacaine and etidocaine may be relatively more cardiotoxic than the less potent and less lipid-soluble agents, such as lignocaine.

The cardiotoxicity of the more potent agents such as bupivacaine appears to differ from that of lignocaine in the following manner:

1 The ratio of the dosage required for irreversible cardiovascular collapse (CC) and the dosage

which produces CNS toxicity (convulsions), i.e. the CC:CNS ratio, is lower for bupivacaine and etidocaine compared with lignocaine.

2 Ventricular arrhythmias and fatal ventricular fibrillation may occur following the rapid intravenous administration of a large dose of bupivacaine but not lignocaine.

3 The pregnant animal or patient may be more sensitive to the cardiotoxic effects of bupivacaine than the non-pregnant animal or patient.

4 Cardiac resuscitation is more difficult following bupivacaine-induced CC.

5 Acidosis and hypoxia potentiate markedly the cardiotoxicity of bupivacaine.

CC:CNS ratio

The ratio of the dosage and blood concentrations of bupivacaine and etidocaine associated with the development of convulsive activity and CC has been reported to be lower in adult sheep than that of lignocaine (Morishima *et al.*, 1985). For example, a CC:CNS dose ratio of 7.1 ± 1.1 existed for lignocaine indicating that seven times as much drug was required to induce irreversible cardiovascular collapse as was needed for the production of convulsions (Fig. 67.10). On the other hand, the CC:CNS ratio for bupivacaine was 3.7 ± 0.5 and for etidocaine 4.4 ± 0.9. Although the CNS was more sensitive to the toxic effects of all three agents, a smaller difference did exist between the dose of bupivacaine and etidocaine that caused convulsions and that which led to irreversible cardiovascular collapse as compared with lignocaine. An examination of arterial drug concen-

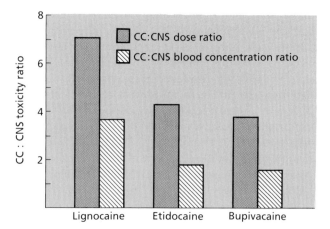

Fig. 67.10 CC:CNS dose and blood level ratio of lignocaine, etidocaine and bupivacaine in sheep.

trations associated with CNS and cardiovascular toxicity revealed that lignocaine possessed a CC:CNS blood level ratio of 3.6 ± 0.3 compared with values of 1.6 to 1.7 for bupivacaine and etidocaine (Fig. 67.10). At the time of cardiovascular collapse, higher concentrations of bupivacaine and etidocaine were present in the myocardium compared with lignocaine. Thus, the enhanced sensitivity of the myocardium to these more potent agents appears to result from greater myocardial uptake.

Ventricular arrhythmias

A number of investigators have reported the development of ventricular arrhythmias in animals exposed to toxic doses of bupivacaine (Reiz & Nath, 1986) (Table 67.4). The incidence of ventricular fibril-

Table 67.4 Ventricular arrhythmias following the use of lignocaine and bupivacaine in various animal preparations

	Ventricular arrhythmias	
Animal model	Lignocaine	Bupivacaine
Unanaesthetized, paralysed cat	6% PVC	100% PVC
Anaesthetized dog	0	0
Unanaesthetized dog	0	40% VT, VF
Unanaesthetized sheep	0	80–100% PVC, VT
Hypoxic, acidotic sheep	0	17–50% VT, VF
Isolated guinea pig heart	0	30–50% PVC bigeminy, trigeminy
Intracoronary injection in anaesthetized pigs	VF at 64 mg	VF at 4 mg
Intracranial injections in cats	17% VT	100% VT
Intracranial injections in rats	55% VT	55% VT
	No deaths	50% deaths

PVC, premature ventricular contractions; VF, ventricular fibrillation; VT, ventricular tachycardia.

lation has been determined in dogs in which convulsant and supraconvulsant doses of various local anaesthetics were administered intravenously. Ventricular fibrillation did not occur in lignocaine-, mepivacaine- or amethocaine-treated dogs, while approximately 20% of animals receiving etidocaine and 50% of those receiving bupivacaine developed ventricular fibrillation. The results suggest that the occurrence of ventricular fibrillation is not related to the basic piperidine ring structure of bupivacaine as mepivacaine, which contains the piperidine moiety, failed to cause these cardiac abnormalities. In addition, a precise correlation does not appear to exist between the frequency of ventricular arrhythmias and the lipid solubility and protein binding of local anaesthetics. Large doses of etidocaine, which is more lipid soluble than bupivacaine and equally protein bound, may cause ventricular arrhythmias and fibrillation but the incidence appears to be lower than that observed with bupivacaine.

It is not certain if the cardiac arrhythmias observed in bupivacaine-treated animals are related to a direct cardiac effect or are secondary to a CNS action or both. Isolated guinea pig hearts perfused with a bupivacaine solution revealed evidence of conduction block and bigeminy and trigeminy, but did not when perfused with lignocaine. In addition, ventricular fibrillation occurred in intact pigs in which bupivacaine was injected directly into the left anterior descending coronary artery. These results suggest that the ventricular arrhythmias are the result of a direct action on the heart. On the other hand, it has been shown that the injection of bupivacaine directly into certain regions of the brain resulted in the development of cardiac arrhythmias. Moreover, bupivacaine did not cause cardiac arrhythmias in dogs anaesthetized with pentobarbitone and intracerebroventricular midozolam terminates arrhythmias produced by bupivacaine given by the same route (Bernards & Artru, 1991). These results are indicative of a relationship between the CNS and cardiotoxic effects of bupivacaine.

Enhanced cardiotoxicity in pregnancy

Several of the cardiotoxic reactions reported following the use of bupivacaine have occurred in pregnant patients. As a result, the 0.75% solution is no longer recommended for use in obstetrical anaesthesia in the USA or UK. Studies in pregnant and non-pregnant sheep have shown that the CC:CNS dosage ratio of bupivacaine decreased from 3.7 ± 0.5 in non-pregnant sheep to 2.7 ± 0.4 in pregnant animals

(Morishima et al., 1985). However, little difference was observed in the CC:CNS blood concentration ratio which varied from 1.6 ± 0.1 in non-pregnant animals to 1.4 ± 0.1 in pregnant ewes. However, the blood concentration of bupivacaine at which circulatory collapse occurred was lower in pregnant animals. No difference in the myocardial uptake of bupivacaine in pregnant and non-pregnant sheep was observed at the time of cardiovascular collapse. Thus, if the pregnant patient is more susceptible to the cardiotoxic effects of bupivacaine, it is not apparently related to a greater myocardial uptake of drug.

Stereoselectivity

Like a number of other local anaesthetics bupivacaine is a racemic mixture of two optically active isomers. In vitro studies have shown that the R(+) enantiomer has greater cardiotoxicity than S(−) bupivacaine (Vanhoutte et al., 1991). Ropivacaine, an analogue of bupivacaine, is currently being evaluated as an alternative and is prepared in the prime S(−) form.

Cardiac resuscitation

Cardiopulmonary resuscitation may be difficult in patients in whom cardiotoxicity has occurred following the administration of a toxic dose of bupivacaine. Studies in acidotic and hypoxic sheep have indicated also that cardiac resuscitation following bupivacaine-induced toxicity is difficult (Covino, 1986b). Recent studies in cats and hypoxic dogs rendered toxic with bupivacaine indicate that resuscitation is possible if massive doses of adrenaline and atropine are employed. In addition, it has been shown that bretylium but not lignocaine could reverse the cardiodepressant effects of bupivacaine in dogs and also raise the threshold for ventricular tachycardia.

Effect of acidosis and hypoxia

Changes in acid−base status alter the potential cardiovascular toxicity of local anaesthetic agents (Covino, 1986b). Isolated atrial tissue studies have shown that hypercapnia, acidosis and hypoxia tend to potentiate the negative chronotropic and inotropic action of lignocaine and bupivacaine. In particular, the combination of hypoxia and acidosis appears to potentiate markedly the cardiodepressant effects of bupivacaine. Hypoxia and acidosis increased markedly the frequency of cardiac arrhythmias and the mortality rate in sheep following the intravenous administration of bupivacaine. Enhanced toxicity in the presence of acidosis does not appear related to a greater myocardial tissue uptake of local anaesthetic because investigations in rabbits demonstrated a decreased cardiac concentration of bupivacaine in the presence of acidosis. Marked hypercapnia, acidosis and hypoxia occur very rapidly in some patients following seizure activity after the rapid accidental intravascular injection of local anaesthetic agents. Thus, the rapid cardiovascular depression observed in some patients following the accidental intravenous injection of bupivacaine may be related in part to the severe acid–base changes that occur during toxic reactions to these agents.

Miscellaneous systemic effects

A variety of miscellaneous systemic actions has been ascribed to local anaesthetic drugs, most of which are related to the generalized membrane-stabilizing property of this class of drugs. For example, local anaesthetics have been reported to possess neuro-muscular-blocking, ganglionic-blocking and anticholinergic activity. There is little evidence to suggest that any of these miscellaneous effects are clinically significant under normal conditions.

A unique systemic side-effect associated with a specific local anaesthetic agent is the formation of methaemoglobinaemia following the administration of large doses of prilocaine. A dose–response relationship exists between the amount of prilocaine administered extradurally and the degree of methae-moglobinaemia. In general, doses of prilocaine of 600 mg are required for the development of clinically significant levels of methaemoglobinaemia. The formation of methaemoglobinaemia is believed to be related to the chemical structure of prilocaine. This agent lacks a methyl group in the benzene ring. The metabolism of prilocaine in the liver results in the formation of o-toluidine, which is responsible for the oxidation of haemoglobin to methaemoglobin. The methaemoglobinaemia associated with the use of prilocaine is reversible spontaneously or may be treated by the intravenous administration of methylene blue.

Allergic effects

The amino ester agents such as procaine have been shown to produce allergic-type reactions. These agents are derivatives of para-aminobenzoic acid which is known to be allergenic in nature. The amino amide local anaesthetics are not derivatives of para-aminobenzoic acid and allergic reactions to the amino amides are extremely rare. Intradermal injections of both amino ester and amino amide local anaesthetics have been made in patients with and without a presumptive history of local anaesthetic allergy. Positive skin reactions were observed in 25 of 60 patients who did not describe any previous allergic symptomatology. In all cases, the cutaneous reactions occurred following the injection of an amino ester type of agent such as procaine, amethocaine and chloroprocaine. No cutaneous reactions occurred following the use of the amino amide agents, namely lignocaine, mepivacaine or prilocaine. Eleven patients were studied with a history of alleged local anaesthetic allergy. Eight of these patients showed a positive skin reaction to procaine, amethocaine or chloroprocaine. However, no positive cutaneous response was seen following the administration of lignocaine, mepivacaine or prilocaine. No signs of systemic anaphylaxis occurred in any of the subjects. It should be remembered that although the amino amide agents appear to be relatively free from allergic-type reactions, solutions of these agents may contain a preservative, methylparaben, whose chemical structure is similar to that of para-aminobenzoic acid. It has been shown that patients in whom methyl-paraben was administered intradermally demonstrated a positive skin reaction.

Local tissue toxicity

Local anaesthetic agents which are employed clinically rarely produce localized nerve damage. Studies on isolated frog sciatic nerve revealed that concentrations of procaine, cocaine, amethocaine and nupercaine required to produce irreversible conduction block are far in excess of the concentration of these agents used clinically. A comparison of the intrathecal administration of lignocaine, amethocaine or etidocaine in rabbits revealed histopathological spinal cord changes following the use of amethocaine 2%, which is considerably greater than the maximum concentration of 1% employed for spinal anaesthesia in humans. In recent years, prolonged sensory motor deficits have been reported in some patients following usually the extradural or subarachnoid injection of large doses of this particular drug (Ravindran et al., 1980; Reisner et al., 1980). Studies in animals have proven somewhat contradictory regarding the potential neurotoxicity of chloroprocaine (Table 67.5). The aetiology of the local neural irritation associated with the use of chloroprocaine solutions is believed to be related to the low pH and presence of the antioxidant, sodium bisulphite, in these solutions.

Table 67.5 Animal studies concerning potential neurotoxicity of 2-chloroprocaine (2-CP) and other local anaesthetics

Type of study	Results
In vitro rabbit vagus nerve	Local irritation with 2-CP, but not lignocaine and bupivacaine
In vivo rat sciatic nerve	No irritation with 2-CP and lignocaine
In vitro rabbit vagus nerve	Irreversible block with commercial 2-CP and Na bisulphite but not with pure 2-CP
Spinal dog	Paralysis with 2-CP, but not with bupivacaine or low pH saline
Spinal rabbit	Paralysis with commercial 2-CP and Na bisulphite but not with pure 2-CP
Spinal sheep	Minimal toxicity with 2-CP, lignocaine, bupivacaine and control solution
Spinal monkey	Minimal toxicity with 2-CP and bupivacaine

Paralysis was observed in rabbits in which intrathecal chloroprocaine solutions which contained sodium bisulphite were employed (Wang *et al.*, 1984). The use of pure solutions of chloroprocaine without sodium bisulphite did not cause paralysis, whereas the sodium bisulphite alone was associated with paralysis. A detailed study has been conducted on the isolated rabbit vagus nerve to investigate the neurotoxicity of the various components of commercial chloroprocaine solutions (Gissen *et al.*, 1984). Commercial solutions of chloroprocaine 3% contain the local anaesthetic agent itself, sodium bisulphite 0.2% and hydrogen ions, which yield a pH of approximately 3.0. Application of commercial chloroprocaine 3% to isolated vagus nerves for 30 min resulted in irreversible conduction block. The use of a chloroprocaine 3% with sodium bisulphite solution buffered to a pH of 7.0 caused reversible conduction block. A chloroprocaine 3% solution with a pH of 3.0 but without sodium bisulphite resulted also in reversible block. Application of a sodium bisulphite 0.2% solution at a pH of 3.0 resulted in irreversible conduction block, whereas the use of a sodium bisulphite 0.2% solution with a pH of 7.0 caused no conduction block. The results of these studies suggest that the combination of a low pH and the presence of sodium bisulphite may be responsible for the neurotoxic reactions observed following the use of large amounts of chloroprocaine solution. Chloroprocaine, itself, does not appear to be neurotoxic.

Skeletal muscle appears to be more sensitive to the local irritant properties of local anaesthetic agents than other tissues. Skeletal muscle changes have been observed with most of the clinically used local anaesthetic agents such as lignocaine, mepivacaine, prilocaine, bupivacaine and etidocaine. In general, the more potent, longer-acting agents such as bupivacaine and etidocaine appear to cause a greater degree of localized skeletal muscle damage than the less potent, shorter-acting agents such as lignocaine and prilocaine. This effect on skeletal muscle is usually reversible, and muscle regeneration occurs rapidly and is complete within 2 weeks following injection of local anaesthetic agents. It may also cause prolonged ptosis after peribulbar block (Rainin & Carlson, 1985).

Complications of regional anaesthesia

Certain regional anaesthetic techniques such as extradural or spinal anaesthesia are associated with sympathetic block that may result in profound hypotension. In general, the degree of hypotension is related to the extent of the sympathetic block.

Extradural anaesthesia

Cardiovascular alterations following extradural block are related to:
1 The level of block.
2 Drug dosage.
3 Specific local anaesthetic agent.
4 Addition of vasoconstrictors.
5 Blood volume status of the patient.

Level of block

Extradural block to the T5 dermatomal level or below is not accompanied usually by significant cardiovascular alterations (Bonica *et al.*, 1970). As the level of anaesthesia extends from T5 to T1, a 20% fall in systemic arterial pressure has been observed. This hypotensive state is related almost exclusively to sympathetic inhibition and peripheral vasodilatation below the level of block which results in a significant decrease in systemic vascular resistance. At dermatomal levels of T1 and above, a reduction in heart rate and cardiac output may occur. The reduction in cardiac output may be related in part to the inhibition of myocardial sympathetic fibres resulting in a decreased cardiac contractility and also in a decrease in venous return from venodilatation and expansion of capacitance vessels.

Drug dosage

Relatively large amounts of local anaesthetic drug are required to achieve a satisfactory degree of extradural block. These local anaesthetic agents are absorbed rather rapidly and significant blood concentrations may be achieved. The absorbed local anaesthetic agent may produce systemic effects involving the cardiovascular system as discussed above. Blood concentrations of lignocaine of less than 4 µg/ml following extradural block resulted in a slight increase in arterial pressure produced by an increased cardiac output (Bonica et al., 1970). Doses of extradural lignocaine which produced blood concentrations in excess of 4 µg/ml caused hypotension resulting in part from the negative inotropic and the peripheral vasodilator actions of the drug.

Specific local anaesthetic drug

Differences in the onset of extradural anaesthesia occur as a function of the specific agent employed. For example, drugs such as chloroprocaine, lignocaine and etidocaine produce a fairly rapid onset of anaesthesia, whilst bupivacaine has been shown to exert a significantly slower onset of action. The more rapidly acting agents produce a more profound degree of hypotension as a result of the more rapid block of sympathetic fibres. In addition, certain agents such as etidocaine can penetrate myelinated fibres more readily and again may be associated with a more profound degree of sympathetic block and hypotension.

Addition of vasoconstrictor agents

Adrenaline is frequently added to local anaesthetics intended for extradural use in order to decrease the rate of vascular absorption and prolong the duration of anaesthesia. Absorbed adrenaline itself may produce transient cardiovascular alterations. An exaggerated hypotensive effect has been reported following the use of adrenaline-containing local anaesthetics for extradural block (Bonica et al., 1972). The absorbed adrenaline is believed to stimulate β_2-adrenergic receptors in peripheral vascular beds leading to a state of vasodilatation and a reduction in diastolic arterial pressure. The β_1-adrenergic receptor stimulating effect of adrenaline results in an increase in heart rate and cardiac output which counteracts the peripheral vasodilator state to some extent. Although absorbed adrenaline may be responsible for the early cardiovascular changes observed following extradural block, the more prolonged hypotension seen after extradural anaesthesia with adrenaline-containing local anaesthetics is related probably to the achievement of a more profound degree of sympathetic block.

Blood volume status of the patient

Cardiovascular depression is more severe and more dangerous following the production of extradural anaesthesia in hypovolaemic patients (Bonica et al., 1972). Extradural anaesthesia in hypovolaemic volunteers was associated with profound hypotension resulting from peripheral vasodilatation and a decrease in cardiac output and heart rate. The addition of adrenaline to the anaesthetic solution resulted in a less profound degree of hypotension in these subjects but was unable to prevent a significant reduction in systemic arterial pressure. The failure of adrenaline to increase cardiac output sufficiently in these subjects to prevent marked hypotension is obviously a result of the diminished circulating blood volume.

Spinal anaesthesia

In general, systemic hypotension occurs following the induction of spinal anaesthesia by block of sympathetic fibres. The degree of hypotension appears to be related almost exclusively to the extent of sensory and sympathetic block. Studies in humans have shown that subarachnoid anaesthesia to the T5 level caused a decrease in stroke volume, cardiac output and peripheral vascular resistance (Ward et al., 1965). The decrease in cardiac output and stroke volume following spinal anaesthesia which extends to the mid-thoracic level, is not believed to be related to a decrease in myocardial contractility but rather to a decrease in venous return. Placement of patients in a slightly head-down position or the infusion of crystalloid solutions are usually sufficient to reverse the hypotensive state. Studies have been carried out in monkeys in which the level of sensory anaesthesia following the intrathecal administration of amethocaine has been correlated with the degree of hypotension (Sivarajan et al., 1975). Anaesthesia to the T10 dermatomal level resulted in a reduction in arterial pressure of approximately 15%. This hypotension was a result almost exclusively of a decrease in peripheral vascular resistance with little change in cardiac output. However, extension of the level of sympathetic and sensory block to the T1 dermatomal level was associated with a 35% decrease in arterial pressure. This exaggerated state of hypotension was caused in part by a decrease in peripheral vascular resistance but also by a significant reduction in cardiac output.

Conclusion

Local anaesthetics may be classified into three groups according to their potency and duration of action. Procaine and chloroprocaine are relatively weak agents of short duration. Lignocaine, mepivacaine and prilocaine are intermediate in terms of potency and duration. Amethocaine, bupivacaine and etidocaine are potent local anaesthetics with a prolonged duration of action. With regard to onset time, chloroprocaine, lignocaine, mepivacaine, prilocaine and etidocaine have a relatively rapid onset of action. Bupivacaine is intermediate whilst procaine and amethocaine demonstrate a long latency period. Anaesthetic activity is determined primarily by physicochemical factors such as pKa, lipid solubility and protein binding. *In vivo* the anaesthetic properties of the various agents can be modified by the dosage administered, addition of vasoconstrictors, site of injection, carbonation and pH adjustment of solutions, use of additives or mixture of agents and the physiological status of the patient such as pregnancy.

The toxicity of local anaesthetics involves primarily the CNS and cardiovascular system. CNS toxicity involves primarily excitation and convulsions. Large doses of local anaesthetics may lead to generalized CNS depression. The rapid intravenous administration or injection of large doses of local anaesthetics can cause hypotension, bradycardia and ultimately cardiac arrest. Certain agents such as bupivacaine may also produce ventricular arrhythmias. In general, the potential for CNS and cardiovascular toxicity is related to the anaesthetic potency of the various agents. Allergic reactions to local anaesthetic agents are limited primarily to the amino ester drugs by the metabolic formation of para-aminobenzoic acid. Methaemoglobinaemia may occur following the administration of large doses of prilocaine.

Complications of regional anaesthesia are most frequent with extradural and spinal anaesthesia. Hypotension is the most common complication produced by sympathetic block associated with these regional anaesthetic procedures.

In general, local anaesthetic agents are very effective and relatively safe drugs when used correctly. However, as with any class of drugs, safe and effective regional anaesthesia requires a knowledge of the pharmacology and toxicity of the various agents, ability to perform regional anaesthesia correctly and a careful evaluation of the clinical status of the patient.

References

Bernards C.M. & Artru A.A. (1991) Hexamethonium and midazolam terminate dysrhythmias and hypertension caused by intracerebroventricular bupivacaine in rabbits. *Anesthesiology* **74**, 89—96.

Block A. & Covino B.G. (1982) Effect of local anesthetic agents on cardiac conduction and contractility. *Regional Anesthesia* **6**, 55—61.

Bonica J.J., Berges P.V. & Morikawa K. (1970) Circulatory effects of peridural block. I. Effects of level of analgesia and dose of lidocaine. *Anesthesiology* **33**, 619—26.

Bonica J.J., Kennedy W.F., Akamatsu T.J. & Gerbershagen H.V. (1972) Circulatory effects of peridural block. III. Effects of acute blood loss. *Anesthesiology* **36**, 219—27.

Bridenbaugh L.D. (1978) Does the addition of low molecular weight dextran prolong the duration of action of bupivacaine? *Regional Anesthesia* **3**, 6.

Bromage P.R. (1965) A comparison of the hydrochloride and carbon dioxide salts of lidocaine and prilocaine in epidural analgesia. *Acta Anaesthesiologica Scandinavica* **16** (Suppl.), 55—69.

Bromage P.R. (1970) An evaluation of two new local anaesthetics for major conduction blockade. *Canadian Anaesthetists' Society Journal* **17**, 557—64.

Brown D.T., Wildsmith J.A.W., Covino B.G. & Scott D.B. (1980a) Effect of baricity on spinal anaesthesia with amethocaine. *British Journal of Anaesthesia* **52**, 589—96.

Brown D.T., Morrison D.H., Covino B.G. & Scott D.B. (1980b) Comparison of carbonated bupivacaine and bupivacaine hydrochloride for extradural anaesthesia. *British Journal of Anaesthesia* **52**, 419—27.

Brown D.T., Beamish D., Wildsmith J.A.W. (1981) Allergic reaction to an amide local anaesthetic. *British Journal of Anaesthesia* **53**, 435—7.

Clarkson C.W. & Hohdeghem L.M. (1985) Mechanism for bupivacaine depression of cardiac conduction: fast block of sodium channels during the action potential with slow recovery from block during diastole. *Anesthesiology* **62**, 396—405.

Concepcion M., Maddi R., Francis D., Rocco A.G., Murray E. & Covino B.G. (1984) Vasoconstrictors in spinal anesthesia with tetracaine. A comparison of epinephrine and phenylephrine. *Anesthesia and Analgesia* **63**, 134—8.

Corke B.G., Carlson C.G. & Dettbarn W.D. (1984) The influence of 2-chloroprocaine on the subsequent analgesic potency of bupivacaine. *Anesthesiology* **60**, 25—7.

Covino B.G. (1986a) Pharmacology of local anaesthetic agents. *British Journal of Anaesthesia* **58**, 701—16.

Covino B.G. (1986b) Toxicity of local anesthetics. *Advances in Anaesthesia* **3**, 37—65.

Datta S., Lambert D.H., Gregus J., Gissen A.J. & Covino B.G.

(1983) Differential sensitivities of mammalian nerve fibers during pregnancy. *Anesthesia and Analgesia* **62**, 1070–2.

DeJong R.H. (1977) *Physiology and Pharmacology of Local Anesthesia* 2nd edn. Charles C. Thomas, Springfield, Illinois.

Duggan J., Bowler G.M.R., McClure J.H. & Wildsmith J.A.W. (1988) Extradural block with bupivacaine: influence of dose, volume, concentration and patient characteristics. *British Journal of Anaesthesia* **61**, 324–31.

Englesson S. (1974) The influence of acid–base changes on central nervous system toxicity of local anesthetic agents. I. An experimental study in cats. *Acta Anaesthesiologica Scandinavica* **18**, 79–87.

Fagraeus L., Urban B.J. & Bromage P.R. (1983) Spread of analgesia in early pregnancy. *Anesthesiology* **58**, 184–7.

Gissen A.J. & Covino B.G. (1985) Differential sensitivity of fast and slow fibres in mammalian nerve. IV. Effect of carbonation of local anesthetics. *Regional Anesthesia* **10**, 68–75.

Gissen A.J., Covino B.G. & Gregus J. (1980) Differential sensitivity of mammalian nerves to local anesthetic drugs. *Anesthesiology* **53**, 467–74.

Gissen A.J., Covino B.G. & Gregus J. (1982) Differential sensitivity of fast and slow fibres in mammalian nerve. III. Effect of etidocaine and bupivacaine on fast/slow fibres. *Anesthesia and Analgesia* **61**, 570–5.

Gissen A.J., Datta S. & Lambert D. (1984) The chloroprocaine controversy II. Is chloroprocaine neurotoxic? *Regional Anesthesia* **9**, 135–45.

Hilgier M. (1985) Alkalinization of bupivacaine for bronchial plexus block. *Regional Anesthesia* **10**, 59–61.

Johns R.A., Di Fazio C.A. & Longnecker D.E. (1985) Lidocaine constricts or dilates rat arterioles in a dose-dependent manner. *Anesthesiology* **62**, 141–4.

Johns R.A., Seyde W.C., Di Fazio C.A. & Longnecker D.E. (1986) Dose-dependent effects of bupivacaine on rat muscle arterioles. *Anesthesiology* **65**, 186–91.

Liu P.L., Feldman H.S., Giasi R., Patterson M.K. & Covino B.G. (1983) Comparative CNS toxicity of lidocaine, etidocaine, bupivacaine and tetracaine in awake dogs following rapid IV administration. *Anesthesia and Analgesia* **62**, 375–9.

Loder R.E. (1960) A local anaesthesia solution with longer action. *Lancet* **ii**, 346–7.

McClure J.H. & Scott D.B. (1981) Comparison of bupivacaine hydrochloride and carbonated bupivacaine in brachial plexus block by the inter-scalene technique. *British Journal of Anaesthesia* **53**, 523–6.

Morishima H.O., Pedersen H., Finster M., Hiraoka H., Tsuji A., Feldman H., Arthur G.A. & Covino B.G. (1985) Bupivacaine toxicity in pregnant and nonpregnant ewes. *Anesthesiology* **63**, 134–9.

Morrison D.H. (1981) A double-blind comparison of carbonated lidocaine and lidocaine hydrochloride in epidural anaesthesia. *Canadian Anaesthetists' Society Journal* **28**, 387–9.

Rainin E.A. & Carlson B.M. (1985) Postoperative diplopia and ptosis: a clinical hypothesis based on the myotoxicity of local anesthetics. *Archives of Ophthalmology* **103**, 1337–9.

Ravindran R.S., Bond V.K., Tasch M.D., Gupta C.D. & Luerssen T.G. (1980) Prolonged neural blockade following regional analgesia with 2-chloroprocaine. *Anesthesia and Analgesia* **58**, 447–51.

Reisner L.S., Hochman B.N. & Plumer M.H. (1980) Persistent neurologic deficit and adhesive arachnoiditis following intrathecal 2-chloroprocaine injection. *Anesthesia and Analgesia* **58**, 452–4.

Reiz S. & Nath S. (1986) Cardiotoxicity of local anaesthetic agents. *British Journal of Anaesthesia* **38**, 736–46.

Rosenberg P.H., Heinowen E., Jansson S.E. & Gripenberg J. (1980) Differential nerve block by bupivacaine and 2-chloroprocaine. *British Journal of Anaesthesia* **52**, 1183–9.

Scott D.B. (1981) Toxicity caused by local anaesthetic drugs. *British Journal of Anaesthesia* **53**, 553–4.

Scott D.B., McClure J.H., Giasi R.M., Seo J. & Covino B.G. (1980) Effects of concentration of local anaesthetic drugs in extradural block. *British Journal of Anaesthesia* **52**, 1033–7.

Sivarajan M., Amery D.W., Lindbloom L.E. & Schwettmann R.S. (1975) Systemic and regional blood flow changes during spinal anesthesia in the Rhesus monkey. *Anesthesiology* **43**, 78–88.

Stewart D.M., Rogers W.P., Mahaffrey J.E., Witherspoon S. & Woods E.F. (1963) Effect of local anesthetics on the cardiovascular system in the dog. *Anesthesiology* **24**, 620–4.

Vanhoutte F., Vereecke J., Verbeke N. & Carmeliet E. (1991) Stereoselective effects of the enantiomers of bupivacaine on the electrophysiological properties of the guinea-pig papillary muscle. *British Journal of Pharmacology* **103**, 1275–81.

Wang B.C., Hillman D.E., Spiedholz N.I. & Turndorf H. (1984) Chronic neurologic deficits and nesacaine-CE — an effect of the anesthetic, 2-chloroprocaine, or the antioxidant, sodium bisulfite? *Anesthesia and Analgesia* **63**, 445–7.

Ward R.J., Bonica J.J., Freund F.G., Akamatsu T., Danziger F. & Englesson S. (1965) Epidural and subarachnoid anesthesia: cardiovascular and respiratory effects. *Journal of the American Medical Association* **191**, 275–8.

Wildsmith J.A.W., Gissen A.J., Gregus J. & Covino B.G. (1985) Differential nerve blocking activity of amino–ester local anaesthetics. *British Journal of Anaesthesia* **57**, 612–19.

Wildsmith J.A.W., Gissen A.J., Takmon B. & Covino B.G. (1987) Differential nerve blockade: esters v amides and the influence of pKa. *British Journal of Anaesthesia* **59**, 379–89.

68

Subarachnoid and Extradural Anaesthesia

J. GREIFF AND M.J. COUSINS

Subarachnoid (intradural, spinal, intrathecal) and extradural (epidural, peridural) anaesthesia are used most commonly to produce anaesthesia for operations on the abdomen, chest and lower extremities. These blocks are also used for pain relief during labour, postoperatively and less frequently, for assessment and treatment of chronic pain states.

Spinal subarachnoid anaesthesia is produced by injection of a local anaesthetic solution into the cerebrospinal fluid (CSF), causing temporary axonal block. The injection is usually performed below the termination of the spinal cord (approximately L2 in adults) to avoid damage. A small volume of local anaesthetic blocks *all* sensation rapidly.

Between the spinal dura and the spinal periosteum lies the extradural space. Extradural anaesthesia is produced by injecting a relatively large volume of local anaesthetic into this space creating neuronal block. Not all sensory modalities may be blocked even with complete block of nocioception (i.e. analgesia not anaesthesia).

Both subarachnoid and extradural administration of opioids may produce selective analgesia (Cousins *et al.*, 1979). Their analgesic effects are mediated predominantly by an action on pre- and postsynaptic receptors on the dorsal-horn neurone. Clonidine and other α_2-agonists have been injected by both spinal routes. Clonidine appears to prolong analgesia when given in combination with either opioids or local anaesthetics (Bonnet *et al.*, 1990; Rostaing *et al.*, 1991).

The important advances in the development of spinal subarachnoid and extradural anaesthesia are summarized in Table 68.1. Subarachnoid anaesthesia for surgery was first described by August Bier of Keil in 1898 using cocaine. The importance of the curves of the vertebral column was realized by Barker (1908) and with the manufacture of hyperbaric and hypobaric solutions of local anaesthetics, spinal anaesthesia became controllable. The popularity of spinal

anaesthesia further increased after the introduction of local anaesthetics with less toxicity and longer durations of action. Greater duration of effect was obtained by the addition of adrenaline to the local anaesthetic solution or by using a continuous spinal technique. By 1940 the three main local anaesthetics in use for subarachnoid anaesthesia were amethocaine (tetracaine), procaine and cinchocaine (dibucaine). The limitations of subarachnoid anaesthesia were soon appreciated. For higher laparotomies the block was often inadequate, causing pain, nausea, hypotension and ventilatory difficulties. Ephedrine or other vasopressors were routinely given because hypotension was feared.

Extradural caudal anaesthesia was described separately by Sicard and Cathelin, both of Paris, in 1901. Lumbar extradural anaesthesia for surgery was first described by Pagès of Madrid in 1921. It was not until the 1960s, however, that a systematic study began, mainly as a result of the work of Bromage (1978). Tuohy's subarachnoid needle was adapted for a continuous extradural technique using a ureteric catheter. In the 1950s, lumbar extradural anaesthesia was used first for obstetric pain relief and became more widely used during surgery and for postoperative pain relief. The use of caudal extradural anaesthesia waned at this time, as it was recognized that the technique required larger doses of local anaesthetic and at least in adults, was less predictable.

In Europe after World War II, the use of subarachnoid anaesthesia declined substantially for two main reasons.

First, 'modern' general anaesthesia was introduced, whereby tracheal intubation could be performed with the aid of the *new* neuromuscular-blocking drugs by trained anaesthetists with an understanding of the physiology of disease.

Second, the adverse publicity surrounding reports of neurological damage associated with subarachnoid

Table 68.1 Important dates in the development of subarachnoid and extradural anaesthesia

1764	Cerebrospinal fluid discovered by Catugno
1853	Invention of hypodermic syringe and needle by Alexander Wood
1860	Cocaine isolated from *Erythroxylen coca*
1884	Cocaine used for topical anaesthesia of the eye by Koller
1885	First spinal anaesthetic by Corning
1886	Heat sterilization described
1891	Lumbar puncture standardized by Quinke as a simple clinical procedure
1898	First planned spinal anesthetic for surgery by August Bier on 16 August
1901	Sicard and Cathelin both independently introduced caudal anaesthesia
1903	Adrenaline used to increase duration and reduce toxicity of spinal anaesthesia
1905	Procaine introduced
1907	Hyperbaric solution of local anaesthetic introduced
1914	Hypobaric solution of local anaesthetic introduced
1921	Lumbar extradural anaesthesia for surgery described by Pagès
1927	Ephedrine used to maintain arterial pressure during spinal anaesthesia
1931	Extradural anaesthesia reintroduced by Dogliotti
1947	First clinical use of lignocaine by Gordh
1949	'Continuous' lumbar extradural analgesia introduced by Cleland
1953	The Woolley and Roe case in the UK
1954	Safety of spinal anaesthesia confirmed by Vadam and Dripps
1979	Description of the combined single-shot subarachnoid and extradural catheter technique by Curelaru

anaesthesia; most notably in England, the Woolley and Roe case (Cope, 1954; Hutter, 1990).

In the last 25 years, spinal anaesthesia has again become popular, rescued by the work of Dripps and Vandam (1954) which demonstrated how safe the technique can be. Subarachnoid and extradural anaesthesia are now established as a substitute for, and an adjunct to, general anaesthesia, being suitable for most gynaecological, as well as some abdominal and orthopaedic surgery. The popularity of the extra-dural technique is partly due to both the ease of catheter insertion and subsequent maintenance of block. More recently, it has been demonstrated that the Whitacre and Sprotte spinal needles have a much lower incidence of postdural puncture headache (PDPH) than Quincke–Babcock spinal needles. Consequently the use of subarachnoid anaesthesia in obstetric anaesthetic practice has increased. Furthermore, the realization that general anaesthesia also has risks and hazards has promoted the techniques of both subarachnoid and extradural anaesthesia.

Equipment

The basic requirements for regional block should be available, including a mobile trolley with shelf space underneath for storage of drugs, sterile packs, needles, syringes and other equipment.

Needles

The needle must have a close-fitting removable stylet. This stiffens the needle and prevents coring of the skin, which in rare cases may lead to an epidermoid spinal cord tumour from the introduction of dermis into the subarachnoid space.

With subarachnoid anaesthesia, for any given needle type the smaller the bore the less likely the patient is to develop PDPH (Geurts *et al.*, 1990). Rounded needles, with a non-cutting bevel, also reduce the incidence of this distressing complication (Shutt *et al.*, 1992).

Spinal needles are usually 9 cm long, and should ideally have a transparent hub so that the flow of CSF can be rapidly identified. The needle should produce minimal trauma and make the smallest possible hole in the dura, for the reasons above. A needle and the various tips described below are shown in Fig. 68.1A.

The Quincke–Babcock spinal needle (so called 'standard' spinal needle) has a sharp point, with a medium-length cutting bevel. Care should be taken when using these needles to ensure that they are inserted so that the bevel is parallel to the longitudinal dural fibres.

The Whitacre spinal needle or the pencil point needle has a completely rounded, non-cutting bevel with a solid tip, the opening being 2 mm proximal to the tip on the side. Various manufacturers have modified the design, such that the steepness of the slope and the opening size/position may vary. The consequence of this is a wide variation in the incidence of PDPH reported in the literature by different authors.

The Sprotte needle is also an adaptation of the Whitacre design, but is different in several ways. First, it has a blunt (non-cutting or bursting) ogival tip; its elongated lateral needle opening gently slopes and is wider than the inner diameter of the needle thus allowing free flow of CSF. In a 24-gauge Sprotte needle, the opening is 1.2 mm from the tip and 1.7 mm long. The needle tip pushes the dural fibres aside, resulting in better dural closure after removal of the needle.

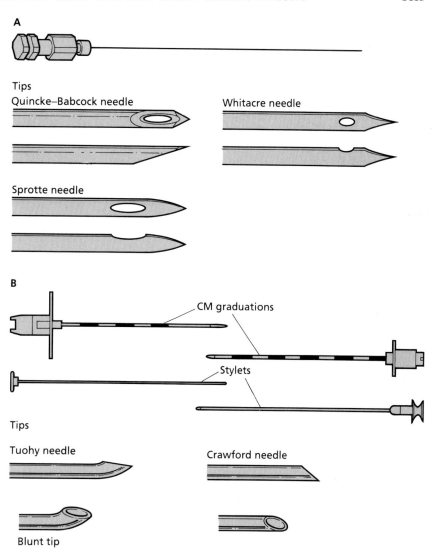

Fig. 68.1 Spinal needle (A) and extradural needles (winged and unwinged) (B) used for subarachnoid and extradural anaesthesia.

Other spinal needles are available but are not discussed here.

The Tuohy needle. For extradural anaesthesia the needle used most frequently in the UK is the *Tuohy needle* (Fig. 68.1B). The Tuohy needle was originally designed for continuous spinal anaesthesia. However because of its *Huber point*, which facilitates the insertion of the extradural catheter. It was also the first needle used for continuous extradural anaesthesia. Its shaft is usually 8 cm long, graduated in centimetres, and available in both 16 gauge and 18 gauge sizes, with and without a 'winged' hub. The needle wall is thin so that it will admit a catheter of reasonable size. The Huber tip is relatively blunt and its shape ensures that the catheter emerges at an angle of 20°, which has the important disadvantage that after insertion the catheter cannot be withdrawn through the needle without the risk of transection.

The Crawford extradural needle (Fig. 68.1B) is a short bevelled (40°) needle, with smooth edges. As the catheter emerges straight from the tip, it impinges on the dura unless the needle is introduced at an angle. The Crawford needle is therefore best suited for the paramedian approach, which permits greater angulation than that obtained from the midline.

Special needles for a *combined subarachnoid/extradural technique* are becoming available from several manufacturers, some of which have a 'back eye' that permits the passage of a spinal needle, and others have a separate channel for each procedure Fig. 68.2A. The combined technique can be accomplished with a standard Tuohy needle, using a long subarachnoid

A
Tuohy with 'back eye' (Sprotte)

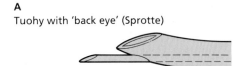

Separate channelled device [Eldor (CSEN)]

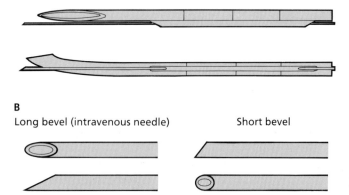

B
Long bevel (intravenous needle)   Short bevel

Fig. 68.2 (A) Combined subarachnoid and continuous extradural systems. (B) Comparison of long- and short-bevel needle points.

needle, such as a 12-cm Sprotte needle, through the Tuohy needle to perform subarachnoid anaesthesia before passing the extradural catheter.

Single-dose caudal blocks can be adequately performed using disposable 22- or 25-gauge short bevelled 4-cm needles (Fig. 68.2B).

Catheters

These are manufactured in two sizes to fit either the 16-gauge or the 18-gauge needle. The 90-cm radiopaque extradural catheter is designed to have the largest internal lumen possible, to reduce resistance to injection, whilst at the same time not having a wall so thin that it kinks or buckles where it enters the extradural space. Modern extradural catheters have two or more side holes within 2 cm from the end, and a closed, rounded tip making puncture of the dura and extradural blood vessels less likely (Fig. 68.3B). Catheters are usually marked from the tip, often at 1-cm intervals, although some makes are only marked at 5-cm intervals (Fig. 68.3A). This enables the anaesthetist to know how much catheter has been inserted, and whether it is intact on removal. At the distal end is a detachable Luer hub, which allows removal of the extradural needle. The Luer hub is attached to a filter, several makes of which are capable of excluding particles down to 22 μm. These filters have not con-

clusively been shown to reduce the incidence of extradural infection. However, particulate matter such as glass from 'snap-neck' ampules is prevented from reaching the extradural space (Katz, 1973).

Contraindications to spinal block

With any procedure the benefits should outweigh the risks; due consideration should therefore be given to the magnitude and frequency of any potential complications as they apply to each particular patient. A list of possible contraindications is summarized in Table 68.2. Clearly abnormality of the clotting mechanism whether by disease or secondary to drugs increases the risk of haematoma formation and subsequent cord compression. However, the place of these techniques in patients taking aspirin or low-dose heparin remains controversial. Needles should not be placed through infected or neoplastic tissue, because spread to the extradural space may result in cord compression.

The technique and anatomy of spinal subarachnoid and extradural injection using the traditional midline approach

As with all regional techniques, the patient should be placed on a tipping trolley or table, venous access

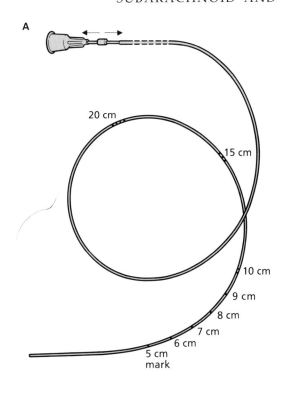

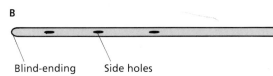

Fig. 68.3 Typical extradural catheter (A) and tip (B).

Table 68.2 Contraindications of subarachnoid and extradural anaesthesia

Relative
Severe headache or backache
Poor-risk patient (possibly)
Neurological diseases or simulators (residual paralysis,
    poliomyelitis)
History of viral disease
Medicolegal considerations
Diseases of the spinal column (arthritis, metastasis,
    osteoporosis)
Blood in CSF (in subarachnoid block) that fails to clear after
    5–10 ml aspirate
Inability to achieve placement of needle after three attempts

Absolute
Patient refusal
Localized infection around puncture site
Generalized infections (septicaemia, bacteremia)
Abnormal clotting
Severe blood loss or shock
Active central nervous system disease, raised intracranial
    pressure
Certain cardiovascular diseases
Miscellaneous conditions or disease states
    Vasomotor instability
    Various simulators of neurologic sequelae
Local anaesthetic drug sensitivity
These techniques should not be performed unsupervised by
    the unskilled

must be obtained with a large-gauge cannula, arterial pressure must be measured, heart rate recorded and continuous ECG monitoring commenced. Resuscitation equipment must be checked and available.

1 The patient is positioned and the midline of the spine and the appropriate interspace is found by inspection and palpation.

In an ideal position, the back of the patient is at and parallel to the edge of the operating table. The knees are flexed and drawn up as much as possible to the abdomen and the head is brought down towards the knees. Special care is required to avoid rotation of the hips and shoulders. The midline cannot be located reliably under the median crease for it may sag downwards (by many millimetres in the obese). The method of Labat, i.e. grasping the spinous process between thumb and forefinger, is recommended (Fig. 68.4).

The easiest and safest extradural and spinal injections are made in the mid-lumbar region. Knowledge

of the surface anatomy and landmarks is therefore crucial. The line drawn between the highest point of the two iliac crests usually passes through the spinous process of the fourth lumbar vertebra (Fig. 68.5). The interspinous space above this spinous process (L3–4) or one higher (L2–3) is the standard site of needle insertion for extradural block in adults, as the spinal cord usually ends at the lower border of vertebra L1. This is not the case in children and is one reason why the caudal route of entry is preferred to the lumbar route in young children. Also, the dural sac terminates at the level of S2 in adults (S3 in small children): a line through the posterior superior iliac spines crosses this level. Attempts at puncture below L4 increases the difficulty of 'midline' extradural block because of the ill-defined interspinous ligament; also, puncture above L2 increases the risk of damage to the conus medullaris, so that the interspace of L2–3 and L3–4 are both the safest and the easiest. Identification of L1 acts as a double check and confirms that the point of entry is safely below the conus medullaris. There is no difference in the potential danger of damaging the cord if one chooses

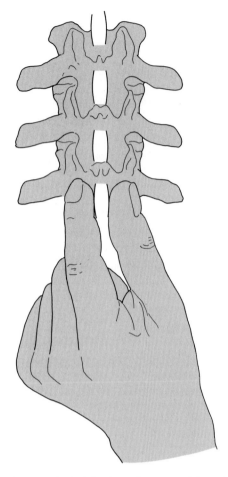

Fig. 68.4 Labat's method of checking the centre of the spinous processes uses the thumb and forefinger to grasp the spinous processes above and below the site of the needle puncture. (Redrawn from Cousins & Bridenbaugh, 1988.)

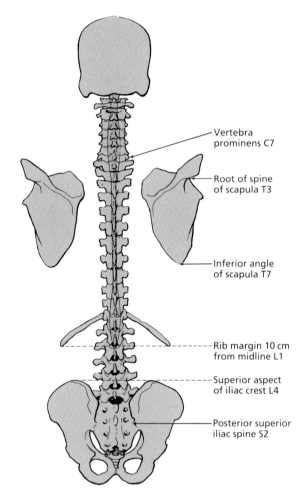

Vertebra prominens C7

Root of spine of scapula T3

Inferior angle of scapula T7

Rib margin 10 cm from midline L1

Superior aspect of iliac crest L4

Posterior superior iliac spine S2

Fig. 68.5 Surface anatomy and landmarks for extradural blockade. The spinous process (vertebra prominens) at C7 is the most prominent spinous process when the neck is flexed. The spinous process at T3 lies opposite the roof of the spine of the scapula (arm by side). The spinous process at T7 lies opposite the inferior angle of the scapula (arm by side). For puncture between C7 and T1 there is direct access to the interlaminal space, but there are other hazards (see text). Puncture below T3 and above T7 is difficult because of angled spinous processes. Puncture below T7 becomes progressively similar to L2–3. Other hazards are the same as those for high puncture (see text). The spinous process at L1 (lower border) is noted by a line meeting the costal margin 10 cm from the midline. The spinous process of L4 (centre) lies at the top of the iliac crests. S2 is noted by the posterior superior iliac spines. Puncture is safest and easiest in the lumbar region. L2–3 and L3–4 are the preferred levels. (Redrawn from Cousins & Bridenbaugh, 1988.)

the T12–L1 interspace or the C7–T1 interspace, both of which can often be technically easy; however, the spinal cord lies directly beneath the extradural space in both instances (Fig. 68.5). Thus, only anaesthetists experienced with extradural techniques require the anatomical landmarks above L1: the inferior angle of the scapula (T7), the root of the spine of the scapula (T3) and the vertebra prominens (C7). Because of the extreme angulation of the spinous processes in the mid-thoracic region, midline puncture is difficult, and the paraspinous (paramedian) approach is preferable. In contrast, there is excellent access to the interlaminar space in the midline at C7–T1 and T1–2; the same applies at the low thoracic region. However, anatomical differences, such as a narrower extradural space, require greater technical skill at these levels and a technique somewhat different from that used usually for lumbar extradural block.

2 The anaesthetist scrubs and dons sterile gloves and gown. The patient should always be accompanied by a nurse or operating department assistant (ODA). A large area of the back around the chosen site is painted with antiseptic and the area draped with sterile towels. The extradural tray may be arranged whilst waiting for the antiseptic to become effective.

In the conscious patient a small weal of anaesthetic solution is raised using a 25- or 27-gauge intradermal needle over the chosen interspace. The subcutaneous tissues are also infiltrated. A small incision in the skin is made using a scalpel blade or large needle. This prevents tough skin from gripping the needle and damping sensation, and also prevents a core of skin from being pushed into the deeper tissues.

3 The needle is pushed slowly forwards at right angles to the back in both planes. A thin flexible spinal needle (25 gauge or smaller) may require an introducer. The first resistance to advancing the needle is the supraspinous ligament (Fig. 68.6).

4 The supraspinous ligament is a strong fibrous cord that connects the apices of the spinous processes from the sacrum to C7, where it is continued upward to the external occipital protuberance as the ligamentum nuchae. It is thickest and broadest in the lumbar region and varies with patient age, sex and body build. In persons who engage in heavy physical activity and elderly patients, the ligament may become ossified, making midline puncture impossible.

The spinous processes are widest in the mid-lumbar region and have only a slight angulation, making insertion of the 16–18 gauge Tuohy needle into the centre of the supraspinous ligament relatively easy compared with elsewhere in the spine. The inferior border of the spinous process lies over the widest part of the interlaminar space (Fig. 68.7). The process becomes somewhat narrower superiorly, so that a needle may be guided by the lateral aspect of the spinous process to enter the mid-point of the ligamentum flavum (Fig. 68.7). In the mid-thoracic region, the spinous processes are much narrower, closer together and angulated sharply downward,

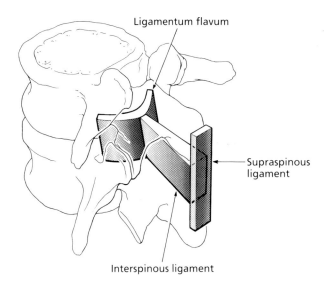

Fig. 68.6 Ligaments encountered during a midline puncture. (Redrawn from Cousins & Bridenbaugh, 1988.)

thus obscuring the interlaminar space (Fig. 68.8). The inferior border of the spinous processes in this region lies opposite the lamina of the vertebral body below. Insertion of an extradural needle may necessitate a paraspinous (paramedian) approach. If the needle is inserted beside the lower border of the spinous process *above* the interspace and angled upward at 130°, the lateral aspect of the process may again be used to guide the needle inward 25° towards the centre of the ligamentum flavum. In the cervical region, the spinous processes widen and become bifid with a wide supraspinous ligament. They are almost horizontal in the lower cervical region and permit easy access to the interlaminar space. The laminae and articular processes form the boundaries of the interlaminar foramen: in the lumbar region,

Fig. 68.7 Lumbar extradural.
(A) Midline. Note insertion closer to the superior spinous process and with a slight upward angulation.
(B) Paraspinous (paramedian). Note insertion beside caudad edge of 'inferior' spinous process, with 45° angulation to long axis of spine below. (Redrawn from Cousins & Bridenbaugh, 1988.)

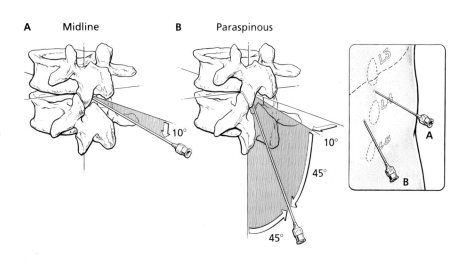

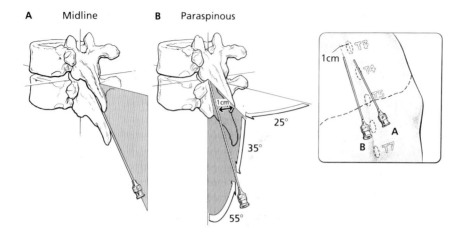

Fig. 68.8 Thoracic extradural. (A) Midline. Note extreme upward angulation required in mid-thoracic region. Therefore, a paraspinous approach may be easier. (B) Paraspinous. Note needle insertion next to caudad tip of the spinous process above interspace of intended level of entry through ligamentum flavum. Upward angulation is 55° to long axis of spine below and inward angulation is 10° to 15°. (Redrawn from Cousins & Bridenbaugh, 1988.)

the foramen is triangular when the lumbar spine is extended, with the base being formed by the upper borders of the laminae of the lower vertebra and the slides, by the median aspects of the inferior articular processes of the vertebra above. However, if the lumbar spine is flexed, the inferior articular processes glide upwards by means of the synovial joints between facets of articular processes, thus enlarging the interlaminar foramen to a diamond shape, and borders of the superior articular process of the vertebra below now form the lower part of the lateral boundaries of the foramen (Fig. 68.5). It is worth noting that, in the lumbar region, the facets of the articular processes articulate at right angles to a circle with its centre in the middle of the vertebral body, so that rotation cannot take place. By contrast, in the thoracic region, the facets articulate in the same plane as such a horizontal circle, so that rotation of one vertebra on another occurs readily. This indicates further, the potentially increased difficulty of puncture in the thoracic compared with the lumbar region.

The lamina itself slopes down and back on its posterior surface, so that it may be contacted by a needle either superficially or deep. The lamina forms only the wide base of the interlaminar space; the remaining boundaries are formed laterally and superiorly by the articular processes (Fig. 68.5).

In the lumbar region, correct needle insertion takes full advantage of the fact that it is both easier and safer to insert the needle at the L2–3 or L3–4 interspace, with the needle entering the extradural space in the midline. The inferior aspects of the spinous processes, in the mid-lumbar region, lie opposite the line across the widest lateral extent of the interlaminar space. Thus, needle insertion should be close to the superior spinous process, as the upper border of the inferior spine lies over the lamina of its underlying vertebral body. A needle inserted with due regard to

this requires very slight upward angulation to give an unobstructed approach to the interlaminar space (Fig. 68.7); this is in comparison with the angulation required to reach the extradural space in the thoracic region (Fig. 68.8). An often neglected surface anatomical aid involves checking that the needle is inserted in the centre of a line running through the middle of the superior and inferior aspects of the spinous processes adjacent to the site of puncture between thumb and forefinger, while the needle is inserted through skin and subcutaneous tissue into the supraspinous ligament (Fig. 68.4). If this is done, the needle should sit firmly in the supraspinous ligament without angulation to either side. Obese subjects may require additional manoeuvres. After penetration, the supraspinous ligament supports the needle at right angles to the skin.

5 The needle is advanced further with the interspinous ligament offering continued resistance. The interspinous ligament runs obliquely between the spinous processes and is continuous anteriorly with the ligamentum flavum and posteriorly with the supraspinous ligament (Fig. 68.6). Its thickness is greatest above L4 in the lumbar region. Although it is a thin ligament, its fibres are attached along the entire superior and inferior surfaces of the spinous processes; thus, in the lumbar region, the ligament is rectangular and provides identifiable resistance to injected air or solution.

6 An increase in resistance is felt when the needle enters the ligamentum flavum, which is composed almost entirely of elastic fibres. Because of its tough elasticity and its thickness of several millimetres in the lumbar region, the ligament imparts a characteristic springy resistance, particularly to a large-gauge needle with a Huber tip (Tuohy needle). The ligament runs from the anterior and inferior aspects of the lamina above to the posterior and superior aspects of

the lamina below. Laterally, the ligament narrows as it blends with the capsule of the joint between the articular processes (Fig. 68.6). Because developmentally, two laminae fuse at each level to form the roots of the spinous process, two ligamenta flava meet in the median plane and here become continuous with the deep fibres of the interspinous ligament. Thus, an extradural needle advancing in the midline encounters continuing resistance that increases immediately as the needle passes into the ligamentum flavum. There is evidence from cadaver dissections that the ligamentum flavum may retain a midline cleft or sulcus in some cases.

7 After a few more millimetres advancement, sudden loss of resistance occurs as the needle tip enters the extradural space. The distance to the extradural space from the skin varies widely. It is most commonly 4 cm (50%) and is 4–6 cm in 80% of the population according to detailed records of 3200 cases. In obese patients, however, this distance may be greater than 8 cm, whilst it is less than 3 cm in some thin patients.

The ligamentum flavum should be entered in the centre of the interlaminar gap, regardless of where the needle enters the skin (midline or paraspinous). Even with midline puncture, failure to control penetration of the ligament results in a second loss of resistance, indicating dural puncture. Entry at the lateral aspect of the interlaminar gap may result also in dural puncture, because the extradural space is narrow at this point; there is also an increased risk of puncturing an extradural vein with return of blood from the extradural needle.

The extradural space should permit easy injection of solution and easy threading of an extradural catheter. Uncontrolled entry or failure to fix the needle securely during subsequent injections or catheter insertions may result in pushing the needle tip forward until it touches the dura. This results in some resistance to injected local anaesthetic and may cause the extradural catheter to puncture the dura if undue force is used when catheter insertion becomes difficult. Many textbooks fail to explain why catheter insertion is impossible, and why further progress of the needle may sometimes be obstructed immediately after an otherwise impeccably correct loss of resistance through the ligamentum flavum. The explanation lies in the anatomy of the lamina and ligamentum flavum; the latter attaches to posterosuperior aspects of the lamina below. Thus, a needle piercing the ligamentum flavum at its extreme inferior aspect may be held up by the upper edge of the sloping lamina. Usually, reinsertion of the needle more towards the centre of the interlaminar space is then necessary.

Less commonly, a needle angled sharply upwards may undergo a clear-cut loss of resistance as its tip penetrates the ligamentum flavum, but attempts to pass a catheter meet with bony resistance. In this case, the Huber tip of an extradural needle still lies partially in the ligamentum flavum immediately adjacent to its attachment to the lamina above. If the extradural needle can be advanced without further resistance, and the catheter then threads easily without aspiration of CSF, this confirms a high entry through the interlamina gap. However, recent evidence indicates that the extradural space narrows superiorly. More rarely, but of great importance, a needle angled acutely laterally may penetrate the ligamentum flavum close to a spinal nerve. Subsequent attempts to pass a catheter may lead to resistance and the immediate report of a unisegmental paraesthesia. This requires repositioning of the needle, because persistence may lead to spinal nerve trauma.

It is unusual not to obtain a jet of CSF back through an 18-gauge (or larger) needle if it pierces the dura. Thus, the syringe should always be disconnected as soon as the loss of resistance through the ligamentum flavum is obtained, or if a subsequent second loss of resistance is noted. The width of the posterior extradural space, beneath the ligamentum flavum, varies considerably, depending on the level of the bony spine at which it is approached and the horizontal point of needle entry; it is widest in the midline in the midlumbar region (5–6 mm) but narrows next to the articular processes. In the mid-thoracic region, it is 3–5 mm in the midline and very narrow laterally. In the lower cervical region, the distance between ligamentum flavum and dura is only 1.5–2 mm in the midline. However, this increases below C7 to 3–4 mm, particularly if the neck is flexed.

The extradural space extends from the base of the skull to the sacrococcygeal membrane and has complicated direct communications with the paravertebral space and indirect communications with the CSF. It leads also directly to the vascular system by way of its large extradural veins, which have no valves and connect with the basivertebral venous plexus, intracranial veins (if flow is reversed by high thoraco-abdominal pressure) and the azygos vein. These are potential direct routes to the brain and heart for drugs, air or other material injected inadvertently into an extradural vein. Within the cranium, there is no extradural space, as the meningeal dura and endosteal dura are closely adherent, except where they separate to form the venous sinuses. At the foramen magnum, these two layers separate; the former becomes the spinal dura, and the latter becomes the periosteum of the spinal canal.

Thus, although local anaesthetics cannot enter between the endosteal and meningeal layer of the cerebral dura, they may diffuse across the spinal dura at the base of the brain into the CSF, and thence to the brain. Between the spinal dura and the spinal periosteum lies the extradural space. The ligamentum flavum completes the posterior wall in direct continuity with the periosteum of the spinal canal. Because the spinal canal is approximately triangular in cross-section and the articular processes indent the triangle, the extradural space narrows posterolaterally and then widens again laterally towards the intervertebral foramina. The safest point of entry into the extradural space is therefore in the midline.

Although the extradural space is nearly circular at the cervical level, it becomes more triangular in the thoracic region and resin injection studies in cadavers have shown that the lumbar extradural space is divided into three compartments: one ventral and two dorsolateral. The dorsal extradural space may be subdivided further by a dorsomedian fold of dura mater (White, 1982).

The dorsal extradural space (studied with computed axial tomography) has a sawtooth shape, with the dorsal extradural space narrowest near the rostral lamina (1.3–1.6 mm) and widest near the caudad lamina (6.9–9.1 mm) of each interspace. This is in keeping with the attachment of ligamentum flavum to the anterior surface of the rostral lamina and the posterior surface of the caudad lamina. It emphasizes the desirability of not entering the extradural space close to the rostral lamina. In addition to nerve roots that traverse the extradural space, there are fat, areolar tissue, lymphatics, arteries and the extensive internal vertebral venous plexus of Batson. The extradural veins are most prominent along the lateral walls of the spinal canal in the lateral position of the extradural space.

Extradural veins. The large valveless extradural veins are part of the internal vertebral venous plexus, which drains the spinal cord neural tissue, the CSF and the bony spinal canal. The major portion of this plexus lies in the anterolateral part of the extradural space. The plexus has rich segmental connections at all levels within intervertebral foramina and extradural space, and within the body of the vertebrae (the basivertebral veins). Superiorly, the plexus communicates with venous sinuses within the cranium. Inferiorly, the sacral venous plexus link the vertebral

plexus to uterine and iliac veins. By way of the intervertebral foramina at each level, the vertebral plexus communicates with thoracic and abdominal veins, so that pressure changes in these cavities are transmitted to the extradural veins, but not to the supporting bony elements of the neural arch and the vertebral bodies. Thus, marked increases in intra-abdominal pressure may compress the inferior vena cava while distending the extradural veins and increasing flow up the vertebrobasilar plexus. This increased flow is accommodated mostly by the azygos vein, which ascends in the right chest over the root of the right lung into the superior vena cava (Fig. 68.9). However, it is also possible for a small dose of local anaesthetic injected rapidly into an extradural vein to be channelled directly up the basivertebral system to a cerebral venous sinus; this is most likely to occur in a pregnant woman in the supine position when the inferior vena cava is obstructed, and intrathoracic pressure increases during active bearing down, so that the azygos flow is temporarily increased. Clearly, local anaesthetic should not be injected into the extradural space under such conditions. More likely, distension of extradural veins, produced by direct inferior vena caval obstruction (e.g. by the uterus) or by increased thoracoabdominal pressure, diminishes also the effective volume of the extradural space, with the result that injected local anaesthetics spread more widely. In addition, the potential absorptive area of venules and capillaries is increased, with increased amounts of drug reaching the heart by way of the azygos vein.

There are three important points with regard to safety:

(a) The extradural needle should pierce the ligamen-

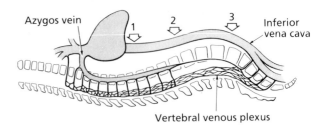

Fig. 68.9 Extradural veins (vertebral venous plexus) and their connections with inferior vena cava (IVC) and azygos vein. Extradural veins are protected from compression by the vertebral canal; thus, obstruction to IVC results in rerouting of venous return by way of extradural veins, and thence to the azygos vein above the level of obstruction. Some common sites of IVC obstruction are shown: (i) below the liver (e.g. severe ascites); (ii) thoracolumbar junction (e.g. abdominal pressure) in prone position; (iii) pelvic brim (e.g. pregnancy). (Redrawn from Bromage, 1978.)

tum flavum in the midline to avoid the large laterally placed extradural veins.

(b) Insertion of extradural needles or catheters, or injection of local anaesthetic should be avoided during episodes of marked increase in size of extradural veins, such as that which occurs with increased thoracoabdominal pressure during straining.

(c) The presence of vena caval obstruction requires a reduction in dose, a decreased rate of injection, and increased care in aspirating for blood before injection.

An intriguing feature of the extradural veins is their importance in draining CSF and in the transfer of local anaesthetic to the CSF. In the region of the dural cuffs, bulbs of arachnoid mater protrude through the dura in the extradural space, where they often invaginate the walls of extradural veins that drain the spinal cord and nerve root area. Although the primary function of these arachnoid granulations is to drain CSF and remove debris from the CSF into the vascular system, they also provide a favourable site for transfer of local anaesthetic into the spinal fluid (Fig. 68.10).

8 From the description so far it is obvious that 'feel' is important in correctly placing the extradural (or subarachnoid) needle. The extradural space may be identified positively by either 'loss of resistance to the injection' of fluid (air or saline) or by a negative-pressure test (usually the 'hanging-drop' negative-pressure test).

In the lumbar region, the major cause of generation of a negative pressure lies in 'coning' of the dura by the advancing needle point. The negative pressure increases as the needle advances across the extradural space towards the dura.

Blunt needles with side openings produce the greatest negative pressure: they produce a good 'coning' effect on the dura without puncturing it and transmit the negative pressure well because of their side opening.

Slow introduction of the needle produces the greatest negative pressure. Even if the needle is halted and the pressure equalized, further advances of the needle continue to produce a negative pressure until the dura is eventually punctured.

Greater negative pressure may be obtained if the dura is not distended (e.g. by gravity in the sitting position or by high abdominal or thoracic pressure).

The absence of an initial negative pressure after entering the extradural space in Bryce-Smith's studies (1950), and in at least 12% of the patients of Usubiaga and colleagues (1967a) in the lying position suggests that negative pressure is an unreliable sign of initial entry into the lumbar space. Further advancement of the needle in the extradural space may be able to demonstrate a negative pressure where it is initially absent. This appears to conflict with the optimal clinical technique of halting the extradural needle as soon as it enters the space. Techniques of lumbar extradural puncture that are based on 'loss of resistance' tests through ligamentum flavum with air-filled or fluid-filled syringes offer a more reliable means of achieving this optimal technique in the

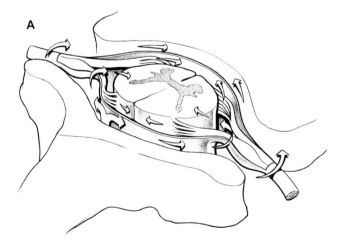

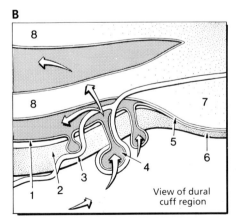

Fig. 68.10 (A) Horizontal spread of local anaesthetic in extradural space. Major spread posteriorly to the region of 'dural cuff' (root sleeve) region is shown, with subsequent entry to cerebrospinal fluid (CSF) and spinal cord. Minor spread into anterior extradural space is also shown. (B) Enlarged view of dural cuff region shows rapid entry of local anaesthetic into CSF by way of arachnoid granulations: (1) arachnoid membrane; (2) dura; (3) extradural vein; (4) arachnoid 'granulation' protruding through dura and in contact with extradural vein; (5) perineural epithelium of spinal nerve in continuity with arachnoid; (6) epineurium of spinal nerve in continuity with dura; (7) dorsal root ganglion; (8) intradural spinal nerve roots. (Redrawn from Cousins & Bridenbaugh, 1988.)

lumbar area (see below). If the anaesthetist finds it easier to use the two-handed grip in the 'hanging-drop' negative-pressure test (Bromage, 1953), it is important to ensure that pressure in the lumbar extradural space is as low as possible by positioning the patient in the lateral position, with a slight head-down tilt, to lower intra-abdominal pressure.

In the thoracic region, the major determinant of negative pressure is the transmission of negative respiratory pressures from the thorax by way of the paravertebral space and intervertebral foramina to the extradural space.

The reliability of a 'hanging-drop' negative-pressure sign in the thoracic region has led to the recommendation that this technique be used at least in the mid-thoracic region. The narrowness of the extradural space in this region and the excellent control afforded by the two-handed grip of the winged 'hanging-drop' needle give support to this recommendation.

If one uses a negative-pressure test routinely for extradural puncture, it is important to be aware of factors that result in marked changes in pressure.

In severe lung disease such as emphysema, negative pressure may be abolished, particularly if the patient is lying down.

Any factor that increases abdominal pressure and/or occlusion of the inferior vena cava may distend the extradural veins (see above) and increase pressure in the lumbar space. This results in only slight changes in the thoracic extradural space, particularly if the patient is sitting.

During labour, baseline lumbar extradural pressures are higher in women in the supine position compared with those in the lateral position. As labour progresses, baseline pressures increase to as high as +10 cmH$_2$O at full dilatation. Also, there are peaks of pressure during each uterine contraction, with increases of 8−15 cmH$_2$O.

Coughing or a Valsalva manoeuvre increases both intrathoracic and intra-abdominal pressure, so that pressures in both thoracic and extradural spaces increase.

Changes in pressure in the extradural space also have implications for the ease of injection and spread of local anaesthetic solutions. Studies by Usubiaga and colleagues (1967b) have helped to explain why successful entry into the extradural space is followed sometimes by 'drip-back' when local anaesthetic is injected subsequently; classic pressure−volume compliance studies showed that compliance decreased with increasing age and that residual pressure after injection of 10 ml of solution at a standard rate had a

positive correlation with age. Thus, some patients with a low compliance in the extradural space are unable to accommodate a large volume of solution if it is injected rapidly. 'Drip-back' is less common in young patients if injection is made slowly because, although there was increased pressure in young patients, Usubiaga and colleagues found that pressure was essentially back to baseline in 30 s.

As expected, Usubiaga and colleagues (1967b) found that spread of analgesia correlated positively with residual extradural pressure and age. These studies tend to support radiological studies, in which 'perio-durograms' with water-soluble contrast media showed a reduced longitudinal spread of injected solutions in young patients because of widely patent intervertebral foramina. In contrast, in elderly patients with relatively obstructed foramina, longitudinal spread was increased. More recent radiological studies have demonstrated minimal leakage of contrast media through intervertebral foramina in young patients. Thus, soft tissue (fat) in the extradural space seems most important in the spread of solutions.

The pedicles that join the laminae to the vertebral bodies complete the bony spinal canal that protects the dural sac. Each pedicle is notched, so that pedicles of adjacent vertebral bodies form the intervertebral foramen. The inferior pedicle of each foramen is notched more deeply. The intervertebral foramina are completed posteriorly by the capsule surrounding the articular processes of adjoining vertebrae, and anteriorly by an intervertebral disc and the lower part of the body above it. Because the extradural space is continuous with the paravertebral space, it is possible to produce an extradural block by injection close to an intervertebral foramen or to penetrate the dura at the dural-cuff region if a needle is inserted into an intervertebral foramen.

The extradural fat extends throughout the spinal and caudal space. It is most abundant posteriorly, diminishes adjacent to the articular processes, and increases laterally around the spinal nerve roots, where it is continuous with the fat surrounding the spinal nerves in the intervertebral foramina and in the paravertebral space. Anteriorly, it is sparse and thus the dura may lie close to the posterior longitudinal ligament. Overall, the amount of fat in the extradural space tends to vary in direct relation to that present elsewhere in the body, so that obese patients may have extradural spaces that are occupied by generous amounts of fat. Mostly, the fat lies free in the extradural space except near the nerve roots, where connective tissue tends to tether it in the intervertebral foramina. Extradural fat is surprisingly vascular, with small capillaries that form a rich network in its substance. The fat itself has a great affinity for drugs with high lipid solubility, such as bupivacaine, etidocaine, fentanyl and some other highly lipid-soluble opioids which may be retained for prolonged periods; uptake of these agents into extradural fat competes with vascular and neural uptake. There is a large variation in compliance between individuals and with increasing age. In children and young adults, it offers little resistance to injection, but in some adults, a low compliance may result in considerable 'drip-back' of injected local anaesthetic.

The dural-cuff region is supplied with a rich lymphatic network that conveys debris rapidly from arachnoid villi out through intervertebral foramina to reach lymph channels in front of the vertebral bodies. 9 An extradural catheter may be threaded down the 16- or 18-gauge Tuohy needle, or direct injection may be made. The speed of injection through needle or catheter should be controlled. A rapid rate of injection may produce neurological signs (Wildsmith, 1986). Slow injection also helps to identify inadvertent intravascular injection before the onset of toxicity. One way to detect this complication is to inject a test dose of adrenaline-containing solution whilst monitoring heart rate (Moore & Batra, 1981).

Incorrect procedure

Incorrect procedure or sometimes inadvertent aberrant needle placement because of anatomical difficulties may result in a different sequence of events from that described above. Failure to define the midline clearly, results in needle entry at the side of the supraspinous ligament. If the anaesthetist persists with this unsatisfactory start, it is likely that the needle may enter interspinous ligament obliquely, resulting in only a transient resistance, followed by loss of resistance, or it may miss the ligament completely, resulting immediately in a feeling of no resistance, in the paravertebral muscles. Both of these situations may be interpreted as rapid entry into the extradural space. However, injection of local anaesthetic is followed by marked 'drip-back' and subsequent attempts to thread an extradural catheter are met with considerable resistance. If the needle is inserted too close to the spinous process (or during any attempt at midline puncture in the mid-thoracic region), it is not uncommon for the needle to contact the spinous process.

Perhaps the most common obstruction to the needle

is the lamina of the vertebral body. Because the posterior surface of the lamina slopes gently down and back from its anterior end to its posterior end (Fig. 68.7), an extradural needle inserted too far laterally may encounter lamina either at a superficial depth or deeper, close to its junction with the ligamentum flavum. Even more extreme lateral insertion or lateral angulation of the needle may result in the needle point contacting the superior or inferior articular processes or the joint space, where their articular facets meet. As the articular facets have a rich nerve supply, needle trauma may result in sudden severe localized pain on one side of the back with accompanying paravertebral muscle spasm on that side. This pain is not dissimilar to that caused by direct contact with a nerve root: 'radicular pain'. Both may result in pain that radiates into the leg. Radicular pain is usually more discrete with only one area involved (e.g. the inside of the knee for L3 or inside of the leg for L4). Facet pain may radiate, although it is somewhat more diffuse.

Additional anatomical and technical aspects of spinal subarachnoid anaesthesia

If subarachnoid anaesthesia is planned, the needle is advanced through the extradural space to puncture the dura and enter the subarachnoid space. Formal identification of the extradural space is undertaken rarely; however, it is a useful exercise for the beginner using a 22-gauge needle.

The test of dural puncture is flow of CSF through the needle. In subarachnoid anaesthesia, CSF must be obtained, but dural puncture is also suspected sometimes during an extradural block, as indicated in Table 68.3.

Combined subarachnoid−extradural techniques

As both subarachnoid and extradural anaesthesia have different advantages and limitations, there may on occasion be some benefit in combining the two techniques giving a degree of flexibility and effectiveness unobtainable by each technique alone. The technique was first described using separate interspaces by Curelaru (1979) and again by Brownridge (1981) in Caesarean section patients, the extradural catheter being placed at L1−2, then subarachnoid anaesthesia being performed at L3−4. The extradural catheter extends analgesia and facilitates postoperative pain relief. The first descriptions using the same interspace were by Coates (1982) and by Mumtaz and colleagues (1982) in orthopaedic patients. The technique can be

Table 68.3 Suspected dural puncture. (Redrawn from Cousins & Bridenbaugh, 1988)

Sign	Cause	Management
Second loss of resistance and fluid flows from needle	Dural puncture	Convert to spinal anaesthetic or move to higher interspace for extradural
Second loss of resistance after identifying ligamentum flavum; no fluid flows from needle, but injected solution: some 'drip-back'	? Entry into subdural space ? Dural puncture	Test 'drip-back' on arm: cold, LA, warm, CSF Drip onto glucose test strip — positive for glucose If drip-back only LA, withdraw needle and reidentify extradural space If 'drip-back' = CSF + LA, move to a rostrad interspace or convert to spinal anaesthetic
One loss of resistance only — 'drip-back' at a shallow level; a deeper level	Interspinous ligament pierced and needle in paravertebral muscle Low compliance of extradural fat Needle only partially through ligamentum flavum	Reinsert needle in midline Test as above, if drip-back only LA: Attempt to pass catheter — easy passage Attempt to pass catheter — does not pass: Superiorly needle can be advanced and then catheter threaded. Inferiorly, needle will not advance
	Needle in CSF	Test for CSF; if positive, move to rostrad interspace or convert to spinal

LA, local anaesthetic; CSF, cerebrospinal fluid. Do not attempt to withdraw needle into extradural space at the same level, as this may result in subdural cannulation.

performed using either a standard or modified Tuohy needle through which a long subarachnoid needle is passed.

The extradural needle is inserted as described above. After the extradural space is identified, the subarachnoid needle is passed through the extradural needle into the extradural space and then through the dura. After injection of local anaesthetic into the subarachnoid space the subarachnoid needle is removed and the extradural catheter is passed in the usual manner.

Since its increase in popularity several companies now supply specially designed packs with the 'back eye' modification to the Tuohy needle (Fig. 68.2). There are several needle modifications, one of which has separate channels for the catheter and subarachnoid needle.

It is claimed that the incidence of postsubarachnoid headache is very low using this technique, possibly because of the ease of subarachnoid injection when the extradural space has been identified by the Tuohy needle. Thus, the rapid onset and reliability of the subarachnoid block is provided with the facility using the extradural catheter, to modify and extend the high-quality analgesia into the postoperative period.

There is some evidence that when extradural injection is made immediately after the subarachnoid injection the initial extension of the subarachnoid block is largely a volume effect, rather than being caused by the additional local anaesthetic *per se* (Blumgart *et al.*, 1992).

In addition to the usual complications associated with subarachnoid and extradural anaesthesia, subarachnoid placement of the catheter is theoretically possible. Whilst this technique adds to the armamentarium of regional anaesthesia, it requires a clear understanding of the equipment used and the aetiology of possible complications and therefore should not be performed by a novice.

Continuous subarachnoid technique

This is achieved by passing a spinal needle as described above, and then threading a catheter directly into the subarachnoid space and removing the subarachnoid needle. This enables a high-quality block to be produced with small doses of local anaesthetic (10–15 times less than with an extradural). In common with the continuous extradural technique the dose can be slowly titrated, minimizing cardiovascular side-effects and the block may be 'topped up' allowing operations that would outlast a single-shot technique to be performed under subarachnoid anaesthesia. Also opioids may be administered for long-lasting postoperative analgesia.

However, there has been a reluctance to pass a

catheter into the subarachnoid space because of the presumed high incidence of postsubarachnoid headache associated with the larger needle required to pass the catheter, and the fear of infection related to the indwelling catheter. Several series have been published with no evidence of infection or undue incidence of postspinal headache (Giuffrida *et al.*, 1972; Denny *et al.*, 1987). Denny and colleagues (1987) reported only one headache in 117 patients using a 18-gauge needle and 20-gauge catheter, although the catheters were only left *in situ* for a few hours, and the mean age was 63 years, with more males than females.

Giuffrida and colleagues (1972) found, using a catheter through a 20-gauge needle, postspinal headache rate of 16% in 74 obstetric patients. Recently, the introduction of microcatheters (32-gauge) associated with fewer PDPH have led to re-examination of this technique. Indeed, with this catheter there is some evidence that the PDPH rate is more dependent on the size of needle used to introduce the catheter, and to the age of the patient than to the presence of the catheter. If these prove safe and reliable, they may permit a continuous spinal technique to be used both during surgery and into the postoperative period (Hurley & Lambert, 1990).

Unfortunately, there have been several case reports of cauda equina syndrome associated with continuous subarachnoid anaesthesia (Rigler *et al.*, 1991). Even though these may have been caused by high local drug and/or dextrose concentrations the future of this technique at present must be in doubt.

Alternative approaches to the extradural space

The technique of spinal injection in the midline has been described. An alternative approach is to use a paraspinous (paramedian or lateral) insertion. The needle should be inserted close to the spinous process because in both lumbar and thoracic regions, the spinous process narrows superiorly, and thus guides the needle to a midline entry through the ligamentum flavum.

Extreme lateral angulation of the needle should be avoided, as it may result in oblique penetration of the ligamentum flavum and vascular or neural damage. In most instances, the needle need not be angulated and merely follows the spinous process. Thus, 'paraspinous' describes the essence of the technique. Indeed, techniques with extreme angulation of the needle should be discarded in favour of the safer paraspinous approach.

In the lumbar region, infiltration is made 1–1.5 cm lateral to the caudad tip of the inferior spinous process of the chosen interspace. A 9–10 cm, 22-gauge spinal needle is used to infiltrate perpendicular to the skin beside the spinal process; this enables the depth of the lamina to be determined before inserting the extradural needle. It is worth noting that for single-shot techniques the extradural space can be identified if an air-filled syringe is attached to the 22-gauge needle and constant pressure is applied to the plunger. However, in most patients, an 18-gauge extradural needle is inserted next beside the spinous process and angled upwards at 45° to the skin (Fig. 68.7); often the spinous process carries the needle slightly inwards, 10–15° to the sagittal plane. This may not always be so, and the needle may pass directly to the ligamentum flavum without any necessity for inward angulation. With this technique, resistance to the advancing needle and syringe plunger is encountered only when the needle tip enters the ligamentum flavum. Thus, careful location of the depth of ligamentum flavum is essential. From this point, the technique is identical to that at the midline.

In the thoracic region, skin infiltration is made 1–1.5 cm lateral to the caudad tip of the spinous process, *cephalad* to the intended level of needle insertion. Infiltration down to the level of the lamina is carried out as described above. The extradural needle is inserted beside the spinous process at 55–60° to the skin (sagittal plane); a steep angle is required to reach ligamentum flavum caudad to the chosen spinous process. For both thoracic and lumbar paraspinous approaches, the Crawford 18-gauge thin-walled needle is suitable for single-shot and catheter techniques. The angulation of the needle may permit easier threading of a catheter if a straight-tipped Crawford needle is used, rather than the Huber tip of the Tuohy needle (Fig. 68.8).

The dural sac ends caudally at the lower border of S2, where it is pierced by the filum terminale. The filum terminale is the terminal thread of the pia mater, which extends from the tip of the spinal cord to blend with the periosteum on the back of the coccyx. The filum terminale anchors the cord and spinal dura, the latter being steadied further in the lower end of the vertebral column by a few fibrous strips from the posterior longitudinal ligament. The spinal dura also provides a thin cover for the spinal nerve roots, becoming progressively thinner near the intervertebral foramina, where it continues as epineural and perineural connective tissue of the peripheral nerves. The dura is the outer of three coverings of the spinal cord (and brain). The middle covering is the delicate non-vascular arachnoid mater.

It is attached closely to the dura and ends with it at S2. Between the dura and the arachnoid lies the (potential) subdural space. A technique for entry into this space with X-ray control has been described. After the needle enters the subarachnoid space with the flow of CSF, one withdraws the needle until the flow stops, and at this point the bevel of the needle should rest in the subdural space.

This space may be entered unintentionally during spinal administration of local anaesthetics. It may explain some failed spinals despite aspiration of 'some' spinal fluid. The case reports of subdural injection indicate unilateral, patchy and inordinately high levels of anaesthesia, but usually after volumes of local anaesthetic intended for extradural anaesthesia.

The dura can be considered as a protective tube that is pierced by and gives a short 'cuff' to each pair of spinal nerves; at this point, the dura becomes markedly thinner and is adherent closely to the dorsal surfaces of the dorsal root ganglia as far as the point where anterior and posterior roots fuse to form the spinal nerve. Within these dural cuffs, there is a small blind pocket of CSF, which is separated from the extradural space only by the greatly thinned dura (Fig. 68.10). Here, the dura is pierced by veins, arteries and lymphatics, running to and from the underlying subarachnoid space. Also, the arachnoid membrane pushes small 'granulations' through the dura; these may either indent extradural veins or come into contact with extradural lymphatics, to facilitate drainage of CSF and elimination of foreign material. This region also provides a ready route for passage of local anaesthetics into the spinal fluid. Although the dura and arachnoid are usually in close apposition, they are separated easily, and it is possible unintentionally to insert a catheter into the subdural space.

The innermost covering of the cord is the delicate though highly vascular pia mater. It invests the spinal cord closely along its length. The space between pia and arachnoid mater is the subarachnoid space and contains the CSF, spinal nerves and a large number of trabeculae which run between the two membranes. The denticulate ligaments which are attached to the dura and help to support the spinal cord are lateral projections of the pia mater.

The dorsal and ventral nerve roots are covered only by pia mater as they traverse the subarachnoid space. They receive a covering of the other two meningeal layers as they pierce the spinal dura and pass through the extradural space. As the dura extends further out to the intervertebral foramina, it becomes thinner. The pia and arachnoid mater extend beyond the dorsal root ganglia as the perineurium of the peripheral nerves.

Spinal cord and nerves

The spinal cord begins at the level of the foramen magnum and ends as the conus medullaris. At birth, the cord ends at the level of L3, but rises with age to end in adults at the lower border of L1 (Fig. 68.11).

There are 31 pairs of spinal nerves. Each is composed of anterior and posterior roots which are formed by coalescence of several rootlets arising from the cord. Beyond the end of the cord, lumbar and sacral nerve roots extend as the cauda equina. The nerves in the cauda equina are covered only by a thin layer of a pia mater and have a large surface area from their cord origin to their exits through the dura. They are therefore especially sensitive to local anaesthetics within the CSF.

Cerebrospinal fluid

The CSF is an ultrafiltrate of blood and is contained within the subarachnoid space of spine and cranium (see Table 68.4). It is clear and colourless in health, with a specific gravity of 1.003–1.009 (mean 1.006) at 37°C and a mean osmolality of 280 mosmoles. The total volume of CSF is 120–150 ml but only 25–35 ml is within the spinal subarachnoid space and most of this volume is below the end of the cord.

CSF is usually homogeneous but if conditions

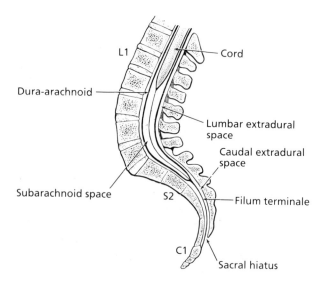

Fig. 68.11 Lumbosacral portion of vertebral column, showing terminal spinal cord and its coverings. (Redrawn from Cousins & Bridenbaugh, 1988.)

Table 68.4 Composition of cerebrospinal fluid

Glucose	1.5–4.0 mmol/litre
Sodium	140–150 mmol/litre
Chloride	120–130 mmol/litre
Bicarbonate	25–30 mmol/litre
Hydrogen ions	32–36 nmol/litre
Protein	0.15–3.0 g/litre

change rapidly (e.g. respiratory acidosis) only cisternal values mirror systemic values and the composition of lumbar CSF changes slowly. CSF is produced at a constant rate of approximately 0.35 ml/min or 500 ml/day and rate of absorption equals rate of formation. Formation of CSF is increased when serum is hypotonic, and reduced when serum osmolality increases. There is an approximately linear relationship with a 1% change in serum osmolality causing a 6.7% change in production of CSF. In conditions where CSF is lost, e.g. PDPH, it is therefore important at least to prevent dehydration but better to infuse intravenous fluids. CSF is produced in the choroid plexuses of the lateral, third and fourth ventricles. There is a concentration gradient of protein from a low level (6–15 mg/dl) in the ventricles to 20–50 mg/dl in the lumbar sac. Anaesthetic drugs have little effect on production of CSF.

The cord is supplied with arterial blood through one anterior and paired posterior arteries (Fig. 68.12). The anterior spinal artery arises above from branches of the vertebral arteries and descends in front of the anterior longitudinal sulcus of the spinal cord. It receives contributions from the spinal arteries which reach the spinal cord by way of the intervertebral foramina and enter the extradural space to reach spinal nerve roots in the region of the dural cuffs. It is thus possible to cause spinal cord ischaemia if a spinal artery is traumatized by a needle inserted towards a spinal nerve root. The spinal cord territory supplied by the anterior spinal artery is most vulnerable, as there is only one anterior artery and the major feeder to this artery usually enters unilaterally (on the left in 78%) by way of a single intervertebral foramen, between T8 and L3. It is termed the artery of Adamkiewicz (radicularis magna). Damage to this vessel may result in ischaemia of the lumbar enlargement of the cord. In a small number of patients, the artery of Adamkiewicz originates at a high level (T5). Iliac tributaries are then larger, but these can be damaged during pelvic surgery or lumbar extradural anaesthesia resulting in a lesion of the conus medullaris.

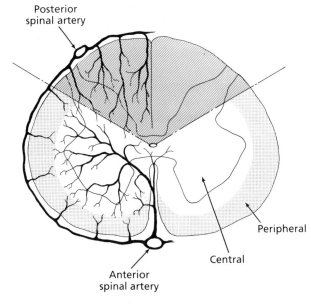

Fig. 68.12 Blood supply of spinal cord, horizontal distribution. The 'central' area, supplied only by anterior spinal artery, is predominantly a motor area (see text). (Redrawn from Cousins & Bridenbaugh, 1988.)

This supports further the practice of ensuring that the needle enters the extradural space in the midline and suggests that the L3–4 interspace is the best choice for beginners.

Anterior spinal artery ischaemia causes a predominantly motor lesion, as the anterior two-thirds of the cord, including the anterior horn cells are supplied exclusively by this artery. The posterior spinal arteries arise from the posterior inferior cerebellar arteries and they descend on the posterolateral surface of the cord lying medial to the posterior nerve roots. They supply the posterior white columns and some of the posterior grey (Fig. 68.12). In contrast to the six or seven vessels feeding the anterior spinal artery, the posterior longitudinal vessels are fed by 25–40 radicular arteries.

Pharmacology of spinal and extradural anaesthesia

Spinal anaesthesia

Baricity

The interrelationship between baricity of the local anaesthetic solution and the posture of patient (first described by Barker) is paramount. A local anaesthetic solution with specific gravity less than that of CSF (hypobaric) tends to rise and if the specific gravity is greater than CSF (hyperbaric) it moves downwards whatever position the patient assumes. Spread is therefore determined by the posture the patient is placed in *after* injection, and a knowledge of the spinal curves is important.

The baricity of various local anaesthetic solutions is summarized in Table 68.5.

The baricity of local anesthetics can be adjusted by adding water, saline or dextrose. Local anaesthetics are made hyperbaric by the addition of dextrose, however concentrations above 8% cannot be recommended as they are also very hypertonic (compared with CSF) and there is some risk of neural damage.

Hyperbaric and isobaric solutions tend to produce blocks of good quality and spread whereas hypobaric solutions produce blocks that are often patchy and of poor quality. Higher blocks are much more reliably obtained using hyperbaric solutions with an appropriate adjustment in posture. Blocks produced by isobaric or hypobaric solutions tend to have a longer duration of action than do those produced by hyperbaric solutions.

It should also be remembered that any injected solution reaches body temperature within 1 min and it is the specific gravity of the solution at body temperature that determines the baricity relative to CSF.

Table 68.5 Local anaesthetic solutions used in spinal anaesthesia

Amethocaine (tetracaine)	Solutions can be hyperbaric (0.5% in glucose 8%, SG 1.0203), isobaric (0.5% in N/2 saline, SG 1.066) or hyperbaric (1% in water, SG 1.0007) Maximal intrathecal dose of 20 mg
Bupivacaine (Marcaine)	Solutions can be (slightly) hypobaric (0.5% in water, SG 1.059) or hyperbaric (0.5% in glucose 8%, SG 1.0278)
Cinchocaine (Nupercainal, dibucaine)	Usually a hyperbaric solution (0.5% in glucose 6%, SG 1.024)
Lignocaine (Xylocaine)	Solutions may be isobaric (2% in water, SG 1.0066) or hyperbaric (5% in glucose 7.5%, SG 1.0333)

SG measured at 37°C; SG CSF 1.0069.

Posture

A patient who is placed supine as soon as the subarachnoid injection has been made develops a block to the mid-thoracic level when a hyperbaric solution is used, but only to the low thoracic segments with hypobaric or isobaric solutions because of the effect of spinal curves. Isobaric solutions (e.g. plain bupivacaine) give a longer duration of block, regardless of posture. In the sitting patient, hyperbaric solutions may be used to create a 'saddle' block. This is a useful block for operations on the perineum, but if a large volume is used or the patient is placed supine too soon (i.e. less than 5 min) the block spreads as if the patient had been supine from the beginning.

Unilateral blocks can be produced by keeping the patient in a lateral position for at least 5 min. This so-called 'hemi-anaesthesia' reduces the physiological consequences of the block. Unfortunately, the block spreads when the patient turns supine and a unilateral block usually becomes bilateral, although the side which was lower is blocked more profoundly (Wildsmith & Rocco, 1985).

Dose of drug

Dose of the drug injected is a third major factor affecting spread of subarachnoid injections. Unfortunately, this factor is not constant but varies within the range of volumes used for spinal anaesthesia. Indeed, dose, volume and concentration are all interrelated and each plays a part. However, there is a critical dose below which a reasonable block cannot be expected. Thus, injection of isobaric amethocaine 0.5% in a dose of 5, 10, or 15 mg produces blocks of similar spread (usually legs and perineum) (Wildsmith *et al.*, 1981). The same phenomenon occurs with bupivacaine 0.5% but not with a 0.75% solution where increasing the dose increases the spread. If the volume of solution is increased but a constant dose is employed, there is only a small increase in spread, at the cost of increased unpredictability of spread. Increasing the dose improves the quality of anaesthesia and prolongs block duration.

Duration

The choice of drug is the main determinant of duration of the block (e.g. lignocaine produces a block lasting approximately 1 h and bupivacaine and amethocaine at least 2 h). Drug dose, however, also affects duration, as does the level of block. If a given dose produces a block to the mid-lumbar level, it lasts longer than if the same dose spread to block up to the mid-thoracic level.

The addition of vasoconstrictors to subarachnoid injections of local anaesthetic, although safe, usually results in under a 10% increase in duration and no alteration in spread of the block. A similar increase can be obtained by increasing the dose of drug by 50% (Wildsmith & Rocco, 1985).

Barbotage

This is the technique of aspirating CSF repeatedly and injecting small volumes of the local anaesthetic (from the French verb *barboter* 'to mix, dabble or paddle'). Greater spread of block is obtained from a given dose, but the result of barbotage is not entirely predictable. Fast injection increases also dispersion of local anaesthetic, but this again is unpredictable. Rapid injection can be considered a form of barbotage and if this is to be avoided for a more predictable spread slow injection (1 ml/10 s) is recommended. Needle size and direction of bevel have little clinical relevance to spread of anaesthesia.

Clinical subarachnoid anaesthesia

The agents available for use are described in Table 68.6. Most studies quote mean level of block. Anaesthetists need to know the minimum level (guaranteed efficacy for surgery) and the maximum level (risk of hypotension from sympathetic block). In practice, only three techniques need to be considered to obtain distinctly different levels of block (Wildsmith & Rocco, 1985; Wildsmith, 1987).

1 For abdominal surgery, block to mid-thoracic

segments is necessary. This is achieved best by injecting a hyperbaric solution (2–3 ml) at the L2–3 or L3–4 interspace and lying the patient supine immediately. The solution runs down the dorsal curve of the spine and excess solution pools opposite the T5 vertebra; it does not spread higher without a steep head-down tilt. The effect of this block on arterial pressure may be profound. Barbotage may increase the height of the block and keeping the patient sitting for a short time after subarachnoid injection may keep the block a few segments lower (e.g. for herniorrhaphy) which may reduce the cardio-vascular consequences.

2 For procedures on the perineum, a saddle block is suitable. This is produced by injecting a small volume (0.5–0.75 ml) of hyperbaric local anaesthetic at the L4–5 interspace and keeping the patient in a sitting position for at least 5 min. Arterial pressure is affected rarely by this block. If the patient is to be placed in the lithotomy position abduction and flexion of the hip may become uncomfortable and the block described in (3) may be more appropriate.

3 For procedures on the lower limb (or perineum) a block to the level of the inguinal ligament is required. This can be achieved by injecting an isobaric solution at the L2–3 interspace. The risk of hypotension is not high, the hip joint is anaesthetized and, unlike the saddle block, there is no special positioning required. Dosages for the various local anaesthetics for different levels of block are given in Table 68.6.

Patient factors influencing local anaesthetic distribution in cerebrospinal fluid

When the technique and agent are held constant several patient factors may influence spread of local anaesthetic in CSF:

1 *Age.* Although the correlation is weak, spread is greater in older patients than in younger ones. Onset of the block is also more rapid with age (Pitkänen *et al.*, 1984).

2 *Height.* The taller the patient the fewer spinal segments are blocked for a given amount of local anaesthetic. Conversely, the dose should be reduced for patients who are less than 150 cm tall (Attygalle & Rodrigo, 1985).

3 *Weight.* A correlation between weight or body mass index (weight/height^2) and height of block has been demonstrated by several authors (McCulloch & Littlewood, 1986; Pitkänen, 1987). A high block can therefore be expected in obese patients (Pitkänen, 1987).

4 *Anatomical configuration.* A kyphosis or lordosis

Table 68.6 Spinal anaesthesia — a guide to dosage and effects

Drug	Dose (mg) To L4	To T10	To T4	Duration (min)
Lignocaine 5%	25–50	50–75	75–100	60–70
Bupivacaine 0.5% (isobaric)	10–15	15–20	—	150–200
Bupivacaine 0.5% (hyperbaric)	4–8	8–12	14–20	90–110
Cinchocaine 0.5%	4–6	6–8	10–15	150–180

See text for appropriate posture, etc. Approximately 10% increase in duration of effect when vasoconstrictors are added to the solution used.

may affect spread of local anaesthetic and may require extra careful positioning of the patient.

5 *Pregnancy, intra-abdominal tumours and ascites.* Increased spread of local anaesthetic results from a decrease in CSF volume in these conditions. This is a result of increased intra-abdominal pressure reducing inferior vena caval blood flow and subsequent development of collateral vessels in the extradural space (Fig. 68.9). As the spinal canal has a fixed volume, venous engorgement in the extradural space is accommodated by reduction in the volume of the subarachnoid space.

Segmental levels

In assessing the level of block, it is important for the anaesthetist to have a method of using simple surface landmarks to indicate level of dermatomal block and hence segmental spinal nerve (and sympathetic) block. Table 68.7 lists the key levels. There is no point in testing for blockade of T1—2 by testing above the nipple line, since this area has double innervation from T1 to T2 and C3 to C4, so that normal sensation remains even when T1—2 are blocked. Thus, residual activity in the cardiac sympathetics T1 and T2 is checked by testing skin sensation on the inside of the arm above the elbow (T2) and below the elbow (T1). Residual motor activity in T1 can be checked also by testing the ability of the patient to hold a sheet of paper between the outstretched fingers (interossei C8, T1). In a lightly anaesthetized patient, spinal reflexes may be useful for testing level of block — epigastric (T7—8), abdominal (T9, T12), cremasteric (L1, L2), plantar (S1, S2), knee jerk (L2—4), ankle-jerk (S1, S2).

The fate of local anaesthetic in the cerebrospinal fluid

Local anaesthetic disappears from the CSF because of uptake by neuronal tissue or vascular absorption. Four factors govern neuronal uptake:

1 Concentration of local anaesthetic in CSF. Uptake is greatest where the concentration of local anaesthetic in CSF is greatest.

2 Surface area of nerve tissue exposed to local anaesthetic. Both nerve roots and the cord take up CSF. The surface of the cord, lying deep to the pia mater is exposed to local anaesthetic, and deeper structures are exposed also through the spaces of Virchow—Robin which accompany blood vessels penetrating the cord.

3 Lipid content of nerve tissue. The local anaesthetic agents are lipophilic and are taken up by myelinated tissue within the subarachnoid space.

4 Blood flow to exposed neural tissue. The local anaesthetics are removed from subarachnoid nerve tissue through the blood; blood flow is therefore the most important determinant of concentration of local anaesthetic in cord or nerve whatever the effects of the other factors. The rate at which the local anaesthetic is removed from the subarachnoid space dictates the duration of block; there is no elimination of local anaesthetic in the CSF. The vessel-rich pia mater carries much local anaesthetic, and the greater the spread of a given dose the shorter the duration of action (because of a larger absorptive area exposed).

Table 68.7 Key levels of dermatomal block. (Redrawn from Cousins & Bridenbaugh, 1988)

Cutaneous landmark	Segmental level	Significance
Little finger	C8	All cardioaccelerator fibres (T1—4) blocked
Inner aspect of arm and forearm	T1 and T2	Some degree of cardioaccelerator block
Apex of axilla	T3	Easily remembered landmark
Nipple line (midway sternal notch and xiphistemum)	T4—5	Possibility of cardioacceleratory block
Tips of xiphoid	T7	Splanchnics (T5—L1) may become blocked
Umbilicus	T10	Sympathetic block limited to lower limbs
Inguinal ligament	T12	
Outer side of foot	S1	No lumbar sympathetic block Most difficult nerve root to block

Vasoconstrictors appear to have little effect on this vasculature. Vessels within the cord help also in the removal of local anaesthetic, but decreases in cord blood flow have little effect on the concentration of local anaesthetic in the systemic circulation.

A significant proportion of a dose injected into the subarachnoid space passes across the dura, down a concentration gradient, and is removed by the mechanisms described below for extradural injections. Other substances injected into the subarachnoid space are also removed by vascular absorption, including the dextrose used to manufacture hyperbaric solutions. At some time after injection (30—35 min for hyperbaric lignocaine), so much dextrose has been eliminated from the CSF that the remaining solution becomes isobaric. At this time a change in position of patient does not affect the spread of anaesthesia; the level of anaesthesia is then said to be 'fixed'.

Sites of action of local anaesthetic after spinal subarachnoid injection

Subarachnoid neural block results from an action of the local anaesthetic on the nerve roots and the dorsal root ganglia; the presence of local anaesthetic in the cord contributes little to the block. The concentration threshold for block (sensitivity) differs between nerve fibre types; the concentration of local anaesthetic in the CSF is reduced with distance from the point of injection. These factors produce *zones of differential block*.

Somatic motor nerves are more resistant to block than sensory nerves; the level of motor block is correspondingly lower than sensory block (approximately two spinal segments). Motor and sensory block from different agents are compared in Fig. 68.13. In addition, different types of sensory nerves have different sensitivity to local anaesthetic, and there is approximately a two segment discrepancy between the levels of analgesia and anaesthesia.

Traditionally, it is taught that the level of sympathetic block is a further two segments higher than the sensory block, thought to result from the preganglion sympathetic nerves being most sensitive to local anaesthetics. Recently, it has become apparent that sensory block may outlast sympathetic block, possibly because of sympathetic pathways within spinal cord or resistance to local anaesthetic block of preganglionic sympathetic β-fibres (Bengtsson *et al.*, 1985).

Extradural anaesthesia

The most important factors influencing spread of local anaesthetic in the extradural space are the volume, concentration, dose of injectate and the site of injection.

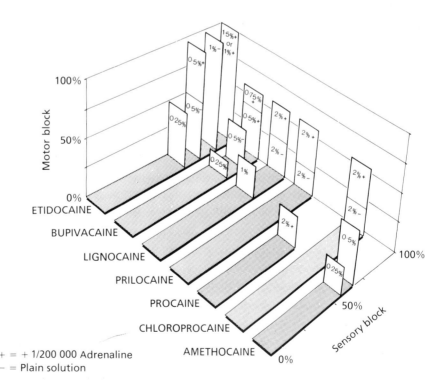

Fig. 68.13 Motor and sensory block percentage success rate. Comparison of agents, concentrations and addition of adrenaline are based on subjective data, so that only approximate comparisons are made. (Redrawn from Cousins & Bridenbaugh, 1988.)

+ = + 1/200 000 Adrenaline
− = Plain solution

Injection site

Speed of onset and intensity of block is greatest at the level of injection. After lumbar extradural injection, there is greater cephalad than caudad spread of analgesia (2:1 segments) and there may also be a delay in onset at the L5 and S1 segments, probably because of the large size of these roots (Galindo et al., 1975). After mid-thoracic extradural injection, there is even spread of analgesia. Repeated doses may cause extensive spread but in addition to L5 and S1, the upper thoracic and lower cervical segments are resistant to block because of their size.

Volume, concentration and dose of injectate

The spread of solutions injected into the extradural space is summarized in Table 68.7. When local anaesthetic solutions are administered, the spread of analgesia for a particular agent is influenced by volume, concentration and dose.

Increasing dosage produces a linear increase in the duration of sensory block, increasing the concentration reduces the onset time and increases the intensity of block. Increasing the volume injected increases the longitudinal spread of solution (and also the duration of block); length of the spinal column (i.e. height) is, therefore, an important influence but not a major factor when lumbar injections are made. For lignocaine 2% and bupivacaine 0.5%, a guide for lumbar administration is to use 1 ml per segment to be blocked for 150 cm (5 ft) of height plus 0.1 ml per segment for each 5 cm (2 in) over 150 cm. Having calculated the required dose, it must be ascertained that this is a safe dose to administer. For extradural anaesthesia in the mid-thoracic region the dose is reduced by one-third.

Age

There is greater spread of local anaesthetic in the extradural space in elderly patients. The consequent declining dose requirements with age can be summarized as:

20–40 years: 1–1.5 ml per segment adjusted for height

40–60 years: 0.5–1 ml per segment adjusted for height

60–80 years: 0.3–0.6 ml per segment adjusted for height

It has been proposed that this phenomenon results from reduced lateral leakage of solution and greater longitudinal spread, but there is conflicting evidence on this subject.

Posture

Whether the patient is sitting or lying has no clinically significant effect generally on cephalad spread although in the obese patient the level of block is lower when the patient is seated. The lateral position does, however, favour spread of analgesia to the dependent side. This is seen in faster onset and longer duration of sensory and motor block (Seow et al., 1983) and greater spread (Husemeyer & White, 1980).

Pregnancy, intra-abdominal tumour or ascites

The potential volume of the extradural space is reduced in these conditions by engorged veins. This makes intravascular injection more likely and increases spread of a given volume. A 30% reduction in volume is recommended.

Speed of injection

Rapid extradural injection must be avoided; it is dangerous and has little effect on spread of analgesia. Rapid injection of a large volume can increase CSF pressure and intracranial pressure (ICP) and compromise spinal cord blood flow. The change in ICP is manifested as headache but cerebral haemorrhage and intraocular haemorrhage have been reported. In addition, slow injection offers the best opportunity to avoid lethal sequelae of intravascular injection of local anaesthetic (see below).

Warming

It has been shown that by injecting warmed (38°C) bupivacaine a reduction in onset time of the order of 20% can be produced (Metha et al., 1987; Howie & Dutton, 1990). This minimal improvement probably does not warrant the practical difficulty of warming both the solution and extradural tray/equipment.

Addition of vasoconstrictor

Great flexibility of sensory and motor block and duration are afforded by careful choice of agent. The addition of adrenaline to solutions of lignocaine both prolongs the block and decreases the rate of absorption (see below); addition of adrenaline to solutions of bupivacaine similarly reduces the peak plasma concentration (Burm *et al.*, 1986). Vasoconstrictors have little effect on the duration of block from the long-acting agents, bupivacaine and etidocaine. The acidity of commercial local anaesthetic solutions containing adrenaline is increased from approximately pH 6 to pH 3 to maintain stability. It has been recommended that because of this, adrenaline should be added freshly, but this, however, increases the risk of inadvertent overdose of adrenaline (0.2–0.25 ml of 1/1000 adrenaline in 50 ml local anaesthetic is suggested). The effect of adrenaline on motor and sensory block is shown in Fig. 68.13.

pH-adjusted anaesthetic solutions

Alkalinization

Local anaesthetics are weak bases and poorly soluble in water. They are usually formulated as hydrochloride salts with a relatively low pH so that the base remains in solution. The lipid-soluble non-ionized free base penetrates the nerve sheath. However, it is only the cationic form that interacts with the axonal membrane to block nerve conduction. The proportion of free base can be increased by adding bicarbonate to the local anaesthetic solution, although the pH should not be raised above 7 as precipitation may occur beyond this.

Significant reductions in onset time have been reported for lignocaine, bupivacaine, mepivacaine and chlorprocaine (Galindo, 1983; DiFazio *et al.*, 1986; Douglas *et al.*, 1986). Not all investigators agree with these findings; Stevens and colleagues (1989) did not find any reduction with bupivacaine. However, the different results may be explained at least in part by the use of different end-points, e.g. pinprick, electrical stimulation, loss of temperature sense. Whilst the results with lignocaine are clinically convincing, further work is required to clarify the (at best) statistically significant reduction in onset time of bupivacaine.

Carbonation

Bromage and colleagues 1967 showed that carbonation of lignocaine reduced the onset time by approximately 33% and carbonation of prilocaine by 25%. However, more recent studies with mepivacaine (Tetzlaff & Rothenstein, 1992) and bupivacaine (Brown *et al.*, 1980) failed to show a significant improvement in the onset time.

Local anaesthetic agents used in extradural anaesthesia

Lignocaine and bupivacaine are used most frequently in the UK. However, ropivacaine, a new amino-amide agent, could become available in the future. In addition, anaesthetists in the USA may use etidocaine and chloroprocaine. Although an excellent agent, prilocaine is not frequently used for extradural blocks.

Lignocaine (Xylocaine, lidocaine) is used in 1–2% formulations. It has a short latency of effect of approximately 10 min and a duration of 1–2 h, depending on strength and the presence or absence of adrenaline. Solutions below 1% produce little motor block and 2% may be required for intense muscle relaxation. With repeated doses, *tachyphylaxis* may develop (see below).

Bupivacaine (Marcaine) is a long-acting agent available widely in 0.25% and 0.5% formulations (and 0.75% in some countries). Whilst some degree of analgesia may persist for several hours, surgical anaesthesia is provided for 1.5 h by bupivacaine 0.5%. Onset is slower than lignocaine, 20–30 min may be required. Analgesia with little muscle relaxation is provided by 0.25%. The drug can be used with or without adrenaline. Bupivacaine 0.75% has a reputation for severe systemic reactions and the manufacturers do not recommend its use in obstetrics. Use of this formulation requires more care but only because it is more concentrated.

Ropivacaine is a new long-acting local anaesthetic with a similar structure and dose–response profile to bupivacaine. It is undergoing Phase III evaluation in 0.5%, 0.75% and 1% formulations. Current work suggests that ropivacaine is less cardiotoxic, causes fewer CNS symptoms on intravenous injection than bupivacaine and may therefore offer an improved margin of safety. Ropivacaine seems to produce less motor block than bupivacaine, and unlike bupivacaine possesses mild vasoconstrictor properties. However, its benefits over bupivacaine will have to prove to be clinically significant to justify the extra cost.

Prilocaine in 1.5%, 2% and 3% formulations with adrenaline has been used for extradural anaesthesia. Speed of onset is similar to that with lignocaine but duration is slightly longer.

Etidocaine in 1.0% or 1.5% solution provides rapid onset of analgesia of long duration. There is good motor block but this may exceed the duration of analgesia.

The addition of adrenaline to prolong block has been described above; other substances have also been added. Carbonated local anaesthetic solutions release base readily, and have a superior penetrating ability resulting in more rapid onset. The addition of potassium also reduces onset time, but the concentration required causes depolarization of nerves, which gives rise to muscle spasms. Adjustment of pH with bicarbonate or carbonation may speed onset of action (see above).

Site of action of extradural anaesthesia

The key data were provided by injecting (^{14}C)-labelled lignocaine into the extradural space of dogs, and then carrying out autoradiography and tissue assays (Bromage *et al.*, 1963). The data suggested that rapid diffusion of local anaesthetic into the CSF at the dural cuff region is the most important determinant of onset of extradural block: peak local anaesthetic concentrations in the CSF are reached within 10–20 min of extradural injection, and concentrations are high enough to produce block in the spinal nerve roots and 'rootlets'. This coincides with the clinical onset of extradural block. The same data also showed that by 30 min after injection, the C_{min} for lignocaine (0.28 µg/mg) had been exceeded in CSF and also in spinal nerves in the paravertebral space (1 µg/mg). Data from other studies in which local anaesthetic was injected directly into the CSF indicate that C_{min} is not exceeded in the dorsal root ganglion or in the more central parts of the spinal cord.

The most likely mechanisms for rapid appearance of local anaesthetic in the CSF relate to the unique anatomy of the dural cuff region. This was reviewed extensively by Shantha and Evans (1972), who observed that arachnoid proliferations and villi are plentiful along both dorsal and ventral roots. Although these 'granulations' are found frequently in quadrupeds, their importance in humans is not certain. They are most plentiful in the region of the dural root sleeves ('cuffs'), immediately proximal to the dorsal root ganglion, where the dura becomes thin and is continuous with the epineurium of spinal nerves (Fig. 68.10). They provide a mechanism by which arachnoid protrudes either partially or completely through the dura into adjacent subdural and extradural spaces. This implies that local anaesthetics may

have to diffuse only across a layer of arachnoid epithelial cells to reach CSF. Even if the granulations are sparse in humans, the dura is thin in the root-sleeve area and it is clear from local anaesthetic and opioid studies that these drugs gain access to CSF rapidly. These anatomical and pharmacological data provide strong evidence that the major sites of action of local anaesthetics after extradural block are the spinal nerve roots and spinal cord.

It is most likely that diffusion into intradural spinal nerve roots plays a major role during the early stages of extradural block. This is in keeping with the rapid onset of a segmental pattern of block. Subsequently, local anaesthetic seepage through intervertebral foramina may contribute by producing 'multiple paravertebral block'. After lumbar extradural block, diffusion through the CSF to the spinal cord (Fig. 68.10) is probably a secondary phenomenon, although it may occur more rapidly when local anaesthetic is injected closer to the spinal cord.

Urban (1973) has reported that regression of analgesia after extradural block follows a circumferential pattern in the sagittal plane rather than the classic segmental pattern seen during onset of block. This is consistent with a persisting action of local anaesthetic on the peripheral spinal cord after the initial effects on spinal nerve roots have abated. Also, Bromage (1974) has observed reflex changes in lower limbs during thoracic extradural block that spares the lumbar segments. Changes typical of an upper motor neurone (long tract) lesion were seen; increased deep-tendon reflexes and an upgoing toe on Babinski's reflex. The peripheral part of the spinal cord in the dorsolateral funiculus contains descending excitatory sympathetic fibres, the descending tracts and medullary reticulospinal fibres. The pyramidal tract synapses in Rexed's Laminae IV, V and VI, which are involved in the modulation of sensory input. It has been hypothesized that local anaesthetics with a high propensity to penetrate the spinal cord may produce a rapid and long-lasting sympathetic block, followed closely by motor block, because of the superficial placement of the appropriate tracts. At the same time, the modulating influences on Laminae V and VI may be blocked with a resultant expansion of segmental receptive fields and a relative 'anti-analgesic' state. This anatomical basis may be an explanation for the 'sensory motor dissociation' exhibited by drugs such as bupivacaine and etidocaine (see below). Currently, no data supports differential penetration of the spinal cord for the various local anaesthetics. Recent support for rapid transport of drugs from extradural space to spinal fluid and spinal cord is provided by studies of extradural opioids.

Some advances in neuroanatomy have helped to explain the segmental onset of extradural block. Studies of the size of dorsal roots indicate a considerable variation in size, with large roots at C8 and S1 and a 'valley' between these two peak sizes in the thoracic region. Studies of the number of myelinated and non-myelinated fibres in ventral roots reveal also a peak at S1 and in the lower cervical region at C5—8. This is in keeping with the relative resistance of the lower cervical region and S1 to neural block. An alternative explanation of the segmental pattern of onset of extradural block was proposed as an initial action on dorsal root ganglia (Frumin et al., 1953, 1954). Although these data are at variance with some subsequent studies, a definitive in vivo study of dorsal root ganglion as a major site of action of extradural local anaesthetics remains to be performed. It has been suggested recently that the pia of the spinal cord and spinal nerve roots is continuous with the perineurium of the spinal nerves. Because the epineurium of spinal nerves is continuous with the dura, this raises the possibility of continuity between the subarachnoid space and a subepineurial space. This would explain reports of transverse myelitis after injection of neurolytic agents directly beneath spinal epineurium. All that is required for rapid spread of injected solution from spinal nerve to CSF is accurate needle placement beneath the spinal nerve epineurium.

Clinical extradural anaesthesia

In addition to choosing the agent and dose, after the extradural space has been located, the injection can be made through the needle, or a catheter can be inserted for repeated or continuous administration of local anaesthetic. Actual spread of analgesia cannot be predicted; thus, a catheter technique is recommended generally, as adequate spread with a single shot requires injection of a generous dose. It may not be easy to thread a catheter into the extradural space, and there is an incidence of outright failure with extradural catheter techniques and a higher incidence of complications. For example, Cousins and Mazze (unpublished data) found a failure rate of 10%, using catheters without stylets in 80 patients. This compares with a rate of failure of 1.2% in 84 cases when injection was made by needle. The major causes of 'catheter failure' were complete in-

ability to thread the catheter (5%), inability to clear the catheter of blood (2.5%) and threading the catheter through an intervertebral foramen (1.3%). The use of stylets to introduce catheters may reduce the incidence of failure to thread the catheter, but may increase the incidence of vascular cannulation. Even if a catheter does not clear of blood completely, a small test dose of adrenaline-containing solution can be injected to test if the catheter is placed within a vessel or outside a vessel that has been traumatized. Threading through a foramen can be reduced by inserting only a minimal amount of catheter. Overall, the irretrievable failure rate of catheters should be close to one in a hundred. Catheters inserted via upward-directed needles in the thoracic region tend to travel straight up the extradural space without deviating through paravertebral foramen. Thus, no catheter failures were encountered in a series of 160 blocks performed between T8 and L1 (Bromage, unpublished data). Only 3—4 cm of catheter should be threaded into the extradural space. This reduces but does not eliminate catheter problems.

Test doses

An effective test dose must be able to demonstrate safely that:
1 The injection is being made into the extradural space and not the subarachnoid space.
2 The injection is not made into a blood vessel in the extradural space.

A 16- or 18-gauge Tuohy needle through the dura usually allows rapid flow of CSF, but not invariably. A tissue plug may prevent it, as may the dura itself if the needle tip is only just piercing it. The test dose must therefore be equivalent to a subarachnoid dose, e.g. 3.5 ml of isobaric bupivacaine 0.5%. Even though the test dose is small, a 'total spinal' following it may occur in some patients, if it is delivered to the subarachnoid space (Galet et al., 1992; Palkar et al., 1992). Questioning the patient about warmth and numbness in the legs reveals misplaced administration readily; a subarachnoid injection results in almost immediate block of β-fibres. Difficulty with injection or 'drip-back' of local anaesthetic after disconnecting the syringe is usually a result of superficial injection (e.g. into interspinous ligament). A recent review of fatalities related to extradural anaesthesia revealed that essential safety checks had been omitted — there is no excuse for this deviation from accepted practice (Prince & McGregor, 1986).

When the injection is made through a catheter,

intravascular administration may occur. Usually, blood flows freely through the catheter when an extradural vein is cannulated. A further check is to aspirate gently with a syringe, but this is not always effective. One way of demonstrating vascular cannulation is to inject slowly (approximately 10 ml/min) an adrenaline-containing test dose (3–5 ml of 1 : 200 000 solution) whilst monitoring pulse rate, ECG and arterial pressure (Moore & Batra, 1981). An increase in heart rate gives a prompt warning and should prevent the problems associated with intravenous injection of toxic quantities of local anaesthetic. Care should be taken even after a test dose appears negative because inadvertent intravascular cannulation may still have been missed (McLean et al., 1992).

If a vessel is cannulated, withdrawing the catheter a little (not through the extradural needle lest it is sheared) and flushing the catheter gently with saline may allow the tip to be withdrawn from the vessel, but remain within the extradural space.

Multiple dosing, infusions and tachyphylaxis

In its simplest application, the catheter is used to consolidate a block for surgery. A single repeat dose of 20% of the total dose, given 20 min after the main dose, consolidates block within the level of block established. Thus, a patchy block with missed segments may be overcome without extending the block. Later, during surgery, a dose of approximately 50% of the main dose, given after the upper level has regressed by one or two segments, restores the block to the initial upper segmental level. This same dose given earlier extends the block.

Mean duration times for a particular anaesthetic dose are shown in Table 68.8. Careful clinical monitoring is necessary to detect signs of regression of block and the requirement for another dose. The intensity of sensory and motor block increases with each successive injection. The analogy of 'repainting the fence' has been suggested by Hingson to describe the deepening of block with repeated doses. With dilute solutions (e.g. lignocaine 1% or bupivacaine 0.25%) motor block is limited but as the number of doses increases, so does the degree of block.

In some circumstances, the duration and degree of block obtained after repeat doses decreases; this is termed tachyphylaxis. It is manifest clinically as increased dose requirements to maintain a given level of block. Tachyphylaxis has been demonstrated clearly during 'continuous' extradural block produced by administration of the short-acting amide anaesthetics (mostly with lignocaine). It has been suggested that repeat injections induce changes in the pH of spinal fluid resulting in diminished efficacy of the local anaesthetic from alterations in the ratio of the ionized : non-ionized fraction, but this is an inadequate explanation. If analgesia from extradural lignocaine is allowed to wear off before a repeat dose is given, tachyphylaxis is more likely. Bromage and colleagues (1969) have reported that if the 'interanalgesic interval' (time from regression of analgesia from one dose to onset of analgesia from the next) is greater than 10 min, tachyphylaxis is likely. Tachyphylaxis increases with lengthening of the interanalgesic interval up to approximately 60 min and then the effect remains constant. At 60 min there is a 30–40% reduction in effect of repeat doses (Fig. 68.14). Another possible factor in increasing

Table 68.8 Clinical effects of local anaesthetic solutions commonly used in extradural block

Drug (min)	Time to + four segments + 1 SD (min)	Approximate time to two-segment regression + 2 SD (min)	Recommended 'top-up' time from initial dose (min)
Lignocaine 2%	15 ± 5	100 ± 40	60
Prilocaine 2–3%	15 ± 4	100 ± 40	60
Chloroprocaine 2–3%	12 ± 5	60 ± 15	45
Mepivacaine 2%	15 ± 5	120 ± 150	60
Bupivacaine 0.5–0.75%	18 ± 10	200 ± 80	120
Etidocaine 1–1.5%	10 ± 5	200 ± 80	120
* Ropivacaine 0.75%	9 ± 10	180 ± 60	120

Note that top-up time is based on duration − 2 SD, which encompasses the likely duration in 95% of the population. In a conscious, co-operative patient, an alternative is to use frequent checks of segmental level. All data are from solutions containing 1 : 200 000 adrenaline (except ropivacaine).

* Ropivacaine is undergoing Phase III trial evaluation and these figures are based on preliminary data.

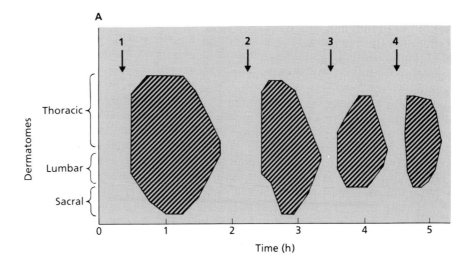

Fig. 68.14 Tachyphylaxis.
(A) Diminished segmental spread and duration of action of repeated extradural injections of the same dose of local anaesthetic, injected at each arrow. Note reinjection has been made at least 30 min after analgesia has regressed two segments. (B) 'Non-analgesic interval'. As the time lag from loss of analgesia to reinjection exceeds 10–15 min, there is a progressive reduction in analgesic effect that reaches a maximum reduction of about 35–40% at 60 min. (Redrawn from Bromage *et al.*, 1969.)

dose requirements is tissue reaction and 'walling off' of the extradural catheter, with a resultant decrease in the amount of local anaesthetic reaching the site of action (Durant & Yaksh, 1986).

Traditionally, extradural analgesia maintained for labour pain or postoperative pain control is *discontinuous*; the patient must complain of pain or discomfort before a repeat dose is given. This would be expected to promote tachyphylaxis, but it seems to be uncommon with the long-acting agents, bupivacaine and etidocaine. This technique does allow the assessment of the patient's neurological status and early diagnosis of any subdural haematoma.

Nevertheless, there is still the humanitarian aspect of only taking 'action on distress' and infusions of local anaesthetic have been introduced in an attempt to provided *continuous* extradural analgesia.

The rate of extradural infusion of local anaesthetic must be a compromise; on the one hand the dose must not exceed the maximum recommended dose; on the other, the volume infused must be sufficient to spread within the extradural space and the concentration must be high enough to block the sensory nerves (C_{min}). Several studies using extradural infusions have claimed good results for both labour (Gaylard *et al.*, 1987) and postoperative pain (Scott *et al.*, 1982). There are several advantages for this method — fewer painful intervals, less motor block, lower risk of infection with a closed system, greater cardiovascular stability and a lower likelihood of a serious complication following accidental subarachnoid or intravenous injection. Despite some encouraging results, this technique has not yet gained widespread acceptance, possibly because occasional top-up injections are still required and a higher total dose of local anaesthetic is administered. Thus, the discontinuous technique of intermittent extradural injection on demand still predominates in obstetric practice and after surgery. An alternative approach is to administer extradural top-up doses regularly by the clock before pain returns. Favourable results have been obtained with regular top-up injections for the relief of postoperative pain. Automatic devices to administer regularly timed extradural injections have been described (Scott *et al.*, 1982).

In a study during labour (Purdy *et al.*, 1987), patients receiving regular extradural injections of local anaesthetic complained of much less pain than those receiving injections on demand, but received only a little more bupivacaine.

Fate of local anaesthetic solutions in the extradural space

The spread of local anaesthetic within the extradural space is summarized in Table 68.9. The local anaesthetic which diffuses across the dura into the CSF is eliminated in the same way as drugs injected directly

Table 68.9 Spread of injected solutions in extradural space

Superior and inferior spread is mainly in the posterior portion of extradural space between dura and ligamentum flavum

Superiorly to foramen magnum. Note the possibility of diffusion of drugs of low molecular weight across dura at base of brain to cerebral CSF, with possibility of access to cranial nerves, vasomotor and respiratory centres and other vital centres

Inferiorly to sacral hiatus, caudal canal and through anterior sacral foramina

Laterally through intervertebral foramina to paravertebral space, to produce paravertebral neural block. Note rapid access to CSF at 'dural-cuff' region to produce spinal nerve root block and subsequent access to spinal cord (see below)

Anteriorly in thin extradural space between dura and anterior longitudinal ligament

Note also:

Access to CSF by slow diffusion across spinal dura, subdural space and subarachnoid membrane into subarachnoid space

Vascular absorption by way of extradural veins may convey drug to heart and brain (see below)

Profuse extradural fat may take up drug

into it. The majority of the local anaesthetic injected is eliminated from the extradural space. Extradural block often requires large doses of local anaesthetic with consequent blood concentrations that are many times higher than those seen after spinal anaesthesia, and often nearly toxic (Tucker & Mather, 1975). A thorough knowledge of the pharmacokinetics and toxicity of local anaesthetics is a prerequisite to the safe utilization of extradural anaesthesia.

Extradural injection deposits local anaesthetic some distance from the neural target, so that diffusion across tissue barriers is important. Thus, local anaesthetics with excellent qualities of penetration of lipid are desirable for rapid and effective extradural analgesia. Because a major site of action is within the dural sac, water solubility is of equal importance (see Chapter 66). Thus, agents with a pKa close to physiological pH (e.g. lignocaine, pKa 7.87) are most effective, in that they readily exhibit both lipid and water solubility. Procaine and amethocaine, with a high pKa (9.04 and 8.46, respectively), suffer in this respect, and perform poorly in extradural block.

Extradural fat provides a potential reservoir for deposition of fat-soluble local anaesthetics. Thus, accumulation of long-acting fat-soluble agents such as bupivacaine, occurs. This is not so for less fat-soluble agents, such as lignocaine. Thus, with repeated injections of bupivacaine, extradural fat concentrations increase but blood concentrations tend to remain the same, provided that dosage is appropriate. Repeated injections of lignocaine result in little accumulation in extradural fat, but progressive accumulation in blood, with a potential for gradually increasing blood concentration.

The extradural venous system provides a rich network of rapid absorption of local anaesthetic. Rapid injection into an extradural vein may despatch local anaesthetic directly to the brain by way of the basivertebral venous system if flow is reversed by the rapidity of injection. Another risk of rapid intravascular injection is high peak concentrations of local anaesthetic in the myocardium. With bupivacaine, this may lead to serious and prolonged 'cardiac toxicity'. The inclusion of adrenaline in local anaesthetic solutions may reduce vascular absorption greatly and thus enhance neural blocking properties and reduce the likelihood of system toxicity.

The time profile of local anaesthetic absorption indicates a peak blood concentration at 10−20 min after injection, so that surveillance is necessary for at least 30 min.

Acid solutions, containing antioxidants to stabilize adrenaline, may release local anaesthetic base with difficulty, and thus spread poorly across lipid barriers. As discussed earlier, alkalinization or the use of carbonated local anaesthetic solutions may improve neural penetration.

Plasma protein binding may influence the amount of free local anaesthetic available for placental transfer, or for action on the CNS, after systemic absorption from the extradural space.

Caudal extradural block

In the past, this approach has been used to produce anaesthesia of lumbar and even low thoracic segments by injecting large volumes of solution (often close to or above a recommended maximum dose). This may be dangerous in adults, but can sometimes be useful in children. In adults, caudal anaesthesia is used almost entirely as an extradural technique to provide analgesia or anaesthesia of the sacral and low lumbar roots. For high blocks, lumbar or thoracic extradural techniques are used.

Anatomy

The five sacral vertebrae are fused, forming the sacrum. The posterior surface of this triangular-shaped bone is convex. Down the middle of the posterior surface runs the sacral crest, composed of three or four remnants of the spinous processes. The laminae of the lowermost vertebra (and sometimes its neighbour) fail to fuse; the resultant gap is the sacral hiatus (Fig. 68.15). The hiatus is bounded laterally by the sacral cornu (these are the remnants of the inferior articular processes of the fifth sacral vertebra) and covered by the sacrococcygeal membrane. This membrane is pierced by the coccygeal and fifth sacral nerves; the first four sacral nerves leave the sacrum through the paired lateral sacral foramina along the length of the sacrum. The dural sac terminates at the level of the lower border of S2 and below this the canal contains a venous plexus (continuation of the internal vertebral plexus), the filum terminale (continuation of the pia mater), the sacral nerves and fatty tissue. The mean total volume of the canal is 32 ml in females and 34 ml in males.

The anatomy of the sacrum and the sacral canal is *extremely variable*, especially in adults. Most of the abnormalities are readily observable or palpable but they contribute to the less-than-100% success rate seen with this block.

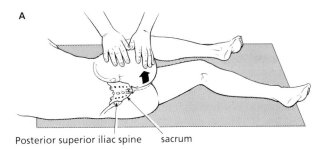

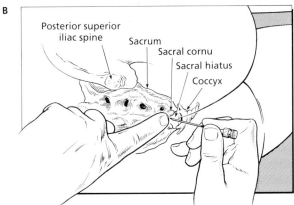

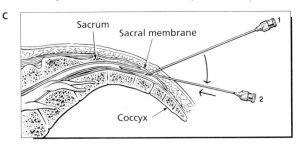

Fig. 68.15 Caudal extradural block. (A) In the lateral Sim's position, an assistant may be required to reposition the gluteal cleft in the midline. (B) Palpation of the sacral hiatus and sacral cornua must not be confused with the sacral foramina. The hiatus should form an equilateral triangle with the posterior superior iliac spines. (C) Initial angle of needle insertion should be about 120° to the skin. After penetration of the sacral (sacrococcygeal) membrane the needle is aligned with the long axis of the canal and inserted 1 cm further. (Redrawn from Cousins & Bridenbaugh, 1988.)

Technique

The patient and anaesthetist should be prepared as for extradural or spinal anaesthesia. The usual position of the patient is lateral with hips and knees flexed (Fig. 68.15A), but alternatives are prone (with a pillow under the hips and toes turned in) and the knee—elbow position. The sacral hiatus must be readily palpable. It lies 3.5—5 cm above the tip of the coccyx and at the apex of the triangle formed by it and the posterior superior iliac spine. Lying between the cornu, it often feels triangular in shape. A small weal of local anaesthetic is raised over this point (too much local anaesthetic and the landmarks are obscured). A short bevelled 22- or 25-gauge needle is inserted at an angle of about 20° to the skin at that point (Fig. 68.15B). The sacrococcygeal membrane is very superficial and a definite 'give' is often felt as it is pierced. The needle is aligned with the anticipated long axis of the canal and advanced no more than 2.5 cm (Fig. 68.15C). In adults, the mean distance from sacrococcygeal membrane to dura is 4.5 cm, but it may be much less and aspiration for CSF must precede injection. It is not unusual for the aspiration to reveal blood (there is a rich venous plexus) and the needle should be repositioned. The local anaesthetic should be injected at the rate appropriate to extra-dural administration (no more than 10 ml/min), and injection of a test dose is recommended. Caudal extradural injection requires very little force. If it does, the needle tip may be deep into the periosteal dura or even within a vertebra. Injection may be easy, but superficial to the sacrococcygeal membrane or within a sacral foramina ('decoy hiatus'). During injection, the free hand can be used to palpate for swelling on the back of the sacrum associated with misplaced injections. After careful aspiration, a test dose of 5 ml of air may be used, palpation being performed to check for superficial crepitus. Another test of placement called the 'Whoosh test' has recently been described, whereby 2 ml of air is injected whilst listening with a stethoscope over the thoracolumbar region for the characteristic 'Whoosh' (Lewis et al., 1992).

A Tuohy needle can be used to place a catheter for continuous techniques. They are often difficult to thread because of the variations in diameter and direction of the sacral canal; an alternative is to insert an intravenous cannula.

Indications

Operations on the perineum are the main indication although the technique is useful for providing post-operative pain control. The use of caudal block in obstetrics and paediatrics is discussed in Chapters 47 and 43, respectively.

Drugs

The choice is dependent on the duration of analgesia required. The absorption, disposition, etc., are similar to that of extradural blocks performed higher up the spine. Typically, 15–20 ml may be expected to block to L1. Lignocaine 1 or 2% with adrenaline or bupivacaine 0.5% provide anaesthesia, whereas bupivacaine 0.25% is adequate for postoperative pain control. Injection of large volumes to increase spread is not recommended. A large and variable amount of the injectate leaks out through the sacral foramina (occasionally visible) and this limits the height of block attained. During injection there should be repeated attempts to aspirate the syringe as the needle tip may have been moved. Direct intravascular injection or rapid absorption of local anaesthetic promoted by rapid forceful injection may result in convulsions or cardiac arrest.

Physiology of spinal subarachnoid and extradural block

Physiological changes may result from:
1 Consequences of neural block — produced mostly by sympathetic block, but sensory and motor block are not wholly benign.
2 Consequences of vascular absorption of drugs used — produced usually by the local anaesthetic agent, but the vasoconstrictor may also have deleterious effects. These consequences are summarized in Table 68.10.

Cardiovascular effects

The sympathetic outflow of the cord is from T1 to L2. Therefore, a block below L2 has little effect on arterial pressure. Block about T2 affects not only sympathetic vasoconstrictor fibres, but also the sympathetic inner-vation of the heart (T1−4). There may still be sympathetic tone below the block, as tracts within the cord are still functioning (note that spinal and extradural anaesthesia does not produce chemical transection of the cord). The majority of spinal and extradural anaesthetics produce effects that lie between these two extremes and have variable effects on the cardio-vascular system (CVS). A block to T10 produces only 'peripheral' sympathetic block and has little effect on the CVS. At this level, only inguinal, perineal and lower limb surgery may be undertaken. Lower ab-dominal surgery (e.g. appendicectomy, Caesarean section and gynaecological surgery) necessitate block to T4.

A small decrease in arterial pressure usually occurs, but the reported incidence of significant hypotension [defined variously as an arterial pressure decrease of greater than 4 kPa (30 mmHg), 20% or 30% of initial pressure] ranges from approximately 3−30%. Obviously the height of block is important but the

Table 68.10 Physiological effects of extradural block. (Redrawn from Cousins & Bridenbaugh, 1988)

Vascular absorption of local anaesthetic or adrenaline	Direct neural blocking effects or indirect results of block
Receptor Beta-stimulation by adrenaline Alpha-stimulation by adrenaline or phenylephrine	*Spinal nerves* (roots and trunks) by axonal block Sympathetic 　Efferent block 　　Peripheral (T1−L2) vasoconstrictor
Smooth muscle Blood vessels, local anaesthetic or adrenaline Heart, local anaesthetic or adrenaline Other organs, local anaesthetic or adrenaline	'Adrenal' (T6−L1) 　　'Central' (T1−4) cardiac sympathetic Sensory 　Afferent block 　　Reduced peripheral sensation
Cardiac muscle By local anaesthetic or adrenaline	Block of visceral pain fibres 　　Reduced efferent neurohumoral responses 　　　to surgical or other stimulus within the blocked area Motor
Neural tissue CNS, by local anaesthetic Conducting system of heart by local anaesthetic	Efferent block 　　Varying degrees of motor paralysis 　　Reflex muscle relaxation without paralysis (deafferentation)
Miscellaneous Neuromuscular junction by local anaesthetic	*Spinal cord* Axons 　Superficial, sensory tracts blocked (e.g. bupivacaine, 　　lignocaine and etidocaine) 　Deep motor paths blocked (e.g. etidocaine) 　　Dorsal horn modulation of pain 　　　transmission (? axons, ? cells) 　　Possibility of 'antianalgesic' effect owing to block of 　　　inhibitory paths Cell bodies: 'selective' block *Secondary changes in parasympathetic activity* Sympathetic block to T5 ↓ venous return may → ↓ vagus Sympathetic block to T1 → unopposed vagus

'category of risk' is also a major factor. There are no data to suggest that hypotension occurs less frequently with extradural or spinal anaesthesia. The level of sympathetic block is the same as (or lower than) sensory with extradural block. In comparison, sympathetic block may be two to three segments higher than sensory level with subarachnoid block.

Vascular absorption of local anaesthetic and vasoconstrictor agent may result in significant haemodynamic changes after extradural but not subarachnoid block. The reason for this lies predominantly in the much larger doses of drugs used and the proximity of the large extradural veins. The more gradual onset of sympathetic block after extradural analgesia compared with subarachnoid block may provide a mechanism for initial responses that are less severe for extradural block. When used extradurally, lignocaine, chloroprocaine and etidocaine have a rapid onset of sympathetic block (especially etidocaine). This is more evident if adrenaline-containing solutions are used. In comparison, onset of sympathetic block is slower with bupivacaine and there is less tendency for rapid development of hypotension. Indeed, sympathetic block may take 25−30 min to develop and even then may be only partial. Animal studies have shown that autoregulation at the level of the precapillary sphincters develops within 30 min of complete ablation of neural activity.

Although controlled studies are not available, experience with large series of thoracic extradural blocks administered in intensive therapy units by continuous catheter techniques supports further the allowance of adequate time for autoregulation. A common management protocol for 'topping up' thoracic extradural block for chest trauma involves keeping the patient supine during, and for 20−30 min after top-up. Using this procedure, serious hypotension is uncommon, whereas topping up in the semi-recumbent position or allowing inadequate time in the supine position after block may result in large reductions in arterial pressure. With continuous extradural infusions, it is only necessary to lie the patient flat while the loading dose is given.

Block below T4

Block restricted to the level of the low thoracic and lumbar region (T5–L4) results in a peripheral sympathetic block with vascular dilatation in the pelvis and lower limbs. If all splanchnic fibres are blocked (T6–L1), pooling of blood in the gut and abdominal viscera may also occur. The peripheral block is manifest as an increase in lower limb blood flow by arteriolar vasodilatation, and pooling of blood in the venous capacitance vessels. Because the latter contain 80% of blood volume, venodilatation has a potential for dramatic changes in venous return, reduction in right atrial pressure and reduced cardiac output. The decrease in venous return has been shown to result in increased vagal tone in young patients. This explains why heart rate remains unchanged or decreased despite hypotension and activation of cardiac sympathetic accelerator fibres.

The patient may compensate for a decrease in mean arterial pressure with a reflex increase in efferent sympathetic vasoconstriction above the level of the block. Thus, blood flow and venous capacitance are reduced in the head, neck and upper limbs. This increased efferent sympathetic activity is mediated predominantly (by means of the baroreceptor) by those sympathetic vasoconstrictor nerves (T1–5) that remain unblocked, and by circulating catecholamines released from the adrenal medulla due to the increased activity in any unblocked fibres in the splanchnic nerves (T6–L1). Although blood vessels in some viscera, such as the kidney, appear to be more responsive to direct neural stimuli, in other vascular beds both neural and hormonal influences have major effects, although at different levels of the vasculature. Major arterioles respond mostly to neural stimuli, while small arterioles and venules near the capillary bed respond predominantly to circulating catecholamines. Thus, while any splanchnic fibres remain unblocked, there is a potential for vasoconstrictor activity below (and above) the level of block, by release of catecholamines from the adrenal medulla. Finally, the ability of precapillary sphincters to achieve autoregulation within a short time of cessation of neural activity provides a further mechanism for regaining vascular tone and minimizing vascular pooling below the level of block.

Increased activity in unblocked cardiac sympathetic fibres (T1–4) may result in increased cardiac contractility and increased heart rate. Similar effects are produced by increased levels of circulating catecholamines. Evidence that the latter are important in maintaining homeostasis in some clinical situations is provided by the surprisingly small changes in heart rate and cardiac output (−16%) with block of C5–T4, but with splanchnic fibres to the adrenal medulla (T6–L1) intact. Although quite large compensatory cardiac effects may be observed in unmedicated volunteers (e.g. a 20% increase in heart rate and cardiac output), these changes are not seen in premedicated patients. In premedicated patients, despite decreased peripheral resistance, unchanged heart rate and cardiac output, mean arterial pressure was reduced by only 10%, because total vascular resistances decreased by only 25% as a result of increased sympathetic activity in unblocked areas. The studies by Germann and colleagues (1979) and others reported changes that are close to those that the anaesthetist may anticipate in clinical practice, although patients in the former study were not rehydrated. The practice of 'preloading' with intravenous balanced salt solution is capable of maintaining mean arterial pressure close to preblock levels in healthy patients, including parturients, provided the level of block is below T4 and inferior vena caval obstruction is avoided. Provided bradycardia is avoided, the healthy supine patient may have little change in arterial pressure. Change in position and ill health may have significant CVS sequelae.

Block below T10

With a lower block, fewer vasoconstrictor fibres are included, and neither the splanchnic nerves nor the nerve supply to the adrenal medulla are affected. Thus, the potential for hypotension is reduced.

Block below L2

There is no sympathetic block and all CVS effects are mediated through absorbed local anaesthetic, etc.

Block above T4

In healthy, supine patients there is often surprisingly little effect with a high thoracic block. However, there are no compensatory mechanisms remaining and the anaesthetist must be able to make physiological adjustments rapidly, i.e. control of blood volume, heart rate, vascular tone and cardiac contractile state.

Effects of local anaesthetic solutions on the cardiovascular system

Plain solutions

Whereas the autonomic effects of extradural and spinal block are similar, because of the much larger doses of local anaesthetic used with the former, the CVS consequences of absorbed local anaesthetic are greater. The slow absorption of local anaesthetic from the extradural space has very different effects to rapid inadvertent intravenous injection.

Extradural block with lignocaine results in plasma concentrations of approximately $3-5\,\mu g/ml$ and little effect on the CVS. Bupivacaine and etidocaine are similarly benign with slow injection. When an extradural dose is injected rapidly intravenously, there may be depression of cardiac contractility and intracardiac conduction, which may occasionally lead to cardiac arrest. With lignocaine, the heart responds rapidly to inotropic support, but if bupivacaine has been injected, prolonged vigorous resuscitation, including large doses of adrenaline and possibly bretylium, may be required to reverse any arrhythmia.

Adrenaline-containing solutions

The cardiovascular effects of low-dose adrenaline are different from those of high doses, which produce tachycardia, hypertension and peripheral ischaemia. Systemic effects of doses of adrenaline in the range of $80-130\,\mu g$, as used in extradural block, are a moderate increase in heart rate, increased cardiac output, decreased peripheral resistance and decreased mean arterial pressure. These changes are, however, greater than if adrenaline without local anaesthetic was administered. This may arise because the degree of sympathetic block is more intense (as with analgesia); the spinal adrenaline itself may cause sympathetic block, and the vasodilator β-adrenergic effects of systemically absorbed adrenaline may counteract compensatory vasoconstriction.

Factors which may modify the cardiovascular effects of extradural and spinal block

Hypovolaemia

Major conduction block should be avoided in patients with uncorrected hypovolaemia. In contrast to the mild changes in normovolaemia, large changes in heart rate, cardiac output and arterial pressures occur. These deleterious changes are reduced by: (i) light anaesthesia, suggesting that the sudden CVS collapse seen (precipitated by bradycardia) is a fainting response to decreased venous return mediated by increased vagal tone; and (ii) adrenaline-containing solutions (the absorbed adrenaline maintaining an adequate heart rate and cardiac output).

In hypovolaemia, the myocardium receives a greater proportion of the cardiac output and may be exposed to a higher concentration of absorbed local anaesthetic. Effects of local anaesthetic on the myocardium are accentuated further by acidosis, which frequently coexists with hypovolaemia and hypotension, although acidosis does not affect the distribution of local anaesthetic to the heart (Nancarrow et al., 1987).

Cardiovascular disease

Patients with cardiovascular disease have poor compensatory capacity and are more prone to the risks of hypotension (Hartung et al., 1986).

General anaesthesia

The effect of general anaesthesia on the CVS changes of extradural and subarachnoid anaesthesia is variable and has been little studied. With an extradural block to mid-thoracic level, a reduction in arterial pressure, heart rate and cardiac output may occur. Whilst arterial pressure is increased by improving venous return (lifting the legs, head-down tilt) the administration of ephedrine improves all variables. A relative bradycardia responds to atropine. The sequence of induction of regional and general anaesthesia does not affect these changes (Germann et al., 1979).

Intestinal obstruction, ascites, large intra-abdominal tumours and surgery

All these conditions increase inferior vena caval obstruction and limit the venous return from below the level of obstruction. When sympathetic block is superimposed, there is an increase in the venous pooling and an exaggerated CVS response. Small carefully titrated doses of ephedrine (5–10 mg) restore venous capacitance to a more normal value. Often these conditions also cause a degree of arterial obstruction and when these are relieved during the course of surgery, precipitous hypotension may result if inadequate fluid replacement has been made. Caval obstruction may result from enthusiastic retraction or packing during abdominal surgery or from poor positioning of the patient on the operating table.

Advanced pregnancy and labour

The result of this is caval and aortic compression. The effects are similar to those of intra-abdominal tumours and are discussed in Chapter 47 (see also Fig. 68.9).

Respiratory effects

Extradural or subarachnoid block *per se* have little effect on respiration, provided that brain perfusion is maintained. The potential for phrenic nerve (C3−5) block is extremely low. With a high block, the diminished input to the reticular activating system may lead to a drowsy patient with quiet regular respiration, and the sedative effect of blood concentrations of local anaesthetic associated with extradural block may contribute to this.

Continuous extradural block for pain relief after surgery improves ability to cough and functional residual capacity in addition to Pao_2 (Spence & Smith, 1971). Studies of diaphragmatic activity following upper abdominal surgery report that extradural block maintains activity closer to normal compared with parenteral opioids (Mankikian *et al.*, 1988).

Visceral effects

Block of sacral segments S2−4 results in bladder atonia. It is temporary and causes no, or minimal increase in postblock bladder dysfunction. Segmental thoracic block may increase bladder-sphincter tone by abolishing reflex sympathetic activity (via T12−L1 segments), predisposing to acute retention. With continuous extradural block, urinary catheterization is often necessary.

Extradural and subarachnoid block from T5−L1 abolishes splanchnic sympathetic supply and because of the intact parasympathetic tone, results in a contracted small bowel, with relaxed sphincters; as there is also relaxation of abdominal muscles operating conditions are also good. There is no evidence that anastomoses are threatened by extradural anaesthesia (Ryan *et al.*, 1992).

Major regional block obtunds the hormonal and metabolic responses to surgery. This effect is short-lived and once the block has worn off the changes are similar to those who received general anaesthesia. A block to T5 (which includes a sympathetic block to this level) abolishes the 'neuroendocrine' response to

surgery temporarily. It is not known what, if any, are the long-term consequences of this. In the short term some advantages have been reported, e.g. reduced catecholamine secretion may reduce the incidence of intraoperative myocardial infarction. Continuation of extradural block into the postoperative period modifies some components of the 'stress' response, e.g. reduced urinary nitrogen loss.

Distribution of blood flow

1 Total peripheral vascular resistance decreases with subarachnoid and extradural block (typically 15−18%). This is a result of differential flow through vascular beds.
2 Pooling in denervated venous capacitance vessels occurs below the level of the right atrium.
3 Blood flow to the brain is maintained whilst the arterial pressure remains within the cerebrovascular autoregulatory range.
4 Myocardial oxygenation decreases, but in parallel with myocardial oxygen demand which is reduced by decreased ventricular work; animal studies indicate overall improved oxygen supply versus demand with a reduction in the size of experimentally produced infarction (Reiz *et al.*, 1982; Davis *et al.*, 1986). Blomberg and colleagues (1990) demonstrated improved myocardial nutritive flow by high thoracic extradural analgesia in patients with severe coronary artery disease.
5 Hepatic blood flow is reduced, hepatic oxygen extraction increases, but in the absence of hypotension, hypoxia does not occur.
6 Renal blood flow is maintained by autoregulation, but even during severe hypotension, blood flow is usually adequate to oxygenate renal tissues so that renal function returns to normal as soon as arterial pressures return to normal.

Temperature control

The vasodilatation of extensive extradural block may predispose to hypothermia in a cold environment. However, this reduction in body temperature occurs slowly and does not explain the rapid onset of shivering that sometimes immediately follows the injection of local anaesthetic into the extradural space. Various causes of shivering have been proposed in association with extradural block:
1 A decrease in core temperature as a result of sympathetic block.
2 An effect of absorbed local anaesthetic on temperature regulatory centres.

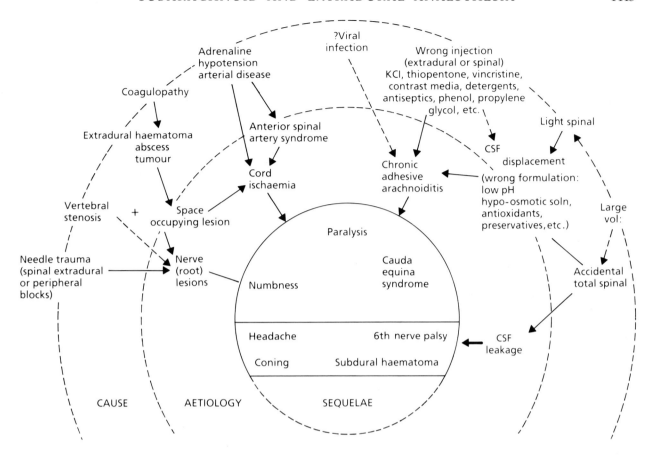

Fig. 68.16 Causation of neurological complications following regional (principally spinal and extradural) block. (Redrawn from Reynolds, 1987.)

3 A differential inhibition of spinal cord afferent thermoreceptor fibres (loss of warm before cold sensation), causing erroneous indication of a reduction in peripheral temperature.

4 A direct effect of cold local anaesthetic solutions on thermosensitive structures within the spinal cord. (Such structures have been demonstrated in animals but not in humans.)

The latter explanation (4) is most likely, although a contribution from one or all of the other factors listed is probable. It has been reported that shivering is more common after bupivacaine, and the slow onset of block would certainly permit a longer period of differential loss of warm sensation with associated shivering.

Neurological deficit

An extensive review has confirmed that the spinal route of administration of local anaesthetic is extremely safe (Kane, 1981). The spinal cord may be damaged by ischaemia, direct trauma or chemicals. Hypotension is the major cause of ischaemia. Consequences vary from absent knee jerks to complete flaccid paralysis. There are often contributing factors such as surgery affecting the cord (e.g. aortic cross-clamping) or vascular lesions, so that all hypotensive episodes must be treated seriously. Trauma and chemicals are infrequent causes of cord damage. However, there is some evidence that local toxicity due to the local anaesthetic caused the cauda equina syndrome cases associated with continuous spinal anaesthesia (see above). In the past, chemicals have been contaminants of local anaesthetic solutions, but they are now administered usually as a result of carelessness. The mechanisms of neurological damage are summarized in Fig. 68.16.

Monitoring for regional block

Venous access with a large-gauge cannula, monitoring of heart rate and arterial pressure are mandatory.

Heart rate should be monitored by ECG before injection of local anaesthetic. Arterial pressure may decrease rapidly and the frequency of measurement should be appropriate for the block. Verbal contact with the patient is a useful monitor of impending problems and complaints, e.g. circumoral tingling, metallic taste or nausea must receive prompt attention. There may be significant changes after repositioning the patient. Oxygenation may be monitored by pulse oximetry. In general, supplemental oxygen should be administered although it may not be necessary for healthy patients with a low level of block.

Sedation

Sedation should be administered carefully. Opioids and benzodiazepines may be used, but these potent drugs are not an alternative to psychological preparation of the patient; 50% oxygen in nitrous oxide (Entonox) by mask is particularly useful.

Management of hypotension

Peripheral venous pooling from sympathetic block reduces preload and hence cardiac output. Myocardial contractility is unchanged by spinal anaesthesia, although it may be reduced after systemic absorption of local anaesthetics from extradural administration. There is controversy over the level to which arterial pressure may decrease before therapy is required; 33% below resting level or an absolute level of 10.6 kPa (80 mmHg) systolic in young, normotensive patients may be safe. In conscious patients, a systolic pressure below 10.6 kPa (80 mmHg) frequently precipitates a vasovagal attack and profound hypotension accompanies the bradycardia, nausea and vomiting. The arterial pressure at which regional cerebral perfusion is compromised is not known but symptoms such as restlessness, breathlessness or nausea may indicate that the critical value has been reached.

Treatment of hypotension comprises restoration of venous return: the Trendelenburg position or elevation of the legs may achieve this, although greater than 20% head-down is counterproductive (and may increase the height of a spinal anaesthetic when a hyperbaric solution is used). Rapid infusion of electrolyte solutions may restore arterial pressure but also increase myocardial oxygen demand in the face of haemodilution, though myocardial flow (and thus myocardial oxygen delivery) may be improved by the resultant reduction in viscosity.

Large infusions of crystalloid may precipitate heart failure or retention of urine when the block regresses. Bradycardia causing hypotension is treated with small doses of atropine, 0.2 mg. When vasopressors are required, drugs with both α- and β-adrenergic effects (e.g. ephedrine) are used to induce vasoconstriction and increase cardiac output (in contrast to pure α-agonist). Vigilant monitoring is required to avoid sudden changes of arterial pressure occurring with position (e.g. lithotomy to supine) both in the operating room and recovery area.

Postdural puncture headache

All patients undergoing spinal anaesthesia should be warned of PDPH. The headache, which may be incapacitating, is bifrontal and occipital and may involve the neck and upper shoulders. It is aggravated by sitting, standing, coughing and straining but subsides completely when the patient lies down. It is often accompanied by nausea, anorexia, photophobia, diplopia, vertigo, neck stiffness and, on rare occasions, cranial nerve palsies. However, serious complications may occur including subdural haematoma (Reid & Thorburn, 1991; Whiteley et al., 1993), and death from medullary and tentorial coning has been reported (Eerola et al., 1981; Hart et al., 1988).

PDPH usually occurs within the first 3 days of puncture and may persist for several weeks or even months causing depression in the patient and anxiety in the anaesthetist. PDPH is thought to be caused by leakage of CSF through a hole in the dura as first suggested by Bier (1899). A compensatory mechanism of reflex cerebral vasodilatation may also cause pain.

The pressure gradient between the subarachnoid and extradural space in the sitting position is approximately 50 cm of water, therefore CSF will pass from the subarachnoid to the extradural space as long as the hole in the dura persists. The rate of CSF loss is therefore dependent on the position of the patient, the size of hole in the dura and the rate of CSF production.

The result of CSF loss is reduced CSF volume and decreased CSF pressure. When sitting or standing, the brain tends to descend as it is deprived of its fluid cushion. Traction occurs in the pain-sensitive meningeal vessels and venous sinuses.

There is a decreasing incidence of PDPH with age, presumably as a result of reduced escape of CSF from the extradural space, increasing extradural pressure, decreasing pain sensitivity and some loss of distensibility of the cerebral pain-sensitive structures. It has been shown by Rasmussen and colleagues (1989) that in elderly patients, the incidence of PDPH is independent of needle size.

It is well known that PDPH is commonest in young women. The incidence and severity is related to the size of the needle puncturing the dura. Headache is common in pregnant patients and one study showed that after subarachnoid anaesthesia, only 33% of headaches were due to PDPH. Twenty-five percent of these were severe (Brownridge, 1984). The reported incidence following subarachnoid anaesthesia varies between 1% and 30% (Gielen, 1989).

The incidence of headache is proportional to the gauge of needle used; rare after dural puncture with a 25-gauge needle, more frequent with 22-gauge needle and common with 18- or 16-gauge extradural needles. Thinner needles make smaller holes. It is not surprising that the greatest incidence (around 70%) of PDPH occurs in obstetric patients whose dura is inadvertently punctured by a large-gauge extradural needle (Crawford, 1980). The incidence of accidental dural puncture during the extradural technique can, with proper training, be reduced to under 0.5% (Reynolds, 1993; Stride & Cooper, 1993).

With subarachnoid anaesthesia, design of the needle tip has an important influence on the incidence of PDPH. Lybecker and colleagues (1990) have suggested that bevel direction parallel to dural fibres may also be important in reducing the incidence of PDPH. Comparative studies have shown that fewer PDPHs occur using Whitacre needles than Quincke needles, despite the larger gauge of the former (Lynch et al., 1992; Shutt et al., 1992). Noel (1990) performing subarachnoid anaesthesia by the paramedian approach with a 22-gauge Whitacre needle reported only one PDPH in a series of 300 patients. Sprotte and colleagues (1987) introduced the 'atraumatic' needle and reported an incidence of PDPH of less than 1%. Ross and colleagues (1992) comparing the use of the 24-gauge Sprotte needle with the 25- and 26-gauge Quincke needles in obstetric anaesthesia showed a PDPH rate of 1.5% in the Sprotte group and 9% and 8% in the 25- and 26-gauge Quincke groups, respectively. Cesarini and colleagues (1990) in a similar study found no PDPH in their Sprotte group and a rate of 14.5% in the 25-gauge Quincke group. In fact, Mayer and colleagues (1992) did not show any difference between the 24-gauge Sprotte and the 27-gauge Quincke needles as regards PDPH, emphasizing the importance of tip design.

Bedrest for 24–48 h postpones the onset, but has no effect on the incidence of PDPH. It is usually self-limiting and control of symptoms is usually achieved by bedrest, and regular administration of simple analgesics. Caffeine (Ford et al., 1989), with its cerebral vasoconstrictor effect, and also vasopressin may prove useful in the treatment of PDPH. Therapies aimed at increasing extradural pressure (e.g. extradural infusion of saline and tight abdominal binding), increasing CSF production (e.g. overhydration of the patient by intravenous or oral fluids at a rate of at least 3 litres/day) and decreasing CSF loss (e.g. by lying flat) are helpful. However, care must be taken to ensure that more serious conditions (see above) are not being masked.

The definitive treatment for severe or refractory headache unresponsive to conservative treatment is extradural injection of autologous blood (extradural 'blood-patch') (Di Giovanni & Dunbar, 1970). Ten to 20 ml of non-anticoagulated autologous blood obtained under aseptic conditions is injected into the extradural space. The success rate is around 90–95% after the first injection and has only a few mild complications of its own (e.g. backache 35%, fever 5%) when infection is avoided. If a PDPH follows accidental dural puncture with a Tuohy needle, then, in the absence of any contraindication, it should be treated promptly with a 'blood patch'.

In conclusion, as Quincke needles are cheap, their use in the elderly patient is probably appropriate because the incidence of PDPH is low. However, in young patients, because of the higher incidence of PDPH, the use of a 24-gauge Sprotte needle (or similar) is beneficial.

Spinal opioids

The spinal route of administration of opioids produces a more selective effect on nocioception than the axonal block of several modalities resulting from local anaesthetics. This method of pain control has developed logically, although the concept progressed rapidly from fundamental experiments in animals to humans (Cousins & Mather, 1984). The 'gate theory of pain' proposed by Melzack and Wall (1965) suggested that pain could be modulated at the spinal cord level. Yaksh and Rudy (1976) reported profound analgesia in rats following spinal administration of opioids. Only 3 years later, reports of subarachnoid and extradural opioid administrations to control cancer pain appeared; prolonged analgesia was obtained with doses a fraction of those used systemically. The first rigorous study of spinal extradural opioid administration for postoperative pain control (Cousins et al., 1979) confirmed that the spinal cord is the site of action and that the systemic blood drug concentration was insufficient to produce analgesia.

The difference in concentration between CSF and blood are high after extradural administration ranging from 50:1 to 200:1 (depending on the opioid and dose), and even higher after subarachnoid dosing. A 0.5 mg subarachnoid morphine dose is huge when compared with the calculated 10 μg which reaches the CNS after an i.m. 10-mg dose, yet despite this, analgesia is not total. Two reasons are suggested to explain this phenomenon. First, a significant proportion of opioid-induced analgesia is mediated through supraspinal opioid receptors (i.e. periaqueductal grey-matter neurones in the midbrain, nucleus raphe magnus and rostral ventral medulla).

Second, spinal opioids through their action pre- and postsynaptically on small cell networks in the dorsal horn, control pain of a constant ongoing nature (e.g. deep and dull forms of somatic pain) better than pain of phasic nature (e.g. sharp pain of acute injury and intermittent visceral injury), where large numbers of afferent neurones are recruited rapidly. In practice, this is manifest as the high success rate seen with spinal opioids for control of cancer pain, some success in postoperative pain and poor results with the pain of surgery, acute labour and primary neurological disease.

There are advantages in combining opioids with local anaesthetics for analgesia via the extradural route. Infusion of bupivacaine 0.125% with fentanyl 5 μg/ml at a rate of 4–7 ml/h generally provides good-quality postoperative analgesia for thoracic and abdominal procedures, with little motor block and little risk of respiratory depression. This enables the patient to cough and cooperate with physiotherapy. Also, as mentioned above, clonidine (α_2-agonist) has been used by both spinal routes and appears to prolong analgesia when used in combination with either opioid, or local anaesthetic agents (Bonnet et al., 1990; Rostaing et al., 1991).

Pharmacology

The distribution of opioids injected spinally is very similar to local anaesthetics. *In vitro* studies suggest the permeability of the dura to opioids varies inversely with the square root of the molecular weight of the drug, but molecular weight is not more important than lipid solubility. *In vivo* transfer of opioid to CNS may occur also by spinal cord blood vessels and by diffusion through the dural-cuff region of neurones. Thus, there is interplay of many physicochemical properties of the agent.

Opioid in the CSF (injected into the subarachnoid or diffused from the extradural space) penetrates the spinal meninges and is taken up by the outer layers of the spinal cord at a rate proportional to the lipid solubility of the agent. For analgesia at a spinal level, both superficial and deeper opioid receptors (i.e. Lamina I and II of the dorsal horn) need to be reached by opioid. Thus, even with spinal subarachnoid injection of morphine, there is a delay of 30 min before full effect is achieved. As with local anaesthetics, vascular uptake is the route of elimination from the CSF and this is proportional to lipid solubility. Thus, lipophilic opioids have the most rapid onset of spinal effect, but are the most rapidly eliminated. Various opioids have been tested by both spinal routes and clinical practice has revealed clear differences between morphine and the 'fentanyl-like' compounds.

Opioids can spread in the spinal subarachnoid space both as a result of diffusion and bulk transport by the circulation of CSF. Because lipophilicity promotes agent uptake, this property is inversely proportional to the cephalad spread of drug within the CSF. It is cephalad spread that allows lumbar administration of morphine to be used in upper-abdominal and thoracic surgery. However, migration of drug to the brain is responsible for most of the serious side-effects.

In opioid-naive subjects, spinal opioids result in a high incidence of non-segmental itching (after about 3 h following lumbar extradural injection of morphine). Nausea and vomiting is a frequent occurrence several hours after injection. The most serious side-effect is delayed respiratory depression, which may be delayed for 3–12 h with morphine, and is presumed to be a result of opioid reaching the brain. Early respiratory depression may occur 0–1 h after extradural or direct subarachnoid injection of lipophilic opioids such as pethidine (see below), alfentanil and even fentanyl. As vascular uptake competes with CNS uptake, it is not surprising that adrenaline enhances analgesia. Adrenaline has inherent analgesic properties at the spinal cord level but delays drug elimination from the CSF also. A consequence of this is more free opioid in the CSF and intensified respiratory depression. Receptor kinetics interplay with lipid solubility. Thus sufentanil has a longer duration of action (approximately 6 h) than fentanyl (2.5–3 h) which, although less lipid soluble, has less intense binding.

As cephalad transport of drug is responsible for the most serious yet unpredictable side-effect of spinal opioids, the more lipophilic agents should be safer. The question of relative safety of morphine (hydrophilic opioid) and pethidine (lipophilic opioid) has been examined in studies to determine the pharmacokinetics of the two agents after both routes of spinal administration (Sjöström et al., 1987a,b). After extradural or subarachnoid administration, peak plasma concentrations of both drugs are attained within 10 min. Pethidine crosses the dura four times faster than morphine, thus the lipophilic drug achieves its peak CSF concentration four times more rapidly than the hydrophilic agent. Similarly, CSF pethidine concentration decreases four times more rapidly than morphine concentration. However, only 4% of the dose of either drug reaches the CSF. The rapid decline in pethidine CSF concentration suggests cephalad transport is unlikely although significant concentrations can be measured at the C7–T1 level 1 h after lumbar administration (Gourlay et al., 1987). It would therefore appear that respiratory depression following pethidine should occur early (at approximately 1 h) and be produced both by systemic absorption and migration in CSF. Some other afferent and motor activity may be affected in addition to block of nocioception and there can be difficulty in initiating micturition leading to urinary retention. This complication has been reported to occur in up to 90% of males given extradural morphine. Pethidine has a marked local anaesthetic action (Way, 1946) and when administered intrathecally can produce segmental somatic block (Famewo & Naguib, 1985).

Spinal opioids in control of acute pain

Postoperative pain

Spinal opioids alone or in combination with local anaesthetic agents can be extremely effective in postoperative pain therapy. There is a plethora of conflicting reports and opinions on which drug, dose and site of injection is best. If the opioid is injected in the middle of the required dermatomal spread, speed of onset of analgesia is determined by the physicochemical properties of the drug. If the opioid is injected distant to the required site of action, onset is related to transport of drugs in the CSF and this may take several hours (Larsen et al., 1985). A larger dose may shorten onset but increases the risk of complications.

There have been few comparisons between drugs and fewer using equipotent doses. Onset of analgesia seems to be slow for morphine (30 min to 1 h), but is similar for most other opioids. Duration of action varies significantly, e.g. morphine (6 mg) 12.3 h,

methadone (6 mg) 8.7 h, fentanyl (100 µg) 5.7 h (Torda & Pybus, 1982).

These figures are not as comparable as it may seem, as doses which are equipotent when given intravenously may not have the same ratio of potency by other routes, e.g. morphine, 4 mg, extradurally is not as effective as methadone, 4 mg. Also, duration of effect is somewhat dose dependent, extradural morphine, 5 mg, 7.5 mg, 10 mg, are all effective after lower-abdominal surgery but the incidence of side-effects is higher with larger doses. A table suggesting initial doses for extradural morphine for postoperative pain has been prepared by Ready and colleagues (1988) (Table 68.11). Subsequent doses should be adjusted after observation of degree of analgesia obtained and the severity of any side-effects (Cousins, 1987). An alternative to morphine is the administration of short-acting opioids with rapid onset by infusion. This technique permits flexibility of the drug administration rate and may avoid 'late' respiratory depression after cessation of therapy. Individualization of dose is stressed: dose–response data suggest that the ratio between analgesic dose and the dose causing life-threatening respiratory depression of spinally administered opioids may be close to two! (Cousins et al., 1988).

There have been no controlled studies comparing spinal subarachnoid and extradural opioids; it appears that the quality of analgesia by the two routes is similar, but using much smaller doses with spinal subarachnoid injection. Unfortunately, ventilatory depression is more common with spinal subarachnoid opioids (Rawal et al., 1987).

The quality of analgesia obtainable with carefully titrated parenteral opioids (e.g. by patient-controlled analgesia) is similar to that from extradural opioids

Table 68.11 Suggested starting dose (mg) of spinal extradural morphine for incisional pain.* (Data from Ready et al., 1988)

Patient age (years)	Non-thoracic surgery (lumbar or caudal catheter)	Thoracic surgery	
		Thoracic catheter	Lumbar catheter
15–44	5	4	6
45–65	4	3	5
66–75	3	2	4
76+	2	1	2

These doses are guidelines only. Safety and effectiveness of these doses may vary considerably between individual patients.
* Undiluted 0.1% preservative-free morphine is used.

but the profile of side-effects is dissimilar. The extra-dural route, however, requires less drug for the same effect and patients are therefore less sedated. Respiratory depression is dose dependent with the parenteral dosing, but is less predictable with the spinal route. However, since the introduction of smaller extradural doses and 'low-dose extradural infusions', respiratory depression has become much rarer.

The Swedish Nationwide Follow-up Survey (Rawal et al., 1987) revealed an incidence of ventilatory depression of approximately 1:1100 (0.09%) after extradural morphine and 1:275 (0.36%) following spinal subarachnoid morphine. This survey includes all patients receiving subarachnoid opioids. If only postoperative patients are studied, the incidence is higher. The study identified old age, poor general condition and the residual effects of anaesthetic drugs as important risk factors for this complication but more than 50% of patients treated for delayed ventilatory depression had received supplementary local anaesthetic. Naloxone readily reverses the respiratory depression, but obviously patients must be managed in a ward where the condition can be recognized. Measuring respiratory rate alone is a poor monitor. Early warning of problems ahead can be obtained from monitoring mental state also. When there has been a sudden deterioration in the conscious level, and/or reduction in respiratory rate, careful titration of naloxone can reverse the adverse effects of the opioid without removing the analgesia.

Ventilatory depression can occur 23 h after spinal subarachnoid opioid administration and may still be 16 h after extradural injection. It has been suggested that when doses of morphine, 4 mg or less, are administered extradurally, surveillance is only necessary for 12 h (Rawal et al., 1987).

Labour pain

Although the first-stage pain can be controlled with extradural opioids alone, active labour cannot. The addition of an opioid to local anaesthetic allows a lower concentration of local anaesthetic to have the desired effect and can abolish the shivering often seen with the local anaesthetic alone: fentanyl, 50–100 µg, or pethidine, 50 mg, in bupivacaine 0.25% are effective (Vella et al., 1985). Mixtures of opioid and local anaesthetic have also been used with success in patients undergoing Caesarean section (Noble et al., 1991). However, respiratory monitoring of the mother should be performed, and if opioids are given before delivery, respiratory monitoring of the neonate is required as well.

Spinal subarachnoid opioids have a high incidence of side-effects (vomiting, urinary retention and itching) when used in labour.

Chronic pain

Spinal opioids can be effective when satisfactory control is not possible by other routes. Their role is controversial and there is only anecdotal evidence that patients who 'fail' with oral opioids obtain better relief from the spinal route. Morphine is administered usually, and 5–10 mg is the usual initial dose range extradurally. Ventilatory depression is not a reported feature of chronic dosing. A physiological explanation lies in the rapid tolerance of brain-stem nuclei to increasing doses of opioids. In in vitro preparations of cells from the locus coereleus (LC), spontaneous discharge of cells can be silenced with morphine. Cells in the LC pretreated with morphine require a manyfold increase in applied morphine to have their activity depressed (Andrade et al., 1983). Fortuitously, tolerance in the more caudad nociceptive circuitry develops much more slowly.

Repeat administration of opioid is possible either through conventional transcutaneous extradural catheters (usually tunnelled to reduce infection risk) or through totally implanted systems requiring repeated percutaneous dosing. Administration through either may be by boluses or continuous infusion. The extradural route is used most frequently because of the absence of dural puncture and hence lower incidence of PDPH and the hope that dura is a barrier to infection. However, spinal subarachnoid administration requires less opioid, migration of catheter tip does not have dangerous sequelae and there is a lower incidence of pain on injection. There is no evidence for the superiority of one route over the other. Totally implanted pump systems such as the 'Infusaid' or 'Synchromed' have been used with spinal subarachnoid catheters most commonly, but may also be used with extradural catheters.

Dose requirements vary widely and generally 'tolerance' develops, necessitating increased doses. Large doses of morphine may give rise to distressing localized convulsive muscle movement and even hyperaesthesia (Yaksh et al., 1986). In clinical practice, tolerance which has developed at the spinal level can be reversed by 'resting' the receptors by administering spinal local anaesthetic or another spinal analgesic drug such as clonidine for a few days. After the receptors are 'rested', spinal opioids can be recommenced at a much lower dose.

Many substances are analgesically active when

administered spinally, e.g. baclofen, calcitonin and dexmedetomidine (a specific α_2-agonist). These are experimental findings useful in deducing pain pathways associated with neurotransmission (Jordan, 1984) but are not recommended at present for routine clinical use until careful studies of neurotoxity, therapeutic index, etc. are available.

Rather than 'flogging' one pain pathway, coadministration of opioids and non-opioids is being studied. Opioid/local anaesthetic mixtures are extremely effective, and in the future non-opioid spinal analgesic agents such as clonidine may be added to spinal opioids or alternated with spinal opioids, as tolerance develops to each drug in turn.

References

Andrade R., Vandermaden C.P. & Aghajanian G.K. (1983) Morphine tolerance and dependence in the locus caeruleus: single cell studies in brain slices. *European Journal of Pharmacology* **91**, 161–9.

Attygalle D. & Rodrigo N. (1985) Control of spinal blockade. A volume expansion technique with hyperbaric cinchocaine. *Anaesthesia* **40**, 1006–8.

Barker A.E. (1908) A report on experiences with spinal anaesthesia in 100 cases. *British Medical Journal* **7**, 453–5.

Bengtsson M., Lofstrom J.B. & Malmquist L.A. (1985) Skin conductance responses during spinal anaesthesia. *Acta Anesthesiologica Scandinavica* **29**, 67–71.

Bier A. (1899) Versuche uber Cocainisirung des Ruckenmarkes. *Dtsch Z Chir* **51**, 361.

Blomberg S., Emanuelsson H., Kuist H., Lamm C., Pontén J., Waagstein F. & Ricksten S. (1990) Effects of thoracic epidural anaesthesia on coronary arteries and arterioles in patients with coronary artery disease. *Anesthesiology* **73**, 840–7.

Blumgart C.H., Ryall D., Dennison B. & Thompson-Hill L.M. (1992) Mechanism of extension of spinal anaesthesia by extradural injection of local anaesthetic. *British Journal of Anaesthesia* **69**, 457–60.

Bonnet F., Buisson V.B., Francois Y. & Saada M. (1990) Effects of oral and subarachnoid clonidine on spinal anesthesia. *Regional Anaesthesia* **15**, 211–44.

Bromage P.R. (1953) The 'hanging-drop' sign. *Anaesthesia* **8**, 237–41.

Bromage P.R. (1974) Lower limb reflex changes in segmental epidural analgesia. *British Journal of Anaesthesia* **46**, 504–8.

Bromage P.R. (1978) *Epidural Analgesia*. W.B. Saunders, Philadelphia.

Bromage P.R., Joyal A.C. & Binney J.C. (1963) Local anaesthetic drugs: penetration from the spinal extradural space into the neuraxis. *Science* **140**, 392–4.

Bromage P.R., Burfoot M.F., Crowel D.E. & Truant A.P. (1967) Quality of epidural blockade III: carbonated local anaesthetic solutions. *British Journal of Anaesthesia* **39**, 197–209.

Bromage P.R., Pettigrew R.T. & Crowell D.E. (1969) Tachyphylaxis in epidural analgesia. I. Augmentation and decay of local anaesthesia. *Journal of Clinical Pharmacology* **9**, 30–8.

Brown D.T., Morrison D.H., Covino B.G. & Scott D.B. (1980) Comparison of carbonated bupivacaine and bupivacaine hydrochloride for extradural anaesthesia. *British Journal of Anaesthesia* **52**, 419–22.

Brownridge P. (1981) Epidural and subarachnoid analgesia for elective Caesarean section. *Anaesthesia* **36**, 70.

Brownridge P. (1984) Spinal anaesthesia revisited: an evaluation of subarachnoid block in obstetrics. *Anaesthesia and Intensive Care* **12**, 334–42.

Bryce-Smith R. (1950) Pressures in the extradural space. *Anaesthesia* **5**, 213–16.

Burm A.G.C., van Kleef J.W., Gladines M.P.R.R., Oltof G. & Spierdijk J. (1986) Epidural anaesthesia with lidocaine and bupivacaine. *Anesthesia and Analgesia* **65**, 1281–4.

Cesarini M., Torrielli R., Lahaye F., Mene J.M. & Cabiro C. (1990) Sprotte needle for intrathecal anaesthesia for Cesarean section: incidence of postdural puncture headache. *Anaesthesia* **45**, 656–8.

Coates M.B. (1982) Combined subarachnoid and epidural techniques. *Anaesthesia* **37**, 89–90.

Cope R.W. (1954) The Woolley and Roe case: Woolley and Roe versus Ministry of Health and others. *Anaesthesia* **9**, 249–70.

Cousins M.J. (1987) Comparative pharmacokinetics of spinal opioids in humans: a step towards determination of relative safety. *Anesthesiology* **67**, 875–6.

Cousins M.J. & Bridenbaugh P.O. (Eds) (1988) *Neural Blockade in Clinical Anaesthesia and Management of Pain* 2nd edn. J.B. Lippincott, Philadelphia.

Cousins M.J. & Mather L.E. (1984) Intrathecal and epidural administration of opioids. *Anesthesiology* **61**, 276–310.

Cousins M.J., Mather L.E., Glynn C.J., Wilson P.R. & Graham J.R. (1979) Selective spinal analgesia. *Lancet* **i**, 1141–2.

Cousins M.R., Cherry D.A. & Gourlay G.K. (1988) Acute and chronic pain: use of spinal opioids. In *Neural Blockade in Clinical Anaesthesia and the Management of Pain* 2nd edn. (Eds Cousins M.J. & Bridenbaugh P.O.) pp. 955–1029. J.B. Lippincott, Philadelphia.

Crawford J.S. (1980) Experiences with epidural blood patch. *Anaesthesia* **35**, 513–15.

Curelaru I. (1979) Long duration subarachnoid anaesthesia with continuous epidural block. *Wjederbelbung und Intensivetherapie* **14**, 71–8.

Davis R.F., De Boer W.V. & Maroko P.R. (1986) Thoracic epidural anesthesia reduces myocardial infarct size after coronary artery occlusion in dogs. *Anesthesia and Analgesia* **65**, 711–17.

Denny N., Masters R., Pearson D., Read J., Sihota M. & Selander D. (1987) Postdural puncture headache after continuous spinal anesthesia. *Anesthesia and Analgesia* **66**, 662–5.

DiFazio C.A., Carron H., Grosslight K.R., Moscicki J.C., Bolding W.R. & Johns R.A. (1986) Comparison of pH-adjusted lidocaine solutions for epidural anesthesia. *Anesthesia and Analgesia* **65**, 760–4.

Di Giovanni A.J. & Dunbar B.S. (1970) Epidural injections of autologous blood for postlumbar puncture headache. *Anesthesia and Analgesia* **49**, 268–71.

Douglas M.J., McMorland G.H., Jefferey W.K., Kim J.H.K., Rose P.L., Gambling D.R., Swenerton J.D. & Axelson J.E. (1986) The effect of pH-adjustment of bupivacaine on epidural anesthesia for Cesarean section. *Anesthesiology* **65**, 380A.

Dripps R.D. & Vandam L.D. (1954) Long-term follow-up of

patients who received 10,098 spinal anaesthetics: failure to discover major neurological sequelae. *Journal of the American Medical Association* **156**, 1486–91.

Durant P.A. & Yaksh T.L. (1986) Epidural injections of bupivacaine, morphine, fentanyl, lofentanil and DADL in chronically implanted rats: a pharmacologic and pathologic study. *Anesthesiology* **64**, 43–53.

Eerola M., Kaukinen L. & Kaukinen S. (1981) Fatal brain lesion following spinal anaesthesia. Report of a case. *Acta Anaesthesiologica Scandinavica* **25**, 115–16.

Famewo C.E. & Naguib M. (1985) Spinal anaesthesia with meperidine as the sole agent. *Canadian Anaesthetists' Society Journal* **32**, 533–7.

Ford C.D., Ford D.C. & Koenigsberg M.D. (1989) A simple treatment of post-lumbar-puncture headache. *Journal of Emergency Medicine* **7**, 29–31.

Frumin M.J., Schwartz H., Burns J.J., Brodie B.B. & Papper E.M. (1953) The appearance of procaine in the spinal fluid during peridural block in man. *Journal of Pharmacology and Experimental Therapeutics* **109**, 102–5.

Frumin M.J., Schwartz H., Burns J.J., Brodie B.B. & Papper E.M. (1954) Dorsal root ganglion blockade during threshold segmental anesthesia in man. *Journal of Pharmacology and Experimental Therapeutics* **112**, 387–92.

Galet A., Fleyfel M., Beague D., Vansteenberghe F. & Krivosic-Harber R. (1992) Rachianesthesies accidentelles en milieu obstetrical. Limites de la dose-test peridurale. *Annales Française Anesthesie Reannimation* **11**, 377–80.

Galindo A. (1983) pH-Adjusted local anesthetics: clinical experience. *Regional Anesthesia* **8**, 35–6.

Galindo A., Hermandez J., Benavides O., Ortega de Munoz S. & Bonica J.J. (1975) Quality of spinal extradural analgesia: the influence of spinal nerve root diameter. *British Journal of Anaesthesia* **47**, 41–7.

Gaylard D.G., Wilson I.H. & Balmer H.G.R. (1987) An epidural infusion technique for labour. *Anaesthesia* **42**, 1098–1101.

Germann P.A.S., Roberts J.G. & Prys-Roberts C. (1979) The combination of general anaesthesia and epidural block. I. The effects of sequence of induction on haemodynamic variables and blood gas measurements in healthy patients. *Anaesthesia and Intensive Care* **7**, 229–38.

Geurts J.W., Haanshcoten M.C., Van-Wijk R.M., Kraak H. & Besse T.C. (1990) Post-dural puncture headache in young patients. A comparative study between the use of 0.52 mm (25-gauge) and 0.33 mm (29-gauge) spinal needles. *Acta Anaesthesiologica Scandinavica* **34**, 350–3.

Gielen M. (1989) Post dural puncture headache (PDPH): a review. *Regional Anesthesia* **14**, 101–6.

Giuffrida J.G., Bizzarri D.V., Masi R. & Bondoc R. (1972) Continuous procaine spinal anesthesia for Caesarean section. *Anesthesia and Analgesia* **51**, 117–24.

Gourlay G.K., Cherry D.A., Plummer J.L., Armstrong P.J. & Cousins M.J. (1987) The influence of drug polarity on the absorption of opioid drugs into CSF and subsequent cephalad migration following lumbar administration: application to morphine and pethidine. *Pain* **31**, 297–305.

Hart I.K., Bone I. & Hadley D.M. (1988) Development of neurological problems after lumbar puncture. *British Medical Journal* **296**, 51–2.

Hartung H.J., Osswald P.M., Bender H.J. & Lutz H. (1986) Severe hypotension and major conduction anaesthesia. In *Anaesthesiology and Intensive Care Medicine* **176**. New Aspects in Regional Anesthesia 4. (Eds Wurst H.J. & Stanton-Hicks M.d'A.) pp. 72–5. Springer-Verlag, Berlin.

Howie J.E. & Dutton D.A. (1990) The effects of warming bupivacaine in patients undergoing elective Cesarean section under epidural anaesthesia. In *Epidural and Spinal Analgesia in Obstetrics* (Ed. Reynolds F.). London, Baillière Tindall.

Hurley J.E. & Lambert D.H. (1990) Continuous spinal anesthesia with a microcatheter technique: preliminary experience. *Anesthesia and Analgesia* **70**, 97–102.

Husemeyer R.P. & White D.C. (1980) Lumbar extradural injection pressures in pregnant women. *British Journal of Anaesthesia* **52**, 55–9.

Hutter C.D. (1990) The Woolley and Roe case. A reassessment. *Anaesthesia* **45**, 859–64.

Jordan C.C. (1984) Current views on the mechanism of opiate analgesics and some novel approaches to analgesic drugs. In *Anaesthesia Review*, vol. 2 (Ed. Kaufman L.) pp. 108–36. Churchill Livingstone, Edinburgh.

Kane R.E. (1981) Neurologic deficits following epidural or spinal anesthesia. *Anesthesia and Analgesia* **60**, 150–61.

Katz H. (1973) Glass-particle contamination of color-break ampules. *Anesthesiology* **39**, 354.

Larsen V.H., Iverson A.D., Christensen P. & Anderson P.K. (1985) Postoperative pain treatment after upper abdominal surgery with epidural morphine at thoracic or lumbar level. *Acta Anaesthesiologica Scandinavica* **29**, 566–71.

Lewis M.P., Thomas P., Wilson L.F. & Mulholland R.C. (1992) The 'Whoosh' test. A clinical test to confirm correct needle placement in caudal epidural injections. *Anaesthesia* **47**, 57–8.

Lybecker H., Möller J.T., May O. & Nielsen H.K. (1990) Incidence and prediction of post dural puncture headache. *Anesthesia and Analgesia* **70**, 389–94.

Lynch J., Arhelger S., Krings Ernst I., Grond S. & Zech D. (1992) Whitacre 22-gauge pencil-point needle for spinal anaesthesia. A controlled trial in 300 young orthopaedic patients. *Anaesthesia and Intensive Care* **20**, 322–5.

Melzack R. & Wall P.D. (1965) Pain mechanisms; a new theory. *Science* **150**, 971–9.

Mankikian B., Cantineau J.P., Bertrand M., Kieffer E., Sartene R. & Viars P. (1988) Improvement of diaphragmatic function by a thoracic extradural block after upper abdominal surgery. *Anesthesiology* **68**, 379–86.

Mayer D.M., Quance D. & Weeks S. (1992) Headache after spinal anesthesia for Cesarean section: a comparison of the 27-gauge Quinke and 24-gauge Sprotte needles. *Anesthesia and Analgesia* **75**, 377–80.

McCulloch W.J.D. & Littlewood D.G. (1986) Influence of obesity on spinal analgesia with isobaric 0.5% bupivacaine. *British Journal of Anaesthesia* **58**, 610–14.

McLean B.Y., Rottman R.L. & Kotelko D.M. (1992) Failure of multiple test doses and techniques to detect intravascular migration of an epidural catheter. *Anesthesia and Analgesia* **74**, 454–6.

Metha P.M., Theriot E., Mehrotra D., Patel K. & Kimball B.G. (1987) A simple technique to make bupivacaine a rapid-acting extradural anesthetic. *Regional Anesthesia* **12**, 135–8.

Moore D.C. & Batra M.S. (1981) The components of an effective test dose prior to epidural block. *Anesthesiology* **55**, 693–6.

Mumtaz M.H., Daz M. & Kuz M. (1982) Another single space technique for orthopaedic surgery. *Anaesthesia* **37**, 90.

Nancarrow C., Runciman W.B., Mather L.E., Upton R.N. & Plummer J.L. (1987) The influence of acidosis on the distribution of lidocaine and bupivacaine into the myocardium and brain of sheep. *Anesthesia and Analgesia* **66**, 925–35.

Noble D.W., Morrison L.M., Brockway M.S. & McClure J.H. (1991) Adrenaline, fentanyl or adrenaline and fentanyl as adjuncts to bupivacaine for extradural anaesthesia in elective Cesarean section. *British Journal of Anaesthesia* **66**, 645–50.

Noel T.A. (1990) Conical needles and transdural fluid leak. *Anesthesia and Analgesia* **70**, 467.

Palkar N.V., Boudreaux R.C. & Mankad A.V. (1992) Accidental total spinal block: a complication of an epidural test dose. *Canadian Journal of Anaesthesia* **39**, 1058–60.

Pitkänen M. (1987) Body mass and spread of spinal anesthesia with bupivacaine. *Anesthesia and Analgesia* **66**, 127–31.

Pitkänen M.T., Haapaniemi L., Tuominen M. & Rosenberg P.H. (1984) Influence of age on spinal anaesthesia with isobaric 0.5% bupivacaine. *British Journal of Anaesthesia* **56**, 279–84.

Prince C. & McGregor D. (1986) Obstetric epidural test doses. *Anaesthesia* **41**, 1240–50.

Purdy G., Currie J. & Owen H. (1987) Continuous extradural analgesia in labour. *British Journal of Anaesthesia* **59**, 319–24.

Rasmussen B.S., Blom L., Hansen P. & Mikkelsen S.S. (1989) Postspinal headache in young and elderly patients. Two randomised, double-blind studies that compare 20- and 25- gauge needles. *Anaesthesia* **44**, 571–3.

Rawal N., Arner S., Gustafsson L.L. & Allwin R. (1987) Present state of extradural and intrathecal opioid analgesia in Sweden. *British Journal of Anaesthesia* **59**, 791–9.

Ready L.B., Oden R., Chadwick H.S., Benedetti C., Rooke G.A., Caplan R. & Wild L.M. (1988) Development of an anesthesiology-based postoperative pain management service. *Anesthesiology* **68**, 100–6.

Reid J.A. & Thornburn J. (1991) Headache after spinal anaesthesia. *British Journal of Anaesthesia* **67**, 674–7.

Reiz S., Balfors E., Sorenson M.B., Häggmark S. & Nyhman H. (1982) Coronary hemodynamic effects of general anesthesia and surgery: modification by epidural analgesia in patients with ischemic heart disease. *Regional Anesthesia* **7** (Suppl.), 8–18.

Reynolds F. (1987) Adverse effects of local anaesthetics. *British Journal of Anaesthesia* **59**, 78–95.

Reynolds F. (1993) Dural puncture and headache. *British Medical Journal* **306**, 874–6.

Rigler M.L., Drasner K., Krejcie T.C., Yelich S.J., Scholnick F.T., DeFontes J. & Bohner D. (1991) Cauda equina syndrome after continuous spinal anesthesia. *Anesthesia and Analgesia* **72**, 275–81.

Ross B.K., Chadwick H.S., Mancuso J.J. & Benedetti C. (1992) Sprotte needle for obstetric anaesthesia: decreased incidence of post dural puncture headache. *Regional Anesthesia* **17**, 29–33.

Rostaing S., Bonnet F., Levron J.C., Vodinh J., Pluskwa F. & Saada M. (1991) Effect of epidural clonidine on analgesia and pharmacokinetics of fentanyl in postoperative patients. *Anesthesiology* **75**, 420–5.

Ryan P., Schweitzer S.A. & Woods R.J. (1992) Effects of epidural and general anaesthesia compared with general anaesthesia alone in large bowel anastomoses. A prospective study. *European Journal of Surgery* **158**, 45–9.

Scott D.B., Schweitzer S. & Thorn J. (1982) Epidural block in postoperative pain relief. *Regional Anesthesia* **7**, 135–9.

Seow L.T., Lips F.J. & Cousins M.J. (1983) Effect of lateral posture on epidural blockade for surgery. *Anesthesia and Intensive Care* **11**, 97–102.

Shantha T.R. & Evans J.A. (1972) The relationship of epidural anaesthesia to neural membranes and arachnoid villi. *Anesthesiology* **37**, 543–57.

Shutt L.E., Valentine S.J., Wee M.Y., Page R.J., Prosser A. & Thomas T.A. (1992) Spinal anaesthesia in Cesarean section: comparison 22-gauge and 25-gauge Whitacre needle with 26- gauge Quincke needles. *British Journal of Anaesthesia* **69**, 589–94.

Sjöström S., Hartvig P., Persson P. & Tamsen A. (1987a) Pharmacokinetics of epidural morphine and meperidine in Humans. *Anesthesiology* **67**, 877–88.

Sjöström S., Tamsen A., Persson P. & Hartvig P. (1987b) Pharmacokinetics of intrathecal morphine and meperidine in humans. *Anesthesiology* **67**, 889–95.

Spence A.A. & Smith G. (1971) Postoperative analgesia and lung function: a comparison of morphine with extradural block. *British Journal of Anaesthesia* **43**, 144–8.

Sprotte G., Schedel R., Pajunk H. & Pajunk H. (1987) An atraumatic needle for single-shot regional anaesthesia. *Regional Anaesthesia* **10**, 104–8.

Stevens R.A., Schubert A., Spitzer L., Chester W.L., Brandon D., Grueter J.A. & Clayton B. (1989) The effect of pH adjustment of 0.5% bupivacaine on the latency of epidural anesthesia. *Regional Anesthesia* **14**, 236–9.

Stride P.C. & Cooper G.M. (1993) Dural taps revisited. A 20 year survey from Birmingham Maternity Hospital. *Anaesthesia* **48**, 247–55.

Tetzlaff J.E. & Rothenstein L. (1992) Alkalinization of mepivacaine does not alter onset of caudal anesthesia. *Journal of Clinical Anesthesia* **4**, 301–3.

Torda T.A. & Pybus D.A. (1982) Comparison of four narcotic analgesics for extradural analgesia. *British Journal of Anaesthesia* **54**, 291–5.

Tucker G.T. & Mather L.E. (1975) Pharmacokinetics of local anaesthetic agents. *British Journal of Anaesthesia* **47**, 213–24.

Urban B.J. (1973) Clinical observations suggesting a changing site of action during induction and recession of spinal and epidural anesthesia. *Anesthesiology* **39**, 496–503.

Usubiaga J.E., Moya F. & Usubiaga L.E. (1967a) Effect of thoracic and abdominal pressure changes on the epidural space pressure. *British Journal of Anaesthesia* **39**, 612–18.

Usubiaga J.E., Wikinski J.A. & Usubiaga L.E. (1967b) Epidural pressure and its relation to spread of anesthetic solutions in the epidural space. *Anesthesia and Analgesia* **46**, 440–6.

Vella L.M., Willats D.G., Knott C., Lintin D.J., Justins D.M. & Reynolds F. (1985) Epidural fentanyl in labour. *Anaesthesia* **40**, 741–7.

Way E.L. (1946) Studies on the local anaesthetic properties of isonipecaine. *Journal of the American Pharmacological Association* **35**, 44–7.

White D.C. (1982) The epidural space. In *Anaesthesia Review*

(Ed. Kaufman L.) pp. 90−9. Churchill Livingstone, Edinburgh.

Whiteley S.M., Murphey P.G., Kirollos R.W. & Swindells S.R. (1993) Headache after dural puncture. *British Medical Journal* **306**, 917−18.

Wildsmith J.A.W. (1986) Exradural blockade and intracranial pressure. *British Journal of Anaesthesia* **58**, 579.

Wildsmith J.A.W. (1987) Intrathecal or extradural: which approach for surgery? *British Journal of Anaesthesia* **59**, 397−8.

Wildsmith J.A.W. & Rocco A.G. (1985) Current concepts in spinal anaesthesia. *Regional Anesthesia* **10**, 119−24.

Wildsmith J.A.W., McClure J.H., Brown D.T. & Scott D.B. (1981) Effects of posture on the spread of isobaric and hyperbaric amethocaine. *British Journal of Anaesthesia* **53**, 273−8.

Yaksh T.L. & Rudy T.A. (1976) Analgesia mediated by a direct spinal action of narcotics. *Science* **192**, 1357−8.

Yaksh T.L., Harty G.J. & Onofrio B.M. (1986) High doses of spinal morphine produce a nonopiate receptor-mediated hyperesthesia: clinical and theoretical implications. *Anesthesiology* **64**, 590−7.

Upper Limb

W.A. CHAMBERS AND J.A.W. WILDSMITH

Regional anaesthetic techniques, used alone or supplemented by sedation or light general anaesthesia, may benefit patients undergoing surgery to the upper limb in a number of ways. Most obviously, the risk of general anaesthesia may be avoided in certain groups (e.g. emergency operation in patients with a full stomach, rheumatoid patients with cervical spine abnormalities, asthmatic patients, etc.), but regional techniques offer more than the mere avoidance of general anaesthesia, e.g. regional anaesthesia can provide very effective postoperative analgesia. If a catheter is inserted, both major (brachial plexus) and minor (e.g. median) nerve blocks may be used to produce analgesia over several days.

Increasing interest in microsurgical reconstruction of the hand and arm after trauma has produced a new indication for brachial plexus anaesthesia, principally because of the sympathetic block and consequent vasodilatation that are produced. This is one of the reasons why brachial plexus block is useful, in patients with renal failure who are having arteriovenous fistulae fashioned for haemodialysis.

Depending on circumstances, it may be possible to choose one of a number of different approaches to produce a regional block. In each case it is necessary to take into account the nerve supply of the operative site, whether or not a tourniquet is to be used, and the likely duration of the procedure. Other important factors are the dose of drug required, the status of the patient and the level of proficiency of the anaesthetist.

Intravenous regional anaesthesia

Injection of a solution of local anaesthetic into an exsanguinated limb was described originally by Bier in 1908, but only became used widely after its reintroduction in the 1960s (Holmes, 1963). Since then, intravenous regional anaesthesia has been used extensively, particularly in accident and emergency departments, where its technical simplicity and reliability are especially suited for many minor procedures to the upper limb. Unfortunately, these features have led to inexperienced clinicians using the technique without understanding its basis and without being able to deal with possible complications. As a result, deaths have been caused by what should be a very safe technique (Heath, 1982).

Intravenous regional anaesthesia (IVRA, Bier's block) provides satisfactory analgesia and muscle relaxation of the hand and forearm in over 95% of patients and it is suitable for many open and closed procedures which are performed distal to the elbow. One of the limiting factors is tourniquet time as some discomfort occurs almost invariably 20−30 min after cuff inflation. This may be alleviated to a limited extent by the inflation of a second cuff immediately distal to the original and deflation of the upper cuff, but even with the use of such a system, it is unwise to embark on a procedure which takes longer than 1 h.

Although IVRA is used normally for relatively minor procedures, usually in outpatients, it can offer particular advantages in other situations. For example, patients who are tetraplegic may require tendon-transfer operations and are at risk of developing postoperative chest infections after general anaesthesia. Thus, local anaesthesia may be preferred. Intravenous regional anaesthesia is tolerated very well by these patients, and tourniquet discomfort from a single cuff is unusual in less than 1 h.

Another special use of IVRA is in operations where it is desirable for the surgeon to observe movement of the hand before the end of the operation. This may be to ensure correct tension in a tendon graft or to ascertain if adequate tenolysis has been performed. Intravenous regional anaesthesia may be used if continued anaesthesia of the hand is obtained with a wrist block. The operation is carried out under IVRA, and the tourniquet is released after suture of any proximal wounds. Movement of the fingers by action of the long flexors and extensors can be observed, any further dissection or adjustment made and the distal wound sutured without discomfort.

Contraindications to IVRA include contraindications to a tourniquet (such as sickle cell disease) and any infective process, the spread of which could be encouraged. It is unwise to use IVRA without other provision for anaesthesia if the intention is to deflate the tourniquet some time before the end of surgery, because the return of sensation may be very rapid. Patients with large lacerations may be unsuitable simply because a large part of the volume injected may escape through the wound.

Technique

The tourniquet should be as simple as possible. The single cuff orthopaedic tourniquet with a 'bicycle-type' pump and high-pressure tubing (Fig. 69.1) has much to recommend it. Double cuffs do not lessen discomfort always and they are potentially dangerous because confusion may lead to accidental deflation of the wrong cuff. Sphygmomanometer cuffs are totally inappropriate and while automatic systems are useful, they can lead to a false sense of security and be confusing to use.

Prilocaine 0.5% (Citanest) is the drug of choice because of its low systemic toxicity. It is available in 50-ml single-dose vials, free of any preservative. The standard adult dose is 40 ml, and this may be reduced in frail or elderly patients. Up to 50 ml (or a standard volume of a more concentrated solution) may be used in healthy subjects with muscular, well-built forearms.

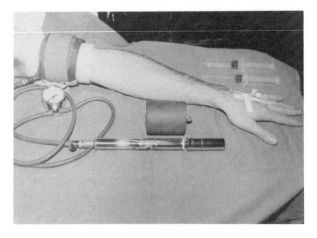

Fig. 69.1 Equipment for intravenous regional anaesthesia.

Intravenous regional anaesthesia should be undertaken with a care that may appear disproportionate to its technical simplicity. The following guidelines are recommended.
1 The patient should be:
   (a) Fasted for at least 4 h before elective surgery whenever possible.
   (b) Placed on a tipping trolley or table.
   (c) Supervised closely by an experienced clinician.
2 Venous access should be established in the opposite arm.
3 Full resuscitation equipment must be available immediately.
4 The tourniquet should be checked for leaks before use and observed constantly.

With the patient supine, the arterial pressure is checked. If it is elevated significantly, the need for the procedure to be performed should be reviewed. An intravenous cannula is placed in a vein on the dorsum of the hand or distal forearm of the limb to be blocked. The tourniquet cuff is applied over a layer of orthopaedic felt on the upper arm and inflated after exsanguination of the limb. Rather than apply an Esmarch bandage over a fracture, it may be kinder to ask the patient to elevate the limb for 2 min while the brachial artery is compressed because this produces almost as good exsanguination (Duggan *et al.*, 1984). The cuff should be inflated to 13.3 kPa (100 mmHg) above systolic arterial pressure, and if there is any doubt about occlusion of the circulation, the tourniquet should be released and the procedure restarted. Once it is certain that the limb has been isolated from the circulation, the chosen volume of prilocaine is injected over 1–2 min. It may be useful to ask an assistant to compress the patient's forearm manually during the injection. This provides an additional safeguard should the tourniquet accidentally deflate at what would be a very critical time and also produces a greater initial concentration of local anaesthetic in the distal part of the limb. Within seconds, the patient may experience paraesthesiae and the skin may appear mottled. Complete sensory block is obtained usually within 10 min, but muscle relaxation may take longer to develop. Throughout the procedure, a careful watch must be kept on the tourniquet which should not be allowed to deflate for at least 20 min after injection of drug. When it is deflated, the patient must be observed closely and kept supine for at least 30 min.

Complications

The major problem is systemic toxicity, and this is

associated usually with inadvertent, premature tourniquet deflation because of failure of equipment or technique. There have been reports (Rosenberg *et al.*, 1983) of convulsions (all with drugs other than prilocaine) despite an adequately applied tourniquet. This can only be explained by leakage of local anaesthetic solution past the tourniquet. It has been demonstrated that very high venous pressure, which could cause systemic leakage, may be produced by rapid injection and poor exsanguination (Duggan *et al.*, 1984). The use of antecubital veins contributes to the risk.

The incidence of toxicity when the tourniquet is released after 20 min or more is variable. Minor symptoms (drowsiness, tinnitus, tingling of the lips) are observed even with prilocaine, but neither major systemic toxicity nor methaemoglobinaemia have been described after IVRA with prilocaine at the recommended dosage.

Nerve damage from tourniquet pressure is extremely rare in association with properly conducted IVRA (Larsen & Hommelgaard, 1987). This complication is more likely when excessive tourniquet times are used and the patient is unlikely to tolerate these with this technique.

Brachial plexus blocks

Although IVRA is useful for minor procedures, brachial plexus blocks have distinct advantages if major surgery is to be carried out using a regional technique. The tissues are not swollen by a large volume of local anaesthetic, and a tourniquet is not necessary. If one is used, the discomfort it causes is minimal. Analgesia may persist well into the postoperative period, and its duration can be varied by using a local anaesthetic agent appropriate to the particular circumstance.

There are disadvantages. A detailed knowledge of anatomy is essential, the procedures take time to perform and the potential for complications is greater.

Anatomy

The nerves of the upper limb derive mainly from the brachial plexus which is formed from the anterior primary rami of the fifth cervical to the first thoracic nerves (Fig. 69.2). Some fibres may be derived also from C4 and T2. The five roots form three trunks, each of which divides into an anterior and a posterior division. These six divisions unite to form three cords, each of which has two terminal divisions which are the nerves that supply most of the upper

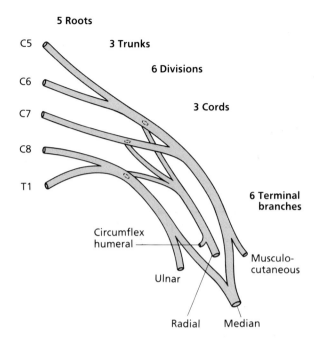

Fig. 69.2 Formative elements of the brachial plexus.

limb. Branches of the formative parts of the plexus supply the deep structures of the shoulder, the skin of this region being supplied by the supraclavicular branches of the cervical plexus. The intercostobrachial nerve (T2) supplies the skin of the inner aspect of the upper arm and, with a branch from the third thoracic nerve, the skin of the axilla. Interbranching within the plexus implies that most of the peripheral nerves carry fibres from several roots. Each nerve supplies a specific area as does each segmental root, but the segmental innervation of deep and cutaneous structures is different.

As they emerge from the intervertebral foramina, the plexus roots lie between the scalene muscles, which join the tubercles of the transverse processes of the cervical vertebrae to the first rib. In the neck (Fig. 69.3), the vertebral artery, the stellate ganglion and the contents of the cervical spinal canal are close relations. The phrenic nerve lies on the anterior surface of scalenus anterior, posterior to the carotid sheath. The recurrent laryngeal nerve lies in the groove between the oesophagus and trachea, and laterally, the external jugular vein crosses the interscalene groove at the level of the sixth cervical vertebra and the cricoid cartilage.

As the plexus approaches the first rib, the trunks are arranged vertically and are named 'superior', 'middle' and 'inferior'. They are close together, and the subclavian artery lies between the plexus and the scalenus anterior muscle. The dome of the pleura is

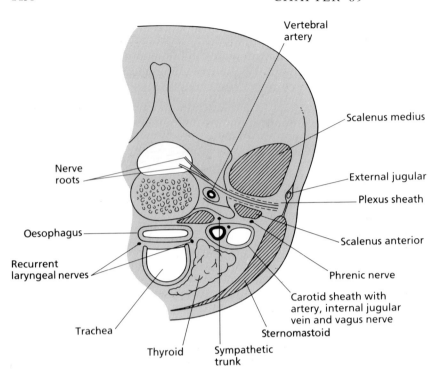

Fig. 69.3 Transverse section of neck to show relations of brachial plexus.

an important inferomedial relation (Fig. 69.4). At the lateral border of the first rib, each trunk branches into its divisions and these pass behind and under the clavicle where the cords are formed. In the axilla, the artery is surrounded completely by the components of the plexus, the cords giving rise to terminal branches behind the lateral border of pectoralis minor. The axillary vein lies medial to the artery and the surrounding plexus, overlapping both partially. The musculocutaneous nerve (from the lateral cord) leaves the plexus and enters the substance of the coracobrachialis muscle high in the axilla.

An important feature (Winnie, 1970) is that the plexus lies within a tube of fibrous tissue which extends from the cervical vertebrae, where it is continuous with the prevertebral fascia, to the distal axilla. Any solution injected into the sheath at any point spreads in both directions. Superiorly, the sheath is continuous with that surrounding the cervical plexus, and this explains why block of the cervical nerves is seen occasionally after interscalene block. Radio-opaque dye studies (Thompson & Rorie, 1983) suggest that the sheath is a multicompartmental structure and this may explain some of the incomplete or delayed blocks which are produced even by experienced clinicians.

Numerous techniques have been described for performing brachial plexus block. From proximal to distal these are:

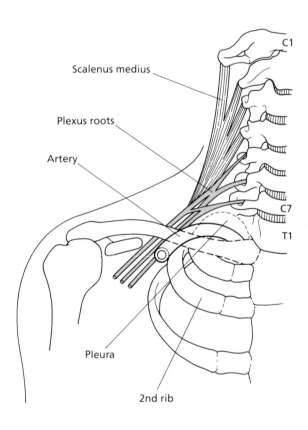

Fig. 69.4 Major relations of the brachial plexus.

1 Interscalene (Winnie, 1970).
2 Parascalene (Vongises & Panijayanond, 1978).
3 Subclavian perivascular (Winnie & Collins, 1964).
4 Supraclavicular (Macintosh & Mushin, 1967).
5 Intraclavicular (Raj et al., 1973).
6 Axillary (de Jong, 1961).

Each of these approaches has its advocates (indeed there are variations on each theme), but it is unnecessary for an individual to master all. The supraclavicular is the classical approach and the others have been introduced in an attempt to produce methods which are easier to learn and without the risk of pneumothorax, the major hazard of the classical method. The supraclavicular and subclavian perivascular techniques produce the most complete limb block (Lanz et al., 1983). The axillary approach does not affect the shoulder, and the interscalene often misses the ulnar aspect of the hand and forearm. The axillary method is somewhat easier to learn and perform than the others, and is perhaps the most suitable for the occasional user.

Latency and duration

Onset may be slow with any of these techniques. Most blocks are well established within 20 min, but they may take much longer on occasion. To some extent, this variation is related to the approach and the drug and concentration used. Testing for sensory loss too early may undermine the patient's confidence and at least 10–15 min should elapse before this is done. Motor block becomes apparent often before sensory loss and the earliest sign of a successful axillary block is often inability to extend the elbow. Movement at the shoulder is first affected by interscalene and subclavian perivascular blocks. If there is no evidence of motor weakness within 10 min of injection, success is unlikely.

Duration is variable even if the same drug and dosage are used. For prolonged operations, discomfort at the tourniquet site may become troublesome despite adequate analgesia in the operating field. Lignocaine has a very brief duration unless used with a vasoconstrictor, but a single injection of plain prilocaine provides at least $1\frac{1}{2}$ h of surgical anaesthesia and bupivacaine 3 h. Longer durations can be achieved by using a catheter technique and bupivacaine may last occasionally for up to 24 h.

Toxicity

Brachial plexus block requires the administration of a large dose of local anaesthetic drug regardless of the approach chosen. Thus, even in the absence of direct intravascular injection, significant plasma concentrations of the local anaesthetic may be produced. The addition of adrenaline (1 : 200 000) produces lower plasma concentrations and is recommended particularly when bupivacaine or lignocaine is used because concentrations near the toxic range may result otherwise (Wildsmith et al., 1977). Similar systemic concentrations are obtained whichever technique is used (MacLean et al., 1987) so the risk of toxicity should not be a consideration when deciding which approach to use.

Assessment and preparation

A patient for surgery under brachial plexus block requires the same investigation and preparation as one having a general anaesthetic. Although regional anaesthesia may offer many benefits, this is not a reason to submit patients to surgery in other than optimum condition. In addition, it can never be guaranteed that a patient will not require general anaesthesia because of failure of the block or unexpected operative findings. Premedication is a matter for individual preference, but the patient should not be sedated so heavily that co-operation is lost.

Needles

Short-bevel needles are preferable, as penetration of the sheath is appreciated more readily and they decrease the incidence of nerve injury (Selander et al., 1977, 1979). It is helpful also to use the immobile needle technique (Winnie, 1969), in which an extension set connects the needle to the syringe. The set is primed with fluid to avoid air embolism and allows the needle to be held motionless during aspiration, injection and changing of syringes. A strict no-touch technique should be adopted, but gloves are unnecessary for a single-injection technique, especially as they may make the palpation of landmarks more difficult. If a cannula is to be inserted, it is probably wiser to 'scrub up' and use gloves and sterile towels. Infection at the site of injection is extremely rare.

Paraesthesiae and nerve stimulators

Before the injection, the patient should be warned about paraesthesiae. It is important to impress on the patient the necessity of reporting paraesthesiae immediately and remaining as motionless as possible at that time. Once paraesthesiae have been elicited, the needle should be held immobile and an aspiration test performed. If blood or air cannot be aspirated, then the solution should be injected slowly. Severe pain during injection indicates that an intraneural injection is being performed. This is extremely rare, but if it is the case, the needle must be withdrawn slightly. Some discomfort on initial injection may be caused by over-rapid distension of the plexus sheath and is avoided if the initial part of the injection is made in small increments.

The use of paraesthesiae to determine accurate needle placement depends on having a conscious, co-operative patient who understands clearly the instructions he/she has been given. The use of a nerve stimulator allows these techniques to be used on patients who cannot co-operate (Yasuda *et al.*, 1980). However, conscious patients may find the nerve stimulator uncomfortable and in experienced hands its use results only in a marginal increase in the rate of successful blocks.

Management

Once a successful block has been established, patient management varies widely. Healthy, young patients undergoing short procedures may be happy to remain fully conscious during the operation. They should be accompanied at all times so that they can converse and describe any problems they experience. At the other extreme, patients undergoing prolonged procedures will almost certainly require some form of sedation or even light general anaesthesia because lying motionless on an operating table for 2 or 3 h can be very uncomfortable, particularly for patients with other skeletal deformities. Care must be taken positioning the patient to prevent damage being caused. It is particularly important not to overextend the arm or to place it on a board which is lower than the level of the operating table. If respiratory-depressant drugs have been administered, oxygen should be given by face mask and saturation monitored with an oximeter. It may be appropriate also to monitor the ECG and arterial pressure in patients with systemic disease.

Postoperative care

It is essential that the arm is cared for properly until the block wears off, because the loss of sensory, proprioceptive and motor function can each lead to damage. Hyperextension, especially if it is ac-companied by external rotation and traction, can lead rapidly to neural injury.

Interscalene block

The interscalene technique is the most proximal approach to the brachial plexus, local anaesthetic being injected between the scalene muscles at the level of the sixth cervical vertebrae. Pneumothorax should not be a risk, but the method has the dis-advantage that the lower roots of the plexus are not blocked consistently. Areas supplied by C5–7, the deep structures of the shoulder, elbow joint and the lateral aspect of the forearm and hand, are blocked reliably. Supplementary blocks may be required for surgery of other parts of the limb, particularly the ulnar aspects of the forearm and hand.

Technique

The patient lies supine with the head resting on one pillow and turned slightly to the opposite side. The arm should be by the patient's side. The lateral border of the sternomastoid is identified. If it is not palpable readily, the patient is asked to lift his/her head just off the pillow as this tenses the muscle. A finger placed in the groove behind the sternomastoid and at the level of the cricoid cartilage lies on the belly of scalenus anterior. The patient is asked to relax completely and the finger rolled laterally over the scalenus anterior until it lies in the groove between the anterior and middle scalene muscles, the interscalene groove. The groove may be made easier to palpate by asking the patient to take a deep breath. The needle is inserted into this groove at the level of the cricoid cartilage. The external jugular vein passes usually near the point of injection and care should be taken to avoid puncturing it.

The needle is inserted at right angles to the skin so that it is directed medially, but also slightly caudally and posteriorly (Fig. 69.5). If it is directed horizon-tally, it may pass between two cervical vertebrae and could puncture the vertebral artery or enter the inter-vertebral foramen. The needle is advanced slowly until paraesthesiae are obtained which radiate to the arm or forearm rather than the shoulder tip or scapula. Paraesthesiae in the latter distribution are caused by stimulation of the suprascapular or supraclavicular nerves, which lie outside the sheath. Subsequent injection is thus ineffective. A click may be felt as the needle pierces the plexus sheath and is a useful guide to correct position. If paraesthesiae are not elicited,

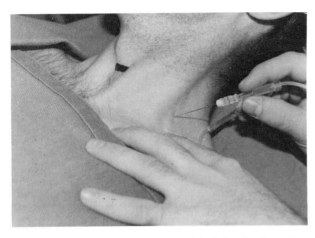

Fig. 69.5 Interscalene block. The tip of the left index finger lies on scalenus anterior.

the needle is withdrawn and its angulation checked. It is important to stress that the plexus is rarely more than 2.5 cm from the skin (Yasuda *et al.*, 1980). Once paraesthesiae have been produced, the neck is compressed firmly by a finger placed above the needle to promote caudal spread. After aspiration, the local anaesthetic solution is injected slowly with repeated aspiration.

Volume requirements

Winnie (1984) has determined the spread of different volumes of solution injected into the brachial plexus sheath with the use of local anaesthetic solutions mixed with radio-opaque dye. Injection of 20 ml of solution at the level of C6 results in a block of the lower cervical plexus in addition to the brachial plexus. However, because the injection is made at such a high level, 20 ml is often insufficient to spread far enough inferiorly to reach the lower roots of the plexus, and anaesthesia may be patchy or absent in the distribution of C8 and T1. If the volume is increased to 40 ml, the entire interscalene space is filled from the transverse processes of the upper cervical vertebrae to the cupola of the lung. Usually, this provides anaesthesia of the entire cervical and brachial plexuses.

Digital pressure applied just above the needle during the performance of an interscalene block inhibits cephalad spread and promotes distal flow of the injected solution. Thus, this manoeuvre reduces the volume necessary to produce a complete block of the brachial plexus.

Complications

Phrenic nerve block has been demonstrated radiographically in 36% of patients with interscalene and subclavian perivascular blocks (Farrar *et al.*, 1981), but this causes symptoms rarely unless the patient has severe respiratory disease. Both techniques are associated also with a low incidence of recurrent laryngeal nerve block. This causes hoarseness which is of no clinical significance, but bilateral blocks would cause laryngeal incompetence. Up to 50% of patients who receive these blocks develop Horner's syndrome, and some patients complain of flushing of the face. Unequal pupils may give rise to concern in a patient who has sustained a recent head injury.

Avoidance of vertebral artery injection by careful aspiration and accurate needle placement is essential, as even a small dose of local anaesthetic given by this route causes severe cerebral toxicity. Extradural and subarachnoid injections are possible also and have been reported. These are avoided by correct needle direction and appreciation of the superficial position of the plexus. Finally, all nerve block techniques can be associated with direct nerve trauma. Constant care is needed so that the wrong solution is not injected and paraesthesiae should be elicited gently (Selander *et al.*, 1979). Short bevel needles are to be preferred (Selander *et al.*, 1977).

Subclavian perivascular block

With this technique, the injection is made into the subclavian perivascular space, i.e. between the lower ends of the scalene muscles and above the first rib. It differs from the classical supraclavicular approach in that the needle is inserted higher in the neck and also further posteriorly and medially. The needle is directed more caudally and should reach the plexus where the trunks lie on top of each other behind the subclavian artery. The lower trunk of the plexus may be missed occasionally as it lies below the subclavian artery, but this can be overcome to some extent by using a generous volume of solution. The risk of pneumothorax is less than with the classical supraclavicular approach, but is still present, so the method is contraindicated in day-patients.

Technique

The interscalene groove is located (see above) and followed downwards until the pulsation of the subclavian artery can be felt. A finger is placed over the artery to mark the site of injection. A needle is inserted in the groove immediately above the artery (Fig. 69.6) and advanced slowly in a caudad direction between the scalene muscles until paraesthesiae are elicited. A click is sometimes felt as the needle penetrates the sheath. If the first rib is contacted before paraesthesiae have been elicited, the needle is withdrawn and redirected more anteriorly or posteriorly. It is important that the needle is not directed medially as this increases the risk of pneumothorax. If the subclavian artery is punctured, the needle should be withdrawn and directed slightly more posteriorly.

Paraesthesiae in the arm or hand indicate that the needle is positioned correctly. Paraesthesiae in any other distribution indicate that the suprascapular, supraclavicular or long thoracic nerves have been stimulated and it is likely that the needle lies outside the sheath.

Volume requirements

Winnie (1984) has again documented the spread of radio-opaque solutions by this approach. Twenty ml provide a block of the entire brachial plexus. However, if the injection is made fairly high in the subclavian, perivascular space, the onset of anaesthesia may be delayed or even absent in the distribution of the inferior trunk, and therefore a slightly larger volume is preferable. If 40 ml of solution are injected, anaesthesia of the lower cervical plexus results.

Complications

Pneumothorax is the principal complication and may become apparent either immediately or up to 24 h later. Any coughing during attempts to obtain paraesthesiae should alert the anaesthetist that the needle tip may be near the pleura. Phrenic, recurrent laryngeal and stellate ganglion block (see above) can all occur although they are seldom significant clinically.

Axillary block

This offers the safest and simplest method of blocking the brachial plexus. It produces consistently good anaesthesia of the medial aspects of the arm, forearm and those parts of the hand supplied by the ulnar and median nerves. The lateral aspects of the forearm and hand, supplied by the radial and musculocutaneous nerves, are blocked in approximately 75% of cases.

Technique

With the patient lying supine, the arm is abducted almost to 90° and rotated slightly externally. It may be helpful to flex the elbow and support the arm on a pillow. If the arm is abducted further, the artery may become more difficult to feel and it is unwise to ask the patient to place his or her palm behind his/her head. The axillary artery is identified as high in the axilla as possible and a needle inserted at an angle of approximately 30° to the skin and directed parallel to the artery (Fig. 69.7). The needle is advanced slowly until it pierces the sheath which lies quite superficially. Evidence that the sheath has been penetrated may take several forms. A 'click' or 'give' may be felt as the needle passes through the sheath and thereafter

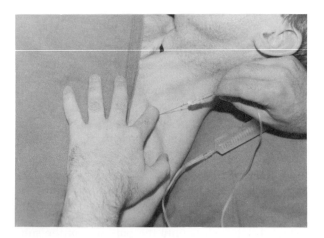

Fig. 69.6 Subclavian perivascular block. The tip of the left index finger is palpating the artery.

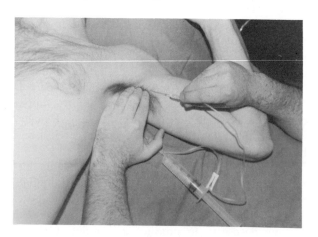

Fig. 69.7 Axillary plexus block. The fingers of the left hand lie over the artery and the needle is inserted just above and parallel to it.

it can be observed pulsating usually if it is supported gently. Although paraesthesiae are not sought deliberately with this technique, they give additional confirmation that the tip of the needle is placed correctly if they are elicited. Similarly, if the artery or vein is punctured, this indicates also that the needle tip is within the sheath. In this case, particular care needs to be taken to avoid intravascular injection, and the needle should be withdrawn slowly until blood can be aspirated no longer.

With the needle in the correct position, and connected to a syringe with an extension set, an aspiration test is performed. The injection is made slowly with repeated aspiration. Pressure on the sheath immediately distal to the injection site aids proximal spread of the solution. Digital pressure is more effective in this regard than the use of a rubber tourniquet around the arm. If aspiration reveals that the needle is intravenous before any solution has been injected, then it may be possible to reposition the needle satisfactorily. If the injection has commenced, considerable damage may be caused to the plexus by traumatizing partially blocked nerves, and it may be wise to abandon the method in favour of another. If a vessel has been punctured, it should be compressed for 5 min after the injection to minimize haematoma formation. A finger placed firmly over the artery distal to the injection site during the injection aids proximal spread of the solution and makes block of those nerves which leave the sheath high in the axilla more likely.

An alternative method is to use a 25-gauge needle and puncture the artery deliberately (Cockings et al., 1987). Once this has been achieved, the needle is advanced slowly while aspiration is continued. As soon as blood can be no longer aspirated (indicating that the needle tip has passed through the artery and is situated posteriorly within the sheath) the needle is fixed and the injection made. Advocates of this method claim that it is more likely to produce block of the radial nerve distribution. In inexperienced hands this may be so, but the deliberate transfixion of a major limb artery seems a high price to pay for this advantage.

Although a needle can be used for axillary block, it is relatively simple to use a cannula technique. The approach is very similar, and once the sheath has been penetrated, the cannula is advanced from the needle. If it is within the sheath, the cannula advances easily and any resistance suggests that it should be withdrawn and reinserted.

Volume requirements

Twenty ml of solution injected into an adult patient without digital pressure does not spread consistently to reach the level of the cords of the plexus. Sensory loss following such a small volume may provide adequate anaesthesia for hand surgery but the block may not be adequate to prevent discomfort from a tourniquet or to prevent the patient from flexing his/ her forearm. If the volume is increased to 40 ml, the solution normally reaches the first rib and thus provides a complete sensory and motor block of the arm (Vester-Anderson et al., 1983). The very large volumes (up to 60 ml) which would be required to produce spread to the cervical portion of the interscalene space are not recommended clinically. Digital pressure applied immediately distal to the injection site prevents distal spread of the solution and encourages proximal flow. This is more effective than the use of a rubber tourniquet because the sheath is situated deeply between coracobrachialis and the long head of triceps. Obstruction to proximal flow can be caused also by the humeral head if the arm remains abducted. Thus, adduction of the arm while maintaining firm digital pressure allows any given volume to reach a higher level within the sheath.

Combined techniques

It is possible to combine two techniques of brachial plexus block to avoid the problems which may arise from insufficient spread of analgesia. This can be achieved by injecting half of the total volume by the axillary approach and half above the clavicle, either in the interscalene groove or by using the subclavian perivascular technique.

Peripheral nerve blocks

The role of individual nerve blocks in the arm is limited. Because of variations in anatomical course and wide cutaneous sensory overlap, multiple injections with supplementary infiltrations are required for major surgical procedures. Patients obviously object to such techniques. The main value of these blocks is in supplementing the major blocks, providing analgesia for short procedures on the hand (particularly if a tourniquet is not required) and also providing analgesia for physiotherapy and manipulation if this is painful.

For all these blocks it is important to avoid intraneural injection, which can be extremely painful and may produce a neuritis. The longer duration of bupivacaine makes it the most suitable drug in many situations, although lignocaine and prilocaine may be used. The abundance of blood vessels in close proximity to nerves at the elbow and the wrist implies that intravascular injection and haematoma formation are potential complications. Even when blocking small nerves, the action of a local anaesthetic drug is seldom instantaneous and up to 15 min should be allowed for its onset.

Clinically, there is little difference between the effect of nerve block at the elbow or the wrist; and thus, only the simpler methods (at the wrist) are described. Block of the ulnar nerve at the elbow is particularly likely to produce neuritis if injections are made where the nerve lies in the groove behind the medial epicondyle and this approach should be avoided if at all possible.

Ulnar nerve block

The palmar branch of the ulnar is blocked at the level of the styloid process. A fine needle is inserted at right angles to the skin, on the radial side of the tendon of flexor carpi ulnaris and the ulnar side of the ulnar artery (Fig. 69.8). The latter can be palpated usually. If paraesthesiae are produced, the needle is held in place and 2—4 ml of local anaesthetic injected. Even if paraesthesiae are not produced, it is usually possible to obtain adequate anaesthesia by injecting 5—10 ml of solution while the point of the needle is moved from contact with deep fascia and bone until it lies subcutaneously. To block the dorsal branch of the ulnar nerve, a ring of local anaesthetic solution is placed subcutaneously around the ulnar aspect of the wrist from the tendon of flexor carpi ulnaris — approximately 5 ml of solution are required.

Median nerve block

At the level of the proximal skin crease at the wrist, the needle is inserted at right angles to the skin immediately radial to palmaris longus, or if it is absent, 1 cm medial to flexor carpi radialis (Fig. 69.9). The nerve is approximately 1 cm deep at this point, but fanwise movements of the needle in a plane at right angles to the long axis of the forearm may be required to obtain paraesthesiae. When these are elicited, 2—5 ml of solution are injected slowly. A further 1 ml may be injected subcutaneously to include the cutaneous branch to the palm of the hand.

Radial nerve block

The terminal part of this nerve can be blocked by infiltrating under the tendon of brachioradialis some 6—8 cm proximal to the wrist, but a simpler and less unpleasant method for the patient is to raise a sub-cutaneous ring around the radial and dorsal aspects of the wrist joint (Fig. 69.10). Approximately 5 ml of solution are used. The ring of infiltration should not extend around the whole circumference of the wrist and care should be taken to avoid damage to the subcutaneous veins.

Digital nerve block

This is very effective for procedures on the finger which are carried out on outpatients. Under no circumstances should solutions containing a vasoconstrictor be used. The needle should be inserted from the dorsal aspect and advanced during the injection until pressure is felt on the anaesthetist's

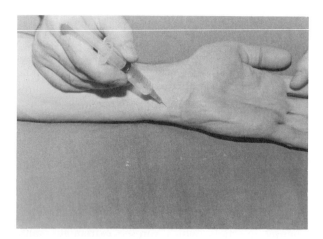

Fig. 69.8 Ulnar nerve block at the wrist.

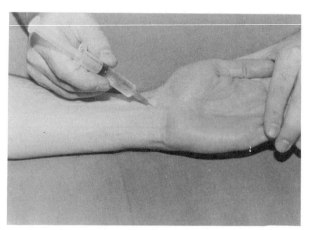

Fig. 69.9 Median nerve block at the wrist.

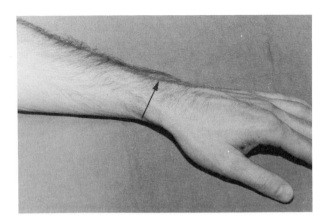

Fig. 69.10 The arrow shows the position and direction of infiltration for radial nerve block at the wrist.

finger which should be placed beneath that of the patient's. One to 2 ml of solution are injected subcutaneously on each side of the base of the finger. The use of larger volumes should be avoided because the increase in local tissue pressure which this will cause may be harmful.

Local infiltration

Many minor surgical procedures such as the excision of small tumours and the suturing of wounds can be performed under infiltration anaesthesia. The use of this method in the hand is limited because of the simplicity with which digital nerve or wrist block can be performed. The technique may be useful for suturing wound edges if it is necessary to release the tourniquet before the end of a procedure carried out under intravenous regional anaesthesia.

Catheter techniques

Postoperative pain after surgery to the upper limb is not usually of sufficient severity or duration to require continuation of local anaesthetic block after the effects of the initial injection have worn off. There are some situations, however, where it is useful to 'top up' a block or even to infuse local anaesthetic. Some operations such as reimplantation of a severed digit will take considerably longer than the normal duration of action of a single bolus. In certain chronic pain conditions it may be desirable to infuse dilute solutions of local anaesthetic for a period of time to allow physiotherapy to be accomplished more effectively.

The axillary route is probably the easiest approach if a catheter is to be inserted, but care must be taken when threading either a catheter or cannula within

the sheath not to damage neural or other structures. Catheters may also be placed near to peripheral nerves at the end of surgery to allow subsequent injection of local anaesthetic agents but this is seldom necessary.

References

Cockings E., Moore P.L. & Lewis R.C. (1987) Transarterial brachial plexus blockade using high doses of 1.5% mepivacaine. *Regional Anesthesia*, **12**, 159–64.

de Jong R. (1961) Axillary block of the brachial plexus. *Anesthesiology*, **22**, 215–55.

Duggan J., McKeown D.W. & Scott D.B. (1984) Venous pressure in intravenous regional anesthesia. *Regional Anesthesia* **9**, 20–2.

Farrar M.D., Schebani M. & Nolte H. (1981) Upper extremity block: effectiveness and complications. *Regional Anesthesia* **6**, 133–4.

Heath M. (1982) Deaths after intravenous regional anaesthesia. (Editorial). *British Medical Journal* **285**, 913–14.

Holmes C.M. (1963) Intravenous regional analgesia. *Lancet* **i**, 245–6.

Lanz E., Theiss D. & Jankovic D. (1983) The extent of blockade following various techniques of brachial plexus block. *Anesthesia and Analgesia* **62**, 55–8.

Larsen U.T. & Hommelgaard P. (1987) Pneumatic tourniquet paralysis following intravenous regional anaesthesia. *Anaesthesia* **42**, 526–8.

Macintosh R. & Mushin W. (1967) *Local Anaesthesia: Brachial Plexus* 4th edn. Blackwell Scientific Publications, Oxford.

MacLean D., Chambers W.A., Tucker G.T. & Wildsmith J.A.W. (1987) Plasma prilocaine concentrations after three techniques of brachial plexus blockade. *British Journal of Anaesthesia* **60**, 136–40.

Raj R., Montgomery S., Nettles D. & Jenkins M. (1973) Infraclavicular brachial plexus block; a new approach. *Anesthesia and Analgesia* **52**, 897–904.

Rosenberg P.H., Kalso E.A., Tuominen M.K. & Linden H.B. (1983) Acute bupivacaine toxicity as a result of venous leakage under the tourniquet cuff during Bier's block. *Anesthesiology* **58**, 95–8.

Selander D., Dhuner K. & Lundborg G. (1977) Peripheral nerve injury due to injection needles used for regional analgesia. *Acta Anaesthesiologica Scandinavica* **21**, 182–8.

Selander D., Edshage S. & Wolff T. (1979) Paraesthesia or no paraesthesia. *Acta Anaesthesiologica Scandinavica* **23**, 27–33.

Thompson G. & Rorie D. (1983) Functional anatomy of the brachial plexus sheath. *Anesthesiology* **59**, 117–22.

Vester-Andersen T., Christiansen C., Sorensen M., Kaalund-Jorgensen H.O., Saugbjerg P. & Schultz-Moller K. (1983) Perivascular axillary block II: influence of injected volume of local anaesthetic on neural blockade. *Acta Anaesthesiologica Scandinavica* **27**, 95–8.

Vongises P. & Panijayanond T. (1978) A parascalene technique of brachial plexus anesthesia. *Anesthesia and Analgesia* **58**, 267–73.

Wildsmith J.A.W., Tucker G.T., Cooper S., Scott D.B. & Covino B.G. (1977) Plasma concentrations of local anaesthetics after interscalene brachial plexus block. *British Journal of Anaesthesia* **49**, 461–6.

Winnie A.P. (1969) An 'immobile needle' for nerve block. *Anesthesiology* **31**, 577–8.

Winnie A.P. (1970) Interscalene brachial plexus block. *Anesthesia and Analgesia* **49**, 455–66.

Winnie A.P. (1984) *Plexus Anaesthesia*, vol. 1. Schultz/Churchill Livingstone, Edinburgh.

Winnie A. & Collins V. (1964) The subclavian perivascular technique of brachial plexus anesthesia *Anesthesiology* **25**, 353–63.

Yasuda I., Hirano T., Ojima T., Ohhira N., Kaneko T. & Yamamuro M. (1980) Supraclavicular brachial plexus block using a nerve stimulator and an insulated needle. *British Journal of Anaesthesia* **52**, 409–11.

Further reading

Eriksson E. (Ed) (1969) *Illustrated Handbook in Local Anaesthesia.* Munksgaard, Copenhagen.

Wildsmith J.A.W. & Armitage E.N. (Eds) (1987) *Principles and Practice of Regional Anaesthesia.* Churchill Livingstone, Edinburgh.

Winnie A.P. (1984) *Plexus Anesthesia*, vol. 1. Schultz/Churchill Livingstone, Edinburgh.

Plexus and Peripheral Blocks of the Lower Limb

F.P. BUCKLEY AND K.J. McGRATH

The leg derives its nerve supply from seven nerve roots (L2–S3), which form the lumbar and sacral plexi, two anatomically separate structures, the anatomy of which is shown in Figs 70.1, 70.2 and 70.9, respectively. These plexi branch into several major peripheral nerves. The dermatomal distributions of the nerve roots and the peripheral nerves supplying the leg are shown in Figs 70.3 and 70.4. The myotomal distributions of the nerve roots supplying the leg is shown in Fig. 70.5. Because the plexi and the peripheral nerves supplying the leg are widely separated anatomically, several different individual nerve or plexus blocks are necessary to produce regional block of the whole leg. This is in contrast to the arm where the whole nerve supply to the arm may be reliably and conveniently blocked by inserting a single needle into the brachial plexus sheath, at a number of locations.

As nerve blocks of the lower extremity are performed relatively infrequently and rely on deep and often indistinct landmarks, these blocks often have a high failure rate in the hands of the novice. To reduce the failure rate, several measures may be used:
1 Do not attempt them in patients with indistinct anatomical landmarks.
2 Provide the patient with sufficient analgesia and sedation to ensure a static and co-operative target.
3 Position the patient carefully and accurately.
4 Identify and mark all anatomical landmarks accurately.
5 If the nerve is to be identified by eliciting paraesthesiae ensure that the distribution of paraesthesiae is consistent with the peripheral, preferably distal, distribution of the nerve.
6 Consider the routine use of a peripheral nerve stimulator (PNS) and an insulated needle to assist in accurate nerve location. Stimulation frequencies of 1.0–2.0 Hz should be used. The general location of the nerve should be initially identified using a stimulation intensity of 2.0 mA. The stimulation intensity should be reduced to 0.4–0.6 mA and the needle repositioned so that a readily discernible twitch in the distal muscles supplied by the nerve is observed. At this stimulation intensity, the needle tip should be within 2–5 mm of the nerve at which point the local anaesthetic may be injected. When the local anesthetic is injected, the anaesthetist should be alert to the need for excessive pressure on the plunger of the syringe and for complaints of pain or parasthesiae immediately upon injection, i.e. within the first 1–2 ml of injection. Each may indicate that the injection is intraneuronal, rather than perineuronal. If such symptoms occur, the needle should be withdrawn 1–2 mm and injection recommenced. The

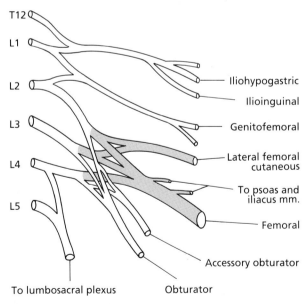

Fig. 70.1 The anatomy of the lumbar plexus. The anterior divisions of the anterior primary rami form the obturator nerve while the posterior divisions (shaded) form the femoral and lateral femoral cutaneous nerves.

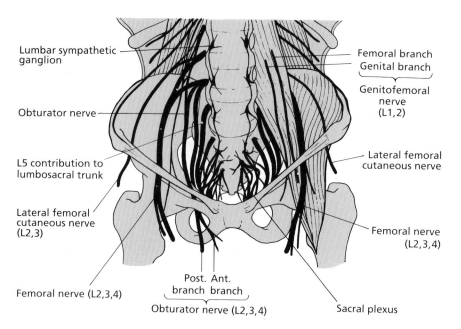

Lumbar sympathetic ganglion

Obturator nerve

L5 contribution to lumbosacral trunk

Lateral femoral cutaneous nerve (L2,3)

Femoral nerve (L2,3,4)

Post. branch Ant. branch
Obturator nerve (L2,3,4)

Femoral branch
Genital branch
Genitofemoral nerve (L1,2)

Lateral femoral cutaneous nerve

Femoral nerve (L2,3,4)

Sacral plexus

Fig. 70.2 The lumbar plexus anatomy on the posterior abdominal wall. On the left the psoas major and minor muscles have been removed to reveal the plexus more completely.

anaesthetist should not be misled by muscle twitches close to the site of needle insertion as these may be caused by direct muscle stimulation. A PNS and insulated needles are valuable tools which permit accurate drug placement and the performance of blocks on patients who are deeply sedated or under general anaesthesia. However, the use of such tools does not compensate for incorrect positioning and inaccurate identification of landmarks.

The solutions which should be used for leg blocks are 2–3% chloroprocaine, lignocaine 1%, mepivacaine 1%, bupivacaine 0.25–0.5% or etidocaine 0.75–1.0%, all with adrenaline. The choice between these agents should be determined by the desired duration of anaesthesia. In the doses described in the text the duration of surgical anaesthesia produced by these agents is: chloroprocaine 1–2 h, lignocaine and mepivacaine 3–4 h and bupivacaine and etidocaine 4–6 h. The duration of the postoperative analgesia produced by these agents is much longer. It may be 15–29 h before the first postoperative analgesic is needed after blocks with bupivacaine (Misra *et al.*, 1991).

Because relatively large masses of drug may be used for leg blocks, care should be taken to stay within the safe maximal dose of any drug for each individual patient. The peak blood concentration of local anaesthetic subsequent to a block may be reduced by the inclusion of adrenaline 1:200000 in the solution (Robison *et al.*, 1991). However, the use of such a concentration of adrenaline in an animal model has been shown to reduce greatly nerve blood

flow for considerable periods of time (Partridge, 1991), and the use of adrenaline may be associated with an increase in nerve damage subsequent to nerve blocks. Thus, in those patients in whom a low nerve blood flow is likely (the elderly patient, the diabetic patient and the arteriopathic patient), smaller concentrations of adrenaline (i.e. 1:400000 or less) may be appropriate.

The lumbar plexus (Figs 70.1 and 70.2)

The lumbar plexus is formed by the roots of L2, 3 and 4. It supplies the skin of the medial, anterior and lateral portions of the thigh and the psoas, quadratus lumborum, quadriceps and adductor muscles. The plexus divides into anterior and posterior divisions within the psoas muscle, the anterior division forming the obturator nerve, and the posterior forming the femoral and lateral femoral cutaneous nerves. As the nerves leave the psoas, they are encased within a fascial sheath which continues with the nerves when they emerge into the leg, a fact which is of particular significance for femoral and 'three in one' blocks (see below).

Lumbar plexus block (psoas compartment block)
(Chayen *et al.*, 1976)

As the lumbar plexus is formed, it lies within its fascia between the quadratus lumborum posteriorly and the psoas anteriorly. The plexus may be blocked by a posterior approach. The landmarks and practical

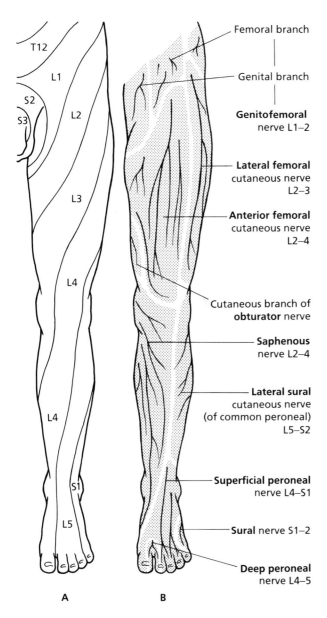

Fig. 70.3 (A) The dermatomal distribution of nerve roots on the anterior surface of the leg. (B) The distribution of cutaneous nerves to the anterior aspect of the leg. The area of distribution of the obturator, lateral femoral cutaneous and saphenous nerves is very variable in extent.

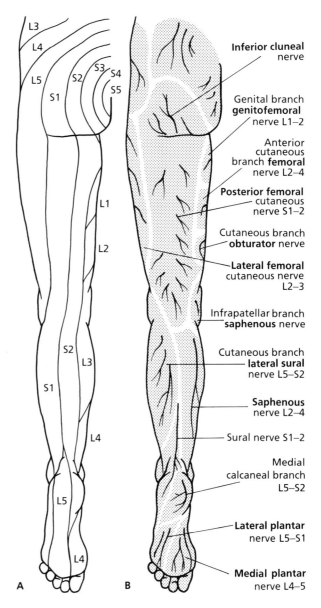

Fig. 70.4 (A) The dermatomal distribution of nerve roots on the posterior aspect of the leg. (B) The distribution of cutaneous nerves to the posterior aspect of the leg.

details of this technique are shown in Fig. 70.6. This block reliably produces anaesthesia in the femoral, obturator and lateral femoral cutaneous nerve distributions, but rarely beyond these (Parkinson *et al.*, 1989). The block may be used in concert with a sciatic nerve block to produce anaesthesia of the whole leg. A catheter may be inserted into the sheath to permit repeated injections of local anaesthetic solution (Brands & Callanan, 1978; Ben-David *et al.*, 1990).

Femoral nerve

The femoral nerve emerges from the lateral border of the psoas muscle in the iliac fossa and runs deep to the iliac fascia in a groove between the psoas and iliacus muscles (Fig. 70.2). It emerges into the thigh lateral to the femoral artery, from beneath the inguinal ligament, enclosed within its fascial sheath. The femoral nerve supplies the muscles of the anterior

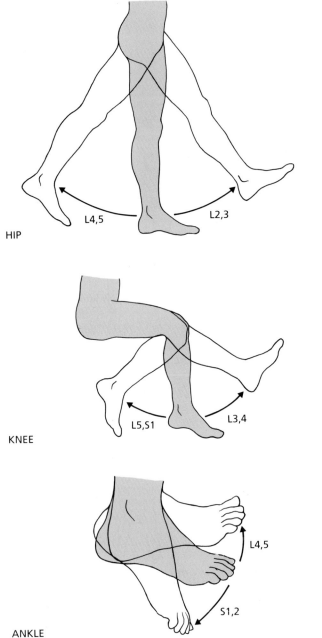

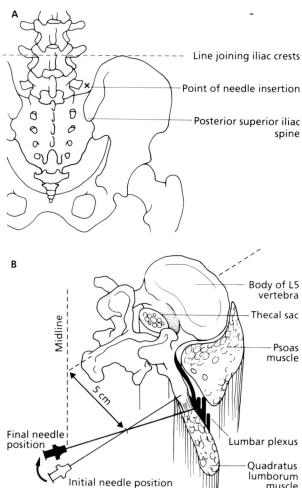

Fig. 70.5 The segmental innervation of the muscles of the leg.

Fig. 70.6 The psoas compartment block. (A) The landmarks. The most superior points of the iliac crests should be identified and a line drawn to join them. Three cm caudad from this line, a second line 5 cm in length should be drawn laterally to the point of needle insertion. This point should overlie the transverse process of L5. (B) The technique. The patient should lie in the lateral position curled up as if for a spinal or extradural block. A 15-cm 22-gauge needle should be inserted perpendicular to the skin at the point shown in (A) until it strikes the transverse process of L5. An air-filled syringe should be attached to the needle, pressure applied to the plunger of the syringe and the needle stepped off the transverse process cephalad and 5° laterally. As the tip of the needle enters the dense fascia on the posterior surface of the quadratus lumborum, tight resistance to injection should be felt. As the needle emerges into the plane which contains the plexus, a distinct loss of resistance should be felt. The plane can then be distended with 20–30 ml of air and 25–30 ml of solution injected (Chayen *et al.*, 1976) or, if a PNS is used, the needle tip adjusted to give optimal twitches in the adductor or quadriceps muscles, and 20–30 ml of solution injected. It is possible to place a needle or catheter close to the plexus at levels above L5 (Brands & Callanan, 1978; Parkinson *et al.*, 1989).

compartment of the thigh and the skin of the anterior surface of the thigh (Figs 70.3 and 70.5). Its terminal branch, the saphenous nerve, follows the long saphenous vein, emerging from beneath the sartorius muscle at the medial side of the knee. The saphenous nerve usually supplies an area of skin on the medial side of the leg to at least the level of the medial malleolus, and frequently beyond, up to the base of the great toe (Fig. 70.3).

Femoral nerve block

The landmarks and technical details of this block are shown in Fig. 70.7. This block produces anaesthesia of most of the anterior surface of the thigh. It may be used alone for anaesthesia of its area of distribution or in concert with other blocks to produce anaesthesia of the whole leg. A catheter may be introduced in a similar fashion to that described in Fig. 70.7 to permit repeated injections of local anaesthetic solution (Rosenblatt, 1980; Lynch *et al.*, 1993).

Lateral femoral cutaneous nerve

This nerve is formed by contributions from L2−3 within the psoas muscle. It emerges from beneath the muscle at the level of the iliac crest, and crosses the iliac fossa. It emerges into the thigh by piercing the inguinal ligament approximately 1−2 cm medial to the anterior superior iliac spine. Approximately 2−4 cm distal to the inguinal ligament, the nerve divides into anterior and posterior branches and emerges from beneath the leg fascia. The area of sensory innervation of the lateral cutaneous nerve is classically described as being the lateral surface of the thigh as far as the knee, but the size of its actual distribution is very variable. It may supply almost the whole of the lateral and anterior surfaces of the thigh (Figs 70.3 and 70.4).

Lateral femoral cutaneous nerve block

The landmarks and the technical details of this block are given in Fig. 70.7. A recently described alternative approach (Brown & Dickens, 1986) is to perform this block at the anterior superior iliac spine. A 22-gauge needle is inserted vertically immediately medial to the anterior superior iliac spine and pressure is applied to the plunger of the syringe. As the needle passes through the external and internal oblique muscles, resistance to injection is felt. This resistance to injection is lost as the tip of the needle enters the canal containing the nerve. Two to 4 ml of solution are injected.

Irrespective of the technique used, blocks of this nerve may be used alone to provide anaesthesia on the lateral side of the thigh (e.g. for harvesting small skin grafts) or in concert with other blocks to produce anaesthesia of the whole leg.

Obturator nerve

The obturator nerve emerges from the medial border

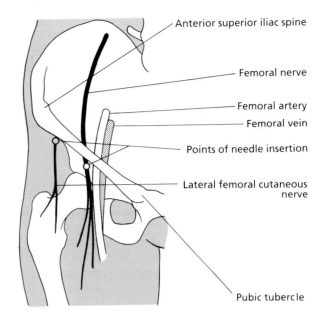

Fig. 70.7 Femoral and lateral femoral cutaneous nerve blocks. The patient should lie in the supine position with the hip slightly abducted and externally rotated. The anterior superior iliac spine and the pubic tubercle are identified. A line joining these two structures overlies the inguinal ligament. The femoral artery is identified at the point where it emerges from beneath the inguinal ligament and this point is marked. Femoral nerve block is accomplished by placing the index finger at the lateral side of the femoral artery to 'guard' it. The point of needle insertion is 2 cm lateral to the point where the artery emerges from beneath the inguinal ligament. A 5-cm 22-gauge needle is inserted perpendicular to the horizontal to pierce first, the fascia lata, which is usually 1.5−3 cm deep in a normal-sized adult, and then the fascia iliaca approximately 0.5 cm deeper. Passing through each fascial layer is usually perceived as a 'pop'. Once the needle tip has passed through the fascia iliaca, the solution may then be injected as a bolus (Khoo & Brown, 1983), or infiltrated as a fan across the path of the nerve. Alternatively, paraesthesiae or, if a PNS is used, a twitch in the quadriceps muscles (not the sartorius muscle — see text) sought and the solution injected. It may be difficult to obtain paraesthesiae or a twitch as at this point in its course the femoral nerve may have divided into a number of branches which slide away from any advancing needle rather easily. An alternative to a discrete femoral nerve block is to use the 'three-in-one' block (see text). The volume of injectate for femoral nerve block is 10−15 ml. For lateral femoral cutaneous nerve block, the point of needle insertion is 2 cm medial and 3 cm distal to the anterior superior iliac spine. A 5-cm 22-gauge needle is inserted perpendicular to the horizontal. Five to 8 ml of solution are injected deep to the fascia which is usually encountered 1.5−2.5 cm deep to the skin. An alternative method of this block is given in the text.

of the psoas muscle at the brim of the true pelvis, crosses the ala of the sacrum and passes along the wall of the pelvis (Fig. 70.2). It emerges into the thigh through the obturator canal at the antero-medial point of the obturator foramen. In the leg, it divides into anterior and posterior divisions, the former supplying the adductors and an area of skin of variable size on the medial side of the thigh, the latter providing motor innervation to the adductors in addition to a small terminal sensory branch to the knee joint.

Obturator nerve block

The landmarks and technical details for performing this block are shown in Fig. 70.8. This is a technically difficult block to perform and is aesthetically unappealing for both operator and patients. It has a high failure rate and thus the use of a PNS is invaluable. If a block of the obturator nerve alone is required (e.g. for diagnostic purposes to ascertain if hip adduction in a patient with neurological disease can be ablated by an obturator nerve block) only an obturator block fulfils the desired purpose. However, if the block is being considered in concert with femoral and lateral femoral cutaneous nerve blocks to provide surgical anaesthesia, it is worthwhile considering using the 'three-in-one' block or the psoas compartment block, which anaesthesizes all three nerves with a high degree of reliability (see below) and are technically easier and quicker to perform than three separate blocks.

'Three-in-one' block (Winnie et al., 1973)

As the femoral, lateral femoral cutaneous and obturator nerves are formed within the psoas, they are enclosed within a fascial sheath which continues to encase the nerves on their journey to the periphery. Placing a sufficient volume of injectate within this sheath and encouraging its proximal spread to the lumbar plexus or nerve roots results in a high incidence of block of all three nerves. Practically, this is achieved by using the landmarks shown in Fig. 70.7 and is performed best with the assistance of a PNS. A 6–8 cm 22-gauge needle is inserted as for a femoral nerve block but at an angle of 45° to the horizontal, aiming the tip of the needle for the manubrium sterni. The nerve is sought, usually being found lateral to this position at a depth of 3–4 cm, and the position of the tip of the needle adjusted to obtain an appreciable twitch of the quadriceps. At this point, the tip of the needle lies under the inguinal ligament and in the centre of the nerve (by moving the needle from medial to lateral, twitches of the vastus medialis and lateralis, respectively, may be obtained as the

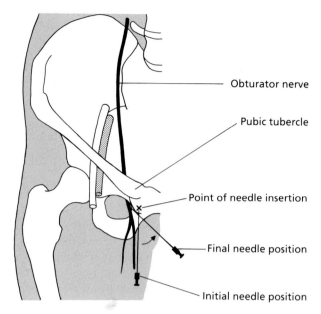

Fig. 70.8 Obturator nerve block. The patient should lie in the supine position with the hip abducted 10–15° and in full external rotation. The pubic tubercule should be identified and marked. A line 3 cm in length drawn caudal to the pubic tubercle and at its termination a further line 2.5 cm in length drawn laterally, to the point of needle insertion. An 8-cm 22-gauge needle should be inserted at 90° to the ischiopubic ramus (usually approximately 45° to the horizontal) parallel to the midline. At approximately 3–4 cm depth, the tip strikes the ischiopubic ramus. The needle is then withdrawn approximately 2 cm and 'walked' laterally and anteriorly until it slides off the lateral surface of the ischiopubic ramus and/or the inferior surface of the iliopubic ramus. The needle tip should then enter the obturator canal and drug may be injected blind, a paraesthesia sought, or a twitch of the adductor muscles obtained if a PNS is being used. See text for recommendations concerning this block. The volume of injectate should be 10–15 ml.

needle sweeps across the nerve). The anaesthetist should be careful not to be mislead by interpreting a twitch of the sartorius muscle, which is often obtained at a point very superficial to the femoral nerve proper, as being a quadriceps twitch. The key to distinguishing between a sartorius twitch and a quadriceps twitch is that the latter produces a very definite, crisp twitch of the patella, whereas the sartorius does not. The position of the tip of the needle should be adjusted so that a twitch of the quadriceps, and the patella, is obtained at a stimulation intensity of 0.4–0.6 mA. To prevent distal spread of the injectate, the sheath distal to the point of injection should be occluded digitally, and occlusion maintained for 5 min, after the injection of 30 ml of solution. This technique results in proximal spread of injectate to the plexus, and even root level, with a high incidence of block of all three major branches of the lumbar plexus (Patel *et al.*, 1986). If a prolonged block is required, an 18-gauge or 20-gauge catheter may be introduced into the sheath using this technique, and analgesia maintained with periodic reinjections, or a constant infusion of local anaesthetic (see below).

The sacral plexus

This plexus is formed by the anterior and posterior divisions of the primary rami of L5 and S1–3 with a small contribution from L4 (Fig. 70.9). These contributions pass over the lateral portion of the sacrum to merge as the sciatic nerve and its branches at the sciatic notch.

The sciatic nerve

The sciatic nerve emerges into the buttock via the sciatic notch, often splitting the pyriformis muscle in the process (Fig. 70.10). It runs caudad on the posterior surface of the gemelli and the quadratus femoris muscles, and is covered posteriorly by the gluteal muscles. The sciatic nerve supplies the sensory and motor innervation to the posterior compartment of the lower extremity. The dermatomal and myotomal distributions and the areas supplied by the sciatic nerve and its branches are shown in Figs 70.3 and 70.4.

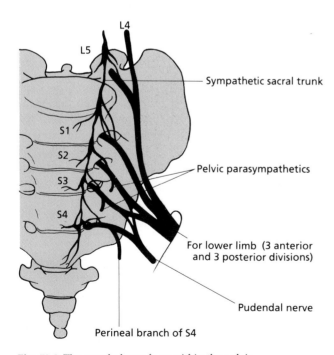

Fig. 70.9 The sacral plexus from within the pelvis.

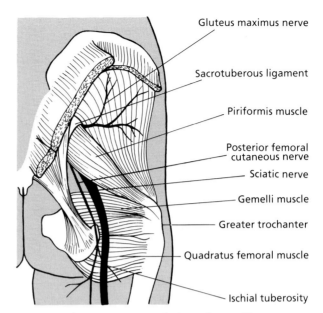

Fig. 70.10 The sciatic nerve in the buttock area. The sciatic nerve emerges into the buttock via the greater sciatic notch, often splitting the pyriformis muscle in the process. It curves over the lateral portion of the sacral spinous process and then runs caudad on the posterior surface of the gemelli and quadratus femoris muscles. It is covered superficially by the glutei.

Sciatic nerve block

The nerve is classically blocked in the buttock by a posterior approach. The landmarks and techniques are detailed in Fig. 70.11. Both of these techniques may be performed with the patient in Sims' position. The more distal block, between the ischial tuberosity and the greater trochanter, may be performed also with the patient in the lithotomy position (Raj *et al.*, 1975).

In the patient who cannot adopt the Sims' or lithotomy position, e.g. a patient with a fractured femur, the nerve may be blocked also by an anterior approach (Fig. 70.12). The anterior technique is difficult to perform and has a high failure rate. Whichever technique is employed, meticulous attention to positioning, identification of landmarks and correct needle placement is essential.

Sciatic nerve blocks may be used in combination with femoral, lateral femoral cutaneous and obturator blocks (or the psoas compartment or three-in-one blocks) to produce anaesthesia of the whole leg, with saphenous nerve blocks for anaesthesia of the leg below the knee, or alone for anaesthesia of the foot. A technique for introducing a catheter close to the sciatic nerve for repeated injections of local

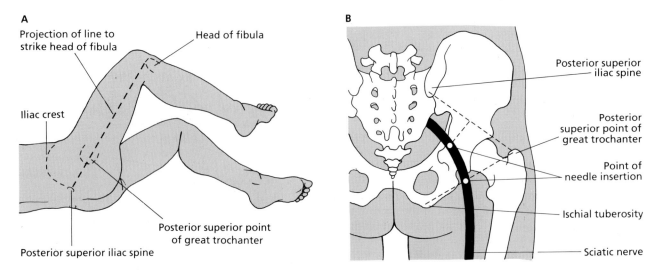

Fig. 70.11 The sciatic nerve block by the posterior approach. (A) The position of the patient. The patient should be placed in the lateral position with the lower leg straight and the upper leg flexed at 45° and adducted so that the knee rests on the bed anterior to the lower leg (Sims' position). The posterior superior iliac spine and the posterior superior end of the greater trochanter should be identified, marked and a line joining those two points drawn. A further refinement of positioning is to place the upper leg so that, when viewed from above, a projection of the line between the anterior superior iliac spine and the greater trochanter strikes the very tip of the head of the fibula. (B) Landmarks and technique of sciatic nerve block by the posterior approach. The patient should be positioned as in (A). For the classical approach (Labat) the posterior superior iliac spine and the posterior superior point of the greater trochanter are identified, marked and a line joining those two points drawn. The mid-point of this line should be marked and a second line drawn at 90° to the first line in a caudad direction. The point of needle insertion is 3–5 cm along this line. (An alternative is to identify the caudal hiatus and draw a line from it to the greater trochanter. Where this line intersects with the perpendicular is the point of needle insertion.) A 10-cm 22-gauge needle is inserted at 90° to the skin in all planes. It should encounter the sciatic nerve as it crosses the lateral portion of the ischial spine. If the nerve is not encountered, a series of needle insertions along the plane of the second line should be performed. A PNS is a helpful tool for nerve block. The solution should only be injected when twitches of the distal musculature supplied by the sciatic nerve, i.e. muscles to the foot and ankle, are produced. For the alternative approach, the ischial tuberosity and the posterior superior end of the greater trochanter should be identified and a line drawn joining those two points. The midline of this line overlies the sciatic nerve as it crosses the quadratus femoris muscle. A 10-cm 22-gauge needle should be inserted at this point at 90° to the skin in all planes. If the nerve is not encountered, a series of passes along the line, at 90° to the course of the nerve, should be made. Again, a PNS is a useful tool. The volume of injectate should be 20–25 ml.

anaesthetic has been described (Smith *et al.*, 1984; Buckley & Cooper, 1992).

Nerve blocks around the knee

Saphenous nerve block

The saphenous nerve is the only component of the femoral nerve which has a distribution below the knee. It emerges from beneath the sartorius muscle on the medial side of the knee and accompanies the long saphenous vein, usually lying just posterior to the vein, over the medial side of the tibia. It is distributed to the medial side of the leg and the dorsum of the foot (Fig. 70.3).

The saphenous nerve may be blocked at a point 4–6 cm distal to the joint line of the knee on the medial side of the tibia. If the long saphenous vein can be identified at this level, a 2–4 ml infiltration on

both sides of the vein blocks the nerve. If the vein cannot be identified, a band of infiltration of 8–10 ml of solution running from the posterior border of the tibia to the tibial tubercule anteriorly blocks the nerve. Saphenous nerve blocks may be used in conjunction with a sciatic block, popliteal fossa block or common peroneal and tibial nerve blocks to produce anaesthesia of the lower leg and foot.

The popliteal fossa blocks (posterior tibial and common peroneal)

At a variable point in its course through the posterior compartment of the thigh, the sciatic nerve divides into its two major terminal branches, the common peroneal and tibial nerves. These nerves become accessible at the apex of the popliteal fossa where they may be blocked. The landmarks and technique are given in Fig. 70.13. This block may be used alone,

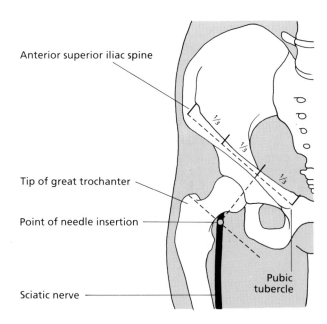

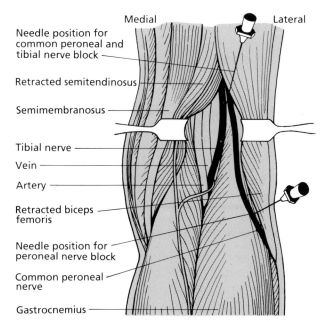

Fig. 70.12 Sciatic nerve block by the anterior approach. The patient should lie supine with the hip abducted at 10° and in full external rotation. The anterior superior iliac spine and the pubic tubercle should be identified, marked and a line joining those two points drawn and divided into three equal lengths. At the junction of the medial and middle thirds, a perpendicular should be drawn caudally and laterally. The superior part of the greater trochanter should be identified, marked and a line drawn parallel to the line between the iliac spine and pubic tubercle, passing through the superior part of the greater trochanter. The point of needle insertion is where this last line and the perpendicular meet. A 15-cm 22-gauge needle should be inserted perpendicular to the horizontal, with air-filled syringe attached and with pressure applied to the plunger of the syringe. The needle usually strikes the medial surface of the femur at a depth of 7–8 cm. The needle should be angled medially to slide off the medial surface of the femur. At this point, the tip of the needle passes through the origins of the adductors and there is resistance to injection. As the needle tip enters the posterior compartment, this resistance to injection is lost and drug may be injected. This block has a fairly high failure rate and the use of a PNS is valuable. The volume of injectate should be 20–25 ml.

Fig. 70.13 Nerve blocks around the knee. The contents of the popliteal fossa with the medial and lateral hamstrings retracted to show the contents. *Popliteal fossa block*: with the patient prone and the knee flexed, the superior end of the diamond-shaped popliteal fossa should be identified and marked. The knee should then be extended and the popliteal artery palpated at the marked apex of the popliteal fossa. If identification of the artery is difficult, a Doppler probe may be helpful. A 10-cm 22-gauge needle is inserted immediately lateral to the artery and advanced until paraesthesiae are obtained or a twitch of the distal muscles, i.e. foot flexors or extensors, produced if a PNS is used. This is usually at a depth of 3–5 cm, and 2–4 cm superficial to the posterior surface of the femur. The volume of injectate should be 10–15 ml. Prior to and during injection careful aspiration of the needle is essential to ensure that injection of solution into the closely adjacent artery and vein does not occur. *Common peroneal blocks*: this nerve should be blocked some 3–5 cm before it curls around the head of the fibula (see text). It can usually be palpated at this point and a 5-cm 22-gauge needle inserted by a posterior or lateral approach. The volume of injectate should be 4–6 ml.

or with saphenous nerve blocks, for lower-leg and foot anaesthesia.

The common peroneal nerve block

This nerve leaves the popliteal fossa, coursing superficial to the lateral head of the gastrocnemius and, having curled around the lateral surface of the fibula some 3 cm distal to the head of the fibula, enters the anterior compartment of the leg.

While it is tempting to block the nerve at the point where it is most easily felt, i.e. just before it winds

around the head of the fibula, this temptation should be resisted. Nerve block at this point may result in drug being injected under pressure into a fascial tunnel which may overlie the nerve at the fibular head. If this occurs there is a substantial potential for nerve damage to occur. The nerve should be blocked by a posterior approach approximately 3–5 cm proximal to the point where it begins to curl around the head of the fibula. A PNS may be used. Three to 5 ml of solution should be used. This block has minimal usefulness on its own, but as it is easily performed, it is useful as a 'back up' where other blocks are not possible, or have failed.

Nerve blocks at the ankle

The nerve supply to the foot is derived predominantly from the branches of the common peroneal and tibial nerves, with a variable contribution from the saphenous nerve. The areas of cutaneous distribution are shown in Figs 70.3 and 70.4. The various nerves and the techniques used to block them are shown in Fig. 70.14. The techniques described in Fig. 70.14 are aimed at the nerves at or above the extensor and flexor retinacula. The various nerves may be blocked also below the retinacula (Sharrock *et al.*, 1986).

Intravenous regional anaesthesia of the leg

Intravenous regional anaesthesia (IVRA) is an appealing, simple technique, but is not applied as readily to the leg as to the arm. If the tourniquet is placed around the thigh, large volumes of injectate, and therefore masses of drug, are necessary to produce

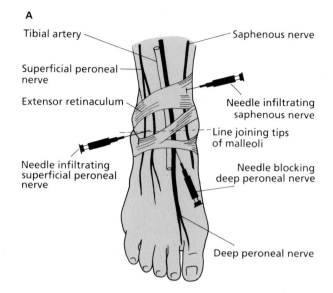

A

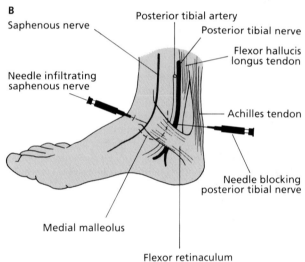

B

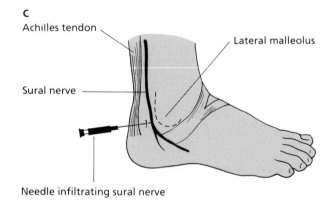

C

Fig. 70.14 (*Right.*) Nerve blocks at the ankle. (A) Anterior view of the ankle. A line should be drawn joining the tips of the two malleoli. The saphenous nerve is blocked 2–3 cm above this line, either by infiltrating on both sides of the long saphenous vein, or by infiltrating a cuff of solution from the anterior to the posterior border of the medial malleolus. Four to 6 ml of solution should be used. The superficial peroneal nerve should be blocked by a band of infiltration along the line joining the two malleoli, superficial to the extensor retinaculum, from the anterior border of the lateral malleolus to the midpoint of the ankle. Four to 6 ml of solution should be used. The deep peroneal nerve should be blocked by infiltrating on the lateral side of the extensor hallucis longus, medial to the anterior tibial artery, either at the level of the line between the two malleoli, or 2.5–3 cm distal to that point. A PNS may be used, the deep peroneal nerve supplies motor innervation to the short toe extensors. Two to 3 ml of solution should be used. (B) Medial view of the ankle. The posterior tibial nerve should be blocked at the upper border of the flexor retinaculum, 2.5 cm proximal to the tip of the medial malleolus. The nerve lies immediately posterior to the tibial artery and anterior to the tendon of flexor hallucis longus. These structures should be identified and, with an index finger 'guarding' the posterior tibial artery, a 2-cm 25-gauge needle inserted from a posterolateral direction. Paraesthesiae may be obtained, or 3–5 ml of solution infiltrated immediately posterior to the artery. The nerve is usually 1–1.5 cm deep to the skin. A PNS may be used, the nerve supplies motor innervation to the intrinsic muscles in the plantar surface of the foot. (C) Lateral view of the ankle. The sural nerve should be blocked by infiltrating a band of solution 2 cm proximal to the tip of the lateral malleolus from the lateral border of the tendo achilles to the posterior border of the lateral malleolus. Four to 6 ml of solution should be used.

satisfactory anaesthesia. With these large masses of drug, toxicity is likely to occur when the drug is released into the systemic circulation at the time of tourniquet release. If the tourniquet is placed above the malleoli, adequate tourniquet occlusion pressures [13.3 kPa (100 mmHg), above systolic pressure], slow injection (over 2–3 min) and modest volumes of drug (20–30 ml lignocaine 0.5%) are used, satisfactory and safe anaesthesia may be produced (Davies & Walford, 1986). Similar precautions to those taken when IVRA is used in the arm should be observed at the time of tourniquet deflation.

Regional anesthesia of the leg in children
(Dalens, 1989; Yaster & Maxwell, 1989)

A discussion of leg nerve blocks in children is outside the scope of this chapter. Local anaesthetic blocks of the nerves to the leg are being increasingly used in children as they can be shown to reduce the need for general anaesthesia, reduce the incidence of morbidity in the immediate postoperative period and provide analgesia which lasts well into the postoperative period. For patient comfort and psychic reasons, regional anaesthesia in children is usually performed with the child deeply sedated or under general anaesthesia. Thus, in order to obtain an acceptable incidence of satisfactory blocks the use of a PNS and insulated needles is almost mandatory. Nerve-blocking techniques must be modestly modified for children and the mass of local anaesthetic reduced consistent with the patient's age and size.

Regional analgesia of the leg for postoperative or post-trauma analgesia

Single-dose regional anaesthetic blocks of the nerves to the leg, using bupivacaine in the doses described in this chapter, produce a relatively pain-free state, i.e. little or no need for supplementary analgesics, for periods of time extending a mean of 12–15 h postblock, with a range of 10–20 h (Misra et al., 1991). Moreover there is a strongly held clinical impression, which remains to be substantiated by scientific study, that subsequent to these blocks wearing off, patients suffer less pain throughout the postoperative period, when compared with patients undergoing similar operations under general anaesthesia and systemic opioid analgesia.

If it is necessary to provide regional anaesthesia beyond the duration of single-shot blocks, this may be achieved by 'continuous' nerve blocks. Techniques have been described for the percutaneous introduction of catheters at or close to the lumbar plexus (Brands & Callanan, 1978; Ben-David et al., 1990), the femoral nerve (Rosenblatt, 1980; Lynch et al., 1993) and the sciatic nerve (Smith et al., 1984; Buckley & Cooper, 1992). These cathether techniques permit local anaesthetic blocks to be conveniently and safely maintained over several days by either intermittent injections of drug at 4–8 hour intervals, or by continuous infusion of drug. The most commonly used drug is bupivacaine, for intermittent injection 15–30 ml of 0.25–0.5%, and for infusions 10–15 ml of 0.25%/h. If such techniques are used, the patients must be carefully monitored for evidence of excessive blood drug levels, though the incidence of CNS problems appears to be low.

The specific technique used in an individual case depends on the operated or injured area. These 'continuous' techniques produce superior analgesia and are especially indicated if it is necessary to move the limb, or joints, e.g. with 'continuous passive motion' as the pain of movement is not well controlled by systemic opioids. Further, as these techniques produce a sympathectomy of the limb, they are indicated when it is necessary to maintain a high blood flow to the damaged area. Examples would be subsequent to operations to reanastomose partially severed limbs or for free-flap grafting operations.

When these long-lasting and 'continuous' nerve-block techniques are used it is essential that the patient also have access to systemic analgesics, e.g patient-controlled analgesia, as the block may not produce perfect analgesia in the damaged area and the patients will often have sources of discomfort outside the blocked area, e.g. sore buttocks, heels.

Following leg amputations, the incidence of phantom-limb pain may be reduced by an extradural local anaesthetic block maintained for a period of time (Bach et al., 1989). Similar benefits (a reduction in analgesic need postoperatively and a reduction in the incidence of phantom-limb pain) following limb amputations may be achieved by 72-h blocks maintained by infusion of 10–15 ml bupivacaine/h via catheters placed on or into the severed nerves at the time of operation (Fisher & Meller, 1991).

Long-lasting nerve blocks, or 'continuous' nerve blocks for leg pain do have some advantages. However, they are not without disadvantages. Some patients are intolerant of having a numb paretic limb that feels like wood. The numb paretic limb must be cared for in such a way that it does not fall heedlessly out of bed, or against other objects, and cause additional damage. The final, and perhaps most important caveat is that some postoperative complications, e.g. an unduly tight cast or a developing compartment syndrome, have pain as their cardinal warning signal. In the numb limb, this warning signal may be concealed. Thus, in the interests of safety, long-lasting blocks should not be used when such complications are likely to occur (a classical example would be a recent mid-tibial shaft fracture from a high-speed injury), and that particular care should be exercised in monitoring both the limb and the patient in circumstances where such blocks are used in the presence of the risk of such a complication.

References

Bach S., Noreng M.F. & Tjelleden N.U. (1988) Phantom limb pain in amputees during the first twelve months following limb amputation, after preoperative lumbar epidural blockade. *Pain* 33, 297–301.

Ben-David B., Lee E. & Croituru M. (1990) Psoas block for surgical repair of hip fracture: a case report and description of a catheter technique. *Anesthesia and Analgesia* 71, 298–301.

Brands E. & Callanan V.L. (1978) Continuous lumbar plexus block. Analgesia for femoral neck fractures. *Anaesthesia and Intensive Care* 6, 265–9.

Brown T.C.K. & Dickens D.R.V. (1986) A new approach to lateral femoral cutaneous nerve of thigh block. *Anaesthesia and Intensive Care* 14, 126–7.

Buckley F.P. & Cooper J.O. (1992) Continuous sciatic nerve block. *Regional Anesthesia* 17, 15, 56.

Chayen D., Nathan H. & Chayen M. (1976) The psoas compartment block. *Anesthesiology*, 45, 95–9.

Dalens B. (1989) Regional anesthesia in children. *Anesthesia and Analgesia* 68, 654–72.

Davies J.A.H. & Walford A.J. (1986) Intravenous regional anaesthesia for foot surgery. *Acta Anaesthesiologica Scandinavica* 30, 145–7.

Fisher A. & Meller Y. (1991) Continuous postoperative regional analgesia by nerve sheath block for amputation surgery — a pilot study. *Anesthesia and Analgesia* 72, 300–3.

Khoo S.T. & Brown T.C.K. (1983) Femoral nerve block the anatomic basis for a single injection technique. *Anaesthesia and Intensive Care* 11, 40–2.

Lynch J., Trojan S., Arhelger S. & Krings-Ernst I. (1993) Intermittent femoral nerve block for anterior cruciate repair. Use of a catheter technique in 208 patients. *Acta Anaesthesiologica Belgica* (In press).

Misra U., Pridie A.K., McClymont C. & Bower S. (1991) Plasma concentrations of bupivacaine following combined sciatic and femoral 3 in 1 nerve blocks in open knee surgery. *British Journal of Anaesthesia* 66, 310–13.

Partridge B.L. (1991) The effects of local anesthetics and epinephrine on rat sciatic nerve blood flow. *Anesthesiology* 75, 243–51.

Parkinson S.K., Mueller J.B., Little W.L. & Bailey S.L. (1989) Extent of blockade with various approaches to the lumbar plexus. *Anesthesia & Analgesia* 68, 243–8.

Patel N.J., Flashburg M.H., Paskin S. & Grossman R. (1986) A regional anesthetic technique compared to general anesthesia for outpatient arthroscopy. *Anesthesia and Analgesia* 65, 185–7.

Raj P.P., Parks R.I., Watson T.D. & Jenkins M.T. (1975) A single position supine approach to sciatic-femoral nerve block. *Anesthesia and Analgesia* 54, 489–93.

Robison C., Ray D.C., McKeown D.W. & Buchan A.S. (1991) Effect of adrenaline on plasma concentrations of bupivacaine following lower limb block. *British Journal of Anaesthesia* 66, 228–31.

Rosenblatt R.M. (1980) Continuous femoral anesthesia for lower extremity surgery. *Anesthesia and Analgesia* 59, 631–2.

Sharrock N.E., Waller J.F. & Fierro L.E. (1986) Midtarsal block for surgery of the forefoot. *British Journal of Anaesthesia* 58, 37–40.

Smith B.E., Fischer H.B.J. & Scott P.V. (1984) Continuous sciatic nerve block. *Anaesthesia* 39, 155–7.

Winnie A.P., Rammamurthy S. & Durrani Z. (1973) The paravascular technique of lumbar plexus block — the '3-in-1' block. *Anesthesia and Analgesia* 52, 989–96.

Yaster M. & Maxwell L.G. (1989) Pediatric regional anesthesia. *Anesthesiology* 70, 324–38.

Surface and Infiltration Anaesthesia

K. HOUGHTON AND J.B. BOWES

Surface or topical application of local anaesthetic agents may be employed to relieve or alleviate pain or to allow pain-free surgery to take place. It comprises the block of touch sensation in skin or mucous membrane. Whilst penetration through intact skin is difficult to achieve, absorption through mucous membrane may be rapid. Although methods such as the application of sprays, cold temperature, counter-irritation, acupuncture and massage may be used also for the transient relief of pain, this section deals only with the use of local anaesthetic techniques.

Drugs suitable for use as surface local anaesthetics

Local anaesthetics are, by definition, drugs which block nerve conduction when applied locally to nerve tissue. In clinical use, their action must be followed by complete recovery of conduction. An agent is suitable for surface anaesthesia only if it is able to penetrate the surface to which it is applied. Penetration through intact skin is generally poor unless high concentrations of certain agents are used and the contact time is long (Covino & Vassallo, 1976; Ritchie & Greene, 1985). In contrast, absorption through mucous membranes may be very rapid and therefore a detailed knowledge of the properties and toxicity of the drugs employed is essential and those with low systemic toxicity are preferred. Agents should not be irritating to the tissues to which they are applied. The pharmacological preparation in which the drug is supplied is relevant in relation to the site where it is applied. The (acidic) salt of the local anaesthetic base is supplied usually in aqueous solution and may be applied by direct instillation, on swabs, as a spray or aerosol, paste, ointment, cream, lotion, suppository or gel.

Objective assessment of the relative efficacy of different agents for surface anaesthesia is difficult because of the variability in the site of application and the diversity of the forms in which an agent may be applied (Covino & Vassallo, 1976). Similarly, the speed of onset of anaesthesia and its duration depends on the agent used, its vehicle and the site to which it is applied. In general, higher doses and concentrations shorten onset time and prolong duration of anaesthesia. Cocaine is the only agent which causes vasoconstriction and this reduces bleeding and improves operating conditions. The addition of phenylephrine 0.005% gives similar conditions but adrenaline is unable to penetrate mucous membranes and is ineffective.

Agents suitable for surface use are shown in Table 71.1. Preparations available in the UK are described below (British National Formulary, 1991).

Lignocaine

Lignocaine is absorbed effectively through mucous membranes, and is the most commonly used agent.

Uses

Mucous membranes, skin and cornea.

Preparations

1 Gel. Lignocaine hydrochloride 1–2% with chlorhexidine gluconate solution 0.25% in a sterile lubricant water-miscible base.
2 Ointment. Lignocaine 5% in a water-miscible base.
3 Aerosol spray. Lignocaine 10% with cetylpyridinium chloride 0.01% in a metered spray container supplying 10 mg lignocaine/dose.
4 Topical solution. Anhydrous lignocaine hydrochloride 4%.
5 Oral solution. Anhydrous lignocaine hydrochloride 2%.

Table 71.1 Local anaesthetic agents for surface use

Agent	Typical conc. used	Max. safe dose mg/kg (max. dose)	Onset (min)	Duration (min)
Lignocaine	2–4%	3 (200 mg)	<5	20–30
Prilocaine	4%	6 (400 mg)	<5	20–30
Cocaine	4%	3 (200 mg)	<5	30–60
Amethocaine	0.2–1.0%	– (40 mg)	3–8	30–60
Benzocaine	1–2%		Slow	Prolonged
Cinchocaine	0.1%	Used rarely	No data	
Eye preparations				
Oxybuprocaine	0.4%			
Proxymetacaine	0.5%			
Colorectal				
Pramoxine	1%			

6 Cream. Lignocaine 50 mg + hyaluronidase 150 μg for application to mucous membranes of the mouth.
7 Eye drops. Lignocaine 4% with fluoroscein.
8 EMLA cream. Lignocaine 2.5% + prilocaine 2.5% as a 5% oil-in-water emulsion cream.

Particular attention should be given to the dose of lignocaine used in sites where absorption is rapid such as the trachea. Its use is contraindicated in patients with myasthenia gravis, complete heart block and in hypovolaemia. It should be used with caution in those with epilepsy, hepatic impairment or abnormal cardiac conduction.

Toxicity

Hypotension, bradycardia, cardiac arrest, sleepiness, agitation, euphoria, respiratory depression and convulsions.

Prilocaine

Prilocaine is similar to lignocaine but less toxic.

Uses

Mucous membranes and skin.

Preparations

1 Prilocaine 3% with felypressin 0.03 units/ml for injection.
2 EMLA cream (see under lignocaine).
3 Although not available commercially in the UK, a topical formulation may be prepared from imported prilocaine powder.

Toxicity

As for lignocaine but in addition, oxidation of haemoglobin by a breakdown product of prilocaine, *o*-toluidine, can occur if high doses are used, causing methaemoglobinaemia.

Cocaine

Cocaine, now used solely for surface anaesthesia, penetrates mucous membranes easily and is extremely effective. It potentiates the action of adrenaline by blocking the re-uptake of transmitter at sympathetic nerve endings and thus cocaine and adrenaline should not be used in combination. It is soluble in water and alcohol. Solutions should be protected from light.

Uses

Nasopharynx, cornea.

Preparations

1 Solution 4–10%.
2 Paste 25%.
3 Eye drops 2–4%.

Toxicity

Excitation of the central and sympathetic nervous systems, depression of the cardiovascular system, respiratory stimulation followed by arrest, pyrexia, clouding of the corneal epithelium; and long-term ischaemia of tissues. Contraindicated in closed-angle glaucoma. Hypersensitivity reactions may occur.

Amethocaine

Amethocaine is an effective surface anaesthetic which is absorbed rapidly through mucous membrane and should not be applied to inflamed, traumatized or highly vascular surfaces, such as the respiratory tract, where lignocaine is safer. Solutions should be protected from light.

Uses

Ophthalmology, skin, oropharynx.

Preparations

1 Eye drops, 0.5% and 1%.
2 Cream. Amethocaine hydrochloride 1% in water-miscible base or in combination with other local anaesthetics.

There are no commercial preparations available for surface or infiltration anaesthesia in the UK.

Toxicity

Cardiac asystole or ventricular fibrillation. Hypersensitivity has been reported. Amethocaine causes stinging in the eye and may produce sensitization of the skin with prolonged use.

Benzocaine

Benzocaine is an agent with low potency and low toxicity. Onset of anaesthesia is slow and of prolonged duration. It is used only for surface anaesthesia where it is absorbed too slowly to be toxic.

Uses

Relief of pain and irritation of the oropharynx and perianal area. It is safe to leave in contact with wounds and ulcerated surfaces.

Preparations

1 Lozenges. Benzocaine, 10 mg, 100 mg.
2 Gel. Benzocaine 1% + cetylpyridinium chloride 0.01%.
3 Ointment (for rectal use). Benzocaine 2% in various compound preparations.
4 Lotion.
5 Spray 5% with triclosan 0.1%.

Toxicity

Prolonged use causes sensitization of skin.

Cinchocaine

Cinchocaine is highly potent, toxic and has a prolonged duration of action.

Uses

Minor skin and anorectal conditions.

Preparations

It is available only for surface use as a 1.1% ointment, or as an ingredient in various compound local anaesthetic creams and suppositories. The 0.1% solution has been reported for use for corneal analgesia. No topical solution is available commercially.

Toxicity

It is more toxic than cocaine or lignocaine.

Miscellaneous

Pramoxine

This agent is too irritating for application to the eye or nose, and its use is limited to preparations for dermatoses and painful perineal and anorectal conditions. It is included in various creams and suppositories in concentrations of approximately 1%.

Oxybuprocaine and proxymetacaine

These are used exclusively for surface analgesia of the eye.

Ethyl chloride

This was used extensively in the past as a local spray for dental extraction where, as a result of its extreme potency, general anaesthesia was known to supervene on occasions! It is now used only occasionally as a spray for incision of small abscesses, before injections, etc. It renders skin anaesthetic by freezing.

Antihistamines

These have some local anaesthetic effect when used topically but are not recommended as they cause sensitization of the skin.

Infiltration anaesthesia

This is the production of regional analgesia by direct infiltration of the incision, wound or lesion. Local anaesthetic solution is injected around and into the site which is to be rendered pain-free in order to prevent the appreciation of pain, although the sensation of touch may persist. No attempt is made to identify individual nerves. Results are most likely to be successful if systematic injection is carried out commencing with dermis, followed by subcutaneous tissue, fascia and then muscle, as appropriate to the plane through which the nerves to be anaesthetized pass (Moore, 1978). Aspiration tests should be performed whenever any quantity of solution is injected in one place to avoid intravascular injection. Various adjuvants may alter the duration of action or rate of spread of the agent used. As only the distal portions of the nerves and nerve endings are blocked, a greater volume of local anaesthetic solution is required when compared with specific nerve blocks and therefore care is needed to avoid toxic doses of both local anaesthetic and vasoconstrictor (if used).

Infiltration anaesthesia in infected areas is likely to be ineffective because of the lower pH of infected tissue which reduces penetration of the local anaesthetic agent. It is considered by some to be contraindicated. A small weal raised over a pointing abscess, however, may prove simple and useful for drainage without serious risk of disseminating infection (Eriksson, 1979).

Complications include neuritis, sloughing of tissue and necrosis of wound edges, particularly if large volumes and vasoconstrictors are used.

A *field block* is produced when a wall of anaesthesia surrounds the operative field (Moore, 1978), thus interrupting the passage of nerve impulses from the operative site to the CNS. Individual nerves are not sought specifically but are anaesthetized in the tissue plane or planes in which they lie. Infiltration should be performed in the area and direction from which the nerves supplying the operative site arise, ensuring that all layers are anaesthetized. Where the nerve supply comes from more than one direction, the site may be outlined geometrically and several points of infiltration used (Fig. 71.1). The latter technique is suitable for skin graft donor areas, biopsies, removal of small lumps, etc.

Drugs suitable for use in infiltration anaesthesia

Lignocaine, prilocaine and bupivacaine are the drugs used most commonly for infiltration anaesthesia. Pro-

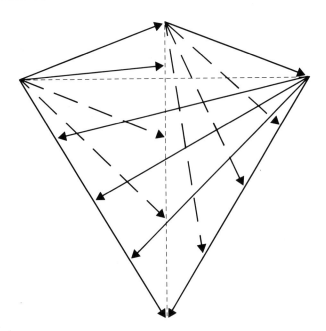

Fig. 71.1 Field block for small operative procedures.

caine is used rarely, as, although it has equivalent potency to lignocaine, it has a shorter duration of action and produces less intense analgesia. It is usually used therefore with adrenaline 1/200 000. It is metabolized to para-aminobenzoic acid which inhibits the action of sulphonamides. Cinchocaine is not used as it produces a high incidence of tissue slough. Amethocaine is more toxic than lignocaine and is now rarely used. A new local anaesthetic, ropivacaine, may also prove suitable for infiltration use. Preliminary trials in animals show that it may be longer acting than bupivacaine (Akerman *et al.*, 1988) and is less cardiotoxic.

Effective infiltration anaesthesia can be obtained with 0.5–1.0% solutions (Table 71.2) (Scott & Cousins, 1980), although higher concentrations are used frequently in dental practice. Onset of analgesia is virtually instantaneous with all agents. Duration of analgesia varies with the agent and increases with higher concentrations and with the addition of other substances (Concepcion & Covino, 1984).

Maximum safe doses depend on the patient's age, weight, physique and clinical condition. The vascularity of the area to which the drug is applied must be considered also. A guide to dosage is given in Table 71.3.

Table 71.2 Local anaesthetic agents for infiltration

| | | | Approx. duration of action (min) | |
Agent	Typical conc. used	Equivalent conc.	−Adren.	+Adren. 1 : 200 000
Short-acting				
Procaine	0.5−2%	2%	15−30	30−90
Chloroprocaine*				
Intermediate				
Lignocaine	0.5%	1%	30−60	120−360
	1%		120	400
Prilocaine	0.5−1%	1%	120	360
Mepivacaine*	0.5−1%	1%	120	360
Long-acting				
Bupivacaine	0.25−0.5%	0.25%	180	420
Etidocaine*	0.5−1%		180	420

* Not available in UK.

Table 71.3 Guide to doses of drugs for infiltration

| | Maximum safe doses (mg/70 kg adult) | |
Agent	−Adren.	+Adren.
Procaine	800	1000
Chloroprocaine	800	1000
Lignocaine	200	500
Prilocaine	400	600
Mepivacaine	300	500
Bupivacaine	150	225
Etidocaine	300	400
Amethocaine	−	200

Substances affecting action of local anaesthetics

Vasoconstrictors

Vasoconstrictors may decrease bleeding, decrease plasma levels of local anaesthetic drug and increase operating time. They are more effective when added freshly to local anaesthetic solutions. They should never be used for infiltration of appendages or digits.

Adrenaline

The addition of adrenaline increases the duration of infiltration anaesthesia of all agents but particularly lignocaine (Covino & Vassallo, 1976) and prilocaine (Hassan *et al.*, 1985). Concentrations of 2−5 µg/ml (1 : 200 000−1 : 500 000) are usual although higher concentrations (12.5 µg/ml or 1 : 80 000) are used frequently in dentistry where the total dose is small. The total dose should not exceed 0.5 mg, but, as plasma catecholamine concentrations vary markedly with the site of application, the safe dose varies also (Cotton *et al.*, 1986). Its use is contraindicated in patients taking tricyclic or related antidepressants (as arrhythmias may result) and in thyrotoxicosis (Boakes *et al.*, 1973).

During halothane anaesthesia the 'safe' dose of adrenaline is said to be 1.0 µg/kg. This is said to be reached with doses of approximately 10 ml of 1 : 100 000 concentration injected every 10 min. The maximum used should be 30 ml/h and carbon dioxide retention should be avoided. Signs of toxicity are pallor, tachycardia and syncope. However, the recommendation should be qualified, as it is known that adrenaline is absorbed much more rapidly from nasal or aural infiltration than from an axillary brachial plexus block (Cotton *et al.*, 1986).

Noradrenaline

Concentrations of 20−40 µg/ml (1 : 50 000−1 : 25 000) may be required for vasoconstriction, but these may cause severe hypertension. It is contraindicated in hypertensive patients and those in whom adrenaline is inadvisable (Boakes *et al.*, 1972, 1973). It is not indicated for routine use.

Phenylephrine

Also an α-receptor stimulant, this may be used in place of adrenaline. It does not cause cerebral stimulation or tachycardia. The usual dose is 0.25−0.5 ml of 1% solution per 100 ml of local anaesthetic solution.

Felypressin

The synthetic polypeptide is related to vasopressin, although it lacks antidiuretic and oxytocic effects and is a less toxic alternative to adrenaline. It is used commonly in combination with prilocaine as it has a more prolonged action than adrenaline, particularly in dentistry. It is safe for use with antidepressants. Typical concentration is 0.03 units/ml.

Dextrans

Dextrans have been used in the past to prolong the duration of local anaesthetics but there is some controversy regarding their efficacy. This is discussed in Chapter 67.

Hyaluronidase

This is an enzyme which inactivates the hyaluronic acid which inhibits diffusion of invasive substances. It appears to be particularly active in subcutaneous tissues and should therefore enhance the rate and distance of spread of local anaesthetic. It is not toxic and may be used concurrently with adrenaline, the addition of which prevents any reduction in duration of anaesthesia caused by enhanced diffusion.

Hypersensitivity has been reported. A dose of 1500 units is a suitable dose to use in any volume of local solution. Its use limits the dosage which can be used because of enhanced absorption, unless adrenaline is used also. It is available as a powder for reconstitution in 1500-unit ampoules.

Individual blocks

Before performing these blocks, the patient should have the procedure explained fully and a suitable premedication such as temazepam 20 mg orally may be prescribed. Resuscitation equipment and oxygen should always be available. If relevant, the skin is prepared.

The techniques employed may not be suitable in children and nervous adults.

Scalp

Uses

Suture or debridement of wounds and removal of small lesions.

Ventriculography, intracranial biopsy, and burr-hole exploration, especially in cases of acute head injury.

As an adjunct to general anaesthesia to reduce blood loss and allow a lighter plane of anaesthesia to be employed.

Anatomy (Williams & Warwick, 1980)

The sensory supply is shown in Fig. 71.2.

The layers of the scalp are shown in Fig. 71.3 and comprise:
1 Skin.
2 Subcutaneous tissue.
3 Epicranial aponeurosis (galea aponeurotica) which is adherent firmly to subcutaneous tissue above and is continuous anteriorly and posteriorly with occipitofrontalis and laterally with temporoparietalis muscle. In combination they form a fibromuscular layer over the upper part of the cranium.

The upper three layers are adherent firmly and remain connected when torn.
4 Subaponeurotic areolar tissue.
5 Pericranium.

Technique

For a limited area of analgesia, solution should be injected in skin and subcutaneous tissue above the aponeurosis, as nerves (and vessels) lie here, followed by infiltration below it in the area required. For a wider area of block, a skull cap distribution of analgesia may be produced by circumferential infiltration along a line passing above the ear from glabella to occiput (Fig. 71.2). It is along this line that the sensory branches of nerves supplying the scalp become subfascial. The landmarks are found by palpation and a circle of anaesthesia produced by systematic infiltration of all layers, accompanied by careful aspiration. In the temporal region, the muscle layer is thicker and the nerves may lie more deeply so more local anaesthetic may be required. Periosteal injection is necessary only if bone is to be removed. Lignocaine or prilocaine 0.5% are suitable and the addition of adrenaline is advisable, as the soft tissues are highly vascular (Macintosh & Ostlere, 1967; Eriksson, 1979; Atkinson *et al.*, 1987).

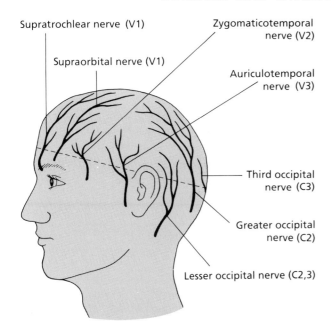

Fig. 71.2 Nerve supply to the scalp with level of circumferential injection for field block of the scalp.

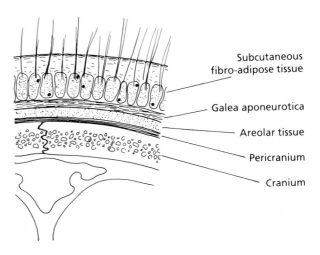

Fig. 71.3 Coronal section through the scalp.

Ear, nose and throat surgery

Advantages of local anaesthesia include avoidance of emergence problems from general anaesthesia, inhalation of blood and sore throat from the use of a throat pack.

Nasal cavities

Uses

Surgery on the nasal septum, submucous resection, cautery or diathermy, polypectomy, turbinectomy.

Anatomy (Williams & Warwick, 1980)

The sensory nerve supply to the nasal cavity and septum originates from the trigeminal nerve (V) via its ophthalmic (V1) and maxillary (V2) divisions (Figs 71.4 and 71.5). The main supply is from:
1 The *anterior ethmoidal nerve* supplying the anterior third of the septum, roof and lateral walls of the nasal cavity. This is a branch of the nasociliary nerve which arises from V1.
2 The pterygopalatine ganglion which arises from V2 gives off the greater and lesser palatine nerves. The nasal branches of the lesser palatine nerves are the *lateral* and *medial posterior superior nasal nerves*. These, together with the *posterior inferior nasal branches* of the greater palatine nerve supply the posterior two-thirds of the lateral wall, roof, floor and septum.

A small supply is received also from:
3 The *infraorbital nerve* (V2) and its branch, the *anterior superior alveolar* (*dental*) *nerve*, supply the vestibule and a part of the septum and floor near the anterior nasal spine and the anterior part of the lateral wall as high as the opening of the maxillary sinus.
4 Branches from the *nerve of the pterygoid canal* (from V2) supply the upper and back part of roof and septum.

Vasomotor sympathetic nerves accompany the sensory fibres and supply the vessels.

Techniques

Packing. The nasal cavities are sprayed with cocaine 4–10% solution and then packed with gauze soaked in cocaine 4–5% solution. Use of a 10% solution with 1:1000 adrenaline has been described, although the powerful vasoconstrictor property of cocaine makes the use of adrenaline superfluous. Adrenaline has the additional disadvantages of potentiating the cardiac sympathomimetic properties of cocaine and of causing reactive vasodilatation when it wears off. The gauze must contact all areas, but in particular the area behind the middle meatus (where it anaesthetizes the greater and lesser palatine nerves) and the cribriform plate (close to the anterior ethmoidal nerve branches). It should remain in place for 10 min. The base of the columella must be injected separately for septal operations.

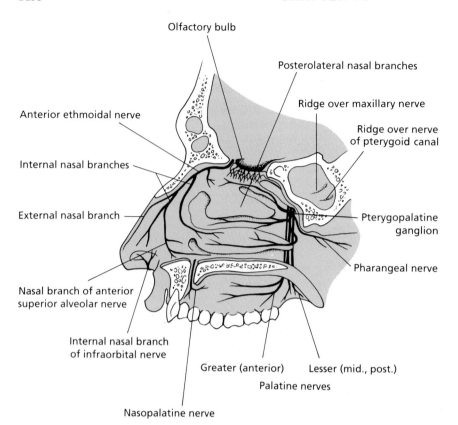

Olfactory bulb

Posterolateral nasal branches

Ridge over maxillary nerve

Ridge over nerve
of pterygoid canal

Anterior ethmoidal nerve

Internal nasal branches

External nasal branch

Pterygopalatine
ganglion

Pharangeal nerve

Nasal branch of anterior
superior alveolar nerve

Internal nasal branch
of infraorbital nerve

Greater (anterior)   Lesser (mid., post.)

Palatine nerves

Nasopalatine nerve

Fig. 71.4 Nerve supply to the lateral wall of the nasal cavity.

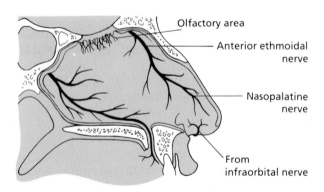

Olfactory area

Anterior ethmoidal
nerve

Nasopalatine
nerve

From
infraorbital nerve

Fig. 71.5 Nerves of the nasal septum.

Direct application. After spraying the cavities with cocaine 4% solution, cocaine paste (e.g. 2 g of a paste containing 25% cocaine and soft paraffin) may be pasted to the areas described above using a wool-covered probe. In particular, the cribriform plate (anterior ethmoidal nerve) and the area behind the middle meatus (where the sphenopalatine ganglion lies) should be pasted. The dose of cocaine is higher than that recommended normally, as absorption is slow in this formulation.

Sluder (1913) described the use of wool mounted on four narrow applicators and then dipped into adrenaline solution and cocaine crystals or cocaine paste. After initial spraying with cocaine, two applicators were placed for 5 min on each side between middle turbinate and septum, one anteriorly and one posteriorly.

For *antral puncture*, applicators with wool soaked in cocaine 4% solution or lignocaine 4% with 2–3 drops (0.15 ml) of adrenaline 0.1% per 5 ml of solution may be placed under the middle and inferior turbinates for 10 min and the mucosa sprayed with lignocaine 10% aerosol spray (Atkinson *et al.*, 1987).

These methods require considerable skill, are time consuming, unpleasant for the patient and may cause mild trauma.

Instillation of solution
1 Moffett (1947) described a method in which Moffett's solution comprising 2 ml cocaine hydrochloride 8%, 2 ml sodium bicarbonate 1% and 1 ml adrenaline 1:1000 is instilled into the nose with the patient adopting three different positions, each of which must be maintained for 10 min.

First, the patient lies on the left side with a pillow under the left shoulder. Using this as a fulcrum, the head is allowed to extend until it is at 45° to the vertical. One-third of the above solution is drawn up and half is instilled into each nostril. The needle used is 5 cm long and angled at 45° with three lateral holes near the blunt end.

Second, a third of the solution is divided between the nares and the patient asked to pinch his/her nose and turn immediately prone.

Third, the patient is positioned as for the first stage but lying on the right side and the final third of the solution instilled. This provides a very satisfactory block with good operating conditions but is time consuming and uncomfortable for the patient. It was modified by Curtiss in 1952.

2 Curtiss (1952) showed radiographically that in each of Moffett's positions, the solution came to lie in the region of the sphenopalatine recess. He showed that the same effect could be obtained by positioning the patient with the head fully extended over the end of the trolley and instilling 2 ml of Moffett's solution into each of the nares. The same type of needle is inserted with the tip directed along the floor of the nose and when the angled part has entered the nose, the direction of the tip is altered to point towards the roof of the nose. When the tip impinges on the bony roof, 2 ml of solution are administered. The same procedure is followed on the other side. The patient remains in position for 10 min.

As with Moffett's method, the pool of solution deposited affects the sphenopalatine ganglion, its branches and the anterior ethmoidal nerve. The main trunk of the maxillary division of the Vth nerve appears to be affected as the area under the inferior turbinate is anaesthetized (this is supplied by the anterior and posterior alveolar nerves). The floor and lateral walls of the antrum are therefore rendered anaesthetic also, allowing antral operations to be performed, e.g. Caldwell–Luc (see below).

3 Macintosh and Ostlere (1967) described a method employing the same position and instilling 2.5 ml of cocaine 5% solution after spraying the mucosa.

4 Bodman and Boyes-Korkis (1960) used 40 ml lignocaine 1.25% with 0.5 ml adrenaline added, with 20 ml being poured into each nostril with the head in hyperextension. The patient breathes through the mouth for 3 min and then sits up and blows excess solution out.

These methods are nerve blocks, albeit administered via the topical route. They are time consuming and uncomfortable for the patient, and toxicity is a risk, particularly if the mucous membrane is inflamed.

Maxillary antrum

Uses

Caldwell–Luc and other antral operations.

Anatomy

The sensory supply is from branches of the infraorbital nerve.

Technique

The gingiva should be sprayed first with lignocaine 4%. Infiltration of the alveolar–buccal mucosa above the premolars with lignocaine 0.5–1% with vasoconstrictor blocks branches of the infraorbital nerve. Further injections may be made into and under the mucous membrane. The nose can be packed with gauze soaked in lignocaine 4% or one of the methods of direct instillation of solution described above may be used. Further solution may be sprayed into the antrum if anaesthesia is incomplete (Oldham, 1968; Bryce-Smith, 1976; Eriksson, 1979; Morrison et al., 1985).

Outer nose and septum

Uses

Operations on the outer nose and septum.

Anatomy

The skin of the nose is supplied by branches of the trigeminal nerve (V).

The skin over the upper part of the nose is supplied by the *nasociliary nerve* (a branch of the ophthalmic nerve, V1). The skin between the palpebral fissure and nostril is supplied by the *infraorbital nerve*, the continuation of the maxillary nerve (V2).

Technique

Subcutaneous infiltration at the tip of the nose and then from the glabella down over the lateral aspects of the nose are made while withdrawing the needle to avoid undue tissue distension. Infiltration can be commenced from either glabella or tip. Four tracks of infiltration are made on each side with lignocaine 1%. The nasal cavities are dealt with separately as are the membranous septum and columella. This technique should not be used in a fractured nose (Eriksson, 1979).

Ear

Uses

Paracentesis of the eardrum, tympanotomy, myringotomy and radical mastoidectomy.

Anatomy (Williams & Warwick, 1980)

The sensory supply to the ear is described below (Fig. 71.6A,B).

Auricle
1 The *great auricular nerve* (a branch of the cervical plexus, C2 and 3) supplying the helix, antihelix, lobule and most of the cranial surface of the auricle.
2 The *lesser occipital nerve* supplying the upper part of the cranial surface.
3 The *auricular branch of the vagus* supplying the concavity and posterior part of the concha.
4 The *auriculotemporal nerve* (a branch of the mandibular nerve) supplying the tragus and adjacent part of the helix.
5 The *facial nerve* which together with the auricular branch of the vagus supplies small areas of skin on both aspects of the auricle, in the conchal depression and over its eminence.

External auditory meatus
1 The *auriculotemporal nerve* supplying the skin of the anterior and upper wall of the meatus.
2 The *auricular branch of the vagus* supplying the posterior wall and floor.

Tympanic membrane
1 The tympanic nerve (a branch of the glossopharyngeal nerve). The auriculotemporal nerve (a branch of the mandibular nerve).
2 The *auricular branch of the vagus.*

Techniques

Paracentesis of the eardrum. Two or three spray doses (20–30 mg) of lignocaine 10% aerosol spray are directed towards the upper wall of the auditory canal and allowed to run down over the eardrum. This can be repeated after 2 min and is then left for 3–5 min. EMLA cream has also been used (Bingham, 1991).

Radical mastoidectomy. Several injections of 1–2 ml of solution made over the mastoid process behind the ear anaesthetizes the great auricular nerve (Fig. 71.6A,

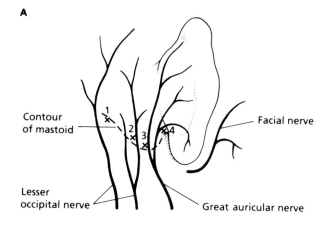

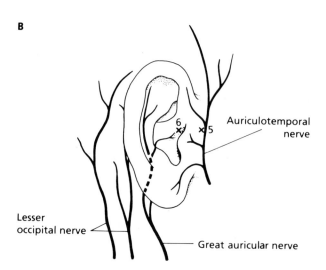

Fig. 71.6 Sensory supply to the auricle showing injection sites for radical mastoidectomy. (A) Cranial aspect; (B) external aspect.

injection sites 1,2,3). Two to 3 ml injected into the skin of the floor of the auditory canal and periosteal injection on the anterior part of the mastoid process (4) blocks the auricular branch of the vagus. Infiltration of the skin and periosteum over the auditory canal in front of the ear blocks the auriculotemporal nerve (Fig. 71.6B, site 5). To include its tympanic branch another injection must be made in the anterior wall of the auditory canal between bony and cartilaginous parts (6).

A few drops of more concentrated topical solution may be instilled into the meatus for surface anaesthesia of the mucous membrane, and tympanic membrane.

Lignocaine 4% may be used for topical application and lignocaine 0.5–1.0% with adrenaline for infiltration.

Tympanotomy. Block of the auriculotemporal nerve and its tympanic branch should be performed as above (Fig. 71.6B, injections 5 and 6). If a wide incision is contemplated, the full block should be performed as for radical mastoidectomy.

Mouth and pharynx

Dental procedures

Uses

Extraction of all teeth except lower molars, some conservation work, periodontal surgery, e.g. gingivectomy.

Anatomy (Williams & Warwick, 1980)

The sensory supply to the teeth is from branches of the trigeminal nerve (V). Maxillary branches supply the upper jaw and mandibular branches supply the lower jaw as follows (Fig. 71.7).

Upper jaw

1 The *superior alveolar nerves* (branches of the infra-orbital nerve, V2) supply the upper teeth, buccal gingiva and periosteum.
2 The *nasopalatine nerve* (one of the posterior nasal branches of the maxillary nerve, V2) supplies the mucosa, gingiva and periosteum of the anterior part of the hard palate.
3 The *greater palatine nerve* supplies the mucous membrane of the hard palate and palatal aspect of gum.

Lower jaw

4 The *buccal nerve* supplies the gum between the second molar and second premolar teeth on the buccal aspect.
5 The *inferior alveolar nerve* supplies the teeth and gums of the lower jaw on the lingual aspect.
6 The *lingual nerve* supplies the lingual gingiva and the floor of the mouth.

Technique

A surface anaesthetic can be applied to the gingiva in the area to be infiltrated.

Because of the tautness of the tissues, it is only possible to use a small volume of local anaesthetic solution, and this must diffuse through periosteum and compact bone to reach the nerve supply to the pulp, periodontum and jaw bone. Using a 26-gauge

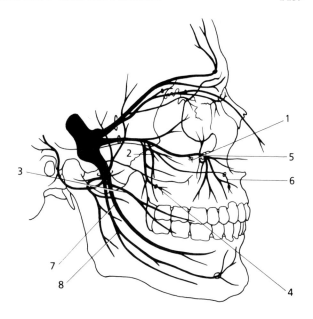

Fig. 71.7 Nerve supply to the upper and lower jaw. 1 and 2, anterior and posterior superior alveolar nerves; 3, buccal nerve; 4, greater palatine nerve; 5, infraorbital nerve; 6, nasopalatine nerve; 7, lingual nerve; 8, inferior alveolar nerve.

needle, solution is injected at the junction of adherent mucoperiosteum of buccal gingiva and mucous membrane of cheek, parallel with the long axis of the tooth. One-half to 1 ml of solution is deposited close to the apex in the buccal fold. Two to 3 ml injected in one site anaesthetizes two to three teeth. It is usually also necessary to anaesthetize the palatal or lingual aspect of the tooth. The mucosa is applied so closely to the periosteum of the hard palate that 0.1 ml of solution is sufficient and should be injected very slowly. One-tenth to 1 ml may be used on the lingual aspect of the lower teeth. For all injections, it is important that the tip of the needle lies just above the periosteum. In the lower jaw, injection must be close to bone to avoid depositing solution in the chin or muscles of the lower lip. All injections should be preceded by aspiration in this vascular area and should be made very slowly to avoid pain and damage to tissues induced by counterpressure. Infiltration blocks do not last as long as nerve blocks as the vascularity of the buccal fold aids rapid transport of solution away from the site of injection.

Anaesthesia may be inadequate for operations on pulp which is more richly innervated than the periodontal gingival and bone tissues. Infiltration blocks are unsuitable for procedures on the lower molars and premolars because of the large mass of mandibular bone. Haematoma and prolonged anaesthesia may result from damage to nerves and blood vessels, which is particularly likely to occur if the needle tip enters a foramen.

Solutions used commonly include lignocaine 2% with 1:80 000 adrenaline and prilocaine 3% with felypressin 0.03 IU/ml (Haglund & Evers, 1984).

Tonsillar block

Uses

Tonsillectomy. Although not used often as the sole anaesthetic, local anaesthesia may be useful with general anaesthesia in adults or children (Boliston & Upton, 1980).

Anatomy

The *tonsillar branch of the glossopharyngeal nerve* forms a plexus around the tonsil with branches of the *middle* and *posterior (lesser) palatine* nerves, which are branches of the maxillary nerve. Filaments are sent to adjacent soft palate and fauces.

Technique

The patient may be given a benzocaine lozenge 30 min before spraying mouth and pharynx with approximately 1 ml of cocaine 4–10% solution or lignocaine 4% or prilocaine 4% (repeated after 5 min).

Infiltration injections are then made (Fig. 71.8):

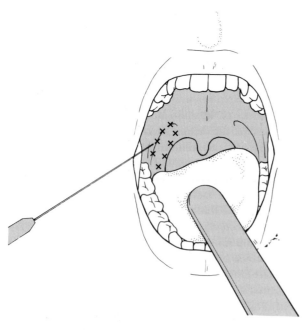

Fig. 71.8 Injection sites for tonsillectomy.

1 Under the mucous membrane of the posterior palatal arch.
2 Under the mucous membrane of the anterior palatal arch, sufficient to make both oedematous.
3 Into remaining peritonsillar tissue, below and above the tonsil. Infiltration into the supratonsillar fossa above is facilitated by drawing the tonsil medially.

Ten to 15 ml of either lignocaine 0.5–1.5% or prilocaine with adrenaline (e.g. 1:200 000) are used for infiltration on each side.

Some operators do not like the loss of cough reflex and the risk of aspiration which may occur with good pharyngeal spraying.

Gastroscopy, oesophagoscopy

Technique

Premedication is helpful, and the patient is asked to suck a benzocaine lozenge 30 min before the procedure. Intravenous sedation with a benzodiazepine, e.g. diazemuls or midazolam in 2 mg increments is often necessary.

Surface anaesthesia of the mouth and pharynx is accomplished by:
1 Spraying with a suitable topical agent, e.g. cocaine 4%, lignocaine 4%, amethocaine 1%.
2 Swallowing a viscous lignocaine preparation (2%) (Williams *et al.*, 1968; Atkinson *et al.*, 1987).

Larynx, trachea and bronchi

Uses

Laryngoscopy, tracheoscopy, bronchoscopy, bronchography and blind nasal intubation.

Anatomy

Larynx, trachea and bronchi. The sensory nerve supply is from the vagus via its superior and recurrent laryngeal branches.

The *superior laryngeal nerve* passes deep to the external and internal carotid arteries and there divides into a small motor external branch and a larger *internal branch* which pierces the postero-inferior part of the thyrohyoid membrane above the superior laryngeal artery and provides sensory supply to the laryngeal surface of the epiglottis, aryepiglottic folds and the interior of the larynx as far down as the vocal cords.

The terminal (inferior) branch of the *recurrent laryngeal nerve* ascends to the larynx in the groove between oesophagus and trachea together with the laryngeal branch of the inferior thyroid artery. It is sensory to the mucosa of the larynx below the cords, and to the trachea and bronchi.

Technique

Sedative premedication may be given 1 h preoperatively and intravenous sedation at the time of the procedure is helpful, although not essential (Pearce, 1980).

The mouth and pharynx are prepared as for oesophagoscopy (see above). For passage of a nasal tracheal tube or flexible bronchoscope, one nostril may be sprayed or packed with local anaesthetic (e.g. with cocaine 5%, lignocaine 4%). The nostril and tube may be lubricated also with lignocaine gel. This may be sufficient for laryngoscopy if inspection of the cords only is intended.

If the cords are to be touched or biopsied, the larynx itself must be anaesthetized. The internal branches of the superior laryngeal nerve may be anaesthetized as they pass beneath the mucosa of the pyriform fossae (Macintosh & Ostlere, 1967) by applying swabs soaked in local anaesthetic solution and held in Krause's forceps (or other curved forceps such as Jackson's or Moynihan's). These are then passed over the back of the tongue until the fossae are reached and held in position there for a short time. The swab should then be palpable through the skin near the tip of the hyoid bone. This procedure is easier if the tongue is held in a gauze swab and brought forward gently. The epiglottis and vocal cords are sprayed, or local anaesthetic solution may be dropped directly onto them under direct vision using a mirror and laryngeal syringe, or injected via the side arm of a flexible bronchoscope. The glottis is rendered anaesthetic by holding a swab soaked in local anaesthetic solution in it for a short time. If solution has been dripped directly onto the larynx this should not be necessary.

Surface anaesthesia of the upper airway may be combined with block of the superior laryngeal nerve performed percutaneously (Gotta & Sullivan, 1981).

The trachea is anaesthetized either by allowing solution dropped onto the glottis to run down the trachea or by injecting 2–4 ml of solution through the cricothyroid membrane into the trachea. Cricothyroid puncture is performed using a 22 gauge needle with syringe attached. The patient lies supine with neck extended and the anaesthetist stands as if for intubation. The cricothyroid membrane is palpated and the needle advanced perpendicularly in the midline until air is aspirated, confirming the presence of the needle tip in the trachea. The solution is then injected at the end of a maximal expiration. Inspiration and coughing then normally ensure spread throughout trachea and bronchial tree (Moore, 1978).

It is possible to produce anaesthesia throughout the respiratory tract using nebulized lignocaine. Methods have been described which utilize either a small disposable type of nebulizer (Vuckovic *et al.*, 1980) or an ultrasonic nebulizer (Christoforidis *et al.*, 1971). The patient mouth-breathes through a mask until 6–10 ml of lignocaine 4% solution is nebulized fully. If a few minutes of positive-pressure breathing via a face mask can be tolerated, solution can be dispensed via a nebulizer and ventilator (e.g. Bird MK 7).

Patients should have no oral intake for 3 h after the procedure to ensure return of laryngeal reflexes.

Absorption from the respiratory tract is rapid, and levels equivalent to intravenous injection may be achieved. Toxic levels of anaesthetic agent may be reached more readily if the mucosa is inflamed or traumatized. Chronic bronchitics may require higher doses for adequate analgesia, and particular care must be taken to avoid toxicity. When any type of spray is used, the accuracy of the dispensing apparatus must be considered. A local technique is contraindicated in patients with a full stomach.

Cricothyroid puncture should not be performed in patients who have a bleeding disorder, local sepsis or tumour. Complications include breakage of the needle during transtracheal injection, subcutaneous emphysema and haematoma, penetration of the posterior wall of the trachea leading to mediastinitis or mediastinal emphysema and vocal cord damage. Inadvertent submucosal injection could produce airway obstruction (Gold & Buechel, 1939; Newton & Edwards, 1979; Prithvi-Raj, 1983; Morrison *et al.*, 1985).

Lignocaine 4% (max. 5 ml) or prilocaine 4% (max. 10 ml) are suitable. Lignocaine 10% aerosol spray may be used with caution.

Tracheostomy

Technique

Infiltration of skin and subcutaneous tissues at the site of the proposed incision followed by infiltration of deeper layers as necessary provides adequate anaesthesia. Transtracheal injection of 2–3 ml of lig-nocaine 4% is advisable to prevent excessive cough-ing on entering the trachea (Morrison *et al.*, 1985).

Eyes

General anaesthesia has become commonly used for all procedures but local anaesthesia is frequently employed, particularly for the elderly high-risk patient and for day cases. The eye is easily amenable to block and local anaesthetic techniques are now gaining in popularity. Full co-operation and immo-bility on the part of the patient are required. The advantages of local anaesthesia are prolonged post-operative analgesia and less nausea and vomiting. There may be less reduction in intraocular pres-sure than with a well-managed general anaesthetic. Anaesthetists are becoming increasingly involved in the performance of these blocks. Premedication helps to produce a calm patient, and an antiemetic is a useful component.

Conjunctiva and cornea

Uses

Tonometry, removal of foreign bodies, syringing and probing of tearduct and as part of the technique for any eye surgery.

Anatomy

The sensory supply to the ocular conjunctiva and the conjunctiva of the upper eyelid arises from branches of the ophthalmic division of the trigeminal nerve. The conjunctiva of the lower eyelid is supplied by branches from its maxillary division.

The cornea is supplied with numerous nerves from branches of the ophthalmic nerve, particularly the long ciliary nerves.

Technique

One to two drops of solution are instilled into the open eye. Discomfort is allowed to settle (30–60 s) and then a further instillation is made. This may be repeated until adequate anaesthesia is obtained.

If solution is syringed into the tearduct, probing can be performed.

A number of local anaesthetic agents are suit-able including lignocaine 4%, prilocaine 4%, oxy-buprocaine 0.2–0.4%, proxymetacaine 0.5% and amethocaine 0.5–1.0%. The latter stings less if used

in solutions containing methyl cellulose, but such solutions increase the viscosity of the preparation and may penetrate the eyeball and should be avoided. Adrenaline may be added to any of these solutions to produce ischaemia although corneal damage can result from vasoconstriction.

Cocaine 2–4% is still used occasionally if pro-longed and intense analgesia is required. It causes vasoconstriction which is useful, but the resultant corneal clouding limits its use. It should not be used in closed-angle glaucoma as it causes mydriasis (Allen & Elkington, 1980; Morrison *et al.*, 1985).

Eyelids

Uses

For removal of superficial lesions, e.g. retention cysts, papillomata, basal-cell carcinomata, for correction of ectropion or entropion and to enable retraction of the eyelids during intraocular surgery.

Anatomy

The upper eyelid is supplied medially by the *supra-trochlear nerve* (a branch of the frontal nerve from V1), the infratrochlear, lacrimal and supraorbital nerves.

The lower eyelid is supplied by the *palpebral branches of the infraorbital nerve* (V2) and the *facial and zygomaticofacial nerves* (the latter being a branch of the facial nerve).

Technique

Both skin and conjunctival aspects of the eyelid must be injected if surgery involves the whole thick-ness of the lid because the tarsal plate in the eyelid limits spread of infiltrated solution. This can be accomplished in one manoeuvre. The needle is inserted at the lateral margin of the tarsal plate and subcutaneous infiltration is first performed with 2–3 ml of solution. The eyelid can then be everted over the needle which is then advanced and when its tip is seen under the conjunctiva, further infiltration can be made subconjunctivally.

Lignocaine or prilocaine 1–2% with adrenaline are suitable. Hyaluronidase aids spread and hastens the onset of anaesthesia (Eriksson, 1979; Allen & Elkington, 1980).

Eyeball

Uses

Intraocular surgery requires anaesthesia of the eyeball in addition to that of the eyelids, cornea and conjunctiva. It is necessary also for enucleation and photoelectric coagulation of the retina.

Anatomy

The nerve supply is from the oculomotor nerve (III) via the *long and short posterior ciliary nerves* and the *ciliary ganglion* which lie within the muscle cone. Some of the short ciliary nerves pass into the ciliary ganglion which lies between the optic nerve (II) and the lateral rectus muscle. Others pass into the long ciliary nerves which lie close to the ganglion and in turn join the nasociliary nerve.

Technique

Block of these nerves abolishes pain and also paralyses the extraocular muscles, an absolute requirement for intraocular surgery as these muscles may cause movement or distortion of the globe and a consequent increase in intraocular pressure. These may all be blocked together by a single infiltration (retrobulbar block), or by the peribulbar (periocular technique) following surface anaesthesia of cornea and conjunctiva.

Retrobulbar block is performed in one of two ways.
1 The patient looks upwards and inwards while a 4—5 cm needle is inserted through a skin weal at the outer inferior angle of the orbit (Fig. 71.9). Alternatively, the needle may be inserted directly through the conjunctiva with the lower eyelid retracted. The needle is advanced for about 3 cm upwards, backwards and medially towards the apex of the orbit. The needle tip should then lie within the cone formed by the extraocular muscles. After aspiration, 2 ml of solution are injected. This is the commonest method employed.
2 The patient looks downwards and the needle is passed through a weal in the centre of the tarsal plate of the upper eyelid and advanced 3 cm backwards and slightly inwards and downwards. Two ml solution are injected.

The block is effective after approximately 5 min. It causes also pupillary dilatation, exophthalmos and a modest decrease in intraocular pressure.

Two ml lignocaine 2% or prilocaine are used

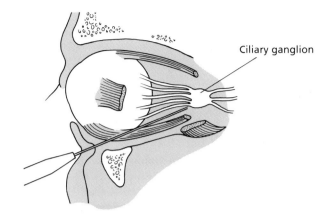

Fig. 71.9 Retrobulbar block. Site and direction of injection.

usually. Four ml may be used for enucleation. The addition of hyaluronidase 6—10 TRU/ml aids diffusion of solution.

The *orbicularis oculi muscle* must be paralysed for all intraocular surgery to prevent movement of the eyelids (blepharospasm). It is innervated by the terminal branches of the facial nerve and these must be blocked near the lateral canthus. A weal is raised at the inferolateral angle of the orbit and the needle inserted at right angles to the skin. Tissues are infiltrated down to bone. The needle is advanced subcutaneously along the lateral and inferior margins of the orbit and further infiltration made (van Lint's method). Alternatively, the facial nerve may be blocked over the condyle of the mandible (O'Brien's method) (Macintosh & Ostlere, 1967; Allen & Elkington, 1980; Morrison *et al.*, 1985).

Retrobulbar block may result in retrobulbar haematoma with resulting marked proptosis. Operation must be deferred until it resolves and this block should not be performed for emergency surgery. Other complications include perforation of the globe, optic nerve damage, central retinal artery occlusion and intradural injection with apnoea and cardiac arrest reported (Fry & Henderson, 1989).

The newer technique of peribulbar block is described in detail in Chapter 38.

Abdomen

Uses

Infiltration of the abdominal wall and rectus sheath block may be used for procedures where profound muscle relaxation is not required and in which there is no great degree of visceral pain. It may be used for Caesarean section in exceptional circumstances

(Ranney & Stanage, 1975), herniorrhaphy (inguinal and femoral), pyloric stenosis in babies and suprapubic cystotomy.

Anatomy (Williams & Warwick, 1980)

The superficial layers of the anterior abdominal wall (from exterior to interior) are:
1 Skin.
2 Superficial fascia from xiphisternum to a point midway between umbilicus and pubis.
3 Superficial (Scarpa's) fascia and deep (Camper's) fascia.
4 Four large flat sheets of muscle (external oblique, internal oblique, transversus abdominis and rectus abdominis) and pyramidalis (Fig. 71.10).

The *external oblique* is the most superficial, with fibres passing downwards and medially from their origins on the lower eight ribs to insert into the anterior superior iliac spine of the iliac crest and into its aponeurosis which ends medially in the linea alba from the xiphoid process to the pubic symphysis. It inserts inferiorly into the pubic symphysis and crest as far as the pubic tubercle. Between this point and the iliac crest insertion on the anterior superior iliac spine, it folds in on itself and forms the *inguinal ligament*.

The *internal oblique muscle* lies beneath the external oblique and arises from the lateral two-thirds of the inguinal ligament, from the iliac crest and from the thoracolumbar fascia between the 12th rib and the iliac crest. Its fibres pass upwards and medially. Superiorly, some fibres attach to the lower three to four ribs but most fibres end in an aponeurosis, the upper two-thirds of which splits at the lateral border of the rectus abdominis and encloses this muscle, reuniting in the midline to help form the linea alba. The anterior layer blends with the aponeurosis of the external oblique and the posterior layer with that of transversus abdominis. The whole lower one-third of the aponeurosis passes anterior to the recti to end in the linea alba. Fibres arising from the inguinal ligament join the aponeurosis of transversus abdominis and form the *conjoint tendon*.

The *transversus abdominis* lies beneath the internal oblique and arises from the lateral one-third of the inguinal ligament, the iliac crest, the thoracolumbar fascia and the lower six costal cartilages. The fibres pass transversely and medially to end in an aponeurosis whose upper two-thirds lie behind rectus abdominis, whilst the lower third passes in front of it. It inserts medially into the linea alba with the lower fibres curving downwards and medially to

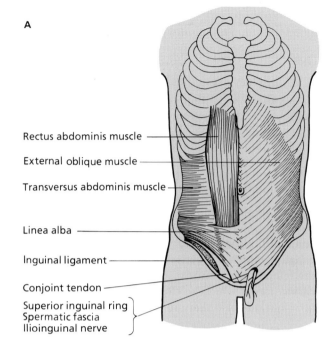

A

Rectus abdominis muscle ——

External oblique muscle ——

Transversus abdominis muscle ——

Linea alba ——

Inguinal ligament ——

Conjoint tendon ——

Superior inguinal ring
Spermatic fascia
Ilioinguinal nerve

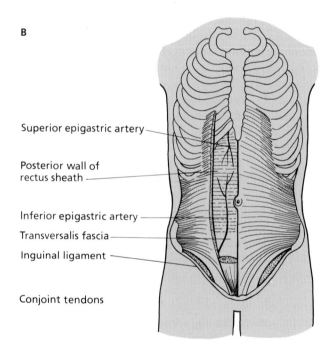

B

Superior epigastric artery ——

Posterior wall of
rectus sheath ——

Inferior epigastric artery ——

Transversalis fascia ——

Inguinal ligament ——

Conjoint tendons

Fig. 71.10 Muscles of the anterior abdominal wall. (A) The external oblique and transversus abdominis muscles; (B) the internal oblique muscles.

form the *conjoint tendon* with the aponeurosis of the internal oblique. This tendon is inserted into the pubic crest.

The two *recti abdomini* are separated by the linea alba and extend from their origins on the fifth, sixth and seventh costal cartilages to the pubis (Fig. 71.11).

The nerve supply to the muscles of the abdominal wall is from T7−12 and L1. The terminal portions of the intercostal nerves 7−12 enter the abdominal wall between the diaphragm and transversus abdominis, and come to lie between the internal oblique and transversus abdominis. They enter the rectus sheath laterally and run within it posteriorly before piercing the recti to supply the overlying skin. L1 makes its contribution inferiorly through the iliohypogastric and ilioinguinal nerves.

Posteriorly, the rectus sheath is pierced by the superior and inferior epigastric vessels.

Techniques

Abdominal field block provides anaesthesia from skin down to peritoneum. The intercostal nerves (T7−12) are blocked as they enter the anterior abdominal wall just below the costal margin. Three weals are raised (Fig. 71.12).
1 Below the xiphisternum.
2 Below the ninth costal cartilage on each side where the rectus muscle crosses it.

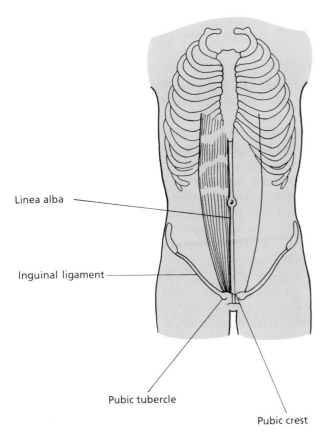

Fig. 71.11 Rectus abdominis muscle showing tendinous intersections.

The muscle is enclosed in the rectus sheath which is formed by the split in the internal oblique aponeurosis which fuses anteriorly with the aponeurosis of the external oblique and posteriorly with that of transversus abdominis as far down as a point midway between umbilicus and symphysis pubis. Below this point, the three aponeuroses all pass anterior to the muscle which is separated from peritoneum by a thin connective tissue layer (transversalis fascia) and fat. Each rectus muscle is intersected within the rectus sheath by three tendinous intersections at the level of the xiphisternum, umbilicus and a point half-way between. They are attached usually to the anterior layer of the rectus sheath but do not pass normally right through the muscle to the posterior layer, and therefore when local anaesthetic is infiltrated, these intersections may limit spread anteriorly but not posteriorly.

The two small *pyramidalis muscles* lie in front of the lower part of the rectus muscles and within the sheath. They arise from the pubis and insert into the linea alba at a point midway between pubis and umbilicus.

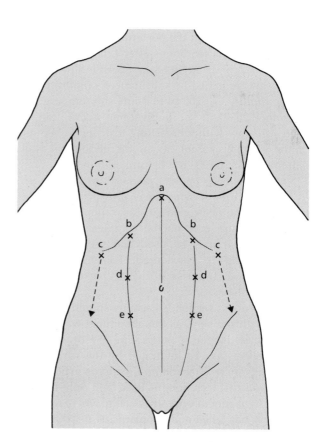

Fig. 71.12 Abdominal field block and rectus sheath block.

3 At the lower borders of the costal margins laterally.

Infiltration is made between these points through subcutaneous tissues and muscle layers to form a continuous line of infiltration along the lower costal margin, bearing in mind that the nerves lie in a plane between the internal oblique and transversus abdominis muscles. Further infiltration is made down the lateral side of the abdominal wall as far as the iliac crest.

Rectus sheath block. If this is also performed, a higher success rate is likely. Rectus sheath block performed alone does not produce relaxation of the other abdominal muscles (external and internal oblique and transversus abdominis). This is performed by raising three weals as for (1) and (2) above (Fig. 71.12), followed by (4) and (5):

4 At the lateral borders of the rectus muscles just above the umbilicus.

5 In the same lateral lines just below the umbilicus.

The needle is advanced at right angles to the skin, and when it is felt that the rectus sheath has been pierced anteriorly, it is advanced a further 0.5 cm, and 5 ml of solution are injected. The needle is then directed upwards and downwards and further solution deposited at each of the three sites. The aim is to deposit solution in the posterior part of the rectus sheath where the tendinous intersections are incomplete. If the costal margin has not been infiltrated, the skin weals are joined by subcutaneous infiltration.

One hundred to 200 ml of dilute solution, e.g. lignocaine 0.25−0.5% or bupivacaine 0.25% can be used with care without reaching toxic levels because of the relative avascularity of the abdominal wall. Adrenaline 1 : 200 000 is a helpful addition.

Success depends largely on injections being made in the correct plane which may prove difficult, particularly in the obese patient. Relaxation of abdominal musculature may not be complete. Near toxic doses of agent may be used and the size of the patient should be considered. Pain from viscera is not obtunded unless a coeliac plexus block is performed also.

For Caesarean section, injections should be made parallel with the skin, as the abdominal wall is thin and there is danger of perforating the uterus. The deeper layers may be infiltrated by the surgeon as surgery advances. Traction on the uterus may still be painful and this technique is used best only to supplement light general anaesthesia, e.g. where tracheal intubation has failed and spontaneous respiration is proceeding (Macintosh & Bryce-Smith, 1962; Bryce-Smith, 1976; Scott, 1983; Atkinson *et al.*, 1987).

Pyloric stenosis in babies (Rammstedt's operation)

Technique

Correction of fluid and electrolyte imbalance must precede surgery and premedication is desirable, e.g. morphine, 0.1−0.2 mg/kg i.m., or chloral hydrate, 30 mg/kg orally. Intravenous access is secured and the baby is bandaged to a cross-splint and maintained in a warm environment. Local infiltration of the abdominal wall is made subcutaneously between umbilicus and costal margin on the right followed by a right or bilateral rectus sheath block, depending on the incision to be used. A rectus sheath block alone may be adequate. The peritoneum may be infiltrated under direct vision by the surgeon.

Lignocaine 0.25−0.5% is suitable, and adrenaline 1 : 400 000 should be used to retard absorption. A volume of 13 ml of 0.25% solution may be used in a 3.5-kg baby (Black & Love, 1957; Leatherdale, 1958).

Suprapubic cystotomy

Technique

A bilateral rectus sheath block performed through weals raised at the lateral margin of the rectus from umbilicus to pubis may be adequate. In addition, the weals may be joined by subcutaneous and intradermal infiltration. A weal is raised also in the midline, 3 cm above the symphysis pubis, and a needle inserted through it in a backwards and downwards direction to enter the retropubic space, where 30 ml of solution are injected (Leatherdale & Ellis, 1958).

Inguinal hernia

Anatomy (Williams & Warwick, 1980)

The sensory supply to the inguinal area is from three nerves, all derived from the lumbar plexus (Fig. 71.13):

1 The iliohypogastric nerve (L1).
2 The ilioinguinal nerve (L1).
3 The genitofemoral nerve (L1 and L2).

The first two arise from the lumbar plexus within psoas muscle, cross quadratus lumborum, pierce transversus abdominis and come to lie between it and the internal oblique near the iliac crest (Fig. 71.14). The iliohypogastric nerve pierces the internal oblique and supplies skin over the lowest part of the abdominal wall and pubis. The ilioinguinal nerve runs parallel to and 1 cm below the iliohypogastric

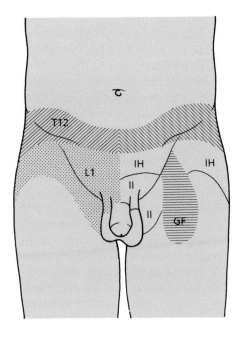

Fig. 71.13 Sensory supply to the inguinal region.

(both now lying between the external and internal oblique muscles). It enters the inguinal canal posteriorly to accompany the spermatic cord or round ligament and becomes superficial after passing through the external ring to supply the skin of the scrotum or labia majora and adjacent thigh.

The genitofemoral nerve divides into a *genital branch* which follows the spermatic cord through the inguinal canal and supplies cremaster muscle plus the skin of the scrotum or labia majora and a *femoral branch* which supplies skin over the upper part of the femoral triangle.

Skin and muscles of the lower abdomen are supplied also by T11 and T12 which run medially from near the iliac crest between transversus abdominis and the internal oblique.

The spermatic cord and testis receive also an autonomic supply.

Technique

Both skin and the hernial sac must be anaesthetized. The iliohypogastric and ilioinguinal nerves, T11 and

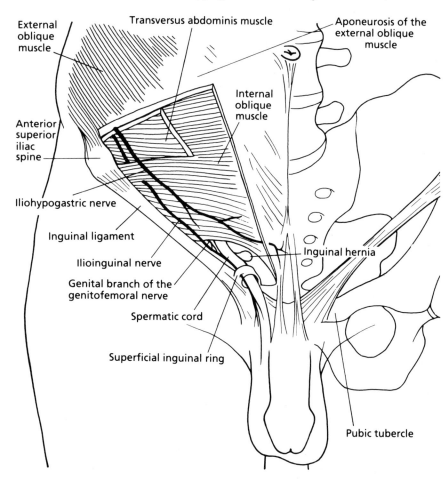

Fig. 71.14 Anatomy of the inguinal region.

T12 may all be blocked by infiltration in the region of the iliac crest. A weal (X, Fig. 71.15) is raised two fingers' breadth medial to the anterior superior iliac spine and a needle inserted perpendicular to the skin until it strikes the medial wall of the iliac bone. Fifteen to 20 ml of solution are infiltrated into the muscle layers as the needle is withdrawn slowly. At the same site, a further 15–20 ml of solution should be injected in a caudal and mediocaudal direction under the aponeurosis of the external oblique (Fig. 71.15, injections a and b). This may be detected more easily if a short-bevelled needle is used, when a click may be felt. Subcutaneous injections can be made also from the same site in a lateral direction towards the inguinal fold and mediocaudally (c and d) towards the midline using a further 10–30 ml of solution.

Another weal (Y) is raised just proximal to the pubic tubercle, and infiltrations made extraperitoneally along the upper border of the pubic bone (e),

then within the external oblique aponeurosis and in a more cranial direction (f). Subcutaneous injections are made at the same site in a fan from the inguinal ligament (g) to midline (h). The injections towards the midline should anaesthetize any overlapping nerve supply from the opposite side. Five ml of solution should be used for each injection.

To anaesthetize the contents of the sac, a percutaneous injection of 20 ml of solution may be made above the mid-point of the inguinal ligament after penetration of the aponeurosis of the external oblique in order to anaesthetize the contents of the inguinal canal. However, this is undertaken best by the surgeon, under direct vision, along the spermatic cord at the superficial inguinal ring or when the inguinal canal has been opened. In the latter case, the sac is opened, the hernia reduced and the neck of the hernia is injected medially and laterally from inside the sac in an outward direction. This renders further manipulation painless. If the hernia is irreducible, the sac may be injected from the outside. Infiltration along the line of incision may also be necessary. Success rate is low in the very obese with irreducible herniae.

Sixty to 90 ml of lignocaine or prilocaine 0.5% may be used. The addition of adrenaline helps to reduce plasma concentrations of local anaesthetic (Bryce-Smith, 1976; Eriksson, 1979).

Femoral herniorrhaphy

Technique

As for inguinal herniorrhaphy with the addition of intradermal and subcutaneous infiltration around the lump. Alternatively, a femoral nerve block anaesthetizes the skin over the thigh.

Urethra

Uses

Bouginage, catheterization, urethrocystography and possibly cystoscopy.

Anatomy

The nerve plexus supplying the urethral mucosa lies directly beneath it. Local anaesthetic placed in contact with the mucosa diffuses easily across it to render the urethra anaesthetic.

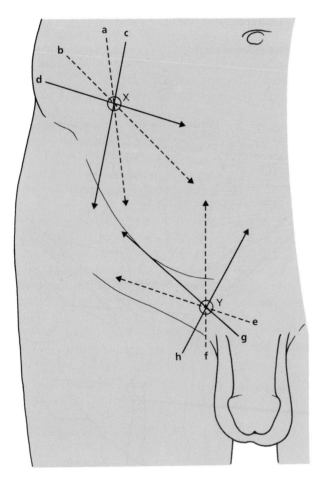

Fig. 71.15 Injections for inguinal herniorrhaphy. (See text for discussion.)

Technique

Male. Glans and foreskin are cleaned and the penis held in a dry swab. Either an aqueous solution of local anaesthetic or a gel may be used, although the latter is more favoured, as it lubricates the mucosa and remains in contact with it for longer. The plastic nozzle of a tube of gel is inserted into the urethra and the contents of the tube squeezed gently into the urethra. After the first few ml, the patient should be asked to strain as if passing urine and the rest of the gel is inserted. This manoeuvre should allow gel to enter the prostatic urethra. A penile clamp should be applied just below the glans and left for 10–15 min. Ten to 15 ml of gel are used.

Female. An applicator (e.g. a throat swab) covered with cotton wool along 4 cm of its length is dipped in gel and inserted into the urethra and left *in situ* for 10 min with the patient lying on her back.

Rupture of the mucosa may occur, making it possible for injection to be made into the circulation if the patient has bulbocavernous reflux. Gels containing methylcellulose have caused serious systemic reactions. Instillations should therefore be made slowly under low pressure and agents of low toxicity used. Bleeding may occur.

Ten to 15 ml of lignocaine gel 1–2% or prilocaine gel 2% are used, or 30 ml of a solution containing cocaine 0.5% and sodium bicarbonate 0.5%.

Pyribenzamine 2% (an antihistamine) may give reasonable analgesia in patients in whom local anaesthetics are contraindicated (Bryce-Smith, 1955; Dix & Tresidder, 1963).

Perineum

Uses

Episiotomy, repair of lacerations, outlet forceps (in combination with pudendal nerve block).

Anatomy

The sensory supply to the vulva is from the *genitofemoral and ilioinguinal nerves* anteriorly and from the *perianal branch of the posterior femoral cutaneous nerve* posteriorly. The perineum is supplied by branches of the *pudendal nerve* (S2, 3, 4).

Technique

For performing an episiotomy, infiltration is made between perineal skin and vaginal mucosa where the incision is to be made. For repair of an episiotomy or lacerations, infiltration should be performed parallel to both perineal skin and vaginal mucosa.

A spray may be applied to vulva and perineum as an adjunct to pudendal nerve block for normal or forceps delivery but this is not employed normally.

Lignocaine 0.5–1.0% for infiltration or a 10% spray should be used. Particular care is needed in calculating dosage in this highly vascular area.

Anus

Uses

Field block of the anal region may be used for lateral sphincterotomy, excision of skin tags, thrombosed haemorrhoids and diagnostic procedures such as proctoscopy, sigmoidoscopy and colonoscopy in patients with painful anal lesions.

Anatomy

The perineal region is supplied by the inferior haemorrhoidal branches of the pudendal nerve (S2, 3, 4).

Technique

To attain satisfactory analgesia, deep injections should be made at 3, 6, 9 and 12 o'clock around the anal margin and approximately 5 ml injected at each site. Subcutaneous circumferential injection is made prior to this through two initial weals on each side of the anus and 2.5 cm from it, using 20 ml of solution. A finger in the rectum should prevent inadvertent perforation of its mucous membrane. Compliance is understandably low even following premedication and intravenous sedation. Techniques have been devised to allow simultaneous injection at all four sites using a four-needle adaptor fitted to a syringe (Dodi, 1986).

Bupivacaine 0.5% with adrenaline 1:200 000 provides a longer period of analgesia than lignocaine or prilocaine.

Miscellaneous

Fracture haematoma block

Uses

Recent fractures, such as Colles', Pott's, metatarsal, metacarpal and femoral fractures. Although analgesia is usually imperfect, this technique may be useful in mass casualty situations.

Technique

A weal is raised over the fracture site and a needle introduced towards the fracture site until aspirated blood confirms that the tip lies in the associated haematoma. Slow injection of solution without vaso-constrictor is made. Volume depends on the fracture site, e.g. 15–20 ml for a Colles' fracture, 20–30 ml for a femoral fracture. Hyaluronidase appears to be a useful addition. Ten min is allowed to elapse before reduction is attempted.

The block should not be performed in the presence of overlying sepsis. Toxicity may occur from rapid absorption of solution.

Lignocaine or prilocaine 1–2% with or without hyaluronidase (1000 units/20 ml solution) are suitable.

Intact skin

Penetration of intact skin by a local anaesthetic depends on the available concentration of its uncharged base form and a high water content. Pharmacologically, this has always proven difficult to achieve as the uncharged base is poorly soluble in water and combination of the active base with water is only possible in an oil-in-water emulsion. In such an emulsion, the maximum achievable concentration of local anaesthetic in a droplet is 20% and this is too low for effective analgesia. This problem has been overcome partly by the formulation of eutectic mixtures of local anaesthetics (EMLA). Lignocaine and prilocaine crystals, when mixed in equal amounts, melt to form an oil (eutectic mixture) at room temperature. When this oil is used in an emulsion, the droplet concentration of local anaesthetic base is raised to 80%, although the total anaesthetic concentration is only 5%. If such a mixture is allowed contact time with skin of 30–60 min, good analgesia can be obtained.

Other local anaesthetic preparations have been assessed (McCafferty et al., 1988) and an amethocaine formulation which may provide analgesia comparable to EMLA (McCafferty et al., 1989) has been used for venepuncture and split-skin grafts (Small et al., 1988).

Uses

The use of EMLA cream has now been described for many other purposes including topical anaesthesia of:

1 Gingival mucosa, for dental work (Haasio et al., 1990).
2 Nasal mucosa, prior to fibreoptic bronchoscopy (Randell et al., 1992).
3 Skin, for venepuncture and superficial skin surgery including skin grafting (Juhlin et al., 1980).
4 Prepuce to allow separation of preputial adhesions in children who may otherwise require circumcision (MacKinlay, 1988; Lafferty et al., 1991).
5 Tympanic membrane for myringotomy and ventilation-tube insertion (Bingham, 1991).

Technique

EMLA cream (lignocaine 2.5% plus prilocaine 2.5% as a 5% oil-in-water emulsion cream) is applied 30–60 min prior to venepuncture over a suitable site and covered with an occlusive dressing. Transient skin blanching, erythema and oedema may occur and methaemoglobinaemia has been reported in an infant when a large area was covered, although toxic plasma levels were not reached (Hallen et al., 1985; Scott, 1986).

Other complications recorded with the use of EMLA are principally related to ingestion of cream +/− occlusive dressing by children and adults whose understanding is limited (Norman & Jones 1990). Secure secondary protective dressings are advocated. Applications of 2 gm over a large area of skin produce serum concentrations of only 0.149 µg/ml (MacKinlay, 1988), which is well below the toxic level (5–6 µg/ml). Amounts of 30 gm have been safely used (Bierkens et al., 1991). However, an experimental study to evaluate the use of EMLA cream in wounds has shown that the cream elicits an exaggerated inflammatory response that damages host defences. The study concluded that the use of the cream in wounds was inadvisable (Powell et al., 1991).

Topical application of amethocaine cream, 2 g (5% w/w), has been shown to produce more rapid and longer lasting effect for equal analgesia when compared with EMLA (Mazumdar et al., 1991). Although no toxic symptoms were demonstrated in the few volunteers studied, plasma levels were measurable in some patients and further evaluation is necessary. Side-effects such as erythema, urticaria and pruritus occur.

References

Akerman B., Hellberg I.-B. & Trossvik C. (1988) Primary evaluation of the local anaesthetic properties of the amino amide agent ropivacaine (LEA 103). *Acta Anaesthesiologica Scandinavica* **32**, 571–8.

Allen E.D. & Elkington A.R. (1980) Local anaesthesia and the eye. *British Journal of Anaesthesia* **53**, 689–94.

Atkinson R.S., Rushman G.B. & Lee J.A. (1987) Regional analgesia. In *A Synopsis of Anaesthesia* 10th edn. John Wright & Sons Ltd, Bristol.

Bierkens A.E., Maes R.M., Hendrikx J.M., Erdos A.F., de Vries J.D.M. & Debruyne F.M.J. (1991) The use of local anesthesia in second generation extracorporeal shock wave lithotripsy: eutectic mixture of local anaesthetics. *Journal of Urology* **146**, 287–9.

Bingham B. (1991) The safety and efficacy of EMLA cream topical anaesthesia for myringotomy and ventilation tube insertion. *Journal of Otolaryngology* **20**, 193–5.

Black G.W. & Love S.H.S. (1957) Anaesthesia for Rammstedt's operation. *Anaesthesia* **12**, 430–4.

Boakes A.J., Laurence D.R., Lovel K.W., O'Neil R. & Verrill P.J. (1972) Adverse reactions to local anaesthetic/vasoconstrictor preparations. A study of the cardiovascular responses to Xylestesin and Hostacain-with-noradrenaline. *British Dental Journal* **133**, 137–40.

Boakes A.J., Laurence D.R., Teoh P.C., Barar F.S.K., Benedikter L.T. & Prichard B.N.C. (1973) Interactions between sympathomimetic amines and antidepressant agents in man. *British Medical Journal* **1**, 311–15.

Bodman R.I. & Boyes-Korkis F. (1960) Anaesthetizing the nose. *British Medical Journal* **2**, 1956.

Boliston T.A. & Upton J.J.M. (1980) Infiltration with lignocaine and adrenaline in adult tonsillectomy. *Journal of Laryngology and Otology* **94**, 1257–9.

British National Formulary (1991) No. 22. British Medical Association and The Pharmaceutical Society of Great Britain.

Bryce-Smith R. (1955) Topical analgesia for the urethra. *British Medical Journal* **1**, 462.

Bryce-Smith R. (1976) In *Monographs in Anaesthesiology*, vol. 5. Practical Regional Analgesia (Eds Lee J.A. & Bryce-Smith R.). Excerpta Medica, Amsterdam.

Christoforidis A.J., Tomashefski J.F. & Mitchell R.I. (1971) Use of an ultrasonic nebulizer for the application of oropharyngeal, laryngeal and tracheobronchial anesthesia. *Chest* **59**, 629–33.

Concepcion M. & Covino B.G. (1984) Rational use of local anaesthetics. *Drugs* **27**, 256–70.

Cotton B.R., Henderson H.P., Achola K.J. & Smith G. (1986) Changes in plasma catecholamine concentration following infiltration with large volumes of local anaesthetic solution containing adrenaline. *British Journal of Anaesthesia* **58**, 593–7.

Covino B.G. & Vassallo H.B. (1976) Clinical aspects of local anesthesia. In *Local Anesthetics. Mechanisms of Action and Clinical Use* pp. 89–92. Grune and Stratton, New York.

Curtiss E.S. (1952) Postural nerve block for intranasal operations. *Lancet* **i**, 989–91.

Dix V.W. & Tresidder G.C. (1963) Collapse after use of lignocaine jelly for urethral anaesthesia. *Lancet* **i**, 890.

Dodi G. (1986) An improved technique of local anal anaesthesia. *Diseases of the Colon and Rectum* **29**, 71.

Eriksson E. (1979) In *Illustrated Handbook in Local Anaesthesia*

2nd edn. Lloyd-Luke, London.

Fry R.A. & Henderson J. (1989) Local anaesthesia for eye surgery. The peri-ocular technique. *Anaesthesia* **45**, 14–17.

Gold M.I. & Buechel D.R. (1939) Translaryngeal anaesthesia: a review. *Anaesthesia* **20**, 181.

Gotta A.W. & Sullivan C.A. (1981) Anaesthesia of the upper airway using topical anaesthetic and superior laryngeal nerve block. *British Journal of Anaesthesia* **53**, 1055–7.

Haasio J., Jokinen T., Numminen M. & Rosenberg P. (1990) Topical anaesthesia of gingival mucosa by 5% eutectic mixture of lignocaine and prilocaine or by 10% lignocaine spray. *Journal of Oral and Maxillo-facial Surgery* **28**, 99–101.

Haglund J. & Evers H. (1984) In *Local Anaesthesia in Dentistry*. Zohlbergs Tryckeri, Malmo.

Hallen B., Carlsson P. & Uppfeldt A. (1985) Clinical study of a lignocaine–prilocaine cream to relieve the pain of venepuncture. *British Journal of Anaesthesia* **57**, 326–8.

Hassan H.G., Renck H., Lindberg B., Akerman B. & Hellquist R. (1985) Effects of adjuvants to local anaesthetics on their duration I. *Acta Anaesthesiologica Scandinavica* **29**, 375–9.

Juhlin L., Evers H. & Broberg F. (1980) A lidocaine prilocaine cream for superficial skin surgery and painful lesions. *Acta Dermatologica Venereologica (Stockholm)* **60**, 544–6.

Lafferty P.M., MacGregor F.B. & Scobie W.G. (1991) Management of foreskin problems. *Archives of Disease in Childhood* **66**, 696–7.

Leatherdale R.A.L. (1958) Anaesthesia for Rammstedt's operation. *Lancet* **i**, 932–5.

Leatherdale R.A.L. & Ellis H. (1958) Prostatectomy: anaesthetic technique and other factors affecting prognosis. *Lancet* **ii**, 1189–92.

Macintosh R.R. & Bryce-Smith R. (1962) *Local Analgesia: Abdominal Surgery* 2nd edn. Churchill Livingstone, Edinburgh.

Macintosh R.R. & Ostlere M. (1967) *Local Analgesia, Head and Neck* 2nd edn. Churchill Livingstone, Edinburgh.

MacKinlay G.A. (1988) Saving the prepuce. Painless separation of preputial adhesions in the outpatient clinic. *British Medical Journal* **297**, 590–1.

Mazumdar B., Tomlinson A.A. & Faulder G.C. (1991) Preliminary study to assay plasma amethocaine concentrations after topical application of a new local anaesthetic cream containing amethocaine. *British Journal of Anaesthesia* **67**, 432–6.

McCafferty D.E., Woolfson A.D., McClelland K.H. & Boston V. (1988) Comparative 'in vivo' and 'in vitro' assessment of the percutaneous absorption of local anaesthetics. *British Journal of Anaesthesia* **60**, 64–9.

McCafferty D.E., Woolfson A.D. & Boston V. (1989) 'In vivo' assessment of percutaneous absorption of local anaesthetic preparation. *British Journal of Anaesthesia* **62**, 17–21.

Moffett A.J. (1947) Nasal analgesia by postural instillation. *Anaesthesia* **2**, 31–4.

Moore D.C. (1978) In *Regional Block* 4th edn. Charles C. Thomas, Springfield, Illinois.

Morrison J.D., Mirakhur R.K. & Craig H.J.L. (1985) In *Anaesthesia for Eye, Ear, Nose and Throat Surgery* 2nd edn. Churchill Livingstone, Edinburgh.

Newton D.A.G. & Edwards G.F. (1979) Route of introduction and method of anesthesia for fibreoptic bronchoscopy. *Chest* **75**, 650.

Norman J. & Jones P.I. (1990) Complications of the use of

EMLA. *British Journal of Anaesthesia* **64**, 403.

Oldham K.W. (1968) A simple technique for anaesthesia of the nose for intranasal surgery. *British Journal of Anaesthesia* **40**, 979–83.

Pearce S.J. (1980) Fibreoptic bronchoscopy: is sedation necessary? *British Medical Journal* **281**, 779–80.

Powell D.M., Rodeheaver G.T., Foresman P.A., Hankins C.L., Bechan K.I., Zimmer C.A., Becker D.G. & Edlich R.F. (1991) Damage to tissue defenses by EMLA Cream. *The Journal of Emergency Medicine* **9**, 205–9.

Prithvi-Raj P. (1983) In *Practical Regional Anaesthesia* (Eds Henderson J.J. & Nimmo W.S.). Blackwell Scientific Publications, Oxford.

Randell T., Yli-Hankala A., Valli H. & Lindgren L. (1992) Topical anaesthesia of the nasal mucosa for fibreoptic airway endoscopy. *British Journal of Anaesthesia* **68**, 164–7.

Ranney B. & Stanage W.F. (1975) Advantages of local anesthesia for Cesarean section. *Obstetrics and Gynecology* **45**, 163–7.

Ritchie J.M. & Greene N.M. (1985) In *The Pharmacological Basis of Therapeutics* 7th edn. (Eds Goodman-Gilman A., Goodman L.S., Rall T.W. & Murad F.). Macmillan Publishing Co. Inc., New York.

Scott D.B. (1983) In *Practical Regional Anaesthesia* (Eds Henderson J.J. & Nimmo W.S.). Blackwell Scientific Publications, Oxford.

Scott D.B. (1986) Topical anaesthesia of intact skin. *British Journal of Parenteral Therapy*, **7**, 134–5.

Scott D.B. & Cousins M.J. (1980) In *Neural Blockade in Clinical Anesthesia and Management of Pain* (Eds Cousins M.J. & Bridenbaugh P.O.) pp. 91–2. J.B. Lippincott Co., Philadelphia.

Sluder G. (1913) Nerve trunk anesthesia and carbolisation in nasal surgery. *Laryngoscope* **23**, 1078.

Small J., Wallace R.G., Millar R., Woolfson A.D. & McCafferty D.F. (1988) Pain-free cutting of split skin grafts by application of percutaneous local anaesthetic cream. *British Journal of Plastic Surgery* **41**, 539–43.

Vuckovic D.D., Rooney S.M., Goldiner P.L. & O'Sullivan D. (1980) Aerosol anesthesia of the airway using a small disposable nebulizer. *Anesthesia and Analgesia* **59**, 803–4.

Williams D.G., Truelove S.C., Gear M.W.L., Massarella G.R. & Fitzgerald N.W. (1968) Gastroscopy with biopsy and cytological sampling under direct vision. *British Medical Journal* **1**, 535–9.

Williams P.L. & Warwick R. (Eds) (1980) *Grays Anatomy* 36th edn. Churchill Livingstone, Edinburgh.

Thorax, Abdomen and Perineum

E.N. ARMITAGE

In clinical practice, local anaesthesia of the thorax, abdomen and perineum is obtained usually with a central block, such as a spinal, extradural or caudal, and the effects of almost all the blocks described in this chapter can in fact be obtained with these regimens. However, central blocks may be contraindicated occasionally or may be difficult to perform, whereas a peripheral block may be appropriate and feasible technically. In such circumstances, the benefits of local anaesthesia to the patient need not be lost if the anaesthetist is capable of performing a suitable peripheral block.

Disadvantages of central blocks

A central block involves the introduction of a needle between two vertebral spines or laminae, through the ligaments connecting them, into the extradural or subarachnoid space. Anatomical abnormality of the bony spine and calcification or ossification of the intervertebral ligaments can make it difficult or impossible to insert the needle. Similar difficulty may be encountered in the grossly obese patient in whom bony landmarks may be impalpable and in whom spinal flexion, which opens up access to the extradural space, is limited. In such cases a peripheral block may be easier.

Although it is possible to confine the effects of a central block to a limited area by careful attention to factors such as the site of needle insertion, the position of the patient and the dose of drug injected, such blocks usually act bilaterally and extend over a greater area than that required for the surgical procedure. Not only is this lack of specificity inelegant, but it is not appreciated by the patient if it causes widespread impairment of sensory and motor function and particularly if it results in urinary retention.

Some degree of autonomic denervation usually accompanies spinal and extradural anaesthesia, and hypotension, produced by sympathetic block, is common. Although this is no longer considered an undesirable side-effect and may actually be an advantage in some cases, it is contraindicated in patients in whom maintenance of cardiovascular stability is paramount. Severe hypotension is not tolerated well by the conscious patient in whom it causes faintness and nausea. In both these groups, therefore, a peripheral block may be preferable because extensive sympathetic denervation is avoided.

Skin sepsis at the site of needle insertion is considered, rightly, to be a contraindication to a nerve block. The skin over the back of the elderly bedridden patient is often unhealthy and if this is the case, central blocks should not be performed. However, it is in patients such as these that regional anaesthesia has so much to offer and a peripheral block may be an acceptable alternative.

Because all central blocks involve the insertion of a needle (and perhaps a catheter) into deep tissues which are surrounded largely by bone, any bleeding in these tissues cannot be controlled directly. This is of little clinical consequence in the presence of normal clotting mechanisms, but patients may already be receiving long-term anticoagulant therapy, such as aspirin, when they undergo surgery and some may require anticoagulants during the operation. Also, it is now common surgical practice to give low-dose subcutaneous heparin before the start of all but the smallest surgical procedures. Although there is evidence from two large series (Rao & El-Etr, 1981; Odoom & Sih, 1983) that central blocks may be performed safely in these three groups, the risk of an extradural haematoma, with its potentially serious neurological consequences, deters many anaesthetists. Furthermore, the preoperative administration of non-steroidal anti-inflammatory drugs (NSAIDs) is becoming popular for the control of some types of postoperative pain. These antiprostaglandin agents can impair platelet function and it remains to be seen whether they are contraindicated when regional techniques are used, and vice versa (Wildsmith & McClure, 1991).

Advantages of specific blocks

Peripheral blocks may be feasible when anatomical abnormalities or skin sepsis preclude a central block, but they have advantages in their own right. They produce a comparatively localized area of anaesthesia which may match the surgical field more exactly. A haematoma produced during the performance of a peripheral block can be controlled almost always by direct pressure. Unwanted side-effects, e.g. hypotension, motor block and disturbance of bladder function, are rare. Thus, patients can stand and walk immediately after surgery. This is an important consideration at a time when day-case surgery is being promoted.

Disadvantages of specific blocks

Whereas central blocks achieve their effects with a single injection, most peripheral blocks require several, and their disadvantages stem mainly from this. Multiple injections may be unacceptable to the patient and, where they are required, the performance of the block and the development of complete anaesthesia may take some time. There is always the possibility that one of the injections may be ineffective, and therefore peripheral blocks requiring multiple injections tend to be somewhat less reliable than central ones. In such cases, the anaesthetist may assess the overall anaesthesia as, say, 80% effective, but the patient is more likely to mark it down as a complete failure. Absorption of a local anaesthetic drug from more than one site, e.g. after multiple intercostal blocks, results in comparatively high plasma concentrations, and systemic toxicity can be a problem.

Large peripheral nerves run with arteries and veins frequently, and attempts to block such a nerve may cause damage to one of the accompanying vessels and may result in a haematoma. Injection of local anaesthetic into one of these vessels is a possible hazard.

For a peripheral block to be successful, local anaesthetic must be deposited close to the nerve. The nerve may be located by probing with a needle until paraesthesiae are elicited, but this method requires a conscious, co-operative patient, and it can be very uncomfortable. It may also damage the nerve.

A nerve stimulator can be used to avoid these disadvantages.

Paravertebral block

Although this block is used rarely in present-day anaesthesia, it is of some historical interest. In 1927, Cleland set out to determine the nerve supply to the uterus. Six years later, after preliminary studies on animals, he was able to conclude that, in the human, the pain of labour from uterine contraction 'is transmitted by afferent fibers through the eleventh and twelfth thoracic roots' and that 'paravertebral block of the eleventh and the twelfth thoracic roots will abolish the pain of uterine contraction ...' (Cleland, 1933).

Anatomy

The paravertebral space is the space which a spinal nerve enters immediately after it has left the intervertebral foramen, and theoretically, therefore, there is a space corresponding to each foramen. However, in practice, only the thoracic and lumbar paravertebral spaces are sufficiently well-defined and accessible to be of use to the anaesthetist. Spaces in the sacral region are of no clinical importance because it is impossible to gain access to them by the posterior approach, and those in the cervical region are more apparent than real because there are no ribs or costotransverse ligaments to bound the space posteriorly and no pleura anterolaterally. Nevertheless, deep cervical plexus block may be thought of as a cervical paravertebral block. The space, seen in transverse section (Fig. 72.1) is triangular with its apex pointing laterally. The base of the triangle is formed by the posterolateral surface of the vertebral body and the intervertebral foramen. The posterior side is made up of the superior costotransverse ligament, which runs from the lower border of a transverse process to the upper border of the rib below. The anterolateral side of the triangle is formed by the pleura.

There is no direct communication between paravertebral spaces because, anterolaterally, the pleura is closely applied to the anterior surfaces of the ribs and, posteriorly, the inferior costotransverse ligament runs forward from the transverse process to its own rib and thus seals off the space above and below (Fig. 72.2). Medially, however, it is possible for injected solution to spread up and down in the loose areolar tissue lining the base of the triangle. A single injection of local anaesthetic can therefore produce anaesthesia of more than one segment.

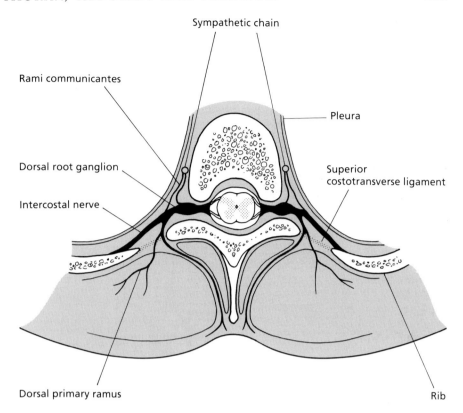

Fig. 72.1 Relations of paravertebral space. (Redrawn from Eason & Wyatt, 1979.)

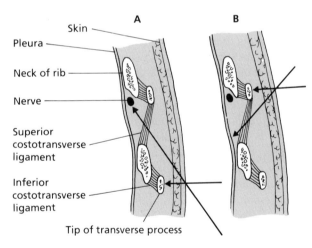

Fig. 72.2 Longitudinal section of paravertebral space. (A) Direction of needle above transverse process or rib; (B) direction of needle below transverse process or rib. (Redrawn from Eason & Wyatt, 1979.)

Purcell-Jones and colleagues (1987) studied the behaviour of radio-opaque solution after paravertebral injection. Using image intensification and computerized tomography (CT) scanning, they found that the spread was unpredictable and in only 10% of cases did the solution remain confined to the para-vertebral space. In most cases, the solution could be seen in the extradural space, sometimes extending bilaterally and spreading over as many as 12 segments. Pleural spread was also demonstrated occasionally.

The spinal nerve enters the paravertebral space through the intervertebral foramen and divides immediately into anterior and posterior primary rami. The posterior ramus runs posteriorly, winds round the medial edge of the superior costotransverse ligament and leaves the paravertebral space. The anterior ramus runs laterally and becomes one of the intercostal nerves. Both rami contain sensory and motor fibres. Rami communicantes are given off and run anteriorly to connect with the sympathetic chain which occupies the anterior angle of the space. Injection of local anaesthetic into the paravertebral space therefore affects sensory, motor and sympathetic fibres (Fig. 72.3).

Indications

Paravertebral block should be considered when unilateral anaesthesia of limited extent is required. Because of the medial communication between paravertebral spaces described above, it is possible to

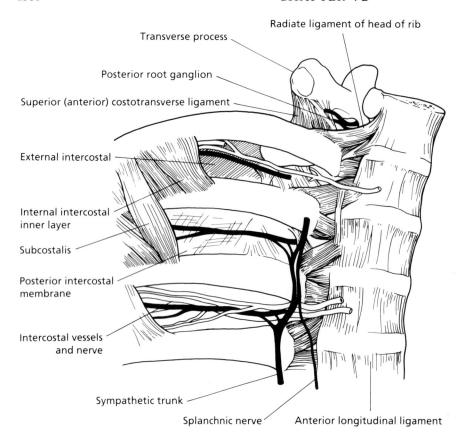

Radiate ligament of head of rib

Transverse process

Posterior root ganglion

Superior (anterior) costotransverse ligament

External intercostal

Internal intercostal inner layer

Subcostalis

Posterior intercostal membrane

Intercostal vessels and nerve

Sympathetic trunk

Splanchnic nerve   Anterior longitudinal ligament

Fig. 72.3 Vertebral end of an intercostal space and the costovertebral ligaments. (Redrawn from Williams & Warwick, 1980.)

produce anaesthesia of at least four segments with a single injection (Eason & Wyatt, 1979). Thus, the technique can provide analgesia for unilateral fractured ribs and for Kocher's subcostal incision for cholecystectomy. It can be used also in cases where access to the extradural space is impossible due to kyphoscoliosis or ossification of the supraspinous and interspinous ligaments; and it has a limited application in certain chronic pain conditions where it is important to know the effect of a comparatively localized segmental block before a more radical neurolytic or surgical procedure is undertaken. However, in view of the unpredictable spread of injected solutions, a diagnostic block in such cases cannot be regarded as reliable and may actually be dangerously misleading (Purcell-Jones et al., 1987).

Paravertebral block may be regarded as midway between extradural and intercostal block not only anatomically, but clinically, in that it usually produces localized, unilateral, segmental anaesthesia without the need for multiple injections.

Technique

The patient may be placed in either the sitting or lateral position. The author finds it easier to visualize

the underlying anatomy when the patient is sitting, and patients themselves often find this position more comfortable. The transverse process must be located. It cannot be palpated, but in the upper and mid-thoracic regions, it lies level with the spine of the vertebra above. A skin weal of local anaesthetic is raised 3 cm lateral to the appropriate vertebral spine. A 3.8-cm 21-gauge needle is inserted through the weal at right angles to the skin, and the deeper tissues are infiltrated until bone is encountered, usually at a depth of about 3 cm. It may occasionally be necessary to use a 5 cm needle in obese subjects.

The choice of needle for the block itself will depend on whether or not a single shot or continuous block is required. For the former, a 9- or 10-cm 18- or 20-gauge needle, with a stilette, is suitable. However, it may be preferable to insert a catheter at the outset, and for this, a Tuohy extradural needle is suitable. The needle is introduced through the skin weal and advanced through the infiltrated tissues until the bone of the transverse process is felt. The depth at which it strikes bone is noted. It is then withdrawn slightly, reangled cephalad and inserted again. This process is repeated until the needle clears the superior edge of the transverse process and lies in the costo-transverse ligament. The stilette is then removed, a syringe of saline is attached to the needle, and the whole assembly is advanced until loss of resistance is felt to pressure on the plunger. This indicates that the needle tip has penetrated the costotransverse ligament and now lies in the paravertebral space. An aspiration test should be performed to exclude air in addition to blood and cerebrospinal fluid (CSF). If a catheter is to be passed, the depth of the space from the skin is noted with reference to the graduations on the Tuohy needle. Eason and Wyatt (1979) recommend that less than 1 cm of catheter should project into the space and an end-hole-only type is therefore required. These authors found that 15 ml of 0.375% bupivacaine anaesthetizes at least four segments.

Complications

Pleural tap and intravenous cannulation can occur, but dural tap has not been reported when the above approach has been used, and hypotension is not a problem even in the presence of high blocks. This is presumably because sympathetic activity on the contralateral side remains unimpaired. However, it should be remembered that diffusion centrally into the extradural space is a theoretical possibility and if this were to occur, bilateral sympathetic block, and bilateral anaesthesia, would result.

Intercostal nerve block

Anatomy

An intercostal nerve is the lateral continuation of a thoracic anterior primary ramus. It is described classi-

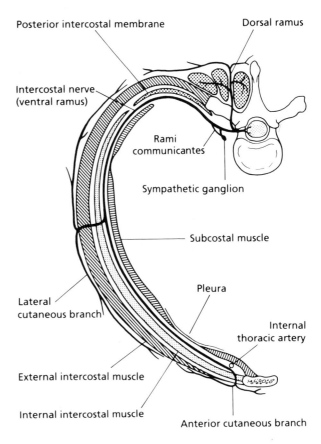

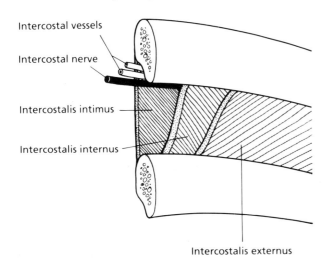

Fig. 72.4 Dissection of part of the thoracic wall showing the position of the intercostal vessels and nerve. (Redrawn from Williams & Warwick, 1980.)

cally as running inferior to its corresponding rib, in the subcostal groove, accompanied by the intercostal artery and vein (Fig. 72.4). In the posterior part of its course, it is bounded laterally by the inferior notched aspect of the rib and the posterior intercostal membrane which lines the medial surface of the external intercostal muscle (Fig. 72.5). Anteriorly, the posterior intercostal membrane is replaced by the internal intercostal muscle. Medially, the intercostal nerve is bounded by the subcostal muscle in the posterior part of its course and by the intercostalis intima anteriorly. The pleura lies medial to both these muscles. Detailed examination of post-mortem specimens has shown that there is considerable variation within this basic arrangement (Nunn & Slavin, 1980). For example, in some cases, the nerve was not a single structure, but consisted of three or four separate bundles, and although the posterior intercostal membrane was always clearly defined and impermeable to India ink injected in the cadaver, the intercostalis intima was found to consist of separate fasciculi between which India ink could pass medially to the subpleural space. It could then track up and down and re-enter adjacent intercostal spaces (Fig. 72.6).

These anatomical studies showed also that at a point 7 cm from the posterior midline, the rib was relatively thick and the pleura lay, on average, 8 mm deep to its lower edge.

Each intercostal nerve has two main branches. The lateral cutaneous branch arises approximately at the mid-axillary line and divides into anterior and posterior branches which supply the skin over the scapula and back and the anterolateral part of the abdominal wall. The anterior cutaneous branch supplies the skin of the anterior abdominal wall. If all the components of an intercostal nerve are to be blocked, it is clear that local anaesthetic must be injected at a point posterior to the origin of the lateral cutaneous branch, i.e. posterior to the mid-axillary line (Fig. 72.5).

Indications

Intercostal blocks can provide unilateral, segmental anaesthesia of the thorax and abdomen without sympathetic block. They are valuable in cases of fractured ribs for initial analgesia and before subsequent chest physiotherapy sessions (Graziotti & Smith, 1988). They are also suitable for a subcostal (Kocher's) surgical incision, and Nunn and Slavin (1980) found that blocks from T5 to T11 inclusive

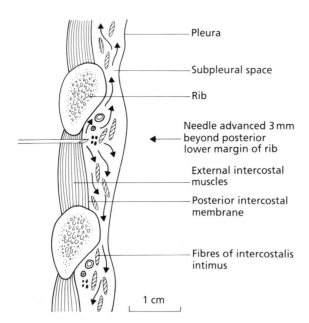

Fig. 72.6 The spread of India ink between pleura and internal surfaces of the ribs. (Redrawn from Nunn & Slavin, 1980.)

produced satisfactory analgesia for at least 5 h after open cholecystectomy. However, unilateral blocks are inadequate for a paramedian incision because the area adjacent to the anterior midline receives its innervation from both sides.

Technique

Bolus injections

The block may be performed with the patient in the prone, sitting or lateral position. The shoulders should be abducted and the arms moved forward to lift the scapula clear of the angles of the ribs. The posterior angles of the ribs are easily palpable in most subjects, but in very obese patients, it may be necessary to locate the rib near the posterior axillary line forward of the anterior border of latissimus dorsi.

A short-bevelled 25-gauge needle is introduced at right angles to the skin and level with the lower half of the rib. When contact with the rib is made, a small amount of local anaesthetic may be injected to render the periosteum insensitive. The depth at which the needle meets bone is noted. The needle is then withdrawn into the subcutaneous tissues and the skin is moved downwards until the needle is judged to be level with the inferior border of the rib. The needle is advanced again and if bone is still encountered, this manoeuvre is repeated until the needle clears the lower border of the rib. The needle is then advanced, in a slightly cephalad direction, 3 mm deeper than its point of contact with the rib. This takes it through the external intercostal muscle and the posterior intercostal membrane, but should leave it well clear of the pleura. An aspiration test is carried out for air and blood before 3–5 ml of local anaesthetic are injected. During aspiration and injection, the patient should be asked to hold his or her breath. This minimizes damage to the pleura and lung if the needle has punctured them accidentally.

Choice of drug

For bolus-dose intercostal block, a long-acting agent such as bupivacaine has advantages, but multiple injections can result in very high plasma bupivacaine concentrations, second only to those obtained after intravenous or tracheal administration (Braid & Scott, 1965). Furthermore, these concentrations are achieved very rapidly. Systemic toxicity is therefore a real possibility, and prilocaine is safer for poor-risk cases and those in whom bilateral block is required.

Continuous catheter technique

Murphy (1983) introduced an extradural catheter through a Tuohy needle into the intercostal space of patients who had undergone cholecystectomy through a subcostal incision. He chose either the T7−8 or T8−9 interspaces, inserted the needle 3 mm under the rib, directed the bevel medially and passed the catheter 3−4 cm into the intercostal space. Twenty ml of bupivacaine 0.5% were injected. The mean duration of the initial dose was approximately 7 h, but top-up injections did not last so long, and in one (and possibly two) cases in his series of 25, the catheter migrated from the intercostal space into the subcutaneous tissues. Graziotti and Smith (1988) inserted a needle under the angle of the sixth rib and passed a catheter 7 cm into the intercostal space. After the injection of 5 ml of contrast medium, the catheter was seen to have passed cephalad, and the dye had spread cephalad and caudad over three ribs. An initial injection of 20 ml of bupivacaine 0.25% was followed by an infusion of 3 ml/h of the same solution. Analgesia of the patient's fractured ribs was excellent and full physiotherapy was possible. After 24 h of this regimen, the serum plasma bupivacaine was 0.4 µg/ml.

Cryoanalgesia

This is performed by the surgeon before the closure of a thoracotomy wound (Glynn *et al.*, 1980). It has the advantage that the intercostal nerves can be identified and exposed, and the cryoprobe can be applied directly to them. The technique is very effective, but it may be 3 months before sensation is fully restored (Palmer, 1987, personal communication).

Complications

There is a risk of *pneumothorax* each time an intercostal block is performed, and several blocks are required usually for surgical analgesia. It is a life-threatening complication and specific measures must be taken to avoid it and to minimize the effects if it occurs. Injections should be made at the posterior angle of the ribs where the intercostal space is at its widest, and the needle should not be advanced more than 3 mm deep to the inferior border of a rib. Stimulation of the pleura with a needle is said to provoke coughing and the needle should be withdrawn if this occurs. The patient should be encouraged to breathe quietly while the needle is being inserted and, if possible, should hold his/her breath during the injection. Bilateral blocks should be avoided. It is unwise to perform intercostal blocks on outpatients even if a chest X-ray taken after the procedure is normal. Symptoms may appear several hours after the block and may be severe before any radiographic abnormality is apparent.

There are several reasons why *systemic toxicity* may occur after intercostal block. Local anaesthetic deposited in the intercostal space is in close contact with the neurovascular bundle and is therefore absorbed readily. However, any solution which tracks medially into the subpleural space is absorbed also very rapidly by the pleura itself. Therefore, a single intercostal injection results in both vascular and pleural absorption. Because multiple blocks are almost always required, high plasma concentrations of local anaesthetic are achieved rapidly. This is a situation which may predispose to the appearance of toxic symptoms, as the latter are determined not only by the absolute plasma concentration, but by the rate at which it has been reached (Scott, 1975).

Moore and colleagues (1976) measured plasma concentrations in patients having bilateral intercostal blocks from T6−T12 inclusively. They injected 5 ml of bupivacaine 0.5% with adrenaline 1:320 000 into each of the 14 intercostal spaces (total 70 ml). Bupivacaine 350 mg was therefore used for the blocks, but a further 10 ml of solution were infiltrated into the skin and subcutaneous tissues, bringing the total to 400 mg. The mean peak arterial and venous plasma concentrations achieved were 3.3 µg/ml (range 1.7−4.0 µg/ml) and 2.5 µg/ml (range 1.4−3.5 µg/ml), respectively. These peaks occurred 10−20 min after injection. No systemic toxic reactions were observed. However, all the patients had received an opioid premedication and were given methohexitone, 100−150 mg, intravenously before and during performance of the blocks.

The systemic effects of adrenaline should be considered also. Eighty ml of bupivacaine with adrenaline 1:320 000 (the total amount used in Moore's cases) contains 0.25 mg of adrenaline, but the commercially prepared solution contains adrenaline 1:200 000. Therefore, 70 ml of bupivacaine with adrenaline (the amount actually needed for the intercostal blocks) contains 0.35 mg adrenaline.

Haemorrhage is a possible hazard when a needle is placed close to a neurovascular bundle. Intercostal vessels which lie snugly in the subcostal groove are protected to some extent, but dissections of the intercostal space show that there is considerable anatomical variation in the individual relationships and sizes of the vessels (Nunn & Slavin, 1980).

Interpleural block

This block was discovered accidentally when an intended intercostal block, performed in a patient who had undergone renal surgery, was observed to give excellent analgesia of more rapid onset and longer duration than would be expected after an intercostal block. Radiography showed the 'intercostal' catheter to be in the pleural cavity.

Embryology, nomenclature and anatomy

In the embryo, the pleura is a layer of mesothelium which is pushed out by, and invaginated in advance of, the developing lung. In the adult, this process results in the pleura consisting of a thin layer of tissue which lines the inner wall of the thorax (parietal pleural) (Figs 72.5 and 72.6), the hilar structures and the surface of the lung (visceral pleura). Interpleural block involves the injection of local anaesthetic solution into the potential space between the parietal and visceral layers of the pleura. Because the pleura is one structure embryologically and the solution is deposited within this structure, some anaesthetists believe that it should be termed an 'intrapleural' injection (Antony, 1991; Miguel & Smith, 1991). However, this is unsatisfactory for two reasons. First, it is the parietal and visceral layers and the space between them which are important anatomically and clinically. Therefore, clinicians are accustomed to thinking of the pleura as consisting of these two layers. Second, the term 'intrapleural' could apply to an injection within the actual tissue of the pleura. The term 'interpleural' is therefore preferred because it was used by the anaesthetists who described the block originally (Reiestad & Stromskag, 1986) and because most anaesthetists are in no doubt that it refers to the space between the parietal and visceral layers of the pleura. Furthermore, Covino (1988) considered the subject of nomenclature and concluded that 'interpleural' was the most appropriate adjective.

Mode of action

The mode of action of interpleural block has not been established definitely. It is assumed that local anaesthetic solution diffuses outwards to reach the intercostal space where it produces multiple intercostal nerve block. However, although this is the probable mechanism, it does not explain why interpleural block should have a more rapid onset than intercostal block, in which local anaesthetic solution is placed in close contact with the nerves and does not have to diffuse across a tissue membrane to reach its site of action.

Indications

Interpleural block was used originally for analgesia after gall bladder, unilateral breast and renal surgery. Twenty ml of bupivacaine 0.5% with adrenaline produced complete analgesia in 78 out of 81 patients, and had a mean duration of 10 h (Reiestad & Stromskag, 1986). It has been used since to provide analgesia after thoracotomy, rib fractures and flail chest, and to control pain resulting from chronic pancreatitis, upper abdominal cancer and reflex sympathetic dystrophies affecting the upper arm, lower face and neck. It is relatively simple technically, avoids or greatly reduces the need for opioids, and may be suitable in cases in which extradural block is contraindicated or in which a more localized area of analgesia is required. Compared with extradural block, it causes less arterial hypotension and no urinary retention, and patients are more mobile.

Interpleural block is less likely to be successful in patients with pulmonary fibrosis and in those with blood or fluid in the pleural space. Although some recent reports claim that it can provide surgical anaesthesia for percutaneous nephrostomy and nephrolithotomy (Trivedi et al., 1990), and for mammographic needle localization and breast biopsy (Schlesinger et al., 1989), it is used mainly for postoperative analgesia.

Technique

A 16-gauge Tuohy needle is introduced, with the bevel facing cephalad and the stilette in place, 8–10 cm from the posterior midline and is passed under the lower border of the eighth rib. A more cephalad rib may be selected if a high block is required. The pleural space is located either by using the negative pressure within it to suck in air from a syringe attached to the Tuohy needle, or by observing the free flow of a saline infusion when the needle enters the pleural space.

Passive loss of resistance to air

The needle is inserted until it is felt to have penetrated the posterior intercostal membrane. The stilette is removed and a glass syringe, with a freely running plunger and containing approximately 4 ml of air, is attached to the needle and the assembly is advanced until the plunger moves inwards. This indicates that the pleural space has been entered and the negative pressure within it has sucked in air from the syringe. The stilette is removed and the needle hub is occluded (to prevent more air entering) until the interpleural catheter is inserted. Approximately 5 cm of catheter is introduced into the pleural space. The needle is removed, a bacterial filter is attached to the catheter and 20 ml of bupivacaine 0.5% with or without adrenaline is injected.

Saline infusion

Scott (1991) has described a technique which takes advantage of the fact that saline flows more freely into the pleural space than into the superficial layers of the chest wall. The essential components are an infusion set and a catheter sheath adaptor consisting of a flap valve and a side port (Fig. 72.7). The adaptor is attached to a Tuohy needle and the assembly is primed with saline from the infusion set, which is connected to the side port.

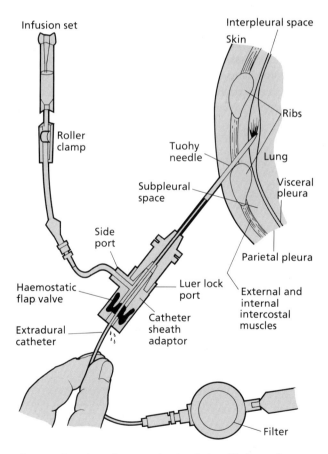

Fig. 72.7 Insertion of an extradural catheter. (Redrawn from Scott, 1991.)

When the needle has been placed in the subcutaneous tissue of the chest wall, the roller clamp of the infusion set is opened fully, but the resistance of the tissues is too high for more than a few drops of saline to enter the drip chamber. If the anaesthetized patient has been ventilated mechanically, ventilation is discontinued until the pleural space has been entered. The conscious patient should hold his/her breath during this period. The needle is advanced through the intercostal muscles, whereupon a slight increase in drip rate is noticeable. The needle is advanced further until the visceral pleura is pierced. Saline now flows freely and this indicates that the pleural space has been entered. The interpleural catheter is introduced through the flap valve so that approximately 5 cm is in the pleural space. The needle and valve are withdrawn and ventilation recommenced.

The saline infusion technique has the advantage that air is excluded from the pleural space, and the flow of saline tends to separate the parietal from the visceral pleura and thus protects the lung tissue from damage by the advancing needle.

Dosage

Reiestad's and Stromskag's (1986) original regimen of 20 ml of bupivacaine 0.5% is commonly used, but there is no consensus regarding the optimal volume, concentration or agent. There is little difference in quality of analgesia between 0.25, 0.375 and 0.5% bupivacaine, although the strongest solution lasts slightly longer (Stromskag *et al.*, 1988). Recommended volumes vary from 8–30 ml (Rosenberg *et al.*, 1987; Seltzer *et al.*, 1987; Durrani *et al.*, 1988).

Plasma concentrations

Twenty ml of 0.5% bupivacaine results in plasma concentrations in the region of 1–2 μg/ml. Arterial concentrations are approximately 10% higher than venous (van Kleef *et al.*, 1990), and bupivacaine with adrenaline produces slightly lower concentrations than the same volume of plain solution (Rademaker *et al.*, 1991). Peak concentrations are reached 15–30 min after injection.

Complications

Production of a clinically significant pneumothorax is obviously a risk with a technique which deliberately breaches the parietal pleura. Brismar and colleagues (1987) reported four of 21 patients who developed this complication. It should be minimized by the use of the saline technique for location of the pleural space. Damage to the lung by a needle which accidentally penetrates the visceral pleura is also a risk. A case of convulsions has been described in which the plasma concentration was found to be 4.9 μg/ml, 5 min after injection (Seltzer *et al.*, 1987).

There is the theoretical possibility that cardiac and respiratory function could be affected if interpleural block resulted in anaesthesia of the cardiac sympathetic and phrenic nerves.

Dorsal nerve of penis (penile) block

Anatomy

The penis consists of the corpus spongiosum, which contains the urethra, and the right and left corpora cavernosa which lie dorsally. Each of the three corpora are enclosed by a tough, inelastic fibrous membrane, the tunica albuginea, and all the corpora are surrounded by a looser layer of fibrous tissue — the fascia penis or Buck's fascia — which is penetrated easily by a needle.

The nerve supply to almost all the penis is derived from the second, third and fourth sacral roots (S2, 3, 4). Fibres travel first in the pudendal nerve and then in one of its terminal branches, the dorsal nerve of the penis. This nerve emerges from the pelvis by penetrating the perineal membrane just inferior to the symphysis pubis (Fig. 72.8). It then runs deep to

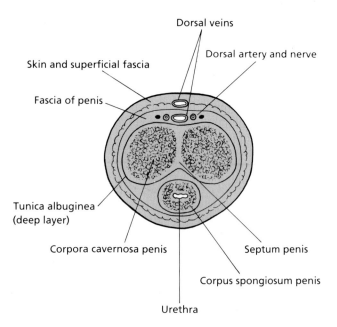

Fig. 72.9 Cross-section of the penis to show the position of the dorsal nerves. (Redrawn from Wildsmith & Armitage, 1987.)

the fascia penis, with the dorsal artery of the penis, along the dorsal surface of the corpus cavernosum which it supplies (Fig. 72.9). Its terminal branches pierce the fascia and supply the skin of the penis and the glans. The autonomic supply to the penis comes from the inferior hypogastric plexus. Fibres may reach the penis by travelling either with the somatic nerves or with the arteries.

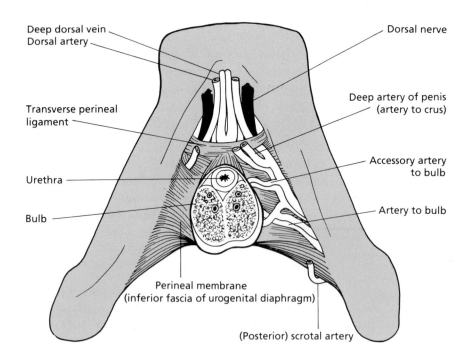

Fig. 72.8 To show the inverted V formed by the right and left pubic arches and the symphysis pubis, the perineal membrane and the emergence of the dorsal nerves inferior to the symphysis. (Redrawn from Boileau, 1951.)

Two important practical points must be considered when penile block is being planned. The penile urethra is supplied throughout its length by the perineal branch of the pudendal nerve. Therefore block of the dorsal nerve does not provide anaesthesia for catheterization. The block is also inappropriate for operations on the base of the penis and the scrotum because these areas are supplied by the genital branch of the genitofemoral nerve.

Indications

Penile block is suitable for operations on the shaft of the penis, the glans and the foreskin. It provides very localized anaesthesia for circumcision, dorsal slit and chordae correction in cases where more extensive blocks, such as a caudal or lumbar extradural, are inappropriate.

Technique

The nerve may be blocked at the root of the penis where it emerges through the perineal membrane. The symphysis pubis is palpated, a skin weal of local anaesthetic is raised over it and a 4 or 5 cm 23-gauge needle is introduced until the symphysis is contacted. A small amount of local anaesthetic may be injected at this point. The needle is then withdrawn into the subcutaneous tissues and the palpating finger moves the skin and needle inferiorly so that when the needle is advanced again, it clears the lower border of the symphysis. After careful aspiration, bupivacaine 0.5% is injected. This process of aspiration and injection is repeated as the needle is advanced down to the dorsal surface of the corpora cavernosa. A total of 10 ml of *plain* solution should be injected. It is essential that adrenaline is *not* used.

Although this approach almost certainly results in a satisfactory block, additional local anaesthetic can be deposited more distally, deep to the fascia penis. The needle is again withdrawn to the subcutaneous tissues, angled distally and advanced until it is felt to have pierced the fascia. Up to 5 ml of solution are injected if no blood appears on aspiration. Finally, the needle is once more withdrawn through the fascia — this sensation is often easier to appreciate than the initial insertion — and a ring of local anaesthetic is infiltrated circumferentially in the subcutaneous layer. This ensures that fibres running superficial to the fascia penis are also anaesthetized.

Therefore, it is possible to block the dorsal nerves at three sites — below the symphysis, and deep and superficial to the fascia penis — with a needle inserted through a single skin weal. A total of 20 ml of solution is required.

Essentially, the same technique may be used in children. Yeoman and colleagues (1983) located the symphysis pubis and then redirected the needle 2 mm inferior to it. They injected bupivacaine 0.5% in a dose of 1 ml for boys up to the age of 3 years and 0.3 ml/year of age thereafter. They had one failure in 19 cases. White and colleagues (1983) used the more distal approach and gave bupivacaine 0.5% in a dose of 0.2 ml/kg body weight. They injected two-thirds of this deep to the fascia penis and the remaining one-third circumferentially in the subcutaneous layers.

Complications

The penis is a highly vascular organ and the most common complication of penile block is haematoma. This may result from damage to the corpora cavernosa [White and colleagues (1983) reported two small haematomas in their series of 27 paediatric cases]. It may result also from puncture of the dorsal vein of the penis when a needle is introduced in the midline. Although bleeding from this vein is not serious and can be controlled easily with pressure, it is superficial and therefore the bruising is obvious to the patient. Identification and avoidance of the dorsal vein prior to insertion of the needle eliminates the problem.

Arterial blood enters the penis through vessels which lie close to the dorsal nerves and run distally with them. These vessels are in effect end-arteries and any vasoconstrictor in the local anaesthetic solution may cause ischaemia and necrosis of tissue distal to the site of injection, with disastrous results. It cannot be emphasized too strongly that only plain solutions of local anaesthetic must be used for penile block.

Coeliac plexus block

Anatomy

The coeliac plexus lies at the level of the junction of the 12th thoracic and the first lumbar vertebrae. It is composed, in part, of two main ganglia which are interconnected and which lie anterior to the crura of the diaphragm and to the aorta at the origin of the coeliac artery, and anterolateral to the vertebral bodies (Fig. 72.10). Preganglionic sympathetic fibres carried in the greater (T5−10), lesser (T10−11) and least (T12) splanchnic nerves relay in the coeliac ganglia, which receive also parasympathetic fibres from the coeliac

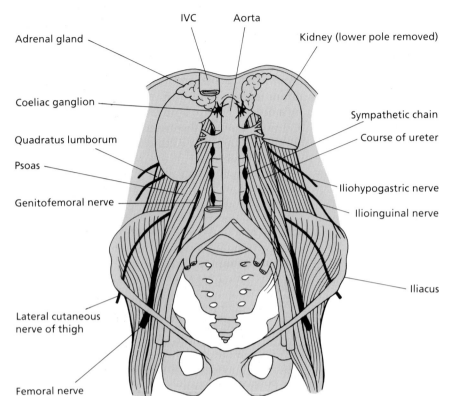

Fig. 72.10 Posterior abdominal wall to show the position and relations of the coeliac plexus. IVC, inferior vena cava. (Redrawn from Wildsmith & Armitage, 1987.)

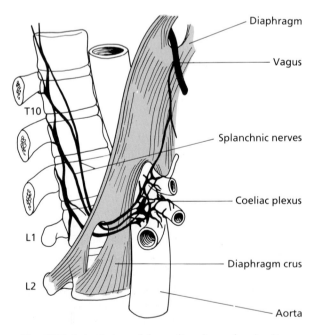

Fig. 72.11 Lateral view of the coeliac plexus showing its relations to the vertebral bodies, diaphragm and vagus. (Redrawn from Wildsmith & Armitage, 1987.)

branch of the right vagus nerve. Postganglionic fibres form a network anterior to the aorta and the whole complex of nerve tissue at this site forms the coeliac plexus (Fig. 72.11). The plexus lies posterior to the stomach, the pancreas and the left renal vein.

Indications

It is occasionally necessary to perform upper abdominal surgery on a patient in whom general anaesthesia is contraindicated. In such a case, extradural anaesthesia provides somatic, motor and sympathetic block, but it leaves the parasympathetic supply to the abdomen unaffected. Coeliac plexus block is therefore required if all sensation is to be abolished. Under these circumstances, the block is performed usually by the surgeon as soon as the abdomen is opened.

It is more commonly used in the treatment of painful conditions, such as malignant disease of the upper abdomen and chronic pancreatitis. Local anaesthetic can be injected initially to see if the benefits are sufficient to justify the later ablation of the plexus with alcohol.

Technique

The coeliac plexus is related to important blood vessels and viscera, so needles and solutions (particularly neurolytic ones) must be placed accurately. Because the plexus is also deeply situated, accuracy can be guaranteed only if the block is performed under X-ray control. A C-arm image intensifier enables the position of the needles to be checked in both posteroanterior and lateral planes.

The patient is placed prone on the X-ray table with a pillow under the chest. The iliac crests are marked. A line joining them crosses the spine of the fourth lumbar vertebra or the interspace below it. From this landmark, the 12th thoracic spine and the 12th ribs are identified and marked (Fig. 72.12).

Skin weals of local anaesthetic are raised approximately 7–12 cm from the midline just inferior to the 12th rib on each side, the greater distance being chosen for the larger patients. A 15-cm 20-gauge needle with stilette is introduced through each skin weal and advanced under the 12th rib, anteriorly, medially and cephalad, until it strikes the body of the 12th thoracic vertebra. Where the needle strikes bone and at any point where it causes localized discomfort, local anaesthetic should be infiltrated. If paraesthesiae are elicited, indicating that a somatic nerve is being stimulated, the needle should be withdrawn and reinserted at a slightly different angle. When the

needle tip contacts the vertebral body, the hub of the needle is held between the thumbs and middle fingers, and the index fingers mark a point along the needle shaft 2–3 cm from the skin. The needle is then withdrawn partially and inserted in the same medial and cephalad directions, but more anteriorly. If bone is encountered again, the position of the index fingers is adjusted so that they are once more 2–3 cm from the skin, and the needle is inserted still more anteriorly. This manoeuvre is repeated until the needle clears the anterolateral border of the vertebral body. The position of the needle must now be checked radiographically and adjusted so that, in the lateral view, it lies approximately 2 cm anterior to the body and, in the anteroposterior view, about one-third of the way across it (Fig. 72.13). When the position of both needles is satisfactory radiographically, aspiration tests should be performed and the position adjusted if blood is obtained.

Correct placement of the needles is confirmed if injected radio-opaque dye spreads up and down in a narrow strip in front of the vertebral body. Any resistance to injection indicates that the needle tip lies in the wall of a major blood vessel, a viscus or a muscle, from which it must be withdrawn before the injection is continued.

Injection in the region of the coeliac plexus causes severe burning abdominal pain. This is usually transient when local anaesthetic is used, but it may be

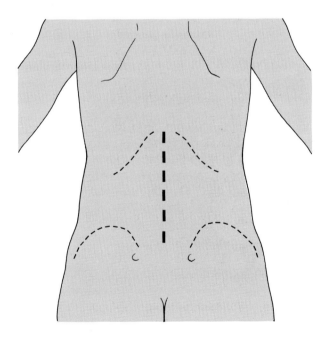

Fig. 72.12 Landmarks and needle alignment for coeliac plexus block. (Redrawn from Wildsmith & Armitage, 1987.)

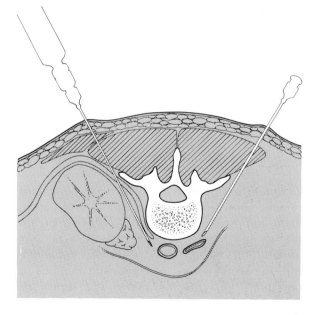

Fig. 72.13 Correct position of needles for coeliac plexus block. (Redrawn from Cousins & Bridenbaugh, 1988.)

necessary to induce general anaesthesia before injection of a neurolytic agent. For a diagnostic block, 25 ml of lignocaine 1% or bupivacaine 0.25% are injected on each side. For neurolysis, 25 ml of 50% alcohol are required on each side and the needles should be cleared of alcohol by the injection of 1 ml of air before they are withdrawn. This prevents necrosis of tissues lying in the track of the needle.

Complications

These may be classified as *technical* and *physiological*.

Technical complications include damage to somatic nerves and dural tap produced by penetration of the intervertebral foramen if initial insertion of the needle is too posterior; haematoma from trauma to the closely related great vessels, and, as a late complication, aortoduodenal fistula resulting from necrosis of the intervening tissue. At least two cases have been reported (Woodham & Hanna, 1989; Van Dongen & Crul, 1991) in which coeliac plexus block, performed with X-ray monitoring, was followed by paraplegia. Damage to the arterial supply to the spinal cord was thought to be the cause. Retroperitoneal fibrosis has been reported in a patient who was treated for chronic pancreatitis with nine coeliac plexus blocks over a 3-year period (Pateman *et al.*, 1990).

The commonest physiological complication is hypotension. This is often first noticed a few minutes after injection, but it can occur also when the patient stands up for the first time after the block, and this must be forbidden unless supervised. Ablation of the coeliac plexus results in impotence, and the patient must be informed of this when neurolysis is being considered.

Lumbar sympathetic block

Anatomy

The sympathetic supply to the lower limb comes from the second, third and fourth lumbar sympathetic ganglia. These ganglia receive preganglionic sympathetic fibres from the lower thoracic sympathetic chain, and preganglionic somatic fibres from the first and second lumbar nerves. Postganglionic sympathetic fibres emerge from the ganglia, run initially with the spinal nerves, continue with the femoral, saphenous and obturator nerves and supply the closely related arteries and their branches. They are vasoconstrictor to the arterioles and pilomotor and sudomotor to the skin within the distribution of the

nerves. It is obvious therefore that block of the lumbar sympathetic ganglia causes absence of sweating, warm dry skin, and vasodilatation in the lower limb. Other postganglionic sympathetic fibres leave the ganglia, but they have no relation with any somatic nerves and run as the hypogastric nerves to enter the hypogastric plexus.

The above anatomical arrangement varies considerably. Accessory ganglia occur sometimes at the level of the first and second lumbar vertebrae, embedded in the body of the psoas muscle, and their presence may result in a block being incomplete in the L1–2 distribution.

The ganglia lie anterolateral to their vertebral bodies and on the medial border of psoas muscle. They are placed less anteriorly than the coeliac plexus. The genitofemoral nerve runs down the surface of psoas and is therefore a lateral relation, with the kidney and ureter more lateral still. On the left side, the aorta lies anteriorly and on the right side, the inferior vena cava (IVC) (Fig. 72.14).

Indications

Chemical lumbar sympathectomy has been advocated for the diagnosis and treatment of a very wide range of symptoms and pathologies, and it has often been used empirically. Its popularity has declined as the measurement of arterial blood flow, the diagnosis of arterial occlusion and the surgical management of

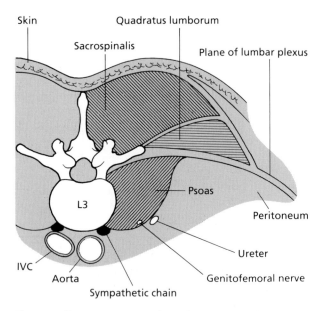

Fig. 72.14 Transverse section through L3 to show the position and relations of the lumbar sympathetic chain. (Redrawn from Wildsmith & Armitage, 1987.)

arteriopathy have improved. It is now used mainly to alleviate the rest pain of chronic, peripheral, obliterative vascular disease, such as atherosclerosis and thromboangiitis obliterans, in patients who are unsuitable for surgery (Reid *et al.*, 1970) and it may improve vasospastic conditions, such as Raynaud's disease, post-traumatic vasospasm, embolism and cold injury.

It is useful also for delineating potentially viable, proximal tissue, capable of responding to the effects of sympathetic denervation, from unsalvageable distal tissue. Therefore, it can help to determine the most suitable site for amputation. Lumbar sympathetic block is performed sometimes to increase the blood supply to the skin flaps after amputation, and to assist the healing of gangrenous areas of skin, 65% of which show some improvement (Lofstrom & Zetterquist, 1969).

The benefits obtained after lumbar sympathetic block depend not only on the increase in total arterial flow to the lower limb, but also on the effects of any redistribution of flow. In the resting limb, most of the increase is to the skin, and this accounts for the finding that over 70% of patients treated for rest pain obtain benefit for at least 6 months (Lofstrom & Zetterquist, 1969) although the muscle blood flow under these conditions may actually decrease (Cousins & Wright, 1971). However, because claudication is improved in up to 20% of patients, some increase in muscle blood flow may apparently occur.

Local anaesthetic block

Local anaesthetic should be used when some indication is sought on whether a more permanent sympathectomy, neurolytic or surgical, is likely to be effective. It can be used also for the treatment of conditions such as phantom limb pain for which a permanent block would be too radical. The block may have to be repeated several times in such cases.

Neurolytic block

Destruction of the sympathetic ganglia with phenol should result theoretically in permanent sympathectomy and relief of symptoms. In practice, some return of sympathetic activity occurs commonly and, because the course of the underlying condition is likely to be one of steady deterioration, symptoms may reappear after a few months. However, neurolytic blocks may be repeated with success and arteriopathic patients can be given long-term relief often before amputation becomes inevitable.

Technique

The procedure is carried out with X-ray monitoring and the patient may be placed prone or in the lateral position. The former facilitates the palpation and drawing of landmarks; the latter is more comfortable for the anaesthetist. The iliac crests are marked. The line joining them crosses the fourth lumbar spine or the interspace below it and from this landmark, the spines of the second, third and fourth vertebrae are identified and marked. A line is drawn, parallel to the vertebral column, 7–11 cm from the midline on the side to be blocked (Fig. 72.15). Three skin weals of local anaesthetic are raised along this line opposite the second, third and fourth vertebral spines and, at each level, the deeper tissues are infiltrated through a longer needle directed medially towards the vertebral body. A 15-cm 20-gauge needle with stilette is inserted through each skin weal and advanced medially and slightly cephalad until bony contact is felt. This should be the vertebral body, but may be the transverse process if contact is made within the first few centimetres. Withdrawal of the needle and insertion with a greater cephalad angle should take the needle clear of the transverse process. When the vertebral body has been located, a small amount of local anaesthetic may be injected, because the contact is often painful and more than one probing may be necessary. The hub of the needle is held between the thumbs and middle fingers while the index fingers mark the shaft about 2 cm from the skin. The needle is withdrawn into the superficial tissues and is reinserted more anteriorly. If it strikes the vertebral body again, the position of the index fingers is adjusted so that they are once more 2 cm from the skin, and the manoeuvre is repeated until the needle tip clears the anterolateral border of the vertebral

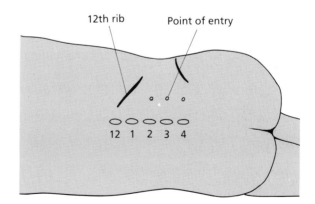

Fig. 72.15 Landmarks and angle of needle insertion for lumbar sympathectomy.

body. The needle is advanced a further 2 cm until the index fingers are flush with the skin. The position of the needle must now be checked radiographically and adjusted until, in the anteroposterior plane, the tip lies one-quarter of the way across the transverse diameter of the vertebral body and, in the lateral plane, level with its anterior border (Fig. 72.16). An aspiration test should be negative and there should be minimal resistance to injection of a small amount of saline.

Although the author prefers to insert needles at the second, third and fourth vertebral level, some anaesthetists take advantage of the fact that solution injected in the correct plane spreads freely up and down, and they therefore insert only one needle, at L3.

If local anaesthetic is to be used, bupivacaine 0.5% or lignocaine 1% is injected in a total dose of 15–20 ml. Before a neurolytic block, there must be radiographic evidence that the solution is confined to the correct plane, so the radio-opaque dye Conray 280 is injected slowly while the patient is screened in the lateral plane. The dye should spread as a thin line up and down from the injection site. Posterior spread may result in damage to somatic nerve roots. Anterior spread indicates that the needle tip has entered the peritoneum and if a full neurolytic dose is deposited there, an aortoduodenal fistula may develop eventually. Spread down the surface of psoas is also unsatisfactory because the genitofemoral nerve may be

affected, causing numbness or paraesthesiae over the front of the upper thigh. In such cases, the dye tracks downwards, but in the lateral view, it tends to run somewhat anteriorly as it does so, while in the anteroposterior view, lateral spread may be seen. Phenol 7.5% in Conray 280 is injected slowly in a total dose of 10–15 ml and its spread is monitored radiographically. The injection must be stopped if the patient complains of pain, and the position of the needle should then be adjusted. At the end of the procedure, the lumen should be cleared by the injection of a small amount of air, so that when the needle is withdrawn, phenol is not deposited along its track.

Complications

If the initial angle of insertion of the needle is too medial, the tip may enter an intervertebral foramen and puncture the dura. This is not an indication for abandoning the block, but it does show that the needle needs to be directed much more anteriorly. Damage to blood vessels and aspiration of blood is common. The aorta on the left side, the IVC on the right and the lumbar vessels on both sides may be punctured. Some bleeding presumably occurs after such damage, so it is essential that the block is not performed on patients with abnormal clotting mechanisms. Significant intravascular injection should be avoided if a careful aspiration test is negative, but it is occasionally seen on screening.

Spinal nerves may be traumatized during insertion of the needle. If paraesthesiae are elicited, the needle should be withdrawn and reangled. The patient should be asked to describe, but not to touch, the area affected, as this gives some indication of the spinal level involved. Phenol may also cause damage to somatic nerves (such as the genitofemoral nerve mentioned above), to the ureter if the needle has been placed too laterally, and to the psoas muscle, though pain on injection gives warning of this.

Caudal (sacral extradural) block

Anatomy

Viewed in the anteroposterior plane, the sacrum is an equilateral triangle with its apex pointing inferiorly. Most of its posterior aspect is bony and is formed by the fusion of the spines, laminae and articular processes of the upper four sacral vertebrae. No posterior fusion takes place at the fifth vertebra at which level the articular processes are represented by

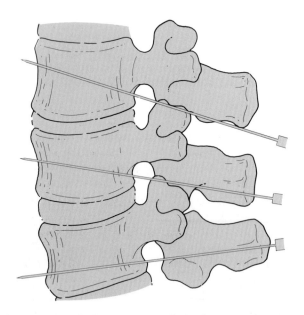

Fig. 72.16 Correct needle position for lumbar sympathectomy. (Redrawn from Wildsmith & Armitage, 1987.)

rounded horns — the sacral cornua. The bony defect, or sacral hiatus, between the cornua and laminae on each side and the vestigial fourth vertebral spine above, is covered by the sacrococcygeal ligament. The lower part of the sacrococcygeal ligament runs from the base of the sacrum to the coccyx. The upper part can be thought of as an isosceles triangle with its apex pointing superiorly, the basal angles being formed by the sacral cornua, and the apex by midline bony fusion at the fourth sacral level (Fig. 72.17).

The extradural space runs from the foramen magnum to the base of the sacrum where it is sealed off by the sacrococcygeal ligament. In most adults, the dural sac ends at the inferior border of the second sacral vertebra, and the spinal cord at the inferior border of the first lumbar vertebra (Fig. 72.18), but in the newborn, the cord and dura extend lower. At all ages, there is much variation and both the cord and dura may be found higher or lower than these points (Lanier *et al.*, 1944). Indeed, all aspects of sacral anatomy may vary, including the level and degree of bony fusion and the prominence and symmetry of the cornua (Trotter & Lanier, 1945; Trotter, 1947).

Because the cord is shorter than the bony spine, the lower lumbar and sacral spinal roots have to run inferiorly in the extradural space, forming the cauda equina, before emerging from their intervertebral foramina at the appropriate level.

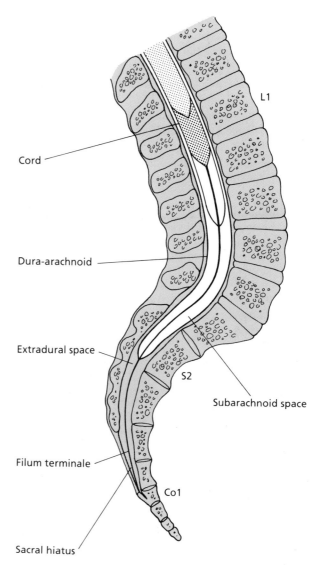

Fig. 72.18 Sagittal section of lumbar and sacral regions of the spine. (Redrawn from Wildsmith & Armitage, 1987.)

Indications

Caudal block is suitable for surgery of the perineum, either as the sole regimen in patients in whom general anaesthesia is contraindicated or, more usually, in combination with light general anaesthesia. Operations such as haemorrhoidectomy, anal dilatation and circumcision are notoriously stimulating, and, when performed under general anaesthesia alone, can induce laryngospasm and marked cardiovascular responses. Caudal block performed before surgery eliminates these problems and allows general anaesthesia to be maintained at a relatively light plane. Extension of analgesia into the postoperative period is an additional benefit.

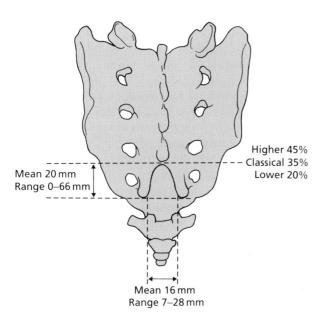

Fig. 72.17 Posterior aspect of sacrum showing cornua and triangular shape of sacral hiatus. (Redrawn from Wildsmith & Armitage, 1987.)

Some relaxation of the anal sphincter is usual after a caudal. This may not always be desirable surgically and the surgeon should be consulted in doubtful cases.

The caudal has a special place in paediatric anaesthesia. This is principally because a child's extradural fat is less dense than an adult's. Injected solution can therefore spread more easily and blocks extending to the umbilicus and higher can be obtained. As a result, inguinal herniotomy, orchidopexy and surgery of the lower limb come within the scope of a paediatric caudal.

Although caudal block has a historical place in obstetric analgesia (Edwards & Hingson, 1942), it has been superseded largely by the lumbar extradural approach, but it is still useful occasionally as a single-injection technique in the second stage of labour.

Technique

The key to successful caudal block is the accurate identification of the sacral cornua. The patient may be placed prone or in the lateral position. Landmarks are easier to feel when the patient is prone because the buttocks tend to fall away from the midline, but the lateral position is more suitable for maintenance of general anaesthesia and the author prefers it. When the triangular outline of the sacrum is visible, the approximate position of the sacral cornua can be estimated. The cornua are not midline structures and palpation should therefore be from side to side. In the obese, considerable pressure may be required for which the thumb is better than the index finger. The sacral cornua were described classically as lying under the proximal interphalangeal joint of the anaesthetist's index finger when its tip was palpating the end of the coccyx, but the anatomy in this region is so variable that this method is unreliable and frequently gives too low a position for the sacral hiatus.

When the cornua have been located, the thumb is drawn cephalad until bone is felt in the midline. This is the apex of the triangle formed by the superior part of the sacrococcygeal ligament. A 19-gauge disposable needle is inserted, immediately caudad to the thumb, at a cephalad angle of about 45°. Resistance is felt after a few millimetres as the needle engages in the ligament, followed by sudden loss of resistance as it penetrates it and enters the sacral extradural space. The angle of insertion is now changed so that it is parallel with the long axis of the sacrum, and the needle is advanced to the hub. An aspiration test should be performed. If the bevel of the needle lies against the intima of a blood vessel, blood does not

necessarily appear. One ml of saline should therefore be injected before aspiration. A caudal need not be abandoned if blood is seen on aspiration, but the needle must be withdrawn or repositioned until the test is negative. Very rarely, the aspiration test may yield CSF. The exact incidence of this complication is unknown, but is probably of the order of 1 : 1000 cases.

Injection should be easy. If resistance is met, the needle should be rotated through 90°, but it should be removed and reinserted if there is persistent difficulty. Lignocaine, prilocaine and bupivacaine are used in their standard concentrations and a volume of 20 ml is adequate for perineal procedures.

If repeated caudal injections are likely to be needed, an 'intravenous' cannula can be inserted, the injection site sealed with an occlusive dressing, and the cannula connected to the syringe by a length of extension tubing and a bacterial filter.

In children, the technique requires some modification. A 21-gauge needle is used for all but the smallest infants in whom a 23-gauge needle is more suitable. When the needle has penetrated the sacrococcygeal ligament, it should not be reangled and advanced to the hub as this is more likely to result in a vascular or dural tap, and the needle does not have to be advanced cephalad for high blocks to be obtained. Advance of 2—3 mm is all that is required.

Paediatric dosage

The spread of a caudal dose of local anaesthetic solution correlates best with the age of a child, but also very satisfactorily with the weight and height (Schulte-Steinberg & Rahlfs, 1970). The equation worked out by these workers (Schulte-Steinberg & Rahlfs, 1977) has been simplified by Hain (1978): volume of drug = [Age (years) + 2 ml] divided by 10, per segment to be blocked, using lignocaine 1% or bupivacaine 0.25%. Although this formula is widely used, it is not entirely satisfactory for infants, some of whom may have been born very prematurely and whose 'age' was obstetrically determined. Another disadvantage is that, because anaesthesia of several segments is invariably required, the arithmetic is not always simple.

The author prefers to use weight as the index and to calculate the volume of drug required to provide anaesthesia in three anatomical areas — lumbosacral, thoracolumbar and lower thoracic. With lignocaine 1% or bupivacaine 0.25%, 0.5 ml/kg body weight is required to block the lumbosacral distribution, 1 ml/kg for the thoracolumbar, and 1.25 ml/kg for the lower thoracic. When this calculation gives a volume greater than 20 ml, one part of saline is added to three parts of drug and the calculated volume of the diluted drug is injected.

Complications and disadvantages

The commonest complication of a caudal block is the inability to locate the sacral cornua and, thus, failure to deposit local anaesthetic in the sacral extradural space. The success rate in adults is rarely higher than 95% and often considerably lower. In children, on the other hand, landmarks are much easier to feel, and blocks are almost always successful.

The sacral extradural space is capacious, and comparatively large volumes of solution are needed to anaesthetize relatively few segments. In adults, this is of no clinical significance if the block is confined to the sacral distribution, but if it is used for anaesthesia of the lumbar segments, systemic toxicity is a potential hazard and the lumbar extradural route is to be preferred.

Accidental intravascular injection can produce a plasma concentration of local anaesthetic high enough to cause a toxic reaction. The author has data which show that intravascular injection can occur even after a negative aspiration test, and plasma concentrations obtained when the injection follows an initial bloody tap tend to be higher than normal.

Some workers use continuous caudal anaesthesia and give top-up injections or infusions during and after surgery. However, many anaesthetists feel that the skin puncture site, being close to the anus, is difficult to keep sterile and is therefore unsuitable for the insertion of a caudal catheter, although there is no good evidence that a caudal carries a higher risk of infection than any other form of extradural.

Paracervical block

Anatomy

Paracervical block anaesthetizes three types of nerve running to and from the uterus in the broad ligament.

The motor supply to the upper uterine segment is derived from sympathetic fibres which travel in the splanchnic nerves and the coeliac, aortic, renal and hypogastric plexuses and then enter the broad ligament, accompanying the uterine vessels, to reach the uterus.

The sensory supply is conveyed by visceral afferents which run with the sympathetic fibres in the broad ligament. They enter the cord at the 11th and 12th thoracic and first lumbar levels. Some sensory fibres, supplying the fundus of the uterus, travel occasionally with the ovarian vessels and are therefore unaffected by paracervical block.

The pelvic splanchnic nerves run in the broad ligament also and contain visceral afferent and efferent fibres. The former are sensory to the cervix and upper vagina, and they enter the cord at the second, third and fourth sacral level.

Paracervical block therefore prevents the pain of uterine contraction, unless a significant proportion of this is transmitted by fibres accompanying the ovarian vessels. It prevents also the pain of cervical dilatation, but sensation to the lower vagina, vulva and perineum is unimpaired.

Indications

Bilateral block provides analgesia for the first stage of labour and may be sufficient also for the second stage, if bilateral pudendal block is added. Because it can be performed easily by the obstetrician, the technique was very popular in the days before extradural services, provided by anaesthetists, were available.

It has no regular place in modern obstetric practice because it has been found to cause fetal bradycardia and depression of the neonate. This was thought initially to result from high concentrations of local anaesthetic reaching the fetal myocardium, but it has been shown that the uterine artery constricts when local anaesthetic is applied directly to it (Cibils, 1976; Greiss et al., 1976) and impairment of uterine blood supply is the more likely cause.

Pudendal nerve block

Anatomy

The pudendal nerve is derived from the second, third and fourth sacral roots. It leaves the pelvis through the greater sciatic notch and, lying medial to the pudendal artery, winds round the lateral side of the ischial spine where it can be blocked. It then runs anteriorly in the pudendal canal, medial to the ramus of the ischium and lateral to the ischiorectal fossa, and emerges at the ischial tuberosity. It supplies the perineum and pelvic floor through its inferior haemorrhoidal and perineal branches, and the penis and clitoris through the dorsal nerve to those organs.

The pudendal nerve is not the only sensory nerve to the perineum. The labia majora are supplied by the terminal branches of the ilioinguinal and genitofemoral nerves, and part of the perineal body is supplied by the perineal branch of the posterior cutaneous nerve of the thigh. These areas are anaesthetized usually by local infiltration, although if the transperineal approach is used for pudendal nerve block, the perineal branch of the posterior cutaneous nerve of the thigh can be blocked where it runs under the ischial tuberosity.

Indications

These are almost entirely confined to obstetrics. Pudendal nerve block provides adequate analgesia for low forceps delivery. It is performed usually by the obstetrician and, in an emergency, is quicker and safer than general anaesthesia. It can be used also for episiotomy and for the repair of perineal lacerations, but supplementary local infiltration may be needed. It has no effect on the pain of uterine contraction or cervical dilatation.

Technique

Transvaginal approach

The patient is placed in the lithotomy position and the ischial spine is palpated through the lateral vaginal wall. The sacrospinous ligament can be felt running posteriorly from the spine. A deep injection is required and the operator has very little space in which to work, so accurate insertion of a long needle is difficult. An introducer, approximately 140 mm long with a blunt, bulbous end, is therefore passed along the palpating fingers until it lies medial and slightly posterior to the ischial spine. A needle long enough to project 10 mm beyond the end of the introducer is then passed through it. With the needle and introducer directed a little laterally, the needle is advanced beyond the end of the introducer so that it penetrates the anterior part of the sacrospinous ligament. After careful aspiration, 10 ml of lignocaine, prilocaine or bupivacaine are injected and the procedure is repeated on the other side.

Transperineal approach

This allows the pudendal nerve to be blocked at the ischial tuberosity in addition to the ischial spine. A skin weal of local anaesthetic is raised midway between the posterior limit of the vagina and the ischial tuberosity, and a 150-mm needle is inserted through it. Palpation of the ischial tuberosity through the vagina assists in directing the needle towards it. Five ml of local anaesthetic injected on the medial

side of the tuberosity will block the pudendal nerve as it emerges from the pudendal canal on the medial aspect of the ischial ramus, and the same amount deposited inferiorly blocks the perineal branch of the posterior cutaneous nerve of the thigh as it runs under the tuberosity. With the palpating fingers now marking the ischial spine, the needle is advanced along the ischiorectal fossa (medial to the tuberosity and ramus) and through the sacrospinous ligament where a further 10 ml of local anaesthetic are injected.

Complications and disadvantages

The pudendal nerve is closely related to the pudendal vessels. Haematoma may result if the latter are damaged and systemic toxicity may occur if an accidental intravascular injection is made. Bilateral blocks are always required, so the risks of complications are compounded.

Pudendal nerve block has no effect on the pain of uterine contractions and although it blocks the sensory supply to the greater part of the perineum, it does not give complete perineal analgesia. Supplementary local infiltration is therefore usually required and Scudamore and Yates (1966) believe that this makes a major contribution to the efficacy of the block.

References

Antony G.P. (1991) Breaking the habit. *Regional Anesthesia* **16**, 299.
Boileau G. (1951) *Grants Atlas of Anatomy* 3rd edn. p. 180. Baillière Tindall, London.
Braid D.P. & Scott D.B. (1965) The systemic absorption of local anaesthetic drugs. *British Journal of Anaesthesia* **37**, 394–404.
Brismar B., Pettersson N., Tokics L., Strandberg A. & Hedenstierna G. (1987) Postoperative analgesia with intrapleural administration of bupivacaine-adrenaline. *Acta Anaesthesiologica Scandinavica* **31**, 515–20.
Cibils L.A. (1976) Response of human uterine arteries to local anesthetics. *American Journal of Obstetrics and Gynecology* **126**, 202–10.
Cleland J.G.P. (1933) Paravertebral anaesthesia in obstetrics. Experimental and clinical basis. *Surgery, Gynecology and Obstetrics* **57**, 51–62.
Cousins M.J. & Bridenbaugh P.O. (Eds) (1988) *Neural Blockade in Clinical Anaesthesia and Management of Pain* 2nd edn. J.B. Lippincott, Philadelphia.
Cousins M.J. & Wright C.J. (1971) Graft, muscle, skin blood flow after epidural block in vascular surgical procedures. *Surgery, Gynecology & Obstetrics* **133**, 59–64.
Covino B.G. (1988) Interpleural regional analgesia. *Anesthesia and Analgesia* **67**, 427–9.
Durrani Z., Winnie A.P. & Ikuta P. (1988) Interpleural catheter analgesia for pancreatic pain. *Anesthesia and Analgesia* **67**,

479—81.

Eason M.J. & Wyatt R. (1979) Paravertebral thoracic block — a reappraisal. *Anaesthesia* **34**, 638—42.

Edwards W.B. & Hingson R.A. (1942) Continuous caudal anesthesia in obstetrics. *American Journal of Surgery* **57**, 459—64.

Glynn C.J., Lloyd J.W. & Barnard J.D.W. (1980) Cryoanalgesia in the management of pain after thoracotomy. *Thorax* **35**, 325—7.

Graziotti P.J. & Smith G.B. (1988) Multiple rib fractures and head injury — an indication for intercostal catheterisation and infusion of local anaesthetics. *Anaesthesia* **43**, 964—6.

Greiss F.C., Still J.G. & Anderson S.G. (1976) Effects of local anesthetic agents on the uterine vasculature and myometrium. *American Journal of Obstetrics and Gynecology* **124**, 889—98.

Hain W.R. (1978) Anaesthetic doses for extradural anaesthesia in children. *British Journal of Anaesthesia* **50**, 303.

Lanier V.A., McKnight H.E. & Trotter M. (1944) Caudal analgesia: an experimental and anatomical study. *American Journal of Obstetrics and Gynecology* **47**, 633—41.

Lofstrom B. & Zetterquist S. (1969) Lumbar sympathetic blocks in the treatment of patients with obliterative disease of the lower limb. *International Anesthesia Clinics* **7**, 423—38.

Miguel R. & Smith R. (1991) Intrapleural, not interpleural analgesia. *Regional Anesthesia* **16**, 299.

Moore D.C., Mather L.A., Bridenbaugh P.O., Bridenbaugh L.D., Balfour R.I., Lysons D.F. & Horton W.G. (1976) Arterial and venous plasma levels of bupivacaine following epidural and intercostal nerve blocks. *Anesthesiology* **45**, 39—45.

Murphy D.F. (1983) Continuous intercostal nerve blockade for pain relief following cholecystectomy. *British Journal of Anaesthesia* **55**, 521—4.

Nunn J.F. & Slavin G. (1980) Posterior intercostal nerve block for pain relief after cholecystectomy. Anatomical basis and efficacy. *British Journal of Anaesthesia* **52**, 253—60.

Odoom J.A. & Sih I.L. (1983) Epidural analgesia and anticoagulation therapy. Experience with 1000 cases of continuous epidurals. *British Journal of Anaesthesia* **38**, 254—9.

Pateman J., Williams M.P. & Filshie J. (1990) Retroperitoneal fibrosis after multiple coeliac plexus blocks. *Anaesthesia* **45**, 309—10.

Purcell-Jones G., Pither C.E., Justins D.M. (1987) Paravertebral block — a misnomer? *Abstracts of Scientific Papers. 6th Annual Meeting of the European Society of Regional Anaesthesia.* p. 82.

Rademaker B.M.P., Sih I.L., Kalkman C.J., Henny C.P., Filedt Kok J.C., Endert E. & Zuurmond W.W.A. (1991) Effects of interpleurally administered bupivacaine 0.5% on opioid analgesic requirements and endocrine response during and after cholecystectomy: a randomized double-blind controlled study. *Acta Anaesthesiologica Scandinavica* **35**, 108—12.

Rao T.L.K. & El-Etr A.A. (1981) Anticoagulation following placement of epidural and subarachnoid catheters: an evaluation of neurologic sequelae. *Anesthesiology* **55**, 618—20.

Reid W., Kennedy Watt J. & Gray T.G. (1970) Phenol injection of the sympathetic chain. *British Journal of Surgery* **57**, 45—50.

Reiestad F. & Stromskag K.E. (1986) Interpleural catheter in the management of postoperative pain. A preliminary report. *Regional Anesthesia* **11**, 89—91.

Rosenberg P.H., Scheinin B.M.A., Lepantalo M.J.A. & Lindfors O. (1987) Continuous intrapleural infusion of bupivacaine for analgesia after thoracotomy. *Anesthesiology* **67**, 811—3.

Schlesinger T.M., Laurito C.E., Baughman V.L. & Carranza C.J. (1989) Interpleural bupivacaine for mammography during needle localization and breast biopsy. *Anesthesia and Analgesia* **68**, 394—5.

Schulte-Steinberg O. & Rahlfs V.W. (1970) Caudal anaesthesia in children and spread of 1 percent lignocaine. A statistical study. *British Journal Anaesthesia* **42**, 1093—9.

Schulte-Steinberg O. & Rahlfs V.W. (1977) Spread of extradural analgesia following caudal injection in children. A statistical study. *British Journal of Anaesthesia* **49**, 1027—34.

Scott D.B. (1975) Evaluation of the clinical tolerance of local anaesthetic agents. *British Journal of Anaesthesia* **47**, 328—31.

Scott P.V. (1991) Interpleural regional analgesia: detection of the interpleural space by saline infusion. *British Journal of Anaesthesia* **66**, 131—3.

Scudamore J.H. & Yates M.J. (1966) Pudendal block — a misnomer? *Lancet* **i**, 23—4.

Seltzer J.L., Larijani G.E., Goldberg M.E. & Marr A.T. (1987) Intrapleural bupivacaine — a kinetic and dynamic evaluation. *Anesthesiology* **67**, 798—800.

Stromskag K.E., Reiestad F., Holmquist E.V.O. & Ogenstad S. (1988) Intrapleural administration of 0.25%, 0.375% and 0.5% bupivacaine with epinephrine after cholecystectomy. *Anesthesia and Analgesia* **67**, 430—4.

Trivedi N.S., Robalino J. & Shevde K. (1990) Interpleural block: a new technique for regional anaesthesia during percutaneous nephrostomy and nephrolithotomy. *Canadian Journal of Anaesthesia* **37**, 479—81.

Trotter M. (1947) Variations of the sacral canal: their significance in the administration of caudal analgesia. *Current Researches in Anesthesia and Analgesia* **26**, 192—202.

Trotter M. & Lanier P.F. (1945) Hiatus canalis sacralis in American whites and negroes. *Human Biology* **17**, 368—81.

Van Dongen R.M.T. & Crul B.J.P. (1991) Paraplegia following coeliac plexus block. *Anaesthesia* **46**, 862—3.

van Kleef J.W., Burm A.G.L. & Vletter A.A. (1990) Single-dose interpleural versus intercostal blockade: nerve block characteristics and plasma concentration profiles after administration of 0.5% bupivacaine with epinephrine. *Anesthesia and Analgesia* **70**, 484—8.

White J., Harrison B., Richmond P., Procter A. & Curran J. (1983) Postoperative analgesia for circumcision. *British Medical Journal* **286**, 1934.

Wildsmith J.A.W. & Armitage E.N. (Eds) (1987) *Principles and Practice of Regional Anaesthesia.* Churchill Livingstone, Edinburgh.

Wildsmith J.A.W. & McClure J.H. (1991) Anticoagulant drugs and central nerve blockade. *Anaesthesia* **46**, 613—14.

Williams P.L. & Warwick R. (Eds) (1980) *Grays Anatomy* 36th edn. Churchill Livingstone, Edinburgh.

Woodham M.J. & Hanna M.H. (1989) Paraplegia after coeliac plexus block. *Anaesthesia* **44**, 487—9.

Yeoman P.M., Cooke R. & Hain W.R. (1983) Penile block for circumcision? A comparison with caudal blockade. *Anaesthesia* **38**, 862—6.

Head and Neck

R.S. NEILL

The classic text, *Regional Anaesthesia* by Labat, written in 1928 includes several chapters on the techniques and indications for regional nerve blocks in the head and neck, ranging from removal of sebaceous cysts to total laryngectomy. With the development of safe and routine tracheal intubation, modern anaesthetic practice has relegated regional nerve block to a minor role in head and neck surgery (Murphy, 1986).

Ophthalmic, ear, nose and throat (ENT), and maxillofacial surgeons continue to use regional anaesthesia for very large numbers of relatively minor surgical procedures, not involving specialist anaesthetists, and where general anaesthesia would be inappropriate (Allen & Elkington, 1980; Jahrsdoerfer, 1981; Martof, 1981; Stromberg, 1985).

During the last decade the pendulum has swung back with an increasing interest and enthusiasm for regional nerve block anaesthesia in obstetrics, general surgery and orthopaedics. An increasing use of daycare facilities has paralleled this renewed interest, with several authors stressing the benefits of regional anaesthesia in this situation (O'Sullivan *et al.*, 1990; Rubin, 1990; White, 1990) and in very large series of patients (Nicoll *et al.*, 1987; Hamilton *et al.*, 1988). In an editorial 'Anaesthetics for cataract surgery — time for change?', Rubin (1990) outlines the advantages to the patient if the anaesthetist is involved in the choice of anaesthetic method, preparation and counselling and monitoring during the procedure. The importance of monitoring if central nervous system (CNS) complications are to be avoided is emphasized by Nicoll and colleagues (1987). Rubin concludes his editorial with the statement 'It would be to the detriment of our patients and specialty if anaesthetists are not involved' (in cataract surgery). This statement might also be applied to the use of regional anaesthesia for other surgery of the head and neck.

Innervation of the head and neck

The structures of the head and neck are supplied by 12 cranial and four cervical nerves. The majority of this supply is of a specialized sensory or secretomotor nature, and has no relevance to nerve block for surgery. A distinctive feature of the nerves to the head and neck is the almost complete separation of sensory and motor function, allowing sensory block to be achieved without motor paralysis. Intraoral blocks may be performed without endangering control of the airway muscles. At other sites it may be important to block both motor and sensory nerves. Anaesthesia for cataract extraction requires block of the orbital branches of the facial nerve to minimize the risk of iris or vitreous prolapse (Feitl & Krupin, 1988; Murphy, 1988).

For the purposes of nerve block for surgery, a detailed knowledge of the sensory supply to the skin of the head and neck and mucous membranes of the airway is required. The anatomical relations of the major motor supply should be known also. Close study of the bony skeleton and dissection specimens help to develop a three-dimensional picture of the anatomy, essential for accurate deposition of the local anaesthetic agent.

Trigeminal nerve

The trigeminal (fifth), the largest cranial nerve, supplies sensation to the face, greater part of the scalp, the teeth, mouth and nasal cavity and through its small motor branch controls the muscles of mastication (Figs 73.1 and 73.2). The trigeminal (Gasserian) ganglion lies in a recess near the apex of the petrous temporal bone.

On leaving the ganglion, the sensory root divides into three divisions: ophthalmic, maxillary and man-

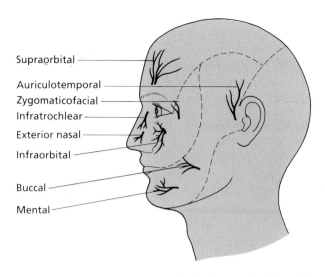

Fig. 73.1 Sensory distribution of the divisions of the V cranial nerve: trigeminal.

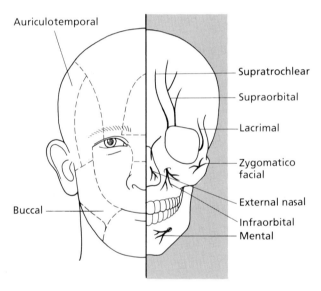

Fig. 73.2 Sensory distribution of the distal branches of the V cranial nerve: trigeminal.

dibular. The motor root lies inferior to the ganglion and joins the mandibular division.

The ophthalmic nerve enters the orbit through the superior orbital fissure and divides into frontal, lacrimal and nasociliary nerves. The terminal cutaneous branches of the frontal are the supraorbital and supratrochlear; of the nasociliary the infratrochlear and external nasal; the lacrimal is inconstant and is replaced sometimes by a branch of the maxillary nerve.

The ophthalmic nerve is joined by sympathetic fibres and fibres from the internal carotid plexus; it has communications with the oculomotor, trochlear and the abducens nerves.

The maxillary nerve leaves the cranial cavity through the foramen rotundum, crosses the pterygopalatine fossa to enter the orbit through the inferior orbital fissure, enters the infraorbital canal, and emerges from the infraorbital foramen as the infraorbital nerve.

An inconstant branch may arise in the infraorbital fissure which emerges as the zygomaticotemporal nerve; a connection between this and the lacrimal nerve may replace one or other of these nerves.

The mandibular nerve is the largest division of the trigeminal. The sensory and motor roots leave the skull through the foramen ovale before uniting and redividing to form the small anterior trunk and larger posterior trunk. At this point the nerve lies in the pterygopalatine fossa, anterior to the neck of the mandible and posterior to the lateral pterygoid plate. The anterior trunk supplies the muscles of mastication and sensation to the skin branch — the buccal nerve.

The posterior trunk is sensory (apart from one branch to the mylohyoid muscle) with three main branches — the auriculotemporal, inferior dental and lingual nerves.

The auriculotemporal emerges from behind the temporomandibular joint to supply sensation to the external auditory meatus and temple. The inferior dental nerve enters the foramen on the medial side of the ramus of the mandible to run through the bone and emerge at the mental foramen, as the mental nerve.

The lingual nerve runs between the ramus of the mandible and the medial pterygoid muscle to lie on the deep surface of the mandible at the third molar, at which point it is covered only by mucous membrane. The lingual nerve supplies sensation to the anterior two-thirds of the tongue and adjacent mucous membrane.

Facial nerve

The facial (seventh) is the motor nerve of the face — supplying the muscles of expression and most importantly the muscles controlling eyelid closure and oral competence.

The nerve runs between the deep and superficial

lobes of the parotid gland. As it does so, it divides into five main branches which fan out to supply their respective areas of the face — temporal, zygomatic, buccal, mandibular and cervical. The mandibular branch runs forward below the angle of the mandible before turning upwards to supply the angle of the mouth (Fig. 73.3).

Glossopharyngeal nerve

The glossopharyngeal (ninth) nerve supplies sensation to the posterior part of the tongue, pharynx and tonsil, secretomotor fibres to the parotid and motor fibres to the stylopharyngeus. It emerges from the jugular foramen in close relationship to the internal jugular vein and internal carotid artery, then runs forward on the stylopharyngeus muscle to pierce the superior constrictor muscle of the pharynx.

Vagus nerve

The branches of the vagus (10th) of importance in the head and neck supply sensory and motor innervation to the larynx.

The superior laryngeal nerve arises from the inferior ganglion of the vagus to run downwards, forwards and medially to the greater cornu of the hyoid where it divides into two branches. The internal branch pierces the thyrohyoid membrane to supply sensation to the larynx above the level of the vocal cords. The external branch is motor to the cricothyroid muscle.

The recurrent laryngeal nerve loops around the aorta on the left and the subclavian on the right before ascending in the groove between the oesophagus and trachea to enter the larynx between the articulation of the inferior cornu of the thyroid and cricoid cartilages. It provides sensation to the larynx below the vocal cords and motor fibres to all the laryngeal muscles except cricothyroid.

Hypoglossal nerve

The hypoglossal (12th) nerve is the motor nerve to the tongue. It leaves the base of the skull related closely to the glossopharyngeal and vagus nerves, lying between the internal jugular vein and internal carotid arteries. At the angle of the mandible, it crosses both internal and external carotid arteries to run downwards and forwards to the greater cornu of the hyoid where it enters the tongue. It supplies branches to the thyrohyoid, styloglossus, hyoglossus, geniohyoid and genioglossus muscles.

Cervical nerves

The skin over a wide area of the scalp, back of the neck and shoulders, the 'cape' area, is supplied by sensory branches of the upper four cervical nerves (Fig. 73.4). Dorsal rami of C2–4 supply the back of the neck and scalp — the greater occipital nerve. Ventral rami of C1–4 form the cervical plexus which may be considered as two separate entities. The deep branches supply the muscles of the neck and the diaphragm. The superficial branches, which pierce

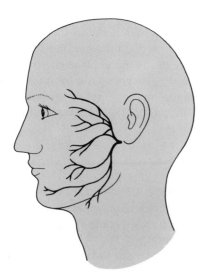

Fig. 73.3 Facial nerve.

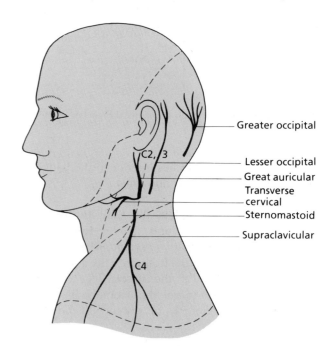

Fig. 73.4 Sensory distribution of the cervical plexus.

the deep fascia at the middle of the posterior border of sternomastoid, fan out to provide sensation from the lower border of the mandible to the level of the second rib. The branches are the great auricular, lesser occipital, the transverse cervical and the supraclavicular.

Clinical applications

The use of regional anaesthesia in the head and neck may produce significant advantage in certain groups of patients.

Outpatient and day-care surgery

The majority of dental surgery is performed on outpatients under local anaesthesia, supplemented frequently by intravenous sedation. When general anaesthesia is employed, nerve block has been advocated as a possible method of reducing intraoperative arrhythmias (Plowman et al., 1974).

This has been confirmed by Rashad and El Attar (1990) who found a statistically significant difference in the incidence of arrhythmias during halothane N$_2$O/O$_2$ anaesthesia when supplemented by nerve block or infiltration compared with placebo. Patients also exhibited faster recovery with enhanced postoperative analgesia.

Day-care cataract surgery using regional anaesthesia is well established in North America (Nicoll et al., 1987; Hamilton et al., 1988) and Rubin (1990) has pleaded the cause for more widespread use in suitable patients in the UK. Szmyd and colleagues (1984) have described a technique for strabismus surgery in adults involving the use of retrobulbar nerve block combined with intravenous sedation. Ocular discomfort occurred 1.5–2 h after the block. Visual acuity and extraocular muscle function were restored fully after 4 h, allowing strabismus to be corrected by adjusting sutures early in the postoperative period.

Attwood and Evans (1985) employed a regional anaesthetic technique for correction of prominent ears in a mixed group of patients in which 20% were under the age of 13 years. The majority were in favour of local rather than general anaesthesia and 30% 'enjoyed' the experience.

White (1990) reports the results of an investigation into perioperative complications conducted by the Federal Ambulatory Surgery Association. The procedures investigated included cervical-node biopsy, jaw wiring, lip-surgery scar revision and blepharoplasty. Complications were lowest, 1:275, when regional or local anaesthesia was used. A significant increase to the level of general anaesthesia, 1:120,

was recorded when regional anaesthesia was accompanied by sedation.

Poor-risk patients

Carefully selected regional anaesthetic techniques can avoid or reduce greatly the need for general anaesthesia. Backer and colleagues (1980) reported no myocardial reinfarction following 288 ophthalmic procedures under local anaesthesia, in 195 patients with a history of a previous myocardial infarction.

Lynch and colleagues (1974) compared general anaesthesia with local anaesthesia for cataract surgery and found a much higher risk of nausea and vomiting following general anaesthesia. This was attributed to the earlier requirement for postoperative analgesia.

Donlon (1986) compared the mortality rates of local and general anaesthetic groups and found them almost equal. However, the patient groups were unequal, as physical status influenced choice and local anaesthesia may be safer in older age groups. Memory performance of patients undergoing extraction of senile cataracts under local anaesthesia with sedation or general anaesthesia was similar 1 week after surgery (Karhunen & Jönn, 1982). Similar results have been reported by O'Sullivan and colleagues (1990) who found no significant difference in morbidity following general or local anaesthesia for day-care cataract surgery. There was no significant difference in cognitive function at day 1 or weeks 2 or 3. Barker and colleagues (1990, 1991) have compared the cortisol, glycaemic and catecholamine responses to cataract surgery during local or general anaesthesia. Local anaesthesia was found to prevent the rise in noradrenaline and glucose found with general anaesthesia and was associated with greater cardiovascular stability.

The ophthalmic surgeon can perform most of his/her surgery with local anaesthesia; however, co-operation of an anaesthetist familiar with these techniques can contribute greatly to the care of patients with eye problems. The choice of anaesthesia can range from local anaesthesia with varying amounts of sedation, to general anaesthesia. If both doctors can perform the regional technique, delays between operations can be minimized (Allen & Elkington, 1980; Jolly, 1980; Nicoll et al., 1987; Hamilton et al., 1988).

Nerve block using small amounts of local anaesthetic with added vasoconstrictor produces effective haemostasis (Keoshian, 1980). The excellent operating conditions can be used as an alternative to induced hypotension in major eyelid surgery in elderly, poor-risk patients (Neill, 1982).

Impaired cerebral circulation

Regional anaesthesia in the awake patient has been advocated as the method of choice for patients requiring carotid endarterectomy following transient ischaemic attacks (Spencer & Eiseman, 1962; Connolly, 1985). The technique permits continuous assessment of neurological status and requirement for shunt (Jopling et al., 1983; Sultz et al., 1990).

Peitzman and colleagues (1982) found the technique safe and reliable with the same rate of neurological complication but a lower rate of non-neurological complications than general anaesthesia. Prough and colleagues (1984) found a low incidence of intraoperative arrhythmias and no perioperative myocardial infarction.

Forssell and colleagues (1989) found a similar incidence of perioperative complications with regional and general anaesthesia. Regional anaesthesia was associated with significantly higher blood pressures. The ability to continuously monitor neurological function led to significantly less use of an intraoperative shunt. Donato and Hill (1992) believe that regional anaesthesia obviates the need for a shunt and its inherent complications in more than 80% of patients.

The sympathetic adrenal responses to carotid endarterectomy performed with either general or local anaesthesia have been investigated by Takolander and colleagues (1990). Significant increases in plasma noradrenaline, heart rate and systolic blood pressure occurred in the local anaesthetic group. General anaesthesia induced a significant degree of hypotension. The conclusion drawn was that both types of anaesthesia have disadvantages in patients with an increased risk of cardiovascular morbidity. Becquemin and colleagues (1991) have concluded that regional anaesthesia was made appropriate for patients with coronary artery disease and at risk of cross-clamping. General anaesthesia was more appropriate in poorly co-operative patients or those with unfavourable operative conditions.

Awake intubation of the trachea

Certain patients have airway abnormalities of such severity that tracheal intubation or tracheostomy should be performed before induction of general anaesthesia. This may be accomplished by a combination of nerve block and topical application of local anaesthetic, using a short-acting agent to limit the time to return of protective laryngeal reflexes (Brown & Sataloff, 1981; Gotta & Sullivan, 1981; Raj, 1983; Murrin, 1985; Donlon, 1986). Awake fibre-optic intubation has been shown to reduce the pressor response to tracheal intubation in normotensive adults (Hawkyard et al., 1992). The authors suggest that this method is of potential value in patients at risk from the pressor response.

Postoperative airway problems

Proximal block of the trigeminal nerve with a long-acting agent offers high quality analgesia and reduced dependence on opioid analgesics to patients in whom the airway may be at risk following major maxillofacial surgery (Murphy, 1988).

Intractable pain

Neurolysis with alcohol or phenol is now reserved for patients with intractable pain from inoperable tumours. Good results can be obtained from proximal block of the trigeminal nerve at the foramen ovale, and cervical plexus at the transverse process (Lipton, 1979; Carron, 1981).

Patients following successful block have a lowered dependence on potent opioid analgesics with an improvement in quality of life (Cousins et al., 1988; Neill, 1992).

Nerve block or local infiltration

Basal-cell carcinoma, the most common skin tumour, occurs frequently on the face and neck. Patients are often frail and elderly, with multiple and extensive lesions, and may be dealt with on an outpatient basis.

Infiltration techniques distend and distort the tissues making accurate definition of the lesion difficult; when multiple lesions are present, the volume of local anaesthetic required may cause anxiety if all lesions are to be removed at one visit. Nerve block supplemented by minimal local infiltration offers a solution (Murphy, 1988).

Volume of local anaesthetic is much reduced, a wide area of anaesthesia is provided with little or no tissue distortion and fear of toxicity removed.

Balanced anaesthesia

Nerve blocks formed the original analgesic component of a balanced anaesthetic (Lundy, 1926). Used thus, the residual effects of the local anaesthetic agent extend into the postoperative period, ensuring a pain-free recovery with reduced requirement for analgesics. Great auricular nerve block with a long-acting agent is of special benefit to children who have had surgical correction of prominent ears.

Careful identification of the branches of the facial nerve is essential during surgery of the parotid gland. The combination of light general anaesthesia and cervical plexus block in a spontaneously breathing patient provides a clear operating field and the ability to assess facial nerve function continuously.

Techniques ranging from profound hypotension to local infiltration of large volumes of vasoconstrictors have been used to control bleeding during corrective rhinoplasty. Regional nerve block in combination with light general anaesthesia can provide comparable conditions to profound hypotension, with little or no tissue distortion from local infiltration (Neill, 1983).

Reconstructive techniques in major intraoral cancer surgery often involve free tissue transfer (Soutar et al., 1983). The reduction in the sympathetic tone produced by a deep cervical plexus block can help in the establishment of an adequate circulation to the transferred tissue (Neill, 1983, 1993).

Possible blocks, problems and hazards

The cranial nerves may be blocked proximally as they leave the base of the skull, but more frequently, block is confined to the distal branches. The anatomical relationship of the nerves to each other and to the major vessels (the carotid artery and internal jugular vein), as they leave the base of the skull creates a significant risk of intravascular injection, haematoma formation and nerve damage.

Retrobulbar nerve block is associated with some potentially catastrophic complications, especially optic nerve damage, central retinal artery occlusion, scleral perforation and intradural injection (Didier et al., 1989; Rigg & James, 1989; Fry & Henderson, 1990; Vestal et al., 1991).

Retrobulbar haemorrhage as a result of accidental puncture of an orbital vein produces proptosis and an increase in intraoperative pressure which necessitates postponement of the surgery (Allen & Elkington, 1980).

The incidence and variety of CNS toxicity following cataract surgery under regional block has been documented by Nicoll and colleagues (1987) and Hamilton and colleagues (1988). The symptoms range from drowsiness, shivering, vomiting and contralateral blindness through to respiratory depression, apnoea, aphasia with or without loss of consciousness, convulsions and cardiopulmonary arrest. Instances of apnoea have also been reported by McGalliard (1988) and Rigg and James (1989). Hamilton (1990) stated that the risk of serious complications associated with traditional retrobulbar nerve block is such that it should no longer be taught or practised and should be replaced by the peribulbar large-volume intraocular technique with orbital compression.

Idiopathic trigeminal anaesthesia has caused trophic ulceration of the ala nasae (McLean & Watson, 1982). This has also followed damage to the infraorbital artery if the needle is introduced deeply into the infraorbital foramen during an infraorbital nerve block (Moore, 1975; Garber, 1980).

Therapy of trigeminal neuralgia by chemical ablation of the affected division of the nerve has been superseded by radiofrequency coagulation (Lipton, 1979; Wise, 1984). Chemical ablation was associated with a 0.9% fatality rate, and a danger of permanent blindness if the injection of the maxillary nerve was misplaced in the infraorbital fissure (Swerdlow, 1988).

Total spinal anaesthesia has followed both trigeminal and anterior ethmoidal nerve block (Nique & Bennett, 1981; Hill et al., 1983). The injections perforated the dura of the foramen ovale and cribiform plate. Both patients recovered following immediate aggressive therapy, and were fortunate that an ablative agent had not been used. Cervical plexus and stellate ganglion blocks carry a significant risk of total spinal anaesthesia or acute cerebral toxicity if the needle enters the dural cuff or vertebral artery. Stannard and colleagues (1990) and Bruyns and colleagues (1991) have reported dural puncture with total spinal block, apnoea and unconsciousness following stellate ganglion block. The report by Durrani and Winnie (1991) of brainstem toxicity with reversible locked-in syndrome occurring after an interscalene brachial plexus block in which local anaesthetic was injected into the vertebral artery should alert anaesthetists to the possibility that not all brainstem toxic reactions lead to unconsciousness. Patients with this syndrome can only communicate by blinking or making vertical eye movements.

The close association of the glossopharyngeal, vagal and hypoglossal nerves at the styloid process creates a significant risk of impairment of motor and sensory supply to the airway from local spread of small volumes of correctly positioned agents. Respiratory obstruction caused the death of a patient who received a vagal nerve block as therapy for a postcricoid carcinoma (Cousins et al., 1988).

Less serious but distressing complications can follow correctly placed nerve blocks. They are self-limiting and related to the duration of action of the anaesthetic agent, e.g. diplopia following maxillary block (Kronman & Kabani, 1984) or Horner's syndrome following a stellate ganglion block. All patients should be given a clear explanation of these complications and reassurance as to the outcome.

Precise anatomical knowledge and meticulous technique can minimize the risk of these mishaps, but few opportunities to acquire these skills exist outside specialist units, and these complex methods offer little advantage over the more distal blocks. These are less demanding technically and may be employed reliably even by the occasional user with benefit to patient and operator, either alone or as a component of balanced anaesthesia (Neill, 1983, 1987).

Techniques of nerve block

Trigeminal

All divisions of the nerve may be blocked as they emerge from the foramina on the base of the skull.

Block of first division (ophthalmic)

The first division is blocked centrally together with the oculomotor, trochlear abducens nerves and ciliary ganglion when a retrobulbar injection is performed. At other times it is sufficient to inject the distal branches to achieve anaesthesia of the cutaneous distribution.

Retrobulbar nerve block (see Chapter 38)

Peribulbar nerve block (see Chapter 38)

Block of second and third divisions (maxillary and mandibular)

These may be blocked using either a lateral or an anterior approach.

Lateral approach

One or both divisions may be blocked from a single entrance point using the landmarks which define the coronoid notch, i.e. the zygomatic arch, the ramus and the coronoid process of the mandible (Fig. 73.5).

To block the maxillary division of the nerve, a 23-gauge spinal needle is introduced through the coronoid notch below the midpoint of the zygomatic arch (Fig. 73.6). It is directed at an angle of 45° to the vertical, aiming for the apex of the bony orbital cone, to strike the medial edge of the lateral pterygoid plate or the body of the maxilla. Care must be exercised to prevent damage to the optic nerve if the needle enters the infraorbital fissure. Following careful aspiration, 2–5 ml of local anaesthetic solution are injected.

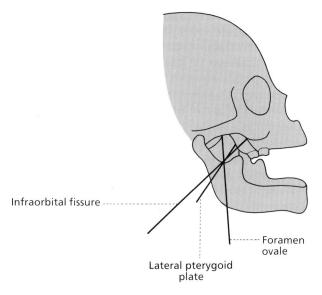

Infraorbital fissure ----------------

Lateral pterygoid plate

Foramen ovale

Fig. 73.5 Block of the V second and third divisions: landmarks.

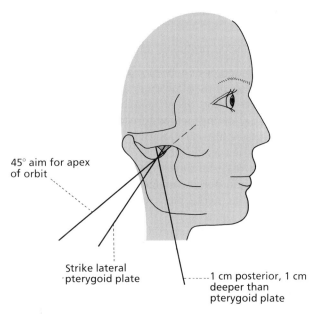

45° aim for apex of orbit

Strike lateral pterygoid plate

1 cm posterior, 1 cm deeper than pterygoid plate

Fig. 73.6 Block of the V second and third divisions: lateral approach.

To block the mandibular division, the same landmarks are used. In this instance, the needle is directed at 90° in both planes to strike the posterior edge of the lateral pterygoid plate. It may then be retracted to the skin and reintroduced aiming for a point 1 cm posterior to and 1 cm more deeply than previously, to slide past the edge of the plate. This step may be omitted (Moore, 1975), as sufficient anaesthetic filters around the pterygoid plate if injection is made at the point of bony contact. Paraesthesiae are not essential for either of these blocks.

Anterior approach

The essential landmarks are the midpoint of the zygomatic arch and the pupil. With the patient's head resting on a 'donut' to provide stability, the midpoint of the zygomatic arch, and a point 3 cm lateral to the angle of the mouth are marked (Fig. 73.7).

Through the latter mark the introducer needle for a 25-gauge spinal needle is inserted. The spinal needle is advanced towards the base of the skull aligning it with the pupil in the vertical plane and 1 cm anterior to the midpoint of the zygoma in the horizontal. The needle strikes the sphenoid anterior to the foramen ovale. It should now be redirected in line with the midpoint of the zygoma and at the same depth should enter the foramen ovale (Fig. 73.7).

This approach to the divisions of the trigeminal nerve has a high risk of serious complications. Involvement of the first division causes loss of corneal sensation, and corneal reflex with the possibility of corneal ulceration. Accidental injection into the cranial cavity can lead to paralysis of other cranial nerves (Nique & Bennett, 1981). Meticulous attention to technique, with careful repeated aspiration is mandatory. Paraesthesiae should be sought always, and it is recommended that this route be used only for treatment of intractable cancer pain.

Glossopharyngeal nerve

This nerve may be blocked, as it lies close to the posterior edge of the styloid process. The block is required infrequently and carries an exceedingly high risk of accidental intravascular injection and spread to hypoglossal, vagus and accessory nerves (Cousins *et al.*, 1988).

Laryngeal nerve

The inferior surface of the epiglottis and the laryngeal inlet derive sensation from the superior laryngeal nerve. Anaesthesia of the area may be achieved by peroral spray or by blocking the nerve as it pierces the thyrohyoid membrane below the greater cornu of the hyoid. To block the nerve, the larynx is displaced laterally to make the hyoid more prominent. A 25-gauge needle is walked off the cornu of the hyoid and 2−3 ml of anaesthetic injected as it penetrates the thyrohyoid membrane.

The inferior surface of the cords and trachea are anaesthetized by injection of 2−3 ml of anaesthetic through the cricothyroid membrane during deep inspiration.

Cervical plexus

The classical method of deep cervical plexus block involves injections on to the transverse processes of C2, 3 and 4 vertebrae.

To locate the relevant transverse processes, a line is drawn from the tip of the mastoid process to the transverse process of C6, which is readily palpable. The transverse processes of C2, 3 and 4 lie approximately 0.5 cm posterior to this line with C2 palpable 2 cm caudad to the mastoid process (Fig. 73.8).

C3 and C4 are palpated a further 1 cm apart and slightly anteriorly. As each landmark is identified, a 23-gauge needle is inserted in a caudad direction to

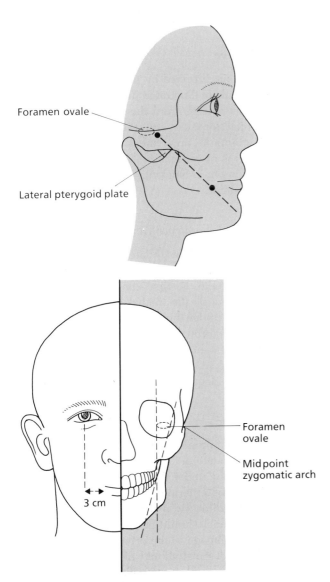

Fig. 73.7 Block of V second and third divisions: anterior approach.

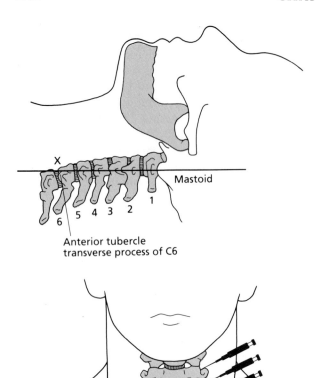

Fig. 73.8 Deep cervical plexus block: injection onto transverse process, needle direction caudad.

rest on the transverse process. This should avoid puncturing the vertebral artery or penetrating the dural space (Winnie *et al.*, 1975). The needle should be kept in contact with bone during aspiration and injection of anaesthetic agent 5—10 ml at each site.

An alternative technique (Winnie *et al.*, 1975) involves a single injection site. Local anaesthetic 10—20 ml is placed at the C4 transverse process. Successful block depends on spread within the fascial sheath. As C4 is a major component of the phrenic nerve, bilateral deep cervical plexus blocks are inadvisable.

Stellate ganglion

This block is requested sometimes as a diagnostic tool or therapeutic aid in circulatory disturbances of the upper limb, e.g. Raynaud's phenomenon. The ganglion lies between the base of the transverse process of C7 and the neck of the first rib behind the carotid sheath. It is related more closely to the pleura on the right than on the left.

The position of C7 transverse process is determined

by placing a mark 3 cm lateral to the middle of the clavicular notch and 3 cm vertical to the clavicle — two fingerbreadths in each direction. Palpation of C6 transverse process should confirm this mark, as it lies 1.5 cm cephalad to C7.

The carotid sheath and sternomastoid are retracted laterally as the needle is inserted perpendicularly through the mark. It impinges normally on the transverse process but should be redirected if paraesthesiae occur in the brachial plexus or if bone is not contacted.

Following the normal careful aspiration, a small amount is injected as a test dose, as a precaution against injection into the vertebral artery, extradural or intradural space.

Techniques of nerve block — distal

Trigeminal nerve

The areas of skin supplied by the terminal branches of the trigeminal are illustrated in Fig. 73.2. The three main branches emerge from the supraorbital notch, the infraorbital foramen and the mental foramen. These exit points lie on a line 1.5 cm from the alar margin which is of especial help in determining the site of injection when blocking these branches in the edentulous patient.

Supraorbital and supratrochlear nerves

Block of both these nerves, bilateral if necessary, can be achieved from a single injection site on the nasal bridge. The needle is first directed downwards and laterally towards the medial canthus, and then directly laterally under the orbital rim to a point 1 cm beyond the supraorbital notch. Injection should be continuous as the needle is advanced, essential if non-aspirating dental cartridge syringes are used. One to 2 ml are adequate for both blocks.

Infraorbital nerve

The infraorbital foramen is located 1 cm below the orbital rim 1.5 cm lateral to the nasal bone. The nerve may be blocked by direct skin puncture at this point or alternatively by entering the buccal sulcus at the upper premolar directing the needle upwards to the orbital rim. A finger should be placed on the orbital rim to prevent damage to the orbit or its contents.

The infraorbital canal should not be entered; it is both unnecessary and potentially hazardous. The floor of the orbit is punctured easily; damage to the infraorbital artery can cause ulceration of the infra-orbital skin (Moore, 1975).

Zygomaticofacial and lacrimal nerves

The zygomatic foramen can be palpated 1–2 cm below the lower lateral orbital margin. The area immediately around the foramen should be infiltrated with 1–2 ml of anaesthetic as the nerve breaks into radiating branches immediately it emerges from the foramen. From the same injection site, infiltration past the lateral canthus to the outer third of the upper eyelid will anaesthetize the lacrimal nerve.

Mental nerve

The mental foramen is situated below the first pre-molar halfway between the gum margin and the lower border of the mandible. In the edentulous patient, the position may be confirmed using the straight-line relationship between the foramina (Fig. 73.9). As with the infraorbital nerve block, the injection may be made through the skin, but the buccal sulcus is used more frequently. The application of anaesthetic gel to this site makes the injection pain-free.

Inferior dental and lingual nerves

These may be injected at the foramen which lies in the centre of the medial aspect of the ascending ramus of the mandible. To locate the foramen, the ramus is palpated with the index finger, the pulp resting on the concavity of the retromolar trigone, the nail identifying the medial ridge. With the barrel of the syringe resting on the contralateral premolars, the needle is directed parallel to the occlusal surface of the mandibular molars to penetrate the mucosa just beyond the midpoint of the palpating finger (Fig. 73.10). As the injection is made, the syringe is swung across to allow the insertion to continue parallel to the mandibular ramus for a distance of 2 cm. Injection of 2 ml will block both nerves.

Buccal nerve

The needle is inserted into the mucous membrane of the cheek at the level of the first mandibular molar and directed backwards. Injection of 2–3 ml is made as the needle is advanced parallel to the lateral aspect of the mandibular ramus.

Akinosi (1977) described a method of mandibular nerve block in which it was not necessary for the patient to open his/her mouth. The injection is made into the tissues between the vertical ramus of the mandible and the maxillary tuberosity (Fig. 73.11). Using this approach, buccal anaesthesia occurs in 80% of cases (Sisk, 1986).

Auriculotemporal nerve

Injection of 2 ml of anaesthetic between the super-

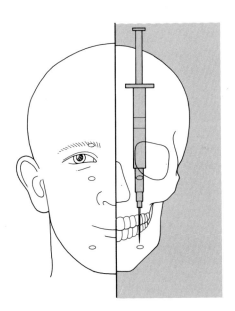

Fig. 73.9 Mental nerve block: approach through buccal sulcus using 'straight-line' relationship between foraminae.

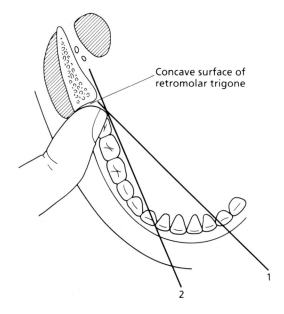

Concave surface of retromolar trigone

Fig. 73.10 Inferior dental nerve block.

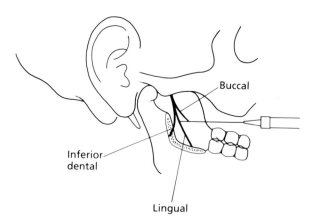

Fig. 73.11 Inferior dental nerve block. (Redrawn from Akinosi, 1977.)

ficial temporal artery and the ear is normally sufficient to produce block of this branch.

Anterior ethmoidal — external nasal nerves, sphenopalatine ganglion

The sensory supply of the mucosa lining the nasal passage is derived from these nerves. The external nasal branches supply the skin on the tip of the nose related to the alar cartilages. Block of the nasal mucosa is achieved normally by packing with cocaine-soaked gauze or mounted pledgets (Q-tips) placed strategically above and below the superior and middle turbinates.

The external nasal nerve is blocked readily with a 1-ml injection at the junction of the bony and cartilaginous nose.

Cervical plexus — superficial block

The superficial branches of the plexus emerge at the midpoint of the posterior border of the sternomastoid muscle. The external jugular vein normally crosses the muscles 1–2 cm below this point. This posterior border of the muscle is identified by asking the patient to raise his/her head, and the injection point marked. Solution is directed upwards and downwards from this point and if made within the correct tissue planes will be seen to 'flow' along the border of the muscle. Five to 10 ml are sufficient and bilateral blocks may be used with safety (Fig. 73.12).

Great auricular nerve

The great auricular nerve divides into pre- and post-auricular branches to supply the greater part of the ear.

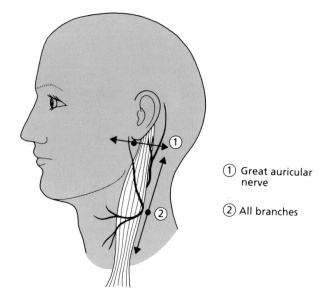

Fig. 73.12 Block of the superficial branches of the cervical plexus.

Both branches may be blocked with a single injection of 2–3 ml infiltrated 2–3 cm from the tip of the mastoid process in anterior and posterior directions (Fig. 73.12).

Anaesthetic agents

Surface anaesthesia. Cocaine 2–10%, lignocaine 4%.

Infiltration anaesthesia. Lignocaine + adrenaline, prilocaine + octapressin, bupivacaine 0.25% or 0.5%.

Nerve block.
1 Anaesthesia. Lignocaine + adrenaline, prilocaine + octapressin, bupivacaine.
2 *Ablation.* Aqueous phenol, alcohol.

Analgesia and sedation

Regional anaesthesia requires the same detailed attention to assessment and preparation as general anaesthesia. Preoperative medication and intraoperative sedation should result in a patient who is calm, drowsy, devoid of anxiety yet capable of arousal and co-operation (Pratt, 1985). This may be achieved using combinations of opioids, short-acting barbiturates, benzodiazepines and butyrophenones given intravenously in very dilute concentration. Individual anaesthetists favour differing combinations of these agents, no one regimen attains universal approval.

Sedation must be regarded always as complementary to the regional nerve block and cannot be used as a substitute for inadequate anaesthesia.

References

Akinosi J.O. (1977) A new approach to the mandibular nerve block. *British Journal of Oral Surgery* **15**, 83–7.

Allen E.D. & Elkington A.R. (1980) Local anaesthesia and the eye. *British Journal of Anaesthesia* **52**, 689–94.

Attwood A.I. & Evans D.M. (1985) Correction of prominent ears using Mustarde's technique: an outpatient procedure under local anaesthetic in children and adults. *British Journal of Plastic Surgery* **38**, 252–8.

Backer G.L., Tinker J.H., Robertson D.M. & Vliestra R.E. (1980) Myocardial reinfarction following local anaesthesia for ophthalmic surgery. *Anesthesia and Analgesia* **59**, 257–62.

Barker J.P., Robinson P.N., Vafidis G.C., Hart G.R., Sapsed-Byrne S. & Hall G.M. (1990) Local analgesia prevents the cortisol and glycaemic responses to cataract surgery. *British Journal of Anaesthesia* **64**, 442–5.

Barker J.P., Vafidis G.C., Robinson P.N. & Hall G.M. (1991) Plasma catecholamine response to cataract surgery. A comparison between general and local anaesthesia. *Anaesthesia* **46**, 642–5.

Becquemin J.P., Paris E., Valverde A., Pluskwa F. & Melliere D. (1991) Carotid surgery: is regional anaesthesia always appropriate. *Journal of Cardiovascular Surgery* **32**, 592–8.

Brown A.C.D. & Sataloff R.T. (1981) Special anaesthetic techniques in head and neck surgery. *Otolaryngologic Clinics of North America* **14.3**, 587–614.

Bruyns T., Devulder J., Vermeulen H., De Colvenaer L. & Rolly G. (1991) Possible inadvertent subdural block following attempted stellate ganglion blockade. *Anaesthesia* **46**, 747–9.

Carron H. (1981) Control of pain in the head and neck. *Otolaryngologic Clinics of North America* **14.3**, 631–52.

Connolly J.E. (1985) Carotid endarterectomy in the awake patient. *American Journal of Surgery* **150**, 159–65.

Cousins M.J., Dwyer B. & Gibb D. (1988) Chronic pain and neurolytic blockade. In *Neural Blockade* 2nd edn. (Eds Cousins M.J. & Bridenbaugh P.O.) p. 1053. Lippincott, Philadelphia.

Didier T., Brasseur G., Retout A. & Charlin J.F. (1989) Perforation du globe oculaire par injection retrobulbaire. *Bulletin Societé Ophthalmologie France* **89** (12), 1405–7.

Donato A.T. & Hill S.L. (1992) Carotid arterial surgery using local anaesthesia: a private practice retrospective study. *American Surgeon* **58**(8), 446–50.

Donlon J.V. Jr. (1986) Anaesthesia for eye, ear, nose and throat. In *Anaesthesia* 2nd edn., vol. 3 (Ed. Miller R.D.) p. 1837. Churchill Livingstone, New York.

Durrani Z. & Winnie A.P. (1991) Brainstem toxicity with reversible locked in syndrome after intrascalene brachial plexus block. *Anesthesia and Analgesia* **72**, 249–52.

Feitl M. & Krupin T. (1988) Neural blockade for ophthalmic surgery. In *Neural Blockade* 2nd edn. (Eds Cousins M.J. & Bridenbaugh P.O.) p. 577. Lippincott, Philadelphia.

Forssell C., Takolander R., Bergqvist D., Johansson A. & Person N.H. (1989) Local vs. general anaesthesia in carotid surgery — a prospective randomised study. *European Journal of Vascular Surgery* **3** (6), 503–9.

Fry R.A. & Henderson J. (1990) Local anaesthesia for eye surgery; the periocular technique. *Anaesthesia* **45**, 14–17.

Garber J. (1980) Neural blockade for dental, oral and adjoining areas. In *Neural Blockade* (Eds Cousins M.J. & Bridenbaugh P.O.). Lippincott, Philadelphia.

Gotta A.W. & Sullivan C.A. (1981) Anaesthesia of the upper airway using topical anaesthesia and superior laryngeal nerve block. *British Journal of Anaesthesia* **53**, 1055–8.

Hamilton R.C. (1990) Complications of retrobulbar and peribulbar blocks (letter; comment). *Regional Anesthesia* **15**(2), 106–7.

Hamilton R.C., Gimbel H.V. & Strunin L. (1988) Regional anaesthesia for 12,000 cataract extraction and intraocular lens implantation procedures. *Canadian Journal of Anaesthesia* **35** (6), 615–23.

Hawkyard S.J., Morrison A., Doyle L.A., Croton R.S. & Wake P.N. (1992) Attenuating the hypertensive response to laryngoscopy and endotracheal intubation using awake fibreoptic intubation. *Acta Anaesthesiologica Scandinavica* **36**, 1–4.

Hill J.N., Gershon N.I. & Cargiulo P.O. (1983) Total spinal blockade during local anaesthesia of the nasal passages. *Anesthesiology* **59** (2), 144–6.

Jahrsdoefer R.A. (1981) Anaesthesia in otologic surgery. *Otolaryngologic Clinics of North America* **14.3**, 699–704.

Jolly C. (1980) Clinical use of nerve blocks in relation to surgery. In *General Anaesthesia* 4th edn., vol. 1 (Eds Gray T.C., Nunn J.F. & Utting J.F.) p. 381. Butterworth, London.

Jopling M.W., De Sanctis C.A., McDowell D.E., Savarin R.A., Martinez O.A. & Gray D.F. (1983) Anaesthesia for carotid endarterectomy a comparison of regional and general techniques. *Anesthesiology* **59**, 217A.

Karhunen U. & Jönn G. (1982) A comparison of memory function following local and general anaesthesia for extraction of senile cataract. *Acta Anaesthesiologica Scandinavica* **26**, 291–6.

Keoshian L.A. (1980) Neural blockade for plastic surgery. In *Neural Blockade* (Eds Cousins M.J. & Bridenbaugh P.O.). Lippincott, Philadelphia.

Kronman J.H. & Kabani S. (1984) The neuronal basis for diplopia following local anaesthetic injections. *Oral Surgery, Oral Medicine, Oral Pathology* **58**, 533–4.

Labat G. (1928) *Regional Anaesthesia; its Technique and Clinical Application* 2nd edn., pp. 75–323. W.B. Saunders, Philadelphia.

Lipton S. (1979) *Relief of Pain in Clinical Practice*. pp. 306–66. Blackwell Scientific Publications, Oxford.

Lundy J.S. (1926) Balanced anaesthesia. *Minnesota Medicine* **9**, 399.

Lynch S., Wolf G. & Berlin I. (1974) 2,200 cases of cataract surgery under general anaesthesia. *Anesthesia and Analgesia* **53**, 909–13.

Martof A.B. (1981) Anaesthesia of the teeth supporting structures and oral mucous membrane. *Otolaryngologic Clinics of North America* **14.3**, 653–8.

McGalliard J.N. (1988) Respiratory arrest after two retrobulbar injections. *American Journal of Ophthalmology* **105**, 90–1.

McLean N.R. & Watson A.C.H. (1982) Reconstruction of a defect of the alanasi following trigeminal anaesthesia with an innervated forehead flap. *British Journal of Plastic Surgery* **35**, 201–3.

Moore D.C. (1975) *Regional Block* pp. 77–111. Charles C. Thomas, Illinois.

Murphy T.M. (1986) Nerve blocks in the head and neck. In *Anaesthesia* 2nd edn., vol. 2 (Ed. Miller R.D.) p. 1044. Churchill Livingstone, New York.

Murphy T.H. (1988) Somatic blockade of head and neck. In *Neural Blockade* 2nd edn. (Eds Cousins M.J. & Bridenbaugh P.O.) p. 533. Lippincott, Philadelphia.

Murrin K.R. (1985) Awake intubation. In *Difficulties in Tracheal Intubation* (Eds Latto I.P. & Rosen M.) p. 90. Baillière Tindall, W.B. Saunders, Eastbourne.

Neill R.S. (1982) Regional anaesthesia for major eyelid surgery in the elderly — an alternative to induced hypotension. *British Journal of Plastic Surgery* **36**, 29–35.

Neill R.S. (1983) Head and neck surgery. In *Practical Regional Anaesthesia* (Eds Henderson J.J. & Nimmo W.S.) p. 165. Blackwell Scientific Publications, Oxford.

Neill R.S. (1987) Head neck and airway. In *Principles and Practice of Regional Anaesthesia* (Eds Wildsmith J.A.W. & Armitage E.N.) p. 168. Churchill Livingstone, Edinburgh.

Neill R.S. (1992) Terminal care of intraoral cancer. *The European Journal of Pain* **13**(1), 8–11.

Neill R.S. (1993) Regional anaesthesia for microvascular surgery. In *Microvascular Surgery and Free Tissue Transfer* (Ed. Soutar D.S.) pp. 17–25. Edward Arnold, Sevenoaks.

Nicoll J.M., Arnachary P., Ahlen K., Baguneid S. & Edge K.R. (1987) Central nervous system complications after 6,000 retrobulbar blocks. *Anesthesia and Analgesia* **66** (2), 1298–302.

Nique T.A. & Bennett C.R. (1981) Inadvertent brainstem anaesthesia following extradural trigeminal V2–V3 blocks. *Oral Surgery, Oral Medicine, Oral Pathology* **51**, 468–70.

O'Sullivan G., Kerr-Muir M., Lim M., Davies W. & Campbell N. (1990) Daycase ophthalmic surgery: general or local anaesthesia? (Letter). *Anaesthesia* **45** (10), 855–86.

Peitzman A.B., Webster M.W., Loubean J.M., Bahnson H.T. & Grundy B.L. (1982) Carotid endarterectomy under regional (conductive) anaesthesia. *Annals of Surgery* **196**, 59–64.

Plowman P.C., Thomas W.J.N. & Thurlow A.C. (1974) Cardiac dysrhythmias during anaesthesia for oral surgery. *Anaesthesia* **29**, 571–5.

Pratt J.M. (1985) Analgesics and sedation in plastic surgery. *Clinics in Plastic Surgery* **12**, 73–81.

Prough D.S., Scuderi P.E., Stullken E. & Davis C.H. (1984) Myocardial infarction following regional anaesthesia for carotid endarterectomy. *Canadian Anaesthetists' Society Journal* **31**, 192–6.

Rashad A. & El Attar A. (1990) Cardiac dysrhythmias during oral surgery: effect of combined local and general anaesthesia. *British Journal of Oral Maxillofacial Surgery* **28** (2), 102–4.

Raj P.P. (1983) Bronchoscopy and tracheal intubation. In *Practical Regional Anaesthesia* (Eds Henderson J.J. & Nimmo W.E.) pp. 289–300. Blackwell Scientific Publications, Oxford.

Rigg J.D. & James R.H. (1989) Apnoea after retrobulbar block. *Anaesthesia* **44**, 26–7.

Rubin A.P. (1990) Anaesthesia for cataract surgery — time for a change? (Editorial.) *Anaesthesia* **45** (9), 717–8.

Sisk A.L. (1986) Evaluation of the Akinosi mandibular block technique in oral surgery. *Journal of Oral Maxillofacial Surgery* **44**, 113–15.

Soutar D.S., Scheker L.R., Tanner N.B.S. & McGregor I.A. (1983) The radial forearm flap; a versatile method for intra oral reconstruction. *British Journal of Plastic Surgery* **36**, 1–8.

Spencer F.C. & Eiseman B. (1962) Technique of carotid endarterectomy. *Surgery Gynecology and Obstetrics* **115**, 115–17.

Stannard C.F., Glynn C.J. & Smith S.P. (1990) Dural puncture during attempted stellate ganglion block. *Anaesthesia* **45**, 952–4.

Stromberg B.V. (1985) Regional anaesthesia in head and neck surgery. *Clinics in Plastic Surgery* **12**, 123–36.

Sultz S., Behar M., Negri M., Hod G., Zaidenstein L. & Bogakowsky H. (1990) Carotid endarterectomy under local anaesthesia supplemented with neuroleptic analgesia. *Surgical Gynaecology and Obstetrics* **170**, 141–4.

Swerdlow M. (1988) Complications of neurolytic blockade. In *Neural Blockade* 2nd edn. (Eds Cousins M.J. & Bridenbaugh P.O.) pp. 719–35. Lippincott, Philadelphia.

Szmyd S.M., Nelson L.B., Calhoun J.H. & Harley R.D. (1984) Retrobulbar anaesthesia in strabismus surgery. *Archives of Ophthalmology* **102** (9), 1325–7.

Takolander R., Bergqvist D., Lennart Hulthen U., Johansson A. & Katzman Der L. (1990) Carotid artery surgery — local versus general anaesthesia as related to sympathetic activity and cardiovascular effects. *European Journal of Vascular Surgery* **4**, 265–70.

Vestal K.P., Meyers S.M. & Zegarra H. (1991) Retinal detachment as a complication of retrobulbar anaesthesia. *Canadian Journal of Ophthalmology* **26**, 32–3.

White P.F. (1990) Outpatient anaesthesia. In *Anaesthesia* 3rd edn. (Ed. Miller R.D.) p. 2025. Churchill Livingstone, New York.

Winnie A.P., Ramamurthy S., Durrani Z. & Radonjic R. (1975) Interscalene cervical plexus block; a single injection technique. *Anesthesia and Analgesia* **54**, 370–5.

Wise R.P. (1984) Pain clinic and operative nerve blocks. In *Wylie and Churchill-Davidson's A Practice of Anaesthesia* (Ed. Churchill Davidson H.C.) p. 893. Lloyd Luke (Medical Books) Ltd, London.

SECTION IV
ACUTE AND CHRONIC PAIN

Assessment of Pain

C.R. CHAPMAN

This chapter is an introduction to the measurement of pain and analgesic states in clinical settings. It is intended for the anaesthetist or pain specialist who wishes to measure pain during a clinical or clinically related study or who plans to assess pain states in patients. A substantial literature exists on the measurement of pain and analgesia in animals, and a smaller but complex literature exists on the measurement of pain in laboratory subjects. These related topics exceed the scope of this chapter, the interested reader should consult the recent volume on pain measurement edited by Chapman and Loeser (1989) and Bromm's earlier edited book (1984).

The objectives of this chapter are: (i) to introduce the basic definitions of pain and the fundamental concepts of measurement; (ii) to discuss three traditions of thought about measurement that have shaped the tools currently used by pain researchers and clinicians; (iii) to review current methods for measuring pain in clinical settings and related research; (iv) to discuss factors that can bias pain measurement; and (v) to offer broad guidelines for choosing among pain-measurement tools for research or clinical-assessment purposes.

Basic definitions and concepts

Pain

Most anaesthetists think of pain as an aversive sensation arising from tissue damage or stress. For most situations in day-to-day clinical life, this is an adequate working definition, but it falters when applied to the distressed patient with labour pain, the querulous postoperative patient or the burn patient terrified of debridement. The concept fails altogether in chronic pain where pain complaint often bears little or no relationship to organic pathology. Experience with awake, suffering patients inevitably convinces even the staunchest purist that human pain is intimately linked with emotion, powerfully altered for better or worse by a patient's expectations and beliefs, and imperfectly correlated with tissue injury. Many chronic pain problems seem to be more under the control of psychological factors rather than physical disease processes.

It is hardly surprising, therefore, that pain research manifests a confluence of clinical wisdom from many settings and of theory from basic science. Consensus exists that sensory processes signalling tissue injury (nociception) are necessary but not sufficient for a working definition of pain. Clinically significant pain involves emotional arousal as well as sensory signalling. Therefore, a comprehensive concept of pain is required in order to design a study or assess patients in pain in a specific clinical setting. There is no single solution for how pain should be defined for there are many types of pain, both acute and chronic in many different patient populations and settings. The exact working definition chosen must fit the circumstances while taking advantage of the state of knowledge in the field.

At present, theory varies with the writer but, in general, current specialists and theorists hold that pain is a complex and multidimensional human perception which involves sensory, affective and cognitive aspects (each of these being complex and multidimensional in themselves). For the purposes of scaling pain in the individual patient, these dimensions manifest themselves via behavioural, physiological or cognitive phenomena. Such phenomena can be considered features or *attributes* of the dimensions they represent, and each requires a separate operation for number assignment. Figure 74.1 illustrates this concept. The problem of assigning numbers to features brings us to the concept of measurement.

Category scale
Please check the category that best describes your pain:

_____ Mild   _____ Horrible

_____ Discomforting   _____ Excruciating

_____ Distressing

Numerical rating scale
Please choose a number from 0 to 100 to describe the intensity of your pain. Zero indicates no pain and 100 means that the pain is as bad as it can be.

Visual analogue scale
Mark the line below to indicate the intensity of your pain.

```
|_____|
No pain                        Pain as bad as
                               it can be
```

Fig. 74.1 Typical scales for subjective pain report (shown with instructions to patient).

Measurement

As ordinary daily life and clinical practice are filled with measurement operations, it may seem superfluous to define measurement. None the less, theorists disagree about what the term should mean (Chapman, 1989). A fundamental issue is whether we should (i) quantify the person who has the subjective state; or (ii) quantify the state itself (Michell, 1986). Pain researchers must decide in a given circumstance whether they intend to measure the person with pain (i.e. pain can be a feature of a patient, just as blood pressure or white cell count are features of an individual) or whether they must measure a pain state to characterize its features (e.g. the qualities and intensity of a specific pain such as postherpetic neuralgia).

Types of pain measurement

The term pain measurement encompasses two conceptual frameworks. Below, I present two pure forms of these concepts as types of measurement; in practice, the two are often confused.

Type I measurement, is objective and typically observational. The scores obtained make it possible to compare patients to one another. The investigator or clinician assigns numbers to persons (patients or subjects) in order to scale them on one or more attributes. Such number assignment allows one to test the effects of therapeutic interventions, describe samples or populations of patients or characterize situations that produce pain. For example, a set of procedures for scoring patients with back pain on pain behaviour was used by Keefe and Block (1982)

to measure each patient in a sample on several pain-related attributes (e.g. groaning and sighing). In Type I measurement, the criteria for scoring are well defined and independent of the patient.

Type II measurement takes place when numbers are assigned to scale the subjective experience of pain itself, i.e. pain is the 'object' being measured and the numbers scale features of the pain such as its intensity or severity. A cardinal characteristic of Type II measurement is that the patient assigns the numbers him/herself because the experience is private and inaccessible to others. This means that the measurement operation is in the hands of the patient rather than those of the investigator or clinician, although the latter can provide guidelines or rules to follow.

The contrast between Types I and II measurement approaches goes beyond the well-worn distinction between objective and subjective; there is a fundamental difference in what is being scaled. In Type I measurement, numbers are assigned to an attribute of the patient, but in Type II measurement, it is the pain itself that is the object of number assignment. Controversy exists about whether the latter should qualify as scientific measurement since the investigator does not carry out a measurement. We normally would not accept a patient's best estimate of a physiological variable as a valid measure, and critics see no reason to suppose that self-report of pain is any more valid than, say, guessing one's own pulse rate. Defendants of Type II measurement point out that such numbers, when carefully collected, are typically consistent, behave as they should across conditions in which injury varies or drugs are given, and conform to theoretical predictions.

In practice, researchers often treat Type II measurements as though they are the results of Type I scaling, i.e. they use such scores to compare patients one with another, evaluate treatment effects, or characterize certain patient populations. Although the numbers are nothing more than scores created by each patient to represent his/her personal experience, they are typically treated like numbers that scale patients relative to one another on an attribute. Dangers are inherent in this practice and, indeed, in any form of casual number assignment.

Basic risks in number assignment

Number assignment does not guarantee that the resulting data have meaning. For example, Chinese medicine assumes that 12 pulses exist, each with several measurable features (six on each wrist). Folklore holds that a physician needs at least a decade to master the skill of reading pulses, but one who perseveres to become a master of oriental medicine can diagnose conditions very accurately. If we develop a 12-pulse coding scheme and recruit a group of 20 masters for a study of, say, migraine headache, Type I number assignment will proceed beautifully. Each of the masters can measure pulses while the patients have headache and while they are pain free, and we can compare the resulting scores across the two conditions. But will we obtain meaningful data? Does our scoring constitute measurement? Can we say that 12 pulses exist because we can assign numbers to them? Elegant number assignment does not ensure valid measurement.

Similarly, a psychiatrist may theorize that anxiety is a feature of pain in certain types of patients and develop a Type II self-report scale in which patients indicate by numbers the anxiety aspect of certain painful events. But patients are not trained in distinguishing between arousal and anxiety, nor do they know the distinction between fear and anxiety (the former has a definite object, the latter is diffuse). The patients will yield numbers and probably be rather consistent, but is the psychiatrist scaling what he/she thinks is being measured? Can we presume that we have scaled what we set out to scale because patients cheerfully co-operated and gave us numbers that fit our expectations? In the end, the scientific value of a set of such scores is constrained by the assumptions the investigator has made in performing measurement.

These examples show that, although assigning numbers is necessary for measurement, it is not sufficient. Proper measurement always requires:
1 *Reliability*. Measurement operations should yield consistent outcomes when carried out under highly similar conditions or when repeated out under highly similar circumstances.
2 *Validity*. Measurement operations should scale precisely what they purport to scale.

While the clinical investigator must be careful to use reliable and valid measurement procedures, he/she must also be pragmatic. Measurement is constrained by the health of the patients under study, limits in manpower or resources, and the nature of the clinical situation. When obtaining data from patients, it is important to impose the smallest possible responder burden and still obtain the highest quality of information possible under the circumstances.

A final consideration (although not a requirement for measurement) is precision: the random error associated with the measurement process should be small. Ideally, measurement should be reasonably sensitive to differences that exist in nature and should faithfully reflect such differences. As we shall see in the following section, the interpretation of these principles in practice depends upon which measurement tradition is followed.

Three traditions of measurement

Michell (1986) reviewed three traditional approaches to measurement of subjective and behavioural variables. His work offers a perspective on the many alternative methods for measurement in today's pain literature and helps the investigator or clinician to reconcile his/her scientific or clinical goals with the pain measurement tools that are currently available. The three traditions are described as classical, operational and representational.

Classical theory

This approach dominates contemporary science and the practice of measurement in the field of pain. Classical theory is concerned with scoring objects according to attributes they possess, i.e. quantifying 'how much' of an attribute an object has. In order to qualify for measurement, an attribute must be quantitative. The classical theorist does not quantify the patient or research subject as an end in itself; rather, the goal is to discover numerical relations between variables by the process of measurement.

The cardinal feature of the classical approach is that measurement links to, and depends upon, scientific theory. This approach argues that no scientist or clinician exists in a conceptual vacuum. A theoretical structure is present whether it is explicit and clearly articulated or implicit. The numbers obtained must have meaning within a definable scientific framework or measurement cannot be said to exist.

Duncan (1975), who exemplifies the classical approach, asserted that science should begin with a highly refined theoretical basis from which one can derive models or predictions. The models specify relationships among theoretical constructs and measures, and must be defined algebraically by a set of structural equations. For Duncan, the purpose of science is to test and refine such models; the goal of research is to produce equations or models that are 'true', i.e. mathematically unambiguous and coherent. The most important guide for identifying an attribute to measure is the theory within which one is working. In this measurement tradition, rating-scale data, test scores and other types of subjective reports have meaning so long as they reflect the structure of *theoretical* variables. Although these variables are not in themselves measurable, the scores obtained are considered to provide valid representations of latent (theoretical rather than actual) variables.

While classicists assume that an attribute to be measured must be quantitative, they put no limits on the evidence necessary for support of this assumption. Therefore they accept numbers that have been generated by the objects of measurement themselves such as pain reports (Type II measures) as long as theory allows one to equate self-reports with attributes that objects possess. Measures, however obtained, are always considered to be unconstrained numbers and any form of statistical manipulation may be imposed on such numbers. The issue of what a self-report of pain really means is one that is to be resolved by theory alone.

Operational theory

The operationalist perspective is six decades old, owing its identity to Bridgman (1927, 1959) who contended that 'Measurement, in its most general sense, may be taken to be description by use of numbers'. For Bridgman, a theoretical concept was equivalent to and defined by a corresponding set of operations and measurement was simply an operation yielding numbers. A variable was nothing more nor less than the operation used to obtain its scores. He cautioned that it was not the business of science to create sham realities by reifying concepts through elaborate theory.

Few, if any, pure operationalists still exist in science and operationalism has minimal influence in pain research. The most limiting feature of the operationalist position is the notion that a single measure obtained from a specific operation provides a valid and specific characterization of the object, event or process. If this were so, we could measure pain or analgesia quite adequately with a single operation, such as recording a spinal nociceptive withdrawal reflex or perhaps a subjective report. Occasionally, someone studying pain or analgesia will use a single-outcome indicator, but this is usually a pragmatic choice rather than a philosophical commitment. Most researchers agree that pain is more than a specific operation that one uses to get pain scores, and patient contact makes this abundantly clear.

Representational theory

Stevens (1946, 1975) strongly influenced the practice of measurement in psychology and related areas through his arguments that numbers represent empirical relations among the objects that are measured. For those who follow this persuasion, measurement produces a numerical representation of empirical fact. Variables and relationships between variables exist in nature, and the purpose of measurement is to characterize these relationships through number assignment. If this is true, then the subject matter of science can be manipulated statistically. Obviously, it is critical that the numbers be faithful representations of the true relationships among the variables in nature.

The representationalists argue that there are different types of relationships between scales. The simplest form of a relationship is classification. One might classify patients with postoperative pain in three categories: abdominal, orthopaedic and head and neck. This type of categorization would be called a *nominal* scale.

Another type of scale is characterized by weak order. One type of object may be said to be greater with regard to one attribute than another. Thus, one might argue that a thoracotomy patient (score = 12) has more postoperative pain than a gastrectomy patient (score = 8) and that the latter has more pain than an appendicectomy patient (score = 4). This statement of rank order is called an *ordinal* scale. The investigator can talk about 'greater than' or 'less than', but can make no more precise statements than those of order. It is meaningless to ask whether the difference in pain level between the thoracotomy and gastrectomy patients is of the same magnitude as that between the gastrectomy and appendicectomy patient. The only information in ordinal data lies in the 'greater than' or 'less than' relationship. The scale would convey exactly the same information about the three patients if the scores were 250, 18 and 1 instead of 12, 8 and 4.

In the third type of scale, the *interval* scale, the numbers assigned to the objects permit one to interpret the differences between scores. The Fahrenheit scale of temperature provides a good example of an interval scale. In this case 0° does not mean a total absence of heat (it is an arbitrary number), but one can say that $40°F - 30°F = 80°F - 70°F$.

Finally, the *ratio* scale is characterized by an absolute zero. The length of a surgical incision provides an example in which zero has an absolute meaning (total absence of surgical insult). The patient with a

20-cm incision has a wound four times as long as the patient whose incision is 5 cm and (although it is pointless) one could calculate the total length of surgical incisions in patients operated upon by surgeon X and compare those with similar scores from a set of matched patients operated upon by surgeon Y. In this case the numbers are meaningful relative to an absolute zero.

The strong influence of the representationalists in measurement derived from their conviction that different types of measurement scales exist (nominal, ordinal, interval and ratio) and that one must classify all scores according to scale type. They have contended that statistical manipulation of the numbers obtained by measurement must be appropriate for the type of scale involved. Although one can perform conventional statistics upon ratio- and interval-level scales, they argue that means and the variances cannot be calculated on ordinal or nominal-level scales. Such manipulation of numbers would distort the relationship between the scores and the actual variables as they exist in nature. On ranked scores, the investigator must use non-parametric statistics suitable for ordinal data. Similarly, calculation of medians for scores which are characterized by nominal scaling would be forbidden and only statistical techniques suitable for categorized data (frequency counts) could be employed. It has often been argued by representationalists that subjective report data derived from rating scales must not be subjected to normal statistical manipulation (cannot be characterized by means, standard deviations, etc.) and can only be treated by statistics designed to handle rank order.

Michell (1986) pointed out that the statistical restriction principles of the representationalists really apply only to representationalists themselves, and that researchers who operate from a basis of classical theory are not obliged to follow them. The classicist would argue that, like the operationalists, the representationalists are guilty of oversimplifying conduct of science. By and large, scientists do not work with numbers as representations of otherwise inaccessible relationships among variables in nature. Rather, scientists operate on the basis of theory (or models) and hypothesize such relationships. The meaning one can derive from a scaling procedure therefore depends on the theory from which one operates and blind commitment to a set of rules about how one handles numbers statistically may impose an unnecessary constraint on scientific endeavour.

Theory and current practices

As the following review indicates, a plethora of procedures for measuring pain exist in current literature. Most reflect classical theory, but the strong influence of the representationalists pervades some of the measurement practices currently in use. It is helpful to recognize the theoretical basis for measurement practices when considering them as candidates for major research or clinical tools.

Procedures for measuring pain

Clinical investigators concerned with pain have attempted to quantify it by using physiological, subjective report and behavioural variables. The scientific and clinical inference permitted by these various approaches depends on the theoretical perspective of the investigator, the measurement tradition in which he/she is working and the limitations inherent in the measurements themselves. An overview of current pain measurement procedures follows and the advantages and limitations of the various approaches are discussed.

Physiological indicators of pain

Pathophysiological correlates

Both acute and chronic pain states may be associated with pathophysiological changes detectable upon medical examination or via medical monitoring (Syrjala & Chapman, 1984; Chapman et al., 1985). Moore and McQuay (1985) described the response of the hypothalamopituitary−adrenocortical axis to surgical insult. Plasma cortisol increases with the start of surgery. The degree of this response is a function of the size of the incision. Heightened plasma cortisol levels continue into the postoperative period for one or more days, but marked decreases in plasma cortisol occur when the anaesthetic is terminated. Large doses of systemically administered opioids such as morphine, fentanyl and sufentanil decrease cortisol responses to surgery and administration of a high dose of naloxone reverses such responses. However, this response is independent of consciousness, and plasma cortisol levels vary with the anaesthetic alone. Thus, although it may be an indicator of stress, it is also a correlate of pain.

Acute-pain states, such as postoperative pain, are often accompanied by motor reflexes that produce muscle spasm or splinting. Surgical trauma to the chest or abdomen, for example, may result in impaired ventilation. Gastrointestinal and genito-urinary inhibition, which encompass both ileus and smooth muscle spasm, reflect autonomic reflexes associated with acute pain (Chapman & Bonica, 1983). In addition, increases in blood pressure and cardiac output and increased respiratory rate are associated with liberation of catecholamines. Thus, variables which are monitored postoperatively may reflect pain.

Pain may be accompanied by trophic changes in certain chronic pain syndromes. In the older patient with clearly defined trigger points and myofascial pain, subtle indicators of autonomic dysfunction such as enhanced pilomotor segmental reflex, vaso- and pseudo-motor disturbances of the skin as well as trophoedematous changes in subcutaneous tissues may be observed (Gunn & Milbrandt, 1978; Gunn et al., 1990).

Neuropharmacological correlates

Intense interest in the endorphins in recent decades has led to the development of elaborate neurophysiological models for the modulation of pain. Several of the biologically active neuropeptides derived from the pro-opiomelanocortic (POMC) gene, including β-endorphin can be detected during acute pain. Some investigators have reasoned that, since β-endorphin is an endogenous opioid, pain intensity should be diminished in its presence. Szyfelbein and colleagues (1985) measured the concentration of endorphins in the plasma of patients in pain and found that endorphin concentration was negatively correlated with acute pain report, i.e. the greater the plasma concentrations of β-endorphin, the lower the reported pain. Because of its inverse relationship to pain report, endorphin plasma concentration may be a better indicator of endogenous pain modulation than of pain itself. An alternative explanation is that the POMC-derived peptides are less analgesic mechanisms than informational substances involved in co-ordination of the complex stress response across the CNS, the neuroendocrine system and the immune system. At any rate, we can be fairly confident that their presence does not provide unequivocal evidence of the existence of pain, since they may appear as part of a global stress reaction.

When pain is chronic, pathophysiological changes sometimes appear at the site of the pain. *Thermography*, the measurement of skin-temperature patterns, attempts to identify such changes and represent them visually. Thermographers contend that skin temperature can be used in the evaluation of certain types of chronic pain (Rubal et al., 1982). Of course, it is well known that dysautonomias including reflex sympathetic dystrophy produce temperature changes in the affected extremities (Bonica, 1980a,b, 1990). Skin temperature is low in the afflicted area in myofascial pain syndromes, certain cancer pain syndromes, and a few other pain problems. This temperature change probably reflects altered sympathetic nervous system function. Conversely, some arthritis conditions may produce abnormal warmth because of acute inflammation.

Neurological measures

Recording of *nerve conduction velocities* in the larger nerves of an extremity can facilitate evaluation of painful and non-painful peripheral neuropathies, entrapment syndromes and nerve injuries. A skin electrode is used to stimulate the nerve and its discharge is recorded distally. Such measures are non-specific since all components of the nerve are activated, and, since nerve endings are not activated, pathology and other factors specific to them cannot be evaluated. Activity in the larger and faster conducting fibres may well obscure responses in the smaller and slower conducting fibres, which carry nociceptive information. Moreover, altered nerve conduction velocities are not synonymous with the presence of pain. Some patients demonstrate abnormal nerve conduction velocities despite being neurologically asymptomatic while others using medication such as phenytoin may show reduced conduction velocities in the absence of structural changes in the peripheral nerves (Thomas, 1984).

Short latency *evoked potentials* are sometimes used to study peripheral neuropathology including pain-related neurological dysfunction (Eisen, 1986). They are also used for surgical monitoring. For example, Campbell and Lipton (1985) recorded intraspinal somatosensory evoked potentials associated with median nerve stimulation during percutaneous cervical cordotomy performed to relieve chronic pain. This type of approach does not easily lead to the independent scaling or even verification of clinical pain since median nerve stimulation is unrelated to clinical pain state. The use of long-latency evoked-potential procedures in human laboratory models in which volunteers undergo painful dental or cutaneous stimulation has been reviewed by Chudler and Dong (1983) and Chapman and Saeger (1985). However, little has been done with these methods with pain patients or in clinically focused research.

Positron emission tomography (PET) seems promising for evaluation of certain pain states. It allows the study of regional cerebral blood flow and regional glucose metabolic rate. PET employs low-intensity radioactive isotopes attached to metabolically active molecules to provide markers for the amount of neurological activity in various parts of the brain. It can be used, for example, to identify seizure foci in patients with partial epilepsy, to identify the brain areas involved in chemically-induced panic attack or to characterize brain activity patterns in schizophrenics. Talbot and colleagues (1991) used scanning technology to show that noxious stimulation activates contralateral anterior cingulate as well as primary and secondary somatosensory cortex. As is the case with other neurological measures, this technology requires concomitant subjective report of pain in order to be valid. If extended studies of thalamus or other brain areas prove promising, PET may help to validate pain complaint in the absence of other organic evidence, but such development is still far off.

Finally, extensive development of *microneurography* and the related procedure of intraneural stimulation appears promising as a technology for assessing chronic pain related to peripheral neuropathy (Ochoa *et al.*, 1985). In this technically demanding procedure, electrodes must be placed accurately upon fibres within a peripheral nerve. By delivering low levels of electrical current to target fibres, a neurologist can activate primary sensory units or sets of units in combination, and abnormal firing patterns may be identified. When this has been successfully accomplished, the neurologist can precisely identify the peripheral origin of a neuropathic pain, and he/she may replicate the pain by electrical stimulation of the involved pathways. Work performed thus far indicates that fibre type is the important determinant of pain rather than pattern of discharge. The quality of pain varies with fibre type whether Aδ or C.

To be meaningful, microneurography data require concomitant verbal report of pain on the part of the patient. The electrical signals obtained do not yield unequivocal evidence about the activation of nociceptive processes or even Aδ- versus C-fibre pain. This approach represents a major advance in pain diagnosis, but it does not offer a definitive or fully objective measure of pain.

Advantages and limitations of physiological approaches

Most physiological indicators of pain are really correlates of nociception. Like alterations in muscle tone, trophoedema and other autonomically mediated indicators occur concomitantly with pain but for the most part do not play a causal role. The value of correlates as measures depends on the theoretical perspective of the investigator or clinician. From the viewpoint of the classical theorist such indicators may prove to be powerful measures given that basic relationships among variables have been clearly established by preliminary work and a well-developed model for these relationships has been defined. In the absence of such resource, they are of limited value.

Measures of neurological function appear to offer considerable promise for the evaluation of certain types of pain. However, the major problems seen in chronic pain clinics (back pain and headache) cannot be evaluated by these approaches. Moreover, neurological methods cannot stand alone. Abnormal neurological function can be observed in the absence of pain, and it is only the coexistence and correspondence of verbal report with neurological abnormality that allows proper diagnosis or scientific inference. This being the case, it is often most cost effective to depend upon verbal report alone.

Self-report measurement procedures

All self-report techniques are Type II measures, i.e. the patient performs the act of number assignment. There are many variations on this approach, and they include both uni- and multidimensional tools. These are evaluated below and examples are provided in Fig. 74.1.

Single-dimension methods

The simplest and most frequently used procedures for subjective pain report are: (i) category scales; (ii) numerical rating scales; and (iii) visual analogue scales. Each of these represents a simple paper-and-pencil instrument which the patient uses to produce a record of his/her pain report. The overwhelming majority of these tools quantify pain intensity.

Category scales make the most minimal demand upon the patient; it is only necessary to choose the best word descriptor for the pain. Testing devices of this sort are sometimes known as verbal rating scales. They are commonly employed for both nominal and ordinal scaling, depending on whether or not the category descriptors connote a ranking among the categories. Sometimes investigators employ category methods to produce interval scales, and Borg (1982) has developed a ratio category scale which combines adjectives and adverbs with the numbers 1 to 10.

An example of an ordinal category scale is provided by Melzack and Torgerson (1971) who introduced a scale which is still used extensively for describing pain intensity (see Fig. 74.1). Any suitable set of categories can be made up depending on what one wishes to measure. Moreover, category scales are not limited to words. A facial expression picture scale involving eight cartoon faces ranked according to expressed displeasure has been developed for pain assessment (Frank *et al.*, 1982). The obvious advantage of the category-scale approach is its simplicity and suitability for all types of patient populations. Its major disadvantage is statistical. It produces simple category data with a limited range. In practice, patients tend to use the middle rather than the ends of category scales and thus the range of responses is further reduced and to some extent distorted.

The numerical rating scale (NRS) (Fig. 74.1). Patients are asked to indicate how intense their pain feels (any dimension can be measured in this way, such as aversiveness) on a scale of 0–10. In effect, this scale uses 10 categories, but the categories are ranked in a way that it implies interval-level scaling. Box scales offer a variation on the standard NRS. The patient encounters the numbers from 1 to 10, each encased in a box. His task is to mark an X in the box containing the number that best represents his/her pain-intensity level. Most patients can comprehend the NRS type of scale and clinicians can administer it easily.

The visual analogue scale (VAS) is perhaps the most intensively studied method. This typically consists of a 10-cm line with verbal anchors at both ends as shown in Fig. 74.1. When a 10-cm line is used, scoring can be accomplished by having the patient mark the line and measuring the length of the line to the mark in metric units. There are many variations of this approach. Tick marks can be placed upon the line or numbers can be placed below the line. The scales can be arranged horizontally or vertically. The important consideration is that the patients understand the two-end points and that they are free to indicate a response at any point in the scale.

Such methods are more demanding of patients than category scales. Researchers have found that 7–11% of patients cannot complete the VAS or find it confusing (Revill *et al.*, 1976; Kremer *et al.*, 1980a) and in one report 26 of 98 patients in a particular sample were unable to complete a VAS (Walsh, 1984). Sometimes patients who have difficulty with the VAS, including elderly patients and those with limited education, can be trained to use it through examples with familiar pain problems.

Carlsson (1983) undertook critical evaluation of the VAS. She examined it as an indicator of both pain state and pain relief in chronic pain patients. Carlsson compared different forms of the scale and found its reliability low as judged from consistency of response to two different forms. This led her to conclude that the validity of the VAS procedure for chronic pain assessment may be unsatisfactory. There are other studies, however, which support both the reliability and validity of the VAS as a measure of pain and change in pain (Revill *et al.*, 1976; Kremer *et al.*, 1980a). Clearly, this tool requires careful planning, a reasonably sophisticated patient population and solid preparatory work on the part of the investigator.

Advantages and disadvantages of unidimensional scaling

The broad advantages of unidimensional scaling methods are their simplicity and efficiency. They provide only a minimal responder burden for patients, the same scale can be used in a wide variety of different settings, most patients can understand the task demand of measuring pain with these technologies, they produce numbers directly and do not require elaborate scoring, and they intrinsically make sense both to the patient and to the data collector (that is, they have high face validity). On the negative side, these methods are subject to subtle distortions and may be misused by patients who appear to understand them but do not. More importantly, they oversimplify the complex human experience of pain. A data collector may ask for sensory intensity but obtain a response that reflects emotional arousal or aversiveness. Despite these limitations, unidimensional self-report methods remain the most efficient and popular way of scaling pain in a clinical setting.

Jensen and colleagues (1986) evaluated several types of scales for assessing pain and concluded that the NRS was the most practical index. They recommended the use of a 01 point scale, which includes 100 points which scale pain in addition to a 0 which indicates no pain. However, the investigator or clinician should consider all three carefully in light of his/her own unique needs and patient population before arriving at a decision. There is no substitute for careful pilot trials which compare the different methods available.

Multidimensional self-report: classical tradition

Comprehensive measurement of pain requires that:

(i) the investigator should adopt or should develop a model for pain perception that involves multiple dimensions; and (ii) use of instruments for the simultaneous measurement of these dimensions (each being an attribute of pain). The most pragmatic approach to this problem is to use several VAS or NRS scales but this is difficult. First, it is impossible to ensure that responses to the different scales are not correlated with one another. Basically, the response to the first scale administered will probably influence the response to following scales. It is important that patients respond to each scale without the opportunity to compare the present response with other, earlier responses (Carlsson, 1983).

Several complex pencil-and-paper tests have been developed to allow simultaneous multidimensional scaling. The best-known and most extensively tested multidimensional scaling tool is the *McGill pain questionnaire* (MPQ). The method is designed to scale pain along three dimensions: sensory, affective and evaluative. Patients encounter 20 sets of words that describe pain and are instructed to select those sets that seem relevant to their pain. They are told to circle the words within each set that best describe the pain. From two to six words reside within each of the sets, and these vary in intensity for the quality described by that set. Sensory qualities are represented by the first 10 sets. The following five indicate affective quality, the 16th set is evaluative and the last four sets are miscellaneous words. There are methods for scoring each dimension and also to obtain a total score.

A supplement to the MPQ, the *Dartmouth pain questionnaire* (DPQ) allows the assessment of three additional factors. These include a general affective dimension, an indication of the time course and intensity of the pain, and a record of behaviours affected by the presence of the pain (Corson & Schneider, 1984). An advantage of the DPQ is its consideration of those remaining positive aspects of functioning in chronic pain patients; most instruments simply assess impairment.

The MPQ possesses high reliability and strong concurrent validity as well as an adequate factor structure (Syrjala & Chapman, 1984; Chapman *et al.*, 1985). Its principal advantage in pain measurement is its comprehensiveness. On the negative side, the MPQ incurs a much greater responder burden than the simpler unidimensional techniques. It takes 5–15 min to complete, and the vocabulary used by the test exceeds the language capability of some patients. Moreover, the scoring procedures, while straightforward, are crude compared to those of most

mental tests of comparable size. Turk and colleagues (1985) have argued that the total score derived from the MPQ is valid as a general measure of pain severity; however, individual scale scores should not be interpreted according to their unique scales because adequate discriminate validity to support such scaling at the level of the three subscales cannot be demonstrated. Walsh (1984) reported that patients who complete the MPQ in the presence of their spouses may give responses that reflect spouse interference or opinion.

Despite criticisms, the MPQ continues as a standard in the area of pain measurement and remains the first choice when the goal is to assess the quality or character of a patient's pain, particularly its sensory aspects and affective impact. Although the responder burden is substantial, the scale can be administered by reading out each word set and having patients indicate responses verbally. This allows even very sick patients to complete the measure. If this alternative is chosen, it is necessary to maintain a standard format (Klepac *et al.*, 1981).

Kerns and colleagues (1985) described the *West Haven-Yale multidimensional pain inventory* (WHYMPI) as an alternative to the MPQ. This test is briefer and more classical in its psychometrics compared with the MPQ. There are three parts to this 52-item test. The first provides five general dimensions of the experience of pain, interference with normal family and work function and social support. The second is concerned with patient perception of how others respond to displays of pain and suffering. The third addresses the frequency with which the patient engages in common daily activities as a function of pain. From the viewpoint of classical measurement theory, this method has been derived from cognitive behavioural models of chronic pain and assesses constructs appropriate to such models. In this sense it is far more focused than the MPQ, but the meaning of the outcome obtained is much more model dependent.

The MPQ, DPQ and WHYMPI have all been designed to address problems of chronic pain. Sometimes the investigator or clinician needs to assess acute or persisting pain problems of a progressive nature such as cancer pain or the pain of an arthritic condition. In these cases, it is not always necessary to conduct extensive evaluation of social contingencies for pain behaviour. A short and efficient measure of worst, average and current pain may be obtained by using the *brief pain inventory* (BPI) developed by Cleeland and colleagues (Daut, *et al.*, 1983; Cleeland, 1985). This instrument also scales pain relief from medication and the extent to which pain interferes with the quality of life.

Multidimensional self-report: representational tradition

Investigators who embrace representational theory when conducting clinical measurement are dissatisfied with most subjective report techniques since they do not follow the representationalist rules for proper scaling nor do they permit the use of normal parametric statistics by the criteria of the representationalist. These investigators have approached multidimensional scaling by using a psychophysical technique known as *cross-modality matching*. With this technique a sensory experience is quantified by matching it to the experience of a precisely controlled stimulus in another sensory modality. One might, for example, produce a safe experimental pain by pressing with controlled force on a finger at the base of the nail and ask the patient to match the intensity of the pain produced to the loudness of a tone that he/she controls by adjusting decibels. A complex psychophysical technology can be used to relate spontaneous pain of natural origin to control stimuli in other sense modalities (Stevens, 1975).

In pain research, words describing pain are typically matched to line length or hand grip, both of these are matched to an experimental pain, and then scaling standards for the relationship for words describing pain to clinical pain are derived. Once this operation has been performed, the technique can be applied to clinical pain assessment. There is no limit on which or how many dimensions of pain one can scale. Gracely and colleagues (1979), for example, used this approach to scale both pain intensity and unpleasantness.

Tursky and colleagues (1982) have used a cross-modality matching approach to develop a procedure for assessing clinical pain, the *pain perception profile*. This method measures sensation threshold, employs magnitude estimation procedures to judge induced pain, scales pain on intensity, reaction and sedation dimensions (employing verbal pain descriptors) and permits the registration of these three dimensions in a diary format for repeated assessment over time. In brief, it assesses pain through the use of psychophysically scaled verbal descriptors. This type of procedure is shorter and less demanding for patients than the MPQ, once the psychophysical scaling has been completed.

Potentially, the data obtained by cross-modality matching should be more reliable and valid than those of these simpler unidimensional self-report scales such as VAS. It is uncertain as to what extent independent validation work needs to be done for different pain populations. Use of this approach would probably necessitate substantial development, including experimental pain testing before one could confidently interpret scores obtained from pain patients. Future development of this approach may yield substantial advances in pain measurement technology, but the disparity in philosophy of measurement between classicists and representationalists may limit its adoption.

Multidimensional behavioural scaling

For the strict behaviourist, measurement of a subjective state is meaningless. Pain can only be defined as a pattern of behaviour. Measurement consists of identifying behaviours and scoring them on the basis of their frequency, speed, rate or accuracy. Since behaviours differ markedly with different pain syndromes, broadly focused tests analogous to the MPQ do not exist within this approach. Methods are highly specific, and back pain has been studied more extensively than other pain problems.

Keefe and Block (1982) and Keefe and Hill (1985) have shown that patients with back pain engage in grimacing, guarding their movements, rubbing the affected body area and sighing. Measures of these behaviours proved reliable and valid in relation to pain reports, and they occurred more frequently in pain patients than in either normals or depressed control patients. Pain behaviour patterns can be quantified in terms of frequency or rate of occurrence and scaled by trained observers either directly or with the use of video-taped records of patients in selected settings involving specific task performance. Behaviour patterns that are non-trivial are invariably complex, and most behavioural observational systems are correspondingly multidimensional. In general, behaviours are tallied over time and scored by frequency counts.

Behavioural observational techniques may include measures derived by mechanical force transducers or other monitors of behaviour. Keefe and Hill (1985) employed a transducer placed in patients' shoes in order to assess walking parameters. During video taping, both patients and normal controls were required to walk a 5-m course. Guarding, bracing, rubbing the painful area, sighing and grimacing were scored by judges. Investigators found that patients walked more slowly than normals, took smaller steps, did not show a normal symmetrical gate pattern, and, in general, exhibited more pain behaviour. This study serves as an excellent demonstration of how behavioural observation may be employed for study of chronic pain.

While these methods are potentially powerful measurement tools, they are extremely specific. Patients with headache, for example, would probably appear indistinguishable from normals on the test basis developed by Keefe and Hill (1985). In light of this limitation, Keefe and colleagues (1985) evaluated pain in patients with head and neck cancer using behavioural techniques. These patients displayed their pain primarily through facial expression rather than through guarded movement or postural changes.

A solution to the problem of overspecificity in behavioural measures might lie with the identification of broad behavioural indicators of pain that are common to different clinical populations. Linton (1985) investigated the general level of activity in chronic back pain patients, hypothesizing that reported pain intensity is inversely related to general-activity level. He quantified this activity by patient self-monitoring or observing behaviour in a test situation. The reported intensity of chronic pain was unrelated to general-activity level, and this suggests that general activity is not a suitable global indicator of pain state.

Multidimensional self-report of behaviours

Type II measures of pain behaviours appeal because it is more efficient and cost effective to ask people about their behaviours and habits than to video-tape and formally score human activity. In some cases investigators ask for reports from the spouse or some other daily observer who lives with the patient. However, the pure behaviourist would be loathe to accept self-report of activities as measures of those activities. It is the business of the behaviourist to score the patient; it is less than legitimate for the patient to score him/herself. Using the spouse to score the patient is viable behaviourism so long as the spouse qualifies as a trained and objective observer. From the classical viewpoint what one makes of a self-reported record of behaviour depends upon the theoretical perspective of investigator. Cognitive behavioural psychologists have elaborate models for how thinking and beliefs affect behaviour; for them, this type of approach can be a rich source of information.

Chronic pain clinics sometimes use a *pain diary* for behavioural self-report. These records typically consist of a log of daily activities broken down to small blocks of time. The activities recorded are pain relevant and would be divided, for example, into sitting, standing and walking and reclining. The patient fills in the specific activity within the appropriate category and indicates the time the activity occurred and how long it lasted. In most cases clinicians also ask the patient to provide an NRS for pain level for each hour and to indicate the medications taken.

There are strong advantages associated with pain diaries. Because these measures are obtained daily, they are neither distorted by memory nor biased by the mental set of the patient. Moreover, the diary relates pain to patterns of normal activity as opposed to contrived activities such as those used in some video-tape observational studies. Extended time patterns involving days or weeks can be derived from examination of pain diaries, as can any relationship between pain, activity and medication intake.

A limitation of the pain diary is that its reliability is unknown and may vary greatly from patient to patient. The record produced day by day is disturbing to some patients because their less-than-ideal habit patterns become apparent over time, and they may refuse to complete it or distort it. Others fill the diary out retrospectively just prior to their appointments, thus defeating the purpose of the measurement.

In using the pain diary or any other similar device, the clinician presumes the patient or the spouse is a reliable historian and capable of accurate record keeping. Ready and colleagues (1982) examined reported medication use in chronic pain patients and found that these patients reported drug usage 50–60% lower than actual drug usage. Kremer and colleagues (1980b) found discrepancies when they compared patient records with staff observations of patient activity or social behaviour. Similarly, Sanders (1983) compared the activity time reported by pain patients with records derived from automatic monitoring of activity in normal controls, psychiatric patients and patients with chronic back pain. All three groups reported less activity than the automated monitoring equipment indicated, but the discrepancy was greatest for the patients with chronic back pain. These studies challenge the validity of self-report methods as indicators of behaviour. Until further information is available or these methods are further refined, they are best regarded as doubtful measurement tools with high liability for patient-response bias.

Health-care-worker patient pain rating

Physicians or other health care workers sometimes

set up a standardized system for health-care-worker patient pain rating. The simplest form of this type of judgement is classification of patients (e.g. cancer patients in a given clinic either have pain or do not have pain as a symptom). Whether this can be termed measurement is debatable, but representationalists may be quick to argue that categorical scaling is the simplest form of measurement. Typically, diagnostic data and medical history are employed to categorize patients with pain. The diagnostic value of physician measures of patients in pain has been investigated by Tearnan and Dar (1986).

In some circumstances it is useful for health care workers to impose a rating upon patients with pain (e.g. none, mild, moderate, or severe pain) based on what the patient does when faced with certain tasks such as lifting a standard weight. This is a form of *ability testing* which is rather crudely scaled. Biases can enter into such measures if the rater knows the patient's diagnosis or medical condition, and it is difficult for raters to avoid stereotyping patients on the basis of age, sex or racial categories. When these methods are used, it is critical that raters be carefully trained with well-defined criteria for judgement.

Multidimensional scaling of pain-related function

The measurement of functional status is a good example of classical measurement. It is difficult to interpret any measures of function apart from a well-defined concept of sickness impact or disability. The presence of persisting pain usually disturbs the ability of the patient to function normally, and this can be quantified if representative behaviours sensitive to pain are identified and measured. For example, patients with low back pain spend more time reclining or in bed because of the pain, restrict normal social and recreational activities, and have difficulty maintaining gainful employment. These disturbances can be defined as sickness impact. They can be measured by the activity diaries like that described above or by any method which systematically scales typical physical, social and psychological limitations imposed by painful illness.

The sickness impact profile (SIP) (Bergner *et al.*, 1981) provides a global well-validated indication of sickness impact. This instrument is not pain specific but rather provides a general indicator of health status and health-related dysfunction. It is designed to be self-administered but can be given via structured interview if necessary. Three dimensions of impact are measured: physical, psychosocial and overall.

Follick and colleagues (1985) found that chronic-pain patients seen at a multidisciplinary pain service showed impaired function on the SIP. The psycho-social dimension of the instrument correlated significantly with scores from the Minnesota multiphasic personality inventory (MMPI) and the physical-dimension score related inversely to independent measures of activity.

Mayer and colleagues (1986) developed a set of rehabilitation-focused tests which consists of mostly *objective physical function measures* suitable for patients with low back pain. These tests in combination with psychological measures provide eight categories of scaling:
1 range of motion;
2 cardiovascular fitness and muscular endurance;
3 gait speed;
4 time on simulated daily activities;
5 static lifting;
6 lifting under load;
7 isometric and isokinetic dynamic trunk strength; and
8 global effort.
Such measures provide a comprehensive assessment of functional capacity which can be obtained repeatedly through the course of treatment and are of use both to the patient and health care worker. The model was employed in a therapeutic trial with a group of patients whose initial unemployment rate was 92% (Mayer *et al.*, 1986). Eighty-two percent of these patients returned to work following treatment with this rehabilitation model combined with psychological intervention. Patients who were successfully rehabilitated maintained high VAS pain reports, indicating that rehabilitation can be achieved without major reduction in reported pain. This outcome stresses the need for comprehensive, multi-dimensional assessment when complex clinical issues are under investigation.

The World Health Organization introduced a model for assessing disease impact (WHO, 1980), and McGrath and colleagues (1990) applied it to chronic pain. The model postulates four planes of experience:
1 the underlying disorder or disease;
2 impairment (includes pain and other symptoms);
3 disability related to the disorder or disease; and
4 handicap — the restriction of social roles — related to the disorder or disease.

Clearly, pain is not the sole determinant of either disability or handicap; these factors interrelate in complex ways, and such interrelationships may vary across cultures and socioeconomic levels. None the less, the emphasis McGrath and colleagues have placed on the broad impact of chronic pain helps to underscore the importance of a comprehensive perspective in assessment of pain in patients.

Bias and pain measurement

The quantification of pain may be systematically inaccurate if any or all of three factors influence the measurement procedures: (i) investigator bias; (ii) patient bias; and (iii) consistent technical errors in data collection or scoring. Both Type I and Type II measures are sensitive to these three sources of bias.

A potential for investigator bias in Type I measures has been noted above for situations in which health care officials rate patients. Knowledge about a patient's history, interaction with a patient or beliefs about the patient's medical condition can affect scoring. The solution to this problem is to ensure that raters perform their tasks objectively and that they have had no prior knowledge about, nor contact with, the patient being evaluated. Strictly defined criteria also help to protect against bias.

Investigator bias may interact with patient bias in Type II measurement when patients' expectations or beliefs are shaped by statements or actions on the part of health care workers. Patients will tend to do what is expected of them in most circumstances, and in chronic pain settings certain kinds of patients will exaggerate pain complaint in an attempt to enhance the credibility of a pain problem which exists in the absence of organic disease.

Patient bias is a continuous concern in Type II measurement since the investigator can exercise no control over the patient's report. Though this type of bias can be offset by clear instructions and guidance, patients' responses will be shaped by their beliefs about their personal health, their expectations surrounding their present situation in a health care setting, and possibly, their personal social or financial goals.

The pain report may vary greatly as a function of the presence or absence of family members. The patient who appears tranquil and resigned on the first day following major surgery is sometimes seen to break into tears and display exaggerated pain behaviour when the spouse enters the room. Pain reports collected in the presence of the spouse may differ markedly from those collected when the spouse is absent.

Patient bias may also arise when they are asked to recall past pain states or to scale pain that is no longer present or has changed. The ability of patients to remember pain while in a relatively pain-free state is

reasonably accurate for approximately a week after surgery (Hunter et al., 1979; Kwilosc et al., 1984). However, when pain continues for a prolonged period and comparisons in pain level are made over time, the pain intensity of the present moment can systematically distort the accuracy of memory for prior pain levels (Eich et al., 1985). This problem presents major obstacles for studies of chronic pain in which the investigator may wish to compare present pain with past pain.

When therapeutic trials are undertaken, systematic biases in reporting pain after treatment occur. These are often referred to as the placebo effect (Shapiro, 1971). In general, the placebo effect refers to the tendency of the patient to report a favourable outcome in order to please the therapist or satisfy the hopes of his/her family. Placebo trials are often included in therapeutic outcome studies in order to gauge the extent to which this source of bias occurs. Ineffectual treatments are sometimes given so that patients may have the opportunity to demonstrate this type of bias.

It has become conventional to use the term placebo effect for any form of bias with represents the patient's beliefs or expectations about the situation and the measurement of pain or its opposite (pain relief). Such bias is affected by any psychological variable impinging upon the patient. There are some patient populations in which the therapeutic opposite of this phenomenon can be observed. Patients who are subjected to surgery which should alleviate a chronically painful condition may insist that the pain is unchanged or even worse following the operation despite correction of the underlying pathology. This is most often observed in patients who have a long history of illness behaviour or a commitment to the illness role. It is sometimes associated with secondary gain such as successful litigation.

Finally, poor instrument design can bias pain measures. Under ideal conditions, a simple instrument such as a VAS should yield a normal distribution of scores characterized by a wide range. Many years ago a colleague of the author designed a VAS which had anchors at both ends of a 10-cm line and small tick marks at 2.5, 5.0 and 7.5 cm. A clinic used this scale routinely for several years until another colleague evaluated the scale in the course of examining the clinic's database. Review of the data indicated that the scores had a trimodal distribution, i.e. instead of marking the score along its full 10-cm length, patients had tended to mark it at one of the three tick marks, and what should have been a normal distribution of scores was reduced to a set of three categories with frequency counts at each. This distortion was systematic, but none the less it was measurement error. Systematic measurement error can therefore contribute major bias in pain studies that have not been carefully planned and adequately piloted.

Pain assessment in paediatrics

Measurement of pain in children is considerably more difficult than in adults and requires attention to developmental stage. Developmental change with age strongly influences behaviour patterns, verbal proficiency and the ability of the child to follow instructions. Since individual children vary in rate of development, it is difficult to assign firm rules about what type of measurement device is suitable for what age. This issue of measuring pain in children is very complex, and a full review goes beyond the scope of this chapter. The interested reader is referred to reviews by Lavigne and colleagues (1986), Thompson and Varni (1986), Ross and Ross (1988) and Goodman and McGrath (1991).

The most difficult problem has been the assessment of pain in infants. In this case the investigator must use gross motor indicators such as generalized body reaction, reflex withdrawal or crying as an indicator of pain. This is far from satisfactory since these are not definitive pain measures and the presence of pain cannot be validated by verbal report. Jeans (1983) suggested that pain in toddlers may be evaluated through more complex behaviour patterns which include pressing the lips together, rocking, rubbing the affected part, kicking, hitting or biting, attempting to escape the situation or opening the eyes wide. Strong models defining pain behaviour in children are lacking, and without them measurement is limited to basic operationalist efforts.

The situation is somewhat better for children older than 3 years, since limited tools for self-report and behavioural observation are available. It is generally accepted that children older than 5 years can reliably complete the VAS and related simple interdimensional scaling instruments (Scott et al., 1977; AbuSaad & Holzmer, 1981). Paediatric investigators find it useful to practise these methods with children on familiar problems before actually using them to scale pain.

Paediatric researchers have designed a number of tools for the use with children. These include a colour-matching procedure in which patients indicate the colour that best represents their pain (Elend, 1981) and a picture scale known as 'Oucher' (Beyer, 1984).

The MPQ has been validated in children 12 and over (Jeans, 1983).

Can an investigator truly measure pain in young children? There is still no definitive answer to this question. Certainly, children are unable to differentiate conceptually between sensory and affective dimensions of pain, and any scores obtained on a single dimension of pain probably reflect a composite expression of distress rather than an accurate quantification of pain intensity. If small children tend not to experience pain as a discrete perception but rather as an element in a poorly differentiated experience of distress, then a precise measure of pain in a child would not be valid.

Scales of behavioural distress have been developed for use with children (Katz et al., 1980; Jay et al., 1983; Jay & Elliott, 1984; LeBaron & Zeltzer, 1984). These methods observe and tally behaviours such as crying, screaming, requests for emotional support, muscular rigidity and verbal expressions. Distress in children can be complicated by parental anxiety. It can be difficult to quantify either distress or pain in a young child independent of its parent. It is sometimes impossible to assess a child in the absence of its parent, or to separate the parent−child suffering unit.

Guidelines for undertaking pain research

Several steps are recommended when initiating pain measurement procedures in a clinical setting. These considerations both facilitate the development of pain measurement and ensure its quality.

Define the population

As a first step an investigator needs to formulate a clear plan that defines which patients should or should not be included in his study. Criteria for inclusion/exclusion typically involve literacy, age, health status, medical history and mental competence. Pain measurement requires that patients understand the instructions given them and are able to perform the necessary tasks. Age is an important factor, particularly in children. Similarly, educational level and grasp of language determine whether measurement will succeed. Finally, patients in different situations have different levels of energy to contribute. Young adults recovering from elective surgery can perform much more demanding tasks than can elderly patients with advanced cancer. Thus, the methods and tools chosen must fit the patients being tested.

When undertaking research, one should define explicit inclusion and exclusion criteria for participation in a study on the basis of ability to be measured. When assessing pain for clinical purposes, it may be valuable to define a minimally demanding alternative strategy. For example, patients who cannot complete the MPQ could probably complete a simple category scale. Pilot data that define the relationship between the complex test scores and the simple test scores will make interpretation of the alternative measures possible.

Define the goals of measurement

In most cases one undertakes measurement to permit the evaluation of a patient, to permit the comparison of one patient with another, or to make possible the comparison of groups or populations of patients. This is Type I scaling. In other cases an investigator seeks uniquely to characterize certain pain syndromes such as pain related to cancer of the pancreas, tic douloureux or thalamic pain. This is Type II scaling. Some measurement tools are much better suited to one type of scaling than the other, and the tools chosen should fit the goal as well as possible. For example, the MPQ is well suited for characterizing a unique pain problem since it records quality differences in pain states while behavioural observation methods offer no data of value for Type II measurement.

Establish a working model for the pain in question

The classical tradition biases of the author cannot be hidden here. It seems inconceivable that either science or clinical evaluation could be undertaken in the absence of some set of assumptions about the nature of pain. Such matters are rarely discussed, but decisions to select or reject a possible tool for pain measurement are often (and appropriately) coloured by what the investigator believes pain is and how the concept of pain fits into his/her beliefs about sickness, suffering and disability in general. By articulating these assumptions, the health care professional can ensure consensus among colleagues engaged as a team in a research or clinical project, identify those tools that are conceptually most meaningful, and avoid the selection of measurement procedures that will lead to fuzzy scientific or clinical inference.

One factor that requires attention in defining the goals of assessment is whether the pain in question is acute or chronic. Acute pain is unstable, varying from moment to moment. Measures of acute pain should be rapidly administered and sensitive to rapid change. Chronic pain, in contrast, is comparatively stable. Minor variations from day to day or moment to moment are of little interest in a study of therapeutic outcome. Changes in acute pain over 2 h following dental extraction in patients with a non-steroidal anti-inflammatory drug versus a placebo are of interest, but changes over 2 h in a patient with chronic pain taking the same drug are not. One needs to know whether the drug alters daily or weekly trends in activity, job performance, family life and recreational habits. Only then can conclusions be drawn about whether the drug is effective for a given type of pain. A clearly thought out model for what constitutes a meaningful outcome is fundamental to definitive research for clinical decision making.

Perform pilot studies

The best of ideas about what should work in one or another situation can fail without reality testing. It is often wise to select several alternatives and pilot them simultaneously in the test situation before making a final decision on the best choice for pain measurement. Sometimes a seemingly good tool is unexpectedly distasteful to patients, hard to understand or difficult to score. Time invested in pilot work is rarely, if ever, wasted.

When conducting pilot studies, it is necessary to assess whether the scores obtained are reliable, i.e. whether similar scores occur in similar situations or with repeated measures of the same person in the same situation (Harms-Ringdahl et al., 1986). The scores should show a good range between patients. If everyone yields low or high scores when pain varies across patients, it is likely that the scaling is not meaningful. Also, a test should be sensitive to differences between patients with obviously different pain levels and the effects of known interventions. Finally, the scores obtained should approximate a normal distribution unless one is undertaking non-parametric scaling.

Anticipate and control sources of bias

One of the ongoing goals of any measurement process is to minimize error. It is probably impossible to devise a system for data collection in a clinical setting that is free from systematic error (bias). It is a good idea to anticipate from the beginning what the most likely sources of bias may be and to conduct continuous surveillance as a data collection proceeds in an attempt to minimize it. Effort expended to control bias is often a seemingly thankless task, but it is usually an important investment of research or clinical resources.

Know the limits of the methods chosen

The scientific or clinical inference that can be derived legitimately from a pain measurement technique may be less than one would like. However, many of the problems that ensue from pain studies or the use of pain measurement techniques in diagnosis are due to overinterpretation of the data. The inference value of a pain score is largely a matter of what it means within the context of an overriding theoretical framework, as discussed above. Much depends on the careful development of a theoretical perspective at the outset of a project. In choosing a pain measurement technology, swift action is always a poor substitute for careful planning.

Conclusions

This chapter has addressed the problem of measuring pain in clinical settings. Review of these approaches and careful consideration of one's goals greatly narrow the range of choices. There is no singular, maximally advantageous method. The important considerations in choosing a test instrument for pain research are:

1 Is the instrument meaningful for the theory, model or set of assumptions used by the investigator or clinician?

2 Will the instrument be sensitive to differences and reliable?

3 Is the responder burden imposed by the instrument appropriate for the patients studied?

Careful planning and pilot work are indispensable in establishing satisfactory procedures for measuring pain.

Acknowledgement

Preparation of this manuscript was supported in part by a grant from the National Cancer Institute (CA 38552).

References

Abu-Saad H. & Holzmer W.L. (1981) Measuring childrens' self-assessment of pain. *Issues in Comprehensive Pediatric Nursing* **5**, 337–49.

Bergner M., Bobbitt R.A., Carter W.B. & Gilson B.S. (1981) The Sickness Impact Profile: development and final revision of health status measure. *Medical Care* **19**, 787–805.

Beyer J.E. (1984) Development of a new instrument for measuring intensity of childrens' pain. IV World Congress on Pain, Seattle, Washington, August 31–September 5, 1984. *Pain* (Suppl.2), 421S.

Bonica J.J. (1980a) *Sympathetic Nerve Blocks for Pain Diagnosis and Therapy: Fundamental Considerations and Clinical Applications*. Breon Laboratories, New York.

Bonica J.J. (Ed.) (1980b) Introduction. In *Pain: Research Publications in Nervous and Mental Disease*, vol. 58. pp. 1–17. Raven Press, New York.

Bonica J.J. (Ed.) (1990) *The Management of Pain* 2nd edn. Lea & Febiger, Philadelphia.

Borg G. (1982) A category scale with ratio properties for intermodal and interindividual comparisons. In *Psychophysical Judgment and the Process of Perception* (Eds Geisler G.-G. & Petzold P.) pp. 25–34. VEB Deutscher Verlag der Wissenschaften, Berlin.

Bridgman P.W. (1927) *The Logic of Modern Physics*. Macmillan, New York.

Bridgman P.W. (1959) *The Way Things Are*. Harvard University Press, Cambridge.

Bromm B. (Ed.) (1984) *Pain Measurement in Man: Neurophysiological Correlates of Pain*. Elsevier Press, Amsterdam.

Campbell J.A. & Lipton S. (1985) Intraspinal somatosensory evoked potentials in man. In *Evoked Potentials: Neurophysiological and Clinical Aspects*. (Eds Morocutti C. & Rizzo P.A.) pp. 37–43. Elsevier, New York.

Carlsson A.M. (1983) Assessment of chronic pain. I. Aspects of the reliability and validity of the visual analogue scale. *Pain* **16**, 87–101.

Chapman C.R. (1989) Concept of measurement: coexisting theoretical perspectives. In *Issues in Pain Measurement* (Eds Chapman C.R. & Loeser J.D.) pp. 1–16. Raven Press, New York.

Chapman C.R. & Bonica J.J. (1983) Acute pain. In *Current Concepts* p. 44. Upjohn Company, Kalamazoo, Michigan.

Chapman C.R. & Loeser J.D. (Eds) (1989) *Issues in Pain Measurement (Advances in Pain Research and Therapy, Vol. 12)*. Raven Press, New York.

Chapman C.R. & Saeger L.C. (1985) The use of evoked potentials in the measurement of analgesic states. In: *Quantitation, Modelling and Control in Anaesthesia* (Ed. Stoeckel H.) pp. 108–22. Thieme Inc., New York.

Chapman C.R., Casey K.L., Dubner R., Foley K.M., Gracely R.H. & Reading A.E. (1985) Pain measurement: an overview. *Pain* **22**, 1–31.

Chudler E.H. & Dong W.K. (1983) The assessment of pain by cerebral evoked potentials. *Pain* **16**, 221–4.

Cleeland C.S. (1985) Measurement and prevalence of pain in cancer. *Cancer Pain* **1**, 87–92.

Corson J.A. & Schneider M.J. (1984) The Dartmouth Pain Questionnaire: an adjunct to the McGill Pain Questionnaire. *Pain* **19**, 59–69.

Daut R.L., Cleeland C.S. & Flanery R.C. (1983) Development of the Wisconsin Brief Pain Questionnaire to assess pain in cancer and other diseases. *Pain* **17**, 197–210.

Duncan O.D. (1975) *Introduction to Structural Equation Models*. Academic Press, New York.

Eich E., Reeves J.L., Jaeger B. & Graff-Radford S.B. (1985) Memory for pain: Relation between past and present pain intensity. *Pain* **23**, 375–9.

Eisen A.A. (1986) Noninvasive measurement of spinal cord conduction: review of presently available methods: *Muscle and Nerve* **9**, 95–103.

Elend J.M. (1981) Minimizing pain associated with prekindergarten intramuscular injections. *Issues in Comprehensive Pediatric Nursing* **5**, 352–72.

Follick M.J., Smith T.W. & Ahern D.K. (1985) The Sickness Impact Profile: a global measure of disability in chronic low back pain. *Pain* **21**, 67–76.

Frank A.J.M., Moll J.M.H. & Hort J.F. (1982) A comparison of three ways of measuring pain. *Rheumatology and Rehabilitation* **21**, 211–17.

Goodman J.E. & McGrath P.J. (1991) The epidemiology of pain in children and adolescents: a review. *Pain* **46**, 247–64.

Gracely R.H., Dubner R. & McGrath P. (1979) Narcotic analgesia: fentanyl reduces the intensity but not the unpleasantness of painful tooth pulp sensations. *Science* **203**, 1261–3.

Gunn C.C. (1989) Neuropathic pain: a new theory for chronic pain of intrinsic origin. *Annals of the Royal College of Physicians and Surgeons (Canada)* **22**, 327–30.

Gunn C.C. & Milbrandt W.E. (1978) Early and subtle signs in low-back sprain. *Spine* **3**, 267–81.

Gunn C.C., Sola A.E., Loeser J.D. & Chapman C.R. (1990) Dry-needling for chronic musculoskeletal pain syndromes — clinical observations. *Acupuncture: The Scientific International Journal* **1**, 9–15.

Harms-Ringdahl K., Carlsson A.M., Ekholm J., Raustorp A., Svenson T. & Torresson H.-G. (1986) Pain assessment with different intensity scales in response to loading of joint structures. *Pain* **27**, 401–11.

Hunter M., Phillips C. & Rackman S. (1979) Memory for pain. *Pain* **6**, 35–46.

Jay S.M. & Elliott C. (1984) Behavioral observation scales for measuring children's distress: the effects of increased methodological rigor. *Journal of Consulting and Clinical Psychology* **52**, 1106–7.

Jay S.M., Ozolins M., Elliot C.H. & Caldwell S. (1983) Assessment of children's distress during painful medical procedures. *Health Psychology* **2**, 133–47.

Jeans M.E. (1983) The measurement of pain in children. In *Pain Measurement and Assessment* (ed. Melzack R.) pp. 183–9. Raven Press, New York.

Jensen M.P., Karoly P. & Braver S. (1986) The measurement of clinical pain intensity: a comparison of six methods. *Pain* **27**, 117–26.

Katz E.R., Kellerman J. & Fingel S.E. (1980) Distress behavior in children with cancer undergoing medical procedures: developmental considerations. *Journal of Consulting Clinical Psychology* **48**, 356–65.

Keefe F.J. & Block A.R. (1982) Development of an observation method for assessing pain behavior in chronic low back pain patients. *Behavioral Therapy* **13**, 363–75.

Keefe F.J. & Hill R.W. (1985) An objective approach to qualifying pain behavior and gait patterns in low back pain patients. *Pain* **21**, 153–61.

Keefe F.J., Brantley A., Manuel G. & Crisson J.E. (1985) Behavioral assessment of head and neck cancer pain. *Pain* **23**, 327–36.

Kerns R.D., Turk D.C. & Rudy T.E. (1985) The West Haven-Yale multidimensional pain inventory (WHYMPI). *Pain* **23**, 345–56.

Klepac R.K., Dowling J., Rokke P., Dodge L. & Schafer L. (1981) Interview vs. paper and pencil administration of the McGill Pain and Questionnaire. *Pain* **11**, 241–6.

Kremer E., Atkinson J.H. & Ignelzi R.J. (1980a) Measurement of pain: Patient preference does not confound pain measurement. *Pain* **10**, 241–8.

Kremer E.F., Block A.J. & Gaylor M.S. (1980b) Behavioral approaches to treatment of chronic pain: the inaccuracy of patient self-report measures. *Archives of Physical Medical Rehabilitation* **62**, 188–91.

Kwilosc D.M., Gracely R.H. & Torgerson W.S. (1984) Memory for post-surgical dental pain. IV World Congress on Pain, Seattle, Washington, August 31–September 5, 1984. *Pain* (Suppl. 2), 426S.

Lavigne J.V., Schulein M.J. & Hahn Y.S. (1986) Psychological aspects of painful medical conditions in children. I. Developmental aspects and assessment. *Pain* **27**, 133–46.

LeBaron S. & Zeltzer L. (1984) Assessment of acute pain and anxiety in children in adolescents by self reports, observer reports, and a behavior check list. *Journal of Consulting and Clinical Psychology* **52**, 729–38.

Linton S.J. (1985) The relationship between activity and chronic back pain. *Pain* **21**, 289–94.

Mayer T.G., Gatchel R.J., Kishino N., Keeley J., Mayer H., Capra P. & Mooney V. (1986) A prospective short term study of chronic low back pain patients utilizing novel objective functional measurement. *Pain* **25**, 53–68.

McGrath P.J., Matthews J. & Pigeon H. (1990) Assessment of pain in children. In *Pain Research and Clinical Management*, vol. 4 (Eds Bond M.R., Charlton J.E. & Woolf C.J.) pp. 509–26. Proceedings of the VIth World Congress on Pain, Elsevier Press, Amsterdam.

Melzack R. & Torgerson W.S. (1971) On the language of pain. *Anesthesiology* **34**, 50–9.

Michell J. (1986) Measurement scales and statistics: a clash of paradigms. *Psychology Bulletin* **100**, 398–407.

Moore R.A. & McQuay, H.J. (1985) Neuroendocrinology of the postoperative state. In *Acute Pain* (Eds Smith G. & Covino B.G.) pp. 133–54. Butterworth, London.

Ochoa J.L., Torebjörk E., Marchettini P. & Sivak M. (1985) Mechanisms of neuropathic pain: cumulative observations, new experiments, and further speculation. In *Advances in Pain Research and Therapy*, vol. 9 (Eds Fields H.L., Dubner R. & Cevero F.) Raven Press, New York.

Ready L.B., Sarkis E. & Turner J.A. (1982) Self-reported vs. actual use of medications in chronic pain patients. *Pain* **12**, 285–94.

Revill S.I., Robinson J.O., Rosen M. & Hogg M.I.J. (1976) The reliability of a linear analogue for evaluating pain. *Anaesthesia* **31**, 1191–8.

Ross D.M. & Ross S.A. (1988) *Childhood Pain: Current Issues, Research, and Management.* Urban and Schwarzenberg, Baltimore.

Rubal B.J., Traycoff R.B. & Ewing K.L. (1982) Liquid crystal thermography. A new tool for evaluating low back pain. *Physical Therapy* **62**, 1593–6.

Sanders S.H. (1983) Automated vs. self-help monitoring of 'up-time' in chronic low back pain patients: a comparative study. *Pain* **15**, 399—405.

Scott P.J., Ansell B.M. & Huskinsson E.C. (1977) Measurement of pain in juvenile chronic polyarthritis. *Annals of the Rheumatic Diseases (London)* **36**, 186—7.

Shapiro A.K. (1971) Placebo effects in medicine, psychotherapy, and psychoanalysis. In *Psychotherapy and Behavior Change* (Eds Bergin A.E. & Garfield S.L) pp. 439—73. John Wiley & Sons, Inc., New York.

Stevens S.S. (1946) On the theory of scales of measurement. *Science* **103**, 667—80.

Stevens S.S. (1975) *Psychophysics: Introduction to Its Perceptual, Neural and Social Prospects*. John Wiley & Sons, Inc., New York.

Syrjala K.L. & Chapman C.R. (1984) Measurement of clinical pain: a review and integration of research findings. In *Advances in Pain Research and (Recent Advances in the Management of Pain)*, vol. 7 (Eds Benedetti C., Chapman C.R. & Moricca G.) pp. 71—97. Raven Press, New York.

Szyfelbein S.K., Osgood P.F. & Carr D.B. (1985) The assessment of pain and plasma β-endorphin immunoactivity in burned children. *Pain* **22**, 173—82.

Talbot J.D., Marrett S., Evans A.C., Meyer E., Bushell M.C. & Duncan G.H. (1991) Multiple representations of pain in human cerebral cortex. *Science* **251**, 1355—8.

Tearnan B. & Dar R. (1986) Physician ratings of pain descriptors: potential diagnostic utility. *Pain* **26**, 45—51.

Thomas P.K. (1984) Clinical features and differential diagnosis. In *Peripheral Neuropathy*, vol. II (Eds Dyck P.J., Thomas P.K., Lambert E.H. & Bunge R.) pp. 1169—90. W.B. Saunders, Philadelphia.

Thompson K.L. & Varni J.W. (1986) A developmental cognitive—biobehavioural approach to pediatric pain assessment. *Pain* **25**, 283—96.

Turk D.C., Rudy T.E. & Salovey P. (1985) The McGill Pain Questionnaire reconsidered: confirming factor structure and examining appropriate uses. *Pain* **21**, 385—97.

Tursky B., Jamner L.D. & Friedman R. (1982) The pain perception profile: a psychophysical approach to the assessment of pain report. *Behavior Therapy* **13**, 376—94.

Walsh T.D. (1984) Letter to the Editor. *Pain* **19**, 96—8.

World Health Organization (1980) *International Classifications of Impairments, Disabilities and Handicaps*. World Health Organization, Geneva.

The Affective Dimension of Pain: Psychobiology and Clinical Implications

C. R. CHAPMAN

Pain is in part an emotion; it is not a simple sensory modality. Unlike touch, temperature, audition and other basic senses, pain possesses a disturbing aversive quality. Its intrusion into ongoing awareness signals threat, produces physiological arousal and disrupts purposeful behaviour. The emotional aspects of pain are more salient clinically than its sensory aspects because patients seek relief, not from the awareness of pain, but from its distress.

This chapter offers an introduction to the emotional dimension of pain, linking nociception to emotion and reviewing current knowledge on the central neurophysiology of emotion. Signals from injured tissues excite more than spinothalamic and thalamocortical processing; they also initiate spinoreticular transmission that, in turn, engages extensive processing in limbic brain and neocortex. In addition, tissue injury signals activate the hypothalamopituitary—adrenocortical (HPA) axis by stimulating the hypothalamus, and this results in sympathetically medicated physiological arousal. Complex neuroendocrine and autonomic processes thus accompany sensory awareness of injury so that pain is the product of sensory and affective processing coloured by awareness of non-volitional physiological arousal. Finally, this chapter addresses therapeutic approaches to the affective dimension of pain and discusses several clinical implications.

Basic definitions

Pain

The affective quality of pain has long been recognized (Bonica, 1990). Aristotle referred to pain as a 'passion of the soul'. In principle, modern theorists concur, emphasizing that pain is a complex experience and only in part a sensation. The International Association for the Study of Pain (IASP) acknowledged the central role of affect in pain in its definition of pain (Merskey, 1979).

'Pain [is] an unpleasant sensory and emotional experience associated with actual or potential tissue damage, or described in terms of such damage.'

This definition implies that the emotional dimension of pain is not a reaction to a completed sensory process. Rather, affective processing occurs in parallel with the sensory processing so that sensation and affect together yield the perception of pain.

Emotion

Although an enormous literature exists on the psychobiology of affect, there is no singular or even preferred definition for emotion. Nor do investigators agree on how many primary emotions, if any, exist. Most of us know emotions as feelings that appear in the course of our interactions with one another, with the world in general, or during our fantasies or imaginings. These feelings are often accompanied by autonomically mediated physiological changes, facial expressions, postural adjustments, alterations in vocal timbre and in social behaviours. Moreover, we know that emotions can accompany the anticipation of a personally significant event as well as the actual occurrence of the event. Panskepp (1986) wisely argued that a definition for emotion is the proper end-point for research rather than a starting point.

An arbitrarily selected definition may be less useful than an overview of current scientific assumptions about emotion. A strong consensus exists in the mainstream literature on the following points:

1 Emotional phenomena have an evolutionary history; consequently, they can be studied in animals as well as in humans.

2 Emotions and emotional expression subserve biological adaptation and survival.

3 Emotions are characterized by positive or negative hedonic qualities (behaviour, approach or avoidance tendencies) and by magnitude of physiological arousal.

4 The central neuroanatomy for emotion corresponds roughly to the limbic brain.

5 Emotions include impulses to act or express one's self.

6 In humans, cognition and emotion are interdependent.

Weak consensus exists on four additional points:

7 Some emotions and emotional behaviours involve activation of underlying, genetically 'prewired' circuits.

8 Emotional processing elicited by a brief stimulus outlasts the sensory processing elicited by that stimulus.

9 As emotions involve complex CNS processing and general physiological arousal, they cannot be characterized adequately by introspection (verbal report) alone.

10 Emotions are essential mechanisms in learning and memory.

These and other concepts in the field of emotion help clarify the IASP definition of pain which refers to pain as an emotional experience. Issues of definition indicate that the emotional processing of noxious events is extremely complex. In addition to neurophysiological and neuroendocrinological mechanisms, it encompasses cognitive processes and behavioural manifestations.

Central mechanisms of affective processing

Neuroscience possesses a great deal of information and theory about emotion and its relation to nociception has become reasonably clear. The following brief review offers a theoretical basis and supporting data for the affective dimension of pain.

Nociception and limbic brain

Noxious stimulation excites spinoreticular pathways (Fields, 1987; Bonica, 1990). Spinoreticular axons possess receptive fields that resemble those of spinothalamic tract neurones projecting to medial thalamus, and they appear to conduct nociceptive information. Most spinoreticular neurones carry nociceptive information and many of them respond preferentially to noxious input (Bowsher, 1976; Willis, 1985; Abou-Samra et al., 1987).

Affective processing of nociceptive signals takes place in reticulocortical pathways. Foote and Morrison

(1987) described four extrathalamic afferent pathways to neocortex: (i) the noradrenergic fibres originating in the locus coeruleus (LC) (the dorsal noradrenergic bundle); (ii) the serotonergic fibres that arise in the dorsal and median raphe nuclei; (iii) the dopaminergic pathways of the ventral tegmental tract that arise from substantia nigra; and (iv) the acetylcholinergic neurones that originate principally from the nucleus basalis of the substantia innominata. Of these, the noradrenergic pathway is most closely linked to emotional states (Gray, 1987). This complex and extensive network of projections, together with hypothalamus, conforms to classical conceptions of limbic brain (Papez, 1937; Isaacson, 1982; Gray, 1987).

Locus coeruleus and central noradrenergic transmission

The LC provides a strong link between nociception and limbic activation. The LC is a bilaterally positioned pontine nucleus, located near the wall of the fourth ventricle (MacLean, 1990). LC neurones respond with phasic activation to sensory stimuli, particularly those associated with threat. Nociception inevitably and reliably increases activity in the LC (Korf et al., 1974; Stone, 1975; Morilak et al., 1987; Svensson, 1987). This occurs even when an animal has been rendered unconscious by anaesthesia. Foote and colleagues (1983) reported that slow, tonic spontaneous activity at LC in rats under anaesthesia altered in response to noxious stimulation. Experimentally induced phasic LC activation produces alarm and fear reactions in primates (Redmond & Huang, 1979; Charney et al., 1990), and lesions of the LC eliminate normal heart rate increases to threatening stimuli (Redmond, 1977).

The LC responds consistently, although not exclusively, to nociceptive sensory input. Increased LC activity also occurs in response to non-painful threatening occurrences such as cardiovascular stimuli (Elam et al., 1985; Morilak, 1987) and peripheral visceral events such as distension of the bladder, stomach, colon or rectum (Elam et al., 1986b; Svensson, 1987). Thus, while it responds to nociception, the LC is not a nociceptive-specific nucleus because several types of threatening stimulation excite it. Amaral and Sinnamon (1977) postulated that the LC represents a central analogue of the sympathetic ganglia. It responds to threatening events, including tissue injury.

The majority of central noradrenergic fibres in the spinal cord, hypothalamus, thalamus, hippocampus and cortex originate from the LC (Levitt & Moore,

1979; Aston-Jones *et al.*, 1985). Research on emotion identifies the dorsal noradrenergic bundle (DNB) as the largest tract and the most important projection for affective processing of nociception. The DNB is an extensive pathway projecting from the LC throughout limbic brain and to all of neocortex (Fig. 75.1). It accounts for about 70% of all brain noradrenaline (Watson *et al.*, 1986; Svensson, 1987). The DNB projects into multiple supraspinal structures including the hippocampus, amygdala, limbic cortex and all of the neocortex. DNB fibres project directly, and indirectly via limbic structures, to the basal ganglia, suggesting that emotional arousal may affect the function of the extrapyramidal motor tract (Wilbur *et al.*, 1988). Through these mechanisms a noxious stimulus can rapidly elicit a CNS reaction, induce alarm and facilitate motor response.

The DNB subserves vigilance and orientation to affectively relevant and novel stimuli, regulates attentional processes and facilitates motor response (Elam *et al.*, 1986a; Foote & Morrison, 1987; Gray, 1987; Svensson, 1987; Calogero *et al.*, 1988). Activation of the DNB and associated limbic structures increases sympathetic nervous system response and elicits emotional behaviours in animals such as defensive threat, fright, enhanced startle, freezing and vocalization (McNaughton & Mason, 1980). Activity in this pathway increases alertness; tonically enhanced discharge corresponds to hypervigilance and emotionality (Foote *et al.*, 1983; Butler *et al.*, 1990).

The LC and DNB together constitute the LC system. This system appears to sustain vigilance for threatening and noxious stimuli. Siegel and Rogawski (1988) linked the LC noradrenergic system to vigilance via rapid eye movement (REM) sleep. They reviewed studies demonstrating that LC noradrenergic neurones maintain continuous activity in the normal waking state and non-REM sleep but during REM sleep these neurones virtually cease discharge activity. Destruction of the DNB increases REM sleep as does administration of clonidine, an α_2-adrenoreceptor agonist.

Siegel and Rogawski (1988) hypothesized that a primary function of the LC noradrenergic system and of REM sleep is to permit sustained periods of high alertness. They contended that '. . . a principal function of noradrenaline in the CNS is to facilitate the excitability of target neurones to specific high priority signals'. Conversely, reduced LC activity periods (REM sleep) allow time for a suppression of sympathetic tone.

Prolonged enhanced tonic activation of the LC may produce a negative emotional state. Orienting responses, startle and environmental searching induced by activity in this system can disrupt both concentration and purposive motor activity, impairing normal behaviour. Depletion of noradrenaline at the LC has been associated with stress-induced depression (Weiss, 1985). Pioneering work on helplessness using animal models (Overmier & Seligman,

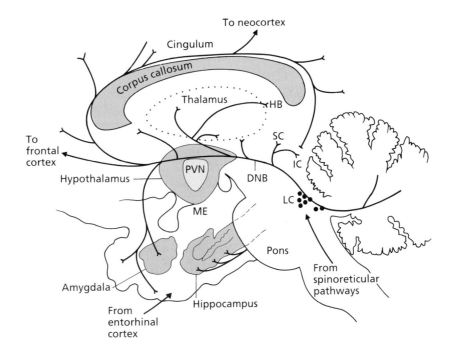

Fig. 75.1 Locus coeruleus (LC) and the dorsal noradrenergic bundle (DNB). Nociceptive signals from spinoreticular pathways excite the primarily noradrenergic locus coeruleus. Projections from this nucleus extend throughout the limbic brain and to the neocortex. HB, habenula; IC, inferior colliculus; ME, median eminence; PVN, hypothalamic paraventricular nucleus; SC, superior colliculus.

1967; Seligman & Maier, 1967) has shown that repeated uncontrollable electrical shock causes behaviourally manifested depression, i.e. decreased motor activity, decreased grooming and poor sleep. Diminished noradrenaline at the LC appears to be the principal change in brain neurochemistry during helplessness, although smaller changes in dopamine and serotonin also occur (Anisman *et al.*, 1980). Changes in central noradrenergic function have been implicated in depression and other affective disorders (Werstiuk *et al.*, 1990).

During painful stimulation, synthesis of noradrenaline at the LC cannot keep pace with the high rate of release. Consequently, the diminished level of noradrenaline reduces the amount of neurotransmitter available for release onto α_2-adrenoreceptors. The α_2-adrenoreceptors function centrally as they do peripherally in haemodynamic stabilization; as autoreceptors they detect the concentration of noradrenaline at the synapse and inhibit further release of the neurotransmitter in response to high concentration (Fillenz, 1990). Figure 75.2 provides a simplified schematic representation of a noradrenergic synapse. A failure in the feedback loop disturbs normal function; LC cell firing rates increase with noradrenaline depletion because the autoreceptor receives insufficient neurotransmitter to activate inhibitory modulation. In distal regions of the brain innervated by the LC noradrenergic system, a corresponding increase occurs in noradrenaline at synapses, pro-

ducing overstimulation. This may be the fundamental mechanism of helplessness depression (Weiss, 1985). Weiss's work (1985) suggests that excessive central noradrenergic activity, produced by compromised ability to inhibit the LC, results in decreased startle thresholds, excessive aversiveness and possibly attentional preoccupation with the offending stimulus.

Van Dongen (1981a) reviewed diseases that disturb the LC and central noradrenergic transmission. He concluded that such pathology results in disorientation, impaired perceptual organization, intellectual and memory deficit, confusion, delusion and hallucination. Van Dongen (1981b) attributed such symptoms directly to LC dysfunction. Charney and colleagues (1990) postulated that the noradrenergic LC system is the fundamental mechanism of panic disorder. These considerations suggest that biologically adaptive hypervigilance is linked to a subjectively aversive state and that excessive activation of central pathways associated with this function can produce behavioural disorders.

In summary, research on the physiological basis of emotion and reviews of pathological processes related to these mechanisms suggest that pain, as an emotion, shares central mechanisms with vigilance and the pursuit of novelty. It points to a single dimension of experience, anchored on one pole by vigilance and on the other by panic. It resembles, and perhaps equates with *threat*. Varying degrees of hypervigil-

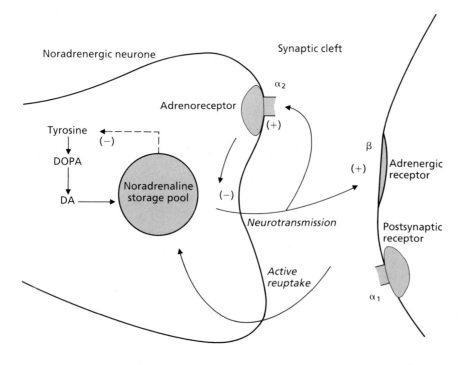

Fig. 75.2 Noradrenergic neurotransmission. Within the axoplasm tyrosine is metabolically transformed to dopa, and then dopamine (DA). Dopamine enters a varicosity where noradrenaline (NA) synthesis occurs and a storage pool forms. Hydroxylation of tyrosine is the rate-limiting step in NA synthesis. During neurotransmission molecules of NA are released into the synaptic cleft where they bind to the β-adrenergic receptor of the postsynaptic cell. The α_2-adrenoreceptor, an autoreceptor, responds to the concentration of NA in the synaptic cleft and inhibits further exocytotic release of NA when synaptic concentrations are high. This feedback loop modulates noradrenergic transmission.

ance and fear exist between the poles. Pribram (1980) emphasized this more than a decade ago: 'The distinction between a feeling of novelty and pain is one of intensity *only* (e.g., electrical stimulations of the amygdala in animals and man produce orienting [interest], avoidance [fear], attack, and escape [pain] as a function of ascending stimulus intensity'. This echoes a concept introduced much earlier by Gastaut (1954).

Cortical processing and cognitions

The neocortex appears to play an important role in the affective dimension of pain. Cortical function forms the cognitive aspects of emotion during pain by labelling feeling states and linking them to language and by associating the immediate meaning of emotion with abstract concepts of past and future. Moreover, the cortex integrates sensory processing with affective processing and other immediate awareness to produce the pain experience.

Current research issues on emotion include the question of whether non-verbal cognitive processes take place and, if so, whether this involves hemispheric specialization. Lesions of the left hemisphere often result in depression (Goldstein, 1948; Robinson *et al.*, 1984; Heilman & Bowers, 1990), suggesting the left hemisphere sustains positive emotional state. Lesions of the right hemisphere can generate positive emotional state in circumstances where this is inappropriate (Denny-Brown *et al.*, 1952; Gainotti, 1972; Starkstein *et al.*, 1989). Moreover, the left hemisphere is more active in negative mood states and the right hemisphere is more active during cheerful mood states (Davidson, 1984). On the basis of multiple studies in this area, Heller (1990) concluded that the right hemisphere is uniquely capable of *interpreting* emotional information in social communication, e.g. facial expression, gesture and vocal tone.

Relationship between cognitive and limbic function

Pribram (1980) linked limbic function to frontal and temporal cortex. This is a bottom-up concept: emotion determines cognition. However, the multimodal neocortical association areas project to limbic structures (Turner *et al.*, 1980), and this may permit abstract concepts of future events or memories of past events to elicit emotional arousal. Higher cognitive processes may well modulate the level of limbic input to consciousness or the entry of information from deeper limbic processing to cortical processing.

The hypothalamopituitary–adrenocortical axis

Threatening environmental or somatic events (and perceived events produced endogenously by cognitive processes) are encoded as neurochemical messages within the CNS; the hypothalamus then transforms these messages into hypophysiotrophic signals. The adenohypophysis further transforms the messages into neurohumoral signals, secreting corticotrophin-releasing hormone (CRH) from the median eminence into the portal circulation. This results in the release of adrenocorticotrophic hormone (ACTH) into systemic circulation; in turn, this stimulates both the synthesis and secretion of adrenocortical steroids. These substances have extensive metabolic effects, and their presence in systemic circulation completes a feedback loop that regulates ACTH release. This axis possesses three major characteristics: (i) its tonic activity manifests a circadium rhythm; (ii) it depends upon feedback control; and (iii) it responds phasically to events that have adaptive significance for the individual.

Figure 75.3 describes the activity of the HPA axis during noxious stimulation. The control centre for the HPA axis is the paraventricular nucleus of the hypothalamus (PVN), and this nucleus responds to noxious stimulation (Kanosue *et al.*, 1984). Nociception-transmitting neurones at all segmental levels of the spinal cord project to medial and lateral hypothalamus and several telencephalic regions (Burtstein *et al.*, 1988). Moreover, neurones in the medullary reticular formation project to hypothalamus via the ventral tegmental tract (Sumal *et al.*, 1983; Bonica, 1990). The medullary neuronal complexes supply 90% of catecholaminergic innervation to the paraventricular hypothalamus via the ventral noradrenergic bundle (VNB) (Assenmacher *et al.*, 1987). Sawchenko and Swanson (1982) identified three noradrenergic and adrenergic pathways to paraventricular hypothalamus in the rat using the Dahlström and Fuxe (1964) designations: A1 region of the ventral medulla (lateral reticular nucleus), A2 in the dorsal vagal complex, and A6 (the LC). The nucleus tractus solitarius (NTS), which receives visceral afferent inputs, includes the A2 cell group and projects to A1. The noradrenergic axons and perhaps others in this tract respond to noxious stimulation (Svensson, 1987) and the hypothalamus itself responds directly to noxious stimulation (Kanosue *et al.*, 1984). Neurones of the PVN also receive sensory information from several reticular areas including ventrolateral medulla, dorsal raphe nucleus, nucleus raphe magnus, LC, dorsomedial nucleus and NTS (Sawchenko & Swanson,

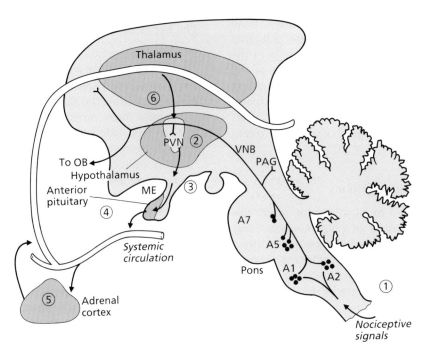

Fig. 75.3 Response of the hypothalamopituitary−adrenocortical axis to noxious stimulation. Feedback-modulated response is depicted in six steps. In the first step signals of tissue injury excite the ventral noradrenergic bundle (VNB), including several medullary and pontine nuclei (designated A1, A2, A5 and A7 in accordance with the nomenclature of Dahlström and Fuxe, 1964). When these signals reach the hypothalamus, they stimulate the paraventricular nucleus (PVN) (Step 2). The PVN produces corticotrophin-releasing hormone. CRH-producing neurones extend from the PVN to the median eminence (ME) where they release CRH into the portal circulation (Step 3). At this point, the tissue-injury signals become neurohumoral rather than neuronal. The anterior pituitary responds to CRH by releasing adrenocorticotrophic hormone (ACTH) into the systemic circulation (Step 4). The adrenocortex responds to ACTH by releasing corticosteroids into the systemic circulation (Step 5). In addition to their extensive metabolic effects, the corticosteroids bind to receptors at the PVN (Step 6), thus closing the feedback loop. This mechanism provides the physiological arousal associated with the affective component of pain. OB, olfactory bulb; PAG, periaqueductal gray.

1982; Peschanski & Weil-Fugacza, 1987; Lopez et al., 1991). Still other afferents project to the PVN from the hippocampus and amygdala. Nearly all hypothalamic and preoptic nuclei send projections to PVN, including the infundibular nucleus. Threatening events, and particularly nociception, excite the HPA axis.

Neurones of the PVN synthesize CRH, a 41-amino acid peptide (Vale et al., 1981). These neurones project to the median eminence, allowing their terminals to secrete CRH directly into portal circulation. The PVN responds to noxious or threatening stimulation by releasing CRH into the portal circulation; this transports CRH to the anterior pituitary (adenohypophysis) where it causes the release of several pro-opiomelanocortin (POMC)-derived biologically active neuropeptides, including ACTH, into systemic circulation (King & Baertschi, 1990). ACTH stimulates the adrenal cortex to release corticosteroids; the most important of these in humans are cortisol (hydrocortisone) and corticosterone. Corticosteroid receptors exist on parvocellular PVN neurones (Fuxe et al.,

1985), and corticosteroids bind to the amygdala, hippocampus and prefrontal cortical areas (Sapolsky et al., 1984; Saphier, 1987).

Corticosteroids play a central feedback role in regulatory processes by exerting an inhibitory influence on the anterior pituitary; this represses the POMC gene expression (Drouin et al., 1989) thereby attenuating ACTH secretion. In binding to hippocampus and amygdala, corticosteroids initiate inhibitory feedback to the hypothalamic PVN and they restrain the activity of the LC (Sapolsky et al., 1984; Fuxe et al., 1985; DeKloet et al., 1987; Saphier & Feldman, 1987).

Finally, the PVN may invoke sympathetic arousal through neural as well as hormonal pathways. It sends direct projections to the sympathetic intermediolateral cell column in the thoracolumbar spinal cord and the parasympathetic vagal complex, sources of preganglionic autonomic outflow (Krukoff, 1990). It has been demonstrated that CRH administration at central sites produces increased plasma noradrenaline levels (Irwin *et al.*, 1988). Noradrenaline has long been recognized as the major transmitter for sympathetic fibres (Von Euler, 1946, 1954) and it serves as a marker for sympathetic nervous system arousal (Svensson, 1987). The adrenal medulla, a transformed sympathetic ganglion, releases adrenaline and noradrenaline in a 4 : 1 ratio into the systemic circulation during HPA-axis activation (Jänig, 1985a).

The HPA does much more than control autonomic nervous system reactivity; it co-ordinates emotional arousal with behaviour. Direct stimulation of the hypothalamus can elicit well-organized patterns of behaviour, including defensive threat behaviours, accompanied by autonomic manifestations (Hess, 1954; Jänig, 1985a,b). The existence of apparent behavioural subroutines suggests that the hypothalamus plays a key role in matching behavioural reactions and bodily adjustments to challenging circumstances or biologically relevant stimuli. Thus, the co-ordination of behavioural readiness with physiological readiness, awareness and cognitive function appears to be an executive responsibility of the HPA system.

Affect, nociception and biological adaptation

Emotion and the affective dimension of pain characterize mammalian species in general and are products of evolution. The experience of threat protects against life-threatening injury, and it fosters adaptive learning.

An animal needs to learn from injurious experiences in order to avoid future life-threatening events. Alterations of a behaviour pattern that occur as a function of the biologically significant consequences for that behaviour pattern demonstrate operant (instrumental) learning. Learning of this sort requires reinforcers: a reinforcer is a stimulus that alters the future emission of a behaviour if its occurrence follows that behaviour. Positive reinforcing events are rewards; negative ones, such as injury, are punishments (i.e. they suppress behaviours). For the behaviourist, the positive or negative nature of reinforcing events, and the importance or magnitude of those events, are represented in consciousness as feelings.

Rolls (1986) described emotions as 'states elicited by reinforcing stimuli'. Put another way, reinforcing events are those which are emotionally significant. Emotional significance may be essential for memory formation (Tucker *et al.*, 1990). Heath (1986) proposed that learning and memory are 'rooted in feeling and emotion' and identified hippocampus, cortical medial amygdala and cingulate gyrus as key areas involved

in painful emotions. These considerations suggest that the affective dimension of pain contributes to adaptation and survival by facilitating learning, memory and related cognitive processes.

Consensus exists that an emotion may function as a cue in memory (Bower, 1981; MacLean, 1990), and emotion appears to govern the retrieval of information from memory stores (Tucker *et al.*, 1990). This suggests that a person's immediate emotion can facilitate access to memory for events that originally entered into long-term storage in the presence of that same emotional circumstance. The importance of past experiences for the perception of pain in the present may therefore depend not only upon one's objective learning history and memory contents, but also upon the emotional state elicited by the immediate situation and the emotional conditions under which initial learning occurred.

Tucker and colleagues (1990) proposed that the limbic structures regulate access to the contents of memory, acting as gatekeepers. Limbic processes determine which elements of immediate perceptual experience gain access to working memory and the opportunity for long-term storage. They argued that the perceived adaptive significance of a perceptual experience determines whether it gains access to long-term storage in memory. The perceived adaptive significance of an experience is an emotion.

The emotional loading of an event, as defined in terms of adaptive significance, may determine the complexity of the brain's response to a stimulus as well as learning and memory. Mesulam (1981) observed that the cingulate cortices of monkeys respond only to stimuli that have adaptive significance for the animals. Some events do not engage the limbic brain, promote learning or form memories; those events have low perceived adaptive significance. Other events with high perceived adaptive significance (emotional colouring) can disrupt ongoing activities.

As the cingulate is characterized by dense noradrenergic innervation (Descarries & Lapierre, 1973), ongoing, tonic activity of the LC system (vigilance, attention, search for novelty) may be altered by the emotional colouring of individual discrete events. This possibility suggests that the extensive LC system may be responsible for the overall emotional 'state' of the individual and that discrete events occurring against the background of the overall emotional state have unique emotional impacts defined by adaptive significance. If this is so, the discrete events could affect the magnitude of arousal of the overall emotional state and, conversely, the background emotional state could alter the perceived adaptive significance of a discrete event.

Whilst these are but hypothetical concepts, they are important for pain because they imply that: (i) a pain can intensify the overall emotional arousal of a patient; and (ii) the ongoing emotional arousal of a patient can alter the perceived adaptive significance of a pain (i.e. the emotional impact of a brief, minor injury). This helps clarify situations in which we observe a poor fit between the true adaptive significance of a minor injurious event and the perceived adaptive significance of that event, as inferred from a patient's seemingly exaggerated emotional expression.

As a subset of emotional expression, pain expression is also governed by social context and sociopsychological factors. The common belief that emotions are private phenomena ignores the powerful social impact of emotional expression. Ethologists and other investigators concerned with emotions and human or animal social behaviour emphasize that signalling (communication) is a fundamental adaptive function of emotion (Ploog, 1986). This research tradition stems from Darwin (1872) who contended that emotions exist to subserve communication through vocalization, startle, posture, facial expression and other behaviours. Social animals use one another or their social group as resources for adaptation and survival. Consequently, human expression of pain, sociobiologically, elicits help and protection, much like the separation cry in infants elicits protection from the mother. Under certain circumstances social rewards for emotional expression during pain may shape the behaviour of the person expressing pain, forming pain habit patterns (Fordyce, 1990).

In summary, the emotional intensity of an experience is essentially a marker of the perceived adaptive significance of the event that produced the experience. Therefore, the affective dimension of a pain is the internal representation of the perceived adaptive significance, or threat, of the injury event that produced the pain. The emotional impact of an injurious event affects the learning associated with that event, the formation of memory and the retrieval of related memory material. The emotional expression of pain in the presence of supporting persons is socially powerful; it draws upon a fundamental sociobiological imperative, communicating threat and eliciting assistance. Positive social consequences for pain expression may foster exaggerated habits of pain expression.

Clinical implications

Pharmacological therapy

The above review suggests that the primary target for control of the affective dimension of pain is noradrenergic hyperactivity in the LC and DNB. Cooper and colleagues (1982) linked this system to affective distress: stress increases activity at the LC as does naloxone-precipitated withdrawal from morphine. During stress, CRH increases the firing rate of the LC (Delgado & Charney, 1991). Prevention or relief of aversiveness during acute pain should therefore target control of central noradrenergic function.

Several approaches exist for controlling noradrenergic function. One is to employ an α_2-agonist such as clonidine. Drugs of this class stimulate presynaptic α_2-receptors which inhibit the release of noradrenaline at the synapse (Fig. 75.2). Therefore, they diminish the activity of the LC and consequently reduce affective arousal via the DNB (Leckman et al., 1980). Another approach is down-regulation of β-receptors. Down-regulation, by definition, decreases the sensitivity of postsynaptic neurones to noradrenaline. The benzodiazepine alprazolam is one of several drugs that down-regulates β-receptors in addition to its better-known GABAergic central inhibition effects (Pandey & Davis, 1983). Moreover, GABAergic neurones modulate LC activity directly (Delgado & Charney, 1991). Benzodiazepines thus offer an approach to controlling central noradrenergic activation.

Tri-cyclic antidepressants offer a third possibility. The precise mood altering mechanisms of these drugs remain at issue. However, both β-receptor down-regulation and presynaptic α_2-receptor agonism offer viable hypotheses; postsynaptic α_1-receptor activation is also a possibility (Gerner & Bunney, 1986). The literature suggests that one can control LC activation through any of these strategies. However, the effects of relevant drugs are far from selective and their side-effect profiles may be complex. The profound cardiovascular peripheral effects of clonidine may limit dosage or work against increasing patient activity levels, for example. The tricyclics have anticholinergic and/or serotonergic as well as noradrenergic effects, and the benzodiazepines, through their GABAergic mechanisms, affect roughly one-third of the synapses in the brain and have widespread central effects.

Finally, opioids affect central noradrenergic processing by acting at the LC. The locus functions in two ways: there is a spontaneous ongoing phasic activity, and the noradrenergic neurones react phasically to potentially injurious or otherwise threatening stimuli. Neurones within the LC possess opioid receptors in high concentration (Herkenham & Pert, 1982; Cooper *et al.*, 1986) and morphine decreases spontaneous discharge in LC neurones (North & Williams, 1985). Valentino and Wehby (1988) demonstrated that morphine inhibited spontaneous LC discharge in rats, both anaesthetized and unanaesthetized, but the effect of morphine was greater by 10-fold in the anaesthetized animals. They could reverse these effects with an opioid antagonist. Valentino and Wehby (1988) proposed that opioids decrease tonic LC activity and, to a lesser degree, diminish the phasic response of LC cells to a discrete stimulus such as foot shock. Ultimately, because the effect of morphine on tonic LC activity is greater than on phasic activity, opioids increase the ratio of evoked (phasic) activity to tonic activity following a stimulus.

As the LC does not perform a sensory function, this does not mean that sensory sensitivity to stimuli increases with morphine. Rather, the brain manifests an overall decrease in ambient vigilance and also in response to discrete stimuli in the presence of morphine. However, the affective response to a discrete stimulus, while diminished under morphine, is less reduced than the background discharge activity of the LC noradrenergic neurones, and so it stands out clearly. Thus, opioids attenuate the affective processing of painful stimuli, just as they reduce sensory awareness, but they do not block affect during pain.

These considerations suggest that the pharmacological tools thus far available for controlling central noradrenergic processing during pain are essentially the familiar alternatives for general sedation.

Psychological therapy

Psychological approaches to pain encompass relaxation, coping skill training, biofeedback and cognitive–behavioural methods, including hypnosis. Interventions such as progressive relaxation can significantly reduce heart rate, muscle tension and respiratory rate in anxious persons (Syrjala, 1990). Therapeutic relaxation techniques include progressive muscle tension and relaxation, instructed deep breathing and autogenic relaxation.

All of these options involve some degree of imagination and mental redirection, usually with guided control of attentional processes. In autogenic training attentional focus and instruction-controlled somatic imagery (e.g. imagined warmth or heaviness in a part of the body) dominate. Cognitive-behavioural

methods typically involve use of positive self-directed statements, relabelling of somatic sensations to make them less threatening and general 'cognitive restructuring' (Turner & Romano, 1990). The latter refers to adjustments of beliefs and expectations so that they foster a stable emotional state and a sense of self-confidence rather than hypervigilance, threat or hopelessness.

Numerous variations and refinements of these approaches appear in the literature; the important point is that a psychological state produced by therapist-guided training can block the hypervigilance and perceived threat associated with LC activation. Threat and profound relaxation are mutually exclusive psychological states.

Psychological techniques generally require patient training, although some patients with meditative skills can master them readily. They are less efficient for day-to-day medical practice than routine sedation, but some patients prefer psychological methods. Some value self-control and others find the mental clouding of sedation undesirable. Cancer patients and others who must encounter repeated painful experiences such as invasive diagnostic or therapeutic procedures, surgery and painful chemotherapy or radiotherapy toxicity sometimes appreciate the opportunity to learn such skills and prefer to cope for themselves.

Indications for intervention

The emotional aspects of pain play a major role in transactions between health care providers and patients. Patients do not seek relief from naked sensations but rather from the accompanying distress. The overwhelming majority of tools and skills in the clinical armamentarium of the anaesthetist are designed to block nociception, interrupt activity in sensory pathways or modulate activity in those pathways. In most cases, prevention or block of nociceptive transmissions suffices. There are, however, marked exceptions.

One exception occurs in control of pain associated with invasive diagnostic procedures (e.g. bone marrow aspiration), minor surgery, and painful interventions such as wound debridement in the burned patient. As regional anaesthetists and especially dentists know, some patients anguish and display pain behaviour despite a competently performed nerve block, and dentists find that multiple repetitions of failed mandibular nerve blocks yields no benefit in such cases.

Such cases can occur if a patient has formed conditioned emotional responses to a past clinical situation in which sensory transmission of noxious stimulation was not blocked or attenuated. The environmental context itself sometimes establishes a hypervigilance for noxious somatic sensations and primes the memory stores for release of pain memories. Specific cues (e.g. the sound or vibration of the dental drill, a certain behaviour or statement by a physician performing a procedure, the sight of a needle being inserted into a vein in one's antecubital fossa) can elicit memories that become immediate emotional and cognitive realities for the patient.

We invariably associate conditioned emotional responses with querulous or difficult patients, but there are many white-knuckled stoics who silently bear up under learned negative affective arousal, manifesting profuse sweating, cardiac acceleration and other indicators of sympathetic nervous system activity. Thus, the anaesthetist sometimes needs to prevent or control the affective dimension of pain, even when he/she can minimize or achieve complete control of nociception.

In situations where pain control is incomplete postoperatively, the nociception leads directly to affective processing via the mechanisms described above. The result is severe distress for the patient. In this case, psychological preparation for surgery or psychological intervention during acute pain can attenuate the distress; it is not necessary to diminish the nociception to achieve this.

Cancer patients experience procedural pains repeatedly. Many require surgical therapy and thus encounter postoperative pain. Treatment toxicities and infections can also inflict pain during the course of treatment. The diseases of cancer produce pain in various ways, but the most common source of pain related to tumour is bone metastasis. During the metastatic progression of disease patients may endure pain at multiple sites. Such nociception produces sustained affective processing. This is complicated by the overarching affective disturbance engendered by personal losses caused by the disease. Patients may suffer degrading changes in physical appearance, lose the ability to participate in treasured recreations or forego the ability to sustain gainful employment, and some reach a point of financial crisis. Perceived helplessness can emerge in cancer patients with poor social support and difficult circumstances. In such cases, when the sensory control of pain is incomplete, once can still intervene by addressing the affective processing component of the pain.

Chronic pain not related to malignant disease encompasses pain related to neuropathic conditions.

This grouping also includes patients who suffer with or become invalid from pain, even though minor or no evidence exists for nociception or neuropathy. Neuropathic pain patients are very difficult to treat via sensory mechanisms since they do not have nociception. Addressing the affective aspect of neuropathic pain may be beneficial; this is an area requiring systematic investigation. Non-malignant chronic pain is also difficult to treat conventionally. By definition, if the pain is chronic, conventional treatments aimed at the sensory basis of the pain do not work.

There are several hypotheses as to how the affective dimension of pain may predominate in some patients with chronic pain:

1 Pain complaint may be a symptom of depression (the patient may have a conditioned association between a somatic awareness and perceived threat, and he/she may express this perception in terms of pain behaviour and pain complaint).

2 Pain is a behaviour that patients repeatedly emit; this behaviour is reinforced by the actions of others (Fordyce, 1990).

Thus, vocalization, postural abnormalities, grimacing and other facial expressions, rubbing, sighing and inhibition of normal activity are all followed by emotionally positive social consequences. This can trap patients in habit patterns characterized by excessive pain expression, help seeking and reduced activity.

Conclusions

In this chapter the author has sought to demonstrate that the emotional aspect of pain is not an ineffable and private epiphenomenon, inaccessible to scientific study. Rather, affect during pain emerges from well-defined brain mechanisms, and it exists to foster survival and adaptation. Emotion, including the affective component of pain, is an internal representation (a feeling) and an outward expression (a pattern of behaviour) of the biological significance of an event or circumstance. The affective component of pain serves no useful purpose in patients undergoing painful procedures, recovering from surgery or experiencing pain from tumour or neuropathy. Indeed, the emotional distress produced by pain degrades rather than supports patient wellbeing.

The affective dimension of pain is the product of complex central processing of noxious signals. The extensive noradrenergic projections of the LC, which ordinarily subserve vigilance, respond to injurious stimuli and produce a sense of threat. In addition, the hypothalamic PVN responds to noxious stimulation, activating the HPA. This produces a global, autonomically mediated physiological arousal with associated metabolic changes which prepare the individual for flight or fight. Emotion and cognition are inseparable and consequently, the affective processing of a noxious event is inextricably interwoven with memory, expectancy and the meaning that the patient imputes to that event.

This complexity offers multiple avenues for intervention: pharmacological interventions can attenuate the affective component of pain. In addition, cognitive–behavioural psychotherapeutic interventions, relaxation training and training in coping skills can help patients gain control over their emotions during pain. By making the emotional component of pain a target in efforts to prevent or control pain, the concerned clinician may well achieve significant control over patient suffering.

Acknowledgements

Preparation of this manuscript was supported in part by a grant from the National Cancer Institute (CA 38552) and by support from the Unrestricted Grants Program of Bristol-Myers Squibb. I am indebted to Dr R.C. Jacobson for technical and artistic guidance in computer development of the illustrations.

References

Abou-Samra A.-B., Harwood J.P., Catt K.J. & Aguilera G. (1987) Mechanisms of action of CRF and other regulators of ACTH release in pituitary corticotrophs. In *The Hypothalamic-Pituitary–Adrenal Axis Revisited*, vol. 512 (Eds Ganong W.F., Dallman M.F. & Roberts J.L.) pp. 67–84. Annals of the New York Academy of Sciences.

Amaral D.B. & Sinnamon H.M. (1977) The locus coeruleus: neurobiology of a central noradrenergic nucleus. *Progress in Neurobiology* **9**, 147–96.

Anisman H., Pizzino A. & Sklar L.S. (1980) Coping with stress, norepinephrine depletion and escape performance. *Brain Research* **191**, 538–88.

Assenmacher I., Szafarczyk A., Alonso G., Ixart G. & Barbanel G. (1987) Physiology of neuropathways affecting CRH secretion. In *The Hypothalamic-Pituitary–Adrenal Axis Revisited*, vol. 512 (Eds Ganong W.F., Dallman M.F. & Roberts J.L.) pp. 149–61. Annals of the New York Academy of Sciences.

Aston-Jones G., Foote S.L. & Segal M. (1985) Impulse conduction properties of noradrenergic locus coeruleus axons projecting to monkey cerebrocortex. *Neuroscience* **15**, 765–77.

Bonica J.J. (1990) *The Management of Pain* 2nd edn. Lea & Febiger, Philadelphia.

Bower G.H. (1981) Mood and memory. *American Psychologist* **36**, 129–48.

Bowsher D. (1976) Role of the reticular formation in responses to noxious stimulation. *Pain* **2**, 361–78.

Burtstein R., Cliffer K.D. & Giesler G.J. (1988) The spinohypo-thalamic and spinotelecephalic tracts: direct nociceptive projections from the spinal cord to the hypothalamus and telencephalon. In *Proceedings of the Vth World Congress on Pain* (Eds Dubner R., Gebhart G.F. & Bond M.R.) pp. 548–54. New York, Elsevier.

Butler P.D., Weiss J.M., Stout J.C. & Nemeroff C.B. (1990) Corticotropin-releasing factor produces fear-enhancing and behavioral activating effects following infusion into the locus coeruleus. *Journal of Neuroscience* **10**, 176–83.

Calogero A.E., Bernardini R., Gold P.W. & Chrousos G.P. (1988) Regulation of rat hypothalamic corticotropin-releasing hormone secretion *in vitro*: potential clinical implications. *Advances in Experimental Medicine and Biology* **245**, 167–81.

Charney D.S., Woods S.W., Nagy L.M., Southwick S.M., Krystal J.H. & Heniger G.R. (1990) Noradrenergic function in panic disorder. *Journal of Clinical Psychiatry* **51** (Suppl. A), 5–11.

Cooper J.R., Bloom F.E. & Roth R.H. (1982) *The Biochemical Basis of Neuropharmacology* 4th edn. Oxford University Press, Oxford.

Cooper J.R., Bloom F.E. & Roth R.H. (1986) *The Biochemical Basis of Neuropharmacology* 5th edn. Oxford University Press, New York.

Dahlström A. & Fuxe K. (1964) Evidence for the existence of monoamine-containing neurons in the central nervous system. *Acta Physiologica Scandinavica* **62**, 1–55.

Darwin C. (1872) *The Expression of the Emotions in Man and Animals*. John Murray, London.

Davidson R.J. (1984) Affect, cognition, and hemisphere specialization. In *Emotion, Cognition and Behavior* (Eds Izard C.E., Kagan J. & Zajonc R.B.) pp. 320–65. Cambridge University Press, New York.

DeKloet E.R., Ratka A., Reul J.M.H.M., Sutanto W. & van Eekelen J.A.M. (1987) Corticosteroid receptor types in brain: regulation and putative function. In *The Hypothalamic-Pituitary–Adrenal Axis Revisited*, vol. 512 (Eds Ganong W.F., Dallman M.F. & Roberts J.L.) pp. 351–61. Annals of the New York Academy of Sciences.

Delgado P.L. & Charney D.S. (1991) Neuroendocrine challenge tests in affective disorders: implications for future pathophysiological investigations. In *Biological Aspects of Affective Disorders* (Eds Horton R. & Katona C.) pp. 145–90. Academic Press, London.

Denny-Brown D., Myer J.S. & Horenstein S. (1952) The significance of perceptual rivalry resulting from parietal lesions. *Brain* **75**, 434–71.

Descarries L. & Lapierre Y. (1973) Norepinephrine and axon terminals in the cerebral cortex of the rat. *Brain Research* **51**, 141–60.

Drouin J., Nemer M., Charron J., Gagner J.P., Jeannotte L., Sun Y.L., Therrien M. & Tremblay Y. (1989) Tissue-specific activity of the pro-opiomelanocortin (POMC) gene and repression by glucocorticoids. *Genome* **31**, 510–19.

Elam M., Svensson T.H. & Thorén P. (1985) Differentiated cardiovascular afferent regulation of locus coeruleus neurons and sympathetic nerves. *Brain Research* **358**, 77–84.

Elam M., Svensson T.H. & Thorén P. (1986a) Locus coeruleus neurons and sympathetic nerves: activation by cutaneous sensory afferents. *Brain Research* **366**, 254–61.

Elam M., Svensson T.H. & Thorén P. (1986b) Locus coeruleus neurons and sympathetic nerves: activation by visceral afferents. *Brain Research* **375**, 117–25.

Fields H.L. (1987) *Pain*. McGraw-Hill, New York.

Fillenz M. (1990) *Noradrenergic Neurons*. Cambridge University Press, Cambridge.

Foote S.L. & Morrison J.H. (1987) Extrathalamic modulation of corticofunction. *Annual Review of Neuroscience* **10**, 67–95.

Foote S.L., Bloom F.E. & Aston-Jones G. (1983) Nucleus locus ceruleus: new evidence of anatomical and physiological specificity. *Physiology Review* **63**, 844–914.

Fordyce W.E. (1990) Contingency management. In *The Management of Pain* 2nd edn. (Ed. Bonica J.J.) pp. 1702–10. Lea & Febiger, Philadelphia.

Fuxe K., Härfstrand A., Agnati L.F., Yu Z.Y., Cintra A., Wikstrom A.C., Okret S., Cantoni E. & Gustafsson J.A. (1985) Immunocytochemical studies on the localization of glucocorticoid receptor immunoreactive nerve cells in the lower brain stem and spinal cord of the male rat using a monoclonal antibody against rat liver glucocorticoid receptor. *Neuroscience Letters* **60**, 1–6.

Gainotti G. (1972) Emotional behavior and hemisphere side of lesion. *Cortex* **8**, 41–55.

Gastaut H. (1954) Interpretation of the symptoms of 'psychomotor' epilepsy in relation to physiologic data on rhinencephalic function. *Epilepsia* (Series III) **3**, 84–8.

Gerner R.H. & Bunney W.E. Jr. (1986) Biological hypotheses of affective disorders. In *American Handbook of Psychiatry* 2nd edn. (Eds Berger P.A. & Brodie H.K.H.) pp. 265–301. Basic Books Inc., New York.

Goldstein K. (1948) *Language and Language Disturbances*. Grune & Stratton, New York.

Gray J.A. (1987) *The Neuropsychology of Anxiety: An Enquiry into the Functions of the Septo-Hippocampal System*. Oxford University Press, New York.

Heath R.G. (1986) The neural substrate for emotion. In *Emotion: Theory, Research, and Experience (Biological Foundations of Emotion)*, vol. 3 (Eds Plutchik R. & Kellerman H.) pp. 91–124. Academic Press, New York.

Heilman K.M. & Bowers D. (1990) Neuropsychological studies of emotional changes induced by right and left hemispheric lesions. In *Psychological and Biological Approaches to Emotion* (Eds Stein N.L., Leventhal B. & Trabasso T.) pp. 97–113. Lawrence Erlbaum Associates, Hillsdale NJ.

Heller W. (1990) The neuropsychology of emotion: developmental patterns and implications for psychopathology. In *Psychological and Biological Approaches to Emotion* (Eds Stein N.L., Leventhal D. & Trabasso T.) pp. 167–211. Lawrence Erlbaum Associates, Hillsdale NJ.

Herkenham M. & Pert C.B. (1982) Light microscopic localization of brain opiate receptors: a general autoradiographic method. A method which preserves tissue quality. *Neuroscience* **2**, 1129–49.

Hess W.R. (1954) *Diencephalon: Automatic and Extra-pyramidal Functions*. Grune & Stratton, New York.

Irwin M., Hauger R.L., Brown M. & Britton K.T. (1988) CRF activates autonomic nervous system and reduces natural killer cell cytotoxicity. *American Journal of Physiology* **255**, R744–7.

Isaacson R.L. (Ed.) (1982) *The Limbic System* 2nd edn. Plenum Press, New York.

Jänig W. (1985a) The autonomic nervous system. In *Fundamentals of Neurophysiology* (Ed. Schmidt R.F.) pp. 216–69. Springer-Verlag, New York.

Jänig W. (1985b) Systemic and specific autonomic reactions in pain: efferent, afferent and endocrine components. *European Journal of Anaesthesia* **2**, 319–46.

Kanosue K., Nakayama T., Ishikawa Y. & Imai-Matsumura K. (1984) Responses of hypothalamic and thalamic neurons to noxious and scrotal thermal stimulation in rats. *Journal of Thermobiology* **9**, 11–13.

King M.S. & Baertschi A.J. (1990) The role of intracellular messengers in adrenocorticotropin secretion *in vitro*. *Experientia* **46**, 26–40.

Korf J., Bunney B.S. & Aghajanian G.K. (1974) Noradrenergic neurons: morphine inhibition of spontaneous activity. *European Journal of Pharmacology* **25**, 165–9.

Krukoff T.L. (1990) Neuropeptide regulation of autonomic outflow at the sympathetic preganglionic neuron: anatomical and neurochemical specificity. *Annals of the New York Academy of Sciences* **579**, 162–7.

Leckman J.F., Maas J.W., Redmond D.E. & Heninger G.R. (1980) Effects of oral clonidine on plasma 3-methoxy-4-hydroxyphenethyleneglycol (MHPG) in man: preliminary report. *Life Sciences* **26**, 2179–85.

Levitt P. & Moore R.Y. (1979) Origin and organization of the brainstem catecholamine innervation in the rat. *Journal of Comparative Neurology* **186**, 505–28.

Lopez J.F., Young E.A., Herman J.P., Akil H. & Watson S.J. (1991) Regulatory biology of the HPA axis: an integrative approach. In *Central Nervous System Peptide Mechanisms in Stress and Depression* (Ed. Risch S.C.) pp. 1–52. American Psychiatric Press, Washington DC.

MacLean P.D. (1990) *The Triune Brain in Evolution: Role in Paleocerebral Functions*. Plenum Press, New York.

McNaughton N. & Mason S.T. (1980) The neuropsychology and neuropharmacology of the dorsal ascending noradrenergic bundle — a review. *Progress of Neurobiology* **14**, 157–219.

Merskey H. (1979) Pain terms: a list with definitions and a note on usage. Recommended by the International Association for the Study of Pain (IASP) Subcommittee on Taxonomy. *Pain* **6**, 249–52.

Mesulam M.M. (1981) A cortical network for directed attention and unilateral neglect. *Annals of Neurology* **10**, 309–25.

Morilak D.A., Fornal C.A. & Jacobs B.L. (1987) Effects of physiological manipulations on locus coeruleus neuronal activity in freely moving cats. II. Cardiovascular challenge. *Brain Research* **422**, 24–31.

North R.A. & Williams J.T. (1985) On the potassium conductance increased by opioids in rat locus coeruleus neurones. *Journal of Physiology (London)* **364**, 265–80.

Overmier J.B. & Seligman M.E.P. (1967) Effects of inescapable shock on subsequent escape and avoidance learning. *Journal of Comparative Physiological Psychology* **63**, 23–33.

Pandey G.N. & Davis J.M. (1983) Treatment with anti-depressants and down-regulation of beta-adrenergic receptors. *Drug Developmental Research* **3**, 393–406.

Panskepp J. (1986) The anatomy of emotions. In *Emotion: Theory, Research, and Experience (Biological Foundations of Emotion)*, vol. 3 (Eds Plutchik R. & Kellerman H.) pp. 125–44. Academic Press, New York.

Papez J.W. (1937) A proposed mechanism of emotion. *Archives of Neurological Psychiatry* **38**, 725–43.

Peschanski M. & Weil-Fugacza J. (1987) Aminergic and cholinergic afferents to the thalamus: experimental data with reference to pain pathways. In *Thalamus and Pain* (Eds Besson J.M., Guilbaud G. & Paschanski M.) pp. 127–54. Excerpta Medica, Amsterdam.

Ploog D. (1986) Biological foundations of the vocal expressions of emotions. In *Emotion: Theory, Research, and Experience (Biological Foundations of Emotion)*, vol. 3 (Eds Plutchik R. & Kellerman H.) pp. 173–98. Academic Press, New York.

Pribram K.H. (1980) The biology of emotions and other feelings. In *Emotion: Theory, Research, and Experience (Theories of Emotion)*, vol. 1 (Eds Plutchik R. & Kellerman H.) pp. 245–69. Academic Press, New York.

Redmond D.E. Jr. (1977) Alteration in the functions of the nucleus locus coeruleus: a possible model for studies of anxiety. In *Animal Models in Psychiatry and Neurology* (Eds Hannin I. & Usdin E.) pp. 293–306. Pergamon Press, New York.

Redmond D.E. Jr. & Huang Y.G. (1979) Current concepts. II. New evidence for a locus coeruleus–norepinephrine connection with anxiety. *Life Sciences* **25**, 2149–62.

Robinson R.G., Kubos K.L., Starr L.B., Rao K. & Price T.R. (1984) Mood disorders in stroke patients. *Brain* **107**, 81–93.

Rolls E.T. (1986) Neural systems involved in emotion in primates. In *Emotion: Theory, Research, and Experience (Biological Foundations of Emotion)*, vol. 3 (Eds Plutchik R. & Kellerman H.) pp. 125–44. Academic Press, New York.

Saphier D. (1987) Cortisol alters firing rate and synaptic responses of limbic forebrain units. *Brain Research Bulletin* **19**, 519–24.

Saphier D. & Feldman S. (1987) Effects of septal and hippocampal stimuli on paraventricular nucleus neurons. *Neuroscience* **20**, 749–55.

Sapolsky R.M., Krey L.C. & McEwen B.S. (1984) Glucocorticoid-sensitive hippocampal neurons are involved in terminating the adrenocortical stress response. *Proceedings of the National Academy of Sciences (USA)* **81**, 6174–7.

Sawchenko P.E. & Swanson L.W. (1982) The organization of noradrenergic pathways from the brain stem to the paraventricular and supraoptic neuclei in the rat. *Brain Research Reviews* **4**, 275–325.

Seligman M.E.P. & Maier S.F. (1967) Failure to escape traumatic shock. *Journal of Experimental Psychology* **74**, 1–9.

Siegel J.M. & Rogawski M.A. (1988) A function for REM sleep: regulation of noradrenergic receptor sensitivity. *Brain Research Review* **13**, 213–33.

Starkstein S.E., Robinson R.G., Honig M.A., Parikh R.M., Joselyn J. & Price T.R. (1989) Mood changes after right-hemisphere lesions. *British Journal of Psychiatry* **155**, 79–85.

Stone E.A. (1975) Stress and catecholamines. In *Catecholamines and Behavior*, vol. 2 (Ed. Friedhoff A.J.) pp. 31–72. Plenum Press, New York.

Sumal K.K., Blessing W.W., Joh T.H., Reis D.J. & Pickel V.M. (1983) Synaptic interaction of vagal afference and catecholaminergic neurons in the rat nucleus tractus solitarius. *Journal of Brain Research* **277**, 31–40.

Svensson T.H. (1987) Peripheral, autonomic regulation of locus coeruleus noradrenergic neurons in brain: putative implications for psychiatry and psychopharmacology. *Psychopharmacology* **92**, 1–7.

Syrjala K.(1990) Relaxation techniques. In *The Management of Pain* 2nd edn. (Ed. Bonica J.J.) pp. 1742–50. Lea & Febiger, Philadelphia.

Tucker D.M., Vannatta K. & Rothlind J. (1990) Arousal and activation systems and primitive adaptive controls on cognitive priming. In *Psychological and Biological Approaches to Emotion* (Eds Stein N.L., Leventhal D. & Trabasso T.) pp. 145–66. Lawrence Erlbaum Associates, Hillsdale NJ.

Turner J.A. & Romano J.M. (1990) Cognitive-behavioral therapy. In *The Management of Pain* 2nd edn. (Ed. Bonica J.J.) pp. 1711–21. Lea & Febiger, Philadelphia.

Turner B.H., Mishkin M. & Knapp M. (1980) Organization of the amygdalopedal projections from modality-specific cortical association areas in the monkey. *Journal of Comparative Neurology* **191**, 515–43.

Vale W., Spiess J.D., Rivier C. & Rivier J. (1981) Characterization of a 41-residue ovine hypothalamic peptide that stimulates secretion of corticotropin and beta-endorphin. *Science* **231**, 1394–7.

Valentino R.J. & Wehby R.G. (1988) Morphine effects of ceruleus neurons are dependent on the state of arousal and availability of external stimuli. Studies in anesthetized and unanesthetized rats. *Journal of Pharmacology and Experimental Therapeutics* **244**, 1178–86.

Van Dongen P.A.M. (1981a) The central noradrenergic transmission and the locus coeruleus: a review of the data and their implications for neurotransmission and neuromodulation. *Progress of Neurobiology* **16**, 117–43.

Van Dongen P.A.M. (1981b) The human locus coeruleus in neurology and psychiatry. *Progress of Neurobiology* **17**, 97–139.

Von Euler U.S. (1946) A specific sympathomimetic ergone in adrenergic nerve fibres (sympathin) and its relation to adrenaline and noradrenaline. *Acta Physiologica Scandinavica* **12**, 73–97.

von Euler U.S. (1954) Adrenaline and noradrenaline. Distribution and action. *Pharmacological Reviews* **6**, 15 22.

Watson S.J., Khachaturian H., Lewis M.E. & Akil H. (1986) Chemical neuroanatomy as a basis for biological psychiatry. In *Biological Phychiatry* vol. 8 (Eds Berger P.A. & Brodie H.K.H.) pp. 3–33. Basic Books, New York.

Weiss J.M. (1985) Neurochemical mechanisms underlying stress-induced depression. In *Stress and Coping* (Eds Field T.M., McCabe P.M. & Schneiderman N.) pp. 93–116. Lawrence Erlbaum Associates, Hillsdale.

Werstiuk E.S., Steiner M. & Burns T. (1990) Studies on leukocyte β-adrenergic receptors in depression: a critical appraisal. *Life Sciences* **47**, 85–105.

Wilbur R., Kulik F.A. & Kulik A.V. (1988) Noradrenergic effects and tardive dyskinesia, akathisia and pseudoparkinsonism via the limbic system and basal ganglia. *Progress in Neuropsychopharmacology and Biological Psychiatry* **12**, 849–64.

Willis W.D. Jr (Ed.) (1985) *The Pain System: The Neurobasis of Nociceptive Transmission in the Mammalian Nervous System.* Karger, New York.

Postoperative Pain

A.J. OGILVY AND G. SMITH

In common with all other types of pain, acute postoperative pain is an extraordinarily complex sensation which may be described as an integration of three components: afferent nociceptive stimulation, interpretation of these signals by higher centres (involving memory and experiences of painful situations) and an emotive or affective component which generally compromises anxiety and/or depression. It is difficult in the human to identify accurately the extent of each component of pain, and it is preferable to regard the patient as a whole who exhibits a spectrum of pain comprising conscious discomfort, autonomic changes and emotional qualities embracing fear, anxiety and depression.

Generally, the factor which separates postoperative pain from other types of pain is the transitory nature of the former, although the intensity of the subjective discomfort may vary from severe to mild or even non-existent. The transitory nature of acute pain renders the condition more easily amenable to therapy than is the case for chronic types of pain.

Treatment of acute pain has failed traditionally to recognize the complex nature of pain. Thus, the standard conventional practice is to prescribe intramuscular administration of fixed dose of opioid on a p.r.n. basis (or as required), i.e. at the discretion of a nurse, on demand by a patient whose pain threshold has been exceeded. This regimen leads to poor control of postoperative pain for the following reasons:

1 Responsibility for the management of the patient is delegated from the anaesthetist to junior medical staff, who in turn delegate responsibility to nursing staff.

2 Nursing staff may vary widely in their level of rapport with the patient. In addition, they may withhold strong opioids because of fear of the side-effects of these drugs, notably physical dependence or addiction and respiratory depression. Whilst there is little evidence to suggest that treatment of acute pain with opioids is likely to produce addiction, respiratory depression is a valid concern none the less.

3 In the absence of personal experience of the severity of postoperative pain, it is difficult for nursing staff to acknowledge the extent of a patient's suffering in the postoperative period.

Furthermore, there are more fundamental reasons why the management of postoperative pain remains difficult as:

1 Analgesic requirements vary widely according to the type and severity of surgery.

2 Analgesic requirements vary widely as a result of variations in pharmokinetics and pharmacodynamics between different patients.

3 Administration of adequate doses of analgesic may be inhibited because of induction of side-effects, notably respiratory depression, nausea and vomiting.

Thus, the disadvantages of the conventional method of administration of intramuscular opioids are: the standard dose prescribed may be too large (side-effects) or too small (no analgesia); the technique results in fluctuating plasma concentrations of the drug; the drug is administered by intramuscular injection which is painful; the onset of analgesia is delayed following the point at which the opioid is administered; and the technique induces a feeling of dependency on the nursing staff (see Fig. 79.5, p. 1643). There are, however some advantages to the conventional method, notably that it represents familiar practice and by and large familiar practices have an inherent safety simply because of accumulated experience: the technique is inexpensive, whilst the gradual onset of analgesia permits the observation of the possible pharmacological overdose.

Causes of variation in extent of postoperative pain

The degree of discomfort experienced by patients in

the postoperative period varies enormously. Thus, following cholecystectomy, it has been reported that some patients require no opioid, whilst others may require as much as 1200 mg of pethidine. This variability reflects the difficulty in quantifying pain (see Chapter 74) and so it is difficult to rank in order of importance.

Type of surgery

The site of operation is probably the most important factor determining the presence and severity of postoperative pain. In general terms, thoracic and upper abdominal operations produce the most severe postoperative pain, almost invariably requiring opioid analgesics for control, whereas minor upper-limb, cutaneous or chest-wall surgery may require no opioid for pain relief. This is illustrated in Table 76.1, which details the frequency of need for postoperative opioids found in a study from Belfast, and in Table 76.2, which notes the number of intramuscular injections of analgesic drugs required in the first 48 h after operation, in a study from Oxford.

It is clear that the duration of pain after surgery is relatively short lived. This is reflected by the fact that in traditional UK practice, the administration of opioids continues for up to 48 h after abdominal surgery, whilst in the USA, it lasts typically for 72 h.

Age, gender and body weight

It is assumed commonly that age, gender and body weight are important factors in pain perception and response to analgesic drugs.

In respect of gender, all studies have suggested that women exhibit higher pain scores than men in chronic pain and experimental pain (Glynn *et al.*, 1976) and also in postoperative pain (Nayman, 1979). However, it has been suggested that these differences are a result of difference in expression of pain suffering by the two sexes. Studies using patient-controlled analgesia (PCA) have demonstrated that there is no sex difference in demand for analgesics (Dahlstrom *et al.*, 1982; Tamsen *et al.*, 1982a,b).

Table 76.2 Percentage of patients who required various numbers of analgesic injections. (Data from Parkhouse *et al.*, 1961)

Operation	Proportion of patients who required no postoperative additional analgesic (%)	Three or more analgesic injections
Minor chest wall	81.7	0
Inguinal hernia	52.4	0
Appendicectomy	25	10%
Lower abdominal surgery	17.6	40% (approx.)
Upper abdominal surgery	10 (approx.)	45−65%

Although it is frequent clinical practice to calculate opioid requirements on a body-weight basis, there is no evidence in adults to suggest that there is any basis for this practice (Cohen, 1980).

Bellville and colleagues (1971) studied the variables of height, weight and age on pain and found that only age correlated with extent of pain and analgesic requirements, confirming the clinical impression that elderly patients require smaller doses of analgesic drugs to achieve adequate pain relief. Although Bellville and colleagues did not think that pharmacokinetic factors were responsible for age-related differences, several workers have reported higher serum levels of morphine in elderly patients as a result of decreased volume of distribution (Berkovitz *et al.*, 1975). Mather and Meffin (1978) have also reported higher concentrations of free drug in elderly patients. In the elderly patient, trait anxiety tends to increase with age, whilst state anxiety decreases, and these have been shown to correlate with postoperative pain (Scott *et al.*, 1983).

Although the cause of increased sensitivity to opioids has not been elucidated, there seems clear agreement that elderly patients obtain effective analgesia for longer periods of time with smaller doses of opioids than young patients.

Table 76.1 Incidence of patients requiring analgesics. (Data from Loan & Dundee, 1967)

Abdominal		Non-abdominal		Thoracic	
Upper	63.2%	Limbs	26.9%	Cardiac	72.5%
Lower	51.3%	Perineal	24.3%	Non-cardiac	74.6%
Inguinal	22.7%	Body wall	20.0%		
		Neck	11.7%		

Psychological factors

Psychological differences between patients may account for much of the variation in response to surgery and also response to opioid analgesics. The psychological factors in postoperative pain have been discussed by Chapman in excellent reviews elsewhere (Chapman, 1985) and in Chapter 75 of this book. In brief, he has classified these factors into two types:

1 Predisposing factors. These consist of personality type, intelligence level, social class and family history.
2 Situational factors.

Amongst the predisposing factors, for personality it has been shown that patients with low pain tolerance demonstrate high scores on anxiety and neuroticism personality scales (Austin *et al.*, 1980a). Furthermore, the studies of Parbrook and colleagues (Parbrook *et al.*, 1973; Boyle & Parbrook, 1977) have shown that there is a correlation between preoperative neuroticism scores and impairment of postoperative vital capacity (VC) and increased incidence of postoperative chest infection.

Anxiety may be considered under two headings: anxiety proneness or trait, and anxiety state (tendency to become anxious in response to circumstances). The study by Scott and colleagues (1983) demonstrated that the level of anxiety state was a linear predictor of postoperative pain.

Of the situational factors involved in the psychological response to surgery, the most important variables comprise the attitudes of the nursing and medical staff, the response of other patients to pain and the ward environment (Dodson, 1985).

Pharmacokinetic factors

There are great variations in the plasma opioid-concentration profile, following intramuscular injection of an opioid. Thus, following the intramuscular administration of pethidine, it has been demonstrated that there may be a two- to five-fold difference in the peak plasma concentrations, and a three- to seven-fold difference in the rate they are attained (Austin *et al.*, 1980a,b) (Fig. 76.1). This variability in response to a standard injection of an opioid is the major reason for the inappropriateness of prescribing intramuscular opioids on a p.r.n. basis.

The pharmacokinetic properties of a drug are usually calculated following changes in blood concentration after an intravenous injection, because of the variability in absorption from an intramuscular injection. The pharmacokinetic parameters of commonly

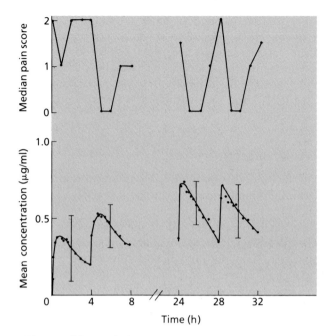

Fig. 76.1 Measured plasma concentration of pethidine (below) and pain score (above) in the postoperative period in response to intramuscular injections of pethidine. Pain score of 0 indicates no pain, while 2 represents very severe pain. (Redrawn from Austin *et al.*, 1980a.)

used opioid drugs are shown in Table 76.3. It may be seen that the pharmacokinetic properties of pethidine, morphine and fentanyl are relatively similar, whilst methadone differs substantially.

In hepatic disease, it has been shown that the β half-life ($t_{\frac{1}{2}}\beta$) of pethidine is approximately doubled because of decreased drug clearance rather than alteration in volume of distribution. Following viral hepatitis, pharmacokinetics may return to normal. It has been shown also that the oral bioavailability of pethidine in cirrhotic patients is increased greatly, although there is relatively little change for morphine or fentanyl (Bentley *et al.*, 1982).

In renal failure, it has been shown that for morphine the terminal half-life ($t_{\frac{1}{2}}\beta$) is the same for patients with end-stage renal failure as it is for normal volunteers (Aitkenhead *et al.*, 1983). However the clearance of one of the active metabolites of morphine, morphine-6-glucuronide, is severely impaired in renal failure and accumulation will occur with repeated administration (McQuay & Moore, 1984). Similarly, the clearance of norpethidine, a metabolite of pethidine and phenoperidine with convulsant actions, is reduced in renal failure and accumulation can result in fitting. Further information on the effect of renal failure on the phar-

Table 76.3 Pharmacokinetic and related data for commonly available opioids

Drug	Intravenous potency ratio	Ionized (%) pH 7.4	Plasma protein binding (%) pH 7.4	$t_{\frac{1}{2}}\alpha$ (min)	$t_{\frac{1}{2}}\beta$ (h)	Clearance (litres/min)	MEAC (ng/ml)
Fentanyl	292	91	83	2.3	2–5	0.8–1.2	1–3
Alfentanil	73	11	91	3	1.3–3.3	0.29	100–300
Sufentanil	4521	80	92	1	2.5	0.73	
Pethidine	0.53	95	65	4.2–11.4	3–7	0.5–1.8	300–650
Morphine	1	76	35	25	1.4–4	0.9–1.5	12–24
Methadone	1	99	85	10	25–45	0.1–0.2	30–70
Buprenorphine	33	91	96	3	2–4.5	1.1–1.5	

macokinetics of opioids can be found in the review of Chan and Matzke (1987).

Age has a marked effect on pharmacokinetic parameters. The half-life of pethidine in humans ($t_{\frac{1}{2}}\beta$) is considerably longer in neonates than in mothers. In patients over 80 years of age, clearance is reduced and the volume of distribution is smaller. Bentley and colleagues (1982) have shown that the $t_{\frac{1}{2}}\beta$ of fentanyl is more than double in elderly patients as a result of decreased drug clearance in the presence of an unchanged volume of distribution. This leads to higher plasma fentanyl concentrations in elderly patients. Other factors causing decreased clearance in elderly patients may be the result of impaired metabolism and/or a decrease in liver blood flow.

Concurrent drug therapy may have a marked effect also on the pharmacokinetics of opioids. Thus, the concomitant administration of phenytoin increases pethidine clearance considerably and reduces the terminal half-life. In contrast with enhanced opioid metabolism produced by phenytoin or phenobarbitone, cimetidine impairs the metabolism of both fentanyl and pethidine. Although cimetidine may decrease liver blood flow, it inhibits Phase I reactions in the liver, notably hepatic oxidative metabolism. Thus, cimetidine impairs the metabolism of both pethidine and fentanyl leading to a prolongation of $t_{\frac{1}{2}}\beta$. Interestingly, cimetidine does not affect morphine metabolism which occurs predominately by glucuronidation, which is not affected by cimetidine.

It has been suggested that under general anaesthesia, a decrease in hepatic blood flow may occur leading to a decrease in clearance. If the volume of distribution is reduced also, then terminal $t_{\frac{1}{2}}\beta$ may remain unchanged as was demonstrated by Mather and colleagues (1975) for patients anaesthetized with halothane.

Other factors affecting pharmacokinetics

Hypothermia leads to hypovolaemia and hypotension resulting in reduced absorption of drugs from injection sites. There is also a reduction in distribution of drug to tissues with reduced blood flow and a tendency to preserve cerebral flow. In addition, hypothermia may lead to a reduction in metabolism causing increased sensitivity to drugs.

In hypothyroidism, metabolism is depressed also, leading to sensitivity to CNS-depressant drugs.

With hyperventilation, there is an increase in pH leading to an alteration in the degree of ionization. For morphine it has been shown that hyperventilation leads to higher concentrations of morphine in the CNS with a slower decline in brain concentration.

Enterohepatic circulation may affect also the pharmacokinetics of several drugs, including pethidine and fentanyl. Both these drugs are excreted in the stomach, and then reabsorbed from the lower gastrointestinal tract, leading to a secondary increase in plasma concentration. Such a mechanism has been alleged to contribute to recurrence of respiratory depression following the administration of fentanyl.

Pharmacodynamic factors

For many years, it was generally held that there was no relationship between the plasma concentration of an opioid and analgesia. This belief stemmed from three reasons:

1 The lack of a suitably sensitive and accurate method for measurement of opioids. This has been corrected by the development of high-pressure liquid chromatography (HPLC) and sensitive radioimmunoassay techniques.

2 As the most common method of pain control was intramuscular injections, there resulted a markedly

fluctuating plasma concentration of opioid with wide interindividual variations (Fig. 76.1).

3 For an individual patient, there is a very steep concentration–response relationship (Fig. 76.2) and the effective plasma concentration associated with analgesia may vary four- to five-fold between individual patients.

With a constant infusion of opioid, depending on the drug, steady-state concentrations are reached eventually, at which receptor–drug concentration is in equilibrium with plasma concentration of the drug. The minimum plasma concentration achieved by this means, at which analgesia is produced, is termed the minimum effective analgesic concentration (MEAC) and values for the commonly available opioids are described in Table 76.3.

The variation of MEAC level between different patients accounts for the widespread variation in drug demand using PCA systems. This varies between 13 and 44 mg/h for pethidine, 30 and 100 µg/h for fentanyl and 0.3 and 9 mg/h for morphine.

Pharmacodynamic variability includes the variability produced by differences in psychological profile (personality, anxiety and neuroticism; see above). A possible link between personality profile and opioid receptor sensitivity is that there may be a variation in endogenous opioid levels in patients of different personality. Lim and colleagues (1983) suggested that 'certain psychological parameters may be related to the ease of activating the endogenous pain suppression system' and by analogy, Tamsen and colleagues have suggested that 'subjective need for analgesics may also be linked to endogenous pain

modulation'. Evidence to support this hypothesis was obtained by Tamsen and colleagues who demonstrated a relationship between concentrations of pethidine in cerebrospinal fluid (CSF) during PCA and the preoperative concentration of endorphins in the CSF (Tamsen *et al.*, 1982c) (Fig. 76.3).

Relationship between plasma drug concentration and analgesic effects

Following the intravenous administration of an opioid, there is a rapid decline in plasma concentration as the drug is redistributed into the volume of distribution (where it is inactive) and also into the biophase, and this is followed by a phase of elimination (Fig. 76.4).

In plasma, opioids are bound to plasma protein, usually by hydrophobic forces, and so the extent of binding is dependent on pH and lipid solubility.

Opioids are weak bases, and thus at physiological pH, they exist in both non-ionized and ionized form. It is only the unbound and non-ionized portion of drug (lipid soluble) which is free to penetrate lipid membranes and this is termed the diffusible fraction. This amounts to 16% of plasma morphine, 2.5% of pethidine and only 1.4% of fentanyl.

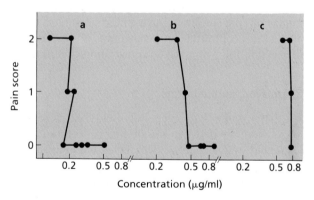

Fig. 76.2 Plasma concentrations of pethidine plotted against pain score for three patients (a, b, c). Note that there is a very steep concentration–response relationship for each patient and that the minimum effective plasma concentration (MEAC) varies four-fold between patients. (Redrawn from Austin *et al.*, 1980a.)

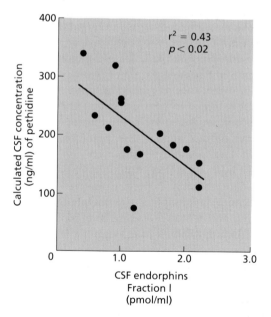

Fig. 76.3 Cerebrospinal fluid concentrations of pethidine in patients during PCA plotted against the patient's preoperative concentration of endorphins in CSF. Note that the higher the resting concentration of endorphin, the lower is the amount of pethidine required in CSF to achieve analgesia. (Redrawn from Tamsen *et al.*, 1982c.)

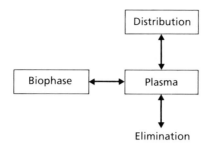

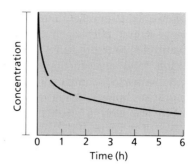

Fig. 76.4 Change in plasma concentration of opioid following bolus intravenous administration. (Redrawn from Hull, 1985.)

The process of diffusion of the opioid from plasma to receptors in the brain is described in Fig. 76.5.

Free base in plasma diffuses through the blood–brain barrier, the extent of diffusion is proportional to the lipid solubility of the drug and the concentration gradient. Within the brain, the extent of binding to receptors depends on receptor affinity and the extent of binding to brain lipid, which is again dependent on lipid solubility.

Thus, for example, morphine possesses a relatively low lipid solubility, resulting in difficult penetration of the blood–brain barrier. However, within the brain, high receptor affinity and low lipid solubility result in a large mass of drug reaching the receptor sites in the biophase (Hull, 1985). In theory, diamorphine which has a higher lipid-solubility than morphine should have a more rapid onset of action. However, this has not been shown to be true under experimental conditions and is probably because it is first converted into the active metabolites which then penetrate the blood–brain barrier.

Physiological effects of pain

The adequate treatment of pain in the postoperative period is important not only from a humanitarian point but also from a physiological aspect. Pain has several detrimental effects, and good pain relief may help to decrease postoperative morbidity.

Cardiovascular system

Pain produces tachycardia and hypertension, leading to an increase in cardiac workload. Although difficult to prove, it is thought that effective pain relief may help to reduce the risk of postoperative myocardial ischaemia or infarction in the high-risk patient.

Pain is often exacerbated by movement and thus will hinder early mobilization postoperatively. Consequently, patients may have a higher risk of developing deep venous thrombosis and subsequent embolic phenomena.

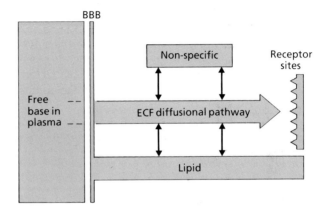

Fig. 76.5 Diagram to describe the diffusion of opioid from plasma to the drug receptors in the brain. BBB, blood–brain barrier; ECF, extracellular fluid. (Redrawn from Hull, 1985.)

Respiratory system

Anaesthesia and surgery are associated with dramatic decreases in functional residual capacity (FRC) resulting in basal atelectasis and the development of pulmonary shunts (Jones et al., 1990). These changes persist into the postoperative period when there is a decrease in tidal volume (V_T), VC and peak expiratory flow rate (PEFR). The deterioration in respiratory function is greater following upper abdominal surgery than lower abdominal or peripheral surgery, and greater after thoracic surgery than abdominal surgery. Postoperative pain hinders patients from coughing effectively and co-operating in chest physiotherapy. It is a common belief that good pain relief reduces the incidence of postoperative pulmonary complications and this has been borne out in practice (Wheatley et al., 1991). Older, obese or patients with respiratory disease are at greater risk of developing complications and should be monitored appropriately in the postoperative period.

Studies examining the effects of different analgesic techniques on postoperative respiratory function have only shown moderate improvements, despite often good pain relief. In a trial comparing two forms of analgesia after open cholecystectomy, excellent pain relief was produced with a thoracic extradural using local anaesthetic and opioid plus systemic indomethacin compared to intermittent intra-muscular opioids (Schulze *et al.*, 1988). However, there was only a small improvement in the peak flows of the extradural group compared to the intra-muscular group (Figs 76.6 and 76.7). These changes cannot be attributed to the effect of a thoracic extra-dural with local anaesthesia on the thoracic cage as studies in volunteers have shown no changes in pulmonary function.

It is probable that the method of pain relief has only a small effect on respiratory parameters post-operatively and that surgical and humoral factors such as an increase in circulating prostaglandins

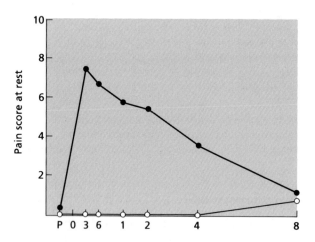

Fig. 76.6 Postoperative pain scores in patients with either conventional intramuscular opioid analgesia (open circles) or extradural local anaesthetic and opioid plus systemic indomethacin (closed circles). (Redrawn from Schulze *et al.*, 1988.)

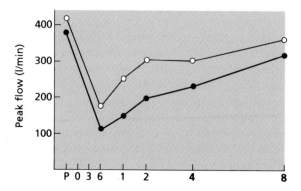

Fig. 76.7 Peak flows in the two groups of patients in Fig. 76.6 showing only a moderate improvement in the extradural group despite excellent analgesia. (Redrawn from Schulze *et al.*, 1988.)

have a significant effect on respiratory function postoperatively.

Gastrointestinal function

Gastrointestinal motility is temporarily impaired after surgery and is due to a combination of surgical and anaesthetic factors. Pain impairs the return of normal gastrointestinal function as do many of the conventional methods of pain relief. Parenteral and extradural opioids decrease gastric emptying whereas it is unaffected by extradural local anaesthetics (Thorén, 1987). A similar effect of parenteral and extradural opioids is seen on colonic motility. For more information readers are referred to the review of Wattwil (1988).

Postoperative mobilization

Adequate analgesia aids early mobilization and several studies have suggested that better analgesia decreases time spent in hospital postoperatively.

Neuroendocrine response

Tissue trauma is associated with a wide range of neuroendocrine changes which are collectively known as the stress response or acute-phase reaction. Clinically, this is recognized as an increase in body temperature, leucocytosis, protein catabolism and negative nitrogen balance. Hyperglycaemia also occurs and there is an overall loss of potassium with sodium and water retention. The magnitude of these changes is generally related to the size of the tissue injury and can be correlated with the increase in acute-phase proteins (e.g. C-reactive protein) after injury.

This endocrine response is activated by nociceptive impulses transmitted along $A\delta$ and C-fibres to the CNS, specifically to the hypothalamopituitary axis. It is also thought that vagal and phrenic afferents may play a small role. This results in an increase of circulating adenocorticotrophic hormone (ACTH), antidiuretic hormone (ADH) and growth hormone and the subsequent release of cortisol and aldosterone from the adrenal cortex. There is also a significant rise in circulating catecholamines due to an increase in sympathetic activity.

It is now apparent that the stress response can be activated and influenced by the release of several cytokines. These polypeptide mediators include interleukin 1 and 6 (IL-1, IL-6), tumour necrosis factor (TNF) and interferons, which are released from a variety of immune cells at the site of injury, and can activate the stress response by acting at various levels of the CNS (Imura, 1991). Other influencing factors include blood loss, nutritional status, cardiovascular changes and concurrent infections and sepsis.

Much debate has been centred on whether this response is of benefit to the modern postoperative patient and many studies have examined the effect of different anaesthetic techniques and postoperative pain relief on their ability to attenuate the response and decrease perioperative mortality (Yeager et al., 1987).

Following abdominal surgery, there is a marked increase in plasma cortisol in patients who receive systemic opioids. However, with an effective high extradural block, there may be no change in plasma cortisol compared with the preoperative baseline values. In contrast, extradural morphine which may produce better analgesia than extradural local analgesia is associated with intermediate levels of plasma cortisol in the postoperative period (Fig. 76.8).

Similar changes are seen with regard to the effects of local anaesthetic subarachnoid block and extradural morphine on sympathoadrenal responses. Figures 76.9 and 76.10 illustrate changes in plasma

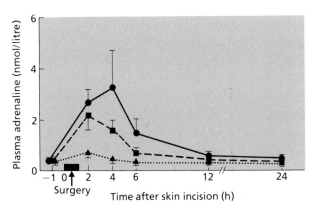

Fig. 76.9 Changes in plasma concentrations of adrenaline in patients following cholecystectomy. ● General anaesthesia; ■ general anaesthesia and extradural morphine; ▲ general anaesthesia and extradural local anaesthesia. Note that block of efferent fibres to the adrenals (T8–L1) inhibits the increase in adrenaline which occurs with general anaesthesia, whilst extradural opioid is associated with intermediate levels of catecholamines but optimal postoperative analgesia. (Redrawn from Rutberg et al., 1984.)

catecholamines following cholecystectomy. In patients receiving intramuscular morphine for postoperative analgesia, there is marked increase in both adrenaline and noradrenaline plasma concentrations,

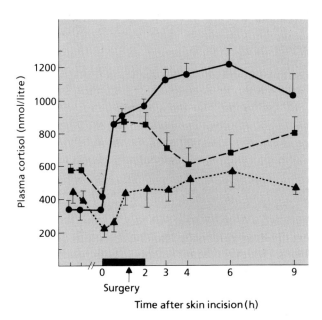

Fig. 76.8 Changes in plasma cortisol in patients during operation (0–2 h) and the postoperative period (2–9 h). ● General anaesthesia with systemic opioids (N = 12); ■ general anaesthesia followed by extradural morphine (N = 12); ▲ high extradural block with local anaesthetics both intra- and postoperatively (N = 12). (Redrawn from Christenson et al., 1982.)

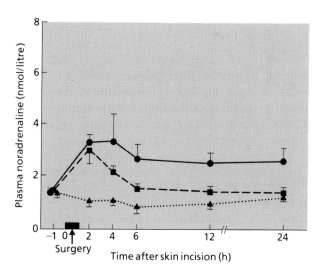

Fig. 76.10 Changes in plasma concentrations of noradrenaline in patients following cholecystectomy. ● General anaesthesia; ■ general anaesthesia and extradural morphine; ▲ general anaesthesia and extradural local anaesthesia. Note that block of efferent fibres to the adrenals (T8–L1) inhibits the increase in noradrenaline which occurs with general anaesthesia, whilst extradural opioid is associated with intermediate levels of catecholamines but optimal postoperative analgesia. (Redrawn from Rutberg et al., 1984.)

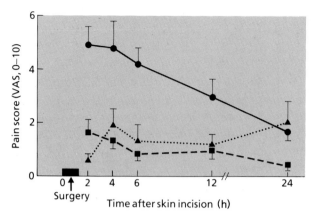

Fig. 76.11 Changes in pain score (visual analogue scale, VAS) in patients following cholecystectomy. ● General anaesthesia; ■ general anaesthesia and extradural morphine; ▲ general anaesthesia and extradural local anaesthesia. Note that extradural morphine produces optimum analgesia followed by extradural local anaesthesia followed by intramuscular morphine. (Redrawn from Rutberg *et al.*, 1984.)

whilst those patients receiving high extradural block with local anaesthetic exhibited very little change in catecholamine concentrations. In contrast, those with extradural morphine exhibited intermediate levels of catecholamines. Despite this, the quality of analgesia was best with extradural morphine (Fig. 76.11).

Combined extradural and general anaesthesia has been shown to be no better in inhibiting IL-6 and TNF release during and after major abdominal surgery compared with general anaesthesia alone (Naito *et al.*, 1992). This is probably due to the failure of dense neural block to inhibit the peripheral release of cytokine mediators which activate the neuro-humoral response via a blood-borne pathway.

However, the magnitude of the stress response is less after peripheral and lower abdominal surgery compared with upper abdominal and thoracic surgery if extradural analgesia is used.

Addition of a NSAID to analgesic regimens has also been ineffective in inhibiting the stress response (Claeys *et al.*, 1992). High-dose methylprednisolone in combination with dense spinal block and a non-steroidal analgesic has been shown to inhibit the increase in acute-phase-reaction proteins after major surgery and provide extremely effective analgesia (Schulze *et al.*, 1992). The mechanism by which steroids exert this effect is by their anti-inflammatory effects and decreased prostaglandin synthesis; how-ever, there was no effect on the IL-6 response in this study.

Table 76.4 Methods of treating postoperative pain

Conventional administration of opioid
Intramuscular on-demand bolus

Opioid agonist/antagonist drugs

Parenteral administration of opioid
Bolus intravenous administration
Continuous intravenous infusion
Patient-controlled analgesia
   Bolus   } intravenous/intramuscular/
   Bolus + infusion } subcutaneous/extradural

Non-parenteral administration of opioid
Buccal/sublingual
Oral
Rectal
Transdermal
Nasal
Inhalation
Intra-articular opioids

Local anaesthetic techniques

Spinal/extradural opioids

Non-steroidal anti-inflammatory drugs (NSAIDs)

α_2-adrenergic agonists
Systemically
Extradurally

Non-pharmacological methods
Cryotherapy
Transcutaneous electrical nerve stimulation (TENS)
Acupuncture
Psychological methods

Whether the use of regional anaesthesia and anal-gesia improves survival in the high-risk patient remains controversial. Dense extradural block may improve postoperative mortality in high-risk patients having lower-abdominal and limb surgery by inhibit-ing the stress response to some extent (Scott & Kehlet, 1988). However, improvements in pain relief and the modification of the stress response after more major surgery and their effects on morbidity and mortality are controversial.

It would appear that excellent pain relief is possible after major operations even without total suppression of the stress response. Readers are referred to the reviews of Kehlet (1989) and Desborough and Hall (1990) for further information.

Methods of treating postoperative pain
(Table 76.4)

Conventional administration of opioids

The failings inherent in the conventional method of administration of opioids by the injection of intramuscular boluses on demand by the patient have been detailed above. In essence, this technique fails to deliver optimum analgesia for many patients as it results in fluctuating plasma concentrations of opioid. In some patients, the troughs are associated with lack of analgesia, and in some the peaks may be associated with unacceptable side-effects such as nausea, vomiting and respiratory depression.

One of the more simple ways of overcoming the problem of inadequate analgesia is to administer opioids on a regular 4-hourly basis. This has been undertaken in several studies resulting in a quality of analgesia approaching that which may be obtained by the use of PCA (Ellis *et al.*, 1982). As an alternative to regular 4-hourly injections of intramuscular opioids, the use of treatment algorithms have been shown to be a more effective way of improving pain relief (Ghould *et al.*, 1992). These charts, in the form of a flow diagram, rely on the regular assessment of the patients degree of pain and side-effects and may allow the administration of very frequent opioids.

Another technique which has been promoted vigorously by the pharmaceutical industry, is the development of opioid drugs which may possess analgesic properties comparable with morphine but with fewer side-effects. This would permit the administration of drugs on a regular basis, resulting in improved analgesia without the development of respiratory depression.

The opioid drugs produce most of their actions by binding with opioid receptors which are now classified into three subtypes: μ, δ and κ. Other receptors have been described including σ- and ϵ-receptors but it is now known that the σ-receptor is not a pure opioid receptor and the ϵ-receptor is thought to be unimportant. Other drugs, including phencyclidine, work via the σ-receptor and some of newer opioids including pentazocine, cyclazocine and nalorphine can produce marked dysphoric reactions by binding to this receptor. The existence of several μ-, δ- and κ-subtypes (e.g. the μ_2-receptor producing respiratory depression) has been suggested on the basis of laboratory investigations, but they are of no clinical significance at present.

Newer synthetic opioids

The newer synthetic opioids are described elsewhere, but for completeness, a list of agents which have been used for postoperative pain is shown in Table 76.5 with an indication of activity at various opioid receptors. The effect of stimulating such receptors is described in Table 76.6.

Table 76.5 Opioid agonist and agonist/antagonist drugs

	μ	δ	κ	σ
Pure agonists				
Morphine	Agonist	Agonist	Agonist	No activity
Codeine	Agonist	Agonist	Agonist	No activity
Pethidine	Agonist	Agonist	Agonist	No activity
Fentanyl	Agonist	Agonist	No activity	No activity
Partial agonists				
Buprenorphine	Partial agonist	No activity	No activity	No activity
Profadol	Partial agonist	No activity	No activity	No activity
Propiram	Partial agonist	No activity	No activity	No activity
Meptazinol	Partial agonist	No activity	No activity	No activity
Agonists/antagonist				
Pentazocine	Antagonist	Agonist	Agonist	Agonist
Cyclazocine	Antagonist	Agonist	Agonist	Agonist
Nalorphine	Antagonist	Partial agonist	Partial agonist	Agonist
Antagonists				
Naloxone	Antagonist	Antagonist	Antagonist	No activity
Naltrexone	Antagonist	Antagonist	Antagonist	No activity

Table 76.6 Opioid receptor subtypes

	Receptor		
	μ/δ	κ	σ
Analgesia	Supraspinal/spinal	Spinal	——
Respiratory depression	++	+	——
Pupil	Constriction	——	Dilatation
Gastrointestinal motility	Reduced	——	——
Smooth muscle spasm	++	——	——
Behaviour	Euphoria ++	Dysphoria	Dysphoria ++
	Sedation ++	Sedation +	Psychotomimetic
Physical dependence	++	+	——

Many of the partial agonist and agonist/antagonist opioid drugs have been assessed in studies examining their efficacy in postoperative pain. However, for those with a marked ceiling effect to respiratory depression, analgesia has usually been found to be inadequate for severe types of postoperative pain. No drug has been found to produce superior analgesia to morphine.

Of the opioid agonist/antagonist drugs, buprenorphine is perhaps one of the most useful as it may be administered by the sublingual route. Using this route it has been shown that satisfactory analgesia may be produced for both upper- and lower-abdominal surgery (Ellis et al., 1982). The major disadvantage of this agent is a considerable degree of sedation which may be undesirable where it is hoped to mobilize patients as soon as possible after surgery.

Reversal of the effects of partial agonist opioids

Pure agonist drugs, such as morphine, pethidine and fentanyl, are considered to be μ-selective but with significant activity on the δ- and κ-receptors. The receptor specificity of the pure opioid antagonist, naloxone, mirrors this profile closely. Thus, all the effects of the agonists are readily reversed by naloxone in a dose-dependent manner typical of competitive antagonism. It should be remembered, however, that the duration of action of a single intravenous dose of naloxone is only approximately 20 min. Repeated doses or a continuous infusion may be necessary when high doses of a long-acting agonist have been administered.

Naltrexone and nalmefene are two new opioid antagonists acting at μ-, δ- and κ-receptors. Both can be given parenterally and naltrexone can also be given orally. Both are considerably longer acting than naloxone. Naltrexone is active for up to 24 h after a single oral dose and has been used to reduce pruritus, nausea and vomiting after extradural opioids.

The situation with partial agonist drugs is somewhat more complex. Typically, they have agonist properties on some of the opioid receptor types but are antagonists on others (Table 76.5). In general, reversal of effect demands the use of a pure antagonist. Morphine in contrast, can be reversed with partial agonists with strong antagonistic properties such as nalorphine.

Thus, pentazocine, butorphanol, meptazinol and nalbuphine may all be antagonized with naloxone despite their differing receptor specificities. Buprenorphine, however, has the property of very slow rate of dissociation from the receptor and is not reversed reliably by naloxone.

The respiratory stimulant doxapram has been used to reverse persisting respiratory depression after general anaesthesia. Its mechanism of action is not entirely clear but is probably due to actions at both central and peripheral chemoreceptors. Other unwanted effects, which appear to be dose related, include tachycardia, hypertension anxiety and intense perineal warmth. Doxapram can be given as an intravenous bolus 0.5−1.5 mg/kg over 30 s or more to produce an increase in ventilation, but its effects are short lived due to its rapid clearance. Therefore an infusion of between 2 and $4 \, mg \cdot kg^{-1} \cdot h^{-1}$ can be used to provide longer-term reversal of respiratory depression.

Several studies have suggested that single doses of doxapram given at the end of anaesthesia may reduce the incidence of postoperative pulmonary complications though the evidence for this is far from conclusive. However, repeated infusions given on subsequent postoperative days may prove to be of some benefit.

Newer parenteral methods of administering opioids

From the discussion on p. 1574, it is clear that in order to obtain effective analgesia the purpose of administering opioids parenterally should be to provide a steady-state plasma concentration of opioid at a level equivalent to the MEAC. However, as the MEAC varies widely between different patients, it is not possible to define the dosage regimen required in advance of assessing an individual's opioid sensitivity. With the bolus and continuous intravenous infusion techniques, assessment of the patient's requirements is in the hands of the observer, nurse or medical attendant. With PCA, a servofeedback loop is produced whereby the patient controls his/her own level of plasma opioid concentration.

Bolus intravenous administration

For many years, it has been common practice to administer small intravenous boluses of opioid in the recovery room to produce analgesia in patients immediately following anaesthesia and surgery. An extension of this practice, which may be undertaken in high-dependency nursing units, is to prescribe small intravenous doses of opioid to be given when necessary by nursing staff in the later postoperative period. Provided that there is a 1 : 1 nursing : patient ratio to detect respiratory depression, this technique may be acceptable. However, it does produce widely fluctuating plasma concentrations of opioid and the advantages of the intravenous infusion and PCA techniques in that these fluctuations are reduced to a certain extent.

Continuous intravenous infusion strategy

Various authors have attempted to assess the patient's opioid requirements by means of small intravenous boluses until adequate analgesia is achieved, and prescribed arbitrarily a fixed continuous intravenous rate dependent upon the initial quantity of opioid administered. Thus, Rutter and colleagues (1980) assessed the initial titration dose and then prescribed 3.5 times this dose over 72 h. Saha (1981) administered papaveretum at a rate of 1 mg/min until analgesia was achieved, and then continued the infusion for 40–50 h at a rate of 1 mg/h, reducing to 0.83 mg/h after 24 h (allowing some flexibility in these rates). Catling and colleagues (1980) achieved analgesia in a similar manner and then gave an infusion of four times the initial analgesic dose per 24 h.

There are various problems associated with this technique, the most important of which is the possibility of inducing respiratory depression. Catling and colleagues (1980) observed in the first 24 h episodes of apnoea associated with significant arterial desaturation. In addition, patients may notice inadequate analgesia on day 1 for reasons that are explained in Fig. 76.12. This shows that the bolus-plus-infusion technique leads to inadequate plasma concentrations of opioid in the early period. In order to prevent this early subanalgesic concentration, it is necessary to fill the central compartment and follow this by a maintenance infusion rate equivalent to the rate of elimination of the opioid. However, it may be seen from this theoretical analysis that the initial bolus has to be so large as to produce very high plasma concentrations, which would lead undoubtedly to apnoea.

More complicated infusion regimens have been devised in order to approach rapidly and then maintain a steady-state plasma concentration in the region of the MEAC level. For further information on this complex topic, the reader is referred to the publications by Stapleton and colleagues (1979), Austin and colleagues (1981) and Hull (1985).

The problems inherent in intravenous infusion techniques based on observer control, notably respiratory depression, are so inherently dangerous in the authors' view that such techniques must be confined to patients observed closely in a high dependency nursing area or the intensive therapy unit.

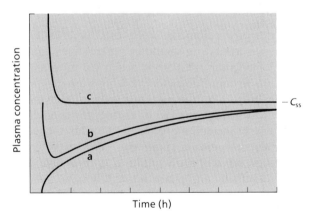

Fig. 76.12 Plasma concentrations of opioid produced by three techniques: (a) following a fixed rate of infusion; (b) after a bolus followed by same infusion rate; (c) after a bolus designed to fill the volume of distribution followed by the same infusion rate which is identical to the rate of elimination. Note that (a) and (b) may be associated with inadequate levels of opioid in the early period, whilst (c) is associated with an extremely high plasma concentration. C_{ss}, steady-state plasma concentration. (Redrawn from Hull, 1985.)

Patient-controlled analgesia

The concept of PCA was first introduced in 1968 by Sechzer when investigating the analgesic response to small intravenous increments of opioid given on patient demand by a nurse observer. It was soon realized that individual requirements for opioids differed considerably but for any one patient were relatively constant. Therefore a system was designed whereby patients could administer their own intravenous pain relief and so titrate the dose to their own 'end-point' of adequate analgesia. A feedback loop is therefore established whereby the patient experiences pain, self-administers a bolus of analgesic and experiences the benefits of their action. They can therefore assess the severity of their pain and adjust the level of analgesia as required. In theory, side-effects should be less, as the plasma level of analgesic will be relatively constant using small intravenous increments, and therefore sudden increases with associated side-effects are avoided (Fig. 76.13).

To establish successful and safe analgesia with PCA requires that the patient fully understands the principal behind the technique. This involves a pre-operative visit explaining when and how to deliver a bolus of pain killer. Next, the choice of drug must be made and a number of parameters set, including the size of bolus dose, the minimum time between boluses (lockout period), maximum dose allowed and whether to provide a background infusion.

Choice of drug

Almost every opioid has been used with PCA. In theory the ideal drug should be potent, have a rapid onset, moderate duration of action (to prevent the need for frequent demands) and have a high therapeutic index. No drug has been shown to have any particular advantages with regard to quality of analgesia or incidence of side-effects. Choice usually depends on personal preference and experience. However, for any one institute it is preferable that medical nursing and pharmacy staff become familiar with one or two drugs with standardized regimens. In the UK morphine is the most popular drug of choice.

Loading dose

To achieve analgesia in the initial postoperative period requires establishing a plasma level of analgesic equal to the minimum effective analgesic concentration. This usually requires a substantial

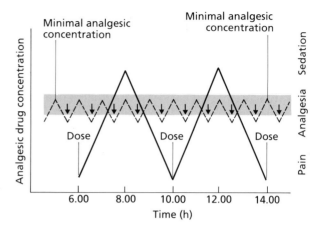

Fig. 76.13 Theoretical relation between analgesic drug concentration, dosing interval, and clinical response for PCA (----) and intramuscular opioid (——). Arrows pointing downwards represent administration of patient-controlled or intramuscular opioid doses. (Data from Ferrante *et al.*, 1988.)

dose of opioid over a relatively short period of time and would be difficult to obtain with the smaller demand dose restricted by the lockout period. Several PCA devices can be programmed to deliver a bolus dose on the first analgesic demand. Empirically, this can be calculated from an estimate of the required plasma concentration and initial volume of distribution; however, this will rapidly redistribute from the central compartment leading to early frequent demands. To overcome this problem, a loading dose infused over a period of time has been suggested to allow for initial redistribution. Both these methods use technical formulae and assume a known MEAC and normal pharmacokinetics in the postoperative patient. A more practical method is to give regular small increments of analgesic in the recovery room until a satisfactory pain relief is established. Subsequently, the patient can then use the PCA device to maintain analgesia.

Demand dose

The size of the demand dose is critical to the success of PCA. The patient must appreciate an improvement in analgesia after each request, otherwise confidence in the system will be lost. Too large a dose produces unwanted side-effects and the system is intolerable or dangerous. For morphine, the ideal demand dose after major abdominal surgery has been estimated to be 1 mg (Owen *et al.*, 1989a). However, with any system regular review and adjustment of dosage may be required to optimize pain relief.

Most demand doses are given as a rapid bolus but

the use of a short infusion has been advocated to avoid sudden peaks in plasma concentration. Experience with alfentanil using demand infusions failed to show any benefits (Owen et al., 1990).

Lockout interval

The aim of the lockout interval is to prevent over-administration of drug and subsequent overdosage. In theory, it should be long enough to allow the previous demand dose to have taken effect. In practice, most opioids have very similar onset times and usually intervals are between 5 and 10 min.

Background infusion

In theory, a background infusion of analgesic should create a buffer to prevent large dips in the plasma concentration of opioid and therefore reduce the number of patient demands to maintain MEAC. This has not been borne out in practice and it is found that patients make the same number of requests either with or without a background infusion (Owen, 1989b). As the analgesic requirements decrease with time postoperatively, a steady-state infusion can increase the risk of side-effects. In an effort to overcome this problem the original on-demand analgesic computer (ODAC) delivered a variable background infusion calculated from the previous hours' total demand dose. This device is no longer commercially available and whether this variable will be incorporated into future designs remains to be seen.

Maximum dose

Many devices can be programmed to limit the maximum dose of opioid that can be delivered at a certain time. This is intended as a safety feature to prevent overdosage. However, it is more logical to accept that patients' analgesic requirements vary considerably and some may require very large amounts to achieve adequate analgesia.

Clinical use

Intravenous PCA is now a standard method of postoperative pain relief in many hospitals. The commonest route of administration is intravenous although the intramuscular, subcutaneous and extradural routes have been used. Despite claims to the contrary, it is generally accepted that intravenous opioid administration using PCA provides better quality pain relief compared with intermittent opioids on a p.r.n. basis. Many controlled trials have shown that intermittent intramuscular opioids can provide good quality postoperative analgesia but most patients prefer and would recommend PCA compared with intramuscular opioids.

Patients using PCA usually titrate their analgesia to a point where they are comfortable rather than totally pain free. The reasons for this are not entirely clear, though many patients expect some pain after surgery or are frightened about possible over-dosage. Although PCA confers a sense of control and autonomy, patients may still feel that personal contact with members of staff is important (Kluger & Owen, 1990).

Patterns of analgesic administration with PCA show that in the initial postoperative period, demands are frequent but then decrease with time. Also, the total analgesic use varies considerably between patients for similar operations, though on the whole opioid use is less with PCA. The incidence of side-effects with PCA opioids is very similar to those experienced with intramuscular injections. The incidence of severe respiratory depression is rare, although has occurred due to incorrect programming or device malfunction.

Several guidelines should be followed to ensure safe and effective use of PCA. Both the patient and the attending staff should understand the principle of the technique. The devices should be tamperproof and demands should only be made by the patient. For regular use on a ward, the number of drugs used and regimens prescribed should be kept to a minimum to avoid staff confusion. Prefilled syringes should ideally be supplied by the pharmacy.

It is important that the pump is connected to an intravenous cannula through a one-way valve to prevent increments of opioid collecting in a giving set which may then be delivered as a large bolus at a later time with possible serious side-effects.

Devices used in patient-controlled analgesia

The first commercially available PCA devices were the Cardiff Palliator and the Janssen ODAC. These have subsequently been replaced by a range of pumps which although identical in principle have increased in sophistication in their programmable parameters.

Most have the standard safety features, including a lock to prevent unauthorized change of dosing parameters or theft of controlled drug. Some pumps are limited by the reservoir size, whereas others can accept several syringe sizes. Other pumps use larger intravenous fluid bags as the drug reservoir which obviously reduces the number of times the pump requires refilling. These sets are also useful if a background infusion is used. Most devices give an audible signal when a successful demand has been given. This has been shown to increase patient satisfaction and reduce anxiety rather than no signal or one every time a demand, either successful or not, is made. Most devices have a continuous display of the set dose, lockout time, number of demands and total dose given and some have the facility to download this information to a printer or computer.

The original ODAC incorporated a respiratory-rate monitor and the pump would not deliver a demand dose if the rate was below a preset limit. Some newer devices can incorporate this function, although respiratory rate is an unreliable measure of respiratory depression.

In addition to the microprocessor-controlled pumps there are now two disposable PCA systems — Baxter and Vygon. Both deliver a preset bolus volume of 0.5 ml so the dose of drug delivered is dependent on the concentration. The Baxter pump has a fixed lockout time of 6 or 15 min, depending on the reservoir used, and the Vygon pump is restricted to a lockout of 5 or 20 min.

In clinical use, the Baxter pump has proved as effective as the more sophisticated devices in controlling postoperative pain. A summary of the available pumps is contained in Table 76.7.

Non-parenteral administration of opioids

Oral administration

The oral route of administration of drugs is the most widely used for all types of medication and most acceptable to the patient. However, apart from minor ambulatory surgery and in the late postoperative period following inpatient surgery, the oral route of administration of opioid analgesics possesses major disadvantages.

1 Absorption occurs from the small intestine and

Table 76.7 Apparatus available for patient-controlled analgesia

Apparatus	Infusion mode	Special features	Reservoir size
Harvard PCA (Bard)	PCA ± background	External printer option LCD display Mains and battery	60 ml syringe only
Harvard PCA1 (Bard)	PCA ± background	LCD display Mains and battery	60 ml syringe only
Bard Ambulatory PCA	PCA ± background	LCD display Battery only Portable	250 ml infusion bag
Graseby PCA	PCA ± background	LCD display Mains and battery	60 ml syringe only
Graseby PCA 3300	PCA ± background	Optional respiratory rate/ SpO_2 monitor LCD display Mains and battery	20, 30, 50 or 60 ml syringes
Abbot Life Provider	PCA ± background	Battery only Portable LCD display	Infusion bags
Abbot Lifecare 4200	PCA ± background	LCD display Mains and battery Printer option	30 ml syringe only
Baxter Travenol (disposable)	PCA only	Lightweight, portable	60 ml
Vygon (disposable)	PCA only	Lightweight, portable	Infusion bag
IVAC	PCA ± background	LCD display Battery only	50 ml syringe only

following surgery there is frequently delay in gastric emptying. Not only does the administration of oral drugs in this situation lead to non-absorption, but there is a danger of dumping a large bolus of drug into the small intestine when gastric motility resumes, leading to the possibility of overdosage. The absorption of morphine sulphate (MST) from the gastrointestinal tract is delayed for 24 h following abdominal surgery. This is illustrated in Fig. 76.14. Thus, MST is *not* recommended for use in the first 24 h following surgery.

2 Oral administration of drugs may be prevented by nausea and vomiting which are common accompaniments of anaesthesia and surgery.

3 Oral administration of opioids leads to metabolism in the gut wall and also in the liver (first-pass metabolism). Thus, the bioavailability of opioids is reduced greatly. Oral bioavailability ratios for commonly available opioids are shown in Table 76.8.

It is concluded, therefore, that the oral route is unsuitable for administration of strong opioids to patients in the early postoperative period, despite the fact that several reports have indicated that satisfactory analgesia may be achieved using this route.

When the need for strong analgesia has decreased however, after 1, 2 or 3 days following surgery, it is common practice to prescribe a mild opioid (such as codeine, dihydrocodeine or dextropopoxyphene), or one of the minor analgesic agents such as acetylsalicylic acid or one of the large number of non-steroidal drugs available. Many of these drugs have been shown to be quite effective after minor orthopaedic surgery.

Sublingual route

The sublingual route possesses two important safety

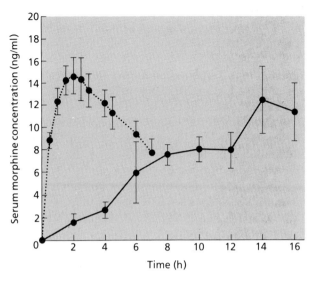

Fig. 76.14 Plasma concentrations of morphine following single administration of MST 20 mg to volunteers (dotted line) and also following regular 4-hourly administration of MST 20 mg to patients following peripheral vascular surgery (solid line). Note that there is a marked delay in the absorption of morphine in patients, and that the peak concentration attained by 16 h is relatively low. (Redrawn from Pinnock *et al.*, 1986.)

features compared with the oral route of administration. Firstly, the tablet may be removed from the mouth in the event of overdosage, and second, for drugs with a high first-pass metabolism, accidental swallowing of tablets does not result in toxicity. The disadvantages of the sublingual route relate to patient tolerance, and absorption may be effected by the rate of production of saliva, chewing or sucking.

The major advantage of the sublingual route is that absorption occurs directly into the systemic circulation and there is no first-pass metabolism (De Boer *et al.*, 1984).

Table 76.8 Oral/parenteral bioavailability ratios of some commonly available opioid drugs. (Data from Hanning, 1985)

Drug	Onset of action (min)	Peak action (min)	Duration of action (h)	Oral/parenteral bioavailability	Oral dose equal to 10 mg morphine intramuscularly (mg)
Morphine	60	60–90	4–5	0.17–0.33	60
MST	60	180	8	0.18	20
Hydromorphone	15–30	30	4–5	0.2	7.5
Pethidine	40–60	60–120	2–4	0.25–0.71	300
Levorphanol	20–60	60–120	8–14	0.5–1.0	4
Methadone	30–60	30–120	4–8	0.45	20
Pentazocine	40–60	60–180	3–4	0.25–0.3	180
Buprenorphine	60–120	120–240	6–8	0.1	4
Meptazinol	60–120	180	5–6	0.2	300
Nefopam	30–60	60–180	6–8	0.3	90

The drug that has been most commonly used by this route for postoperative pain is sublingual buprenorphine, which has a sublingual/parenteral bioavailability of approximately 30%, which is far greater than by the oral route. Thus, swallowing results in considerable deactivation of the tablet and lessens any possibility of toxicity.

Absorption of sublingual buprenorphine is relatively rapid, and blood concentrations 3 h after administration are similar following sublingual and parenteral administration.

Sublingual buprenorphine (as 0.4 mg on a regular 6-hourly basis) has been used successfully as the sole analgesic for major abdominal surgery and it has been shown to produce analgesia comparable with that following PCA with pethidine or regular 4-hourly intramuscular morphine. The major disadvantages of buprenorphine are a relatively high degree of sedation and nausea (Ellis et al., 1982) and its taste.

Rectal route

The rectal route possesses the following advantages:
1 Absorption from the lower part of the rectum bypasses first-pass metabolism, although in the upper part, absorption through the superior rectal vein leads to first-pass metabolism. In general, therefore, bioavailability is higher than that following the oral route although there may be considerable interindividual variations depending on the siting of the suppository in the rectum.
2 Absorption is unaffected by gastric emptying, nausea and vomiting, and administration may be discontinued by removal of the suppository.

The major disadvantages are that the rate of onset of analgesia is slow, and aesthetic considerations render the technique relatively unpopular in the UK and North America.

The rectal route of administration has been used with sustained-release preparations impregnated with morphine, and it has been suggested that this may be a suitable technique for maintainance of relatively low levels of analgesia, i.e. it might be useful for producing a low sustained plasma concentration of morphine, which may be augmented by further systemic administration (Hanning et al., 1988).

Transdermal opioids

Topically applied opioids can be absorbed transdermally into the systemic circulation and therefore provide analgesia. The rate of absorption is dependent on the degree of lipid solubility of individual drugs and skin perfusion. Fentanyl patches delivering 100 μg/h have been shown to produce equivalent plasma concentration as an intravenous infusion delivering the same dose but obviously require an intravenous loading dose to achieve a sufficiently high initial plasma concentration (Duthrie et al., 1988). However, such patches do not deliver enough fentanyl to provide adequate analgesia after upper-abdominal surgery but do reduce opioid requirements given by other routes (Rowbotham et al., 1989). Drug absorption is also decreased if skin perfusion is reduced due to hypovolaemia, hypotension or hypothermia.

Other drugs given by this route include morphine, which has a slower absorption due to its lower lipid solubility. However, the rate of absorption can be increased by the application of a small electric current across the skin in a process termed iontophoresis.

Inhaled opioids

The lungs provide a large surface area over which drugs can be rapidly absorbed. Fentanyl and morphine have been given as nebulized solutions to achieve pain relief postoperatively (Worsley et al., 1990). The bioavailability of nebulized opioids is considerably smaller than when given by other routes as some drug is lost on exhalation, or adheres to the apparatus. However, despite relatively low plasma levels, compared with those after intravenous administration, satisfactory analgesia can be obtained and it may be that the mode of action of opioids given by this route differs from that produced by more conventional means.

Intra-articular opioids

Following injury, peripheral opioid receptors can be found in nociceptor nerve endings in inflamed tissue. On the basis of this finding, several studies have shown the benefits of intra-articular morphine in reducing pain and conventional opioid requirements after arthroscopic and open-knee surgery (Joshi et al., 1993). The doses given in these trials have been relatively small (1−5 mg) and the analgesic effects cannot be attributed to significant plasma levels (Stein et al., 1991). Using this method, significant analgesia has lasted up to 2 days postoperatively. Whether this technique can be used for other joint surgery remains to be seen.

Intranasal opioids

Fentanyl and butorphanol have been given by a metered nasal spray to provide rapid-onset analgesia postoperatively (Striebel *et al.*, 1992). This is a relatively simple and effective means of providing analgesia due to the rapid uptake of these lipid-soluble opioids across the nasal mucosa. Potential developments in this area include PCA using nasal opioids in an aerosol capable of delivering metered doses with a predetermined lockout period.

Local anaesthetic techniques (Table 76.9)

Since the publication of the first edition of this book there has been increased enthusiasm for the use of somatic nerve blocks to provide postoperative analgesia. Using bupivacaine, useful postoperative analgesia may be produced for 8–12 h following injection. A single administration is particularly useful for outpatient anaesthesia, especially in children.

In paediatric practice it is now common to administer a local anaesthetic somatic nerve block, or extradural block, after induction of anaesthesia. The type

Table 76.9 Local anaesthetic techniques used for postoperative pain relief

Upper extremity
Axillary brachial plexus block
Interscalene or supraclavicular block
Individual nerve blocks

Lower extremity
Femoral nerve block
Sciatic nerve block
Femoral/sciatic/obturator 'three-in-one block'
Psoas compartment block
Caudal

Thoracic
Extradural
Intercostal
Interpleural

Abdominal
Extradural
Intercostal
Interpleural
Rectus sheath block
Mesosalpinx block
Intraperitoneal

Penis
Caudal
Penile block

of blocks which are particularly useful in paediatric day-case surgery include:
1 Ilioinguinal block (for herniotomy and orchidopexy).
2 Penile dorsal nerve block (for circumcision).
3 Caudal block (for lower-abdominal and lower-limb surgery).

For further information on postoperative pain relief and the use of local anaesthetic blocks in the paediatric population the reader is referred to Chapter 77.

In adults, 'single-shot' somatic nerve blocks with bupivacaine are used frequently to provide postoperative analgesia for 8–12 h, by brachial plexus block for upper-limb surgery, caudal block for haemorrhoidectomy and intercostal nerve blocks for thoracotomy or cholecystectomy.

Whilst these techniques may provide excellent analgesia after surgery, it is only for a relatively short time and further prolongation of analgesia is required in the majority of patients. One of three approaches may be used to achieve this end:
1 Prolongation of the local anaesthetic agent — the duration of action of local anaesthetic agents can be prolonged by addition of adrenaline. However, overall increase in duration varies between individual local anaesthetics and the route by which they are given. Ropivacaine is a new amide local anaesthetic agent with more vasoconstrictor activity than bupivacaine and may provide longer-lasting anaesthesia.
2 Repeated somatic nerve block.
3 Placing a catheter close to the nerves which require block.

Catheter techniques

Insertion of catheters for prolonged anaesthesia has been advocated for the following situations:

Axillary blocks. It has been suggested that a catheter is placed into the brachial plexus sheath following identification by use of either a nerve stimulator or tactile perception of penetration of the sheath. Initial doses administered through the catheter are similar to those using a single-injection technique (40–50 ml) and repeated doses use slightly smaller volumes. The problems of this technique include systemic toxicity, nerve injury, haematoma (all very small) and a relatively high incidence of kinking of the catheter.

Interscalene and supraclavicular perivascular blocks. Several authors have described the insertion of catheters into the brachial plexus sheath via the supraclavicular or interscalene route. Intermittent injections of 20–30 ml of bupivacaine 0.25% are administered at 6–8-hourly intervals.

Intercostal nerve blocks can be achieved by several techniques:
1 Useful analgesia has been demonstrated after thoracotomies using a catheter placed intraoperatively in an extrapleural pocket over several costovertebral joints. Local anaesthetics injected then block the underlying intercostal nerves (Sabanaythan *et al.*, 1990).
2 Although techniques have been described for placing cannulae percutaneously into intercostal nerve spaces, such techniques have not superseded that of intermittent administration of intercostal nerve blocks.

For upper paramedian incisions, intercostal bilateral blocks from T5 to T11 are necessary and, because the major complication of intercostal nerve block is pneumothorax, such a technique is not advocated. However, for subcostal incision, unilateral block of T5 to T11 is required.

Interpleural block. This block involves injecting a relatively large volume of local anaesthetic between the visceral and parietal pleura. The anaesthetic solution has been shown to spread over the surface of the lung and produces a rapid-onset block of many intercostal nerves. Several techniques have been described to identify the potential space between the two layers of pleura and most use the principle of a hanging-drop method, similar to that used to identify the extradural space. By using an indwelling catheter, repeat injections can be given thereby increasing the length of analgesia (Lee *et al.*, 1990). This form of analgesia is particularly effective for providing unilateral anaesthesia over the chest wall, abdomen and flanks and has been successfully used after mastectomies, cholocystectomies and nephrectomies. Potential hazards include lung trauma and pneumothorax and local anaesthetic toxicity due to rapid absorption from the interpleural space.

Paravertebral block. This technique is a useful alternative to multiple intercostal blocks because it requires only a single injection of 15 ml of bupivacaine to block up to four intercostal nerves. Spread of local anaesthetic solution into the extradural space is possible with this technique with subsequent extradural block.

Femoral nerve and 'three-in-one' blocks. Catheters can be introduced into the femoral nerve sheath and continuous anaesthesia of the femoral nerve and lumbar plexus achieved with intermittent or continous infusions of local anaesthetic. This is a useful technique for providing analgesia after operations on the femur or front of the thigh. It does not provide total analgesia for hip or knee surgery as the sciatic nerve is usually unblocked with this technique.

Psoas compartment block. This is an alternative method of producing anaesthesia of the lumbar plexus by injecting a large volume of local anaesthetic into the space between the psoas and quadratus muscles. This can be achieved either as a single shot or with a catheter allowing repeat injections (Ben-David *et al.*, 1990).

Local anaesthetic blocks after laparoscopic surgery

Laparoscopic surgery is becoming very common especially as a day-case procedure in gynaecological surgery. Intraperitoneal instillation of large volumes of local anaesthetic under the subdiaphragmatic area can reduce the incidence of shoulder-tip pain (Narchi *et al.*, 1991) associated with these operations. Mesosalpinx blocks are particularly effective at reducing pelvic pain after laparoscopic sterilization and if combined with a rectus sheath block can reduce abdominal-wall pain also (Smith *et al.*, 1991).

Extradural and subarachnoid local techniques

Subarachnoid and extradural local anaesthetic blocks have been described in detail elsewhere (Chapter 68).

Because single-shot extradural and subarachnoid injections produce analgesia of only a relatively short duration (4–8 h and 2–4 h, respectively, with bupivacaine) these techniques are seldom employed for postoperative pain relief. However, the insertion of a catheter into the subarachnoid or extradural space permits continuous analgesia to be provided for 2–3 days postoperatively. Prolonged use of subarachnoid catheters has recently been associated with the development of cauda equina syndrome and their use in the USA for prolonged analgesia is no longer advocated. It is therefore unlikely that they will become an established method of analgesia in the UK. Thus, for all practical purposes, extradural techniques for postoperative analgesia are confined to:
1 Thoracic extradural catheters.

2 Lumbar extradural catheters.

3 Caudal extradural catheters or single-shot techniques.

Details of the physiological effects, and description of insertion of extradural catheters are provided in excellent accounts by Bowler and colleagues (1986) and Stanton-Hicks (1985). The following is a brief summary of these accounts and for more information the reader is referred to the original articles.

Physiological effects of extradural block

For practical purposes, extradural blocks may be categorized into high blocks (above T5) or low blocks (below the level of T5). The heart receives sympathetic innervation from T1 to T5, the lower limbs from T10 to L2, the adrenal medulla from T8 to L1, the abdominal viscera from T6 to L2, the liver from T7 to T9 and the kidneys from T10 to L1.

With high sympathetic blocks, there is very little change in cardiac output and mean arterial pressure in the conscious normovolaemic patient but a reduction in systemic vascular resistance (SVR). With low blocks, there is reduction in blood flow in the upper limbs accompanied by vasoconstriction and an increase in blood flow in the lower limbs as a result of vasodilatation, leaving central venous pressure (CVP), cardiac output and SVR, and mean arterial pressure more or less unchanged. With hypovolaemia, however, high blocks are associated with dramatic reductions in cardiac output and mean arterial pressure. In contrast, the patient with the low block is capable of compensating for small reductions in blood volume.

In patients free from respiratory disease and pain-free, low extradural blocks have little effect on lung volumes, FRC, expiratory reserve volume (ERV), residual volume (RV) and V_T remaining more or less unchanged. With high blocks, there is a decrease in ERV with little change in inspiratory capacity.

In contrast, for patients in pain, extradural block improves VC, FRC and Pao_2. However, there is little difference in the improvement produced by extradural block or optimum administration of systemic opioids. High extradural block causes a reduction in pulmonary artery pressure, with an increase in alveolar deadspace leading to slight hyperventilation and maintenance of $Paco_2$. Perhaps the greatest benefit of extradural block is maintenance of respiratory function in the absence of respiratory depression or sedation, thus permitting improved patient co-operation with physiotherapy.

Techniques for postoperative pain control

For post-thoracotomy pain, a catheter should be inserted at the level of incision, for upper-abdominal surgery at T6−T10, for lower-abdominal surgery at T10−L1 and for the lower limbs at L3−4. Low concentrations of local anaesthetic solution should be used in order to obviate motor block; thus, bupivacaine is used normally in a concentration of 0.25%, although the lumbar region may require higher concentrations because the nerve roots are of larger diameter.

For bolus administration, the volume of solution infused varies from 4−7 ml but by continuous infusion from a motor syringe pump, a rate of 7−22 mg/h may be utilized (Stanton-Hicks, 1985).

The contraindications and potential complications of extradural catheter techniques are described in Chapter 68.

Wound infusions

The technique of injecting local anaesthetic solution into the edges of a surgical incision was described in 1935, but there has been recently a resurgence of interest in this technique.

This form of analgesia is particularly worthwhile when a particular nerve block is not feasible, and is worth remembering for day-case surgery analgesia. Alternatively, catheters can be placed during the closure of the wound and used for repeat injections during the postoperative period.

Provided that bacterial filters are used, there would appear to be little danger of wound infection. Adrenaline should be avoided as theoretically, it may reduce blood supply to the tissues.

The technique abolishes only somatic pain and has little effect on visceral pain but, none the less, good results have been claimed for this technique following abdominal surgery. It is likely that some of the analgesia produced by wound infiltration is due to the anti-inflammatory effects of local anaesthetics as well as their effects on conduction block.

Spinal opioids

The identification of opioid receptors within the spinal cord in 1973 by Pert and Snyder introduced the possibility of using locally applied opioids to the cord either extradurally or intrathecally as a method of analgesia. The perceived advantages were that segmental analgesia could be established at the cord level without the side-effects of systemic opioids which are mediated at supraspinal-level opioid receptors. Also, spinal opioids do not produce sympathetic or motor block and so might be preferable to local anaesthetics.

Opioid receptors are found in high concentrations around the C-fibre terminal zones in Lamina 1 and in the substantia gelatinosa of the dorsal horn in the spinal cord. Endogenous and exogenous opioid agonists reduce the transmission of nociceptive inputs by presynaptic inhibition of neurotransmitter release (e.g. substance P) from afferent nociceptive fibres within the dorsal horn. They also cause pre- and postsynaptic inhibition of interneurone transmission between the nociceptive fibres and ascending fibres in the spinothalamic tracts (Fig. 76.15). Some opioids including pethidine and fentanyl are also thought to have a local anaesthetic action when used spinally.

Spinal opioids can be administered intrathecally or extradurally as either a single dose or as an infusion. To achieve analgesia the opioid must be absorbed into the dorsal horn from the CSF. The amount of drug taken up by the cord and the rate of absorption depends on the physical properties of the individual drugs. Speed of onset is proportional to the lipid solubility and degree of ionization. Lipid-soluble drugs such as fentanyl and sufentanil are easily absorbed into the cord, producing rapid analgesia limited to the spinal segments around the point of injection. Morphine has a relatively low fat solubility and therefore remains in the CSF for a longer time than the more lipid drugs. Spinally mediated analgesia with morphine is therefore slower in onset but more extensive because of spread of morphine away from the site of injection.

Opioids given by the extradural route first have to cross the dura before they can be absorbed into the dorsal horn from the CSF. Dural permeability is related to the molecular weight and shape of the molecule as well as its lipid solubility and degree of ionization (Table 76.10). The relative importance of these characteristics is unclear, though some studies suggest that the elongated opioids such as fentanyl have better dural penetration. Some uptake into the CSF also occurs by absorption into arachnoid granulations and radicular arteries. In addition to uptake into the CSF, extradural opioids can be absorbed into the extradural fat, reducing the concentration available for dural spread, or can be absorbed into the systemic circulation therefore producing systemic effects.

Clinical experience with intrathecal opioids

Intrathecal opioids have been used to produce good quality analgesia after a variety of operations including cardiothoracic and major abdominal surgery (Gjessing & Tomlin, 1981). Advantages include excellent analgesia with low doses and no haemodynamic or motor effects associated with local anaesthetics. The most popular drugs used by this route are morphine, diamorphine and pethidine which can produce analgesia for up to 20 h depending on the

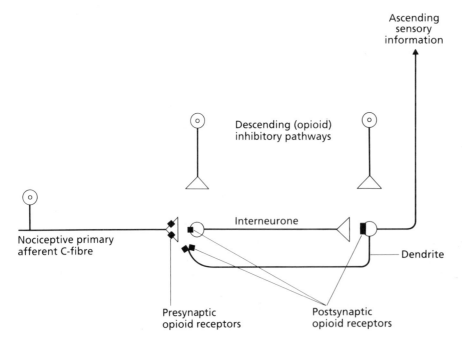

Fig. 76.15 Site of action of spinal opioids.

Table 76.10 Characteristics of opioids used by the spinal route

Drug	Lipid solubility	Mol.wt (daltons)	Percentage non-ionized at pH 7.3	Comments
Morphine	Low	285	21.3	Late respiratory depression common
Pethidine	↓	247	4.1	Late respiratory depression uncommon
Fentanyl	High	336	7.8	Early respiratory depression more likely Late respiratory depression unlikely but reported

dose used. Shorter-duration opioids probably do not have a place in intrathecal use as repeat administration is impractical, although they do produce a rapid-onset segmental block. Indwelling intrathecal catheters can be used to give repeat injections, but popularity for this technique has diminished for the reasons mentioned above.

A major disadvantage of intrathecal opioids is estimation of the correct dose. Higher doses produce better and longer-lasting analgesia with greater distribution along the spinal cord but have a higher incidence of side-effects due to rostral spread. Late-onset respiratory depression has occurred up to 20 h after morphine given intrathecally and is caused by relatively large concentrations reaching supraspinal opioid receptors by rostral spread in the subarachnoid space. Several other factors known to increase the risk of respiratory depression are shown in Table 76.11. Because of this potentially lethal complication, all patients should be closely monitored after spinal opioids. Other less-troublesome side-effects can also occur after spinal opioids and are listed in Table 76.11.

The ideal dose for any opioid used intrathecally is unknown and probably differs between patients and for different procedures. Most studies have shown that 0.5–1.0 mg of morphine will produce good analgesia after major abdominal surgery and doses as small as 0.06–0.12 mg have been effective for pain relief after cholecystectomy with minimal side-effects.

Clinical experience with extradural opioids

Extradural opioids used either alone, or in combination with local anaesthetics, have become more popular in recent years as a method of treating postoperative pain. Many different drugs have been given via the extradural route and most have been shown to provide effective analgesia with lower doses than required by conventional administration or PCA.

Table 76.11 Complications associated with the use of spinal opioids

Respiratory depression
Early: from systemic absorption
Late: from rostral spread in CSF augmented by:
   Dose
   Age
   Posture
   Aqueous solubility
   Additional systemic opioid
   Intermittent positive-pressure ventilation (IPPV)
   Increased abdominal pressure

Nausea/vomiting
Similar incidence to that following intramuscular administration

Itching
More common with morphine than fentanyl/diamorphine
Mechanisms possibly central and only relieved potentially by naloxone, antihistamine

Urinary retention
Incidence varies
Improved by naloxone

Sedation
Associated invariably with severe late form of respiratory depression

No one drug has been shown to have any particular advantages and most are now given by a constant infusion although some experience with PCA exists. The less lipid-soluble drugs such as morphine can be given via a lumbar catheter to provide thoracic analgesia by spread of these drugs within the CSF (Fromme et al., 1985). In theory, drugs such as fentanyl need to be administered at the level of the spinal cord where they are required to provide analgesia as there is relatively little spread within the CSF. Controversy exists as to whether there is any benefit in using the highly-lipid-soluble opioids as they have been shown to be rapidly absorbed in the systemic circulation after extradural administration and therefore will exert a significant systemic effect as well as one at the dorsal horn (Camu & Debucquoy, 1991; Glass *et al.*, 1992). Such systemic absorption probably explains why lumbar extradural fentanyl is as effective for pain relief after thoracic surgery as thoracic extradural fentanyl (Coe *et al.*, 1991).

Many different doses of extradural opioids have been used in an attempt to achieve the balance of good spinally mediated analgesia without the supra-spinal side-effects. Bolus doses of morphine, 1–10 mg, and diamorphine, 0.5–5 mg, have been reported, although many would consider the larger doses extreme in view of the greater risk of side-effects. An advantage of the extradural route is that infusions can be given and the dose adjusted according to response (Table 76.12). Dose requirements vary between patients and smaller doses should be used in elderly or infirm patients, or when used in combination with local anaesthetics (see below).

Side-effects of spinal opioids

The side-effects produced by spinal opioids are shown in Table 76.11, the frequencies of which vary considerably depending on the route of administration and the dose given. The most significant side-effect is respiratory depression, which occurs most commonly after morphine. Early respiratory depression from vascular absorption has been described with fentanyl but late respiratory depression is probably unlikely but has been described.

With all opioids, early respiratory depression may occur as a result of vascular absorption. Late respiratory depression produced by rostral spread within the CSF is extremely unpredictable and may occur at any time up to 24 h after administration of the drug. Respiratory depression can also be very insidious in onset and very difficult to recognize with intermittent observations of respiratory rate. Studies using continuous pulse oximetry have shown that periodic dramatic decreases in arterial saturation can occur with any form of opioid analgesia and that hypox-

aemia is more likely during sleep. Several studies have shown that extradural opioids produce longer periods of mild postoperative hypoxaemia compared with intramuscular or PCA methods of administration (Wheatley *et al.*, 1990). Whether intermittent boluses of extradural opioid are preferable to continuous infusions of opioid and local anaesthetic as regards postoperative hypoxaemia is unresolved (Madej *et al.*, 1992). However, it would appear that some patients normally experience episodic hypoxaemia during sleep and these may be at greater risk of hypoxaemia postoperatively. Supplemental oxygen is therefore of value in any patient receiving opioids postoperatively and many recommend that it be continued for several nights after operation (Hanning, 1992).

Opioid-induced respiratory depression and also coma can be reversed by naloxone (occasionally this may require very large doses). However, because of the relatively short duration of action of naloxone, patients may relapse back into respiratory failure and coma and a continuous infusion may be required.

In general, it is possible to give naloxone in such a dosage as to reverse respiratory depression without reversing analgesia. For an infusion the recommended doses of naloxone range from 0.6 mg/h to $5 \mu g \cdot kg^{-1} \cdot h^{-1}$. The use of the longer-acting opioid antagonists naltrexone and nalmefene may have a useful role in this situation.

There are several factors which are known to increase the incidence of respiratory depression following spinal opioids:

1 Posture. Rostral spread may be encouraged by the supine posture, particularly if there is an element of straining or coughing.

2 The use of further systemic opioids.

3 Increasing age of the patient. Doses should be reduced in elderly and infirm patients.

4 Dosage of drug. The higher the initial bolus dose of drug placed in the extradural or subarachnoid space, the higher is the CSF concentration.

5 Lipophilicity of the drug.

6 Thoracic administration. The distance for the

Table 76.12 Doses of spinal opioids

Drug	Extradural bolus	Extradural infusion	Intrathecal
Morphine	2–5 mg	$0.5–2 mg \cdot kg^{-1} \cdot h^{-1}$	0.5–1 mg
Diamorphine	1–5 mg	$0.4–0.8 mg \cdot kg^{-1} \cdot h^{-1}$	0.5–1 mg
Fentanyl	1–2 μg/kg	$1–2 \mu g \cdot kg^{-1} \cdot h^{-1}$	——
Pethidine	0.75 mg/kg	——	0.1 mg/kg
Alfentanil	15–30 μg/kg	$15–30 \mu g \cdot kg^{-1} \cdot h^{-1}$	——

opioid to migrate rostrally is considerably shorter than that for the drug administered by the lumbar route.

Because of the potentially serious complications associated with spinal opioid administration, many feel that patients should be nursed on high dependency or intensive care units if they have this form of analgesia. However, many units which regularly use them routinely nurse these patients on normal postoperative wards with adequate monitoring, oxygen therapy and regular assessments by nursing staff following strict treatment protocols.

For further information on spinal opioids readers are referred to the reviews by Morgan (1989) and Green (1992).

Non-steroidal anti-inflammatory drugs

The use of non-steroidal anti-inflammatory drugs (NSAIDs) in the treatment of postoperative pain is becoming more popular due to increased understanding of the role of inflammatory mechanisms in tissue injury and their effects on nociception. Their advantages include the lack of opioid related side-effects, including respiratory depression, sedation and dependence.

After tissue injury the threshold to painful stimulus is markedly reduced both at the site of injury (primary hyperalgesia) and in the surrounding area (secondary hyperalgesia). Primary hyperalgesia is due to the sensitization of nerve endings by neurotransmitters and inflammatory mediators released at the site of injury, including metabolites of arachidonic acid formed via the cyclo-oxygenase pathway. Secondary hyperalgesia is due to dynamic changes in the processing of nociceptive information at the level of the spinal cord and in the periphery.

NSAIDs decrease pain by a central analgesic action and by inhibiting cyclo-oxygenase, therefore reducing prostaglandin-mediated inflammation at the site of injury. They may also stabilize phagocytic polymorphoneutrophils and reduce their release of proteolytic enzymes and reactive oxygen species and so decrease tissue inflammation.

There are several different classes of NSAIDs which differ in their relative analgesic and anti-inflammatory actions. Particular NSAIDs that are proving more popular for postoperative pain relief are those which can be given by the intravenous, intramuscular and rectal routes thereby allowing administration when the oral route is unavailable.

In general, NSAIDs are able to provide good analgesia after minor operations when given as the sole analgesic (McLoughlin et al., 1990). After major surgery they can provide a useful supplement to other analgesic techniques and have been shown to reduce the opioid requirements after major surgery (Kinsella et al., 1992). Better and more consistent analgesia may be obtained with NSAIDs if they are given as a constant intravenous infusion rather than intermittent intramuscular injections.

Possible side-effects associated with NSAIDs include gastric ulceration, decreased renal function and an increased bleeding tendency. Several studies have shown that short-term use of these drugs provides useful analgesia with no effect on morbidity (Dahl & Kehlet, 1989). However, consideration must be made before using these drugs in patients with a history of gastric ulceration, renal insufficiency, cardiac failure or hypovolaemia or other conditions when adequate renal blood flow may be dependent on prostaglandin-mediated vasodilatation. Aspirin is now contra-indicated in children under 12 years due to an association with Reye's syndrome. However, the use of other NSAIDs still continues in this population of patients. For further information on NSAIDs refer to Chapter 10.

Alpha-2 agonists

The application of α_2-agonists in anaesthetic practice is rapidly becoming apparent (Maze & Tranquilli, 1991). Clonidine has been shown to improve pain relief and decrease traditional analgesic requirements either when given systemically during operation (De Kock et al., 1992) or extradurally, either alone (Carabine et al., 1992) or with local anaesthetic/opioid mixtures (see p. 1596). Although the exact mechanism of action is unclear, it probably involves activation of descending inhibitory nor-adrenergic pathways at a spinal and supraspinal level independent of the method of administration. Side-effects include sedation, respiratory depression and urinary retention and careful postoperative monitoring should be used if these agents are given. The ideal dose of clonidine to improve analgesia and avoid side-effects has not been determined. Dexmedetomidine is a newer more specific α_2-agonist than clonidine and this may have a role in the future.

Other methods of treating postoperative pain

Cryoanalgesia

Because the intercostal nerves are readily accessible

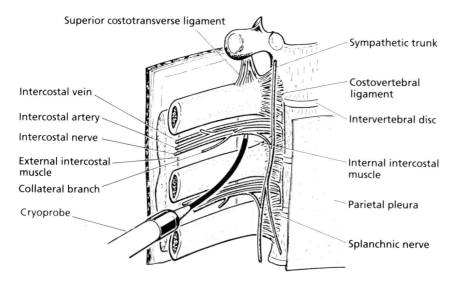

Fig. 76.16 Application of a cryoprobe to the intercostal nerve at thoracotomy to produce postoperative somatic analgesia. (Redrawn from Maiwand *et al.*, 1986.)

during thoracotomy, it has been common practice for the thoracic surgeon to perform intercostal block with local anaesthetics, before closing the thoracotomy incision. Alternatively, several units now employ routinely cryotherapy of the intercostal nerves at the time of surgery (Fig. 76.16).

Depending on the duration of freezing, numbness can be produced for a period of 30–200 days after application. Excellent postoperative analgesia can be obtained using this technique. However, supplementation with opioids is frequently necessary in the early postoperative period. Potential side-effects include the development of hyperaesthesia in the dermatomal distribution of the nerve treated. In addition, prolonged analgesia in the region of the nipple of younger women is particularly distressing (Maiwand *et al.*, 1986).

Non-pharmacological methods of pain control

Stimulation-produced analgesia (transcutaneous nerve stimulation)

The modes of action of transcutaneous nerve stimulation (TNS or TENS) and acupuncture are probably similar. The techniques act probably by stimulation of non-pain afferent fibres (Aα-fibres) which activate directly modulation systems at the spinal cord level.

For postoperative pain control, TENS is used frequently in the form of two electrodes placed on each side of the incision. However, electrodes may be placed also over the dermatome where pain is perceived. It has been suggested that the more effec-tive sites for TENS electrodes correspond to established acupuncture points.

It is generally agreed that TENS does not produce satisfactory postoperative analgesia. However, it may produce a modest reduction in the overall requirements for systemic opioids, although the effect is not apparent in every patient. Its advantages are that it is non-invasive and drug-free.

Acupuncture

There have been relatively few studies of the use of acupuncture in the treatment of postoperative pain in Western Europe and its use is confined largely to the chronic pain clinic.

Psychological methods

A variety of psychological methods have been described in the management of acute postoperative pain and these have been shown to be associated with improvement in the postoperative experience. The reader is referred to articles by Chapman (1985) and Chapter 75.

It would be true to say that good doctors have always employed such methods in the treatment of pain. In essence, a patient's surgical experience will be rendered much more pleasant and less distressing if he/she is encountered by a courteous and kindly doctor, who provides a full and rational explanation of the surgical experience, and who will reassure the patient that all his/her anxieties and somatic pain will receive prompt, immediate and effective therapy. In addition, the patient should be looked after by highly trained nursing staff of a similar disposition to that of the attending doctor and receive similar support and encouragement from friends and relatives. Positive encouragement from patients who have been through the same experience provides further reassurance and support.

This overall description of what constitutes good medical practice has been analysed into several components:

1 *Cognitive technique*. This comprises the provision of adequate explanations and coaching.

2 *Social modelling*. This term is applied to the technique whereby patients are introduced to others who have coped successfully with the same procedure.

3 *Biofeedback*. This term describes the use of distraction, suggestion and relaxation, which can help to reduce analgesic requirements. The technique requires considerable training, whereby the patient learns to relax muscles and reduce tension by providing cognitive and behavioural help.

Hypnosis

This technique has been used to only a small extent in acute postoperative pain, with claims for reduced analgesic requirements postoperatively.

Pre-emptive analgesia

There is now good experimental evidence that painful stimuli can produce changes in CNS function, which alter the perception of acute pain and may lead to the sensation of pain long after the noxious stimulus has been removed. The exact mechanisms which cause these effects are complex and have not been completely elucidated (Woolf, 1989). Most evidence suggests that noxious inputs cause the release of several excitatory amino-acids and neuropeptides from C-fibre neurones within the dorsal horn. This then leads to a state of hyperexcitability within the dorsal horn neurones (wind up), which results in a decreased threshold for firing of these neurones.

In addition there is an expansion of the receptive fields of the neurones within the dorsal horn and this explains the phenomenon of secondary hyperalgesia around the site of injury (see below).

N-methyl-D-aspartate (NMDA) receptors within the spinal cord may have an important modulatory role in this sensitization because antagonists to these receptors have been shown to inhibit or reduce dorsal horn wind up. Other receptors which may attenuate these changes in the dorsal horn include μ-opioid receptors, and σ-receptors, which are intrinsically linked to the NMDA receptors. Conversely, κ-receptor agonists (dynorphine) antagonize the analgesic effects of μ-receptor-mediated spinal analgesia and may contribute to spinal sensitization. Changes in second-messenger systems or gene expression within nociceptive pathways may herald longer-term changes in the transmission and perception of pain.

Clinically, several changes in pain perception may occur at and around the site of the injury, which might be explained by the alterations in central processing of nociceptive inputs. These include the experience of pain to normally non-painful stimuli (allodynia), and a reduced threshold to a painful stimulus at the site of injury and in the adjacent area (primary and secondary hyperalgesia). More long-term effects may occur and include the development of a 'pain memory' and includes such conditions as phantom limb syndrome after the amputation of a painful limb.

Thus, it can be seen that the nervous system is not a fixed 'hard wired' circuit, but exhibits plasticity whereby acutely painful conditions can produce significant changes in its processing of nociceptive information. Whether these mechanisms occur after a surgical insult in humans is unclear. However, one study has shown that central hyperexcitability occurs postoperatively (Dahl *et al.*, 1992a).

The concept of pre-emptive analgesia is based on the theory that inhibition or attenuation of the initial nociceptive input occurring during surgery will prevent spinal sensitization and will reduce the amount of pain suffered postoperatively (McQuay, 1992). Therefore the concept of timing of analgesia is considered to be extremely important (Wall, 1988).

An initial study showing that preoperative extradural block with local anaesthetics reduced postamputation pain at 6 months and 1 year postoperatively (Bach *et al.*, 1988) fuelled enthusiasm for the concept of pre-emptive analgesia. A trial showing that premedication with an opioid and the use of a local anaesthetic block increased the time to first analgesia request after orthopaedic surgery (McQuay *et al.*, 1988) and also demonstrated the efficacy of early effective analgesic regimens. However, it is unknown if the same results would have been obtained if these methods of pain relief had been used after surgery had begun.

At present, only a few well-controlled trials using different methods of pre-emptive analgesia have been performed. These include the use of extradural fentanyl (Katz *et al.*, 1992) pre- and post-thoracotomy incision, which only reduced pain scores in the early postoperative period with no significant differences between the two groups after 12 h. The effect of extradural morphine/bupivacaine infusion administered either before surgical incision or at the end of surgery has been shown to produce no difference in pain scores or opioid requirements after major abdominal surgery (Dahl *et al.*, 1992b). Other studies using peripheral nerve blocks or NSAIDs have either failed to show an improvement or have only measured pain for a very short time postoperatively with very minor improvement.

Therefore, the clinical benefit of pre-emptive analgesia on postoperative pain perception remains to be convincingly demonstrated. Questions that remain to be answered include what type of analgesia will be the most effective at preventing spinal sensitization and how long it should be continued into the postoperative period to prevent it occurring. Also, the effect of different operations on spinal cord processing is unknown.

For further information on pre-emptive analgesia, the reader is referred to the review of Dahl and Kehlet (1993).

Balanced (combined) analgesia

Postoperative pain relief using a single drug is unlikely to succeed in producing satisfactory pain relief unless large doses are used with the increased risk of side-effects. As nociceptive impulses can be blocked at several sites along the pain pathway, a logical step is to use combinations of drugs which act at these different sites to produce a balanced form of analgesia (Dahl *et al.*, 1990). An additional benefit is that as combinations of drugs may act synergistically their individual doses can be reduced thereby decreasing the incidence of side-effects.

The theoretical possibilities that exist therefore include (Fig. 76.17):

1 Inhibition of peripheral nociceptive mechanisms with NSAIDs, steroids, peripherally applied opioids and other anti-inflammatory drugs.

2 Neural block of Aδ- and C-nociceptor fibres with peripheral, extradural or spinal local anaesthetics.

3 Activation of descending inhibitory pathways with opioids (acting at a spinal and supraspinal level), α$_2$-agonists and NMDA antagonists.

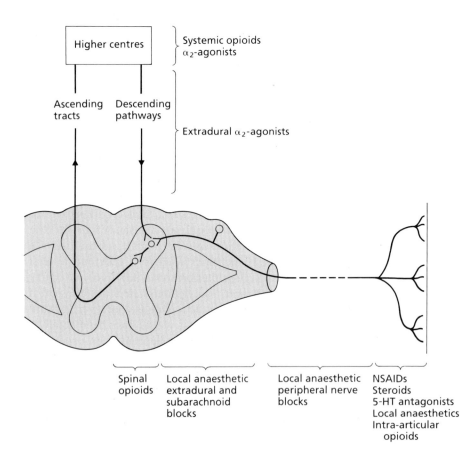

Fig. 76.17 Potential sites of action of different analgesics in balanced analgesia.

Most experience is with using combinations of low-dose extradural opioids and local anaesthetic infusions. An extradural infusion of bupivacaine, 18.75 mg/h, and diamorphine, 0.5 mg/h, has been shown to be more effective than either of the two drugs given separately after major gynaecological surgery with no increase in side-effects (Lee *et al.*, 1988). Although extradural infusions of opioids alone are extremely effective, the addition of local anaesthetic has been shown to prevent pain on movement and coughing compared with single-drug infusions after major abdominal surgery (Dahl *et al.*, 1992c).

The addition of non-steroidals to any analgesic regimen should inhibit peripheral inflammatory-mediated pain at the site of injury in addition to producing centrally mediated analgesia. NSAIDs have been shown to reduce PCA and intramuscular opioid requirements after several types of operation (see above) but their efficacy when used with effective extradural regimens is unproven (Bigler *et al.*, 1992).

Clonidine has been used to improve analgesia when given in combination with extradural opioids and local anaesthetics (Mogenson *et al.*, 1992) and also with PCA opioids (see above).

Future developments in this field will be estimation of the optimal doses of analgesics used in combination to provide maximal analgesia with minimal side-effects. It is probable that these combinations will differ between operations. Newer drugs that may be incorporated into analgesic regimens may include steroids and other anti-inflammatory agents.

Recommendations for improving postoperative pain relief

In recent years there has been an increased awareness of the general poor quality of analgesia available to patients in the postoperative period as highlighted in a report on pain after surgery by the Royal Colleges of Surgeons and Anaesthetists. This influential document outlines the reasons for the failure of traditional analgesic methods and indicates how postoperative pain relief can be improved without it becoming a large drain on financial or staffing resources.

The aims and recommendations of the working party report are to:
1 Improve education of hospital staff with regard to postoperative analgesia.
2 Regularly assess and record pain in postoperative patients.
3 Appoint individuals responsible for the management of pain-relief policies on postoperative wards.
4 Establish acute-pain teams in all hospitals.

5 Improve analgesia by utilizing existing methods to their maximum effect and introduce newer methods with due regard to safety.
6 Audit and continuously appraise analgesic methods employed.
7 Establish appropriate facilities for the safe provision of adequate postoperative analgesia in all hospitals.
8 Provide properly trained staff and resources for the above services.

Additional recommendations include conducting further research into safer and more effective methods of pain relief including counselling and psychological methods, monitoring of patients in the postoperative period and assessing the safety and efficacy of newer methods of pain relief.

Acute pain services

Many of the problems of traditional analgesic methods are that they are prescribed in the operating theatre by an anaesthetist who invariably will not administer them or assess their effects in the postoperative period. This duty is left to nursing and junior medical staff who are unsuitably trained in the assessment of pain and will usually underadminister analgesia for fear of dangerous side-effects. The prescription of different drugs and regimens by different physicians leads to confusion amongst nursing staff.

Centres providing an acute pain service have considerably improved the quality of analgesia in the postoperative period. Most pain teams are based on the system first described by Ready and colleagues (1988) in the USA and usually consist of anaesthetic, nursing and pharmacy staff.

In general, these teams are responsible for the day-to-day treatment of postoperative pain on surgical wards. This is accomplished by increasing education of nursing and medical staff in the more effective use of conventional analgesic methods in addition to more modern techniques, including extradurals and PCA. Most units adopt specific analgesic policies to reduce confusion and increase compliance by staff. These can range from the increased use of nerve blocks during operations, a more logical approach to intramuscular opioid administration or the introduction of PCA or extradural techniques.

An important aspect of the educational role of pain teams is the training of staff to assess and record postoperative pain and to monitor regularly for side-effects. The use of algorithms is particularly useful in improving the effectiveness and safety of analgesic therapies. Although it is generally considered safe to use PCA opioids on normal surgical wards, the use of extradural opioids outside the intensive or high-dependency unit is controversial. However, several hospitals have found them a very effective and safe method of analgesia in properly selected patients on wards with staff trained in their use (Ready *et al.*, 1991; Wheatley *et al.*, 1991).

Anaesthetists are a logical choice to supervise a pain team with their knowledge of analgesic drugs and the methods to administer them safely. Most hospitals have found that an acute pain service can be formed with a relatively small investment in terms of additional personnel. This usually includes a dedicated member of the nursing profession to co-ordinate the training of staff and the introduction of new methods onto surgical wards.

Choosing an analgesic regimen

Several factors should be considered before a decision is made on the type of analgesia to be used for a particular patient postoperatively. These include the general health of the patient, the operation site and the duration and amount of pain expected post-operatively. Other factors such as experience of the medical and nursing staff with equipment and more complicated types of analgesic regimens (e.g. extra-dural infusions) should also be taken into account.

Experience of acute pain teams has shown that PCA with opioids can provide good quality analgesia after many types of operations and is the usual main-stay of therapy. Extradural opioid and local anaes-thetic infusions provide extremely effective analgesia although have a higher risk of potentially serious side-effects and therefore can only be used under the supervision of trained staff. Most units reserve this form of analgesia for patients in whom particularly good analgesia is important such as patients with respiratory disease undergoing abdominal or thoracic surgery.

NSAIDs can be used alone for analgesia after many minor operations or as a supplement after more major surgery.

References

Aitkenhead A.R., Vater M., Cooper C.M.S. & Smith G. (1983) Pharmacokinetics of single dose i.v. morphine in normal volunteers and patients with end stage renal failure. *British Journal of Anaesthesia* **55**, 905.

Austin K.L., Stapleton J.V. & Mather L.E. (1980a) Multiple intramuscular injections: a major source of variability in analgesic response to meperedine. *Pain* **8**, 47–62.

Austin K.L., Stapleton J.V. & Mather L.E. (1980b) Relationship between blood meperidine concentrations and analgesic response: a preliminary report. *Anesthesiology* **53**, 460–6.

Austin K.L., Stapleton J.V. & Mather L.E. (1981) Pethidine clearance during continuous intravenous infusions in post-operative patients. *British Journal of Clinical Pharmacology* **1**, 25–30.

Bach S., Noreng M.F. & Tjéllden N.U. (1988) Phantom limb pain in amputees during the first 12 months following limb amputation, after preoperative lumbar epidural blockade. *Pain* **33**, 297–301.

Bellville J.W., Forrest W.H., Miller E. & Brown B.W. Jr (1971) Influence of age on pain relief from analgesics *Journal of the American Medical Association* **217**, 1835–41.

Ben-David B., Lee E. & Croitoru M. (1990) Psoas block for surgical repair of hip fracture: a case report and description of a catheter technique. *Anesthesia and Analgesia* **71**, 298–301.

Bentley J.B., Borrel J.D., Nenad R.E. & Gillespie T.J. (1982) Age and fentanyl pharmacokinetics. *Anesthesia and Analgesia* **61**, 968–71.

Berkovitz J.B., Ngai S.H., Yang J.C., Hemstead J. & Spector S. (1975) The disposition of morphine in surgical patients. *Clinical Pharmacology and Therapeutics* **17**, 629–35.

Bigler D., Møller J., Kamp-Jensen M., Berthelsen P., Hjortsø N.C. & Kehlet H. (1992) Effect of piroxicam in addition to continuous thoracic epidural bupivacaine and morphine on postoperative pain and lung function after thoracotomy. *Acta Anaesthesiologica Scandinavica* **36**, 647–50.

Bowler G.M.R., Wildsmith J.A.W. & Scott D.B. (1986) Epidural administration of local anaesthetics. In *Acute Pain Management* (Eds Cousins M.J. & Philips G.D.) pp. 187–235. Churchill Livingstone, Edinburgh.

Boyle P. & Parbrook G.D. (1977) The interrelation of personality and postoperative factors. *British Journal of Anaesthesia* **49**, 259–64.

Camu F. & Debucquoy F. (1991) Alfentanil infusion for post-operative pain: a comparison of epidural and intravenous routes *Anesthesiology* **75**, 171–8.

Carabine U.A., Milligan K.R., Mulholland D. & Moore J. (1992) Extradural clonidine infusions for analgesia after total hip replacement. *British Journal of Anaesthesia* **68**, 338–43.

Catling J.A., Pinto D.M., Jordon C. & Jones J.G. (1980) Respiratory effects of analgesia after cholecystectomy: comparison of continuous and intermittent papaveretum. *British Medical Journal* **281**, 478–80.

Chan G.L.C. & Matzke G.R. (1987) Effects of renal insufficiency on the pharmacokinetics and pharmacodynamics of opioid analgesics. *Drug Intelligence and Clinical Pharmacy* **21**, 773–83.

Chapman C.R. (1985) Psychological factors in postoperative pain. In *Acute Pain* (Eds Smith G. & Covino B.G.) pp. 22–41. Butterworths, London.

Christenson P., Brandt M.R., Rem J. & Kehlet H. (1982) Influence of extradural morphine on the adrenocortical and hyper-glycaemic response to surgery. *British Journal of Anaesthesia* **54**, 23–7.

Claeys M.A., Camu F. & Maes V. (1992) Prophylactic diclofenac infusions in major orthopaedic surgery: effects on analgesia and acute phase proteins *Acta Anaesthesiologica Scandinavica* **36**, 270–75.

Coe A., Sarginson R., Smith M.V., Donnelly R.J. & Russell G.N. (1991) Pain following thoracotomy: a randomised, double-blind comparison of lumbar versus thoracic epidural fentanyl. *Anaesthesia* **46**, 918−21.

Cohen F.L. (1980) Postsurgical pain relief: patient's status and nurses' medication choices. *Pain* **9**, 265−74.

Dahl J.B. & Kehlet H. (1989) Non-steroidal anti-inflammatory drugs: rationale for use in severe postoperative pain. *British Journal of Anaesthesia* **66**, 703−12.

Dahl J.B. & Kehlet H. (1993) The value of pre-emptive analgesia in the treatment of post-operative pain − a critical analysis. *British Journal of Anaesthesia* **70**, 434−79.

Dahl J.B., Rosenburg J., Dirkes W.E., Mogensen T. & Kehlet H. (1990) Prevention of postoperative pain by balanced analgesia. *British Journal of Anaesthesia* **64**, 518−20.

Dahl J.B., Erichsen C.J., Fuglsang-Frederiksen A. & Kehlet H. (1992a) Pain sensation and nociceptive reflex excitability in surgical patients and human volunteers. *British Journal of Anaesthesia* **69**, 117−21.

Dahl J.B., Hansen B.L., Hjortsø N.C., Erichsen C., Møiniche S. & Kehlet H. (1992b) Influence of timing on the effect of continuous extradural analgesia with bupivacaine and morphine after major abdominal surgery. *British Journal of Anaesthesia* **69**, 4−8.

Dahl J.B., Rosenberg J., Hansen B.L., Hjortsø N.C. & Kehlet H. (1992c) Differential analgesic effects of low-dose epidural morphine and morphine-bupivacaine at rest and during mobilization after major abdominal surgery. *Anesthesia and Analgesia* **74**, 362−5.

Dahlstrom B., Tamsen A., Paalzow L. & Hartvig P. (1982) Patient controlled analgesic therapy, part IV: pharmacokinetics and analgesic plasma concentrations of morphine. *Clinical Pharmacokinetics* **7**, 266−79.

De Boer A.G., De Leede L.G.J. & Breimer D.D. (1984) Drug absorption by sublingual and rectal routes. *British Journal of Anaesthesia* **56**, 69−82.

De Kock M.F., Pichon G. & Scholtes J.L. (1992) Intraoperative clonidine enhances postoperative morphine patient-controlled analgesia. *Canadian Journal of Anaesthesia* **39**, 537−44.

Desborough J.P. & Hall G.M. (1990) The stress response to surgery. *Current Anaesthesia and Critical Care* **1**, 133−7.

Dodson M.E. (1985) *The Management of Postoperative Pain* p. 274. Edward Arnold, London.

Duthrie D.J.R., Rowbotham D.J., Wyld R., Henderson P.D. & Nimmo W.S. (1988) Plasma fentanyl concentrations during transdermal delivery of fentanyl to surgical patients. *British Journal of Anaesthesia* **60**, 614−18.

Ellis R., Haines., Shah R., Cotton B.R. & Smith G. (1982) Pain relief after abdominal surgery − a comparison of intramuscular morphine, sublingual buprenorphine and self-administered pethidine. *British Journal of Anaesthesia* **54**, 421−8.

Ferrante M.F., Orav J.E., Rocco A.G. & Gallow J. (1988) A statistical model for pain in patient-controlled analgesia and conventional intramuscular opioid regimes. *Anesthesia and Analgesia* **67**, 457−61.

Fromme G.A., Steidl L.J. & Danielson D.R. (1985) Comparison of lumbar and thoracic epidural morphine for relief of post-thoracotomy pain. *Anesthesia and Analgesia* **64**, 454−5.

Glass P.S.A., Estok P., Ginsberg B., Goldberg J.S. & Sladen R.N. (1992) Use of patient-controlled analgesia to compare the efficacy of epidural to intravenous fentanyl administration. *Anesthesia and Analgesia* **74**, 345−51.

Ghould T.H., Crosby D.L., Harmer M., Lloyd S.M., Lunn J.N., Rees G.A.D., Roberts D.E. & Webster J.A. (1992) Policy for controlling pain after surgery: effect of sequential changes in management. *British Medical Journal* **305**, 1187−93.

Gjessing J. & Tomlin P.J. (1981) Postoperative pain control with intrathecal morphine. *Anaesthesia* **36**, 268−76.

Glynn C.J., Lloyd J.W. & Folkard S. (1976) The diurnal variation in the variation of pain. *Proceedings of the Royal Society of Medicine* **69**, 369−72.

Green D.W. (1992) The clinical use of spinal opioids. In *Anaesthesia Review*, vol. 9 (Ed. Kaufman L.) pp. 80−111. Churchill Livingstone, Edinburgh.

Hanning C.D. (1985) Non-parenteral techniques. In *Acute Pain* (Eds Smith G. & Covino B.G.) pp. 180−204. Butterworths, London.

Hanning C.D. (1992) Prolonged postoperative oxygen therapy. *British Journal of Anaesthesia* **69**, 115−16.

Hanning C.D., Vickers A.P., Smith G., Graham N.B. & McNeil M.E. (1988) The morphine hydrogel suppository: a new sustained release rectal preparation. *British Journal of Anaesthesia* **61**, 221−8.

Hull C.J. (1985) The pharmacokinetics of opioid analgesics with special reference to patient controlled administration. In *Patient Controlled Analgesia* (Eds Harmer M., Rosen M. & Vickers M.D.) pp. 7−17. Blackwell Scientific Publications, Oxford.

Imura H. (1991) Cytokines and endocrine function; an interaction between the immune and neuroendocrine systems. *Clinical Endocrinology* **35**, 107−15.

Jones J.G., Sapsford D.J. & Wheatley R.G. (1990) Postoperative hypoxaemia: mechanisms and time course. *Anaesthesia* **45**, 566−73.

Joshi G.P., McCarrol S.M., Brady O.H., Hurson B.J. & Walsh G. (1993) Intra-articular morphine for pain relief following anterior cruciate ligament repair. *British Journal of Anaesthesia* **70**, 87−8.

Katz J., Kavanagh B.P., Sandler, A.N., Nierenberg H., Boylan J.F., Friedlander M. & Shaw B.F. (1992) Preemptive analgesia − clinical evidence of neuroplasticity contributing to postoperative pain. *Anesthesiology* **77**, 439−46.

Kehlet H. (1989) Surgical stress: the role of pain and analgesia. *British Journal of Anaesthesia* **63**, 189−95.

Kinsella J., Moffat A.C., Patrick J.A., Prentice J.W., McArdle C.S. & Kenny G.N.C. (1992) Ketorolac trometamol for postoperative analgesia after orthopaedic surgery. *British Journal of Anaesthesia* **69**, 19−22.

Kluger M.T. & Owen H. (1990) Patients' expectations of patient controlled analgesia. *Anaesthesia* **45**, 1072−4.

Lee A., Simpson D., Whitfield A. & Scott D.B. (1988) Postoperative analgesia by continuous extradural infusion of bupivacaine and diamorphine. *British Journal of Anaesthesia* **60**, 845−50.

Lee A., Boon D., Bagshaw P. & Kempthorne P. (1990) A randomised double-blind study of interpleural analgesia after cholecystectomy. *Anaesthesia* **46**, 1028−31.

Lim A.T., Edis G., Kranz H., Mendelson G., Selwood T. & Scott

D.F. (1983) Postoperative pain control: Contribution of psychological factors and transcutaneous nerve stimulation. *Pain* **17**, 179–88.

Loan W.B. & Dundee J.W. (1967) The clinical assessment of pain. *Practitioner* **198**, 759–68.

Madej T.H., Wheatley R.G., Jackson I.J.B. & Hunter D. (1992) Hypoxaemia and pain relief after lower abdominal surgery: comparison of extradural and patient-controlled analgesia. *British Journal of Anaesthesia* **69**, 554–7.

Maiwand M.O., Makey A.R. & Rees A. (1986) Cryoanalgesia after thoracotomy. *Journal of Thoracic and Cardiovascular Surgery* **92**, 291–5.

Mather L.E. & Meffin P.J. (1978) Clinical pharmacokinetics of pethidine. *Clinical Pharmacokinetics* **3**, 352–68.

Mather L.E., Tucker G.T., Pflug A.E., Lindop M.J. & Wilkerson C. (1975) Meperidine kinetics in man. Intravenous injection in surgical patients and volunteers. *Clinical Pharmacology and Therapeutics* **17**, 21–30.

Maze M. & Tranquilli D.V.M. (1991) Alpha-2 adrenoceptor agonists: defining the role in clinical anesthesia. *Anesthesiology* **74**, 581–605.

McLoughin C., McKinney M.S., Fee J.P.H. & Boules Z. (1990) Diclofenac for day-care arthroscopy surgery; comparison with standard opioid therapy. *British Journal of Anaesthesia* **65**, 620–3.

McQuay H.J. (1992) Pre-emptive analgesia. *British Journal of Anaesthesia* **69**, 1–3.

McQuay H.M. & Moore A. (1984) Be aware of renal function when prescribing morphine. *Lancet* **ii**, 284–5.

McQuay H.J., Carroll D. & Moore R.A. (1988) Postoperative orthopaedic pain — the effect of opiate premedication and local anaesthetic blocks. *Pain* **33**, 291–5.

Mogensen T., Eliasen K., Ejlersen E., Vegger P., Nielson I.K. & Kehlet H. (1992) Epidural clonidine enhances postoperative analgesia from a combined low-dose epidural bupivacaine and morphine regimen. *Anaesthesia and Analgesia* **75**, 607–10.

Morgan M. (1989) The rational use of intrathecal and extradural opioids. *British Journal of Anaesthesia* **63**, 165–88.

Naito Y., Tamai S., Shingu K., Matsui T., Segawa H., Nakai Y. & Mori K. (1992) Responses of plasma adrenocorticotropic hormone, cortisol and cytokines during and after upper abdominal surgery. *Anesthesiology* **77**, 426–31.

Narchi P., Benhamou D. & Fernadez H. (1991) Intraperitoneal local anaesthetic for shoulder tip pain after day case laparoscopy. *Lancet* **338**, 1569–70.

Nayman J. (1979) Measurement and control of postoperative pain. *Annals of the Royal College of Surgeons* **61**, 419–26.

Owen H., Plummer J.L., Armstrong I., Mather L.E. & Cousins M.J. (1989a) Variables of patient controlled analgesia 1. bolus size. *Anaesthesia* **44**, 7–10.

Owen H., Kluger M.T. & Plummer J.L. (1989b) Variables of patient controlled analgesia 2: concurrent infusion. *Anaesthesia* **44**, 11–13.

Owen H., Brose W.G., Plummer J.L. & Mather L.E. (1990) Variables of patient controlled analgesia 3. Test of an infusion demand system using alfentanil *Anaesthesia* **45**, 452–5.

Parbrook G.D., Steel D.F. & Dalrymple D.G. (1973) Factors predisposing to postoperative pain and pulmonary complications: a study of male patients undergoing elective gastric

surgery. *British Journal of Anaesthesia* **45**, 21–33.

Parkhouse J., Lambrechts W. & Simpton B.R.J. (1961) The incidence of postoperative pain. *British Journal of Anaesthesia* **33**, 345–53.

Pert C.B. & Snyder S. (1973) Opiate receptors: demonstration in nervous tissue. *Science* **179**, 1011–14.

Pinnock C.A., Derbyshire D.R., Achola K.J. & Smith G. (1986) Absorption of controlled release morphine sulphate in the immediate postoperative period. *British Journal of Anaesthesia* **58**, 868–71.

Ready L.B., Oden R., Chadwick H.S., Benedetti C., Rooke G.A., Caplan R. & Wild L.M. (1988) Development of an anesthesiology based postoperative pain management service. *Anesthesiology* **68**, 101–6.

Ready L.B., Loper K.A., Nessly M. & Wild L. (1991) Postoperative epidural morphine is safe on surgical wards. *Anesthesiology* **75**, 452–6.

Rowbotham D.J., Wyld R., Peacock J.E., Duthrie J.R. & Nimmo W.S. (1989) Transdermal fentanyl for the relief of pain after upper abdominal surgery. *British Journal of Anaesthesia* **63**, 56–9.

Rutberg H., Hakanson E., Anderberg B., Jorfeldt L., Martensson J. & Schildt B. (1984) Effects of the extradural administration of morphine, or bupivacaine, on the endocrine response to upper abdominal surgery. *British Journal of Anaesthesia* **56**, 233–8.

Rutter P.C., Murphy F. & Dudley H.A.F. (1980) Morphine: controlled trial of different methods of administration for postoperative pain relief. *British Medical Journal* **1**, 12–13.

Sabanaythan B.J., Mearns A.J., Bickford-Smith P.J., Eng J.B., Berrisford R.G., Bibby S.R. & Majid M.R. (1990) Efficacy of continuous extrapleural intercostal nerve block on postthoracotomy pain and pulmonary mechanics. *British Journal of Surgery* **77**, 221–5.

Saha S.K. (1981) Continuous infusion of papaveretum for relief of postoperative pain. *Postgraduate Medical Journal* **57**, 686–9.

Schulze S., Roikjaer O., Hasselstrøm L., Jensen N.H. & Kehlet H. (1988) Epidural bupivacaine and morphine plus systemic indomethacin eliminates pain but not systemic response and convalescence after cholecystectomy. *Surgery* **103**, 321–7.

Schulze S., Sommer P., Bigler D., Honnens M., Shenkin A., Cruickshank A., Bukhave K. & Kehlet H. (1992) Effect of combined prednisolone, epidural analgesia and indomethacin on the systemic response after colonic surgery. *Archives of Surgery* **127**, 325–31.

Scott N.B. & Kehlet H. (1988) Regional anaesthesia and surgical morbidity. *British Journal of Surgery* **75**, 299–304.

Scott L.E., Clum G.A. & Peoples J.B. (1983) Preoperative predictors of postoperative pain. *Pain* **15**, 283–93.

Sechzer P.H. (1968) Objective measurement of pain. *Anesthesiology* **29**, 209–10.

Smith B.E., MacPherson G.H., de Jonge M. & Griffiths J.M. (1991) Rectus sheath and mesosalpinx block for laparoscopic sterilization. *Anaesthesia* **46**, 875–7.

Stanton-Hicks M.J. (1985) Subarachnoid and extradural analgesic techniques. In *Acute Pain* (Eds Smith G. & Covino B.G.) pp. 228–56. Butterworths, London.

Stapleton J.V., Austin K.L. & Mather L.E. (1979) A pharmacokinetic approach to postoperative pain: continuous infusion of pethidine. *Anaesthesia and Intensive Care* **7**, 25–32.

Stein C., Comisel K., Haimerl F., Yassouridis A., Herz A. & Peter K. (1991) Analgesic effect of intraarticular morphine after arthroscopic knee surgery. *New England Journal of Medicine* **325**, 1123–6.

Striebel H.W., Koenigs D. & Kramer J. (1992) Postoperative pain management by intranasal demand-adapted fentanyl titration. *Anaesthesiology* **77**, 281–5.

Tamsen A., Hartvig P., Fagerlund C. & Dahlstrom (1982a) Patient controlled analgesic therapy, part II: individual analgesic demand and analgesic plasma concentrations of pethidine in postoperative pain. *Clinical Pharmacokinetics* **7**, 164–75.

Tamsen A., Bondensson U., Danlstrom B. & Hartvig P. (1982b) Patient controlled analgesic therapy, part III: pharmacokinetics and analgesic plasma concentrations of ketobemidone. *Clinical Pharmacokinetics* **7**, 252–66.

Tamsen A., Sakurada T., Wahlstrom A., Terenius L. & Hartvig P. (1982c) Postoperative demands for analgesics in relation to individual levels of endorphins and substance P in cerebrospinal fluid. *Pain* **13**, 171–83.

Thorén T. (1987) Effects on gastric emptying of thoracic epidural analgesia with morphine or bupivacaine. *Anesthesia and Analgesia* **67**, 687–94.

Wall P.D. (1988) The prevention of postoperative pain. *Pain* **33**, 289–90.

Wattwil M. (1988) Postoperative pain relief and gastrointestinal motility. *Acta Chirurgica Scandinavica Supplementum* **550**, 140–5.

Wheatley R.G., Somerville I.D., Sapsford D.J. & Jones J.G. (1990) Postoperative hypoxaemia: comparison of extradural, i.m. and patient-controlled opioid analgesia. *British Journal of Anaesthesia* **64**, 267–75.

Wheatley R.G., Madej T.H., Jackson I.J.B. & Hunter D. (1991) The first year's experience of an acute pain service. *British Journal of Anaesthesia* **67**, 353–9.

Woolf C.J. (1989) Recent advances in the pathophysiology of acute pain. *British Journal of Anaesthesia* **63**, 139–46.

Worsley M.H., Macleod A.D., Brodie M.J., Asbury A.J. & Clark C. (1990) Inhaled fentanyl as a method of analgesia. *Anaesthesia* **45**, 449–51.

Yeager M.P., Glass D., Neff R.K. & Brinck-Johnsen T. (1987) Epidural anaesthesia and analgesia in high-risk surgical patients. *Anesthesiology* **66**, 729–36.

Paediatric Analgesia

L. R. McNICOL

That a major textbook on anaesthesia should have a section dedicated to pain relief in paediatric practice is a recognition of the problems that exist in providing adequate analgesia for this specialized group of patients. Although older children and adolescents have in general been treated as adults, smaller children, especially neonates and infants, have to be considered separately because of psychological, behavioural, physiological and anatomical differences which make assessment and treatment of pain much more difficult. Although some children, especially those suffering from childhood cancers, do suffer chronic pain, the greatest problem from the anaesthetic point of view is the management of acute pain — postoperative pain. The treatment of chronic pain in paediatric practice is very similar to that in adults.

Neonates

It is only in recent years that it has been accepted that very small children do suffer from unrelieved postoperative pain. There is no doubt that it was convenient to dismiss any pain suffered by neonates in the postoperative period on the grounds that 'neonates do not feel pain'. There is no doubt that some surgeons and anaesthetists working in paediatric hospitals genuinely did believe at one time that neonates did not feel pain but there are others who have used this dictum as an excuse to avoid the complicated pharmacological and physiological difficulties associated with treating pain in children so young.

It is now firmly accepted that neonates *do* feel pain and that this can be recognized by experienced nurses and doctors working regularly in a paediatric environment. However, care must be taken not to equate neonatal perception of pain with that of older children and adults as it is clear that this differs greatly from other age groups. Gross and Gardner (1980) have commented that as newborns develop, so do their reactions to a set painful stimulus, twice as much being required to produce a response in a 1-day-old as in a 3-month-old baby. There are several factors which account for the assumed reduction in pain perception by neonates (Table 77.1).

The importance of immature pain receptors in the neonatal period is not obvious. However, myelinization of the CNS is not completed until about 18 months of age and transmission of pain through the central pathways is delayed; indeed, not all central pathways are fully developed in neonates, the thalamocortical radiations not being completed until the end of infancy. Thus, rate of conduction of nerve impulses is markedly reduced in neonates, especially preterm neonates, and indeed, this is such a consistent finding that the rate of nerve conduction is a useful tool for estimating gestational age of a child when this is in doubt. It is interesting to note that despite these differences in early anatomy of nerves, there is little difference in the time for spinal reflexes to occur between neonates and older children as the actual distance travelled by a nerve impulse is less in neonates because the nerve is shorter. The third factor modifying the perception of pain by neonates is of great interest. Both parturient mothers and their neonates have been found to have elevated plasma β-endorphin concentrations (Csontos et al., 1979). Although the level of this neurotransmitter in the newborn is high immediately after birth and may be assumed to be a result of placental transfer, it remains

Table 77.1 Factors modifying neonatal pain perception

1 Immaturity of pain receptors
2 Incomplete myelinization of CNS
3 Increased β-endorphin levels in plasma and CSF

high for the first 4 or 5 days of life, indicating that it is in fact being produced by the neonate. The reasons for this at present remain obscure although it can be postulated that it is a protective mechanism in response to the trauma of birth. However, the net effect of these high levels is that with a less well-developed blood−brain barrier, as is found during the neonatal period, the β-endorphin may have a greater tendency for central depression. Thus, while it is accepted that neonates do feel pain, it has to be said that the intensity and quality of this pain is different from that perceived by older children and adults. Indeed, it may be analogous to the pain perceived by adults with a demyelinating disease or a peripheral neuropathy.

Recent years have seen many studies aimed at proving that neonates suffer from pain and also at assessing this pain (Table 77.2).

Clinical and behavioural methods of estimating pain are by far the most important as these are the methods which are routinely used in neonatal units. These observations have all been made in the presence of a known painful stimulus, commonly circumcision without general anaesthesia and heel lancing (Table 77.3).

In 1987 Anand and colleagues showed that neonates and preterm neonates produced a stress response after major surgery. They noted increased outputs of catecholamines and steroids which could be modified if fentanyl $10 \mu g/kg$ was added to the general anaesthetic technique. This group of workers also showed that for less major surgery, the stress response could be modified in neonates by simply including halothane as part of the anaesthetic technique (Anand

Table 77.2 Methods for assessment of neonatal pain

1 Clinical
2 Behavioural
3 Endocrine
4 Skin conduction
5 Voice spectographic analysis

Table 77.3 Neonatal response to pain (pooled data)

1 Undue wakefulness/sleeping
2 Prolonged periods of crying
3 Grimacing
4 Purposeless movements of all four limbs
5 Increased heart rate
6 Increased respiratory rate
7 Decreased Spo_2

et al., 1988). Although skin-conductance levels have been shown to increase during a standard painful stimulus in the absence of other physiological or behavioural changes in neonates and voice spectrographic analysis can identify the type of cry associated with pain, both these techniques are of limited practical value.

The treatment of neonatal pain depends very much on the severity of the surgical procedure. The basis of good postoperative analgesia for this group of children is to establish a degree of intraoperative analgesia using a local anaesthetic technique which lasts into the postoperative period and if this is effective, many children who undergo minor surgery require no further analgesia and respond well to warmth, early feeding and swaddling. The pharmacological agents of choice for this group of children are either paracetamol or codeine phosphate and ideally these drugs should be administered before any intraoperative local analgesia wears off. Under such circumstances it is rare for a child to require more than one dose of these systemic analgesics. Hopkins and colleagues (1991) have investigated the pharmacokinetics of paracetamol in a group of children who had elevated temperatures after cardiac surgery, 12 of whom were neonates. Paracetamol was administered either as a triglyceride suppository or orally and these authors noted that plasma concentration did not exceed $20 \mu g/ml$ even after doses close to $25 mg/kg$ were administered, much less than the proposed level of $120 \mu g/ml$ at which paracetamol concentrations are likely to cause hepatic damage. However, plasma elimination half-life and the area under the curve were significantly increased in neonates compared with older children and the authors concluded that there may be a possibility that this drug could accumulate in neonates after regular dosing and as such it is best to limit it to a total daily dose of $60 mg/kg$. Codeine phosphate in a dose of $1 mg/kg$ intramuscularly or orally is enthusiastically used by the Great Ormond Street Group of anaesthetists (Hatch & Sumner, 1989). They stress, however, that it should be used in single doses only and that it must not be administered intravenously as it occasionally causes a profound reduction in cardiac output.

The local anaesthetic techniques which may be used for minor surgical procedures in neonates vary but should be kept as simple as possible, good analgesia being possible with basic techniques such as infiltration (Fell et al., 1988) and instillation (Casey et al., 1990) of bupivacaine and also the application of topical local anaesthetic agents to mucosal surfaces; e.g. lignocaine either as a gel, ointment or aerosol applied to the glans penis after circumcision but before the child awakens can provide a short period of analgesia postoperatively during which it is possible to commence a child on systemic analgesics. Tre-Trakarn and Pirayavarporn (1985) have used this technique in older children and found it to be as effective as a block of the dorsal nerve of the penis (DNP) or morphine. For relieving postcircumcision pain in neonates, Kirya and Werthmann (1978) advocate the use of DNP block and are confident that under such circumstances the procedure should be 'painless'. Arthur and McNicol (1986) use bupivacaine 0.5% for such blocks, stressing that no vasoconstrictor should be added to the anaesthetic solution. In recent years there have been many studies of spinal anaesthesia as an alternative to general anaesthesia for children at risk from postoperative apnoea and bradycardias. These children are mainly 'graduates from the special care baby unit (SCBU)' — premature and ex-premature children. The incidence of inguinal hernia is 16% in these children. Repair is necessary at an early age in order to avoid the complications of incarceration and strangulation, and while no definite answer has been reached regarding the benefits of spinal anaesthesia compared with general anaesthesia for this group of children, an interesting off-shoot has been the excellent postoperative analgesia which can be achieved using some of these techniques. They may last for 2–3 h into the postoperative period, during which time systemic analgesics can be administered if necessary. Indeed, if bupivacaine is injected into the wound intraoperatively by the surgeon, postoperative analgesia lasting 4–6 h can be achieved. Many different local anaesthetic agents and combinations of local anaesthetic agents have been recommended for spinal anaesthesia but the easiest to use is possibly that recommended by Mahé and Ecoffey (1988) using plain isobaric bupivacaine 0.5% in a dose of approximately 0.8 mg/kg of body weight. It should be remembered that the spinal cord ends at the lower border of the third lumbar vertebra in neonates and as such, a low approach to spinal anaesthesia is mandatory.

Local anaesthetic agents have to be used with care in neonates as differences in metabolism and protein binding result in high free concentrations. Neonates and infants up to 6 months of age have less than half the adult levels of pseudocholinesterase and clearance of the ester group of local anaesthetics may be reduced with subsequent prolongation of action. For example, the plasma half-life of chloroprocaine in umbilical cord plasma has been reported to be twice that of the maternal half life — 43 s compared to 21 s. The metabolism of the amide group of local anaesthetics depends on oxidative pathways in the liver involving cytochrome P450. The level of this enzyme has been found to be almost the same in neonates as in adults, but with the exception of lignocaine the capacity of both age groups to metabolize amide local anaesthetics is not the same. The metabolism of mepivacaine, for example, is greatly reduced in the neonate and up to 90% of this local anaesthetic agent is excreted unchanged in the urine and dealkylation of bupivacaine cannot occur until several hours after birth. With the exception of bupivacaine, the amide local anaesthetics have relatively high hepatic clearance and the hepatic blood flow is therefore the factor which most limits clearance. As this is reduced in neonates and young infants less than 3 months of age, larger fractions of local anaesthetics are unmetabolized and remain active in the plasma than in the adult. It is interesting to note that after the first few months of life children eliminate drugs at a greater rate than adults and this may be due at least in part to the fact that the liver is relatively much larger in children as a percentage of body weight and also contains more metabolic sites for the breakdown of local anaesthetics (Boreus, 1982).

It is generally believed that non-protein-bound (free) concentrations of drugs relate to pharmacological and toxic effects more closely than do total concentrations, especially for lignocaine and bupivacaine. Thus, variations in the extent of plasma binding in different subjects may be associated with very different total concentrations. Therefore neonates and infants may be at increased risk of toxic effects of amide local anaesthetics because of lower levels of albumin and α_1-acid glycoprotein (AAG). Both these proteins are important for the binding of local anaesthetics although their binding properties are very different. Albumin has a low affinity for local anaesthetics and almost never becomes saturated; AAG, on the other hand, has a high affinity for such drugs and a greater number of molecules are bound per mole compared to albumin. However, AAG soon becomes saturated and when this threshold is reached, the free fraction of drug increases very rapidly when the total concentration in the plasma increases. These protein concentrations are very low at birth, albumin being 60–80% of adult levels and AAG 50%. Adult levels are not reached until between 6 and 12 months of age. Age is not the only factor which influences protein binding; metabolic and respiratory acidosis increase the free fraction of lignocaine and bupivacaine and an anaesthetic technique associated with hypoventilation in a small infant may lead to a sudden increase in the risk of toxicity of local anaesthetics and as such a technique may also result in increased cerebral blood flow, the risk of CNS toxicity of local anaesthetics is very real. This may be compounded if neonates are suffering from jaundice, as bilirubin competes with local anaesthetic for albumin resulting again in higher, free local anaesthetic levels. Thus, the total dose of local anaesthetic administered to neonates should be less than recommended adult doses and it is the author's practice to restrict the maximum dose of bupivacaine to 1.5 mg/kg of body weight.

For surgical procedures which may result in moderate pain, local anaesthetic techniques may also be used to establish intraoperative and early postoperative analgesia. The author has recommended that bupivacaine 0.25% with adrenaline be injected underneath the rectus sheath intraoperatively during pyloromyotomy (McNicol et al., 1990). Markedly less disturbances in pulse and heart rate, and behaviour were found in a group of children who received this treatment compared with a control group who did not, and although these differences were most evident in the immediate postoperative period, they were still present 24 h postoperatively. An alternative to peripheral nerve blocks, infiltration and spinal anaesthesia for operations on the lower abdomen in the neonates is a caudal extradural block. However, this does require a large volume and dose of local anaesthetic, although Peutrell and Hughes (1993) have reduced this to an absolute minimum by using a caudal extradural catheter with its tip in the lumbar extradural space. With paediatric spinal needles now in a highly sophisticated state of development and spinal anaesthesia firmly established, it is the author's opinion that a small volume of local anaesthetic injected into the subarachnoid space is more efficient and safer than a caudal extradural in this age group.

It is now recognized that neonates undergoing major surgery deserve the same standard of analgesia as any other patient and morphine is still the most widely opioid used for this purpose. However, there is no doubt that neonates are extremely sensitive to opioids in general for a variety of reasons

Table 77.4 Causes of neonatal sensitivity to morphine

1 Elimination half-life ($t_{\frac{1}{2}}\beta$) increased
2 Clearance (Cl) reduced
3 Blood–brain barrier less effective
4 Endogenous β-endorphins increased
5 $\mu_1 : \mu_2$-receptor ratio altered

(Table 77.4). Booker (1989) has reviewed the age-related differences in the pharmacokinetic parameters of opioids and comments that although the apparent volume of distribution (V_d) of morphine in the neonate is not dissimilar from that of adults (3.4 litres/kg) the elimination half-life is 629 min, approximately three-and-a-half times as long as that of adults, and that the clearance at $7 ml \cdot kg^{-1} \cdot min^{-1}$ is half adult values. The reasons for these differences are not entirely clear, but neonates do exhibit many physiological differences from older children and adults which may account for these pharmacokinetic findings. In adults approximately one-third of an intravenous dose of morphine is protein bound. Protein binding of many drugs, including morphine, is much reduced in the neonate leading to increased concentrations of the free drug and when all plasma-protein-binding sites are occupied, the addition of more of the drug increases the unbound fraction by a disproportionate amount thus making more drug available to the tissues. As mentioned above adult levels of albumin are not reached until about 3 months of age but in addition, during the early neonatal period, variable amounts of fetal albumin may persist and this has a lower affinity for drugs than adult albumin. Marked differences in the metabolism and excretion of morphine exists between neonates and adults. Drugs cleared by the liver are classified conventionally into those whose clearance is dependent largely on hepatic blood flow and those dependent on metabolism by the liver cells. For drugs which have a high hepatic extraction ratio such as morphine, the elimination half-life tends to reflect hepatic blood flow and is relatively unaffected by microsomal activity. Thus, the relatively reduced hepatic blood flow which is present in neonates and in infants less than 3 months of age may account in part for the delay in clearance. In addition, conjugation of morphine with glucuronic acid is reduced in neonates and indeed does not reach adult values until about 3 years of age. The importance of the immature neonatal kidney with respect to the metabolism and elimination of morphine is not clear and indeed in the past was discounted. However, Booker (1989) draws attention to the fact that extrahepatic metabolism of morphine may be a real possibility (McQuay & Moore, 1984) and is dependent on normal mature renal function. He concluded that an adequate urinary output is probably important for the elimination of active (and inactive) metabolites and termination of clinical effect. In addition to these pharmacokinetic variabilities, neonates are sensitive to morphine for several pharmacological reasons.

The immature neonatal blood–brain barrier may allow increased passage of some drugs across it including morphine and this may be compounded by the presence of increased endogenous β-endorphin levels in the first few days of life. Finally experimental studies suggest that the proportion of μ_1-receptors (analgesia) is low at birth and that μ_2-receptors (respiratory depression) are relatively high thereby increasing the risk of respiratory depression (Leslie et al., 1982).

As a result of this increased sensitivity to morphine, it is conventional to discuss its administration in two groups of neonates — those breathing spontaneously and those having respiratory assistance. Although these two groups of children may exist as a result of the severity of the operative procedure performed on them or because of pre-existing cardio-respiratory problems, there are some paediatric anaesthetists who feel that it is quite legitimate to electively ventilate the lungs of a neonate solely to ensure that it receives adequate analgesia. Only neonates who can be guaranteed intensive postoperative monitoring and a 1:1 nurse:patient ratio should be given morphine, thus limiting its administration to children in neonatal high-dependency units or intensive care units. Booker (1989) drew attention to the fact that in addition to the problems of a prolonged elimination half-life in neonates there are also great variations in serum concentrations following any μg/kg dose and that plasma morphine concentrations can also increase despite cessation of an infusion; thus, these children require close supervision. Anecdotal incidents abound about neonates developing apnoea after administration of morphine and Purcell-Jones and colleagues (1987) have described some of these problems. Hatch and Sumner (1989) observed the safety of a continuous infusion of morphine, $5–10\,\mu g \cdot kg^{-1} \cdot h^{-1}$ (one-quarter to one-half the dose of older children), in spontaneously breathing newborns although it is the author's practice to try to restrict this to $5\,\mu g \cdot kg^{-1} \cdot h^{-1}$. Neonates receiving respiratory support can be managed with an infusion of morphine running at about $10\,\mu g \cdot kg^{-1} \cdot h^{-1}$, which on occasion may be increased to $15\,\mu g \cdot kg^{-1} \cdot h^{-1}$. As with morphine infusions in all age groups, the aim should be to assess the patient continually and attempt to reduce the infusion rate.

Fentanyl is an alternative to morphine in this group of children but the highly variable disposition of this drug in neonates compounds the difficulty in predicting full and permanent ventilatory recovery. However, there is no doubt that neonates are extremely sensitive to fentanyl and in the author's opinion it has little to offer over morphine for routine postoperative analgesia. Marlow and colleagues (1990) have used alfentanil successfully without evidence of accumulation as a bolus dose of 20 μg/kg administered slowly over 30 min followed by an infusion running at $5\,\mu g \cdot kg^{-1} \cdot h^{-1}$ and this may allow rapid recovery after cessation of the infusion.

Infants

Most paediatric anaesthetists tend to treat the analgesics requirements of infants between 5 and 6 months and 1 year similarly to those of adults. Between the 1st month of life and the 5th or 6th month of life, there is an intermediate period during which they show increasing resistance to morphine and the opioids but nevertheless have to be observed for signs of respiratory depression should these drugs be used. For minor surgery the basis is a good intraoperative local anaesthetic block lasting into the early postoperative period and simple systemic analgesia should be commenced before the block wears off. Again, paracetamol, dihydrocodeine and codeine phosphate are the drugs of choice. For major surgery a morphine infusion can be commenced intraoperatively and can be established in the early postoperative period as a local block wears off. Half the adult dose ($10\,\mu g \cdot kg^{-1} \cdot h^{-1}$) is adequate for children breathing spontaneously and this may be administered intravenously or subcutaneously. Provided adequate nursing staff are available, it is possible to manage these children in an ordinary surgical ward. Postoperative monitoring is essential and should include not only pulse oximetry but also clinical observations charted regularly on a 'subcutaneous morphine chart' (see below).

Children from about 5 or 6 months of age can generally be treated as adults as far as their morphine requirements are concerned and a dose of $20\,\mu g \cdot kg^{-1} \cdot h^{-1}$ (Bray, 1983) following an intraoperative local anaesthetic block produces excellent analgesia in spontaneously breathing patients. Despite this age group's apparent resistance to morphine compared with younger infants, it is essential that they are closely monitored in the postoperative period.

Older children

From the end of infancy up until about 7 years of age children pass through various stages of development during which their perception of pain and their reaction to it change. Marked behavioural changes are evident in younger children, evident as crying, tantrums, rocking, teeth clenching and even head banging. Not uncommonly, appetite is adversely affected, there may be regression of acquired social habits, bedwetting may recur and skills such as holding utensils and using them correctly may be temporarily lost. Preschool age children who are extremely dependent on the presence and support of parents may benefit greatly from parental presence in the immediate postoperative period.

From about the age of 5, children verbally complain and leave the observer in no doubt that they are suffering pain and visual analogue scales are of some use in this age group (Fig. 77.1). Other scales have used different colours to signify severities of pain, red being associated with severe pain by most children and others have used toys climbing up visual analogue scales, the monkey at the top of the pole being in more pain than the monkey at the bottom. Although these tools are used mainly for research, nevertheless they have proved useful and it would appear that round about 7 years of age childrens' perception of pain is similar to that of adults, i.e. they are able to quantify it accurately and indeed, it would appear that the assessment of pain in this age group by external adult observers tends to underestimate that which the child is feeling. For younger children, pain/discomfort scales such as that described by Hannallah and colleagues (1987) are not only useful for comparing analgesic regimens in comparative studies, but also when used routinely indicate when an individual child requires postoperative analgesia.

As with other age groups, the mainstay of postoperative analgesia in older children is to establish an effective local anaesthetic block intraoperatively. These are discussed in detail elsewhere and recent advances in these techniques have been reviewed by the author (McNicol, 1991). Systemic analgesia, either oral or parenteral, by single shot or infusion depending on the severity of the operation, can be commenced before the block wears off and an alternative to paracetamol and codeine for the relief of minor or moderate pain are the non-steroidal anti-inflammatory drugs (NSAIDs). Maunuksela and colleagues (1988) used indomethacin intravenously as a 350 μg/kg bolus followed by an infusion of 70 μg·kg^{-1}·h^{-1}, converting to oral indomethacin at 3 mg·kg^{-1}·day^{-1} in an attempt to control pain following tonsillectomy. Although they showed a morphine-sparing affect with this regimen, no improvement in the quality of pain relief could be detected using a pain score. Moore and Hargreaves (1985) used ibuprofen in liquid form to relieve pain after dental extractions and found it to be more effective than either paracetamol or a paracetamol—codeine compound agent. Most recently, diclofenac has been singled out for special attention from other NSAIDs. Bone and Fell (1988) used this drug in a dose of 2 mg/kg administered rectally to control pain after tonsillectomy in a group of children aged between 3 and 13 years and found it to be as effective as intramuscular papaveretum 200 μg/kg with less central sedation. Similarly Watters and colleagues (1988) used it administered intramuscularly in a dose of 1 mg/kg after induction of anaesthesia, to provide analgesia the equal of pethidine after adenotonsillectomy, again maintaining an acceptable level of sedation postoperatively.

Moores and colleagues (1990) compared 2.5 mg/kg of diclofenac administered rectally with a caudal extradural block using bupivacaine 0.25%, 1 ml/kg, for the control of pain following inguinal herniotomy. Although the children who received the extradural block were assessed as having superior analgesia immediately after surgery, the diclofenac group had better pain relief later on in the postoperative period and the authors have postulated that this may be due to the presence of a metabolite. The main disadvantages of electing to use diclofenac are that when used intramuscularly it causes pain on injection and when used intravenously it is associated with an unacceptably high rate of thrombophlebitis. However, Campbell and colleagues (1990) has used it in a dose of 1 mg/kg dissolved in dextrose 5%, 1 mg/ml i.v., in a group of adolescents after oral surgery with an effect equal to that of 2 μg/kg of fentanyl and without producing any thrombophlebitis. It has to be said that this route of administration is not recommended by the manufacturers of diclofenac (Geigy). Nevertheless, further studies on this method of adminis-

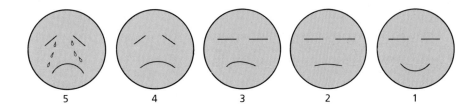

Fig. 77.1 'Happy/sad face' visual analogue scale designed for paediatric use. (Redrawn from Maunuksela *et al.*, 1987.)

tration are continuing and Berry and colleagues (1991, personal communication) have used it in similar dosage and concentration dissolved in dextrose 5% to produce highly effective analgesia following tonsillectomy and adenoidectomy in children. Again there was neither evidence of thrombophlebitis nor of increased intraoperative or postoperative bleeding as a result of platelet inhibition by diclofenac.

Extradural analgesia

Although single-shot caudal analgesia is popular and firmly established in paediatric practice, techniques of continuous extradural block are becoming more popular even in neonates and preterm neonates and are run for some period postoperatively. The technique of passing an epidural catheter by way of the sacral hiatus was pioneered in 1989 by Bosenberg and colleagues. This is an interesting technique as a catheter passed into the extradural space by this route may reach almost any level because the extradural fat in children is gelatinous, offering minimal resistance. Bosenberg originally used this technique in infants undergoing correction of biliary atresia and Busoni (1990) has used it for similar procedures and other lower abdominal operations for children in whom the postoperative course was particularly easy and satisfactory. Van Niekerk and colleagues (1990) have used this technique in 20 premature high-risk infants as part of a balanced anaesthetic technique. All of these children were extremely premature and small, their weights ranging from only 950 gm to 2750 gm. The catheters were left in place in 17 of these infants and they received continuous postoperative analgesia with nicomorphine. Nine of these children were on the verge of respiratory failure and Van Niekerk commented that had not a balanced anaesthetic technique been used, these children would have undoubtedly required prolonged postoperative ventilation with all the risks that this entails in the premature. In order to ensure correct placement of the extradural catheters, contrast medium was injected; this indeed proved to be an essential part of the technique as it was evident from the radiographs that in one patient, the catheter had penetrated the dura, in another it was located in an extradural vessel and in a third it was curled up within the extradural space.

Although other approaches to the extradural space are more popular in children older than 1 year, nevertheless, they can be used with care in smaller children; in a series of 650 consecutive extradural blocks, Dalens and Chrysostome (1991) included 95

infants. Fifty of this group were less than 6 months of age and 15 had thoracic extradural block successfully — 27 lumbar extradurals and eight extradurals via sacral intravertebral spaces. Although these authors used narrow 20-gauge extradural needles for the majority of these blocks and 'infant' 24-gauge nylon catheters were passed through these needles, the diameter of the needle is probably not crucial as larger needles may safely be used in paediatric practice. However, the length of the needle used is more crucial and it is much easier to perform an extradural block in small children if a short needle is used as the distance from the skin to the ligamentum flavum is only of the order of 1 cm in newborn children.

In children older than 1 year, continuous lumbar and thoracic extradurals are becoming more popular in paediatric practice as part of a balanced anaesthetic technique, continuing into the postoperative period to provide analgesia after major surgery or in high-risk patients. Most studies have been performed on lower-abdominal operations and on orthopaedic procedures on the pelvis and lower limbs, although good upper-abdominal pain relief can be achieved with high 'lumbar' extradurals or thoracic extradurals. It is possible to block as high as T4 in children less than 5 or 6 years of age without adversely affecting arterial pressure or cardiac output (Dohi et al., 1979) possibly because compared with other age groups, the sympathetic nervous system is relatively immature and capacitance vessels on a weight-related basis are not so fully developed. However, in children older than 6 years of age, unpredictable hypotension may occur after a high block as occurs in adult practice.

Although the level of analgesia after caudal extradural block can be fairly accurately predicted there are no set formulae for achieving a set spread of analgesia after lumbar or thoracic extradurals. Murat and colleagues (1987) recommended the use of bupivacaine 0.25%, 0.75 ml/kg, for children weighing less than 20 kg or 1 ml for every 10 cm of height for children taller than 100 cm. This provides blocks of the order of 10—12 segments when injected at a lumbar intravertebral space.

Continuous lumbar extradural block, although recommended by some paediatric anaesthetists for virtually any procedure involving dermatomes below T5, is probably best restricted to children undergoing major abdominal procedures and orthopaedic procedures or children with pulmonary or muscle diseases where complete pain control can be achieved without having to resort to opioids. When adequate analgesia has been established, it can usually be maintained if bupivacaine 0.125–0.25% is infused at a rate of about $0.1\,\text{ml}\cdot\text{kg}^{-1}\cdot\text{h}^{-1}$.

Continuous thoracic extradural blocks are also becoming more popular in paediatric practice and in Dalens' and Chrysostome's series of 650 extradural blocks, 76 or 11.7% were thoracic. Murat (1990) observed that this technique should be reserved for major surgical procedures in poor-risk children. It is Murat's practice to explain the technique in detail to parents and to obtain informed consent with a note on the patient's record outlining the 'real benefit' of the technique. Typical indications for this block are upper abdominal procedures such as Nissen's fundoplication for hiatus hernia, nephrectomy and reconstructive renal surgery, hepatectomy and surgery for biliary atresia and resection of large abdominal masses such as Wilm's tumours. For children weighing less than 30 kg Murat recommends bupivacaine 0.25%, 0.5–0.75 ml/kg. This anaesthetizes approximately 12 spinal segments. She observed that in adults the dose required for anaesthesia of a given number of segments by the thoracic approach is about two-thirds of that required by the lumbar, because the thoracic dural space is narrower. However, this is not true for children, especially the very young, in whom both the anatomy of the extradural space and the nature of the gelatinous extradural fat encourages spread of local anaesthetics. It is Murat's practice therefore initially to inject 0.5 ml/kg and top up with further injections if necessary. For control of postoperative pain, some paediatric anaesthetists top up thoracic extradurals intermittently rather than run a continuous infusion; the dose is normally of the order of half the original dose. Again it is worthy of note that cardiovascular changes are minimal in children under the age of 6 years even when the block extends as high as T4. This has been illustrated by Arthur (1980) who used thoracic extradural blocks postoperatively after repair of coarctation of the aorta in an attempt to control the secondary hypertension commonly seen after this procedure; despite large volumes of bupivacaine and a level of block higher than T4, arterial pressure remained high (Fig. 77.2).

Although the use of extradural opioids is firmly established in adult practice, it is still uncommon in paediatric anaesthetics. Dalens and Chrysostome (1991) added 25–50 µg/kg of preservative-free morphine to the local anaesthetic and considerably increased the period during which the patients were pain-free, over 93% not complaining of pain for 16 h following the extradural injection. However, this was associated with an increased incidence of adverse effects. Treatment aimed at decreasing the occurrence of these side-effects was not always effective. Small doses of droperidol and a low-dose continuous infusion of naloxone resulted in a comparable decrease in pruritis and also reduced the incidence of nausea and vomiting whereas naloxone alone prevented urinary retention and delayed respiratory depression. However, droperidol had no effect on the duration of postoperative pain relief whereas naloxone infusions slightly, but significantly, reduced it. It is now generally recognized that low doses of opioids combined with dilute concentrations of local anaesthetics appear to act synergistically and a high therapeutic ratio can be obtained with a reduction of the side-effects commonly seen if both types of drugs are used individually — i.e. less motor block, urinary retention, pruritis and delayed respiratory depression. Berde and colleagues (1990) used extradural bupivacaine and fentanyl infusions in children to prevent pain after urologic surgery. Fentanyl, approximately 2 µg/ml, in bupivacaine 0.1–0.125% was given at an approximate rate of $0.22\,\text{ml}\cdot\text{kg}^{-1}\cdot\text{h}^{-1}$ and although the common side-effects of both drugs were noted to some extent, these were not as frequent as when each of these agents are used alone in greater concentrations.

A natural progression in the management of postoperative pain would seem to be combining patient-controlled analgesia (PCA) with extradural anaesthesia either using local anaesthetics or anaesthetics in combination with opioids. Bellamy and

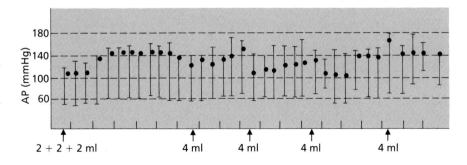

Fig. 77.2 Thoracic extradural block: effect on systemic arterial pressure in a child aged 3 years 10 months (17 kg) following surgery for coarctation of the aorta. Large doses of bupivacaine were administered as indicated and subsequent blood pressure measurements, taken every 5 min following a top-up, remained elevated. (Redrawn from Arthur & McNicol, 1986.)

colleagues (1990) have assessed the feasibility of this technique in a small group of children. (It should be noted that these authors have assessed 10 000 patient hours using this technique of patient-controlled extradural infusion in adults.) They inserted extradural catheters after induction of anaesthesia and each patient received 20–30 µg/kg of preservative-free morphine sulphate 1 h before the end of surgery combined with 1.25 µg/kg boluses of preservative-free morphine sulphate by means of a PCA system. Preservative-free morphine sulphate was also given as a background infusion of $5 \mu g \cdot kg^{-1} \cdot h^{-1}$. Side-effects were low and patient satisfaction high in this small study.

Although continuous extradural techniques are safe and effective in paediatric practice, in the absence of sedation, the child may object to the presence of intravenous infusions, nasogastric tubes, urinary catheters and wound dressings (Wolf & Hughes, 1993). In order to prevent these being ceremoniously removed one by one, an opioid or sedative may have to be administered. In many ways, this defeats the initial purpose of using extradural analgesia. As a result, some anaesthetists are using systemic opioids more frequently as continuous infusions or as part of PCA rather than continuous local anaesthetic techniques.

Opioid infusions in paediatric practice

Morphine is the drug most commonly used. A continuous infusion can be administered either intravenously or subcutaneously in a dose of $20 \mu g \cdot kg^{-1} \cdot h^{-1}$. Lloyd Thomas (1990) in a comprehensive review of pain management in children noted that although morphine has been administered continuously subcutaneously in children suffering from terminal malignancies in a dose of $30–60 \mu g \cdot kg^{-1} \cdot h^{-1}$, it has not been applied to relieve postoperative pain. He suggested that the dose required should be little more than that administered intravenously. This is now the author's first choice for postoperative pain relief following surgical procedures which produce moderate to severe pain (McNicol, 1993). A 24-gauge cannula (Neoflon) is inserted subcutaneously usually over the deltoid muscle (Fig. 77.3) and connected by an extension tube to a 50 or 60 ml syringe in an infusion pump which contains 1 mg/kg of body weight of morphine made up to 20 ml with normal saline. If run at a rate of 0.4 ml/h, 20 µg/kg of morphine are delivered each hour and it is normal practice to prescribe a rate of 0.3–0.6 ml/h that can be adjusted by the nursing

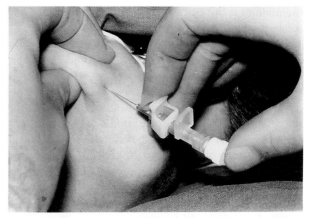

A

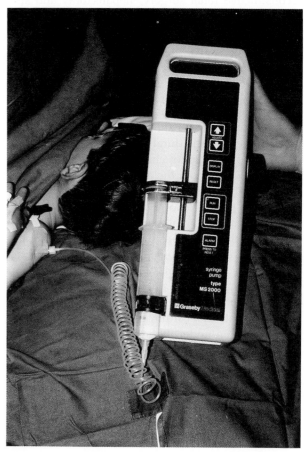

B

Fig. 77.3 (A) A 24-gauge cannula (Neoflon) is inserted subcutaneously after the induction of anaesthesia. (B) The cannula is firmly secured and attached via extension tubing to a syringe pump.

staff. An important part of this technique are the postoperative observations made by the nursing staff on a Royal Hospital for Sick Children (McNicol) chart (Fig. 77.4). In addition to clinical observations, pulse

Subcutaneous morphine infusion   (Please file completed chart in casenotes)

Name: *Unit no:*   *DOB:*   *Age:*   *Weight:*

Operation: *Date:*

Morphine concn: (1 mg/kg in 20 ml 0.9% saline)   *Infusion site:* Deltoid
rate from: ml *to:*   ml   Pectoral
                                                                           Abdominal
Any adjustments: (specify type, reason and time made)

Record hourly:

Time	Resp. rate	O₂ sat.	Sedation score Eyes open: 0=Spontaneously 1=To speech 2=To shake 3=Unrousable (Call doctor)	Pain score 0=No pain A=Asleep 1=Not really sore 2=Quite sore 3=Very sore (crying) (Call doctor)	Nausea score 0=None 1=Nausea only 2=Vomiting ×I in last hour 3=Vomiting >1 in last hour (Call doctor)	Rate of infusion ml	Vol. left in pump ml

Fig. 77.4 Postoperative observations chart for children receiving continuous subcutaneous infusions of morphine. (Redrawn from McNicol, 1993.)

Call doctor if severe pain (score 3), patient unrousable (sedation score 3), excessive nausea and vomiting (nausea score 3), SaO₂ <90, respiration rate less than 10 if over 5 years, less than 20 if under 5 years, or pump alarming.

Contact duty anaesthetist bleep 2602 if help needed,

or Dr   Home no.:

oximetry is mandatory; under these circumstances it is our practice to manage these patients postoperatively in the normal surgical ward. Although respiratory rate and oxygen saturations are minute-to-minute aids to assessing respiratory depression, more important emphasis is placed on conscious level. Ideally, the children should be sleepy but easy to rouse. There should be a named doctor who may be contacted in the event of any abnormalities being noted.

The advantages of subcutaneous morphine administration are that it is administered through a dedicated cannula, does not depend on the patency of small cannulae in small veins and there is less chance of sudden depression of respiration because of inadvertent large doses being injected as may occur with intravenous infusions.

PCA is now firmly established in paediatric practice. Our practice follows that recommended by Lawrie and colleagues (1990). A bolus dose of 20 μg/kg is injected with a lockout period of 5 min with or without a background infusion ($4 \mu g \cdot kg^{-1} \cdot h^{-1}$),

which may improve sleep pattern without an increase in side-effects (Doyle *et al.*, 1993). This can be used on the normal postoperative ward provided that careful observations are made and charted (Morton, 1993) — see Royal Hospital for Sick Children (Morton) chart (Fig. 77.5). In general, PCA is only successful in children from about 5 years of age onwards (Fig. 77.6) and of normal intelligence, although parent and nurse-assisted PCA may be more common in the future provided strict criteria for top-up doses are laid down.

Using similar charts for two different techniques in the same hospital has made it possible to compare the effects of subcutaneous morphine infusions with PCA administered either by a Graseby system or by cheaper disposable systems (Irwin *et al.*, 1992). With the regimens noted above very similar pain relief and sedation was achieved with subcutaneous morphine infusions using less morphine ($20 \mu g \cdot kg^{-1} \cdot h^{-1}$) compared with $30 \mu g \cdot kg^{-1} \cdot h^{-1}$ for PCA in the first postoperative day.

PCA protocol
(Please place completed chart in casenotes)

Name: Unit no: DOB: Age: Weight:

Operation: Date:

Morphine concn:
(l mg/kg in 50 ml 0.9% saline, i.e. 20 μg·kg^{-1}·ml^{-1})

Bolus dose 1 ml: (i.e. 20 μg/kg)

Lockout interval: 5 min   Background infusion 0.2 ml/h: (i.e. 4 μg·kg^{-1}·h^{-1})   yes/no

Any adjustments: (specify type, reason and time made)

Record hourly:

Time	Spo$_2$	Resp. rate	Sedation score Eyes open: 0 = Spontaneously 1 = To speech 2 = To shake 3 = Unrousable (Call doctor)	Pain score at rest	Pain score on movement (deep breath in and cough) 0 = No pain A = Asleep 1 = Not really sore 2 = Quite sore 3 = Very sore (crying) (Call doctor)	Nausea score 0 = None 1 = Nausea only 2 = Vomiting × 1 in last hour 3 = Vomiting > 1 in last hour (Call doctor)	Total dose since reset mg	No. of presses and percentage good (press verify) ml	Vol. left in syringe ml

Call doctor if severe pain (score 3), patient unrousable (sedation score 3), Spo$_2$ < 90, respiration rate less than 10 if over 5 years, less than 20 if under 5 years, excessive nausea or vomiting, drip blocked/tissued or pump alarming.

Contact duty anaesthetist bleep 2602 if help needed,
or Dr   Home no.:

Fig. 77.5 Postoperative observation chart for children receiving patient-controlled analgesia. (Redrawn with permission of Dr N.S. Morton and Dr E.I. Doyle.)

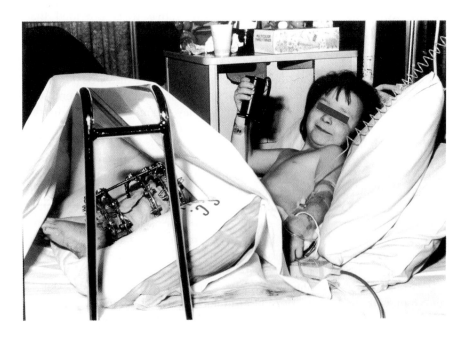

Fig. 77.6 Five-year-old girl on patient-controlled analgesia 24 h following a leg-lengthening procedure. This was commenced in the ward before an intraoperative single-shot extradural block wore off.

Conclusion

It is the author's practice to establish intraoperative and early postoperative pain relief with an appropriate local anaesthetic block, either simple peripheral block or a single-shot extradural. Depending on the severity of the operation and the age of the child this is followed by either simple oral analgesics or NSAIDs before the block wears off. If the operative procedure is associated with severe pain, a subcutaneous infusion of morphine is commenced towards the end of the operation and this should be well established before the block wears off. Alternatively, PCA may be used if the patient is old enough and can understand what is required. Suggested case examples are shown in the Appendix.

The regular charting of clinical signs, pain and nausea scores are an important by-product of the regular use of morphine infusions and PCA, as nursing staff quickly become skilled at assessing pain and analgesic requirements and if used for all types of postoperative analgesia can form the basis of the paediatric acute pain team.

Appendix

There are many methods of postoperative analgesia recommended for children and those below are examples aimed at highlighting some useful techniques.

Case histories

1 Ex-premature baby born at 28 weeks, now 8 weeks of age (2.5 kg) for repair of right inguinal hernia.
Anaesthetic:
Spinal — 0.45 ml plain isobaric bupivacaine plus intraoperative infiltration of wound with 0.75 ml bupivacaine 0.25%.
Postoperative analgesia:
Paracetamol elixir, 48 mg (2 ml) orally, 6-hourly (restrict to three doses/24 h).

2 Term baby now 3 weeks old (4.5 kg) for pyloromyotomy.
Anaesthetic:
General — intermittent positive-pressure ventilation (IPPV)/relaxant plus inhalation agent. Intraoperative infiltration of wound with 3 ml bupivacaine 0.25%.
Postoperative analgesia:
(a) Paracetamol elixir, 72 mg (3 ml), 6-hourly (restrict to three doses only).

(b) Codeine phosphate, 4 mg, intramuscularly (one dose only).

3 Six-month-old 7 kg infant with Hirschsprung's disease for 'pull through' procedure.
Anaesthetic:
General — IPPV/relaxant plus inhalation agent. Caudal extradural 6 ml 0.25% plain bupivacaine.
Postoperative analgesia:
Subcutaneous morphine infusion, 7 mg, in 20 ml normal saline at 0.3−0.6 ml/h or intravenous infusion, 7 mg, in 50 ml at 0.5−1.0 ml/h. Commence before block wears off.

4 Six-year-old (20 kg) outpatient for repair of left inguinal hernia.
Anaesthetic:
General — intravenous induction (EMLA cream) spontaneous respiration via laryngeal mask airway. Iliohypogastric/ilioinguinal nerve blocks after induction with 4 ml bupivacaine 0.5%.
Postoperative analgesia:
Paracetamol elixir, 360 mg (15 ml), before block wears off and 6-hourly p.r.n.

5 Three-year-old (12 kg) for bilateral pyeloplasties.
Anaesthetic:
General — IPPV/relaxant plus inhalation agent. Single-shot lumbar extradural 8 ml bupivacaine 0.25% after induction of anaesthesia.
Postoperative analgesia:
Subcutaneous morphine infusion, 12 mg, in 20 ml normal saline at 0.3−0.6 ml/h, commenced before block wears off.

6 Eight-year-old (25 kg) for femoral lengthening.
Anaesthetic:
General — intravenous induction, spontaneous respirations via laryngeal mask airway. Caudal extradural 20 ml plain bupivacaine 0.25% after induction of anaesthesia.
Postoperative analgesia:
PCA. Morphine sulphate, 25 mg, in 50 ml normal saline. Bolus = 1 ml = 500 μg = 20 μg/kg, lockout = 5 min. No background infusion.

7 Fourteen-year-old (35 kg) for posterior fusion of idiopathic scoliosis.
Anaesthetic:
General — IPPV/relaxant/opioid (fentanyl) plus inhalation agent.
Postoperative analgesia:
Morphine titrated slowly in recovery room until

patient comfortable then PCA 35 mg morphine in 50 ml normal saline. Bolus = 1 ml = 700 µg = 20 µg/kg. Lockout 5 min, background infusion 0.2 ml/h (4 µg · kg^{-1} · h^{-1}).

8 Five-year-old (18 kg) for reimplantation of ureters.
Anaesthetic:
General — IPPV/relaxant plus inhalation agent. Continuous lumbar extradural commenced after induction of anaesthesia. 12–13 ml plain bupivacaine 0.25% before operation.
Postoperative analgesia:
Continuous lumbar extradural commenced in ward.
   (a) Bupivacaine 0.125–0.25% at 2 ml/h; or
   (b) Bupivacaine 0.1–0.125% plus 2 µg/ml fentanyl, at 4 ml/h.

9 Six-year-old (20 kg) for tonsillectomy.
Anaesthetic:
General — IPPV/relaxant (? spontaneously) with inhalation agent. Diclofenac, 20 mg, intramuscularly after induction of anaesthesia.
Postoperative analgesia:
   (a) Dihydrocodeine syrup, 18–20 mg, orally 4–6 hourly; ±
   (b) Diclofenac, 25 mg, rectally, *nocte*.

References

Anand K.J.S., Sippell W.G. & Aynsley-Green A. (1987) Randomised trial of fentanyl anaesthesia in preterm babies undergoing surgery: effect on the stress response. *Lancet* **i**, 243–8.

Anand K.J.S., Sippell W.G. & Schofield N.M. (1988) Does halothane anaesthesia decrease the metabolic and endocrine stress response of newborn infants undergoing surgery? *British Medical Journal* **296**, 668–72.

Arthur D.S. (1980) Post-operative thoracic epidural analgesia in children. *Anaesthesia* **35**, 1131.

Arthur D.S. & McNicol L.R. (1986) Local anaesthesic techniques in paediatric surgery. *British Journal of Anaesthesia* **58**, 760–78.

Bellamy C.D., McDonnell E.J., Colclough G.W., Walmsley P.N., Hine J.M., Jareky T.W. & Vanderveer B.L. (1990) Epidural infusion/PCA for pain control in paediatric patients. *Anesthesia and Analgesia* **70** (Suppl.), 19.

Berde C.B., Sethna N.F., De Jesus J.M., Yemen T.A. & Mandell J. (1990) Continuous bupivacaine–fentanyl infusions in children undergoing urologic surgery. *Anesthesia and Analgesia* **80** (Suppl.), 22.

Bone M.E. & Fell D. (1988) A comparison of rectal diclofenac with intramuscular papaveretum or placebo for pain relief following tonsillectomy. *Anaesthesia* **43**, 277–81.

Booker P. (1989) Intravenous agents in paediatric anaesthesia. In *Textbook of Paediatric Anaesthesia* (Ed. Sumner E.L. & Hatch D.J.) pp. 61–90, Baillière Tindall, London.

Boreus L.O. (1982) *Principles of Paediatric Pharmacology*. Churchill Livingstone, Edinburgh.

Bosenberg A.T., Bland B.A.R., Schulte-Steinberg O. & Downing J.W. (1989) Thoracic epidural anaesthesia via caudal route in children. *Anesthesiology* **69**, 265–9.

Bray R.J. (1983) Post-operative analgesia provided by a morphine infusion in children. *Anaesthesia* **38**, 1075–8.

Busoni P. (1990) Continuous caudal block. In *Regional Anaesthesia in Children* (Eds St Maurice C. & Schulte-Sternberg O.) pp. 88–97. Mediglobe, Fribourg.

Campbell W.I., Kendrick R. & Patterson C. (1990) Intravenous diclofenac sodium. *Anaesthesia* **45**, 763–6.

Casey W.F., Rice L.J., Hannallah R.S., Broadman L., Norden J.M. & Guzzetta P. (1990) A comparison between bupivacaine instillation versus ilioinguinal/iliohypogastric nerve block for post-operative analgesia following inguinal herniorrhaphy in children. *Anesthesiology* **72**, 637–9.

Csontos K., Rust M., Holt V., Mahr W., Kromer W. & Teschemacher H.J. (1979) Elevated plasma β-endorphin levels in pregnant women and their neonates. *Life Sciences* **25**, 835–44.

Dalens B. & Chrysostome Y. (1991) Intervertebral epidural anaesthesia in paediatric surgery: success rate and adverse effects in 650 consecutive procedures. *Paediatric Anaesthesia* **1**, 107–17.

Dohi S., Naito H. & Takahashi T. (1979) Age related changes in blood pressure and duration of motor block in spinal anaesthesia. *Anesthesiology* **50**, 319–22.

Doyle E., Harper I. & Morton N.S. (1993) Patient-controlled analgesia (PCA) with low dose background infusions after lower abdominal surgery in children. *British Journal of Anaesthesia* (In press).

Fell D., Derrington M.C., Taylor E. & Wandless J.G. (1988) Paediatric post-operative analgesia: a comparison between caudal block and wound infiltration of local anaesthetic. *Anaesthesia* **43**, 107–10.

Gross S.C. & Gardiner G.G. (1980) *Child Pain: Treatment Approaches in Pain: Meaning and Management* pp. 127–42. JPMS Books, New York.

Hannallah R.S., Broadman L.M., Belman B.A., Abramowitz M.D. & Epstein B.S. (1987) Comparison of caudal and ilioinguinal/iliohypogastric post orchidopexy pain in paediatric ambulatory surgery. *Anesthesiology* **66**, 832–4.

Hatch D.J. & Sumner E. (1989) Neonatal physiology and anaesthesia. In *Textbook of Paediatric Anaesthesia* (Eds Sumner E. & Hatch D.J.) pp. 255–73. Baillière Tindall, London.

Hopkins C.S., Underhill S. & Booker P.D. (1991) Pharmacokinetics of paracetamol after cardiac surgery. *Archives of the Disabled Child* **65**, 971–6.

Irwin M., Gillespie J.A. & Morton N.S. (1992) Evaluation of a disposable patient controlled analgesia device in children. *British Journal of Anaesthesia* **68**, 411–13.

Kirya C. & Werthmann M.W. (1978) Neonatal circumcision and penile dorsal nerve block — a painless procedure. *Journal of Paediatrics* **92**, 998–1000.

Lawrie S.C., Forbes D.W., Akhtar T.M. & Morton N.S. (1990) Patient controlled analgesia in children. *Anaesthesia* **45**, 1074–7.

Leslie F.M., Tso S. & Harlbutt D.E. (1982) Differential appearance of opiate receptor subtypes in neonatal rat brain. *Life Sciences* **31**, 1393–6.

Lloyd-Thomas A.R. (1990) Pain management in paediatric patients. *British Journal of Anaesthesia* **64**, 85–104.

McNicol L.R. (1991) Anaesthetic practice and pharmacology with a focus on the application of nerve blocks and epidural anaesthesia in paediatric patients. *Current Opinion in Paediatrics* **3**, 455–62.

McNicol L.R. (1993) Continuous subcutaneous morphine for children. *British Journal of Anaesthesia* (In press).

McNicol L.R., Martin C.S., Smart N.G. & Logan R.W. (1990) Perioperative bupivacaine for pyloromyotomy pain. *Lancet* **335**, 54–5.

McQuay H. & Moore A. (1984) Metabolism of narcotics. *British Medical Journal* **228**, 237–40.

Mahé V. & Ecoffey C. (1988) Spinal anaesthesia with isobaric bupivacaine in infants. *Anesthesiology* **68**, 601–3.

Marlow N., Weindling A.M., Van Peer A. & Heykents J. (1990) Alfentanil pharmacokinetics in pre-term infants. *Archives of the Disabled Child* **65**, 349–51.

Maunuksela E.L., Olkkola E.T. & Korpela R. (1987) Measurement of pain in children with self reporting and behavioural assessment. *Clinical Pharmacology and Therapeutics* **42**, 137–47.

Maunuksela E.L., Olkkola E.T. & Korpela R. (1988) Does prophylactic I.V. infusion of indomethacin improve the management of post-operative pain in children? *Canadian Journal of Anaesthesia* **35**, 123–7.

Moore P.A. & Hargreaves J.A. (1985) Post extraction pain relief in children: a clinical trial of liquid analgesics. *International Journal of Clinical Pharmacology, Therapy and Toxicology* **23**, 573–7.

Moores M.A., Wandless J.G. & Fell D. (1990) Paediatric postoperative analgesia: a comparison of rectal diclofenac with caudal bupivacaine after inguinal herniotomy. *Anaesthesia* **45**, 156–8.

Morton N.S. (1993) Development of a monitoring protocol for safe use of opioids in children. *Paediatric Anaesthesia* **3**, 179–84.

Murat I. (1990) Continuous thoracic epidural block. In *Regional Anaesthesia in Children* (Eds Sainte-Maurice C. & Sculte-Sternberg O.) pp. 113–18. Mediglobe, Fribourg.

Murat I., Delleur M.M., Esteve C., Egy J.E., Raynaud P. & Sainte-Maurice C. (1987) Continuous extradural anaesthesia in children. *British Journal of Anaesthesia* **69**, 1441–50.

Peutrell G.M. & Hughes D.G. (1993) Epidural anaesthesia through caudal catheters for inguinal hernias in awake ex-premature babies. *Anaesthesia* **48**, 128–31.

Purcell-Jones G., Dorman F. & Sumner E. (1987) The use of opioids in neonates. A retrospective study of 933 cases. *Anaesthesia* **42**, 1316–20.

Tre-Trakarn T. & Pirayavardorn S. (1985) Post-operative pain relief for circumcision in children: comparison among morphine, nerve block and topical analgesia. *Anesthesiology* **62**, 519–22.

Van Niekerk J., Bax-Vermiere B.M.J., Jeurts J.W.M. & Kramer P.P.G. (1990) Epidurography in premature infants. *Anaesthesia* **45**, 722–5.

Watters C.H., Patterson C.C., Mathews H.M.L. & Campbell W. (1988) Diclofenac sodium for post-tonsillectomy pain in children. *Anaesthesia* **43**, 641–3.

Wolf A.R. & Hughes D. (1993) Pain relief for infants undergoing abdominal surgery: comparison of infusions of i.v. morphine and extradural bupivacaine. *British Journal of Anaesthesia* **70**, 10–16.

Common Conditions in the Pain Clinic and Their Management

H.J. McQUAY

This chapter describes the clinical management of conditions which occur commonly in the pain clinic. The technical details for drug management, procedures and alternative measures are described elsewhere; this chapter is intended to suggest which of these measures is appropriate and when, taking a conservative view.

Which are the common pain conditions? The prevalence of chronic pain (pain resistant to 1 month of treatment) in the population at large is not known. Within the pain clinic population, 25% of patients have pain associated with malignancy, 75% have 'non-malignant' pain.

An outline of the commoner causes of pain associated with malignancy is given on p. 1621. In practice, the simple distinction between malignant and non-malignant is not very helpful, both because the treatment methods may be the same, and also because the differential diagnosis for many pain conditions includes both malignant and non-malignant causes (cf. back pain and facial pain, pp. 1623 and 1628 respectively). Therefore, the common pain conditions (prevalence greater than 3%; Table 78.1) are described after discussing separately pains of malignant or non-malignant origin.

Pain associated with malignancy
(Chapters 75 and 79)

Not all patients with cancer have pain, but the prevalence increases with the progression of disease, so that with advanced disease 60–90% of patients have significant pain (Twycross & Lack, 1983; Foley, 1985).

Management of acute cancer-related pain associated with diagnosis or treatment involves identifying the cause, and treating the pain, which is often self-limited. The methods needed are often analogous to those used in postoperative pain.

Chronic cancer-related pain may be related to tumour progression (62%), tumour treatment (25%), or may be a pre-existing chronic pain (10%) (Foley, 1985) unrelated to the tumour. Transient relief in cancer pain may be achieved by the same blocks which are used in non-malignant pain, such as extradural local anaesthetic — extradural steroid may be very effective. These 'simple' measures are often forgotten. Longer-term relief can be achieved by using an extradural (or intrathecal) catheter and infusing a combination of local anaesthetic and opioid. Other procedures used to obtain longer-term relief include injections using neurolytic solutions, cryoanalgesia or radiofrequency, percutaneous cordotomy or hypophysectomy (see Chapter 81 for technical details). Pain due to malignancy is often managed on a co-operative basis between general practitioner, oncology and radiotherapy departments, hospice and pain clinic. While the specific role of the pain clinic is to provide pain-relieving procedures, most patients benefit from the combination of these procedures with skilful analgesic management, radiotherapy and appropriate control of symptoms other than pain. In our local experience patients referred primarily because of pain tend to come to the pain clinic rather than the hospice; shared care with the hospice then makes available the full range of community and social support.

The pattern of referral of malignant-pain problems to pain clinics falls into two main categories. The first relates to problems which are thought to be amenable to nerve-blocking procedures; the referral may come at an early stage in the patient's illness, or when they are terminally ill. The educative role of pain clinics is important here, because others involved in the patient's care are sometimes unaware of what is possible. The second category is the despairing referral, often at a late stage in the illness, when the pain is not responding well solely to drug manage-

Table 78.1 Data from 1115 patients with chronic non-malignant pain. (From McQuay *et al.*, 1985)

Pain condition*	Percentage of total	Sex ratio (M : F)	Age (years) (mean and range)	Duration of pain (years) (mean and range)
Low back pain	26	1 : 1.7	51.8 (23−>80)	8.8 (0.5−32)
Postherpetic neuralgia	11	1 : 1.6	73.0 (35−>80)	2.6 (0.5−20)
Post-traumatic neuralgia	9	1 : 1.2	50.0 (19−>80)	4.8 (0.5−36)
Atypical facial pain	6	1 : 2.0	48.2 (22−79)†	4.3 (0.5−17)
Intercostal neuralgia	5	1 : 1.5	55.0 (25−>80)†	4.3 (0.5−30)
Trigeminal neuralgia	5	1 : 2.4	64.3 (32−>80)	9.3 (0.5−52)
Perineal neuralgia	4	1 : 1.9	64.5 (32−>80)	6.8 (0.5−35)
Abdominal neuralgia	4	1 : 1.2	56.2 (26−>80)	5.6 (1−24)
Stump/phantom pain	3	1 : 0.4	62.6‡ (28−>80)	12.5 (1−61)
Osteoarthritis hip	3	1 : 1.2	74.4 (30−>80)	4.3 (0.5−15)
Sympathetic dystrophy	2.4	1 : 1.1	59.1 (27−>80)	4.2 (1−6)
Coccydynia	2.3	1 : 4.2	53.8 (26−73)	5.7 (0.5−31)†
Cervical spondylosis	2.1	1 : 1.5	52.6 (37−>80)	5.9 (0.5−17)
Other conditions	18.5			

* All conditions with >2% incidence; †, significant difference ($p < 0.05$) in mean age or mean pain duration (female > male); ‡, significant difference ($p < 0.01$) in mean age or mean pain duration (female > male) (Student's 't' test). Other conditions include osteoarthritis (unspecified), osteoarthritic spine, causalgia, other nerve neuralgia, cord damage, thalamic syndrome, disseminated sclerosis, occipital neuralgia, claudication and neuroma.

ment. It is important that we teach the referring doctors and nurses the factors which predict poor control with conventional analgesic management. The commoner pain conditions associated with malignancy are discussed later. Oral analgesic management, and the special case of the dying patient, are covered in Chapter 79.

Non-malignant pain

The prevalence of the various pain conditions at the Oxford Unit is shown in Table 78.1 (McQuay *et al.*, 1985). The population served by the Oxford Region is 2.3 million. Table 78.1 summarizes the information (age, sex, duration of pain at first attendance) for diagnostic categories with prevalence greater than 2%. The pain condition with highest prevalence (26%) was low back pain; only postherpetic neuralgia also had prevalence greater than 10%. For the purposes of this chapter, 'common' non-malignant pain conditions were those with greater than 3% prevalence in Table 78.1; clinical features and outline of management of those conditions are described on p. 1623.

The list of conditions in Table 78.1 is long; the doctor must therefore be able to manage a variety of conditions which are not common. The length of the list of diagnostic categories implies that no single clinic will see large numbers of patients with the low prevalence conditions. Management strategy is then necessarily empirical because such small numbers make controlled studies very difficult to perform.

Non-malignant pain management presents great resource problems, because for many conditions there is no cure, but treatment may provide short-term relief. Many of these patients have normal life expectancy, and will continue to seek such short-term relief because it improves their quality of life. The ethos of the pain clinic, often the last medical resort, is very important to these patients and to their management (Editorial, 1982).

Patient assessment

The most important principle is that the patient and the physician are best served if the physician believes the patient's report (Foley, 1985). Pain is necessarily subjective, and there are few objective signs which the doctor can use to judge the severity of reported pain. Many patients have no visible handicap and their problems may be ill-understood, even disbelieved, at work and at home. Much time and energy is wasted on procedures designed to 'catch the patient out'. Chronic pain changes people, affecting their personal and working lives, and ultimately their personalities. Often such changes are reversible with successful treatment. Labelling patients as malingerers or the pain as psychogenic may be easier than admitting that there is no successful treatment.

The pain history

The extra emphasis of a pain history compared with a 'normal' medical history is summarized in the following series of questions.

Site of pain.
Where do you feel this pain?
Does it go anywhere else?
Is it numb where you feel the pain?

Character of pain.
What sort of a pain is it?
Burning/shooting/stabbing/dull, etc.

History of pain.
How long have you had this pain?
How did it start?
Did it come on out of the blue or was it triggered by something?

Relieving factors.
Does anything make it better? (Position, drugs, distraction, alcohol, etc.)

Accentuating factors.
Does anything make it worse?
(Position/exercise/weather, etc.)

Pattern.
Is there any pattern to the pain? (Frequency/severity.)
Is it worse at any particular time of day?

Sleep disturbance.
Do you get off to sleep with no trouble?
Does the pain wake you up?

Activities.
What does the pain stop you doing which you would otherwise do?

Previous treatments.
What methods have been tried already?
Did they help the pain?

Asking if sensation is normal in the painful area and if the pain is shooting or stabbing in character may help to identify the pains variously known as dysaesthetic, deafferentation or neuropathic. It is important to distinguish these because they are unlikely to respond to conventional analgesics. These pains often have little pattern, but are less troublesome when the patient is distracted.

It is important to enquire specifically about the efficacy of each particular drug class (major and minor analgesics, anticonvulsants, etc., Table 78.2). This information prevents the inept prescription of drugs which have failed previously, and may give important clues as to the kind of pain and its sensitivity to different classes of drug.

It is also important to know the dose size, frequency, duration of prescription and the side-effect problems for each drug which has been prescribed. Dose-response relationships apply in analgesic management, and therapeutic failure should not be presumed if the dosage was inadequate; a good example is the use of carbamazepine in trigeminal neuralgia. Is the patient taking drugs other than analgesics? Anticoagulation, for instance, is not only an (almost) absolute contraindication to pain management by injection procedures, but also interacts with some anti-inflammatory drugs.

It is important to be sure if nerve blocks used previously were technically effective (e.g. did the patient have any numbness after an extradural which included local anaesthetic?), before dismissing them as being of no help to this patient. Equally, other measures, such as transcutaneous nerve stimulation, may not have been used correctly, and may succeed if the patient receives proper instruction in their use.

Some index of function is necessary as a baseline so that improvement or deterioration may be monitored. Useful clinical outcome measures are notoriously difficult; using simple pain charts and indices of activity can work well.

Examination and investigations

Specific features of physical examination and investigations will be mentioned with the pain conditions.

Table 78.2 Treatment options

Analgesics	*Conventional*	
	Minor non-opioid	Aspirin, paracetamol, non-steroidal anti-inflammatory (NSAI), nefopam
	Minor opioid and combination	Codeine, dihydrocodeine, dextropropoxyphene, alone or in combination with minor non-opioid
	Major opioid	Morphine, buprenorphine, etc.
	Unconventional	
	Anticonvulsant	Carbamazepine, valproate, phenytoin, clonazepam
	Antidepressant	Amitriptyline, dothiepin
	Others	Steroid, baclofen, clonidine
Nerve block or surgery	Reversible	e.g. Local anaesthetic ± steroid, cryoanalgesia
	Irreversible	e.g. Ablative nerve blocks, surgical procedures, radiofrequency
Alternatives	Transcutaneous nerve stimulation, hypnosis, acupuncture, etc.	

As patients with chronic pain may be seen over years, accurate serial record of physical signs is important in deciding whether or not a new pathology has developed or whether or not new or repeat investigations are required.

Treatment options

The major options are summarized in Table 78.2.

Analgesics

Drugs are the mainstay of chronic pain treatment. The simplest classification is conventional analgesics, from aspirin through to morphine, and unconventional, antidepressants and anticonvulsants (Table 78.2). Acute pain can be managed with the conventional analgesics and one of the many differences between acute and chronic pain is that chronic pain may not be so straightforward. About one-third of our patients in both malignant and non-malignant categories have pains which respond poorly, if at all, to conventional analgesics. For example, carbamazepine is a classic 'unconventional' analgesic used successfully in the management of trigeminal neuralgia. A simple rule of thumb is that pains in numb areas, known variously as neuropathic and deafferentation pains, are unlikely to respond well to opioids (McQuay, 1988). Good examples of deafferentation pain are phantom limb pain and the pain after brachial plexus avulsion, and an example of a central neuropathic pain is poststroke pain

(thalamic pain). Opioids may make patients with these pains feel better, but the analgesic effect will be poor. This distinction must be sought in the history, from the character of the pain and from previous response to conventional analgesics. Is this a pain in a numb area? How has it responded to adequate doses of conventional analgesics?

Within the conventional analgesics, non-steroidal anti-inflammatory drugs (NSAIDs) at maximum recommended dose produce about 30% more analgesia than aspirin or paracetamol 1000 mg. The combination of opiate and non-opiate produces additive analgesia; the two mechanisms may combine to give better pain control in contexts such as bony pain. Within the NSAID class it is necessary to find the best drug (best analgesia with minimal adverse effects), for each individual patient.

Using major opiates in non-malignant pain is controversial, because of fear of addiction. This is extremely unlikely, but there is no point in prescribing drugs which the patient or others involved in their care do not appreciate. A simple rule is that where the pain is sensitive to opiates, and there is no other effective remedy, opiate prescription may be tried, but only with the agreement of all concerned. The opiate would be used by non-injection route unless impracticable.

For pains insensitive to opiates, the choice between antidepressants and anticonvulsants is empirical. For burning pains, low-dose antidepressants are the first choice, preferably a non-selective tricyclic such as amitriptyline, at a dose of 25 mg *nocte* titrated as necessary to 150 mg *nocte*. The analgesic effect occurs within a week, so that dose increments can be made quickly. For shooting pains, anticonvulsants work best, and first choice is sodium valproate (200 mg b.d. or 500 mg *nocte*).

Nerve blocks

Nerve blocks may be classified into two categories — reversible, e.g. local anaesthesia or cryoanalgesia, and irreversible, e.g. ablative nerve blocks and surgical or radiofrequency procedures (Table 78.2). When the effect of reversible procedures wanes, the pain is unchanged. If pain recurs after an irreversible procedure, it may have altered character, e.g. anaesthesia dolorosa.

The common nerve-block procedures are summarized in Table 78.3. There is a trend away from procedures which destroy nerves, based on the concept that continued (peripheral) pain results in a 'memory' of the pain centrally in the nervous system. Disrupting the peripheral painful input may then make little difference. Continued painful stimuli alter the nervous system. Pain which had a peripheral origin

Table 78.3 Common nerve blocks. (From Foley, 1985)

Block	Common indications
Trigger point	Focal pain (e.g. in muscle)

Peripheral	Pain in dermatomal distribution
	    Intercostal
	    Sacral nerves
	    Rectus sheath

Extradural	Uni- or bilateral pain (lumbosacral, cervical, thoracic, etc.) Midline perineal pain

Intrathecal	Unilateral pain (neurolytic injection for
	    pain due to malignancy limbs, chest,
	    etc.)
	(Midline perineal pain)

Autonomic
    Intravenous
    sympathectomy
	Reflex sympathetic dystrophy

Stellate ganglion	Reflex sympathetic dystrophy Arm pain Brachial plexus nerve compression
Lumbar sympathetic	Reflex sympathetic dystrophy Lumbosacral plexus nerve compression Vascular insufficiency lower limb Perineal pain
Coeliac plexus	Abdominal pain

may become 'central' (Wall, 1989). An example is phantom limb pain; the peripheral neural basis for the pain no longer exists, but yet the pain is felt. This concept of nervous system plasticity affects management in several ways (McQuay & Dickenson, 1990). With established chronic pain, conventional analgesics may be relatively ineffective, because the neural basis of the pain has changed and no longer responds to those remedies. Plasticity also implies that attacking the cables which carry the (original) pain message may be ineffective in the short term if those cables are no longer the bearers of the message, and ineffective in the long term if the system can 'rewire'. These ideas are supported by both experimental work and clinical observation. Pre-emptive strategies, such as blocking pain before amputation to reduce phantom limb pain incidence, and the idea of modulating the painful input, for instance, by sustained local anaesthetic block as an alternative to irreversible attack on the cables, are being used increasingly.

The major indication for nerve-blocking techniques is lack of response to pharmacological management and/or unacceptable side-effects. Many of these blocks may be performed 'diagnostically' with local anaesthetic, as a preliminary to making a more permanent block with cryoanalgesia, radiofrequency lesions, phenol or surgery. Use of steroid may convert the diagnostic block to a therapeutic block, e.g. extradurals in low back pain. Repeated blocks with local anaesthetic may in themselves be therapeutic (Arner *et al.*, 1990).

The technical aspects and the potential morbidity of these blocks are familiar to most anaesthetists. Image intensification should increase efficacy and reduce the incidence of adverse events for procedures such as lumbar sympathectomy (Boas, 1983) and coeliac plexus block. Many of these procedures are performed on an outpatient basis, and the time between the block and when the patient goes home should be sufficient for any complications (most of which are 'early', e.g. pneumothorax after intercostal or stellate blocks) to be apparent *before* the patient leaves. Two complications present particular problems. Hypotension occurs during the first few hours after coeliac plexus block; patients may need to be admitted for this procedure. Lumbar sympathectomy with neurolytic agents may cause a troublesome neuralgic pain, often in the groin or on the anterior aspect of the thigh. Although this may be a severe pain, occurring in as many as 10% of patients, it is self-limiting (6–8 weeks), and transcutaneous nerve stimulation may give very effective relief.

The place of many of these blocks in pain management is very ill-defined, because, despite widespread use of the techniques, careful studies of quality and duration of relief and morbidity compared with other methods have not been performed. Improvement in pain control generally, with better use of drugs, has reduced the need for these blocks. The use of continuous spinal infusion of a combination of local anaesthetic and opioid is superseding neurolytic procedures (Sjöberg et al., 1991).

Using intercostal neuralgia as an example, diagnostic intercostal blocks with local anaesthetic would confirm that the pain could be controlled by blocking the relevant nerves. Extended duration of relief could then be achieved by cryoanalgesia to those intercostal nerves. If intercostal block did not work, then extradural block with steroid would follow. In general, neurolytic blocks in non-malignant pain are not recommended, because they do not last forever, and if the pain recurs, it may be more difficult to manage. In cancer pain with limited prognosis, then, in the intercostal example, if the pain did not respond to intercostal block, an intrathecal neurolytic block may be used. For severe pains (particularly pelvic or perineal), these can be most rewarding; the limitation is the potential for motor and sphincter damage. This risk is higher with bilateral and repeat procedures and low-level blocks. Extradural neurolytics have limited efficacy. While claims have been made that the paravertebral approach is preferable, patchy results may be attributed to unpredictable injectate spread. We have found the results of spinal infusion of a combination of local anaesthetic and opioid to be superior, providing good analgesia with minimal irreversible morbidity.

Similar distinction between malignant and non-malignant pain holds for coeliac plexus block in pancreatic pain. Pain associated with pancreatic cancer responds well to coeliac plexus block, and it may also help those with abdominal or perineal pain from tumour in the pelvis. In chronic pancreatitis, results are much less convincing.

Pain conditions associated with malignancy

The specific role of the pain clinic in pain associated with malignancy is the provision of nerve-blocking procedures. The use of neurolytic procedures has become much less common for patients who are still mobile and continent. This is because spinal infusion of local anaesthetic and opioid can provide better analgesia with minimal adverse effects. The place of the neurolytic blocks in pain management is becoming restricted to patients who are confined to bed and who have lost sphincter control.

Pharmacological management

Oral drug therapy is discussed in Chapter 79. In the pain clinic, many patients are not terminal, and patients referred for a specific nerve block may also be helped by sensible use of analgesics (in addition to other supportive measures). The pain clinic doctor must be familiar with oral opioid analgesic use, both in the ambulant patient and the terminal case.

It is important to remember that not all pains are sensitive to opioids (Jadad et al., 1992). A careful history (noting response at each site of pain to analgesics) is required. Any increase in dose required to sustain analgesia should be noted, with the time intervals. Patients may be referred to the pain clinic for therapeutic trial of opioids given spinally, and patient selection for extradural or intrathecal catheterization for opioids requires careful attention to these details for the procedures to be worthwhile (Jadad et al., 1991). In general, we have found the use of spinal opioids alone to be merely a more complicated procedure than subcutaneous opioids. The use of local anaesthetic combined with opioid has altered our practice radically, because it can produce analgesia for pains poorly responsive to opioids alone. The logic, then, is that pains poorly responsive to oral opioids are unlikely to improve simply by changing the route by which the opioid is given. Spinal use of local anaesthetic and opioid can produce the necessary analgesia.

Lack of response to pharmacological management and/or unacceptable side-effects are major indications for nerve-blocking techniques in pain due to malignancy. The anticonvulsant and antidepressant drugs (Table 78.2) may be useful alternatives if a block is impossible, or to manage pain at other sites.

Nerve blocks

Technical details of the ablative nerve-blocks are discussed in Chapter 81.

Head and neck

Swallowing difficulties may limit oral opioid intake, and in this group subcutaneous, spinal and intracerebroventricular opioid infusions have been used. Pain in the trigeminal nerve distribution, accompanied at worst by trismus, dysphagia or halitosis may be helped by blocking the relevant nerve branch. Mandibular or maxillary blocks are the most useful.

Chest wall

Intercostal diagnostic blocks with local anaesthetic may be used and, to extend duration of relief, cryo-analgesia has superseded the use of neurolytics. If the pain does not respond to intercostal block, an intrathecal neurolytic block may be used. Extradural neurolytics have limited efficacy. While claims have been made that the paravertebral approach is preferable, patchy results may be attributed to unpredictable injectate spread.

Abdomen

Abdominal pain associated with pancreatic cancer responds well to coeliac plexus block (Jones & Gough, 1977), and this block may also help those with abdominal or perineal pain from tumour in the pelvis. Postural hypotension, however, can be an unwelcome long-term adverse effect. The procedure may be technically more difficult, and less successful, if there is anatomical disruption. Abdominal pain from tumour in general is not an easy pain to manage with opioids alone, and opioids, in conjuction with coeliac plexus block (if feasible), may provide better pain control. The splanchnic approach, placing the solutions dorsal rather than ventral to the diaphragmatic crura, has been claimed to enhance the technical precision of the block (Boas, 1983). The good results with the classic method (technically improved by use of image intensification or CT-scan imaging) are unlikely to be improved by the newer approaches, but morbidity might be further reduced.

Sympathetic blocks (lumbar sympathectomy) may also be of value in rectal pain. Rectal 'phantom' pain after resection is not uncommon, and both this phantom pain and tenesmus may respond to sympathectomy. Pain in the distribution of the sacral nerves may respond to sacral extradural block with local anaesthetic and steroid; individual sacral nerves may also be blocked diagnostically at the foramina. Cryoanalgesia can be used to extend the duration of relief.

The ultimate management for such pain remains the intrathecal neurolytic block. For severe pelvic or perineal pain, these can be most rewarding. However, bilateral pain requires bilateral blocks with a higher risk of bladder dysfunction.

Pain from bony metastases

Isolated metastases which occur in areas already maximally radiated, or unresponsive to radiation, may respond to 'simple' blocks, such as extradural local anaesthetic and steroid for spinal metastases. Spinal continuous infusion may be necessary for pain in arm or leg long bones, particularly if the pain is movement related. In general, movement-related pain is very difficult to manage (Banning et al., 1991); oral analgesic regimens adequate to control the pain on movement tend to anaesthetize the patient when they are not moving. Cordotomy may be most useful for unilateral pelvic, hip or leg pain. Hypophysectomy used to be used to manage the pain of multiple bony metastases; it is being superseded by hemi-body radiation or strontium.

Pain from nerve plexus compression

Local spread of tumour, metastases or tumour treatment may result in compression of either lumbosacral or brachial plexus. Pelvic tumour (cancer of colon, rectum, cervix, etc.) can produce direct nerve compression or compress the lumbosacral plexus at various levels. Carcinoma of the breast (and radiotherapy), together with carcinoma of the lung (Pancoast's) are the commonest causes of brachial plexus involvement in the pain clinic.

The pain which results may be the most difficult of all to treat. In an advanced stage, the pain is often in a numb (deafferented) area. One example is a breast cancer patient presenting with a swollen painful arm. Initial investigation should determine whether tumour spread has occurred (potentially treatable) or whether radiation fibrosis is the cause. In its early stages, the swelling may be reduced by the simple techniques used to control lymphoedema; results in late cases are poor. The pain from a Pancoast's tumour may be more restricted to (a) particular dermatome(s). In either condition, poor management with conventional analgesics may be improved by using an anticonvulsant and antidepressant regimen. If such regimens fail, our initial choice would be spinal infusion of local anaesthetic and opioid, with intrathecal neurolytic block for the relevant dermatome if indicated clinically. Cordotomy is often not feasible if the pain is higher than the C6 level, and extradural neurolytic injection gives poor results. The response to intrathecal neurolytics is better for tumour damage than for radiation fibrosis.

Lumbosacral plexus involvement may present as root pain, pain from peripheral nerve involvement or pain in widespread areas of numbness. Successful peripheral nerve diagnostic block with local anaesthetic may be extended (as with cryoanalgesia). Cordotomy is practicable in this region for root pain or more widespread pain. However, spinal infusion of local anaesthetic and opioid or intrathecal neurolytic block are the major options.

Common pain conditions

Chronic back pain

Chronic back pain is by far the commonest condition seen in the pain clinic (about 25% of non-malignant cases; Table 78.1). The patients fall into three main categories:

1 Pain due to malignancy.

2 Pain which has not responded to conservative measures.

3 Pain recurring despite previous surgery.

The major pitfall is to miss a treatable cause of the pain in the rush to treat the symptoms. In the failed conservative management category, the most difficult decision may be what changes in signs and symptoms warrant further investigation. Pain despite surgery should become less common as awareness increases that pain alone may not justify laminectomy, because 40% of these patients have recurrent pain after one year (Martin, 1981; Benzon, 1986). While such patients are still being referred, it is important to remember that some may still have a surgically remediable lesion.

The next section outlines some common and some obscure causes of back pain which may trap the unwary. There are many different ways of classifying back pain. This section uses the common categories presenting at the pain clinic. For more general purposes the fundamental distinction of three main presenting problems (mechanical back pain, possible spinal pathology, nerve root pain) should be used (Waddell, 1982). Management of the pain is then discussed.

Causes (Table 78.4)

Prolapsed intervertebral disc

Site. Pain in the back (lumbago) with pain down the leg (sciatica) if severe.

Features. Often occurs once or twice a year, with or without a history of provocation, and often settles on its own (conservative management). The pain is

Table 78.4 Causes of back pain in the pain clinic

Major
Prolapsed intervertebral disc
Facet joint degeneration
Pain recurring after previous surgery
Arachnoiditis

Pitfalls
Cauda equina claudication
Cauda equina tumours
Pelvic lesions
Arteriovenous malformations of the cord

Tumour
Primary, e.g. myeloma
Secondary (breast, prostate, melanoma, etc.)
Compression of lumbosacral plexus

Tuberculosis, osteomyelitis, ankylosing spondylitis

thought to come from swollen nerve roots and subsequently the disc retracts with the development of scarring after months.

A herniated disc compressing a nerve root may produce limitation of one specific movement only, straight leg raising of the good leg may produce crossed pain in the bad leg and there may be a positive femoral stretch test.

Facet joint degeneration

Site. Back pain with or without leg pain.

Features. The pain is said to be due to degeneration of the facet joints. Some distinction from disc disease may be possible from the history. Facet joint degeneration may give pain on sitting, which may then be relieved by standing up and walking (the opposite of the usual history for disc problems). On examination, pain from the facet joints may be elicited by lying the patient prone and extending the facet joints by lifting the legs.

Pain recurring after previous surgery

Patients referred to the pain clinic because of back pain recurring after surgery present special diagnostic problems. The causes of such recurrences include the following.

Recurrent prolapsed intervertebral disc. Does the patient have a recurrent disc? The patient may have a good original story, positive myelogram, disc protrusion removed at operation and have done well for several months, or indeed, years. Then history repeats itself (Martin, 1981), and the pain (and any radiation) may be the same as before the operation.

The disc which was causing the pain was not removed at operation. Straight X-ray of the lumbar spine should reveal the level of the operation.

The disc removed was not the cause of the pain. If a prolapsed intervertebral disc was found on myelography, and then was removed at operation, and yet the pain persisted, that disc may not have been the cause of the pain. Original investigations (myelography) must include the conus in order to exclude other causes of the pain coexisting with disc lesion.

Patients in this category may respond to facet joint procedures, suggesting that this may have been the cause of the original pain.

Postoperative complications causing pain. Such complications include dural damage, arachnoid hernia, nerve root pressure, sciatica and sterile osteitis. Patients referred soon (6 weeks) after operation may have sterile osteitis, which presents as severe lumbar back pain associated with the slightest movement. Translucency at the upper and lower margins of the adjacent vertebral bodies, raised erythrocyte sedimentation rate (ESR) and white cell count confirms the diagnosis. The condition settles with rest and leads to bony fusion. When fusion occurs, the pain does not recur.

Arachnoiditis

Intrathecal adhesions, which occur after a variety of intrathecal insults, may result in the clinical syndrome of arachnoiditis, which can cause grave long-term problems (Shaw *et al.*, 1978). The causes include:
1 Myelography.
2 Bleeding.
3 Rough or recurrent surgery.
4 Infection.
5 Idiopathic.

Fifty percent of the patients develop symptoms and/or signs within 1 year; in a small number (15%) 10 years may elapse before problems develop (Shaw *et al.*, 1978). In Shaw's and colleagues' series of 80 patients, 43 had had myelography, and in many this had been a technically difficult procedure. Fifty-one had undergone spinal surgery and 25% of the patients had progressive disease. In a clinic with a high proportion of 'failed surgery' back pain patients, arachnoiditis may be a common problem.

Site. Back pain, with root signs in 50%.

Features. Classically, the pain of arachnoiditis is a burning constant pain with sciatic distribution to one or both legs, with signs of gradual and progressive loss of leg reflexes. In reality, the pain may be difficult to distinguish from that caused by other back problems and the signs may be unconvincing. The diagnosis rests on the history, examination and myelographic evidence, where at least two of the following changes should be sought (Shaw *et al.*, 1978) to support the diagnosis.
1 Partial or complete block.
2 Narrowing of the subarachnoid space.
3 Obliteration of the nerve root sleeves and thickening of the nerve roots.
4 Irregular distribution and loculation of the contrast medium.
5 Fixity of previously inserted contrast medium.
6 Pseudocyst formation.

The pitfalls

Cauda equina claudication is caused by spondylosis producing narrowing of an already narrow lumbar canal, occurs mainly in those over 60 years old, and there is often a long history. The pain is sciatic, with pins and needles on standing and walking, relieved by sitting and lying down. The pain is often made worse by bending forward (flexion presumably accentuating the narrowing). It may be distinguished from claudication *per se* because resting relieves claudication, but may not do so in the cauda equina condition. Some patients may be able to walk further by bending forward. Cycling often does not bring on the pain. On examination, one or both ankle jerks may be absent. On investigation, myelography shows complete block or marked stenosis.

Cauda equina tumours have the reputation of being classic diagnostic pitfalls (Fearnside & Adams, 1978). The patients are often labelled hysterics. The site of pain is in the back with a sciatic component in 50%. There is a progressive history, the pain being worse at night. The patient has to get out of bed and then sit in a chair for the rest of the night. The pain may be made worse by jolting or jarring rather than by the twisting or bending which often elicits pain from disc problems. There may be micturition difficulties some time before motor or sensory signs are found. The clinical diagnosis rests largely on the history; there may be few neurological signs.

Primary or secondary malignancy in the pelvis may produce back pain with or without leg pain. This may come from the disease mass or from lumbar plexus invasion. Arteriovenous malformation of the spinal cord can produce back pain, with or without leg pain. The pain may be worse on walking. Neurological signs appear progressively, and myelography may be reported as normal. Tumour and infection around the spine can produce back pain: causes include primary myeloma, bony secondaries, extradural tumour, tuberculosis, osteomyelitis and ankylosing spondylitis. The symptoms, signs and investigations to distinguish these diagnoses are discussed by Waddell (1982).

Management of back pain

History

In taking the pain history, potentially the most useful questions for distinguishing the causes of the pain are those relating to potentiating and relieving factors (Fig. 78.1).

It is useful to have some idea of which activities are limited by the pain; improvement in such indices may be the best guide as to treatment efficacy.

The drug history may give a guide as to the type of pain. The patients usually have tried non-opioid analgesics, and often report that 'they just take the edge off the pain'. They may have distinct preferences between the drugs because of differential

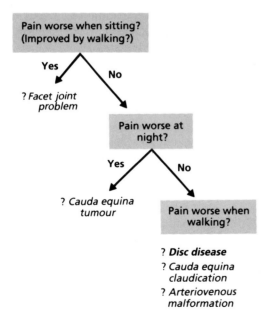

Fig. 78.1 Causes of back pain — clues from the history.

incidence of side-effects. This information is important when trying to choose the most effective drug, and particularly when injections fail to help. Some patients with arachnoiditis find little benefit with conventional analgesics, and this may point to a deafferentation type of pain.

Examination

The serial measurement and recording of neurological signs is important in these patients so that change can be monitored objectively.

The simple reminders of sensory innervation are that L1, L2 and L3 supply the anterior aspect of the thigh, L4 the medial malleolus and toes, and S1 the lateral malleolus. More weight should be placed on numbness with tingling than on the finding of numbness alone.

L2 and L3 are involved in hip flexion, L3 and L4 in knee extension (knee jerk), other hip and knee movements being L5. Ankle movements involve S1 and S2 (ankle jerk S1).

Gauging the limitation of straight leg raising (SLR) may require common sense. Gross limitation of SLR is incompatible with the ability to sit comfortably at 90° with legs outstretched.

Investigations

Straight X-ray of spine; check facet joints (exclude, e.g. tumour, infection, spondylolisthesis).

There is disagreement as to whether or not myelography, computerized tomography (CT) or magnetic resonance imaging (MRI) scans are 'best' in helping to decide if surgery is indicated. The lowest rate of false-positive findings occurs with myelography with screening. If abnormality at the conus is suspected then radiculograms are inadequate. The combination of myelography and CT scanning may still be the final arbiter in problem cases.

Type and timing of treatment

The philosophy presented is to use the low-morbidity outpatient extradural (lumbar or sacral) steroid or facet joint (where these are appropriate; see Fig. 78.2) injections as first-line treatment. This is justified for the back-pain sufferer because even short-term benefit from injections may be better than poor relief with drugs, and drugs often cause more side-effect problems than the injections. There are some careful studies of the efficacy of extradural steroids (for reviews see Kepes & Duncalf, 1985; Benzon, 1986),

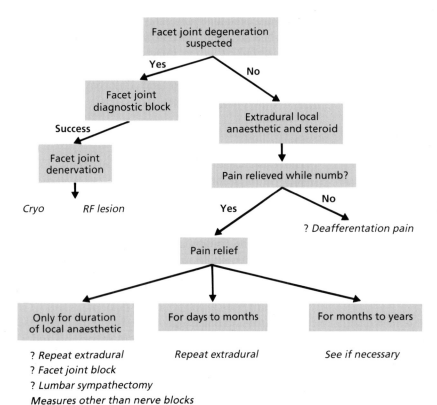

Fig. 78.2 The type and timing of treatment (if no surgically remediable lesion and no contraindication to injection).

which justify the technique. Better results may be achieved the earlier the patient is treated (Benzon, 1986), and when there is good evidence that the pain results from nerve-root irritation. Used as a first-line injection treatment for back pain in the Oxford Unit (mean duration of pain 9 years at first visit, Table 78.1), we would expect about 50% of the patients to have short-term (4–8 weeks) benefit, and 10% to have pain relief for 6 months or more. These figures improve in direct relation to the duration of the pain and are better in patients who have not had back surgery.

It may take as long as a week for benefit from the steroid to be felt (Benzon, 1986). If the injection produced incomplete or short-lived relief, then it is worth repeating, and a course of three injections is recommended. No additional benefit accrues from more than three injections.

The steroid should be diluted in 5–10 ml diluent to prevent any toxicity from the glycol or phenol derivatives in the ampoule of steroid. The use of local anaesthetic with the steroid provides a technical 'marker' for correct extradural injection, so that a failure of the technique is not attributable to technical failure in placement.

Facet joint injection with local anaesthetic and steroid as a diagnostic/therapeutic procedure may be

indicated by a history of pain worse when sitting, and pain on lateral rotation and spine extension. Short-lived success (less than 6 weeks) with local anaesthetic and steroid may be improved by use of cryoanalgesia or radiofrequency blocks to the nerves. Recent studies suggest that whether or not the injection is actually in the facet joint makes little difference (Lilius et al., 1989), and indeed cast some doubt on long-term utility (Carette et al., 1991).

If sciatic pain is the predominant feature, sacral foramen block may be the best block to use. Some patients with long back-pain histories, and particularly where arachnoiditis is suspected, may have symptoms and signs suggestive of deafferentation. Diagnostic lumbar sympathectomy with local anaesthetic may help such pains. Short-lived success may be prolonged with chemical sympathectomy.

Drug therapy of back pain is often unsatisfactory. The pain may be both sufficiently severe and sufficiently sensitive to justify the use of strong opioid analgesics, but this is rarely a socially acceptable solution. Non-opioid analgesics may be used in conjunction with injections, or if injections have failed to help. In many patients such drugs provide inadequate relief even at maximum permitted dosage. Effervescent paracetamol and ibuprofen (fewest NSAID side-effects) may be the most useful.

Where the pain is clearly a deafferentation pain, then the unconventional analgesic regimens of anticonvulsants and antidepressants should be used (valproate, 200 mg b.d., and amitriptyline, 25 mg *nocte*, as first-line).

Those who do not respond

Some back pain patients, particularly those who have had back surgery, respond poorly, which is disheartening for both patient and doctor. It is important that they receive honest advice and treatment, and that patients who still have surgically remediable disease are identified (a tiny minority). Those with arachnoiditis are at risk of progressive disease.

Alternative methods such as transcutaneous nerve stimulation, acupuncture or psychological/behavioural therapies are often tried at this point, which is probably an unfair test of any treatment, and all this can achieve is short-term relief in a subgroup, but again unsustained. There is no simple way to manage these 'failed' back pain patients. It may be difficult to protect them from the worst excesses which may be offered as they go desperately from place to place seeking help. Their heterogeneity implies that no single new treatment or drug is likely to be successful.

Postherpetic neuralgia

Background

Postherpetic neuralgia (PHN), in common with other neuralgias, is a pain in the distribution of a nerve. It follows an acute herpetic (shingles) attack, the pain of PHN being caused by destruction of cells in the posterior nerve root. If enough are destroyed, there is sensory loss directly proportional to the degree of dysaesthesia. The natural history of PHN is intriguing and important for management.

Shingles

Shingles is an infection with the varicella zoster DNA virus. Some 90% of the urban population have had chickenpox by early adulthood, and a prolonged carrier state results with intracellular latency in the dorsal root ganglion. Reactivation of the latent virus causes shingles. The overall incidence of 3–4 : 1000 masks the difference with increasing age; it is rare in children (less than 1 : 1000 up to age 9 years) and much commoner in those over 80 years old (10 : 1000) (Hope-Simpson, 1965). While adults do not catch

zoster by contact, children can acquire chickenpox by contact with zoster. In the general population shingles is commonest in the thoracic region (more than 50%), with 10–15% of cases occurring in the trigeminal distribution (most common in first division).

Incidence and natural history of postherpetic neuralgia

The incidence of PHN in general practice was 10–15% of patients who had pain which lasted more than 1 month and 5–7% who had pain for more than 3 months. One-third of patients who were more than 80 years old when they contracted shingles then had PHN (Hope-Simpson, 1965). PHN is thus more common in elderly patients, but so is the incidence of shingles; it is unclear if elderly patients run an increased risk of PHN independent of their increased risk of shingles.

PHN in the pain clinic reflects the increased incidence with increasing age (Table 78.1), so that 90% of pain clinic PHN patients are more than 60 years old. PHN in the trigeminal nerve distribution is more likely to be referred to the pain clinic than PHN affecting other sites (30% trigeminal PHN in the pain clinic, 10–15% in general practice).

The 'classic' accounts of the natural history of PHN claimed that it did not last more than 6 months (Burgoon *et al.*, 1957). Median pain duration at first clinic visit was more than 2 years (Table 78.1), and 15% of patients attending have had their PHN for more than 5 years, so that those accounts were incorrect.

Pain of postherpetic neuralgia

There is rarely diagnostic difficulty with PHN. The site of the pain is in the distribution of the shingles, and the scarring is often visible to confirm the diagnosis if this is in doubt. PHN patients are not usually wakened at night by their pain.

Four qualities of pain may be distinguished, and this may be helpful in management.
1 Burning pain; a dysaesthetic pain which is initiated by light touch, clothing, etc., 'hypersensitive'. Seen in about 25% of pain clinic PHN patients.
2 Constant deep aching pain with no dysaesthesia (50% incidence).
3 Crawling or scratching pain, just under the skin surface.
4 Stabbing or shooting pain (30% incidence).

There may be visceral involvement in the acute attack, the viscera involved being those supplied with afferent fibres by the posterior nerve roots corresponding to the affected skin areas (Wyburn-Mason, 1957). Symptoms such as constipation, indigestion, frequency or dysuria, depending on the affected nerve, may persist, akin to PHN.

Management

The depressing statement that 'the good results reported by one author are not confirmed subsequently by others, and no single method of therapy has produced more than temporary enthusiasm' (de Moragas & Kierland, 1957) is unfortunately still true for PHN. There is a strong feeling that the success of any remedy is in inverse relation to the duration of the pain. Claims for putative remedies must be examined in this light.

Does treating the pain of shingles prevent PHN?

It has long been held that effective management of the pain of the acute shingles attack reduces the incidence of PHN. While sympathetic blocks (stellate, lumbar sympathetic or extradural) can undoubtedly be effective in relieving the pain of acute zoster (Harding et al., 1986), there is as yet no controlled evidence to show if such pain relief prevents the development of PHN. A control group in whom the intervention is not made is required.

The use of antiviral agents such as topical idoxuridine 35 or 40% in dimethyl sulphoxide or acyclovir, 800 mg 4 hourly, orally can help 'abort' the acute zoster attack if given early (McKendrick et al., 1986). It is not yet known if curtailing the acute attack in this way results in lower PHN incidence.

Injections to relieve PHN

Evidence from controlled studies to support particular remedies is in short supply. While sympathetic, regional or even local nerve blocks may provide short-term relief, there is little evidence that they alter the natural history of the disease process. If the affected area still has sensation, diagnostic nerve blocks with local anaesthetic may produce short-term relief, and this may be extended by measures such as cryoanalgesia. Neurolytic agents are not indicated because initial short-term relief may be followed by pain worse than that which the patient had initially. The relevant blocks include:
1 *Sympathetic system*: stellate ganglion block for head and neck, lumbar sympathetic or extradural for trunk and lower limb.
2 *Peripheral nerve*: subcutaneous infiltration of local

anaesthetic and steroid, repeated weekly for 3 weeks.
The subcutaneous infiltration may be most effective in treating hyperaesthetic burning pain.

Pharmacological management

Conventional analgesics have a very limited role in PHN. The pain does not appear to be sensitive to opioids.

Of the unconventional analgesics, widespread use of the tricyclic antidepressants in PHN is supported by the positive results obtained in controlled studies (Watson et al., 1982). Amitriptyline is the drug of choice, with an initial dose of 25 mg *nocte* reduced to 10 mg in elderly or infirm patients. Its use may be difficult in elderly men with prostate problems.

Persistent shooting or stabbing pain may respond to anticonvulsants, and valproate, 200 mg b.d., or clonazepam, 500 µg *nocte* (rising to b.d.), may be helpful.

Local anaesthetic creams or topical non-steroidal agents are of limited benefit, but may help the hyperaesthetic pain.

Alternative methods

Transcutaneous nerve stimulation may be helpful in the dysaesthetic pain, as indeed may a simple vibrator applied to the junction of the skin areas with normal and abnormal sensation.

Facial pain

The commoner causes of facial pain in the pain clinic are listed in Table 78.5.

PHN affecting the trigeminal division is not uncommon but rarely presents difficulties with diagnosis. Two other neuralgias affecting the face, trigeminal neuralgia and atypical facial pain, are relatively common in the pain clinic. Distinguishing them should not be difficult, but often cases of atypical facial pain are referred to the clinic as trigeminal neuralgia resistant to carbamazepine.

Table 78.5 Common causes of facial pain

Trigeminal neuralgia
Atypical facial pain
Postherpetic neuralgia
Post-traumatic neuralgia
Malignancy
Temperomandibular dysaesthesia

Trigeminal neuralgia

Background

This is the prototypic cranial neuralgia. It is a primary neuralgia although many attempts have been made to explain its pathology on the basis of a somatic cause. Tumour, vascular malformations, dental disease, sinusitis or multiple sclerosis (3%) can cause trigeminal neuralgia, but the aetiology of the bulk of the cases is unknown (White & Sweet, 1969). An abnormality in the pattern of the afferent transmission to the trigeminal nucleus is one explanation. Vascular elongation, local demyelination with age, local compression or crossaxonal discharges have all been proposed as causes of the abnormal transmission.

The condition occurs more often in middle-aged patients and is twice as common in females as in males. This pattern of incidence is the same in the pain clinic; the striking feature is the long duration (mean 9 years) of pain prior to the first visit.

Patients may be referred to a pain clinic with trigeminal neuralgia because the diagnosis is in doubt, because straightforward management with carbamazepine has failed, because of tolerance, side-effects or allergy, or because previous invasive measures have failed.

Site and features of the pain

The pain is, for practical purposes strictly unilateral (White & Sweet, 1969); multiple sclerosis patients constitute the bulk of the 2% of patients with bilateral disease. Trigeminal neuralgia is twice as common on the right side. Combining published figures (8124 cases) the commonest (32%) pain referral was to both the mandibular and maxillary divisions. The figures for divisions 1, 2 and 3 separately were 4%, 17% and 15%, respectively. Seventeen percent had pain in all three divisions (White & Sweet, 1969). The pain may remain unchanged, but usually there is a spread to involve another division.

The pain in the face is characteristically sharp, severe (paroxysmal) and brief, lasting no more than a few seconds. Tic douloureux describes the facial contortions which may accompany the pain. A high frequency of these attacks may lead to a persistent pain which is duller in nature.

The pain may be brought on by thermal, tactile or proprioceptive stimuli, but not by nociceptive stimuli. These intermittent attacks may last for 6–8 weeks. Long spontaneous remissions of months or even years may occur in the early stages, but tend to be shorter as the disease progresses. The severity and frequency of the attacks thus increase over the years.

The history and examination must exclude other potential pathology. There should be no abnormal neurological signs in trigeminal neuralgia, and pain relief with carbamazepine is taken to be diagnostic.

Pharmacological management

Patients are often taking (or have already tried) the anticonvulsant carbamazepine when they come to the pain clinic. If the drug is well tolerated but ineffective, increasing the dose in divided doses to daily maximum of 1500 mg should be tried. If the drug is poorly tolerated (nausea and vomiting, ataxia, skin rash or blood dyscrasia) phenytoin, 100 mg t.d.s., may be tried instead, or in addition to the lowest-tolerated carbamazepine dose.

Peripheral nerve blocks

The role of nerve blocks is to provide pain relief when pharmacological management is unsuccessful, or as an adjunct to allow dose reduction. Individual divisions of the fifth nerve may be blocked with local anaesthetic where they leave the skull and enter the face and mouth (infraorbital, supraorbital, inferior dental and mental nerves). In addition to their diagnostic value, it is not uncommon for these blocks to break a cycle of pain. Relief may then be obtained for much longer than the duration of local anaesthetic. Because the natural history of the disease is one of spontaneous remissions, it is difficult to quantify this relief in the absence of untreated controls; when such relief occurs the patient and the doctor accept it gratefully.

Short-lived success with local anaesthetic may be prolonged with cryoanalgesia (Barnard et al., 1981). In Barnard's study of 24 patients, median duration of relief was 186 days (range 0–1236), contrasting with median duration of sensory loss of 67 days (range 14–80) which indicates the 'reversible' nature of the cryoanalgesia lesion. There were no complications in that series.

Cryoanalgesia, 'peripheral' radiofrequency lesions, neurolytic injections or avulsion and/or nerve section should not be regarded as curative; they are ineffective long term. Relapse rates are higher the longer the follow-up. The advantage of cryoanalgesia is that the patient is no worse if the pain returns, and the cryoanalgesia can be repeated successfully. This is not always the case with the other measures.

Surgical and other more central procedures

Over the years, many surgical procedures have been used to treat trigeminal neuralgia. However, it takes years to establish the success of a novel procedure, because of the extended follow-up required to assess recurrence rate. Procedures need also to be judged on operative morbidity and mortality and long-term morbidity (sensory or motor loss, anaesthesia dolorosa, damage to other cranial nerves). It is a difficult balance. A patient being referred for such procedures may rightly expect to be cured. Unfortunately, the operations with the lowest recurrence rates are likely to be those with the highest complication rates. Some of the procedures are listed in Table 78.6.

Of these probably the most predictable manoeuvre to ablate tic douloureux is sensory root rhizotomy, usually performed in the middle cranial fossa and although there may be some sparing of sensation, corneal ulceration, drooling and trophic lesions of the skin may occur. The recurrence rate with this procedure is low (4% at 4 years). The most serious morbidity is anaesthesia dolorosa, a constant burning pain in the numb area. The incidence of this complication is probably 5–10%, and the only treatment is symptomatic.

Vascular decompression procedures are currently fashionable, and time will tell if the low complication rate is balanced by a high recurrence rate (?50% at 4 years). If that proves to be the case such major surgery may not be justified. Radiofrequency lesions at the Gasserian ganglion, where the electrode is inserted through the foramen ovale under X-ray control, use controlled temperatures to destroy smaller pain fibres selectively. If sensation is preserved, recurrence rates for the first division may be as high as 25%, and there is also a risk of anaesthesia dolorosa (0.3–3%). The injection of glycerine into Meckel's Cave appears

Table 78.6 Nerve block and surgical procedures for trigeminal neuralgia

---

Peripheral nerve section or injection

Middle fossa
Section
Injection
Decompression
Radiofrequency

Posterior fossa
Section
Decompression

Medullary tractotomy

---

not to have been as successful as the early reports claimed.

Different clinics have different views on management, usually held very firmly, but trigeminal neuralgia is a condition where the medical aphorism that the patient should not be made worse is particularly appropriate. The strategy proposed is that failed medical management is an indication for peripheral nerve diagnostic injection, with sustained relief if necessary provided by cryoanalgesia. If these peripheral measures fail, then radiofrequency lesion of the Gasserian ganglion or rhizotomy should be considered.

Atypical facial pain

The diagnosis of atypical facial pain is made often by exclusion of other causes of facial pain. Classically it affects middle-aged women (Miller, 1968). Pain clinic patients in whom this is the ultimate (correct) diagnosis may have been referred because they were thought to have trigeminal neuralgia, which had failed to respond to carbamazepine, or because their facial pain was wrongly associated with dental problems, and had continued despite extraction(s). It should not be a difficult diagnosis to make, but the major confusion is with trigeminal neuralgia.

Site and features of the pain

While the site of pain is in the face, it may not tie in with the distribution of any particular nerve, and it may cross the midline.

The features of the pain are that it is a dull pain (cf. the sharp pain of trigeminal neuralgia), which may be persistent or recurrent, uni- or bilateral, in the absence of any muscular or joint problems, and with no abnormal neurological signs, akin to trigeminal neuralgia. Although the pain is episodic, it is unlike that of trigeminal neuralgia in that it builds up gradually to a climax and it may last for hours and even days. It is anatomically imprecise and covers a much larger territory than that supplied by an individual cranial nerve. The pain is never 'electric' and is usually described as tearing or crushing.

The pain may be associated with other symptom complexes, such as spastic colon, dysfunctional uterine bleeding, headaches and low back pain. These complexes may recur sequentially or simultaneously in response to stress.

It is wise to look for a hidden cause and here teeth, sinuses and eyes may be incriminated. At least three 'parallel' conditions may be associated with atypical facial pain. Temperomandibular dysaesthesia (facial arthromyalgia) may be difficult to distinguish from atypical facial pain but there is usually a history of pain in muscles and/or joints, clicking, sticking or trismus, and a feeling of buzzing or fullness in the ear. On examination there may be ridged buccal mucosa, crenated tongue, or masseteric hypertrophy, and arthritic change may be seen on X-ray of the condylar surface. Atypical odontalgia may be distinguished from atypical facial pain because the continuous or throbbing pain is felt in the teeth (tooth), is hypersensitive to all stimuli and may move from tooth to tooth. Glossodynia or oral dysaesthesia is the sensation of a dry mouth, burning tongue and gums, with denture intolerance, disturbance of taste and salivation and no organic pathology.

Management and course

The pathogenesis remains mysterious, but the patients need to be reassured that it is a 'real pain', and is best managed medically rather than by surgery, which may make it more refractory. The association with adverse life events (80% of patients) emphasizes that this condition may affect the emotionally fit as a stress response.

Tricyclic antidepressants are the treatment of choice. Treatment with dothiepin (75−150 mg *nocte*) proved effective and well tolerated (Feinmann *et al.*, 1984). It is not clear if there is any difference between the various antidepressants. Treatment should be maintained for 3 months. Trifluoperazine, 2−4 mg *mane*, may then be prescribed in addition if relief is poor. One-third of patients needed short courses (3 months or less) in response to stress, and 40% needed 18−24 months maintained therapy. Four years on from diagnosis, 70% of the patients were pain-free, but half needed intermittent medication and 10% still needed continuous treatment.

Post-traumatic neuralgia (including postoperative wound pain)

Pain after trauma and pain in or near the operative scar, occurring for months and even years after surgery, can be extremely difficult to manage. Because the principles of management are similar they are discussed together.

Post-traumatic neuralgia may occur in a context where the patient is seeking compensation for the accident. Much has been made of the intransigence of the neuralgia until the compensation is settled; unfortunately for many patients, the pain remains long after the compensation is paid. The aetiology of postoperative wound pain is unknown. Why are some patients affected and not others? As always when this is the case, doctors ascribe a psychogenic overlay.

Site and features of the pain

Post-traumatic neuralgia

The pain may be in any part of the body, and may be associated with damage to bone, nerve, muscle or other tissue. Specific information to be sought in the history and examination includes nerve damage to the affected area at the time of injury and the current neurological status of the painful area. Is it numb? Are there painful pins and needles? Is there any difference in temperature between affected and unaffected areas?

Postoperative wound pain

Three particular postoperative situations seem most likely to result in postoperative wound pain, thoracotomy (particularly thoracoabdominal incisions), nephrectomy and inguinal herniorrhaphy, but pain at or around scars from other operations is also seen.

The quality of the pain is often described as burning, even if the area still has normal sensation (unusual). Commonly there is no hyperaesthesia. The aura of the pain (the extent of the area affected) may increase as time elapses.

Management

Pharmacological

Conventional analgesics may have a very limited role in both post-traumatic and postoperative neuralgias referred to the pain clinic, indeed the patient was in all likelihood referred because such regimens had failed to help significantly.

The use of antidepressants and anticonvulsants is more likely to help, particularly if the pain is burning and occurring in an area of altered sensation. A starting regimen might be amitriptyline, 25 mg *nocte*. Alternatives are valproate, 200 mg b.d., or clonazepam, starting at 500 μg *nocte*, and increasing the dose in the absence of side-effects to 1.5 or 2 mg t.d.s.

Peripheral nerve blocks

Diagnostic blocks with local anaesthetic should be tried when appropriate in these conditions. For the postoperative pains intercostal blocks for thoracotomy or nephrectomy and ilioinguinal blocks for herniorrhaphy may produce relief. If the relief is short lived, then the duration may be extended by repeating the block with cryoanalgesia. This may (especially for the ilioinguinal nerve) be best achieved with surgical exposure under direct vision rather than with a percutaneous approach.

Autonomic nerve blocks

Stellate ganglion (for head, neck, upper limbs and upper chest wall) or lumbar sympathectomy may be the first-line of management, particularly in post-traumatic neuralgia, and the greatest chance of success is if the pain is in an area of altered sensation.

Extending the duration of pain relief with successful 'single-shot' stellate ganglion block may be achieved by repeating the block every 3—7 days on up to 10 or more occasions. If there is undoubted success with local anaesthetic blocks but this cannot be sustained despite repeated injections, then surgery may be appropriate, perhaps the best results being achieved with a transthoracic approach using the operating microscope.

Short-lived relief from lumbar sympathectomy with local anaesthetic may be prolonged by using phenol.

Perineal neuralgia

Perineal neuralgia with no malignant cause occurs most commonly in women, often postmenopausal. Again it is a most difficult pain to treat successfully. The aetiology is unknown, but pelvic varicosities are thought to be a cause of pelvic pain (Beard *et al.*, 1986), but the symptoms and signs (or lack of) in perineal pain would seem to be distinct from the pelvic pain syndrome (Beard *et al.*, 1986).

Site and features of the pain

The pain is described variously as a 'tugging', 'pulling' or 'crawling' sensation, commonly in the clitoral area. Many women with this condition prefer to stand, because the pain is worse when they sit.

Management

Pharmacological

Conventional analgesics are rarely effective, and unfortunately antidepressants and anticonvulsants do not help most patients. Women are often prescribed local hormone therapy; few seem to be helped.

Nerve blocks

Sacral extradural with local anaesthetic may be tried diagnostically. Many of these patients will still have their pain even when the relevant area is numb from the local anaesthetic. If the local anaesthetic does help the pain, the duration of relief may be prolonged with sacral extradural cryoanalgesia.

Lumbar sympathectomy may be a logical procedure if the cause is pelvic varicosities, but has not proved successful.

Phantom and stump pain

Background

Phantom pain

The proportion of amputees suffering from phantom pain is high (78% of the 55% responding to a survey of 5000 amputees; Sherman *et al.*, 1984), although previous reports had given much lower incidence of pain. There seem to be few predictors of disabling phantom pain; age at amputation, years since amputation, reason for amputation, site of amputation and pain before surgery were similar in those with and without problematic phantom pain (Sherman *et al.*, 1984).

The aetiology of the pain is unknown. It is thought that preventing pain before surgery may reduce the incidence of phantom pain (Bach *et al.*, 1988).

Stump pain

Pain in the stump may occur early after surgery due to surgical postoperative complications, but pain clinic patients with stump pain tend to be late referrals with well-healed stumps, and the origin of the pain is attributed to neuroma development.

Management

Phantom pain

At least 50 different methods of treating phantom limb pain are currently in use, but only 1% of patients had long-term benefit (Sherman *et al.*, 1984). Whichever method is used, best results come with early treatment.

Pharmacological

Neither minor (including NSAID agents) nor major conventional analgesics are of great analgesic benefit, but opiates may make the patient feel better. The use of anticonvulsants has been more successful, but with no controlled evidence to support their use. Severe shooting or lancinating pains are most likely to respond, and clonazepam, 500 µg *nocte*, rising to 1.5–2 mg t.d.s. if the drug is well tolerated may be the most effective of this group.

Nerve blocks

Sympathetic blocks with local anaesthetic may be used diagnostically, and short-lived relief may be prolonged with repeat local anaesthetic blocks or chemical sympathectomy. Despite pain-clinic claims for the efficacy of these procedures, there is little evidence for long-term benefit.

Surgery

Surgical procedures seem to be the least successful.

Stump pain

Stump pain often coexists with phantom pain (Sherman *et al.*, 1984), and treatment of the phantom with anticonvulsants may also help the stump pain. A purely 'local' stump pain with neuroma development may benefit from local anaesthetic injection to the site, repeated if required, and with either percutaneous or direct vision cryoanalgesia to extend the duration of relief.

Conclusions

What function is served by pain clinics? There are those who argue that a good doctor, whatever his/her specialty, should be able to treat pain. The reality is that this does not always happen, and the pain clinic provides a focus, a 'critical mass' of experience, where, by combining pharmacology, nerve blocks and other measures, patients may be helped. Pain management is not an exact science, but will become more of one when underlying mechanisms are understood (cf. phantom pain), and as the methods used to provide a rational basis for treatment in other branches of medicine are applied.

What is the role of the anaesthetist in chronic pain management (Diamond, 1991)? Many patients benefit from their skills with nerve-blocking procedures, and many anaesthetists enjoy the contrast between their pain clinic work and their theatre sessions. Anaesthetists in theatre have to be expert in the pharmacology of the drugs which they use; equally, pain work requires pharmacology, but with the twist

that not only are some of the drugs rarely seen in the operating theatre, but the major route is oral rather than intravenous.

How do we progress? It is unfortunate that, at a time when basic scientists are fascinated by pain mechanisms and pharmacology, clinical progress with chronic pain control has been limited largely to better use of oral opiates, attributable to the teachings of the hospice movement. The nerve-blocking procedures, which were historically the reason why anaesthetists became involved in pain control, are unfashionable. The reason is the lack of careful data comparing quality and duration of relief, both between different nerve-blocking techniques and between nerve blocks and other measures. Without such data, not only is management necessarily empirical, but the spectre of litigation may deprive patients of potentially beneficial treatment. It is incumbent on pain clinics which use blocks to gather this information.

References

Arner A., Lindblom U., Meyerson B.A. & Molander C. (1990) Prolonged relief of neuralgia after regional anesthetic blocks. A call for further experimental and systematic clinical studies. *Pain* **43**, 287–97.

Bach S., Noreng M.F. & Tjellden N.U. (1988) Phantom limb pain in amputees during the first 12 months following limb amputation, after preoperative lumbar epidural blockade. *Pain* **33**, 297–301.

Banning A., Sjögren P. & Henriksen H. (1991) Treatment outcome in a multidisciplinary cancer pain clinic. *Pain* **47**, 129–34.

Barnard D., Lloyd J.W. & Evans J. (1981) Cryoanalgesia in the management of chronic facial pain. *Journal of Maxillofacial Surgery* **9**, 101–2.

Beard R.W., Reginald P.W. & Pearce S. (1986) Pelvic pain in women. *British Medical Journal* **293**, 1160–2.

Benzon H.T. (1986) Epidural steroid injections for low back pain and lumbosacral radiculopathy. *Pain* **24**, 277–95.

Boas R.A. (1983) The sympathetic nervous system and pain relief. In *Relief of Intractable Pain* (Ed. Swerdlow M.) pp. 215–37. Elsevier, Amsterdam.

Burgoon C.F., Burgoon J.S. & Baldridge G.D. (1957) The natural history of herpes zoster. *Journal of the American Medical Association* **164**, 265–9.

Carette S., Marcoux S., Truchon R., Grondin C., Gagnon J., Allard Y. & Latulippe M. (1991) A controlled trial of corticosteroid injections into facet joints for chronic low back pain. *New England Journal of Medicine* **325**, 1002–7.

de Moragas J.M. & Kierland R.R. (1957) The outcome of patients with herpes zoster. *Archives of Dermatology* **75**, 193–5.

Diamond A. (1991) The future development of chronic pain relief. *Anaesthesia* **46**, 83–4.

Editorial (1982) Pain clinics. *Lancet* i, 486.

Fearnside M.R. & Adams C.B.T. (1978) Tumours of the cauda

equina. *Journal of Neurology, Neurosurgery and Psychiatry* **41**, 24–31.

Feinmann C., Harris M. & Cawley R. (1984) Psychogenic facial pain: presentation and treatment. *British Medical Journal* **288**, 436–8.

Foley K.M. (1985) The treatment of cancer pain. *New England Journal of Medicine* **313**, 84–95.

Harding S.P., Lipton J.R., Wells J.D.C. & Campbell J.A. (1986) Relief of acute pain in herpes zoster opthalmicus by stellate ganglion block. *British Medical Journal* **292**, 1428.

Hope-Simpson R.E. (1965) The nature of herpes zoster: a long-term study and a new hypothesis. *Journal of the Royal Society of Medicine* **58**, 9–20.

Jadad A.R., Popat M.T., Glynn C.J. & McQuay H.J. (1991) Double-blind testing fails to confirm analgesic response to extradural morphine. *Anaesthesia* **46**, 935–7.

Jadad A.R., Carroll D., Glynn C.J., Moore R.A. & McQuay H.J. (1992) Morphine responsiveness of chronic pain: double-blind randomised crossover study with patient-controlled analgesia method. *Lancet* **339**, 1367–71.

Jones J. & Gough D. (1977) Coeliac plexus block with alcohol for relief of upper abdominal pain due to cancer. *Annals of the Royal College of Surgeons of England* **59**, 46–9.

Kepes E.R. & Duncalf D. (1985) Treatment of backache with spinal injections of local anesthetics, spinal and systemic steroids. A review. *Pain* **22**, 33–47.

Lilius G., Laasonen E.M., Myllynen P., Harilainen A. & Grönlund G. (1989) Lumbar facet joint syndrome. *Journal of Bone and Joint Surgery* **71**, 681–4.

McKendrick M.W., McGill J.I., White J.E. & Wood M.J. (1986) Oral acyclovir in acute herpes zoster. *British Medical Journal* **ii**, 1529–32.

McQuay H.J. (1988) Pharmacological treatment of neuralgic and neuropathic pain. *Cancer Surveys* **7**, 141–59.

McQuay H.J. & Dickenson A.H. (1990) Implications of nervous system plasticity for pain management. *Anaesthesia* **45**, 101–2.

McQuay H.J., Machin L. & Moore R.A. (1985) Chronic non-malignant pain: a population prevalence study. *Practitioner* **229**, 1109–11.

Martin G. (1981) The management of pain following laminectomy for lumbar disc lesions. *Annals of the Royal College of Surgeons of England* **63**, 244–52.

Miller H. (1968) Pain in the face. *British Medical Journal* **2**, 577–80.

Shaw M.D.M., Russell J.A. & Grossart K.W. (1978) The changing pattern of spinal arachnoiditis. *Journal of Neurology, Neurosurgery and Psychiatry* **41**, 97–107.

Sherman R.A., Sherman C.J. & Parker L. (1984) Chronic phantom and stump pain among American veterans: results of a survey. *Pain* **18**, 83–95.

Sjöberg M., Applegren L., Einarsson S., Hultman E., Linder L.E., Nitescu P. & Curelaru C. (1991) Long-term intrathecal morphine and bupivacaine in 'refractory' cancer pain. I. Results from the first series of 52 patients. *Acta Anaesthesiologica Scandinavica* **35**, 30–43.

Twycross R.G. & Lack S. (1983) *Symptom Control in Far Advanced Cancer: Pain Relief*. Pitman, London.

Waddell G. (1982) An approach to backache. *British Journal of Hospital Medicine* **28**, 187–233.

Wall P.D. (1989) Introduction. In *Textbook of Pain* (Eds Wall P.D. & Melzack R.) pp. 1–18. Churchill Livingstone, London.

Watson C.P., Evans R.J., Reed K., Merskey H., Goldsmith L. & Warsh J. (1982) Amitriptyline versus placebo in post-herpatic neuralgia. *Neurology* **54**, 37–43.

White J.C. & Sweet W.H. (1969) *Pain and the Neurosurgeon* pp. 123–78. Thomas, Springfield.

Wyburn-Mason R. (1957) Visceral lesions in herpes zoster. *British Medical Journal* **i**, 678–81.

The Management of Pain in Cancer

R.G. TWYCROSS

Published data suggest that 75% of patients with advanced cancer have pain (Bonica, 1990). Some reports indicate that many do not receive adequate relief (Bonica, 1985) but others have stated that pain can be controlled completely in 80–90% of patients and that 'acceptable relief' is possible in most of the rest (Twycross & Lack, 1983; Foley, 1985; Rappaz *et al.*, 1985; Ventafridda *et al.*, 1987; Takeda, 1989). The reasons for the difference between demonstrated possibility and general performance include (World Health Organization, 1986):

1 Lack of recognition that established methods already exist for cancer pain management.

2 Lack of systematic teaching of medical students, doctors, nurses and other health-care workers about cancer pain management.

3 Fears concerning addiction in both cancer patients and the wider public if strong opioids are more readily available for medical purposes.

4 Non-availability of necessary pain relief drugs in many parts of the world.

5 Lack of concern by many national governments.

Caring for cancer patients is emotionally demanding for several reasons — notably an instinctive fear of death and, in consequence, a reluctance to care for those who remind us of our common destiny. A failure to understand this and to take corrective measures hinders good pain control.

Causes of pain in cancer

Pain is a complex 'somatopsychic' experience (Chapter 75). In advanced cancer, a sense of hopelessness and the fear of impending death adds to the suffering of the patient. In these circumstances, the concept of 'total pain' is helpful (Saunders & Baines, 1983; Mount, 1984). This takes cognizance of psychological, social and spiritual factors in addition to the physical.

Case history

A 55-year-old man with recently diagnosed cancer of the oesophagus was still in pain despite receiving slow-release morphine, 6000 mg (100 mg × 60) twice a day. Following inpatient admission to a hospice, he became pain-free on 30 mg twice a day and diazepam 10 mg at bedtime. He was able to return home and convert the spare bedroom into a workshop where he spent many happy hours creatively and productively. The key to success was *listening*, *explaining* and *setting positive rehabilitation goals*.

Diagnostic probabilities

Pain in cancer may be:

1 Caused by the cancer itself (this is by far the most common).

2 Related to the cancer or debility (e.g. muscle spasm, constipation, bedsores).

3 Related to cancer treatment (e.g. chronic post-operative scar pain, chemotherapy mucositis).

4 Caused by a concurrent disorder (e.g. arthritis, spondylosis).

Many patients with advanced cancer have multiple pains which relate to several of these categories. A prospective survey of 100 cancer patients with pain revealed a total of 303 anatomically distinct pains, an average of three per patient (Twycross & Fairfield, 1982). Eighty had two or more pains; 34 had four or more (Fig. 79.1). Cancer was the sole cause of pain in only 41 patients (Table 79.1). In nine patients none of the pain was caused by cancer; in two of these, constipation was the sole cause of pain. Myofascial trigger point pain occurred in 12 patients and accounted for 24 pains.

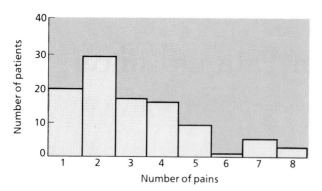

Fig. 79.1 Number of pains experienced by 100 consecutive cancer patients with pain on admission to Sir Michael Sobell House. (Redrawn from Twycross & Fairfield, 1982.)

Pain syndromes in cancer patients

A series of specific pain syndromes unique to cancer have been described (Foley, 1979; Portenoy, 1989; Bonica, 1990). Although some are uncommon, an awareness of these syndromes is necessary for the correct diagnosis to be made without undue delay (Tables 79.2 and 79.3).

Pathophysiology of cancer pain

From a pathophysiological point of view there are two main types of cancer pain:
1 Nociceptive.
2 Neuropathic.

Nociceptive pain is produced by the activation of specific peripheral receptors (nociceptors), whereas neuropathic pain occurs as a result of injury to or dysfunction of the peripheral nervous system or CNS. Neuropathic pain differs from nociceptive pain in several ways (Zimmerman, 1983; Bowsher; 1990):
1 It does not involve activation of nerve endings (nociceptors).
2 It relates to central neuronal dysfunction secondary to partial or total loss of afferent input.
3 It is associated with sensory loss.

Table 79.1 Causes of 303 pains in 100 cancer pain patients. (Data from Twycross & Fairfield, 1982)

Cancer	63%
Muscle	13%
Spondylosis ⎫	
Osteoarthritis ⎭	8%
Constipation	4%
Chronic postoperative	3%

Neuropathic pain is often not abolished by conventional analgesics, including morphine (Arner & Meyerson, 1988). Surgical section of peripheral or central pathways does not always help (Tasker, 1987). On the basis of studies of intravenous opioid infusions, it has been claimed that neuropathic pain is opioid responsive (Portenoy *et al.*, 1990). However, in the patients studied, 'maximum pain relief' was concomitant with 'maximum sedation', thereby casting doubt on the interpretation of the relief obtained.

Animal studies have demonstrated that, after peripheral nerve injury, the damaged neurones become hypersensitive to mechanical and α-adrenergic stimulation, and show spontaneous electrical activity (Tasker & Dostrovsky, 1989; Wall, 1989). Subsequently, changes may be detected in the cell bodies in the dorsal root ganglia where abnormal 'cross-talk' occurs between neighbouring neurones. The end result of these changes is a new CNS steady state in which there is: (i) spontaneous activity; (ii) hyperexcitability; and (iii) an expanded receptive field.

Nerve injury, however, does *not* always result in pain. For example, postherpetic neuralgia is rare in young adults. Further, even with apparently identical lesions, only a minority of patients develop neuropathic pain. A genetic factor has been postulated to explain this (Devor & Raber, 1990).

Characteristics

An associated sensory deficit has given rise to a working definition of neuropathic pain, namely, *pain in an area of abnormal or absent sensation* (Glynn, 1989). Although not strictly true (sensory loss is also associated with nerve compression pain), this description serves to alert the doctor to the possibility of neuropathic pain whenever pain and altered sensation coexist.

Peripheral neuropathic pain ('deafferentation pain') typically has the following characteristics:
1 Superficial burning pain with a neural distribution ± shooting pain.
2 Allodynia (pain caused by a non-noxious stimulus).
3 Partial sensory deficit (pinprick and temperature most constantly affected). There may be an associated aching pain, which sometimes is predominant (Kastrup *et al.*, 1986).

Allodynia is pathognomonic of neuropathic pain, though is not invariably present. It may be of three varieties which may coexist in the same patient:
1 Mechanical (pain triggered by touch, wind or clothing).

Table 79.2 Selected pain syndromes caused by cancer. (Adapted from Foley, 1979; Portenoy, 1989; Bonica, 1990)

Syndromes	Pathophysiology	Characteristics of pain	Concomitants
Tumour invasion of bone			
Base of skull			
Occipital condyle	Metastasis to occipital condyle	Severe localized unilateral occipital pain exacerbated by neck flexion	Dysfunction of cranial nerve XII: paralysis of tongue, weakness of sternocleidomastoid, stiff neck
Jugular foramen	Metastasis to jugular foramen	Occipital pain radiating to the vertex and to one or both shoulders and arms, exacerbated by head movement	Dysfunction of CN IX−XII: hoarseness, dysarthria, dysphagia, trapezius muscle weakness and often ptosis
Clivus syndrome	Metastasis to clivus of sphenoid bone and basilar portion of occipital bone	Progressively severe vertex headache exacerbated by neck flexion	Dysfunction of CN VII−XII: begins unilaterally but extends bilaterally
Sphenoid sinus	Metastasis to the sphenoid sinus on one or both sides	Severe bifrontal headache radiating to both temples with intermittent retro-orbital pain	Nasal stuffiness or sense of fullness in the head, diplopia
Cavernous sinus	Metastasis to cavernous sinus	Unilateral frontal headache and aching pain in supraorbital and facial regions	Dysfunction of CN III−VI: diplopia, ophthalmoplegia, papilloedema
Vertebrae			
Fracture of odontoid process	Metastasis of odontoid process of axis→ compression of spinal cord	Severe neck pain radiating to occiput and vertex of skull, exacerbated by movements of neck	Progressive sensory, motor and autonomic dysfunction beginning in upper limb
C7−T1 metastasis	Haematogenous spread of cancer of breast and bronchus; or tumour in paravertebral space→ spread to adjacent vertebra and extradural space	Constant aching pain in paraspinal area radiating to both shoulders; unilateral radicular pain radiating to shoulder and medial (ulnar) aspect of arm	Tenderness on percussion of spinous process; paraesthesia and numbness in ulnar distribution of limb; progressive weakness of triceps and hand; Horner's syndrome if sympathetic involvement
L1 metastasis	Common site of metastasis from breast, prostate and other tumours	Aching pain in midback with reference to one or both sacroiliac joints; radicular pain with girdle-like distribution in groins	Pain may be exacerbated by lying down
Sacral metastasis	Common site of metastasis from breast, prostate and other tumours	Aching pain in the sacral and/or coccygeal region exacerbated by sitting and relieved by walking	Perianal sensory loss; bowel and bladder dysfunction; impotence
Cord compression and meninges			
Extradural spinal cord compression	Tumour compression of spinal cord, usually as a result of vertebral metastasis and collapse	Aching pain and tenderness in the region of involved vertebrae, radicular pain, and garter or cuff distribution of pain in legs	Motor weakness progressing to paraplegia; sensory loss; loss of bowel and bladder function
Leptomeningeal carcinomatosis	Tumour infiltration of the cerebrospinal leptomeninges	Headache, with or without neck stiffness; and pain in the low back and buttocks	Malignant cells in cerebrospinal fluid

Table 79.3 Selected pain syndromes caused by cancer treatment. (Adapted from Foley, 1979; Portenoy, 1989; Bonica, 1990)

Syndromes	Pathophysiology	Characteristics of pain	Concomitants
Postoperative syndromes Post-thoracotomy Postmastectomy Postradical neck resection	Severance of nerves during operation → neuropathic response	Continuous burning or aching pain ± bouts of stabbing pain in the areas supplied by affected nerves, exacerbated by touch and movement	Allodynia in the scar; hypaesthesia in the adjacent area. Neuroma only rarely present
Postamputation pain	Neuropathic	Constant aching or burning pain in stump and/or in phantom limb	Palpation of trigger points in stump precipitates or exacerbates pain
Postchemotherapy Peripheral neuropathy	Caused by vinca alkaloids	Constant symmetrical burning pain in the hands and/or feet	Allodynia
Steroid pseudorheumatism	Caused by rapid withdrawal of corticosteroids	Diffuse myalgia and arthralgia	Fatigue and general malaise
Aseptic necrosis of humoral/femoral head	Complication of chronic corticosteroid therapy	Aching pain in shoulder or knee	Limitation of joint movement
Mucositis	Ulceration of buccal and pharyngeal mucosa	Severe pain exacerbated by drinking, eating and talking	
Postradiation therapy Radiation fibrosis of brachial or lumbosacral plexus	Fibrosis of connective tissue surrounding nerves with consequent neural injury	Increasingly severe burning pain in the arm or leg	Allodynia; numbness; motor weakness (usually C5–6 distribution in the arm)
Radiation myelopathy	Damage to spinal cord; causes pain in less than 20%	Pattern similar to spinal cord compression; local back pain, radicular pain and/or neuropathic pain referred distally	Other sensory and motor symptoms and signs of myelopathy

2 Cold (pain exacerbated by cold).
3 Movement (related to dysfunction of the muscle spindles).

There may also be evidence of sympathetic dysfunction manifest as (Bowsher 1990):
1 Cutaneous vasodilatation.
2 Increased skin temperature.
3 Altered pattern of sweating.

Neuropathic pain with sympathetic involvement is, however, distinct from sympathetic maintained pain (Churcher & Ingall, 1987; Churcher, 1990). This rare type of neuropathic pain also tends to be superficial and burning, and associated with a sensory abnormality (Table 79.4). In addition, there may be radiographic evidence of osteoporosis and of hot spots on isotope bone scans which may be mistaken for osteolytic metastases. Both pain and sensory abnormalities are corrected by sympathetic block.

Neuropathic pain in cancer is usually the result of either treatment (Table 79.3) or malignant infiltration of a nerve.

Assessment

Doctors caring for cancer patients should, as far as possible, acquire the skill of determining the cause of the pain on the basis of diagnostic probabilities and pattern recognition. Invasive investigations are increasingly contraindicated as patients become more terminally ill. A comprehensive list of possible causes of pain is unnecessary because, inevitably, it would be too long to be helpful. What is required is an informed imagination, making use of the data presented above. An awareness of the common muscular pain syndromes is necessary to prevent many erroneous conclusions. Similarly helpful is some knowl-

Table 79.4 Superficial burning pain. (From Twycross & Lack, 1990)

	Somatic neuropathic pain	Sympathetic-mediated pain
Cause	Nerve destruction	Nerve irritation (?)
Pattern	Dermatomal (if peripheral)	Vascular
Concomitants		
Stabbing pain	Common	Unusual
Allodynia	+	+/−
Hyperpathia	+/−	+/−
Deep pressure	Comforts	Tender near joints (common)
Pinprick	Diminished (usually)	Diminished (usually)
Muscle atrophy	+	+/−
Muscle fatigue	−	+/−
Trophic changes	Late	Early*
Limb temperature	Normal/cold	Usually colder†
Tricyclic drug	Good relief (often)	Little or no relief
Sympathetic block	No relief	Partial or complete relief‡

* Trophic changes may affect skin, subcutaneous tissues and/or nails; may be atrophic (e.g. shiny taut skin, hair loss) or hypertrophic (e.g. hyperkeratosis); † if in doubt, temperature changes can be confirmed with a thermocouple. Valid only if the pulses are equal in both the affected and normal limbs, and no history of deep venous thrombosis. In some patients the temperature may vary with warm episodes and sweating; ‡ sensory abnormalities revert to normal.

edge of the patterns of metastatic spread (Figs 79.2 and 79.3). If wrongly assumed to be cancerous in origin, the pain tends to be invested with all the negative implications of cancer pain. Such investment will make the pain worse.

Case history

A 63-year-old woman complained of weight loss, epigastric pain and insomnia of several months' duration. At laparotomy, she was found to have

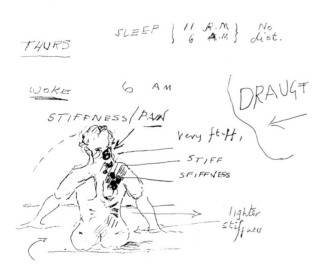

Fig. 79.2 A pain self-portrait by a 65-year-old male patient with pancreatic cancer. Sites of pain indicate that pain was probably muscular/myofascial in origin. Explanation, massage and diazepam at night were prescribed. (From Twycross & Lack, 1986.)

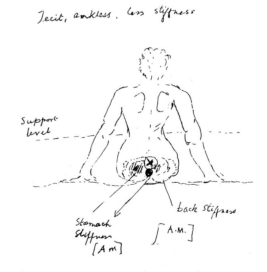

Fig. 79.3 A pain portrait by a patient with pancreatic cancer. Myofascial pains have now resolved. New pain probably also non-malignant, related to lying in bed for long periods. Again, analgesics were not prescribed. Explanation, sheepskin and progressive mobilization resulted in relief. (From Twycross & Lack, 1986.)

carcinoma of the pancreas with liver metastases. When seen 10 days postoperatively by a hospice doctor she was receiving 25 mg of morphine sulphate by mouth every 4 h. This failed to provide adequate relief (Fig. 79.4). She was drowsy, mentally distressed and complained of continued insomnia. It was explained that some of her pains were muscular and that she probably also had pain from a cracked rib. She was advised that an abdominal incision (particularly with deep tension sutures) could be uncomfortable on movement for several weeks, but that it would improve progressively. It was pointed out that certain pains respond better to aspirin and non-drug measures than to morphine. She was also told that some of the abdominal pain was probably caused by constipation. She was prescribed regular aspirin every 4 h, and the nurses advised about the nature of the rib pain. The morphine was reduced and a specific night hypnotic introduced. A laxative was prescribed and rectal measures planned for the following day. The next day she was dramatically improved after a good night's sleep and had much less pain. Her morphine was reduced further and after 3 days she was taking only 5 mg every 4 h with 15 mg at night.

This case history reinforces the following points:
1 Not all pains in cancer are malignant in origin.
2 Cancer patients with pain often have more than one pain.
3 Muscular pains may be as severe as (or even more severe than) much cancer-caused pain.
4 Some pains, however intense, do not benefit from incremental doses of morphine.

5 Careful clinical assessment is necessary before commencing treatment.
6 Explanation is an essential modality of treatment.
7 Reassessment after initiating treatment is necessary to confirm or modify the initial assessment.
8 Reassessment may also lead to changes in treatment in the light of initial results and/or adverse drug effects.

Management of pain

The use of analgesics and pain management are not synonymous. Not only is pain a complex somato-psychic experience, but all pains do not respond equally to analgesics. Thus, the use of analgesics should be regarded as part of a multimodality approach to treatment (Table 79.5).

From a therapeutic point of view, pain in cancer falls into three categories:
1 Opioid-responsive pains, i.e. pain that is relieved by opioids.
2 Opioid semiresponsive pains, i.e. pain that is relieved by the concurrent use of an opioid and an adjuvant drug.
3 Opioid-resistant pains, i.e. pain that is not relieved by opioids but is by other drugs.

The term 'opioid responsive pain' is used to describe pains that respond increasingly well to increasing doses of opioid analgesics. In other words, if moderately severe, the pain responds to codeine and, if very severe, to morphine. This classification is important because it reminds doctors that opioids

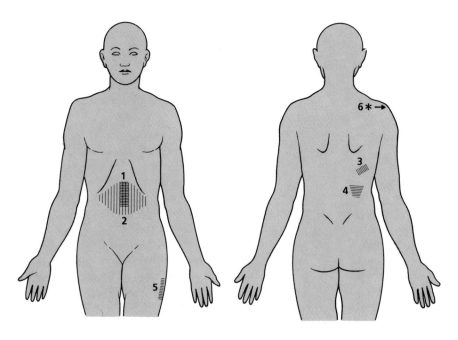

Fig. 79.4 Based on a pain chart of a 63-year-old woman with cancer of tail of the pancreas, 10 days postoperatively. 1 Intermittent stabbing pain (postoperative wound pain). 2 Diffuse upper abdominal discomfort (probably constipation — colonic pain). 3 Rib pain (? cracked). 4 Muscle spasm. 5 Meralgia paraesthetica. 6 TP pain (supraspinatus). (Redrawn from Twycross & Lack, 1986.)

Table 79.5 Pain control in cancer. (From Twycross & Lack, 1986)

Examination	To establish trust	
Explanation	To reduce psychological impact of pain	
Modification of pathological process	Radiation therapy Hormone therapy Chemotherapy	Surgery Correction of hypercalcaemia Pituitary ablation with alcohol
Elevation of pain threshold	Relief of other symptoms Sleep Rest Sympathy Understanding Companionship Creative activity	Reduction in anxiety Elevation of mood Relaxation Analgesics Anxiolytics Antidepressants

Interruption of pain pathways	*Local anaesthesia*
	Lignocaine
	Bupivacaine
		Neurolysis
		Chemical:
		  Alcohol
		  Phenol
		  Chlorocresol
		Cold (cryotherapy)
		Heat (thermocoagulation)

Modification of lifestyle	Avoid pain-precipitating activities	
Immobilization	Rest Cervical collar Surgical corset	Moulded plastic splints Slings Orthopaedic surgery

are of limited value for certain pains, and that sometimes they are contraindicated (Table 79.6). However, the classification is true only for opioids given by mouth or by conventional parenteral routes. Anecdotal evidence suggests that by a spinal route — extradural or intrathecal — 'opioid resistant' pains may be more opioid responsive (Ottesen *et al.*, 1990).

Opioid-responsive pains

Visceral pains are in this category, as are many deep soft-tissue pains. Five important concepts govern the use of analgesics in the management of opioid-responsive pains:
1 'By the mouth'.
2 'By the clock'.
3 'By the ladder'.
4 'For the individual'.
5 Adjuvant medication.

'By the mouth'

Morphine and other strong opioids are effective by mouth. Thus, apart from the last few hours or days of life, few patients require injections to control pain.

However, because of reduced bioavailability, the oral dose is 2−3 times larger than the equianalgesic dose by injection (Hanks *et al.*, 1987). Patients with intractable vomiting in addition to pain require parenteral medication — both antiemetic and analgesic. When vomiting has been controlled, it is generally possible to revert to the oral route. Suppositories are a useful alternative, particularly in the home. The dose of morphine *per os* and *per rectum* is the same (Pannuti *et al.*, 1982; Kaiko *et al.*, 1989).

'By the clock'

To allow pain to re-emerge before administering the next dose causes unnecessary suffering and encourages tolerance. 'As required' medication has no place in the treatment of persistent pain (Fig. 79.5). Whatever the cause, continuous pain requires regular prophylactic therapy. The next dose is given before the effect of the previous one has worn off and, therefore, before the patient may think necessary.

For codeine and morphine an 'every four hours' regimen is optimal. If a strong analgesic other than morphine is used, the doctor must be familiar with its pharmacology (Table 79.7). Pethidine is generally

Table 79.6 Types of pain and implications for treatment

Type of pain	Mechanism	Example	Opioid responsiveness	Drug treatment
Nociceptive	Stimulation of nerve endings			
Visceral		Hepatic capsule pain	+	Analgesics
Somatic		Bone pain	+/−	Analgesics
Nerve compression*		Nerve root compression	+/−	Analgesics; corticosteroids
Muscle spasm			−	Muscle relaxants
Neuropathic				
Peripheral	Injury to peripheral nerve**	Neuroma; nerve infiltration, e.g. brachial or lumbar plexus	⎫ ⎬ − ⎭	Tricyclic antidepressants; Anticonvulsants; Local anaesthetic congeners
Central	Injury to CNS	Thalamic tumour; poststroke pain		(Corticosteroids‡) (Opioids§)
Sympathetic-mediated	Partial injury to sympathetic nerves†	Some postsurgical neural injury pains	−	

* Caused by stimulation of nervi nervorum in the nerve sheath. ** Characterized by superficial burning pain and/or stabbing pain with sensory loss in a dermatomal pattern. † Characterized by superficial burning pain in a *non-dermatomal* pattern. Often called reflex sympathetic dystrophy. Some neuropathic pains have a sympathetic component (e.g. Pancoast syndrome). ‡ May cause reversion of mixed nerve compression — neuropathic pain to more opioid responsive nerve compression pain. § In cancer, often mixed nerve compression — neuropathic pain, and therefore partly opioid responsive. Neuropathic pain associated with degenerative neurological disorders is sometimes responsive to opioids.

effective for only 2−3 h, though is commonly given every 4−6 h. On the other hand, levorphanol and phenazocine are satisfactory when given every 6 h; and buprenorphine and methadone every 8 h. Methadone has a plasma half-life of more than 2 days when taken regularly by mouth, and there is a likeli-

Table 79.7 Approximate oral analgesic potency ratios

Pethidine	1:8	Dextromoramide	(2)**
Dipipanone	1:2	Methadone	(3−4)†
Papaveretum	2:3	Levorphanol	5
Oxycodone	7:8	Phenazocine	5
Morphine	1*	Hydromorphone	6‡
Diamorphine	1.5	Buprenorphine	(60)§

* Oral morphine, 3 mg, or oral diamorphine, 2 mg, = injected diamorphine, 1 mg. ** Dextromoramide, a single 5 mg dose is equivalent to morphine, 15 mg, in terms of peak effect but is generally shorter acting. The overall potency ratio has been adjusted accordingly. † A single dose of methadone, 5 mg, is equivalent to morphine, 7.5 mg. It has a prolonged plasma half-life which leads to accumulation when given repeatedly. This means that it is several times more potent when given regularly. ‡ Not available in the UK. § Buprenorphine must be taken sublingually.

hood of cumulation leading to worsening adverse effects, particularly in elderly and debilitated patients.

'By the ladder'

The three standard analgesics are aspirin, codeine and morphine (Fig. 79.6). Other analgesics should be considered as alternatives of fashion or convenience. Appreciating this helps to prevent switching from one analgesic to another in a desperate search for some drug that may suit the patient better. If a non-opioid−weak opioid preparation, such as aspirin−codeine or paracetamol−dextropropoxyphene, fails to relieve the pain, it is usually best to move directly to a small dose of oral morphine sulphate than, for example, to prescribe dihydrocodeine.

It is necessary to be familiar with one or two alternatives for patients who cannot tolerate the standard preparations. Aspirin has two alternatives — paracetamol which has no anti-inflammatory effect, and the non-steroidal anti-inflammatory drugs (NSAIDs). For Step 2, the author uses dextropropoxyphene in preference to codeine. It is less consti-

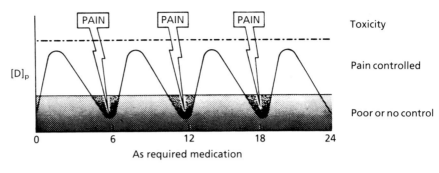

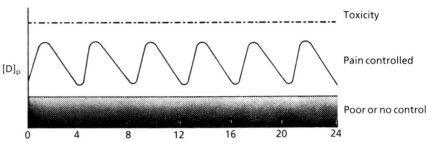

Fig. 79.5 Diagram to illustrate the results of 'as required' compared with regular 4-hourly morphine sulphate. $[D]_p$ = plasma concentration of drug. (Redrawn from Twycross & Lack, 1983.)

pating and, in the UK, the compound tablet with paracetamol (co-proxamol) has a considerably greater 'codeine-equivalent' content than other weak opioid compound tablets.

Oral codeine is about 1:12 as potent as oral morphine and dihydrocodeine about 1:10. Although dextropropoxyphene is less potent than codeine in single doses (Beaver, 1984), it has a prolonged plasma half-life and may, in practice, be regarded as equipotent with codeine when given regularly.

The use of morphine is determined by analgesic need and not, for example, by the doctor's estimate of life expectancy — which is often wrong. The correct dose of morphine is that which gives adequate relief for 4 h without unacceptable side-effects. 'Maximum'

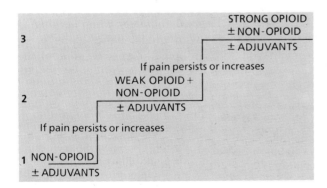

Fig. 79.6 The analgesic ladder for cancer pain management. (Redrawn from the World Health Organization, 1986.)

or 'recommended' doses, derived mainly from post-operative parenteral single-dose studies, are not applicable for cancer pain.

The following points should be noted:
1 It is pharmacological nonsense to prescribe simultaneously two weak opioids or two strong opioids.
2 It is sometimes justifiable for a patient on a strong opioid to be given another weak or strong opioid as a second 'as needed' analgesic for occasional, troublesome pain. Generally though, if pain breaks through the 'analgesic cover', patients should be advised to take an extra dose of their regular medication.
3 Avoid short-acting preparations such as pentazocine (weak opioid), pethidine (intermediate) and dextromoramide (strong opioid).
4 Do not prescribe a mixed agonist—antagonist (e.g. pentazocine) with a strong opioid agonist (i.e. morphine). It is unnecessary and may result in unintended antagonism.

'For the individual'

Morphine may be given either as an aqueous solution of morphine sulphate, as ordinary tablets or as slow-release tablets. The latter are available as 10, 30, 60, 100 and 200 mg strengths. Most patients changing from a weak opioid commence on 60 mg a day, i.e. aqueous morphine sulphate, 10 mg every 4 h, or slow-release morphine, 30 mg every 12 h. As the effective dose of oral morphine ranges from as little as 5 mg to more than 1g every 4h (Fig. 79.7), the top of the ladder is not reached simply by prescribing morphine.

However, most patients never require more than 100 mg every 4h; the majority continue to be well controlled on doses as small as 10–30 mg (or slow-release morphine, 30–100 mg, twice a day).

Adjuvant medication

Laxatives are always necessary when a patient is prescribed morphine, unless there is a definite reason for not doing so, e.g. steatorrhoea or an ileostomy (Twycross & Harcourt, 1991). Experience at many centres strongly suggests that a combination of a contact laxative (peristaltic stimulant) and a surface-wetting agent (faecal softener) achieves the best results, e.g. standardized senna (up to 75 mg a day) and docusate (up to 600 mg a day). Combination preparations reduce the number of tablets/capsules the patient has to swallow [e.g. co-danthrusate (UK) and casanthranol-docusate (USA)]. More than 33% of inpatients with terminal cancer continue to need rectal measures (suppositories, enemas or manual evacuations) in addition to oral laxatives (Twycross & Lack, 1986).

About 60% of patients prescribed morphine need an antiemetic. Haloperidol, 1–1.5 mg stat. and at bed-time, is the antiemetic of choice if nausea or vomiting is opioid-induced. In some patients haloperidol is ineffectual because of morphine-induced delayed gastric emptying. Thus, if a patient does not respond to haloperidol and the pattern of vomiting is suggestive of gastric stasis, a prokinetic antiemetic (meto-clopramide or domperidone) should be substituted.

If the patient is very anxious, an anxiolytic should be prescribed (e.g. diazepam 5–10 mg at bedtime). If a patient remains depressed after 1–2 weeks of much improved pain relief, an antidepressant should be considered. Many patients benefit from the use of a night sedative (e.g. temazepam, chloral hydrate).

At some centres, morphine is always prescribed for cancer pain with a second drug, either cocaine (a stimulant) or a phenothiazine (an anxiolytic–sedative). Sometimes both are given — which is pharmacological nonsense. Increasing the dose of morphine may be hazardous in these circumstances if, by increasing the volume of the mixture taken, the dose of the adjunctive drug is increased automatically. Depending on the adjunctive drug, this could lead either to agitation or to somnolence. It is better to give adjunctive drugs separately; then the dose of each drug can be adjusted individually according to need.

Discomfort is worse at night when the patient is alone with his/her pain and fears. The cumulative effect of many sleepless, pain-filled nights is a sub-stantial lowering of the patient's pain threshold with a concomitant increase in pain intensity. Sometimes, it is necessary to use morphine at night in patients well controlled by a weak opioid during the day; or to use a considerably larger dose of morphine at bedtime to relieve pains which are particularly troublesome when lying down for a prolonged period.

Opioid semiresponsive pains

Bone pain

Pain caused by bone metastases is often only opioid semiresponsive. Some soft-tissue pains are also in this category. Best results are obtained with a combi-nation of a NSAID and morphine. Many osseous metastases produce a prostaglandin (PG) which causes osteolysis (Galasko, 1981). The PG also lowers the 'peripheral pain threshold' by sensitizing the nerve endings (Ferreira, 1972). NSAIDs inhibit the synthesis of PGs and thereby alleviate pain.

Response to PG inhibitors is variable. Even so, an NSAID should be used routinely when seeking to relieve bone pain with drugs, either alone or in combination with an opioid. Generally, one of the

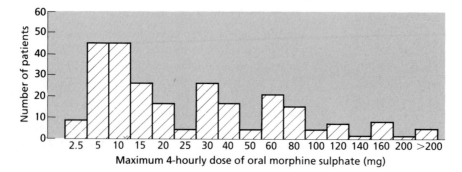

Fig. 79.7 Maximum doses of oral morphine sulphate given every 4 h to 254 cancer patients at Sir Michael Sobell House, Oxford, 1982. Median dose 15 mg; maximum dose 1800 mg. 67% = 30 mg; 91 ≤ 100 mg; 2 ≥ 200 mg.

newer twice-daily NSAIDs should be prescribed (e.g. flurbiprofen, naproxen or diflunisal).

Nerve compression pain

Pain caused by nerve compression is often not controlled with morphine alone. In this situation a corticosteroid should be prescribed, e.g. dexamethasone, 4–8 mg daily. Commonly, marked improvement occurs within 48 h. If the nerve compression relates to an identifiable bone metastasis or soft-tissue mass, radiotherapy should be considered. It is normally possible to reduce the dose of morphine and dexamethasone after radiotherapy.

For patients who do not respond adequately to the combined use of morphine and dexamethasone, a neurolytic or neuroablative procedure should be considered. The need for these, however, has decreased dramatically in countries where oral morphine has been made available. At the Palliative Care Service, National Cancer Institute, Milan, fewer than 10% of pain patients now need such procedures (Ventafridda, 1989). In a series of 158 patients admitted to a palliative care unit in Britain, neurolysis (coeliac-axis plexus block) was used on only one occasion (Walker *et al.*, 1988).

Other corticosteroid-responsive pains

A corticosteroid drug should be considered as a 'coanalgesic' whenever there is a large tumour mass within a relatively confined space, i.e. headache associated with raised intracranial pressure, spinal cord compression, head and neck tumours (sometimes), and intrapelvic tumours (sometimes). A tumour is often surrounded by inflamed oedematous tissue, and pressure on neighbouring veins and lymphatics may lead to further local or regional swelling. Corticosteroids reduce the inflammation and thereby reduce the total tumour mass (Fig. 79.8).

Corticosteroids reduce the production of PGs by inhibiting phospholipase activity, thereby preventing the formation of arachidonic acid from cell-membrane phospholipids. Arachidonic acid is the stem precursor substance of PGs. There is, therefore, a theoretical case for using both corticosteroids and NSAIDs in the management of certain pains, e.g. bone metastasis. However, more tablets may lead to reduced compliance and more adverse effects. Sometimes, however, maximal relief is obtained, only by using an opioid, NSAID and a corticosteroid concurrently, e.g. intrapelvic malignancy invading muscle and bone, and compressing nerves.

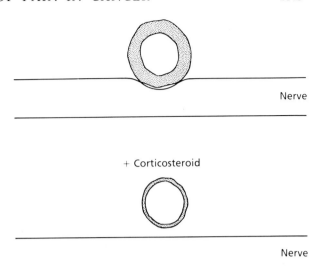

Fig. 79.8 Presumed mechanism of action of corticosteroids in relief of nerve compression pain. Total tumour mass = neoplasm + surrounding hyperaemic oedematous tissue. General anti-inflammatory effect of corticosteroid reduces total tumour mass, resulting in reduction of pain. (Redrawn from Twycross & Lack, 1983.)

Opioid-resistant pains

Muscle pain

Muscle cramp is a universal experience. The pain is extremely intense for a short time. It is coped with partly by saying, 'it is only cramp'. Unless recognized for what it is, however, cramp in cancer patients conveys a different message, namely, 'My God, it's the cancer'. Such a response inevitably magnifies the pain and perpetuates it. Cramp is usually secondary to underlying bone pain and/or skeletal deformity. Myofascial trigger point-(TP) related pains also occur. Treatment comprises explanation, physical therapies (local heat and massage), diazepam and relaxation therapy. In addition, for TP-associated cramp, injection of the TP with local anaesthetic (e.g. 0.5% bupivacaine) should be considered. *Morphine is not indicated for muscle spasm and TP-related pains, however severe.*

Neuropathic pain

The following represents a practical synopsis. For an extensive discussion the reader is referred to other sources (McQuay, 1988; Wall & Melzack, 1989; Bonica, 1990). As always treatment begins with explanation: 'Nerve damage pain does not respond to ordinary pain killers such as aspirin, codeine and morphine.'

'Need to phase out unhelpful medication and start some new tablets, to be taken at bedtime.'

A tricyclic antidepressant is recommended for superficial burning pain; and an anticonvulsant for stabbing pain in the absence of burning pain. With mixed burning—stabbing pains, start with tricyclic and *add* an anticonvulsant after 1—2 weeks if the stabbing pain is still troublesome.

Many of the controlled studies relate to the use of amitriptyline and carbamazepine. However, dothiepin or desipramine and sodium valproate are probably equally effective and tend to cause less adverse effects (Bowsher, 1990; Kishore-Kumar *et al.*, 1990). As with the tricyclic drugs, sodium valproate may be given in a single bedtime dose aiding compliance and capitalizing on its sedative effect.

The dose of tricyclic drug depends on the age and size of the patient. For an average-sized patient of up to 70 years, the following regimen is appropriate:

Nights 1 and 2:   dothiepin, 50 mg.
Night 3 onwards: dothiepin, 75 mg.

In older patients, it may be better to start with 25 mg and to take 10 days to reach 75 mg. In the very frail, 50 mg may be the maximum tolerable dose. Subsequent dose alterations depend on response. A few patients need 100—150 mg. Adverse effects limit dose escalation in poor responders.

One centre recommends distigmine, 5 mg once or twice a day, in addition to a tricyclic drug, claiming greater benefit (Hampf *et al.*, 1989). Distigmine is an anticholinesterase and its use has the added benefit of counteracting the mouth-drying action of the tricyclic drug.

Sodium valproate is given in a dose of 200—500/600 mg at bedtime, after a similar incremental pattern. Many centres still use carbamazepine. If used, the dose must be built up slowly from an initial dose of 200 mg twice a day at the rate of 200 mg/week. It should be given several times a day, which is a potential disadvantage. When given with a tricyclic drug, the metabolism of both drugs is slowed, which implies that smaller doses of both are needed.

Several centres now use oral local anaesthetic congeners (e.g., mexilitine and flecainide). These are marketed as antiarrhythmic drugs, but often relieve neuropathic pain (Dejgard *et al.*, 1988; Dunlop *et al.*, 1988). Flecainide and mexilitine, in common with tricyclic drugs, possess Class 1 antiarrhythmic properties. In some circumstances they may become proarrhythmic. Concomitant use with a tricyclic drug may increase this risk and should normally be avoided.

Relief from neuropathic pain may be achieved in 1—2 weeks, though occasionally it takes much longer. The patient and family should be warned about the probable time scale. The first aim is improved sleep, with consequential correction of fatigue and mental exhaustion. In some patients, the worst pain intensity may initially remain unchanged but the periods of less-intense pain lengthen. Recognizing this boosts morale, which thereby has a positive impact on pain intensity.

Opioid-responsive pains — but do *not* use opioids

There is a fourth category of pains, namely, those that may respond to opioids but which should be treated more specifically. Indeed, 'blind' treatment with opioids may make matters ultimately worse, despite initial relief.

Functional bowel pains

Irritable bowel syndrome occurs in about 10% of cancer patients (as in the general population) and calls for appropriate measures (Read, 1985). Colic associated with constipation should be treated by treating the constipation, and also rectal spasm caused by faecal impaction. A third pain syndrome associated with constipation is that of right iliac fossa pain. In this, the descending colon (and sometimes the transverse colon) is easily palpable as it is full of hard faecal lumps. The caecum feels distended and is tender on palation. The pain is that of gaseous caecal distension secondary to constipation. Identical caecal symptoms and signs are also seen in obstruction of the colon. Careful history taking and assessment normally indicates which is the more likely of the two diagnoses. Sometimes, because of the intensity of the discomfort, a weak opioid preparation (e.g. co-proxamol) may be necessary for several days while the constipation is being corrected.

Intestinal colic associated with obstruction responds to opioids. Sometimes, however, an antispasmodic is preferable. Mild recurrent colic often responds to agents such as mebeverine, propantheline, or hyoscine butylbromide (Buscopan). Unpredictable, occasional severe colic may be treated with sublingual hyoscine hydrobromide (Quick Kwells), 0.3 mg, as required. This acts within minutes of administration.

Squashed stomach syndrome

This is frequently seen in advanced cancer and warrants special mention. In this syndrome, epigastric pain is caused by relative gastric distension. This often occurs in patients with a grossly enlarged liver, whether or not there is any associated gastric abnormality. It is important to recognize the postprandial discomfort for what it is, because explanation to the patient is crucial in management. Some patients, particularly those with an oesophageal tube, also experience retrosternal pain as a result of acid-induced oesophagitis. The aim of treatment is to prevent distension. This requires a combination of dietary and pharmacological measures (Table 79.8).

Fears about opioid use

Respiratory depression

It is often stated that morphine is a dangerous drug because of the risk of respiratory depression. In pain patients this is not so, however, because pain is the physiological antagonist to the central depressant effects of opioids. In contrast with postoperative opioid use, the cancer patient in pain:

1 Has usually been receiving a weak opioid for some time (i.e. is not opioid naive).
2 Takes medication by mouth (slower absorption and lower peak concentration).
3 Titrates the dose upwards step by step (less likelihood of an excessive dose being given).

Moreover, the fact that a double dose of morphine at bedtime causes no excess night mortality indicates that there is a reasonable safety margin (Regnard & Badger, 1987).

On the other hand, if the patient's pain is treated successfully by neurolytic or neuroablative techniques, life-threatening respiratory depression may

occur if the dose of morphine is not reduced equally dramatically (Hanks et al., 1981). A reduction to 25% is recommended. If the nerve block is successful, it is possible to discontinue the morphine completely over the next week or so. However, if only partly successful, it may be necessary to increase the dose again to 50–60% of the original dose, or even more.

In short, morphine is a safe drug provided the patient is not dying from exhaustion as a result of weeks or months of intolerable pain associated with insomnia and poor nutrition. In this circumstance, almost anything which eases the patient's mental or physical distress is likely to 'tip the scales' further in the direction of death. On the other hand, circumstantial evidence suggests that the correct use of morphine prolongs the life of a cancer pain patient as he/she is free of pain, better able to rest, sleep and eat, and is generally more active.

Tolerance

In the past, predictions about dose 'escalation' were made on the basis of animal and volunteer studies. These subjects, however, were not in pain and the emphasis was on inducing tolerance and physical dependence as rapidly as possible by using maximum-tolerated doses. Although such studies may be useful in predicting abuse liability, they are irrelevant to clinical practice. Several studies have reviewed the long-term opioid requirements of cancer pain patients (Twycross, 1974; Twycross & Wald, 1976; Twycross & Lack, 1983). They demonstrate that the longer the duration of treatment:

1 The slower the rate of increase in dose.
2 The longer the periods without a dose increase.
3 The greater the likelihood of a dose reduction.
4 The greater the likelihood of stopping medication altogether.

Thus, when used within the context of comprehensive biopsychosocial care, morphine may be used for long periods in cancer patients without concern about tolerance. Moreover, although physical dependence may develop after several weeks of continuous treatment, this does not prevent a downward adjustment of dose should the pain be relieved by non-drug measures (e.g. radiation therapy or neurolytic block).

With the exception of constipation and miosis, tolerance to the unwanted side-effects of morphine appears to develop more readily than tolerance to analgesia. Should tolerance develop, however, an upward adjustment of dose is all that is necessary to regain pain control. It must be emphasized that the main reason for increasing the dose is not tolerance

Table 79.8 Squashed stomach syndrome

Symptoms	Treatment
Early satiation	Explanation
Epigastric fullness	Dietary advice ('small and often')
Epigastric discomfort/pain Flatulence Hiccup Heartburn	Antiflatulent (e.g. Asilone, 10 ml, after meals and bedtime)
Nausea Vomiting	Metoclopramide (after meals and bedtime or every 4 h if also receiving morphine)

but progression of the disease (Twycross, 1974; Kanner & Foley, 1981).

Psychological dependence ('addiction')

The fear of causing psychological dependence is still a potent cause of underprescription and underuse of strong opioid analgesics (Hill, 1987). Published data indicate that this fear is unfounded and unnecessary. The incidence of opioid dependence in some 40 000 hospitalized medical patients was examined in a retrospective study (Porter & Jick, 1980). Among nearly 12 000 patients who received at least one strong opioid preparation, there were only four reasonably well-documented cases of dependence in patients who had no history of drug abuse. The dependence was considered major in only one instance.

The diversion of strong opioids for illicit use by non-patients is a parallel concern, particularly of governments and law-enforcement agencies. Experience in Sweden helps to allay this fear. The medicinal use of morphine and methadone in Sweden increased 17 times between 1975 and 1982 (Agenas et al., 1982). While the increased use presumably led to better cancer pain control, there was no associated increase in illicit drug use or diversion of strong opioids to established addicts.

Drowsiness

In most patients this is an initial side-effect which lasts only 3–7 days on a steady dose. Elderly patients and their families, in particular, need to be warned about this as it may be associated with an element of confusion and/or unsteadiness. If severe, it may be an indication that the dose of morphine is excessive and a trial reduction should be made. Alternatively, it may suggest changing from a night sedative such as nitrazepam (with a prolonged half-life) to temazepam; or discontinuing a concurrently prescribed phenothiazine (particularly chlorpromazine) and using haloperidol if a neuroleptic or an antiemetic is needed.

After the first few days, some less physically active patients continue to experience drowsiness when sitting or reclining in chair or bed. This inactivity drowsiness is usually not a problem. It helps pass what might otherwise be a long day and conserves limited energy for when other family members are home or friends visit.

Alternative routes of administration of opioids

Injection

In the UK, when injections are necessary, subcutaneous diamorphine is often used instead of morphine. Diamorphine hydrochloride is highly soluble (1 g in 1.6 ml), which implies that large amounts dissolve in 1 ml or less. It is, however, no more efficacious than morphine sulphate, merely more soluble (Twycross, 1977). Some patients with inoperable bowel obstruction need parenteral medication for several weeks. The use of a battery-driven portable syringe driver facilitates administration via a continuous subcutaneous infusion, using a combination of diamorphine and an antiemetic (Oliver, 1985; Jones & Hanks, 1986).

Suppository

Morphine sulphate suppositories provide another alternative mode of administration. Fifteen mg and 30 mg suppositories are commercially available in the UK, and a pharmaceutical company makes suppositories of other strengths on receipt of a special order from a local pharmacy or hospital. The same dose is given *per rectum* as *per os*.

Oxycodone pectinate suppositories (30 mg) are made by Boots. These may be given only every 8 h. Oxycodone and morphine are approximately equipotent (i.e. oxycodone pectinate, 30 mg every 8 h, is about equivalent to aqueous morphine sulphate, 15 mg every 4 h).

Spinal morphine

Extradural and intrathecal morphine is used in selected patients (Ventafridda et al., 1986). It is indicated in patients with localized regional pain who cannot tolerate morphine systemically, because of excessive sedation and/or dysphoria (Ottesen et al., 1990).

Alternatives to morphine

The regular use of morphine sulphate solutions or tablets (every 4 h) or slow-release tablets (e.g. MST-Continus every 12 h) is regarded by the author as the treatment of choice for cancer patients in pain who require a strong opioid. Other strong opioids are available but none has any clear advantage compared with morphine. It is necessary to have an alternative for the small minority of patients who cannot tolerate morphine because of a functional gastric outflow obstruction that is not responsive to a prokinetic agent (i.e. metoclopramide or domperidone).

Phenazocine

The author uses phenazocine in morphine intolerant patients. Each 5-mg tablet is equivalent to 20–25 mg of morphine sulphate by mouth. Thus 'one tablet every 4 h' may be excessive. The tablets can, however, be halved and need not be taken more than four times a day. This implies that 2.5 mg four times a day is about equivalent to 10 mg of morphine sulphate every 4 h. In some centres, phenazocine is being used successfully every 8 h (Baines, personal communication). Although not manufactured specifically for sublingual use, the tablets dissolve readily in the mouth. Phenazocine appears to be equipotent whether swallowed or taken sublingually. Phenazocine is useful also in the patient who has deeply rooted irrational fears about morphine, and who firmly declines to take it.

Buprenorphine

Sublingual buprenorphine is widely used. It is a partial μ-agonist and should be considered as an alternative to morphine (Table 79.9). As with morphine, a proportion of patients experience troublesome nausea and vomiting, and virtually all become constipated with regular use.

Supervision

All cancer patients receiving analgesics need close supervision to achieve maximum relief with minimum adverse effects. Treatment review is sometimes necessary within hours; certainly after 1–2 days; and always at the end of the first week. Subsequent follow-up varies according to psychological and therapeutic needs. New pains may develop and old pains re-emerge. A fresh complaint of pain demands reassessment; not just a message to increase pain medication, though this may be an important short-term measure.

Expectations

Of 205 patients treated according to the World Health Organization method for relief of cancer pain, 86% had complete relief, 11% had 'acceptable relief', and 3% had partial relief (Takeda, 1989). However,

Table 79.9 Guide to the use of sublingual buprenorphine

A semisynthetic thebaine derivative with potent partial μ-agonist properties

An alternative to oral morphine in the low-medium part of morphine's dose range

In low doses, buprenorphine and morphine are additive in their effects; at high doses, antagonism by buprenorphine may occur

Buprenorphine is available as a sublingual tablet; ingestion reduces bioavailability

Needs to be given only every 8 h; to give more often is to make life unnecessarily harder for a hard-pressed patient

With daily doses of over 3 mg, patients may prefer to take fewer tablets more often, i.e. every 6 h

Analgesic ceiling at a daily dose of 3–5 mg. This is equivalent to 180–300 mg of morphine

Buprenorphine is *not* an alternative to codeine or dextropropoxyphene. Like morphine, it should be used when a weak opioid has failed

Assuming previous regular use of codeine or dextropropoxyphene, patients should commence on 0.2 mg ever 8 h with the advice that: 'If it is not more effective than your previous tablets take a further 0.2 mg after 1 h, and 0.4 mg every 8 h after that'

When changing to morphine, multiply total daily dose by 60. If pain previously poorly controlled, multiply by 100

Adverse effects need to be monitored as with morphine: nausea, vomiting, constipation, drowsiness

There is never need to prescribe both buprenorphine and morphine. Use one or the other; then unintended antagonism cannot occur

whereas relief is obtained within 2 or 3 days in some patients, in others it may take 2–3 weeks of inpatient treatment to achieve satisfactory control, particularly with those whose pain is made worse by movement and in the very anxious and depressed. Even so, it should be possible to achieve some improvement within 24–48 h in all patients. Although the ultimate aim is complete freedom from pain, there is less disappointment but, paradoxically, more success if in practice the aim is 'graded relief'. Furthermore, as some pains respond more readily than others, improvement must be assessed in relation to each pain.

The initial target should be a night free of pain with adequate sleep. Many patients have not had a good night's sleep for weeks or months and are exhausted and demoralized. To sleep through the night pain-free and wake refreshed is a boost to both the doctor's and the patient's morale. Next, one aims for relief at rest in bed or chair during the day; finally, for freedom from pain on movement. The former is always eventually possible; the latter is not. However, the encouragement that relief at night and when resting during the day brings, gives the patient new hope and incentive and enables him/her to begin to live again despite a variable amount of activity-precipitated discomfort.

Conclusion

In the majority of cancer patients it is not difficult to achieve good or even complete relief. It does, however, require a doctor who:

1 Appreciates that pain is a somatopsychic experience.

2 Carefully evaluates the cause(s) of pain.

3 Adopts a multimodality approach, combining non-drug with drug measures.

4 Differentiates between 'opioid-responsive' and 'opioid-resistant' pains.

5 Uses the correct drug in the correct dose at the correct time intervals.

6 Recognizes that the effective dose of a strong opioid varies widely.

7 Closely monitors patients receiving opioids, and carefully controls adverse drug effects, particularly constipation.

8 Works closely with, and listens to, the nurses and other care-givers.

References

Agenas I., Gustafsson L.L., Rane A., Sawe J. & Sjoberg C. (1982) Analgetikaterapi for cancerpatienter. *Lakartidningen* **79**, 287−9.

Arner S. & Meyerson B.A. (1988) Lack of analgesic effect of opioids on neuropathic and idiopathic forms of pain. *Pain* **33**, 11−23.

Beaver W.T. (1984) Analgesic efficacy of dextropropoxyphene and dextropropoxyphene-containing combinations: a review. *Human Toxicology* **3**, 191S−220S.

Bonica J.J. (1985) Treatment of cancer pain: current status and future needs. In *Advances in Pain Research and Therapy*, vol. 9. (Eds Fields H.L., Dubner R. & Cervero F.) pp. 589−616. Raven Press, New York.

Bonica J.J. (1990) *The Management of Pain* 2nd edn. Lea & Febiger, Philadelphia.

Bowsher D. (1990) How physiology of neurogenic pain dictates management. *Geriatric Medicine* Sept, 33−40.

Churcher M.D. (1990) Cancer and sympathetic dependent pain. *Palliative Medicine* **4**, 113−16.

Churcher M.D. & Ingall J.R.F. (1987) Sympathetic dependent

pain. *The Pain Clinic* **1**, 217−18.

Dejgard A., Petersen P. & Kastrup J. (1988) Mexiletine for treatment of chronic painful diabetic neuropathy. *Lancet* **1**, 9−11.

Devor M. & Raber P. (1990) Heritability of symptoms in an experimental model of neuropathic pain. *Pain* **42**, 51−67.

Dunlop R., Davies R.J., Hockley J. & Turner P. (1988) Analgesic effect of oral flecainide. *Lancet* **1**, 420−1.

Ferreira S.H. (1972) Prostaglandins, aspirin-like drugs and analgesics. *Nature New Biology* **240**, 200−3.

Foley K.M. (1979) Pain syndromes in patients with cancer. In *Advances in Pain Research and Therapy*, vol 2 (Eds Bonica J.J. & Ventrafridda V.) pp. 59−75. Raven Press, New York.

Foley K.M. (1985) The treatment of cancer pain. *New England Journal of Medicine* **313**, 84−95.

Galasko C.S.B. (1981) The development of skeletal metastases. In *Bone Metastasis* (Eds Weiss L. & Gilbert H.A.) pp. 83−113. G.K. Hall, Boston, Mass.

Glynn C. (1989) An approach to the management of the patient with deafferentation pain. *Palliative Medicine* **3**, 13−21.

Hampf G., Bowsher D. & Nurmikko T. (1989) Distigmine and amitriptyline in the treatment of chronic pain. *Anesthesia Progress* **36**, 58−62.

Hanks G.W., Twycross R.G. & Lloyd J.W. (1981) Unexpected complication of successful nerve block. *Anaesthesia* **36**, 37−9.

Hanks G.W., Hoskin P.J., Aherne G.W. & Turner P. (1987) Explanation for potency of repeated oral doses of morphine? *Lancet* **2**, 723−4.

Hill S.C. (1987) Painful prescriptions. *Journal of the American Medical Association* **257**, 2081.

Jones V.A. & Hanks G.W. (1986) New portable infusion pump for prolonged subcutaneous administration of opioid analgesics in patients with advanced cancer. *British Medical Journal* **292**, 1496.

Kaiko R.F., Healy N., Pav J., Thomas G.B. & Goldenheim P.D. (1989) The comparative bioavailability of MS Contin tablets (controlled release oral morphine) following rectal and oral administration. In *The Edinburgh Symposium on Pain Control and Medical Education* (Ed. Twycross R.G.) pp. 235−41. Royal Society of Medicine, London.

Kanner R.M. & Foley K.M. (1981) Patterns of narcotic drug use in cancer pain clinic. *Annals of New York Academy of Sciences* **362**, 162−72.

Kastrup J., Angelo H.R., Petersen P., Dejgard A. & Hilsted J. (1986) Treatment of chronic painful diabetic neuropathy with intravenous lidocaine infusion. *British Medical Journal* **292**, 173.

Kishore-Kumar R., Max M.B., Schafer S.C., Gaughan A.M., Smoller B., Gracely R.H. & Dubner R. (1990) Desipramine relieves postherpetic neuralgia. *Clinical Pharmacology and Therapeutics* **47**, 305−12.

McQuay H.J. (1988) Pharmacological treatment of neuralgic and neuropathic pain. In *Cancer Surveys*, vol. 7 (Ed. Hanks G.W.) pp. 141−59. Oxford University Press, Oxford.

Mount B.M. (1984) Psychological and social aspects of cancer pain. In *Textbook of Pain* (Eds Wall P.D. & Melzack R.) pp. 460−71. Churchill Livingstone, Edinburgh.

Oliver D.J. (1985) The use of the syringe driver in terminal care. *British Journal of Clinical Pharmacology* **20**, 515−16.

Ottesen S., Minton M. & Twycross R.G. (1990) The use of

epidural morphine at a palliative care centre. *Palliative Medicine* **4**, 117−22.

Pannuti F., Rossi A.P., Iafelice G., Marraro D., Camera P., Cricca A., Strocchi E., Burroni P., Lapucci L. & Fruet F. (1982) Control of chronic pain in very advanced cancer patients with morphine hydrochloride administered by oral, rectal and sublingual route. Clinical report and preliminary results on morphine pharmacokinetics. *Pharmacological Research Communications* **14**, 369−80.

Portenoy R.K. (1989) Cancer pain: epidemiology and syndromes. *Cancer* **63**, 2298−307.

Portenoy R.K., Foley K.M. & Inturrisi C.E. (1990) The nature of opioid responsiveness and its implications for neuropathic pain: new hypotheses derived from studies of opioid infusions. *Pain* **43**, 273−86.

Porter J. & Jick H. (1980) Addiction rate in patients treated with narcotics. *New England Journal of Medicine* **302**, 123.

Rappaz O., Tripiana J., Rapin Ch-H., Stjernsward J. & Junod J.-P. (1985) Soins palliatifs et traitement de la douleur cancereuse en geriatrie. *Revue Therapeutique/Therapeutische Umschau* **42**, 843−8.

Read N.W. (1985) *Irritable Bowel Syndrome*. Grune and Stratton, London.

Regnard C.F.B. & Badger C. (1987) Opioids, sleep and the time of death. *Palliative Medicine* **1**, 107−10.

Saunders C. & Baines M. (1983) *Living with dying. The Management of Terminal Disease*. Oxford University Press, Oxford.

Takeda F. (1989) The management of cancer pain in Japan. In *The Edinburgh Symposium on Pain Control and Medical Education* (Ed. Twycross R.G.) pp. 17−21. Royal Society of Medicine, London.

Tasker R. (1987) The problem of deafferentation pain in the management of the patient with cancer. *Journal of Palliative Care* **2** (2), 8−12.

Tasker R.R. & Dostrovsky J.O. (1989) Deafferentation and central pain. In *Textbook of Pain* 2nd edn (Eds Wall P.D. & Melzack R.) pp. 154−80. Churchill Livingstone, Edinburgh.

Twycross R.G. (1974) Clinical experience with diamorphine in advanced malignant disease. *International Journal of Clinical Pharmacology, Therapy and Toxicology* **9**, 184−98.

Twycross R.G. (1977) Choice of strong analgesic in terminal cancer: diamorphine or morphine? *Pain* **3**, 93−104.

Twycross R.G. & Fairfield S. (1982) Pain in far-advanced cancer. *Pain* **14**, 303−10.

Twycross R.G. & Harcourt J.M.V. (1991) Use of laxatives at a palliative care centre. *Palliative Medicine* **5**, 27−33.

Twycross R.G. & Lack S.A. (1983) *Symptom Control in Far-advanced Cancer: Pain Relief*. Pitman, London.

Twycross R.G. & Lack S.A. (1986) *Control of Alimentary Symptoms in Far-advanced Cancer*. Churchill Livingstone, Edinburgh.

Twycross R.G. & Lack S.A. (1990) *Therapeutics in Terminal Cancer* 2 edn. Churchill Livingstone, Edinburgh.

Twycross R.G. & Wald S.J. (1976) Longterm use of diamorphine in advanced cancer. In *Advances in Pain Research and Therapy*, vol. 1 (Eds Bonica J.J. & Albe-Fessard D.G.) pp. 653−61. Raven Press, New York.

Ventafridda V. (1989) Continuing care: a major issue in cancer pain management. *Pain* **36**, 137−43.

Ventrafridda V., De Conno F., Tamburini M. & Pappalettera M. (1986) Clinical evaluation of chronic infusion of intrathecal morphine in cancer pain. In *Advances in Pain Research and Therapy*, vol. 8 (Eds Foley K.M. & Inturrisi C.E.) pp. 391−405. Raven Press, New York.

Ventafridda V., Tamburini M., Caraceni A., De Conno F. & Naldi F. (1987) A validation study of the W.H.O. method for cancer pain relief. *Cancer* **59**, 851−6.

Walker V.A., Hoskin P.J., Hanks G.W. & White I.D. (1988) Evaluation of WHO analgesic guidelines for cancer pain in a hospital-based palliative care unit. *Journal of Pain and Symptom Management* **3**, 145−9.

Wall P.D. (1989) Introduction. In *Textbook of Pain* 2nd edn (Eds Wall P.D. & Melzack R.) pp. 1−18. Churchill Livingstone, Edinburgh.

Wall P.D. & Melzack R. (eds) (1989) *Textbook of Pain* 2nd edn. Churchill Livingstone, Edinburgh.

World Health Organization (1986) *Cancer Pain Relief*. World Health Organization, Geneva.

Zimmerman M. (1983) Deafferentation pain. In *Advances in Pain Research and Therapy*, vol. 5 (Eds Bonica J.J., Lindblom U. & Iggo A.) pp. 661−2. Raven Press, New York.

Acupuncture, TENS, Hypnosis and Behavioural Therapy

J.E. CHARLTON

Drug therapy is the chief method of pain relief for both acute and chronic pain. Problems with drugs in the form of side-effects or lack of appropriate response have led to some disenchantment and a search for other methods of pain relief. Destructive procedures such as neurolytic blocks or neurosurgery may provide an answer for some carefully selected patients but carry serious risks of morbidity and mortality and are inappropriate for acute pain relief.

There is a variety of relatively non-invasive methods of pain relief which provide alternatives to conventional therapy. Examples are acupuncture, transcutaneous electrical nerve stimulation (TENS), hypnosis, biofeedback and various psychologic and psychiatric techniques. All these techniques are important in the management of chronic pain and may have some application to acute pain relief.

Acupuncture

Throughout history humans have learned to fight pain with pain. As a rule, brief moderate pain tends to abolish severe prolonged pain. Procedures such as cupping, cauterization and the application of 'counter-irritants' are found in most cultures. The fact that they have survived thousands of years suggests that they must be more effective than placebo. None of these therapies has been subjected to clinical trial, but work done with acupuncture and TENS suggests that there is every reason to believe that they have survived because they are effective. They have the advantage that they do not necessarily need to be administered by a physician but can be carried out by less highly trained personnel or by the patient and family. In addition, they do little harm.

Classical acupuncture

Acupuncture has been practised in China for at least 2000 years, and is linked inextricably with classical ideas of health and disease. The ancient Chinese believed that the universe was permeated with a vital life-force or energy (called Ch'i) which circulated continuously through all living organisms. In humans, the energy was thought to follow specific pathways or meridians upon which the acupuncture points lie. Classically, there are 12 bilaterally symmetrical meridians and two non-paired midline control meridians, each representing internal organs as visualized by traditional Chinese medicine.

If the circulation of Ch'i along the meridians was altered by any disease process, either physical or emotional, an increase or deficit of Ch'i resulted. The resultant imbalance revealed itself eventually as pain or disease. This imbalance could be corrected by the insertion of acupuncture needles into specific points along the meridians near the surface of the body. The selection of the appropriate acupuncture points was made after studying the patient and by taking into account various philosophical and theoretical concepts. Many years of study are required to master all the subtleties of traditional acupuncture.

Modern acupuncture

The meridians are unrelated to any known nervous, circulatory or lymphatic system. However, many acupuncture points are close to branches of cutaneous nerves, nerves to muscles and main nerve trunks (Kaada, 1976). In addition, more than 60% of acupuncture points correspond to known trigger points and it has been suggested that they may represent the same phenomenon and may be explained in terms of the same underlying neural mechanisms (Melzack et al., 1976). This does not seem likely as trigger points have a physical existence whereas acupuncture points do not.

Acupuncture points have a functional electrical

existence in that they are sites of low skin resistance (and therefore high conductivity) and can be identified using a skin resistance meter. It has been suggested that the low skin resistance is caused by local changes in sympathetic tone (Nakatani & Yamashita, 1977). The most effective acupuncture points are located often where nerves enter muscle (Gunn, 1978). Acupuncture points are generally stimulated with fine 30-gauge, solid stainless-steel needles. There are no convincing data to show that variations in gauge or in the type of metal make any difference to the clinical effect. Methods of stimulating acupuncture points range from simple digital pressure, through the spectrum of high technology to lasers. None has been shown to be any better than electrical stimulation alone.

After the appropriate acupuncture point has been selected, the needle is inserted deep into the muscle. This is best achieved by holding the needle at the mid-point of the shaft between thumb and forefinger and using a quick twirling motion. The needle is then advanced into the muscle until the point is reached and the patient experiences the sensation of 'Teh Chi'. This is a feeling, variously described as tingling, soreness, numbness or heaviness, which is essential if acupuncture is to be successful. If it is not obtained, the needle should be reinserted, and it should be noted that this characteristic sensation is almost impossible to obtain at non-acupuncture points.

Electroacupuncture

Modern acupuncture practice utilizes electrical stimulation of the needle with a pulse generator. Most deliver pulsed direct current with a square wave and have the options of varying frequency, pulse width and voltage. Most modern practitioners prefer to use low-frequency stimulation (2–4 Hz) (Omura, 1975), and it is alleged that this produces much longer-acting pain relief than that provided by high-frequency stimulation, albeit at the cost of a slower onset time. The intensity of stimulus is usually of the order of 200 μA, but this may vary widely. Stimulation is applied for approximately 20 min and, when effective, treatment may have to be repeated on several occasions to produce an effect of prolonged duration.

Mechanisms of action

The gate-control theory of pain (Melzack & Wall, 1965) may explain some of the effects of acupuncture, but not others. It explains why stimulation in the same dermatome may be effective, but it does not explain why stimulation at distant sites may be equally as effective. However, it does offer a theoretical explanation why acupuncture is frequently unsuccessful in relieving pain characterized by large fibre destruction such as trigeminal or postherpetic neuralgia.

Acupuncture has been shown to release endorphins and other peptides and to be reversed by naloxone (Melzack, 1973), but this does not imply that this is the mechanism of action of acupuncture; it may only represent a small part.

In a study using mice, naloxone has been shown to block acupuncture analgesia, whilst sham electro-acupuncture produced no analgesia and naloxone infusion alone had little effect (Pomeranz & Chiu, 1976). The same authors have shown a similar effect in anaesthetized cats (Cheng & Pomeranz, 1979).

A double-blind study of experimental tooth pain showed that acupuncture analgesia could be produced by manual stimulation of needles in the hand, and that this could be reversed by intravenous naloxone (Mayer et al., 1977).

It has been shown in other studies that acupuncture does not induce significant analgesia in all human volunteers, and may cause temporary hyperalgesia in some individuals. Only 42% of subjects were able to increase their pain threshold by 20% or more above baseline after 20 min of acupuncture (Benedetti & Murphy, 1985). Practical experience would suggest that similar results are obtained in treatment of both acute and chronic pain, and it is this lack of a predictable, uniform and intense analgesia which leads to ambivalence by Western physicians and their patients with regard to its use.

Indications

Acupuncture is used in the treatment of acute and chronic pain of musculoskeletal and neurogenic origin. Neck and back problems, myofascial pain and acute strain/sprain injuries have been successfully treated with acupuncture. There have been reports also of the successful treatment of postoperative pain, although in general this has been disappointing. There are theoretical grounds for its use in cases where opioids are contraindicated or where conventional analgesia might diminish the level of consciousness.

Results

It is impossible to give accurate figures on the success

of acupuncture analgesia in either acute or chronic pain. Many claims have been exaggerated which leads to cynicism on the part of physicians who do not practise acupuncture therapy.

In order for acupuncture to be successful, several important points must be borne in mind. First, the patient must be motivated psychologically for the acupuncture therapy to be successful. This appears to be essential, as several studies have shown total failure of acupuncture analgesia for acute pain in unmotivated patients, and in chronic pain patients with an associated depression (Frost *et al.*, 1976; Hossenlopp *et al.*, 1976). Second, only a small percentage of patients respond to acupuncture treatment. Acupuncture may not produce anaesthesia or true analgesia but only a modest reduction in painful sensations. Third, the physician should have no false illusions or hopes on the efficacy of acupuncture and should communicate his/her doubts beforehand to the patient.

Acupuncture has large limitations, and it is unrealistic to expect good results in severe pain from acupuncture therapy except in a few individuals. The difficulties of assessing the results of acupuncture therapy have been summarized by one of its protagonists (Lewith, 1984). Many of the reports cited by Lewith are unconvincing and a more recent attempt has been made to improve the standards by which acupuncture is studied (Vincent & Richardson, 1986). The same authors have reviewed the clinical use of acupuncture where adequate controls are available (Richardson & Vincent, 1986). This has led to better designed clinical trials which have shown encouraging benefit in intermittent pain syndromes such as migraine (Vincent, 1989). Practical experience and further information is obtained best by attending a good practical course.

Complications

Acupuncture treatment has few complications provided adequate care is taken in sterilizing skin and equipment. The patient may have a syncopal attack and a haematoma may occur at the site of needle insertion. However, more serious complications have occurred including pneumothorax and damage to the spinal cord.

Physiotherapy

Physiotherapy plays a vital role in the management of both acute and chronic pain. The restoration of normal function is the most important goal of any pain management programme, and analgesic measures are usually directed at making it possible for the patient to begin the necessary activity. It can be argued that many of the techniques used in physical therapy will eliminate or reduce pain.

A comprehensive list of the various treatments available is beyond the scope of this chapter, but obvious examples include the use of heat and cold, massage, traction, manipulation and electrical stimulation. For a review of this topic the reader is referred to Lehmann and de Lateur (1985).

Heat and cold

Heat treatment can be given by superficial or deep heat. Most patients with chronic pain are aware of the effects of superficial heat, applied locally in the form of a hot water bottle, or generally in the form of a hot bath or shower. Deep heat can be applied by one of three methods: short-wave diathermy, microwave diathermy or ultrasound. The energy of short-wave diathermy is transferred into the deeper tissue layers by a high-frequency electromagnetic current (27.12 MHz), whereas microwave diathermy energy is propagated by means of electromagnetic radiation at a frequency of 2456 and 915 MHz. Under optimal conditions, short-wave diathermy causes an increase in tissue temperature to a depth of 3 cm, whereas microwave diathermy causes an increase to a depth of 5 cm (Griffin & Karselis, 1978). Ultrasound comprises the use of high-frequency acoustic vibration at 0.8—1.0 MHz. All three methods may produce valuable pain relief in both acute and chronic pain states, particularly in musculoskeletal pain.

Local heat can produce many different responses including changes in neuromuscular activity, blood flow, capillary permeability, enzymatic activity and pain. Distant heat causes less marked changes, but none the less alters muscular function, blood flow and local reflexes. The mode of action of the benefit has not yet been demonstrated clearly but would appear to include improved blood supply and suppression of sympathetic overactivity.

Cold therapy has been used for the relief of pain since ancient times. In recent years, it has become used increasingly in the form of ice packs, vapocoolant sprays and ice massage. It is most useful in acute musculoskeletal pain associated with sports injuries or trauma. Pain can be alleviated frequently and to some extent prevented by early application of cold in the form of an ice pack. Not only may this help pain, but it also reduces bleeding and oedema by causing vasoconstriction.

Massage, traction and manipulation

Massage also has been used for centuries in many different cultures for the purpose of pain relief. There are many different sorts of massage, but all are essentially a form of stimulation technique aimed at muscle relaxation and improvement in local blood flow. It is not clear if benefit is achieved by local reflex activity or by mechanical stimulation.

Lumbar and cervical traction are used frequently for musculoskeletal disorders and problems arising from discs and degenerative joint disease. The purpose of traction is to distract the vertebrae and relieve muscle spasm, by doing so it is believed that pain arising from nerve root compression and from the facet joints may be relieved.

Similar properties are claimed for the manipulation which has also been employed for many centuries in the successful treatment of acute and chronic pain. The efficacy of spinal manipulation for patients with back or neck pain has been reviewed by Koes and colleagues (1991). They concluded that efficacy of manipulation could not be shown convincingly, although some results were promising. Manipulative medicine takes many forms, osteopathy, chiropractic as well as 'orthodox' medical manipulation and for a helpful introduction to this subject the reader is referred to Paterson and Burn (1985).

Electrical stimulation

Therapeutic electrical stimulation in physiotherapy is usually either low-frequency, alternating or faradic current, or direct current of a wide range of frequencies, termed galvanic current. These are distinct from TENS with portable stimulating units which is considered separately below.

The same type of conditions that benefit from treatment by ultrasound or short-wave diathermy may be expected to improve with electrical stimulation techniques. Galvanic stimulation with high-voltage high-peak current generators is alleged to provide better results as the current is believed to penetrate deeper and to cause less painful contractions during stimulation.

Transcutaneous electrical nerve stimulation

There are historical precedents extending back to the Ancient Greeks for the therapeutic use of electricity. The first clinical report was that of Scribonius Longus who used the electrical discharge of the torpedo fish to treat headache and arthritis. Electrostatic generators and Leyden jar condensers reawakened an interest in electrotherapy in the late Middle Ages, and the invention of the battery provided another impetus in Victorian times. However, little work that was of clinical use emerged until two decades ago.

The use of TENS in clinical pain relief is a direct result of the publication in 1965 of Melzack's and Wall's 'Spinal gate-control theory'. This theory suggested that the dorsal horn of the spinal cord was an important modulator of pain transmission. One of the most important predictions of the gate-control theory was that signals in the large primary afferent fibres (the A-fibres) would, by stimulating inhibitory circuits in the dorsal horn, suppress the onward transmission of signals in the small unmyelinated primary afferent fibres (the C-fibres).

This supposition was put to the test by Wall and Sweet (1967) who showed that clinical and experimental pain could be reduced by prolonged stimulation of peripheral nerves by percutaneous electrodes, without untoward effects. Since then, a great deal of research has been performed on the clinical application of electrical stimulation, which now includes not only TENS, but also direct peripheral nerve stimulation, extradural and direct spinal stimulation, and even direct stimulation of the pain regulating areas of the brain. However, the discussion in this chapter is confined to TENS.

Theory

Peripheral nerve stimulation utilizes the large myelinated afferent nerve fibres to activate local inhibitory circuits within the dorsal horn of the spinal cord. These inhibitory circuits reduce the transmission of painful impulses through the spinal cord. TENS produces non-painful paraesthesiae and is used usually in a segmental fashion as inhibition of nociception mediated by the large A-fibres is segmental. This is in contrast with acupuncture and similar counterirritant techniques which are extrasegmental and use painful stimuli. Polysegmental inhibitory circuits do exist, but require generally much higher-intensity stimuli to become activated, as they are usually mediated by the smaller Aδ- and C-afferents (Woolf, 1985).

The long-term relief of pain by TENS is more difficult to explain. Melzack (1973) has suggested two mechanisms. First, a painful joint relieved of pain by stimulation becomes more mobile and is able to undergo more activity, thus restoring large-fibre input and 'closing the gate'. Second, pain may form part of a central 'memory', with self-perpetuating neural circuits in the periaqueductal grey region forming the 'central biasing mechanism'. TENS may break into this closed loop system and allow a reduction in the pain experienced.

Equipment

The equipment required for electrical stimulation is a pulse generator, an amplifier and a system of electrodes. Most modern stimulators are small and relatively inexpensive. They use rechargeable batteries and may power up to four electrodes.

In most stimulators the frequency range is from 1–100 Hz. Most patients find that stimulation at a fairly high frequency (70 Hz) is the most comfortable and effective. Stimulation at low frequency (2 Hz) requires a higher intensity and may produce painful muscle contractions. There appear to be fundamental differences between high- and low-frequency stimulation. High-frequency stimulation produces fast onset of pain relief, which lasts only a short period of time and is not reversed by naloxone. Low-frequency stimulation has a slow onset of pain relief, a long aftereffect and is reversed by naloxone. An attempt has been made to utilize both forms of stimulation with the 'burst' stimulator which delivers short trains of high-frequency bursts repeated at low frequency. This method of delivery makes it possible to use higher intensities of stimulation without distress to the patient (Erikssen et al., 1979).

There has been much research claiming to identify the optimal waveform, but in practice rectangular pulses are easiest to generate and are quite satisfactory for clinical use. It has been suggested that those waveforms that have the most influence on circulation are the most effective in relieving chronic pain. The standard pulse width varies between 0.1–0.5 ms. A higher pulse width than this may stimulate motor or Class III fibres and produce unwanted activity and unpleasant sensations for the patient.

The output intensity control on most TENS units provides an output up to 50 V. Although only about 20 mV is necessary to excite large myelinated fibres, TENS units can produce at least 1000 times this level. This is necessary as a large amount of current is distorted and lost in the tissues between the electrode and the target nerve. In the normal configuration of electrode, electrode gel and skin, resistance would be around 1 kohm and the peak current 50 mA if the maximal output is 50 V.

The most important principle is that the current density produced by the apparatus should be able to excite the target nerve in a controllable fashion and without damage to the skin. Many types of electrode have been used, the most common being soft, carbonized, silicone rubber. These are strong, inert and will conform to most of the body contours. Electrodes should be at least 4 cm^2 in area, as too high a current density in a small electrode may cause skin irritation. Conversely, large electrodes may not deliver sufficient current to stimulate the nerves effectively because of decline in current density with length (Brennan, 1976). Electrolyte gel should always be used to lower the high skin impedance and obtain a good contact, thus minimizing the possibility of skin damage. Self-adherent electrodes are available now that obviate the need for electrode gel and are more convenient for prolonged use.

Clinical use

The basic aim of TENS is to stimulate the large sensory myelinated fibres without discomfort to the patient and without muscle contraction. This is achieved most readily by positioning the electrodes proximally over the nerve supplying the painful area. This is not always possible, nor is it always successful and it is important to realize that it may take some time to find the most effective site for stimulation. It is best to work in a logical fashion, commencing along the length of the appropriate sensory nerve and following with stimulation at the point of maximum intensity of the pain, then dermatomally, over trigger points and on the contralateral side.

It is important to choose a site where the stimulus can be felt by the patient. The aim being to produce what is termed the 'maximum comfortable paraesthesia'. The patient is asked to increase the level of stimulation until it is painful; the highest intensity below that which is not painful is the maximum comfortable paraesthesia. It is most unlikely that the patient will gain any benefit if an adequate paraesthesia is not experienced. It is equally important to allow the patient sufficient time to get used to the apparatus. Many patients are overawed by the machine and do not use it unless they have received a comprehensive explanation and demonstration. It has been argued that patients should be admitted to hospital for an adequate trial to be carried out (Wynn-Parry, 1980).

Patients should be encouraged to experiment with electrode position and with the settings on the machine. For chronic pain a minimum of 3 h stimulation per day is recommended, and this should be continued for 4–6 weeks. With chronic pain there is frequently a gradual development of pain relief which may not be noticeable immediately and the patient should be encouraged to persevere with treatment even though the initial response is unfavourable. There is also a small group of patients who find the sensation produced by the stimulator unpleasant and who cannot tolerate it. There are no predictors of the type and intensity of stimulus that will produce relief, nor predictors for the type of condition or patient that responds. Some patients obtain pain relief only while using the stimulator; others may gain none whatsoever during stimulation but experience long periods of relief after stimulation. Johnson and colleagues (1991) carried out an in-depth study of the long-term clinical use of TENS in chronic pain patients. They confirmed the lack of correlation between patient, stimulator and outcome variables, but concluded that TENS was a most valuable treatment in many chronic conditions.

Acute pain

TENS has been used to treat a wide variety of acute pains, with varying degrees of success. Probably the most appropriate and successful use of TENS is in acute musculoskeletal injuries. Outstanding pain relief can be obtained in many conditions where there is associated muscle spasm, such as acute low back pain, whiplash injuries and sports injuries. TENS has been reported as highly effective in the management of fractured ribs (Myers et al., 1977), acute orofacial pain (Hansson & Ekblom, 1983) and childbirth (Augustinsson et al., 1977). Subsequent work suggests that whilst it may be effective for the early part of labour it is ineffective for the pain of the second stage of delivery.

The majority of studies of TENS in acute pain have been undertaken on postoperative pain. However, there are few really good studies of its effect. There are technical problems with the structure of controlled double-blind trials with a treatment method that requires a comprehensive explanation to be effective and also produces a characteristic sensation that has to form part of the explanation. None the less TENS has been shown to be effective in several reasonable studies (Pike, 1978; Rosenberg et al., 1978; Schuster & Infante, 1980; Ali et al., 1981; Tyler et al., 1982). Not only did the patients complain of less pain, but also postoperative opioid requirements were reduced.

Other studies have demonstrated a reduction in postoperative ileus (Ledergerber, 1978), but this was not seen by others (Vanderark & McGrath, 1975; Rosenberg et al., 1978). Patients having TENS for postoperative pain relief also showed less depression of Pao_2, vital capacity and functional residual capacity (Ali et al., 1981).

There is still a need for further controlled studies of TENS in postoperative pain. Despite the obvious advantages of TENS in that it is simple to use, cheap, portable, continuously available and non-addictive it has not gained a great deal of acceptance, and the suspicion is that this is because it is not effective. There is some evidence that if opioids have been used preoperatively TENS is ineffective (Solomon et al., 1980).

Chronic pain

There is no doubt that TENS is a very effective way to treat a wide variety of painful conditions. It is most useful in the control of pain of neurogenic origin such as peripheral nerve damage, plexus injuries (Wynn-Parry, 1980), causalgia (Meyer & Fields, 1972), phantom limb pain (Miles & Lipton, 1978), post-herpetic neuralgia (Nathan & Wall, 1974) and post-thoracotomy neuralgia. In addition, root compression, radiculopathies, postlaminectomy syndrome and many other forms of low back pain respond to TENS (Procacci et al., 1982). Chronic pain states that are unlikely to respond to TENS are psychogenic pain (Nielzen et al., 1982), pain with multiple sites and aetiologies, and those that are difficult to localize, such as visceral pain.

TENS becomes less effective with the passage of time. Various authors have noted a high initial success rate, of the order of 70%. This declines to approximately 60% after 1 month and a stable long-term success rate of the order of 20–30% is achieved usually. Some of the early success can be attributed to a placebo effect, but this is usually transient, and the results are more impressive when the wide variety of clinical conditions that have been successfully treated is considered. Woolf (1985) has reviewed the literature and lists those conditions where TENS has been of benefit and of little or no help.

Complications

There are few side-effects. The most common problems are allergic responses to either tape or electrode gel and less commonly, the electrode itself. It is possible to produce superficial erythema with over-zealous stimulation over a partially denervated area or where insufficient gel has been applied. Some patients experience an increase in their pain when TENS is used.

The use of stimulators in patients with cardiac pacemakers is an absolute contraindication. Theoretical risks may be present if stimulation is applied over the carotid sinus or the gravid uterus, although no problems have been reported so far. Stimulators are relatively contraindicated where the patient may have difficulty either understanding or using the machine, e.g. at the extremes of age or where mental or physical handicap prevent full control. The most common problem is for a patient to fall asleep wearing a stimulator and to change position, with a consequent improvement in the electrical contact which may prove quite a shock to the system.

Hypnosis

Hypnosis has been used for the control of acute and chronic pain for more than 100 years. Despite some widely publicized successes, it remains little used except by a small number of talented practitioners. In the past, proponents of hypnotherapy tended to present their findings in an overenthusiastic and uncritical way, which led to indiscriminate use and an inevitable disappointment with the results. However, many practitioners may use hypnotic techniques unknowingly, e.g. during the induction of anaesthesia or during dentistry.

Definitions

The nature of hypnosis cannot be defined readily. It has been described as an altered state of awareness during which the patient experiences increased suggestibility, and during which the patient's conscious and unconscious mind is more likely to accept ideas uncritically (Hilgard & Hilgard, 1975). Another description suggests that hypnosis is a communication of ideas and understanding to a patient in such a way that he/she will be more receptive to suggestions, thereby becoming motivated to explore their ability to control psychological or physiological responses and behaviour (Erickson, 1968).

Although hypnosis is an altered state of consciousness, the hypnotized individual does not lose consciousness and control. He/she is aware all the time, sometimes in a heightened fashion. As the patient is in control, it is possible to terminate the hypnotic state at any time if so desired, and contrary to popular belief, the patient will not begin spontaneous recitals of personal and intimate information. Hypnotic susceptibility is the subject of continuing debate. Approximately 66% of the population have some hypnotic capacity, whilst approximately 10% are extremely susceptible. To assess this, there are several standard scales for predicting the subject's susceptibility. Difficulties in predicting susceptibility and the variability in effect are two of the biggest problems that occur in the clinical use of hypnosis.

Clinical use in acute pain

Hypnosis has been used in a very wide range of medical and behavioural problems. Among the best-known uses for hypnosis is pain relief. There is reasonable evidence that hypnosis can modify experimental pain (Orne, 1974). However, such pain relief is usually short lived, and this is frequently so where acute pain is concerned, such as that of an operation. In general, it is not feasible to use hypnosis predictably to permit painful surgery. However, there are plenty of anecdotal reports of major procedures being performed with the only analgesia being provided by hypnosis. The author has witnessed a patient use autohypnotic techniques whilst undergoing an intramedullary nailing of a fractured femur; a procedure that included reduction of the fracture and intramedullary reaming. At no stage during or after this procedure was there any complaint of pain or demand for analgesia.

Hypnosis can be most useful in the susceptible individual for less painful procedures such as dentistry and where frequent painful procedures have to be carried out such as dressing changes or the debridement of burns.

Clinical use in chronic pain

Chronic pain, by definition, lasts a long time and for hypnosis to have a useful part to play it must form part of a broader co-ordinated approach that uses conventional therapy in addition to psychotherapeutic interventions. Various hypnotic control strategies have been described and the following are examples.

Suggestions of deep relaxation are frequently effective in pain control, as anxiety and pain are usually interrelated and relaxation will bring about a reduction in anxiety and accompanying muscle tension. This technique is utilized in relaxation training (p. 1659).

Direct suggestions of decreased pain may be given; for example, 'Your unconscious mind will now help you to become more comfortable'. Suggestions may be given to the patient that the pain is decreasing slowly or diminishing.

Displacement of pain to another part of the body may often help. For instance, a pain in the chest can relocated to a hand or finger where it is less troublesome.

Dissociation can be used to separate the patient from painful circumstances. They may be asked to imagine themselves floating above the pain or being in a different place and observing the procedure from afar.

Transformation of the pain into a sensation that can be tolerated such as a feeling of warmth or tingling.

Time distortion enables a painful procedure to pass by more quickly.

It is most likely that the hypnotized patient experiences benefit by entering a deep state of relaxation, which may short-circuit the continuum of stress/ anxiety/pain. In addition, there may be other advantages such as involving the patient in their own care which, in turn, may lead to the patient developing a sense of control over the pain. Other benefits may accrue from the necessarily close relationship between the patient and the hypnotherapist, whereby hidden factors that have a significant influence upon the pain may be brought out, such as the influence of family and workmates, or fears about security and health (Chapter 75).

If hypnosis is to be used successfully, the patients must be assessed thoroughly and the expectations of both patient and physician must be realistic. Scepticism on the part of pain clinic staff can be an obstacle to successful treatment (Finer, 1979). Since it is not easy to attain an uncritical acceptance of any treatment in most pain clinics, especially when there is more and more emphasis on the 'scientific' approach, it is unsurprising that hypnotherapy forms only a small part of their work (Pilowsky, 1986). Despite this, controlled trials of the successful use of hypnotic techniques for the management of chronic pain have been reported (Large & Peters, 1991).

Motivation and compliance are important if success is to be achieved, but once a patient derives some benefit from hypnosis continuation is not a problem usually. In addition, once success has been experienced, these techniques are learned easily by the patient and can be applied at any time without the need for professional help. Finally, it should be emphasized that hypnosis is used best as part of an overall treatment strategy that involves other methods of pain relief, and that hypnosis does not produce changes in pain or behaviour that the patient is not willing to modify (Orne & Dinges, 1984).

Relaxation training

The object of relaxation training is to decrease levels of stress, anxiety and muscle tension. It is customary to begin with an attempt at educating the patient on his/her condition and the technique to be employed, with an emphasis upon positive results. The next step is to have the patient assume a comfortable position in a comfortable environment (quiet room and lighting, non-restrictive clothing). Relaxation is taught by a cognitive technique such as by having the patient repeat silently words, sounds or images. These focus the attention upon the differences in sensation from alternatively relaxed and contracted muscle groups and lead to the patient being able to relax tense muscle groups by following simple steps. These manoeuvres can be used by the patient at home with the aid of prerecorded tapes.

Biofeedback

This treatment method is analogous to that of other behavioural approaches and is rarely used in isolation. Biofeedback has been used most commonly to treat headache.

There are four types of biofeedback being used at present. Electromyographic feedback is used to reduce muscle tension. EEG feedback is used to increase α-wave activity in the brain, as this is thought to be incompatible with pain. Skin temperature feedback is used to alter sympathetically mediated blood flow and temporal-artery blood-flow feedback is used to control temporal artery flow in migraine.

There are many reports of benefit, but at least one excellent review has cast doubt upon what, if anything, biofeedback may achieve (Turner & Chapman, 1982a).

Meditation techniques

Meditation techniques are frequently quoted as being of value in the management of pain (Choi, 1987). Unfortunately, science has not yet found any method of measuring the validity of meditation as a treatment method.

Behavioural therapy

Basic concepts

When dealing with pain it is important to recognize that pain is a subjective phenomenon, whatever its cause. The pain that is suffered by patients with psychiatric or psychologic problems is no different from that described by patients with purely organic disease. The concept of 'psychogenic' pain should be discarded as it implies that somehow the pain is not genuine, yet the distress suffered by the patient with psychiatric or behavioural problems is indistinguishable from that experienced by the patient with purely organic disease.

It is important to recognize and look for psychiatric and psychologic problems in any patient presenting with pain. Anxiety about the reason for pain is a natural response, as is depression when faced with the prospect of unrelieved or partially relieved pain associated with either acute or chronic disease. Anxiety and depression are frequently expressed in terms of physical illness of which pain is a common symptom. Failure to recognize this may lead to misdiagnosis and consequent mistreatment.

Emotional components of pain

The gate-control theory of pain (Melzack & Wall, 1965) has recognized the influence that higher centres may have upon the appreciation of pain and superseded previous pain models that emphasized sensory physiology alone. There is now an established neurophysiological basis for the different psychological components of pain and the neurophysiological mechanisms for many emotional states are becoming delineated. Attention has been directed to the unpleasant affective qualities of pain and the roles of anxiety in acute pain and depression in chronic pain, and in general these affective qualities vary with the chronicity of the pain.

Acute versus chronic pain

Acute pain is usually characterized by tissue damage, and this causes action to minimize the damage, which itself has strong affective qualities such as fear and anxiety. The greater the pain, the greater the anxiety. By definition, acute pain is transient and reduces as healing takes place.

Chronic pain is sometimes defined as pain that serves no useful purpose and is quite capable of destroying the physical and emotional wellbeing of the individual, with further malign effects upon the patient's family and friends. It is important to recognize the difference between acute and chronic pain, as treatment of an individual with chronic pain by methods that are suitable only for acute pain relief may lead to further problems. For example, if strong analgesics are prescribed for long periods of time, and the individual is recommended to undergo extensive periods of inactivity and convalescence, this will inevitably lead to cessation of normal activity such as work or caring for the family.

Pain expression

Pain is an intensely personal experience and methods of evaluating pain accurately are still being developed. One of the most well-known attempts to measure pain systematically is the McGill pain questionnaire (Melzack, 1975) (Chapter 74). This instrument permits the patient to describe pain in three dimensions: sensory, affective and evaluative. By including the emotional aspects of pain, this questionnaire contributes to the accuracy of diagnosis, as recognizing the way certain pains are described may suggest the diagnosis.

In addition, it is important to recognize pain behaviour, and note the discovery that behaviours that occur for one set of reasons can persist for a different set of reasons. For example, when an injury is followed by a period of rest, freedom from work and household responsibilities, sympathetic attention and a continuation of income in the form of sickness benefit there is a strong risk that the patient will become trapped in the role of the invalid (Fordyce, 1984).

Psychiatric/psychologic considerations

Most patients presenting in a chronic pain relief clinic will have an organic problem with some evidence of emotional disturbance. The task is to decide which is the most important component. The bulk of psychiatric disease seen in pain clinics falls into one of two major categories; reactive depression or a larger group with essentially neurotic conditions such as anxiety, often with hysterical symptoms or personality abnormalities (Merskey, 1984). Both these groups of conditions present with pain frequently, as it is much more acceptable for the patient to complain of pain than to say that depression and anxiety are overwhelming his/her life.

Psychiatric or psychologic screening tests are useful in establishing a diagnosis. However, a positive result on a screening test does not mean that the patient has anxiety or depression, it merely implies that further help should be sought from an appropriately trained individual to determine the contribution of anxiety or depression to the whole problem. No matter what diagnosis is reached eventually, the pain is always 'real' pain to the individual and every effort should be made to communicate to the patient that the physicians believe that this is so. There can be little worse than the all too commonly held belief that pain is 'imaginary' or 'all in the mind'.

Placebo

It has generally been considered since the work of Beecher (1955) that a placebo effect can be found in 35% of patients with postoperative or acutely painful conditions. This is rarely so in patients with chronic pain. However, it should be emphasized that a placebo responder is no more than that; an individual who responds to placebo. This is a normal response, and not evidence of psychiatric or psychological problems.

Acute pain

Factors affecting the appreciation of acute pain

There do not seem to be any predictors for the amount of pain that an individual experiences postoperatively. It is likely that psychological variables may account for some of the puzzling differences in the response of patients to surgery. These may be classified into two groups: predisposing factors and situational factors. The former are factors over which physicians have no control such as personality type, intelligence level, social class and family history. These have been reviewed well by Bond (1980).

Situational factors may have a great impact on the pain response and may be modified by appropriate therapeutic intervention. Chapman (1977) has proposed a multidimensional model for acute pain that takes into account the emotional and social aspects of the response to pain in addition to other factors. Examples of factors that influence the perception of pain are previous experience, the meaning of the surgery, present social circumstances and cultural background. Techniques that can be used to control or lower the amount of pain are social modelling, relaxation training and the provision of information to the patient in the preoperative period.

Hospital stress

Stress is a pattern of responses which occur when the individual is threatened. These responses may be both physiological and psychological. There can be no doubt that the simple act of being admitted to hospital is extremely stressful as it entails vast changes in social routines, diet and surroundings. There may be confusion and uncertainty about the intended procedure with an associated helplessness. This will be even worse if there are language difficulties or if the patient is from a very different cultural background.

Anxiety is a very complex phenomenon which plays a major role in the perception of pain postoperatively. In general, there is a direct relationship between preoperative anxiety and the amount of distress suffered after operation. Anxiety can be measured easily with standard questionnaires and can be related to pain (Speilberger et al., 1973). The concept of state and trait anxiety is a useful one. State anxiety measures the response to a specific event such as surgery, whereas trait anxiety is the patient's predisposition to become anxious in any stressful situation. Patients with high trait-anxiety scores preoperatively can be expected to show high state anxiety and high levels of pain and distress postoperatively. The clinical implications of this have been demonstrated by Boeke and colleagues (1991). They showed that high levels of state anxiety preoperatively were associated with increased length of hospital stay following gall-bladder surgery.

Any individual who has undergone major surgery may find him/herself physically helpless. Helplessness is a well-known source of stress and if the condition is prolonged for any length of time, it may lead to depression. It has been estimated that a hospital stay of 3 weeks or more predisposes to depression and a prolonged period of helplessness is a potent factor in inducing this state. Studies carried out on patients with chronic pain have shown that helpless patients suffer from higher levels of depression, anxiety, vulnerability and hostility (Wade et al., 1992).

The reasons for the surgery and the postoperative consequences are powerful stressors. The surgery may be associated with benefit, such as the delivery of a baby, or the cure of painful condition. However, there are circumstances when the surgery may have catastrophic consequences such as the confirmation of an inoperable malignancy or the loss of a limb. Preoccupation with the effects of surgery upon future life, work or recreation may lead easily to great distress which must be anticipated and handled in a sympathetic and speedy fashion.

Psychological preparation for surgery

There is excellent evidence that preoperative psychological preparation can reduce the pain and anxiety associated with surgery. Several methods are available of which the commonest are cognitive, behavioural and social modelling. Cognitive methods require the presentation of information about the operation and its likely effects, coupled with instructions on methods of coping with the pain. Examples of this are the preoperative visit by the anaesthetist or explanations by ward or intensive-therapy staff on what the patient may expect on return from their operation. Behavioural methods utilize relaxation training and breathing exercises.

Social modelling is commonly used in paediatric patients and involves the use of film or videotape to show children what they may expect on admission to hospital. Other examples are self-help groups in which patients who have undergone a particular procedure provide practical advice on the proposed operation and its long-term effects to those awaiting the same type of surgery.

Chronic pain

Many patients with chronic pain present with a confusing combination of organic and emotional problems. This is made worse frequently by other difficulties relating to excessive treatment and medication, and these in turn may be related to associated problems regarding family, work, compensation or legal action. No single therapeutic approach is appropriate for all these problems, and behavioural management of chronic pain problems forms merely part of an overall strategy that may include other methods of treatment such as drug therapy, nerve blocks or neurosurgery.

Specific techniques for the psychological management of pain

Analytic psychotherapy of the 'notebook and couch' variety is used rarely in the treatment of chronic pain. It is more common to use what may be described as 'support psychotherapy' (Pilowsky & Bassett, 1982). This treatment seeks to maximize the patients own coping mechanisms and is coupled with cognitive strategies aimed at increasing the patients insight into his/her condition and the various treatments

that have been offered, or are about to be offered, There are extensive reviews of these therapies by Tan (1982), Turner and Chapman (1982b) and Jensen and colleagues (1991). Jensen and colleagues reviewed the relationships between the patients' beliefs, coping mechanisms and adjustment to chronic pain. They found that those patients who maintained a positive attitude to their problems were able to function much better than those who adopted the sick role and who believed and behaved as though they were disabled. A carefully conducted study by Pilowsky and Barrow (1990) demonstrated that psychotherapy is not an inert component of pain management and may have a measureable effect on activity and productivity. There is a need for further studies that examine how psychotherapy reacts with other methods of treatment.

The development of behavioural programmes for the management of chronic pain largely results from the work of Fordyce (1976). These 'operant' programmes stem from the idea that chronic pain patients display or operate 'pain behaviours' that they use to manipulate their own lives and those of close relatives or friends. For example, moaning, limping or grimacing will make it more likely that they are believed to be in pain, and thus sympathy, time off work and household tasks, prescription of medicines and financial reward in the form of sickness benefit are all easier to obtain and maintain. These positive benefits tend therefore to reinforce these behaviours and make them more frequent.

Equally, such behaviours tend to make it easy to avoid aversive situations such as unpleasant tasks or undesired responsibilities. Thus, the goal of operant programmes is to decrease the number and frequency of learned pain behaviours and replace them with behaviours that are incompatible with the sick role — well behaviours. For these programmes to be effective, inpatient admission for up to 16 weeks is required. They consist of a structured programme of therapy designed to maximize the patients' activities and minimize pain behaviour.

Thus, when the patient displays pain behaviour either by movement or complaint this is ignored by the staff; when patients are indulging in well behaviour, by taking part in exercise classes or occupational therapy, they are rewarded by attention and support. This part of the programme is associated usually with the setting of targets to increase the amount of activity undertaken by the patients, vocational training, counselling sessions with the family and the systematic reduction of the amount of medicines taken (Buckley et al., 1986). Incentives are given to encourage participation and the achievement of targets in the form of passes for weekend leave or visits from family and friends.

Doubts have been cast on the value of operant programmes (Merskey, 1984). It has been suggested that it is unlikely that the pain may be alleviated merely by ignoring pain behaviour, especially if there is a physical basis for it, and that it requires a change in the physical status of the patient for improvement to occur. This may be produced by improvements in the patients' fitness following an increase in activity. However, there is no doubt that patients complain of less pain, take less medicine and are able to do more after treatment on an operant programme. Long-term results seem to indicate that although the patients complaints of pain tend to recur, the long-term gains are maintained in terms of higher activity levels, decreased drug intake and better work records than similar patients who were treated by conventional means. The overall results are a little difficult to assess as the majority of programmes include other treatment methods in addition, such as TENS, biofeedback or relaxation training. It would appear that operant programmes, when coupled with other non-invasive therapy represent a most effective, if costly, way of improving the life of the patient with chronic pain.

References

Ali J., Yaffe C. & Senette C. (1981) The effect of transcutaneous electric nerve stimulation on postoperative pain and pulmonary function. *Surgery* **89**, 507–12.

Augustinsson L., Bonlin P., Bundsen P., Carlsson C.A., Forssman C., Sjoberg P. & Tyreman N.D. (1977) Pain relief during delivery by transcutaneous nerve stimulation. *Pain* **4**, 59–65.

Beecher H.K. (1955) The powerful placebo. *Journal of the American Medical Association* **159**, 1602–5.

Benedetti C. & Murphy T.M. (1985) Non-pharmacological methods of acute pain control. In *Acute Pain* (Eds Smith G. & Covino B.) pp. 260–1. Butterworths, London.

Boeke S., Duivenvoorden H.J., Verhage F. & Zwaveling A. (1991) Prediction of postoperative pain and duration of hospitalisation using two anxiety measures. *Pain* **45**, 293–7.

Bond M.R. (1980) Personality and pain: the influence of psychological and environmental factors upon the experience of pain in hospital patients. In *Persistent Pain*, vol. 2 (Ed. Lipton S.) pp. 1–25. Academic Press, London.

Brennan K.R. (1976) The characterization of transcutaneous stimulating electrodes. *IEEE Transactions on Biomedical Engineering* **23**, 337–40.

Buckley F.P., Sizemore W.A. & Charlton J.E. (1986) Medication management in patients with chronic non-malignant pain. A review of the use of a drug withdrawal protocol. *Pain* **26**, 153–65.

Chapman C.R. (1977) Psychological aspects of pain: patient management. *Archives of Surgery* **112**, 767–72.

Cheng R. & Pomeranz B. (1979) Electroacupuncture analgesia is mediated by stereospecific opiate receptors and is reversed by antagonists of Type I receptors. *Life Sciences* **26**, 631–9.

Choi J.J. (1987) Meditation. In *Pain Management. Assessment and Treatment of Chronic and Acute Syndromes* (Eds Wu W. & Smith L.G.) pp. 216–44. Human Sciences Press, New York.

Erickson M.H. (1968) An introduction to the study and application of hypnosis for pain control. In *Hypnosis and Psychosomatic Medicine* (Ed. Lassner J.) pp. 125–40. Springer-Verlag, New York.

Erikssen M.B.E., Sjolund B.H. & Nielzen S. (1979) Long term results of peripheral conditioning stimulation as an analgesic measure in chronic pain. *Pain* **6**, 335–47.

Finer B. (1979) Hypnotherapy in pain of advanced cancer. In *Advances in Pain Research and Therapy*, vol. 2 (Eds Bonica J.J. & Ventafridda V.) pp. 223–30. Raven Press, New York.

Fordyce W.E. (1976) *Behavioural Methods for Chronic Pain and Illness*. Mosby, St Louis.

Fordyce W.E. (1984) Behavioural science and chronic pain. *Postgraduate Medical Journal* **60**, 865–8.

Frost E.A.M., Hsu C.Y. & Sadowsky D. (1976) Acute and chronic pain: a study of the comparative values of acupuncture therapy. In *Advances in Pain Research and Therapy*, vol. 1 (Eds Bonica J.J. & Albe-Fessard D.G.) pp. 823–9. Raven Press, New York.

Griffin J. & Karselis T. (1978) *Physical Agents for Physical Therapists*. Charles C. Thomas, Springfield, Illinois.

Gunn C.C. (1978) Motor points and motor lines. *American Journal of Acupuncture* **6**, 55–8.

Hansson P. & Ekblom A. (1983) Transcutaneous electrical nerve stimulation (TENS) as compared to placebo–TENS for the relief of acute orofacial pain. *Pain* **15**, 157–65.

Hilgard E.R. & Hilgard J.R. (1975) *Hypnosis in the Relief of Pain*. William Kaufman, Los Altos.

Hossenlopp C.M., Leiber L. & Mo B. (1976) Psychological factors in the effectiveness of acupuncture for chronic pain. In *Advances in Pain Research and Therapy*, vol. 1 (Eds Bonica J.J. & Albe-Fessard D.G.) pp. 803–9. Raven Press, New York.

Jensen M.P., Turner J.A., Romano J.M. & Karoly P. (1991) Coping with chronic pain: a critical review of the literature. *Pain* **47**, 249–83.

Johnson M.I., Ashton C.H. & Thompson J.W. (1991) An in-depth study of long-term users of transcutaneous electrical nerve stimulation (TENS). Implications for clinical use of TENS. *Pain* **44**, 221–9.

Kaada B. (1976) Neurophysiology and acupuncture: a review. In *Advances in Pain Research and Therapy*, vol. 1 (Eds Bonica J.J. & Albe-Fessard D.G.). pp. 733–41. Raven Press, New York.

Koes B.W., Assendelft W.J.J., van der Heijden G.J.M.J., Bouter L.M. & Knipschild P.G. (1991) Spinal manipulation and mobilisation for back and neck pain: a blinded review. *British Medical Journal* **303**, 1298–303.

Large R. & Peters J. (1991) A critical appraisal of outcome of multidisciplinary pain clinic treatments. In *Proceedings of the VIth World Congress on Pain* (Eds Bond M.R., Charlton J.E. & Woolf C.J.) pp. 417–27. Elsevier, Amsterdam.

Ledergerber C.P. (1978) Postoperative electro-analgesia. *Obstet-*

rics and Gynecology **151**, 334–8.

Lehmann J.F. & de Lateur B. (1985) Ultrasound, shortwave, microwave, superficial heat and cold in the treatment of pain. In *Textbook of Pain* (Eds Wall P.D. & Melzack R.) pp. 717–24. Churchill Livingstone, Edinburgh.

Lewith G.T. (1984) Can we assess the effects of acupuncture? *British Medical Journal* **288**, 1475–6.

Mayer D.J., Price D.D. & Raffii A. (1977) Antagonism of acupuncture analgesia in man by the narcotic antagonist naloxone. *Brain Research* **121**, 368–73.

Melzack R. (1973) *The Puzzle of Pain*. Penguin, Harmondsworth.

Melzack R. (1975) The McGill pain questionnaire: major properties and scoring methods. *Pain* **1**, 277–99.

Melzack R. & Wall P.D. (1965) Pain mechanisms — a new theory. *Science* **150**, 971–9.

Melzack R., Stilwell D.M. & Fox E.J. (1976) Trigger points and acupuncture points for pain: correlations and implications. *Pain* **3**, 3–23.

Merskey H. (1984) Psychological approaches to the treatment of chronic pain. *Postgraduate Medical Journal* **60**, 886–92.

Meyer G.A. & Fields H.L. (1972) Causalgia treated by selective large fibre stimulation of peripheral nerves. *Brain* **95**, 163–7.

Miles J. & Lipton S. (1978) Phantom limb pain treated by electrical stimulation. *Pain* **5**, 373–82.

Myers R.A.M., Woolf C.J. & Mitchell D. (1977) Management of acute traumatic pain by peripheral transcutaneous electrical stimulation. *South African Medical Journal* **52**, 309–12.

Nakatani Y. & Yamashita K. (1977) *Ryodoraku Acupuncture*. Ryodoraku Research Institute, Tokyo.

Nathan P.W. & Wall P.D. (1974) Treatment of post-herpetic neuralgia by prolonged electrical stimulation. *British Medical Journal* **iii**, 645–7.

Nielzen S., Sjolund B.H. & Erikssen B.E. (1982) Psychiatric factors influencing the treatment of pain with peripheral conditioning stimulation. *Pain* **13**, 365–71.

Omura Y. (1975) Electro-acupuncture: its electrophysiological basis and criteria for effectiveness and safety. Part 1. *Acupuncture and Electrotherapy Research* **1**, 157–81.

Orne M. (1974) Pain suppression by hypnosis and related phenomena. In *Advances in Neurology*, vol. 4 (Ed. Bonica J.J.) pp. 563–72. Raven Press, New York.

Orne M.T. & Dinges D.F. (1984) Hypnosis. In *Textbook of Pain* (Eds Wall P.D. & Melzack R.) pp. 806–16. Churchill Livingstone, London.

Paterson J.K. & Burn L. (1985) *An Introduction to Medical Manipulation*. MTP Press, Lancaster.

Pike P.M. (1978) Transcutaneous electrical stimulation: its use in management of postoperative pain. *Anaesthesia* **33**, 165–71.

Pilowsky I. (1986) Current views on the role of the psychiatrist in chronic pain. In *The Therapy of Pain* (Ed. Swerdlow M.) pp. 31–55. MTP Press, Lancaster.

Pilowsky I. & Bassett D. (1982) Individual dynamic psychotherapy for chronic pain. In *Chronic Pain: Psychosocial Factor in Rehabilitation* (Eds Roy R. & Tunks E.) pp. 107–24. Williams and Wilkins, Baltimore.

Pilowsky I. & Barrow C.G. (1990) A controlled study of psychotherapy and amitryptiline used individually and in combination in the treatment of chronic intractable, 'psychogenic' pain. *Pain* **40**, 3–19.

Pomeranz B. & Chiu D. (1976) Naloxone blockade of acupuncture analgesia: endorphin implicated. *Life Sciences* **19**, 1757–62.

Procacci P., Zoppi M. & Maresca M. (1982) Transcutaneous electrical stimulation in low back pain: a critical evaluation. *Acupuncture and Electrotherapy Research* **7**, 1–6.

Richardson P.H. & Vincent C.A. (1986) Acupuncture for the treatment of pain: a review of evaluative research. *Pain* **24**, 15–40.

Rosenberg M., Curtis L. & Bourke D.L. (1978) Transcutaneous electrical nerve stimulation for the relief of postoperative pain. *Pain* **5**, 129–35.

Schuster G.D. & Infante M.C. (1980) Pain relief after low back surgery: the efficacy of transcutaneous electrical nerve stimulation. *Pain* **8**, 299–302.

Solomon R.A., Viernstein M.R. & Long D.M. (1980) Reduction of postoperative pain and narcotic use by transcutaneous electrical nerve stimulation. *Surgery* **87**, 142–6.

Speilberger C.D., Gorsuch R. & Lushene R. (1973) *The State–Trait Anxiety Inventory*. Consulting Psychologists Press, Palo Alto.

Tan S.-Y. (1982) Cognitive and cognitive behavioural methods for pain control. *Pain* **12**, 201–28.

Turner J.A. & Chapman C.R. (1982a) Psychological interventions for chronic pain: a critical review. I. Relaxation training and biofeedback. *Pain* **12**, 1–21.

Turner J.A. & Chapman C.R. (1982b) Psychological interventions for chronic pain: a critical review. II. Operant conditioning, hypnosis and cognitive–behavioural therapy. *Pain* **12**, 23–46.

Tyler E., Caldwell C. & Ghia J.N. (1982) Transcutaneous electrical nerve stimulation: an alternative approach to the management of postoperative pain. *Anesthesia and Analgesia* **61**, 449–56.

Vanderark G. & McGrath K. (1975) Transcutaneous electrical stimulation in treatment of postoperative pain. *American Journal of Surgery* **130**, 336–40.

Vincent C.A. (1989) A controlled trial of the treatment of migraine by acupuncture. *Clinical Journal of Pain* **5**, 305–12.

Vincent C.A. & Richardson P.H. (1986) The evaluation of therapeutic acupuncture: concepts and methods. *Pain* **24**, 1–14.

Wade J.B., Dougherty L.M., Hart R.P. & Cook D.B. (1992) Patterns of normal personality structure among chronic pain patients. *Pain* **48**, 37–43.

Wall P.D. & Sweet W.H. (1967) Temporary abolition of pain in man. *Science* **155**, 108–9.

Woolf C.J. (1985) Transcutaneous and implanted nerve stimulation. In *Textbook of Pain* (Eds Wall P.D. & Melzack R.) pp. 679–90. Churchill Livingstone, Edinburgh.

Wynn-Parry C.B. (1980) Pain in avulsion lesions of the brachial plexus. *Pain* **9**, 41–53.

Ablative Nerve Blocks
and Neurosurgical Techniques

K. BUDD

In the treatment of chronic pain, it may seem reasonable to suppose that destruction of the afferent sensory pathways from the area in which the pain is produced would have the desired effect of preventing access of nociceptive impulses to the sensorium and its appreciation as pain. Many techniques both surgical and non-surgical have been introduced during the past 50 years for this purpose, and whilst some remain in contemporary use, none has achieved universal popularity. Although ablative techniques in general are used less frequently, for some well-defined indications they retain major clinical usefulness and may be the treatment of choice. The patient only benefits significantly, however, when such techniques are performed with care following well-established procedural guidelines.

Because the side-effects of many of these techniques include conditions worse than the original painful state, every effort should be taken to avoid not only these complications for the patient but also the possibility of consequent litigation against the practitioner.

Neurolysis

Interruption of nerve pathways (neurolysis) may be achieved using a variety of methods. These may induce either temporary or permanent cessation of nervous transmission: the former is utilized mainly for diagnostic procedures, the latter is the main therapeutic modality used in the treatment of chronic pain as an alternative to drug therapy. Neurolytic methods include:

For temporary neurolysis:
1 Pressure applied to the nerve.
2 Local anaesthetic applied to the nerve.

For permanent neurolysis:
3 Application of chemicals to the nerve.

4 Application of cold to the nerve.
5 Application of heat to the nerve, nerve root or tract.
6 Surgical section of the nerve, nerve root or tract.

In the majority of cases, permanent neurolysis should be preceded by a temporary block with local anaesthetic in order that the degree of pain relief and its extent may be appreciated by both patient and doctor, and potential side-effects such as numbness and muscle weakness may be experienced by the patient. In the light of all these factors, informed discussion may take place between patient and doctor before the decision is taken to produce permanent neurolysis.

Neurolytic agents

Chemical agents

The commonly used neurolytic chemicals are phenol, alcohol and chlorocresol.

Phenol

Phenol is a weak acid with both bactericidal and neurolytic properties. Even in concentrations as low as 1%, neurolysis may be achieved, but in clinical practice the concentration used varies between 5 and 10% in aqueous solution. The neurolytic effect is more pronounced on small Aδ- and C-fibres which conduct pain, whereas the larger fibres with motor function are affected much less. This differential action is valuable, as pain may be relieved without disturbance of motor function and sensory modalities other than pain (Nathan & Sears, 1960).

Clinically, the effect of phenol appears to be exclusively on small fibres, but histological evidence shows that the effect is exerted on fibres of all sizes although a larger proportion of the smaller-diameter ones are affected. The eventual outcome is dictated, however, by the concentration of solution, nature of solvent and duration of contact with nervous tissue. As a neurolytic agent, phenol is quicker in action than alcohol but less predictable in its spread and effect. A significant advantage is that it is less likely to produce chemical neuritis than is alcohol.

Phenol solutions are thought to spread along the perineural sheath and nerve destruction is followed by gradual regeneration of the fibres over 5–20 weeks (Khalli & Ditzler, 1968). If phenol is placed inadvertently on a mixed somatic nerve, transient evidence of complete nerve block is seen, but appreciable reversal occurs within 1–2 weeks, and there is a high likelihood of complete motor function being restored. This is not usually the case with alcohol when motor function returns rarely to pretreatment values.

Toxic effects with phenol are seen infrequently with the small doses used in clinical practice. However, following inadvertent intravascular injection, patients may complain of faintness and dizziness accompanied by excitement. This progresses rapidly to depression of the vital centres leading to loss of consciousness, circulatory and respiratory collapse.

In the adult, the toxic dose for phenol is 8–15 g (Esplin, 1970) but in normal clinical practice this figure is never approached. Bryce-Smith (1966) recommends that the maximum amount injected in one bolus should be 66 mg. In doses less than this, patients may experience tenderness at the site of injection for several days and may exhibit also mild, influenzal-like symptoms for 48 h, but serious complications are rare. When used intrathecally, phenol is dissolved in glycerine or a radio-opaque medium in order to render the resulting solution hyperbaric (SG 1025 compared with cerebrospinal fluid SG 1005–1009). Phenol produces an immediate local anaesthetic effect with recovery occurring over the subsequent 15–30 min followed by permanent nerve destruction (Nathan & Scott, 1958; Editorial, 1964). Patchy degeneration occurs in nerve fibres of all sizes, the principle site of action being the nerve roots between the cord and the dural cuff. The cord itself is undamaged, but degeneration in the the posterior columns has been reported following repeated injections.

Ethyl alcohol

This is the most reliable agent for the production of peripheral nerve neurolysis (Dam & Larsen, 1974). It was used first to treat the pain of trigeminal neuralgia in 1888 (Pitres & Vaillard, 1888) and although its popularity has waned because of a high incidence of postinjection neuritis, some authorities advocate its use as the treatment of choice for the block of autonomic ganglia (Mehta, 1973).

When ethyl alcohol is injected intra- or perineurally, coagulation necrosis occurs characterized by diffuse eosinophilic staining with complete loss of detail in axons, myelin sheath, nodes of Ranvier and Schwann cells (Pizzolato & Mannheimer, 1961). Under similar conditions, phenol produces almost identical damage but regeneration of the axon occurs within 2 months. By injection, alcohol is extremely irritating to tissues, and causes pain, burning and local tenderness. In order to minimize these effects, the injection should be placed accurately so that the minimum volume is used. Nevertheless, the incidence of postinjection neuritis is significant and has resulted in loss of popularity of this agent.

When injected either peripherally or intrathecally, alcohol is used undiluted. As it has a lower specific gravity than cerebrospinal fluid (0.805 compared with 1.005) in the intrathecal space, the hypobaric alcohol floats upwards onto the specific nerve roots thereby allowing the patient to be positioned with the painful side uppermost.

Dilute solutions of alcohol are used occasionally for ablation of the coeliac plexus. Fifty percent alcohol in saline or bupivacaine is used commonly, but, as the injection is painful, it is necessary to perform this block under general anaesthesia or heavy sedation. With the dilute solutions, chemical neuritis is seen in up to 15% of patients (Brown, 1981).

Chlorocresol

Chlorocresol is a more potent agent than phenol and has been used only in the extradural and intrathecal spaces (Maher, 1963) as a 2% solution in glycerine and a 5% solution in glycerine, respectively. It is one of the more effective agents for the treatment of cancer pain and has a greater ability to penetrate cancerous tissue surrounding nerve roots than does phenol or alcohol.

After injection of chlorocresol into the extradural or subarachnoid spaces, pain relief is delayed usually for up to 24 h and, unlike phenol, it is not associated with immediate sensory changes or the onset of paraesthesiae. Until the full effect has been produced, the patient may complain of dull pain, sluggish limb movement and diminished sensitivity to heat and cold in the affected segments.

In the intrathecal space, chlorocresol appears to diffuse more widely than phenol, and is used therefore in a smaller dose, 0.35 ml of 2% solution in glycerine being equivalent to 0.5 ml of 5% phenol solution in the same solvent. Localization of the block with chlorocresol is more difficult than with alcohol or phenol because of the absence of immediate sensory changes but the neurolysis is of a more intense nature after it has developed.

Other neurolytic agents

Ammonium chloride

This agent has been used intrathecally in concentrations varying from 0.5 to 20%. Although excellent neurolysis is obtained with the higher concentrations, the injection is painful and the active agent may require dilution with local anaesthetic (Dam, 1965). Reduction in concentration produces adequate results in terms of neurolysis without discomfort (Mehta, 1973). After intraneural injection, severe injury and degeneration is produced, but regeneration may be complete within 60 days (Pizzolato & Mannheimer, 1961).

Silver nitrate

In resistant cancer patients, silver nitrate may be added to solutions of phenol in glycerine to increase penetration. Maher (1957) has recommended the addition of 0.6 mg silver nitrate to 1 ml of a 4% solution of phenol in glycerine. Because of apparent lack of damage to sacral outflow and consequent sphincter sparing, the main uses are in the lower thoracic and lumbosacral areas. Excellent penetration may be achieved although it may take up to 5 days for the peak effect to become established (Maher, 1969). The use of silver nitrate in cervical and upper thoracic regions is not advocated because of the toxic properties of the agent. Based on pathological studies, Nathan and Scott (1958) suggested that silver nitrate is dangerous at all levels.

Glycerine

The injection of glycerine into the trigeminal cistern may abolish completely typical trigeminal pain. In many patients, this pain relief is accompanied by very little disturbance of facial sensation (Hakanson, 1981). Long-term follow-up of this treatment shows a relapse rate of 31%, suggesting that this is safe and effective therapy (Hakanson, 1983). Glycerine does not appear to have the same neurolytic action when injected around a peripheral nerve or intrathecally.

Hypertonic saline

This has been used intrathecally to treat the pain of both benign and malignant disease, with claims for a 50% permanent improvement (Hitchcock & Pradinin, 1973). However, pain, hypertension and muscle fasciculations produced on injection make the concomitant use of general anaesthesia necessary.

Sclerosant solution

This solution has been used for injection into strained ligaments and joint capsules for the relief of pain. It acts by destruction of fine nerve endings. It is claimed also to tighten flaccid ligaments, possibly by the formation of scar tissue. The solution contains: phenol 2%, dextrose 20%, glycerine 25% and water to 100%. As the solution is an irritant to tissues and may produce pain on injection, it may be combined with local anaesthetic agents prior to use or its injection preceded by infiltration of the tissue with local anaesthetic solution (Barber, 1971).

The application of cold — cryotherapy

Although the principle of using extreme cold to produce insensibility to pain has been known and used for centuries (Armstrong-Davidson, 1965), its clinical application to produce analgesia was not introduced until 1976 (Lloyd et al., 1976).

The cryoprobe comprises a fine needle probe with built-in thermocouple. It utilizes the Joule–Thompson effect with either nitrous oxide or carbon dioxide as the expanding gas, thereby reducing the temperature at the tip of the probe to −70°C (Fig. 81.1). When introduced into the body, by freezing tissue water the iceball formed at the tip of the probe grows to encompass the selected nerve (Fig. 81.2),

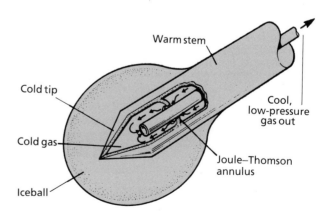

Fig. 81.1 Principle of cryoprobe. (Courtesy of Spembly Ltd.)

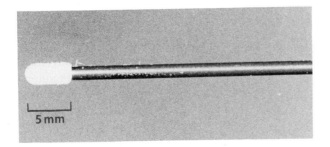

Fig. 81.2 Cryoprobe tip with iceball. (Courtesy of Spembly Ltd.)

thereby disrupting the neural tissue but with minimal effects on endoneurium and other connective tissue. This lesion produces a break in the functional continuity of the nerve and hence analgesia which may last up to 6 months. The incidence of postlesion neuralgia is less with cryotherapy than with other neurolytic techniques (Carter *et al.*, 1972; Loyd *et al.*, 1976; Barnard, 1980).

A lesion may be produced either by picking up the exposed nerve on the tip of the probe (e.g. when the nerve is exposed at surgery) for postoperative analgesia (Katz *et al.*, 1980; Maiwant & Make, 1981; Orr *et al.*, 1983) or percutaneously using the stimulator built into the probe to locate the probe tip on or close to the selected nerve (Fig. 81.3). The lesion is made using two, 2-min freeze cycles separated by a 1-min warming period. This technique appears to give

better results both in terms of degree and duration of analgesia than a single freeze of equivalent duration (Jones & Murrin, 1987).

There are few side-effects following cryotherapy, and these are limited usually to soreness at the site of insertion of the probe and occasional neuritic pain along the course of the nerve. On the rare occasion that the latter does not resolve spontaneously, infiltration of the site of the cryolesion with bupivacaine and methylprednisolone is beneficial. Alternatively, oral medication with an anticonvulsant (carbamazepine or sodium valproate) in combination with a tricyclic antidepressant (amitriptyline or nortriptyline) may produce remission within 2 weeks (Budd, 1981).

The application of heat

Cautery was used by the ancient Egyptians to coagulate tissue and was favoured also by the Arab school of surgery (Ellis, 1984).

Electrocautery was introduced in 1896 and was used first in 1926 for neurosurgical operations by Harvey Cushing.

In spite of various refinements in surgical diathermy, it was not until 1965 that radiofrequency current was used to produce therapeutic lesions in appropriate areas of the CNS (Mullan *et al.*, 1965).

Nervous tissue is resistant to temperatures up to 42.5°C. At 42.5–44°C there is temporary disturbance

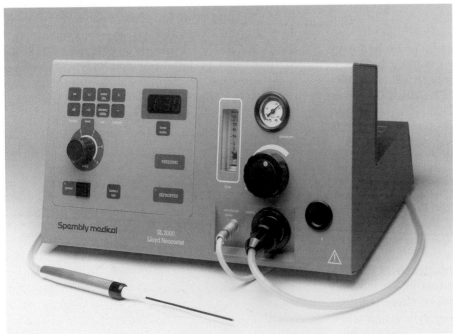

Fig. 81.3 Cryotherapy apparatus. (Courtesy of Spembly Ltd.)

of function, and above 45°C there are irreversible changes. This effect is not spread uniformly and the initial lesions at temperatures above 45°C tend to be confined to the smaller nerve fibres including Aδ- and C-fibres. Consequently, a heat lesion has a central area of total destruction surrounded by a zone that is damaged selectively. If the central temperature is high, the central area of the lesion is large in comparison with the peripheral zone. If the central temperature is low, the extent of the selectively damaged zone is relatively more important.

For any given electrode current, thermal equilibrium is established in approximately 60 s. Lesion size may be controlled by limiting the current to an exposure of approximately 60 s or by generating higher currents for periods shorter than 30 s. The most satisfactory method of controlling the size of lesion is by maintaining a constant electrode tip temperature for a period of 1–2 min. By doing so, time-dependent factors are eliminated as thermal equilibrium is established, and lesion size depends directly on the measured temperature (Fig. 81.4).

The electrode current required to produce a given tip temperature depends on tip diameter and area and on the thermal characteristics of the target site. Consequently, accurate measurement of temperature is the single most important requirement of a lesion generator. This is achieved by building a thermistor or thermocouple into the tip of the electrode. Lesion generators deliver an alternating current with a frequency above 250 kHz to avoid the unpleasant sensory responses which occur at lower frequencies (Alberts *et al.*, 1972). A wide power range and fine output resolution are provided to give accurate temperature control. Variables which may be measured include temperature, current, voltage and impedance. Facilities are inbuilt also for electrical stimulation (Fig. 81.5). In general, the technique for producing a lesion in either a peripheral or central structure consists of positioning the insulated cannula in or close to the target area under X-ray control. The electrode is inserted through the cannula and the position of its tip determined finally both radiologically and by electrical stimulation (Fig. 81.6). An increase in tissue electrical impedance may be used also during percutaneous cordotomy to indicate passage of the electrode from cerebrospinal fluid (CSF) into the cord. Because of the need for patient co-operation, such procedures are undertaken using local anaesthesia, neuroleptanalgesia or intermittent general anaesthesia.

The most common side-effects caused by radiofrequency lesions are neuritic pain and hyperaesthesia in the treated dermatome. Fortunately, this tends to resolve spontaneously within 4–5 weeks and needs treatment rarely. Specific side-effects related to the site of lesion are discussed later in this chapter.

The use of surgery

Since the introduction of new therapeutic agents and techniques, particularly radiofrequency lesions, the need for surgical interruption of nerve pathways has diminished greatly. However, there is still occasionally a need for surgical neurectomy, applied usually to peripheral nerves when all other forms of neurolytic manoeuvres have failed to relieve pain. Even in such cases, surgery may fail.

Common neuroablative techniques
(Table 81.1)

Peripheral nerve

The entrapment of a perforating cutaneous nerve in the abdominal wall may occur spontaneously or following previous surgical intervention. In the former case, compression of the nerve takes place in the posterior rectus sheath as a result of scar formation following a small herniation of the fatty plug through which the nerve passes (Applegate, 1972). In such a case, the patient presents with constant or intermittent abdominal pain which may be localized or widespread. Often it radiates into the loin or chest wall

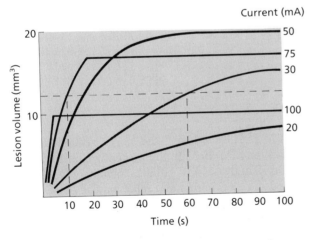

Fig. 81.4 Relationship between lesion size, current and duration of current flow. The horizontal dotted line represents the volume of optimal lesion. The vertical dotted line indicates the time taken to achieve this at varying levels of current. At 75 and 100 mA the tissue boiled; this insulation caused cessation of current flow.

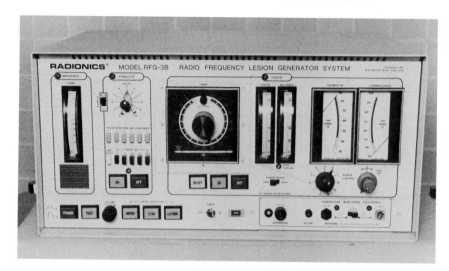

Fig. 81.5 Radiofrequency lesion generator. (Courtesy of Radionics Ltd.)

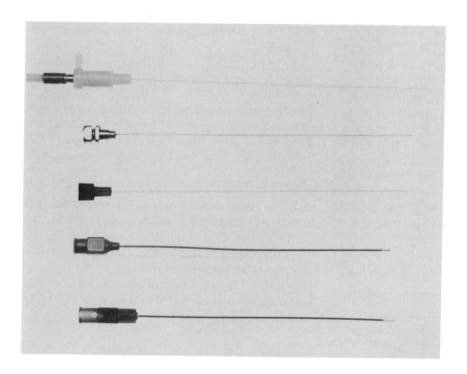

Fig. 81.6 Radiofrequency needles and electrode. Top, electrode; centre, two stilettes; bottom, two needles. (Courtesy of Radionics Ltd.)

along the segmental distribution of the nerve. Diagnosis is made by locating a discrete tender area, deep in the rectus muscle at its outer border and confirmed by the abolition of pain temporarily following injection of local anaesthetic.

Permanent cure may be obtained by the injection of a neurolytic agent, e.g. phenol 5% aqueous solution, 2–3 ml. This may require repeated injections and if pain persists, cryotherapy or radiofrequency lesions should be instituted. Occasionally, some cases are resistant to these treatments and are referred for surgical exploration and open neurectomy; the rectus

muscle is reflected and the nerve sectioned as it passes forward through the posterior rectus sheath.

Surprisingly, a few patients obtain only a short period of relief. Permanent relief may be obtained by the insertion of an extradural catheter behind the rectus muscle and the infusion by pump of aqueous phenol over the course of 48 h (phenol 7% aqueous, 20 ml in 48 h).

Intercostal neuralgia may be treated following an initial diagnostic block with local anaesthetic using a neurolytic subcostal block with either phenol 7% aqueous or absolute alcohol or by a direct cryo- or

Table 81.1 Possible levels of neuroablation

Peripheral nerve
Receptor containing tissue or end-organ
Nerve trunk
Nerve plexus
In the paravertebral space
Extradurally
Subdurally or within the subarachnoid space

Nerve root
Intra- and extradurally
Dorsal root ganglion

Cord
Ascending tracts
Spinal decussation

Intracranial
Brainstem
Thalamus
Hypothalamus
Pituitary
Sensory cortex
Frontal lobes
Cranial nerves intra- or extracranially

Autonomic system
Symphathetic chain
Parasympathetic outflow

radiofrequency lesion following electrical stimulation to confirm the diagnosis and correct placement of the probe.

Following the use of any of these neurolytic techniques, there may be intermittent pain and hyperaesthesia in the distribution of the lesioned nerve for several days after treatment. This settles invariably without further treatment. Rarely, the neuritis may persist for several months before settling spontaneously.

Nerve plexus

Apical tumours of the lung (Pancoast tumour) spread occasionally to involve the adjacent brachial plexus with consequent pain in the arm, reduced mobility and lymphoedema.

In many of these patients, the prognosis is poor and pain relief is extremely important. It is essential to explain to the patient that neurolytic techniques result in the loss of both sensation and mobility in the arm and it is important to ensure that the patient understands and consents to this.

Phenol 5% aqueous, 15 ml, may be injected into the brachial plexus, usually by the supraclavicular route. Repeated injections may be required until adequate analgesia is obtained; alternatively, an extradural catheter may be inserted into the plexus to enable multiple injections to be given.

If the tumour involves only the lower cords of the plexus, a percutaneous cervical cordotomy or multiple dorsal root ganglion lesions should be considered (see below).

Other alternatives include the use of neurolytics (either alcohol or phenol) intrathecally or extradurally via a catheter.

Side-effects of the intraplexus neurolytic include failure to relieve pain, with or without motor impairment and chemical neuritis with increased pain or pain of a different nature — a burning dysaesthesia — that may be unresponsive to oral or parenteral analgesics.

Pneumothorax is a complication of the technique, and the production of a persistent sinus along the track of the needle or catheter may be seen occasionally.

Nerve root

Dorsal root ganglion lesion

This procedure is used mainly for pain in the distribution of one or possibly two nerve roots on one side of the body. Destruction of the cell bodies of the neurones avoids regeneration and produces analgesia in the distribution of the nerve.

Following a prognostic block using local anaesthesia, a radiofrequency probe is introduced under X-ray control into the appropriate intervertebral foramen. The dorsal root ganglia (DRG) are situated posteriorly in the intervertebral foramina and on an anteroposterior view are at the level of a line joining the articular spaces of the facet joints.

Radio-opaque dye is injected to outline the nerve root (Fig. 81.7) and correct localization checked by electrical stimulation (100 Hz at 1.0 V or less) which causes paraesthesiae in the area affected by the pain or reproduces the pain itself. Local anaesthetic is instilled through the probe and the lesion made (80°C for 60 s).

Basically, the technique is similar at all spinal levels (Figs 81.8 and 81.9), but below L5 it may be necessary to make burr holes to obtain access to the ganglia of the sacral roots.

The main side-effect is neuritis which may be severe and require medication with anticonvulsant drugs. If untreated, the condition abates within 6–8 weeks.

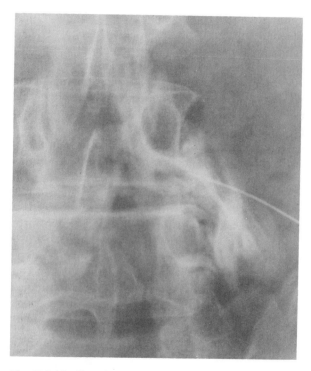

Fig. 81.7 Needle in lumbar intervertebral foramen. Contrast is seen outlining nerve root, dorsal root ganglion and flowing into the extradural space.

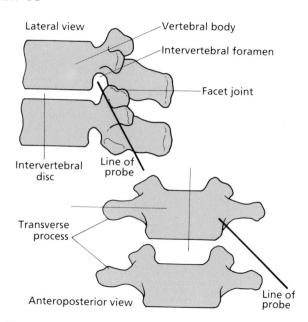

Fig. 81.9 Position of probe for dorsal root ganglion lesion. Diagrammatic representation taken from X-rays.

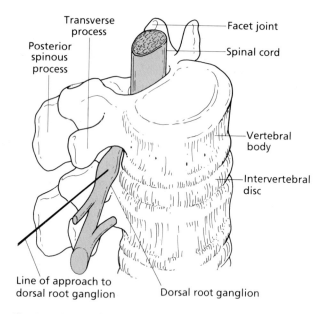

Fig. 81.8 Approach to the dorsal root ganglion.

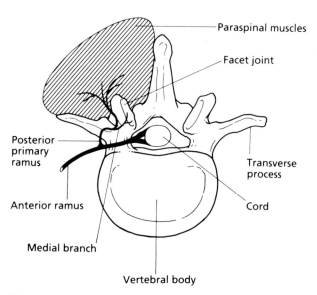

Fig. 81.10 Nerve supply to a lumbar facet joint.

Posterior primary ramus

The medial branch of the posterior primary ramus provides the articular branches to the facet joints (Fig. 81.10). These joints may undergo similar degener-

ative and post-traumatic changes affecting any synovial joint. This results in pain not only in the back in the distribution of the posterior ramus but also in part or all of the distribution of the anterior primary ramus.

Radiofrequency denervation of these joints may be undertaken if local anaesthetic diagnostic block caused temporary pain relief. Under X-ray control, the probe is inserted to a position at the cephalad or caudad (Fig. 81.11) end of the joint in order to lesion

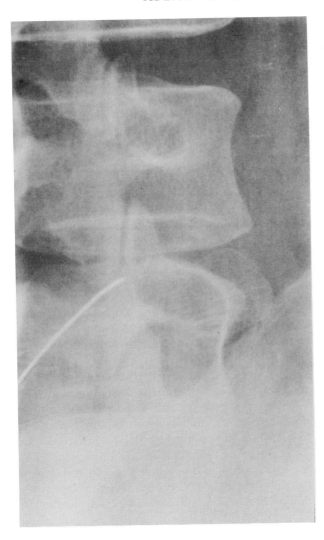

Fig. 81.11 Probe at lower pole of facet joint prior to performing a lesion.

the nerve supply to both aspects. Alternatively, the probe is inserted in the groove at the base of the transverse process in which the nerve runs before supplying the joint.

The radiofrequency probe is adjusted to produce a temperature in the range 80–90°C for 60–160 s. With the standard probe of 4 mm tip, the longer lesion time at the higher temperature produces a lesion of 5 mm in its longer diameter (Sluijter & Mehta, 1981).

Side-effects are rare; transient back ache is the most common.

Extradural

The use of extradural neurolytics is restricted usually to those patients who have malignant disease causing pain. The technique has been advocated for patients with severe postherpetic neuralgia but the results do not confirm early optimism for this therapy.

The neurolytic agent may be administered as a single injection using aqueous phenol if spread over several segments is required, or phenol in glycerine if a localized effect is required at one segmental level (Swerdlow, 1974). Catheterization of the extradural space is recommended for repeated injections until optimal results are produced; slow, constant infusion of neurolytic using a syringe-driver may also be useful.

In the lower lumbar or sacral regions, the minimum quantity of neurolytic should be used to obviate spread onto the sacral roots subserving sphincter control to avoid rendering the patient incontinent.

Following resection of rectal cancer, the presacral plexus may have been damaged and urinary sphincter control may be affected readily by small amounts of neurolytic. The most common presentation is with urinary retention which settles usually after a few days.

Other side-effects include painful neuritis, burning dysaesthesia in the affected nerves together with distressing numbness which, in some patients, may be worse than the original pain.

Subdural and subarachnoid

The extraarachnoid subdural space has been used as the site of deposition of neurolytic solutions in patients with malignant disease (Maher & Mehta, 1977). The technique described was for use in the cervical spine with phenol 5% in glycerine, but it appears to have no advantages compared with the easier subarachnoid block.

The aim of subarachnoid block is destruction of segmental nerves at the dorsal roots but there may be damage to ventral roots and cord also. The indication for its use is malignant disease where life expectancy is short and pain is severe.

Hyperbaric phenol in glycerine is used if the patient is able to lie with the painful side dependent; if not, hypobaric alcohol is used to float in the CSF.

Following dural puncture, the position of the patient is adjusted with the aid of small amounts of contrast medium injected into CSF. The position of the patient is altered until the correct flow pattern is achieved. The neurolytic is injected, but the patient must remain motionless until the agent fixes to tissues.

The maximum volumes of agents recommended to prevent undue spread (Swerdlow, 1974) are phenol, 0.5 ml, and alcohol, 1.0 ml. It may be necessary to repeat this procedure several times to cover all the segments involved, especially if the pain is bilateral. This technique is more suitable, therefore, for unilateral, sacral or perineal pain caused by malignant disease infiltrating the pelvis or lower lumbar and sacral spine. Lumbar puncture is performed with the patient sitting, and before instillation of hyperbaric neurolytic solution, the patient is tilted backwards to 45° so that the agent runs down the posterior dural wall, investing only the dorsal sensory roots. During this manoeuvre the sacral motor roots are at risk; sphincter disturbances may occur — frequently transient but occasionally permanent. Perineal numbness and paraesthesiae may be unpleasant, particularly if unanticipated, because of failure to perform a previous local anaesthetic block.

The most common side-effects are related to sensory root damage and include numbness, paraesthesiae and hyperaesthesiae, all of which are usually temporary. Motor paralysis and sphincter disturbances occur rarely, usually with lower lumbar and sacral blocks. Uncommonly, anterior and posterior spinal artery thrombosis may occur causing partial or profound neurological damage. Direct damage to nerve roots by the needle used for the injection may also cause motor and sensory deficit but this persists rarely for more than a few days. Neuritis has been reported following the use of subarachnoid alcohol and headache and neck stiffness have been experienced particularly after cervical neurolytic injections (Swerdlow, 1983).

Cord

Percutaneous cervical cordotomy

Surgical section of the anterolateral quadrant of the spinal cord was introduced at the beginning of this century. The open method has been superseded almost entirely by the percutaneous cervical radiofrequency heat lesion in the relevant area of the lateral spinothalamic tract (Rosomoff *et al.*, 1965) (Fig. 81.12) to produce analgesia on the contralateral side to the lesion.

There are three approaches to the anterolateral aspect of the cervical cord: laterally through the C1—2 intervertebral space (Rosomoff *et al.*, 1965) (the most common), through a cervical intervertebral disc space (Linn *et al.*, 1966) and a posterior approach between the base of the skull and C1 (Hitchcock, 1969).

Percutaneous cervical cordotomy is suited ideally for patients who have a life expectation not exceeding 2 years, as the average duration of effect of the

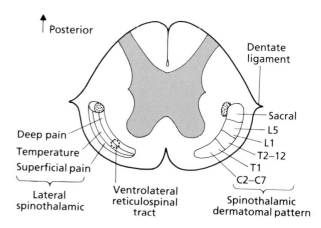

Fig. 81.12 Cross-section of human spinal cord at C2 level.

technique is 2 years (Nathan, 1963). It is not a stressful procedure and can be used even in very ill or frail patients. All patients suffering inoperable malignant conditions with pain below the L5 dermatome should be considered for treatment by this method. For those with a normal life expectancy the only patients suitable for cordotomy are elderly patients with severe pain in the lower half of the body (Lipton, 1984).

With the supine patient sedated sufficiently to produce comfort, immobility and ability to respond to questions, the needle (Fig. 81.13) is inserted under X-ray image intensification control through the C1—2 interspace until its tip lies anterior to the dentate ligament (Fig. 81.12). Contrast medium is injected to outline the anterior surface of the cord, the dentate ligament and the posterior dura. A position of the needle 1—2 mm anterior to the dentate ligament and 2—3 mm posterior to the anterior cord surface is ideal. The electrode is inserted through the needle and connected to the impedance meter. When the uninsulated tip of the electrode is in CSF, impedance is low; on entering cord tissue the change in impedance is in the order of 300—1000 ohms. When there is a satisfactory impedance recording, the lesion generator is switched to the stimulus mode. As the voltage is increased, pulsations at 2 Hz are seen in the neck and trapezius muscles on the ipsilateral side. Stimulation at 100 Hz produces sensory hallucinations at approximately one-tenth of the voltage used at 2 Hz stimulation. When all conditions are satisfied, i.e. X-ray position, correct impedance measurement and stimulation producing sensations in the painful part of the body, a small test lesion is made using a current of no more than 20 mA for 30 s. The degree of tract ablation is checked by careful mapping of the hyperaesthetic region on the contralateral body surface. During the passage of current it

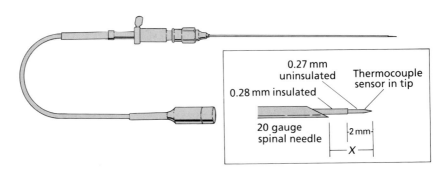

Fig. 81.13 Cordotomy cannula and electrode with details of tip. X, variable electrode extension depending on sizing clamp setting. (Courtesy of Radionics Ltd.)

is essential that corticospinal tract function of the ipsilateral side is evaluated by testing grip strength, etc.

In general, the lesion is produced gradually as a series of bursts of radiofrequency current each no longer than 30 s until the hypalgesic area corresponds to that in which pain is felt. Once the area of analgesia is achieved, the final power and time of coagulation used are repeated three times with intervals of 1 min to allow heat to dissipate. Horner's syndrome occurs on the ipsilateral side and transitory weakness of the ipsilateral leg develops, returning to normal in a few days.

Decreased or absent thermal sensation occurs also over the whole of the analgesic area and may extend for a few segments beyond.

The main side-effects are motor weakness (40% of these patients have to alter their lifestyle; 2% have permanent weakness), late developing dysaesthesia in the treated area, and occasional disturbance of respiration in patients who have pre-existing respiratory problems, particularly in carcinoma of lung. Impotence, headache, ataxia, hemiparesis and micturition disturbance have been described following cordotomy, but are rare. The frequency of all side-effects and complications is increased dramatically if the cordotomy is bilateral.

Cranial nerves

Trigeminal nerve

The classical facial pain experienced in the distribution of one or more of the divisions of the trigeminal nerve is trigeminal neuralgia or 'tic douloureux'. The pain is usually transient and described often as 'lancinating'. It is felt mainly in the second and third divisions of the nerve. The pain radiates frequently from one or more trigger points, one of which is often the nasolabial fold. The pain may be induced

by touching the trigger area, eating and drinking, talking and cold winds.

Many patients respond to therapy with anticonvulsant drugs, but destructive therapy of peripheral branches of the nerve or the ganglion may be necessary because of lack of drug efficacy, inability of the patient to tolerate the drug, drug-induced blood dyscrasias and breakthrough pain. If ablative therapy is considered, investigations must be undertaken to exclude defined pathology. These include plain X-rays of the skull including a submentovertical projection and computerized tomography (CT) scan to exclude tumours of the base of skull and some vascular lesions.

If the patient is young, a neurological opinion should be sought to exclude multiple sclerosis or other possible CNS pathologies, particularly if remote neurological signs are evident on routine examination.

Ablative procedures should be considered also if the trigeminal pain results from inoperable malignant disease.

There are two main approaches to the treatment of trigeminal neuralgia: ablative lesions of the peripheral branches or direct approach to the ganglion within the skull. The former may be achieved mainly at the exit foramina of the three divisions of the nerve from the skull using neurolytic chemicals (alcohol, phenol), cryolesions, radiofrequency lesions or surgical neurectomy. These produce not only analgesia in the selected division but also complete anaesthesia which may be extremely distressing.

Lesions of the ganglion may be induced with either glycerine or radiofrequency. The use of glycerine has an advantage that it is a relatively minor procedure giving pain relief in approximately 65% in the long term with only slight disturbance of facial sensation (Hakanson, 1983).

Under X-ray control the trigeminal cistern is punctured percutaneously by the anterior route via the foramen ovale. Following drainage of CSF, a small (0.5 ml) volume of contrast medium (metrizamide) is injected to verify the position of the tip of the needle within the cistern. Glycerine, 0.2–0.3 ml, is injected and the patient maintained in the sitting position for at least 1 h (Fig. 81.14).

The most common side-effect is headache, occurring almost immediately after the injection of glycerine. This usually resolves rapidly with the use of simple analgesics, e.g. paracetamol.

The radiofrequency coagulation technique utilizes the same approach as that for the instillation of glycerine, but is performed usually under general anaesthesia. After insertion through the foramen ovale, the probe (Fig. 81.15) is advanced under or through the ganglion into the sensory roots in the subarachnoid space of the trigeminal cave. The patient is allowed to waken, a 100 Hz stimulating current is applied to the probe and its position adjusted until the patient experiences paraesthesiae in the area of the face in which the neuralgia is experienced. Brief sleep is induced whilst the first lesion is made (usually 60 s at 65°C). The patient is wakened and the face tested with pinprick and cotton wool. The ideal is to produce diminution of sensation in the area over which pain is felt, and further lesions may be made by increasing the temperature of the probe tip to 80 or 90°C until this is achieved. If pain is experienced mainly in the first division, it may be difficult to angle the probe through the foramen ovale to reach the specific root fibres. To overcome this problem, a side-extension-tip probe has been developed which, when inserted through the can-

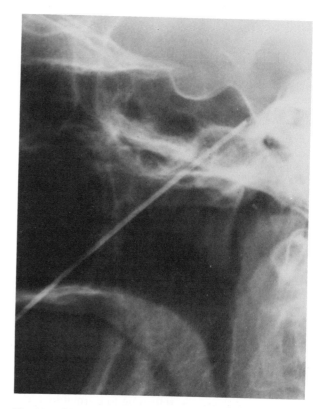

Fig. 81.14 Needle in Gasserian ganglion.

nula, curves to one side allowing the relevant fibres to be lesioned (Fig. 81.16).

The side-effects of thermocoagulation include numbness in the treated portion of the face and, rarely, keratitis if the first division is treated. Anaesthesia dolorosa may occur also, but the radiofrequency

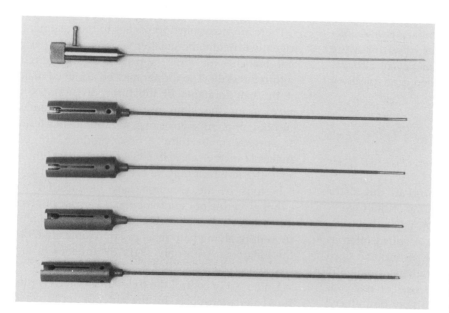

Fig. 81.15 Trigeminal probes with 2 mm, 5 mm, 7 mm and 10 mm uninsulated tips.

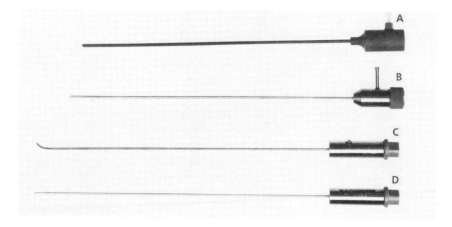

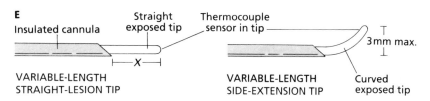

Fig. 81.16 Trigeminal lesion unit with side-extension tip. (A) Cannula (insulated); (B) stilette; (C) variable-length side-extension tip; (D) variable-length straight tip; (E) details of (C) and (D).

E

Insulated cannula | Straight exposed tip | Thermocouple sensor in tip | 3mm max.

VARIABLE-LENGTH STRAIGHT-LESION TIP

VARIABLE-LENGTH SIDE-EXTENSION TIP | Curved exposed tip

technique is less likely to produce this complication than open surgical rhizotomy or neurolytic injection into the ganglion (Miles, 1980; Rizzi *et al.*, 1985; Schrotter, 1985).

Glossopharyngeal nerve

Glossopharyngeal neuralgia is an episodic pain of marked intensity, described as hot, burning, sharp or knife-like. Pain is felt in the base of the tongue, larynx, tonsillar region, face, neck or scalp. Constant, dull, aching sensations may persist between attacks which may be triggered by eating, swallowing, chewing or talking (Rushton *et al.*, 1981). A variety of other symptoms may accompany attacks including hiccups, cardiac arrythmias, laryngeal stridor and coughing. Initially, treatment comprises therapy with anticonvulsant drugs, but in unresponsive cases, ablation of the nerve may be produced in the post-tonsillar space. Following initial diagnostic block with local anaesthetic, nerve ablation may be carried out using either cryotherapy or radiofrequency coagulation.

The needle or probe is introduced through the anterior pillar or the tonsil on the affected side to a depth of 5 mm, and the lesion made using either two 2-min freeze cycles for a cryolesion or a 90°C × 80 s thermal lesion (Fig. 81.17). The procedure is relatively free from side-effects with the exception of occasional transient neuritis and sore throat.

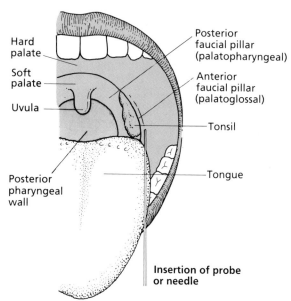

Fig. 81.17 Glossopharyngeal nerve lesion through tonsillar pillar.

Pituitary ablation

Pituitary ablation has been used to treat patients with pain produced by advanced malignant disease, especially those with bone metastases from breast, prostate and renal tumours unresponsive to drug therapy.

The gland has been subject to destruction by

surgery, ionizing radiation, radioactive implants, injection of alcohol and, more recently, by cryo- or radiofrequency lesions.

All techniques produce pain relief in 70% of cases for approximately 3–4 months although some patients have freedom from pain at 1 year. The exact mechanism of analgesia is unknown, but as pain relief is experienced immediately after the ablative procedure, it is unlikely to be mediated hormonally.

For chemical, thermal or cryodestruction of the pituitary gland, the cannula or probe may be passed through the nose and through the sphenoid bone into the pituitary fossa, under biplanar X-ray control (Moricca, 1977; Duthie, 1983).

The incidence of side-effects and the need for hormone replacement vary according to the operator and technique used. The most dangerous complication is blindness, which is the main reason for loss of popularity of this technique.

There is a suggestion that pituitary ablation may have a small role in the treatment of pain from non-cancerous sources (Gallimore & Duthie, 1987).

Autonomic system

There is a sound clinical basis for the use of autonomic block in the treatment of many specific painful disorders (Table 81.2).

In general terms, ablation should be preceded always by a diagnostic block with local anaesthetic.

Ablative procedures should be performed always with the aid of X-ray image intensification, and the use of contrast medium. Full resuscitation facilities should be available.

The most commonly used ablative agents are alcohol and phenol. The former is more painful on injection and causes significantly more neuritis.

More recently, both cryolesions and radiofrequency lesions have been used, particularly in the lumbar sympathetic chain. The areas in which the sympathetic chain may be ablated are:

Stellate ganglion. This is approached most readily from the front using a paratracheal approach. The sympathetic chain lies on both C6 and C7 transverse processes and can be reached easily using a short 3-cm needle (Boas, 1983).

Upper thoracic chain. This may be approached posteriorly with the patient in the prone position. The levels destroyed most frequently are T2, T3 and T4 (Wilkinson, 1984).

Splanchnic nerve ablation. This provides good analgesia for upper abdominal malignant disease and chronic pancreatitis with an efficacy equal to that of coeliac plexus block but it utilizes less neurolytic solution and produces much less neuritis and hypotension (Fig. 81.18).

Coeliac plexus block. This is the traditional technique for upper abdominal malignant disease (with alcohol

Table 81.2 Clinical objectives of sympathetic block. (After Boas, 1983)

Sympathetic dystrophy
Diagnostic confirmation
Treatment

Improvement in blood flow
Vasospastic disorders
Acute cold trauma, thromboembolic ischaemia
Postsurgical vasodilatation
Arteriosclerotic disease

Visceral pain
Diagnosis
Long-term treatment

Differential diagnosis
Sympathetic pain or peripheral neuralgia
Somatic or visceral pain

Hyperhydrosis and postherpetic neuralgia
Treatment

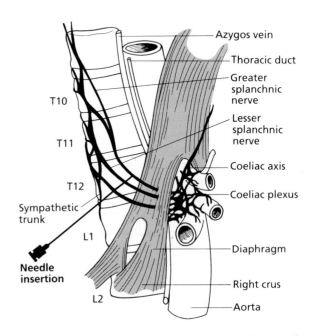

Fig. 81.18 Splanchnic nerve block — anatomy and approach.

or phenol). Large volumes of neurolytic are required and this may be associated with a high incidence of side-effects. The procedure should be performed under general anaesthesia.

Lumbar sympathectomy. This is the standard ablative procedure for the treatment of ischaemic rest pain in the lower limbs, and is used also for pelvic malignancy or causalgia in the perineum. The use of neurolytic solutions is being replaced gradually by thermal lesioning of the sympathetic chain at L2, 3, 4. (Figs 81.19 and 81.20).

Surgery

Surgery for the relief of pain should be considered only when all other appropriate therapies have been utilized appropriately. The risks of destructive surgery include neurological deficit and incapacity; in time, the pain is likely to return but residual dysfunction may persist. It is possible to attempt further destruction of nervous tissue on a second occasion, but pain recurs usually following a shorter period of remission, and the degree of residual dysfunction may be increased.

These risks are often acceptable in patients in the terminal stages of malignant disease. In those with a normal life expectancy, surgical techniques should be considered only when the relatively non-destructive techniques have failed and the patient has become desperate. Operative intervention may take place at three levels of the pain transmission system (Fig. 81.21).

1 In the region of the first-order neurone. This

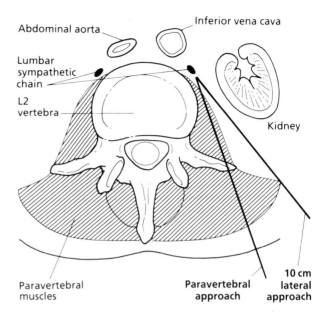

Fig. 81.20 Lumbar sympathectomy — anatomy and approaches.

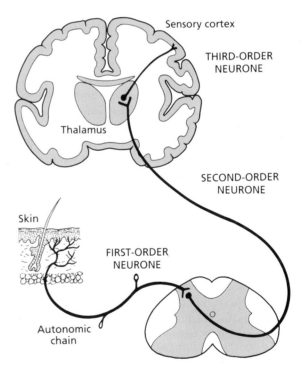

Fig. 81.21 Levels of surgical intervention in the CNS for the relief of pain.

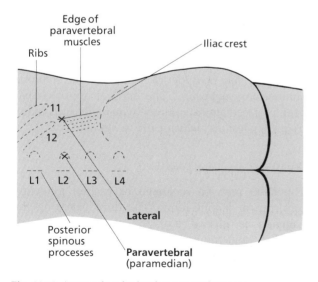

Fig. 81.19 Approaches for lumbar sympathectomy.

includes the area of the receptor apparatus of the peripheral nerve and the afferent spinal nerve root.
2 In the region of the second-order neurone. This includes the dorsal horn, spinal decussation, cord and midbrain up to the synapse in the thalamus.

3 In the region of the third-order neurone. This includes the postsynaptic thalamic regions to the sensory cortex, frontal lobes, limbic system, pituitary and hypothalamus.

In addition to the above neuronal pathways, the autonomic system may be subjected to surgical ablative procedures for the relief of certain chronic painful conditions, hyperhydrosis, etc.

Surgery has a higher success rate for neuronal destruction than other forms of ablation, but it possesses also greater morbidity and mortality. It cannot be performed at many intracranial sites.

First-order neurone

Excision of skin

The removal of damaged peripheral sense organs has been practised in such conditions as postherpetic neuralgia and following burns. Reinnervation of the subsequent scarred tissue results frequently in a patchy, dysaesthetic area which is more painful than the original lesion. Because of this poor long-term prospect, the technique is performed rarely.

Section of the peripheral nerve

Peripheral nerves may be exposed and sectioned easily. However, there are few indications for this intervention mainly because of the speed at which regeneration occurs, resulting in restoration of the pain. The commonest indication is when ablation of another modality such as muscle tone is required, and sectioning of the peripheral nerve produces analgesia and loss of tone, e.g. multiple sclerosis with painful muscle spasms responds to nerve ablation. Nerve section may be employed also when other forms of neurolysis have failed. Nerve injection, cryotherapy and radiofrequency lesions may not alleviate the pain of abdominal wall nerve entrapment, and section of the segmental nerves as they perforate the posterior rectus sheath produces pain relief. In the debilitated patient who cannot tolerate intracranial surgery for relief of trigeminal neuralgia, section of the appropriate nerve under local anaesthesia as it emerges from the skull, e.g. via the supraorbital or infraorbital foramina, is the treatment of choice.

Root section

Surgery on the root may be performed in a number of locations (Fig. 81.22).

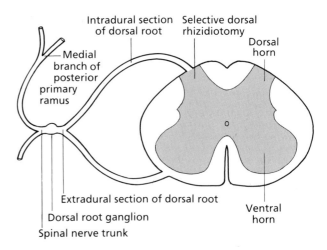

Fig. 81.22 Locations for root surgery.

Posterior primary ramus

The innervation of the posterior articular facet joints of the spine is by the medial branch of the posterior primary ramus. Attempts to denervate these structures were described first in 1971 by Rees using a long scalpel blade percutaneously to sever the articular branches. This technique has been replaced by the use of either radiofrequency or cryotherapy (Shealy, 1975; Sluijter & Mehta, 1981). Occasionally, during surgery for disc exploration, the nerve supply to degenerate facet joints may be sectioned under direct vision rather than perform a facetectomy.

Spinal nerve root

If a painful dermatome requires denervation, an extradural approach is probably the most logical. Thirty percent of afferent sensory fibres enter the spinal cord via the ventral root, even though their cell bodies are in the DRG (Coggeshall *et al.*, 1974).

From a technical aspect, intraspinal approaches are easier and may be undertaken through the standard laminectomy exposure. The surgical approach has been replaced almost entirely by percutaneous radiofrequency lesions, which carry fewer side-effects.

Dorsal root ganglionectomy

The DRG may be sectioned or excised following exposure at laminectomy. The dura overlying the ganglion is incised and the ganglion removed, thereby preventing regeneration. The technique suffers from the problems of all sensory root sections; apart from single root-pain syndromes such as chronic disc prolapse, at least two nerve roots above and below the painful segments should be sectioned in addition to the painful segment innervation, as there is considerable sensory overlap. The anaesthesia accompanying division of many roots (especially when involving a limb) makes the operation unattractive.

Extradural root section

The dorsal root may be sectioned proximal to the ganglion through an intraspinal, extradural approach. A hemilaminectomy and facetectomy are performed to expose the relevant root sheath. After identification of the root sheath, it is opened for 5–8 mm just proximal to the ganglion, thereby exposing the dorsal and ventral fibres separated by the dural septum. The ventral roots may be identified by electrical stimulation and the production of muscle contractions. If a 'wake-up' anaesthetic technique is used, stimulation of the dorsal fibres in the awake patient confirms the contribution that the root is making to the pain.

Following accurate identification, the dorsal fibres are cut.

Intradural root section

Intradural roots are conveniently sectioned in the cervical and thoracic segments as the nerve roots exit at levels corresponding to cord level. For intradural section, the correct vertebral level must be ascertained by radiography. After hemilaminectomy, the dura is opened together with arachnoid and the dorsal rootlets at the correct level identified, sometimes by electrical stimulation in doubtful cases. The relevant rootlets are then divided.

Six adjacent thoracic roots may be sectioned without significant loss of function, but in the cervical and lumbar regions, the number of roots sectioned is governed by the potential loss of limb function.

After the section of a single dorsal root of brachial or lumbar plexus, no proprioceptive deficit and only minimal hypoaesthesia was seen in a series of spinal rhizotomies (White & Kjellberg, 1973). It was recommended also that in the cervical plexus C6 or C7 or else both C5 and C8 should be spared to protect proprioception in the upper limb, and at least one root of L2–4 in cases of extensive lumbosacral rhizotomy. Section of both L5 and S1 may interfere with proprioception in the foot.

Selective dorsal rhizidiotomy

At the junction of each dorsal rootlet with the spinal cord, small afferent fibres tend to cluster in the ventrolateral section of the junction, and they may be divided here by a small incision where they penetrate Lissauer's tract (Sindov et al., 1974). There are no major limitations to the number and levels of rootlets which may be treated. Identification of rootlets may be made easier, particularly in the lumbosacral region, by electrical stimulation of the corresponding ventral roots observing for muscle contractions.

Spinal root surgery is useful often for pain associated with tumours of the apex of the lung with involvement of the brachial plexus. Selective rhizidiotomy may be used to prevent total denervation of the arm. It is also the procedure of choice in patients with pelvic malignant disease causing perineal and leg pain as useful afferent function may be preserved.

In general terms, spinal root surgery produces better results in malignant disease than in nonmalignant situations, although the long-term results are not good in both groups.

In benign conditions, the most consistent results are obtained with root surgery in occipital neuralgia, which may be relieved often permanently by section of the first three cervical dorsal roots.

Postsurgical incisional pain, circumscribed posttraumatic pain and idiopathic intercostal neuralgia may often be managed effectively by either root section or ganglionectomy. Two roots above and below those involved should be sectioned.

Idiopathic coccydynia responds well to bilateral sacrococcygeal root section; the long-term results are good unless there is also pain in the back and/or leg (Albrektsson, 1981).

Conspicuous failures for root surgery include postherpetic neuralgia, postlumbar-disc-surgery pain and arachnoiditis.

Side-effects of root surgery include failure to achieve adequate analgesia, loss of proprioceptive facility in arms or legs after multiple root sections, loss of sphincter control and impotence after sacral root operations (in addition to the usual complications of open surgery) (Dubuisson, 1984).

After rhizotomy, numbness may be a problem in patients who have not been exposed previously to this by a local anaesthetic block. Genital hypoaesthesiae occur after sacral root surgery and may be made even more distressing if accompanied by impotence or sexual dysfunction.

Severe pain in deafferented dermatomes (anaesthesia dolorosa) may occur following rhizotomy or, more frequently, following ganglionectomy. Transitory paraplegia may follow bleeding into extradural or subarachnoid spaces but irreversible damage to the cord may be produced if this is not diagnosed early or if there is devascularization of the cord—spinal artery syndrome.

Because of the major nature of the surgery and the high failure and complication rate, open surgery to the spinal roots is being replaced almost completely by the use of radiofrequency lesioning of structures.

Cranial nerve surgery

Trigeminal nerve

Surgical treatment for trigeminal neuralgia is reserved for patients who fail to respond to anticonvulsant drug therapy or who are unable to tolerate these drugs. There also is a small group of patients whose pain relief following other forms of interventional therapy is transient (radiofrequency lesions, glycerine injections and pressure applied to the Gasserian ganglion by balloon). In such patients, the operation of suboccipital craniectomy with microvascular decompression of the trigeminal nerve is appropriate (Jannetta, 1976). The procedure is performed under general anaesthesia using a small, lateral suboccipital craniectomy and the trigeminal nerve exposed by retracting the cerebellum. Up to 90% of patients have impingement by a small artery or vein upon the nerve, and in 1—3%, a tumour or bony abnormality is found. Approximately 5—10% have no apparent pathology. Any tumour is removed and any vessel is eased from the nerve and kept separate by the insertion of a piece of sponge or muscle.

In the group of patients without pathology, a sub total rhizotomy is performed on the main sensory root preserving some touch sensation over the face and the corneal reflex. The small fibres carrying touch and corneal sensation diverge from the main sensory root just before its entry into the pons and are identified at this point. Following rhizotomy, long-term success rate is 80%, morbidity 5—10% and mortality 1—2% (Loeser, 1984). Peripheral nerve avulsions should be offered only when gangliolysis has failed and the patient cannot or will not tolerate the intracranial procedure. They result in dense sensory loss and provide pain relief for only 1—2 years. Repeated avulsions are even less likely to be successful.

Patients who have failed to obtain relief from any of these techniques may be offered descending trigeminal tractotomy. This is performed through a C1—2 laminectomy and results in loss of pain and temperature sensation on the ipsilateral side of the face but does not alter touch perception.

Geniculate neuralgia

Geniculate neuralgia has characteristic paroxysms of pain felt deep within the ear. This may be relieved by severing the fibres of the nervus intermedius through a posterior fossa approach (Sachs, 1968).

Glossopharyngeal neuralgia

Glossopharyngeal neuralgia is a severe tic-like pain experienced in the tonsillar region and back of the tongue or larynx. It is induced by swallowing or talking. On rare occasions, the pain may be associated with syncopal attacks, presumably because of involvement of branches from the carotid sinus.

This condition responds frequently to anticonvulsant drug therapy. Resistant cases may be treated surgically by severing the ninth nerve in the neck near the styloid process. The best results are obtained using a posterior fossa exposure and section of the glossopharyngeal rootlets intracranially after separation of these from the vagus.

Autonomic faciocephalgia

Autonomic faciocephalgia (or, as it is more commonly termed, sphenopalatine neuralgia) is a diffuse pain experienced often in the upper half of the face and associated with unilateral lacrimation and nasal discharge. Many cases respond to ergotamine preparations (as does migraine) but intractable cases may be treated by trigeminal nerve section or section of the petrosal nerves through an extradural temporal approach (Gardner et al., 1947). Section of the nervus intermedius may be more effective (Sachs, 1968).

Second-order neurone

Anterolateral cordotomy

The cord is exposed by laminectomy at either the upper thoracic level for lower trunk and leg pain or in the upper cervical segment for pain extending up to the fifth cervical dermatome.

Access to the contralateral anterolateral quadrant is obtained by gripping and dividing a digitation of the dentate ligament and using it to rotate the cord. The anterolateral tract is cut between two consecutive roots. In this quadrant, the spinothalamic tract exhibits some somatotopic stratification with lower sacral and coccygeal dermatomes being represented superficially and posteriorly whilst higher dermatomes are represented more deeply (Fig. 81.23).

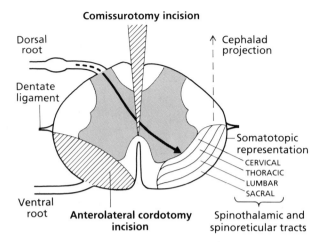

Fig. 81.23 Direct surgical approaches to the cord in the cervical and upper thoracic regions.

The analgesia produced is always temporary and lasts for a maximum of 2 years. Consequently, anterolateral cordotomy is usually reserved for patients with a life expectancy limited by malignant disease.

Repeated cordotomy is associated with progressively reduced analgesia both in level and duration. There is an increase also in the risk of neurological morbidity.

Even in the best series, ipsilateral hemiparesis occurs in approximately 15%, postoperative dysaesthesia in 5% and disturbance of sphincter control and sexual function in 5% of patients. These disturbances increase to approximately 20% if bilateral cordotomy is performed; in addition this carries the risk of damage to respiratory function and the possible emergence of 'Ondine's syndrome'.

The introduction of the percutaneous radiofrequency procedure has replaced the surgical method almost totally.

Spinal commisurotomy

Spinal commisurotomy is the division of the spinothalamic fibres as they cross the midline of the cord prior to their ascent in the anterolateral tract (Fig. 81.23).

As the fibres cross only gradually, often taking several segments, it may be difficult to determine the length of incision required to produce adequate analgesia. Consequently, a long, multiple laminectomy must be performed. This may explain why the duration of effect does not equate with that following cordotomy (King, 1977).

Brainstem tractotomies

These are major operations designed to section the spinothalamic tract at various locations in the midbrain to obtain analgesia without the additional anaesthesia seen with other destructive procedures. Medullary spinothalamic tractotomy involves exposing the medulla between the superior roots of the accessory nerve and the inferior olive, at which point the tract is deep to the spinocerebellar tract. Trigeminal tractotomy is designed to divide the descending spinothalamic tract of the trigeminal nerve in the medulla. The operation is a posterior fossa exploration with division of the tract, which is within the medullary substance lateral to the line of the cuneate nucleus and behind the line of exit of the spinal accessory nerve rootlets.

Brainstem tractotomy is designed to section the spinothalamic tract in the dorsolateral tegmentum between the superior and inferior colliculi. Morbidity is high with many persistent side-effects, including dysaesthesia and diplopia. These operative procedures are rarely performed because of the high morbidity and failure rates.

Third-order neurone

The use of surgery in the region of the third-order neurone is confined almost entirely to the thalamus where stereotactically controlled heat lesions, radiofrequency lesions or cryolesions are induced.

At least part of the spinothalamic tract ends in the region of the ventral posterolateral nucleus of the thalamus and lesions of this locus do not produce analgesia but rather sensory deficits. Indirect pain pathways via the reticular formation connect with the more medial areas of the thalamus and lesions in the centremedian, parafascicularis and intralaminar areas tend to relieve pain without producing sensory deficit. Lesions in the more posterior parts such as the pulvinar, produce analgesia also without sensory deficit but often produce hemiparesis.

Spiegel has summarized the value of thalamic lesions (Spiegel & Wycis, 1966):
1 Pain may be relieved by lesions in either the medial or the lateral pain-conducting systems.
2 Improved results occur by attacking both systems.
3 Successful procedures should produce analgesia for more than 5 years.
4 If long-lasting analgesia is required, these procedures should be undertaken only as a last resort in view of extensive lesions.

There remain three types of surgery on the third

neurone for which certain claims have been made but which are used rarely.

Leucotomy

Frontal leucotomy consists of the interruption of the frontothalamic pathways in the basomedial frontal lobe. The greater the degree of interruption, the greater is the likelihood of pain relief but, at the same time, the greater the modification of affect. This latter effect has rendered the procedure of debatable value and ethically dubious.

Hypothalamotomy

The hypothalamus has numerous direct connections with the thalamus and direct and indirect connections with many parts of the sensory system. Stereotaxic lesions in the posterior medial hypothalamus have been claimed (Sano, 1973) to produce good results in painful malignancy. Ipsilateral lesions were found to

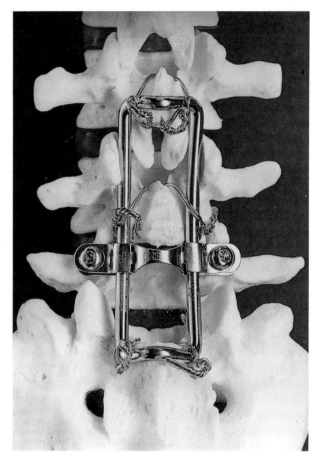

Fig. 81.25 Hartshill rectangle with pedicle screw-bridge modification showing fixation of lumbar spine. (Permission of Mr J. Dove and Surgicraft Ltd.)

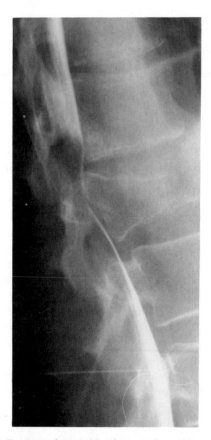

Fig. 81.24 Fracture of second lumbar vertebra with posterior displacement and cord compression (myelogram). (Permission of Mr J. Dove and Surgicraft Ltd.)

be effective in head and neck pain whilst contralateral lesions appeared better for pain relief below that level.

Cortical ablation

Cortical ablation of the parietal sensory cortex followed reports of analgesia being associated with pathological lesions of this area. Long-term results have not been encouraging but Lebal (1973) claims the technique is useful when applied to the frontal cortex.

Surgery of the autonomic system

Surgery of the autonomic system is confined mainly to situations where repeated percutaneous attempts at neurolysis by chemical, cryo- or radiofrequency lesion have failed to produce lasting analgesia.

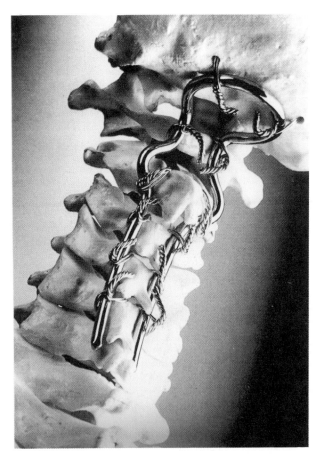

Fig. 81.26 Hartshill–Ransford loop. Posterior cervical spinal fixation. (Permission of Mr J. Dove and Surgicraft Ltd.)

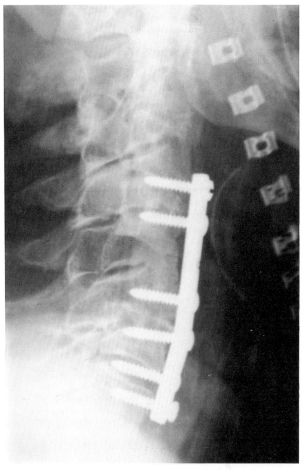

Fig. 81.27 Banks–Dervin rod. Anterior fixation for metastatic involvement of C6 vertebral body. (Permission of Mr J. Miles, FRCS.)

Internal fixation of the unstable spine

Instability of the spine is not an uncommon cause of both severe acute and chronic pain.

Trauma is the commonest cause of acute spinal instability whilst malignant disease both primary and secondary, infection and rheumatoid arthritis more frequently produce chronic instability often with an insidious onset and increasing severe and unremitting pain (Fig. 81.24).

Bed rest and simple analgesics had been the treatment of preference for many years, but internal fixation of the mobile segment of the spine has more recently become a routine method, some would say the method of choice (Dove, 1989).

Internal fixation was first used in 1910 by Lange (1910) using steel bars; more recently, Harrington (1973) popularized the use of combinations of compression and distraction hooks and rods.

Significantly less traumatic techniques were introduced by Luque (1982) who used double L-shaped rods and sublaminar wires. Technical difficulties, however, prompted the combination of the L-rods to form a single rectangle (Dove, 1987).

The Hartshill rectangle (Fig. 81.25) has been used successfully at all levels in the spine and modifications have been introduced especially for the treatment of occipitoatlantoaxial instability, the Hartshill–Ransford loop (Fig. 81.26) (Ransford *et al.*, 1986).

Other types of fixation have also been found to be effective and may be used either anteriorly or posteriorly (Miles *et al.*, 1984; Redfern *et al.*, 1988) (Fig. 81.27).

Internal fixation of the spine is a relatively atraumatic procedure which will produce dramatic improvement in the patient's state with, frequently, complete remission of pain.

In cases of acute or chronic spinal instability where severe pain and/or impending cord damage is present, such techniques of fixation should always be seriously considered.

References

Alberts W.W., Wright E.W., Feinstein B. & Gleason C.A. (1972) Sensory responses elicited by subcortical high frequency electrical stimulation in man. *Journal of Neurosurgery* **36**, 80–2.

Albrektsson B. (1981) Sacral rhizotomy in cases of anococcygeal pain. *Acta Orthopaedica Scandinavica* **52**, 187–90.

Applegate W.V. (1972) Abdominal cutaneous nerve entrapment syndrome. *Surgery* **71**, 118–24.

Armstrong-Davison M.H. (1965) Refrigeration anaesthesia. In *The Evolution of Anaesthesia* pp. 162–70. Sherratt, London.

Barber R. (1971) Sclerosant therapy. In *Textbook of Orthopaedic Medicine*, vol. 2, 8th edn. (Ed. Cyriax J.) p. 286. Cassell, London.

Barnard J.D.W. (1980) The effect of extreme cold on sensory nerves. *Annals of the Royal College of Surgeons of England* **62**, 180–7.

Boas R.A. (1983) The sympathetic nervous system and pain relief. In *Relief of Intractable Pain* (Ed. Swerdlow M.) pp. 215–38. Elsevier, Amsterdam.

Brown A.S. (1981) Current views on the use of nerve blocking in the relief of chronic pain. In *The Therapy of Pain* (Ed. Swerdlow M.) pp. 111–34. MTP Press Ltd, Lancaster.

Bryce-Smith R. (1966) Local and regional analgesia. *Postgraduate Medical Journal* **42**, 367–9.

Budd K. (1981) Non-analgesic drugs in pain management. In *Persistent Pain*, vol. 3 (Eds Lipton S. & Miles J.) pp. 223–40. Academic Press, London.

Carter D.C., Lee P.W.R., Gill W. & Johnson R.J. (1972) The effect of cryosurgery on peripheral nerve function. *Journal of the Royal College of Surgeons of Edinburgh* **17**, 25–31.

Coggeshall R.E., Applebaum M.L., Fazan M., Stubes T.B. & Sykes M.T. (1974) Unmyelinated axon in human ventral roots, a possible explanation for the failure of dorsal rhizotomy to relieve pain. *Brain* **98**, 157–61.

Dam W.H. (1965) Therapeutic blocks. *Acta Chirurgica Scandinavica* **343**, 89S.

Dam W.H. & Larsen J.V.V. (1974) Peripheral nerve blocks in the relief of intractable pain. In *Relief of Intractable Pain* (Ed. Swerdlow M.) p. 133. Excerpta Medica. Amsterdam.

Dove J. (1987) Luque segmental spinal instrumentation: the use of the Hartshill rectangle. *Orthopedics* **10**, 955–61.

Dove J. (1989) Internal fixation of the cervical spine: the Hartshill system. In *Cervical Spine II* (Eds Louis R. & Weidner A.) pp. 79–86. Springer-Verlag, Marseille.

Dubuisson D. (1984) Root surgery. In *Textbook of Pain* (Eds Wall P.D. & Melzack R.) pp. 590–600. Churchill Livingstone, London.

Duthie A.M. (1983) Pituitary cryoablation. *Anaesthesia* **38**, 495–7.

Editorial (1964) *Lancet* **ii**, 896.

Ellis H. (1984) *Famous Operations*. Harwal, Pennsylvania.

Esplin D.W. (1970) Antiseptics and disinfectants: fungicides: ectoparasites. In *The Pharmacological Basis of Therapeutics* 4th edn (Eds Goodman L.S. & Gilman A.) p. 1036. Macmillan, London.

Gallimore A.P. & Duthie A.M. (1987) Pituitary cryotherapy: its use in the treatment of chronic non-malignant pain. *The Pain Clinic* **1**, 259–60.

Gardner W.J., Stowell A. & Dutlinger R. (1947) Petrosal nerve section for facial pain. *Journal of Neurosurgery* **4**, 105–6.

Hakanson S. (1981) Trigeminal neuralgia treated by injection of glycerol into the trigeminal cistern. *Neurosurgery* **9**, 638–9.

Hakanson S. (1983) Retrogasserian glycerol as a treatment of tic douloureux. In *Advances in Pain Research and Therapy*, vol. 5 (Ed. Bonica J.J., Lindblom U. & Iggo A.) New York, Raven Press.

Harrington P.R. (1973) The history and development of Harrington instrumentation. *Clinical Orthopaedics* **93**, 110–12.

Hitchcock E.R. (1969) An apparatus for stereotactic spinal surgery. *Lancet* **i**, 705–6.

Hitchcock E.R. & Pradinin M.N. (1973) Hypertonic saline in the management of intractable pain. *Lancet* **i**, 310.

Jannetta P.J. (1976) Microsurgical approach to the trigeminal nerve for tic douloureux. *Progress in Neurological Surgery* **7**, 180–200.

Jones M.J.T. & Murrin K.R. (1987) Intercostal block with cryotherapy. *Annals of the Royal College of Surgeons of England* **69**, 261–2.

Katz J., Nelson W., Forest R. & Bruce D.L. (1980) Cryoanalgesia for post thoracotomy pain. *Lancet* **ii**, 512–13.

Khalli A.A. & Ditzler J.W. (1968) Neurolytic substances in the relief of pain. *Medical Clinics of North America* **52**, 161–71.

King R.B. (1977) Anterior commissurotomy for intractable pain. *Journal of Neurosurgery* **47**, 7–12.

Lange F. (1910) Support for the spondylitic spine by means of buried steel bars attached to the vertebrae. *American Journal of Orthopaedic Surgery* **8**, 344–6.

Lebal J. (1973) Limited frontal lesions, open and stereostatic. *Symposium sur la Doleur* pp. 24–5. Paris.

Linn P.M., Gildenberg P.L. & Polakoff P.P. (1966) An anterior approach to percutaneous lower cervical cordotomy. *Journal of Neurosurgery* **25**, 553–60.

Lipton, S. (1984) Percutaneous cordotomy. In *Textbook of Pain* (Eds Wall P.D. & Melzack R.) pp. 632–8. Churchill Livingstone, Edinburgh.

Lloyd J.W., Barber J.D.W. & Glynn C.J. (1976) Cryoanalgesia: a new approach for pain relief. *Lancet* **ii**, 932–3.

Loeser J. (1984) Face pain. In *Textbook of Pain* (Eds Wall P.D. & Melzack R.) pp. 426–34. Churchill Livingstone, Edinburgh.

Luque E.R. (1982) The anatomic basis and development of segmental spinal instrumentation. *Spine* **7**, 256–9.

Maher R.M. (1957) Neurone selection in relief of pain: further experiences with intrathecal injections. *Lancet* **i**, 16–18.

Maher R.M. (1963) Intrathecal chlorocresol in the treatment of pain in cancer. *Lancet* **i**, 965.

Maher R.M. (1969) Some aspects of the management of cancer pain. *Update* **1**, 751.

Maher R.M. & Mehta M. (1977) Spinal (intrathecal) and extradural analgesia. In *Persistent Pain*, vol. I (Ed. Lipton S.) pp. 61–99.

Maiwant O. & Make A.R. (1981) Cryoanalgesia for relief of pain after thoracotomy. *British Medical Journal* **282**, 1749–50.

Mehta M. (1973) Pharmacology of neurolytic agents. In *Intractable Pain* p. 55. W.B. Saunders, London.

Miles J. (1980) Trigeminal neuralgia. In *Persistent Pain*, vol. 2 (Ed. Lipton S.) pp. 203–22. Academic Press, London.

Miles J., Banks A.J., Dervin E. & Noori Z.F. (1984) Stabilisation of the spine affected by malignancy. *Journal of Neurology, Neurosurgery, Psychiatry* **47**, 897–904.

Morrica G. (1977) Pituitary neuroadenolysis in the treatment of intractable pain from cancer. In *Persistent Pain*, vol. I (Ed. Lipton S.) pp. 149–73. Academic Press, London.

Mullan S., Hekmapatnah J., Dobson G. & Beckman F. (1965) Percutaneous intramedullary cordotomy utilising the unipolar anodal electrolytic lesion. *Journal of Neurosurgery* **22**, 531–8.

Nathan P.W. (1963) Results of anterolateral cordotomy for pain in cancer. *Journal of Neurology, Neurosurgery and Psychiatry* **26**, 353–62.

Nathan P.W. & Scott P.G. (1958) Intrathecal phenol for intractable pain: safety and dangers of the method. *Lancet* **i**, 76.

Nathan P.W. & Sears T.A. (1960) Effects of phenol on nerve conduction. *Journal of Physiology* **150**, 565–6.

Orr I.A., Keenan D.J., Dundee J.W., Patterson C.C. & Greenfield A.A. (1983) Post thoracotomy pain relief: combined use of cryoprobe and morphine infusion technique. *Annals of the Royal College of Surgeons of England* **65**, 366–9.

Pitres A. & Vaillard L. (1888) Des nevrites provoques par le contact de l'alcool pur ou dilue avec les nerfs vivant. *C R Societee Biologigue* **5**, 550–1.

Pizzolato P. & Mannheimer W.H. (1961) *Histopathologic Effects of Local Anaesthetic Drugs*. Thomas, Illinois.

Ransford A.O., Crockard H.A. & Pozo J.L. (1986) Cranio-cervical instability treated by contoured loop fixation. *Journal of Bone, Joint Surgery* **68B**, 173–7.

Redfern R.M., Miles J. *et al.* (1988) Stabilisation of the infected spine. *Journal of Neurology, Neurosurgery, Psychiatry* **51**, 803–7.

Rees W.E.S. (1971) Multiple bilateral subcutaneous rhizolysis of segmental nerves in the treatment of the intervertebral disc syndrome. *Annals of General Practice* **26**, 126–7.

Rizzi R., Terrvoli A. & Visentin M. (1985) Long term use of alcoholization and thermocoagulation of the trigeminal nerve for cancer pain. *The Pain Clinic* **1**, 223–33.

Rosomoff H.L., Carroll F., Brow J. & Sheptak P. (1965) Percutaneous radiofrequency cervical cordotomy technique. *Journal of Neurosurgery* **23**, 639–44.

Rushton J.G., Stevens T.C. & Miller R.H. (1981) Glossopharyngeal (vagoglossopharyngeal) neuralgia. *Archives of Neurology* **38**, 201–5.

Sachs E. (1968) Posterior fossa approach to nervus intermedius section. *Journal of Neurosurgery* **28**, 54–7.

Sano K. (1973) Thalamotomy and hypothalamotomy. *Symposium de la doleur*. pp. 24–5. Paris.

Schrotter O. (1985) Results of thermocoagulation in trigeminal neuralgia. Comparison of preoperative treatment with carbamazepine alone versus additional denervation procedures. *The Pain Clinic* **1**, 233–9.

Shealy C.N. (1975) Percutaneous radiofrequency denervation of spinal facets. *Journal of Neurosurgery* **43**, 448–51.

Sindov M., Fischer G., Goutelle A. & Mansuy L. (1974) La radicellotomie posterieurre selective. Premiers resultata dans la chirurgie de la doleur. *Neurochirurgie* **20**, 391–408.

Sluijter M.E. & Mehta M. (1981) Treatment of chronic back and neck pain by percutaneous thermal lesions. In *Persistent Pain*, vol. 3 (Eds Lipton S. & Miles J.) pp. 141–79. Academic Press, London.

Spiegel E.A. & Wycis H.T. (1966) Present status of sterioencephalotomies for the relief of pain. *Confinia Neurologica* **27**, 7–17.

Swerdlow M. (1974) Intrathecal and extradural block in pain relief. In *Relief of Intractable Pain* (Ed. Swerdlow M.) pp. 148–75. Excerpta Medica, Amsterdam.

Swerdlow M. (1983) Intrathecal and extradural block for pain relief. In *Relief of Intractable Pain* (Ed. Swerdlow M.) pp. 175–214. Elsevier. Amsterdam.

White J.C. & Kjellberg R.W. (1973) Posterior spinal rhizotomy: a substitute for cordotomy in the relief of localised pain in patients with normal life expectancy. *Neurochirurgica* **16**, 141–70.

Wilkinson H.A. (1984) Radiofrequency percutaneous upper thoracic sympathectomy. *New England Journal of Medicine* **311**, 34–6.

SECTION V
INTENSIVE CARE

Principles of Intensive Care

A.R. AITKENHEAD AND I.K. FARQUHAR

Intensive care is the term used to describe the greatest available level of continuing patient management. In addition to nursing care, observation and monitoring, this usually involves active treatment; thus, in some centres the term intensive therapy is used. The intensive care unit (ICU) is an area where facilities are concentrated for treatment of the critically ill patient and exceed those available in an ordinary ward. Some hospitals contain a high-dependency unit (HDU), which is an area of care intermediate between that available in a general ward and the high level in an ICU. In addition, some theatre recovery wards provide a standard of care for postoperative patients similar to that provided in an HDU. In some centres, a number of separate ICUs exist for specialized fields of medicine, e.g. cardiothoracic surgery, neurosurgery, paediatrics, transplant surgery. However, in the majority of hospitals in the UK and many other countries, one general ICU deals with critically ill patients of many types.

This chapter discusses administration, assessment of severity of illness, patient monitoring and infection in relation to the general ICU, although many aspects are applicable also to more specialized units.

Administration

Intensive care unit design

Location and size

The siting of an ICU is determined by both building and clinical considerations. The Department of Health and Social Security (DHSS) guidelines (DHSS, 1970) suggest that the ICU should be situated near the operating theatres in order to share engineering services. This is also convenient clinically, as many patients are admitted directly from the operating theatre. However, the unit should also be readily accessible to other areas from which admissions are common, especially the accident and emergency department, medical and surgical wards, and the theatre recovery area. It is also preferable if the ICU is situated close to laboratories and imaging departments so that appropriate investigations may be performed with the minimum of delay.

It is recommended that 1–2% of the total number of acute beds in a hospital should be allocated to the general ICU, in addition to regional or subregional specialized units for cardiothoracic, neurosurgical and burns patients. Small units (less than four beds) may not be viable, and large units (more than 10 beds) are difficult to manage (Ledingham, 1977). If more beds are required, it may be desirable to divide the unit into more specialized areas (e.g. paediatric, neurological), although it is useful to group these units close to each other in order to share medical, technical, laboratory and engineering services. Normally, it is best to keep the ICU separate from the coronary care unit, although in smaller hospitals it may be necessary to combine them in order to make efficient use of available resources.

Accommodation (Intensive Care Society, 1984)

The patient area should consist of a large open ward containing four to 10 beds, with at least one side room. Side rooms make efficient nursing difficult, but are essential for patients who require isolation. A floor area of at least $20\,m^2$ is recommended for each bed in the open patient area in order to accommodate the bed, essential equipment and storage cupboards; a floor area of $30\,m^2$ is required in each side room. Ideally, each single room should be equipped with reversible ventilation, to minimize cross-infection. Facilities for renal dialysis should be available in one side room.

In addition to the area available for patient care,

space should be allocated for storage, offices and other facilities (Table 82.1).

A management base is required within or immediately adjacent to the patient area. This should be positioned so that all patients are visible. It should house telephones, an intercom connecting it with the offices and rest room, a central monitoring station and a computer terminal. Drug cupboards and refrigerator, blood refrigerator, emergency trolley and defibrillator should be within easy reach.

The entire area should be ventilated with air filtered to extract particles larger than 5 μm. Because of the heat generated by equipment, air conditioning should be provided, and temperature and humidity should be adjustable. Windows should be provided in the patient area and in the staff rest areas, as lack of natural daylight has adverse psychological effects on both patients and staff (Wilson, 1972). The type of artificial light should be appropriate for ready recognition of cyanosis.

Services

Each bed station should be equipped with wall outlets for vacuum, oxygen and medical air; nitrous oxide or Entonox (50% nitrous oxide : 50% oxygen) may be desirable also. The recommended supply pressures and minimum flow rates are shown in Table 82.2. At least two vacuum outlets should be provided in order

Table 82.2 Recommended supply pressures and flowrates for piped medical gases and vacuum

Facility	Pressure (kPa)	Pressure should be maintained when all outlets are being used at a flowrate of (litres/min)
Oxygen	414	20
Air	414	20
Nitrous oxide, (Entonox)	414	10
Vacuum	−67	40

to accommodate the potential need for low-pressure continuous drainage and high-pressure intermittent suction, e.g. for tracheal aspiration. There should be at least three outlets for both oxygen and medical air in order to power ventilators and to supply both flowmeters and gas-mixing devices. Only one nitrous oxide or Entonox outlet is required per bed, but each must be accompanied by an active scavenging point for waste gas.

A spotlight or anglepoise lamp and at least 16 electric sockets are required at each bed station. In order to minimize electrical accidents, all electrical outlets in the patient area should be on the same phase and should have a common ground earth. All electrical power to the patient area should be supplied by a standby power source, which should be tested

Table 82.1 Space allocation for intensive therapy unit facilities

Purpose	Floor area	Notes
Storage for consumables	>30 m²	Should include shelves, cupboards, drawers
Storage for equipment	>30 m²	Should include shelves, cupboards, drawers, bins
Storage for linen	>10 m²	
Dirty utility sluice		
Nurses' office	>15 m²	Telephone, intercom, notice boards
Medical office	>15 m²	Telephone, intercom
Staff restroom		Telephone, intercom, facilities for beverages
Staff changing rooms		Lockable lockers, showers, toilets
Doctor's bedroom	>15 m²	Bed, wash basin, shower, toilet, wardrobe, telephone, intercom
Laboratory	>15 m²	Power points, sink, specimen fridge
Workshop	>10 m²	Bench, compressed gas outlets, power points, sink
Relatives' rooms		At least two waiting areas, one suitable for interviews
Kitchen		
Reception area		
Cleaners' room	>4 m²	
Procedures room		All facilities, screened walls if image intensifier to be used
Seminar room	>30 m²	Projection facilities
Computer room/technician's office	>10 m²	Bench, electrical sockets
Receptionist's office	>15 m²	Filing cabinets, typewriter

monthly. The delay between mains failure and restoration of supply from the standby generator should be no more than 5 s. Emergency lighting and electrical sockets for ventilators, computers and other equipment sensitive to power failure should be protected by a battery power source which restores power immediately if the mains voltage fails; these emergency sockets must be marked clearly. A television aerial socket and radio outlet should be provided at each bed. Many patients in the ICU are alert mentally, although immobile.

One hand-wash basin should be available for each bed to minimize cross-infection; heated water traps are recommended to sterilize water in the effluent pipe.

Bed layout

Much of the equipment required is located at the head of the bed, and this can create problems of access. The traditional bed position is with the head of the bed located in close proximity to the wall. Equipment is mounted on or close to the wall so that electrical and gas supplies can be obtained from wall sockets or outlets. However, there are several disadvantages associated with this arrangement. In modern hospitals, the wall may have to be reinforced before heavy equipment, e.g. physiological monitors, can be supported. The attendants must walk around the foot of the bed in order to move from one side of the patient to the other, and there is a tendency for the nurse to make observations and recordings from the foot of the bed, thereby reducing verbal and visual contact with the patient. In addition, access to the head of the bed, e.g. for resuscitation, insertion of venous catheters or tracheal intubation, requires the bed to be moved away from the wall.

An alternative layout employed in some units offers significant advantages in terms of access, but is more expensive and requires a larger floor area. The bed is situated with the head approximately 1 m from the wall, allowing free access to the patient's head (Kerr et al., 1985). All services are supplied from the wall along a boom, or run under the floor to a 'bollard' situated at the side of the bed; a similar arrangement, which permits even greater access than the 'bollard', can be achieved using a 'stalactite' structure attached to the ceiling, although plugs and sockets may be beyond the reach of smaller members of staff. The installation of either system improves access for all nursing and medical procedures, and the nurse may observe the patient from a position close to the head, improving communication and contact. In addition, a work surface and storage area can be situated behind the bed.

Storage space is essential at each bedside. Shelves are required for syringes, needles, suction catheters, disposal bins, etc., and cupboards or drawers may be used to store linen, sterile packs for eye and mouth care, and other items of equipment which are in frequent use. If these items are readily available, the nurse has to leave the patient less frequently. A degree of privacy is necessary, and some form of screening must be provided during bedbaths and other intimate nursing procedures. Charts for recording the patient's observations and results of laboratory investigations should be easily accessible to the nurse and visiting medical staff, but not visible to the patient.

Staffing

Nursing staff

Nurses are the most important staff in the ICU. Although it is appropriate for student nurses to receive some training in intensive care nursing, they should attend only in a supernumerary capacity. The number of trained nurses on the establishment depends on several factors (Intensive Care Society, 1984).

Dependency categories

The most seriously ill patients, e.g. those with multiple organ failure or multiple injuries, may require more than one nurse. All patients who require mechanical ventilation, those with an insecure airway or those receiving continuous drug infusions, should have one nurse in attendance at all times. Patients who are 'recuperating' from more serious illness, or those admitted for routine monitoring, parenteral nutrition or correction of fluid and electrolyte imbalance, require less nursing care, and one nurse may be able to care for two patients simultaneously. The pattern of admissions varies from unit to unit, and calculation of an average 'dependency score' (average number of nurses required for each patient) for an individual unit is based on careful record keeping.

Occupancy

It is clearly impractical to calculate the number of nursing staff on the basis of maximum bed occupancy. The demand varies for general ICU beds, and at times of low bed occupancy, nurses are under-occupied, and may be assigned to other parts of the hospital. This is generally poor for morale. The calculation must therefore take account of the average bed occupancy in conjunction with the average 'dependency score' of each occupied bed. A calculation based on these average values results in a sufficient number of nurses to cope with demand for 50% of the time. In order to meet demand for 95% of predicted needs, the calculation should be based on the mean + 2 standard deviations.

Effective working time

Allowances must be made for the limited hours worked by nurses (currently 37.5 h per week in the UK), and for annual and study leave, and predicted sickness leave.

Support nurses

If each nurse at the bedside is to stay with the patient, additional nurses are required to undertake administration, teaching, relief for meal breaks, to collect drugs and equipment from stores and to assist with lifting and turning. One additional nurse is required normally on each shift for three nurses at the bedside.

For an average general ICU, with a 'dependency weighted occupancy' (DWO) (average dependency score × average bed occupancy) of 50–75%, the total number of nurses required to ensure that bedside demand is met on 95% of occasions is:

$$\text{Total beds} \times (\text{mean DWO} + 2\text{SD}) \times 5.5$$

To allow for support nurses, this value should be multiplied by 1.33. The nursing establishment should include one sister or charge nurse per bed to ensure that at least one is available to work each day.

Other staff

Auxiliary nurses may be employed to assist trained staff in lifting, changing linen and running errands. A ward clerk/receptionist is invaluable, and cleaning staff are required. In addition, other categories of staff should be available as required. There should be permanent cover by technical staff, who are responsible for maintenance and cleaning of equipment, and a technician, or a member of laboratory staff, to ensure quality control of on-site biochemical analyses. Physiotherapy is required for all patients in the ICU, and should be provided by those experienced

in this specialized type of work. A dietician and radiographer must also be on call at all times, and it is helpful if a pharmacist with knowledge of the requirements of an ICU is available. Additional staff may be called upon for electrocardiography, ultrasound imaging, electroencephalography, etc.

Medical staff

Consultant staff

Consultant medical staff with responsibility for the ICU require a combination of enthusiasm, medical knowledge, technical expertise and diplomatic skill. The consultant's parent specialty is relatively unimportant, provided that he/she has sufficient experience and training. Most ICU consultants in the UK are anaesthetists, probably because of flexibility of sessional commitments, experience in ventilation and cardiovascular monitoring techniques and the fact that anaesthesia is at present the only specialty which currently provides ICU training for all junior staff. Often, critically ill patients develop progressive organ failure, irrespective of the initial pathology. Treatment therefore involves management of multi-system failure, and consequently, an important role of the ICU consultant is to co-ordinate treatment by identifying each patient's requirements and to call upon the services of appropriate specialists for advice.

A consultant experienced in ICU should be on call for the unit at all times. In many units, between three and five consultants share responsibility; a larger number dilutes the experience gained, whilst a smaller number results in an unacceptable on-call commitment, particularly during holiday absences. One consultant should be in administrative charge. It is important that a working relationship is established with referring consultants. In some centres, the latter retain 'control' over patients admitted to the unit, although they may visit the patient only once or twice each week. This is unsatisfactory as it results in time wasted in contacting the consultant and causes confusion among the nurses. Whilst the referring team must be consulted on major policy decisions, diagnosis and specialized management, it is more efficient if the ICU consultant is able to undertake the general management of the patient, and to deal immediately with sudden changes in the patient's condition without recourse to the referring consultant. In general, this policy becomes acceptable to most consultants from other specialties after confidence has been gained in the management of patients by the ICU team.

Junior staff

Junior medical staff should be responsible only for the ICU, have no commitments elsewhere in the hospital and should be resident on the unit. They may be drawn from any specialty, but previous experience in maintenance of the airway and in resuscitation is essential. In most units, the ICU resident post is part of the anaesthetic department rotation. Junior staff should spend a block of at least 3 months working on a unit in order to achieve basic proficiency.

The ICU resident is responsible for examination of each patient on admission, and at least once each day. With appropriate guidance, he/she should also be responsible for all aspects of treatment, and all requests for investigations and changes in treatment prescribed by visiting medical teams should be channelled through the resident.

In larger units, a senior registrar may be a member of the ICU team. Although most ICU senior registrars at present are undertaking higher professional training in anaesthesia, this may change in future. The senior registrar assumes a higher degree of responsibility than the ICU resident. He/she should be involved in policy decisions and administration.

Other medical staff

Even the most experienced ICU consultant cannot manage all the possible conditions with which the critically ill patient may present. Thus, he/she should seek advice from a wide variety of specialists when the need arises.

Medical staff training

Currently, there is no accepted standard of training in the UK for the ICU consultant. In the USA, a multidisciplinary approach to ICU training has been adopted whilst two independent types of ICU have emerged in Australia — one managed by anaesthetists and the other by physicians.

In the UK, intensive care is not recognized by the Department of Health as an independent specialty. The majority of new consultant posts in general intensive care are appointed within departments of anaesthesia, although 25% of units have a surgeon or physician in charge. In addition, there are several categories of specialist unit (e.g. cardiothoracic, neurosurgical, poisons, burns). In order to rationalize intensive care training in the UK, an inter-faculty/collegiate liaison group has considered the problems (Hanson, 1985). It was suggested that full-time intensive care specialists should not evolve, but that intensive care should be conducted by consultants of different backgrounds after completion of a recommended pattern of training. The liaison group proposed a minimum training period of 7 years after registration. At the level of Senior House Officer or Registrar, training in intensive care should be incorporated into basic specialist training (BST) programmes of anaesthetists, physicians and surgeons, who would proceed to take the appropriate higher qualifications in their parent specialty. A total of 2 years would be spent in recognized posts in intensive care; in many cases, this would require extension of the BST period. Overseas experience in appropriate units would be recognized. Research projects would be encouraged, and it has been suggested that presentation of a dissertation should be an essential part of training. At some time during training, a period of 1 year would be spent in medical training by anaesthetists, and 6 months in an anaesthetic training post by physicians.

The scheme is a source of controversy; some critics believe that anaesthetists should continue to predominate in intensive care (Stoddart, 1986), whilst others suggest that the ICU should be managed by full-time specialist 'intensivists' (Dudley, 1987).

Admission policy

The purpose of the ICU is to provide a level of care unattainable in other areas of the hospital for patients who are suffering an acute illness from which they have a realistic chance of recovery. In many cases, these criteria are met when a request is made for admission. For example, a patient with Guillain–Barré syndrome who develops ventilatory failure can be treated only where facilities for long-term artificial ventilation are available, but is likely to recover after the acute illness and should then return to a normal life. Difficulties may arise, particularly if there is pressure for ICU beds, when patients are referred only for 'high-dependency' care, or when a request for admission is made for a patient with severe chronic disease.

The admission policy for high-dependency patients is determined usually by the average demand for ICU beds. Some units admit high-dependency patients routinely, whilst others are seldom able to do so. High-dependency patients require relatively little nursing care, and it may be appropriate to admit patients routinely after major surgery (particularly if a facility for 24-h recovery is not available), for simple monitoring (e.g. central venous pressure), for supervision of parenteral nutrition, etc. However, nurses in the general wards become progressively less experienced in the management of this type of patient, and are less able to cope satisfactorily on occasions when the unit is busy and admission is not possible.

The admission of patients with severe chronic disease and with a limited life expectancy generates major moral and ethical questions. It is possible in a very small number of patients to predict that there is virtually no chance of survival (see 'Scoring systems' below), although in these circumstances many doctors find it difficult to withhold treatment. The overall mortality of unstable patients is high. In one study, it was found that mortality within 1 month was 56%, and a further 17% died within 1 year; less than half of those who survived returned to a normal life 1 year after their illness (Cullen, 1977). Patients who present with an acute illness, but whose life expectancy is limited, e.g. patients with incurable malignant disease or chronic incapacitating respiratory or cardiac disease, have a high mortality, and may require treatment for many days or weeks. Only a small proportion survive to return home; their remaining life may be short and its quality severely impaired. For the remainder, the suffering and indignity are unnecessary, and the stress on relatives is enormous (Jennett, 1984).

A similar dilemma is presented by patients with acute complications of severe but potentially curable diseases, particularly in the younger patient. The mortality in patients with acquired immune deficiency syndrome (AIDS) who require admission to ICU is 80% (Deam et al., 1988). At present, the survivors are thought to have limited life expectancy.

In the past, admission policy in some units was based primarily on age. There is conflicting evidence on the relationship between age and outcome from ICU admission. Cullen (1977) found an inverse relationship, although the quality of life for ICU survivors was not influenced by age; in a later study, age was not found to have influenced outcome significantly among patients admitted to a medical ICU (Fedullo & Swinburne, 1983). The decision to admit a patient is also influenced by attitudes towards the termination of treatment in those who fail to progress. Patients who do not improve despite continuing high levels of therapeutic intervention over many days have a very high mortality (Cullen, 1977).

In the USA, it has become necessary to resolve many of these very difficult decisions in courts of law. In some states, only a court can decide that

treatment can be terminated. In the UK, decisions regarding termination of treatment are taken usually by all the consultants involved with the care of the patient, after consultation with relatives. Admission of patients who may benefit little from ICU treatment may be determined also by discussion among all parties involved. As health care resources become more limited, and medical and technological advances decrease the number of patients deemed 'incurable', less flexible guidelines may become necessary in future.

Scoring systems

General ICUs admit patients with a wide variety of conditions and complications. Thus, it is difficult to compare morbidity and mortality among different units. Many of the new forms of treatment and apparatus used are enormously expensive. In the USA, intensive care budgets amount to over 20% of total hospital costs, and 1% of the gross national product (Berenson, 1984). The mean daily cost of patients who die in ICU is 55% higher than that of survivors (Ridley et al., 1993).

Little information is available on the efficiency of ICUs. Although individual units may maintain records of admissions, brief details of therapeutic manoeuvres and patient outcome, these figures are seldom published. In addition, because of differences in admission policies and treatment regimens, and the wide variation in the type of illness precipitating admission to a general ICU, results from a small number of units cannot be extrapolated to provide figures representing the country as a whole.

Many of the newer forms of therapy, and some invasive monitoring techniques, have not been evaluated adequately for a number of reasons:
1 Many units are small, and most general units admit patients with a wide variety of pathologies.
2 Because of differences in the severity of disease, the patient's individual response, the presence of concurrent chronic disease and the stage of illness at which the patient is referred for treatment, it is difficult to compare patients with the same disease process.
3 There may therefore be a variety of methods of treatment for each disease within a single unit.
4 Multicentre trials necessary to obtain sufficient numbers of patients for adequate controlled clinical trials have proved impractical for the above reasons.

Finally, there is concern that the advanced technology and expertise which is able to maintain life by artificial support of the pulmonary, cardiovascular and renal systems may be used to prolong life in an undignified manner in patients whose prognosis is hopeless (Jennett, 1984). Unfortunately, despite the increasing information provided by the widespread implementation of numerous scoring systems, it remains extremely difficult to predict outcome in individual cases (see below).

Scoring systems have been used for some years for patients with certain types of illness, e.g. Glasgow coma score for patients with severe head injury, injury severity score and trauma score for patients with severe trauma. These have proved useful in defining relationships between treatment and outcome. For example, Watt and Ledingham (1984) demonstrated that increased mortality among trauma patients in ICU was related to the introduction of etomidate for sedation rather than to differences in severity of illness.

Types of scoring system

Patients admitted to ICU may be categorized into populations on the basis of the benefit that is expected as a result of intensive care (Jacobs et al., 1989). The first group is expected to benefit, the second is not expected to benefit because the patients are not sick enough to require the interventions unique to intensive care, while the third group is not expected to benefit from intensive care because the patients are either so sick on admission that they could never benefit from intensive care or have deteriorated to the extent that the application of intensive care can only prolong the process of dying.

In order to make the best use of the limited resources available, it is appropriate to attempt to identify these groups. This could reduce the rate of admission of patients to ICU who had no need for it and allow identification of patients whose prognosis was hopeless as early as possible in order to allow institution of appropriate care.

A number of 'scoring systems' have been designed in order to attempt to quantify the 'illness' of critically ill patients. These have been based upon different criteria. One of the earliest systems, the therapeutic intervention scoring system (TISS) (Cullen et al., 1974) scored patients on the basis of their therapeutic requirement. The mortality prediction model (MPM) (Lemeshow et al., 1985), the acute physiology and chronic health evaluation system (APACHE) (Knaus et al., 1981b), the simplified acute physiology score (SAPS) (Le Gall et al., 1984) and the scoring of organ system failure (Knaus et al., 1985b) all attempt to

quantify physiological disturbance. These scoring systems may be applied to a range of conditions. However, a number of other scoring systems have evolved which are applicable in specific conditions such as pancreatitis (Ranson et al., 1974, 1976), adult respiratory distress syndrome (ARDS) (Murray et al., 1988), sepsis (Elebute & Stoner, 1983; Stevens, 1983), head injury (Teasdale & Jennett, 1974; Marrubini, 1984) and pneumonia (Durocher et al., 1988). The scoring of trauma patients by the abbreviated injury scale (AIS), and the manipulation of this data to produce the injury severity score (ISS), represent attempts to quantify the severity of anatomical injury, whereas the trauma score (Champion et al., 1981) is a system for facilitating rapid assessment of physiological disturbance in trauma patients. New scoring systems continue to be developed.

The combination of the trauma score and the ISS has been used to predict mortality in trauma patients (the TRISS methodology) (Boyd et al., 1987). All of the non-disease-specific scoring systems have been used, alone or in combination, to provide estimates of mortality and though their primary role has been to allow stratification of patients into groups by severity of illness for research, audit and billing purposes, it has always been an implicit part of the development of the systems that they might one day assist in the decisions concerning individual patients.

Only the generally applicable scoring systems will be discussed further here.

Therapeutic intervention scoring system

The basis of the TISS is that increasing severity of illness usually results in more therapeutic intervention. A panel of intensive-care physicians and nurses selected 57 therapeutic interventions and then graded them by nursing time and effort (Cullen et al., 1974). Values were assigned to the interventions on a scale of one to four, e.g. ECG monitoring and intracranial pressure monitoring scored 1 and 4 points, respectively. A patient's TISS score was the sum of the points for all the interventions undertaken in a given period of time (usually 24 h). It was suggested that the TISS score be used for assessing the necessary staffing levels for intensive care facilities, for classification of patients by severity of illness and for cost analysis. Originally published in 1974, the system was updated in 1983 to reflect the changes in intensive care therapy. TISS scores are dependent upon availability of specific treatment and on medical treatment protocols, both of which may vary from hospital to hospital; thus, it is inappropriate to use the TISS system to make comparisons between units.

The acute physiology and chronic health evaluation score

In 1981 Knaus and colleagues published the APACHE scoring system (Knaus et al., 1981b). This system was based on allocation of a score for abnormalities of 34 physiological variables. Ranges of values above and below the normal range were defined for each variable, and the ranges were assigned weights on an integer scale of 0 to 4 — the higher the value, the greater the deviation from normal. Some variables, thought to be of lesser importance, scored less than 4 at their most abnormal. The acute physiology score (APS) was calculated by summing the weights for the most abnormal value of each variable in the first 24 h of the intensive care admission. In addition to the APS, a letter subscript (A–D) was added to denote preadmission health in the previous 3–6 months. These variables, their weightings and the chronic health criteria were chosen by a consensus conference of seven critical care physicians. The APACHE system was validated initially in 582 patients, and the APS was shown to correlate with the TISS score. Using a decision criterion of 0.5 (i.e. patients with a greater than 50% risk of death were predicted to die, those with a risk of less than 50% were predicted to live), the APS has a sensitivity of 49%, a specificity of 97% and a positive predictive value of 79% for predicting mortality. In this study, 13 of 63 patients predicted to die survived, a false-positive rate of 10%.

APACHE II

In 1985, a revised system was published (Knaus et al., 1985a). The new system scored 12 variables rather than 34, facilitating data gathering, and gave increased weight to the Glasgow coma score (GCS) and to acute renal failure (Table 82.3). Points for age and chronic health status were incorporated directly into the score; non-operative or emergency postoperative admissions received an extra weighting in the chronic health evaluation as compared with elective postoperative cases.

Calculation of the risk of death for an individual involves summing the APS score, age points and the chronic health evaluation (weighted appropriately) to give the APACHE II score. This is inserted into an equation, which includes further weighting for either the specific disease state or, if this is unclear, the single organ system failure which was principally to

Table 82.3 Variables used in calculation of APACHE II score

Acute physiology score

Variable	Maximum score for	
	Low value	High value
Rectal temperature	4	4
Mean arterial pressure	4	4
Heart rate	4	4
Respiratory rate	4	4
Oxygenation		
$(A-a)Do_2$ if $F_IO_2 > 0.5$		4
Pao_2 if $F_IO_2 < 0.5$	4	
Arterial pH	4	4
Serum sodium	4	4
Serum potassium	4	4
Serum creatinine (double score if acute renal failure)	2	4
Haemoglobin	4	4
White blood count	4	4
Glasgow coma score (GCS)	Score = 15 − GCS	

Age

Age (years)	Points
<44	0
45–54	2
55–64	3
65–74	5
>75	6

Chronic health

If history of severe organ system insufficiency or if immunocompromised, then:
1 For non-operative or emergency postoperative patients, 5 points
2 For elective postoperative patients, 2 points

blame for admission to ICU; this is because differences were identified in death rates for equivalent APACHE II scores in different disease states. A further correction factor is added depending on whether the patient is non-operative or postoperative, and if emergency surgery was required. The result of the calculation is a probability of death, given as a percentage. Using a decision criterion of 0.5, the APACHE II system showed an overall sensitivity of 47%, a specificity of 94.9% and a positive predictive value of 69.6% for prediction of mortality. The cost of treatment on the day of admission to ICU has been shown to correlate with the APACHE II score (Ridley et al., 1993).

Organ system failure scoring

Knaus and colleagues also developed objective criteria for defining failure in five organ systems (Knaus et al., 1985b). They developed mortality prediction data from 5677 patients and derived mortality rates in relation to the number and duration of organ system failures, and stratified for age less than or greater than 65 years. They found that a single organ failure for 1 day led to a predicted mortality of 16% or 32% for patients less than or greater than 65 years of age, respectively, whereas failure of three or more organ systems for 5 or more days was uniformly fatal in both age groups. Chang and colleagues (1988a) studied the use of daily APACHE II scoring in predicting mortality and utilized the definitions of organ system failures defined by Knaus, multiplying the APACHE II score by (1 + organ failure coefficient). The organ failure coefficients were obtained by dividing Knaus's mortality rates for days of organ failure by 1000.

APACHE III

A further revision of the APACHE system is in progress. A detailed proposal has been published (Zimmerman, 1989). This system, which will become available as a commercial product, is intended to improve on the predictive power of the APACHE II system. It has been suggested that it will be sufficiently accurate to allow decisions regarding institution or termination of treatment to be made in individual patients on the basis of the APACHE III score (Knaus & Wagner, 1989); however, accompanying editorials expressed some reservations over this proposition (Cullen, 1989; Shoemaker, 1989; Teres, 1989).

Simplified acute physiology score

The SAPS system was evolved in response to the complexity of the original APACHE score. It was felt that variations in the mean number of data collected per patient might introduce a systematic bias, because missing values are interpreted as normal. Le Gall described the SAPS system (Le Gall et al., 1984), which utilized 13 of the original APS variables, and added age. The same weighting system was used as in the APS, and the worst value of each variable in the first 24 h of admission was used to calculate the score.

Mortality prediction model

The MPM consists of two models, one based on admission data and one based on data available 24 h after admission to intensive care (Lemeshow et al., 1985). The variables used were extracted by linear discriminant function analysis and subsequent multiple logistic regression from a minimum of 227 which were measured in each patient. The resulting models each consisted of seven variables (not all the same) which were all significant predictors of mortality, and calculation of each of the models gives a probability of mortality without additional manipulation. The models were later validated in 1997 patients (Teres et al., 1987); it was found that only the admission model predicted mortality accurately. Using a decision criterion of 0.5, the admission model was found to have a sensitivity of 50%, a specificity of 95% and a positive predictive value of 71% in predicting mortality.

Problems of scoring systems

There are a number of potential concerns relating to the calculation and implementation of the scoring systems described above; some of the problems inherent in such systems have been detailed by Marrubini (1984). For instance, the significance of a given score is uncertain, as it may result from a huge number of combinations of scores for individual variables, which represent different patterns of physiological disturbance. The original consensus conference for the APACHE system tried to allocate weights to derangement of physiological variables such that equal weights for different variables would indicate equivalent physiological disturbance: '... a weight of 4 given for a mean arterial pressure of less than 50 mmHg is roughly equivalent to a 4 given for a pH of less than 7.15'. This 'equivalence' has not been verified.

It has been demonstrated that level of consciousness is one of the most important determinants of outcome for critically ill patients (Teres et al., 1982), and this has been reflected by the increased weighting for the GCS in APACHE II. However, up to 70% of admissions to intensive care units are postoperative, and in a large percentage of these patients, the trachea has been intubated. The presence of a tracheal tube prevents assessment of speech, and the residual effects of anaesthesia affect other components of the GCS (Rutledge et al., 1991). These factors make the scoring of level of consciousness uncertain, and the worst GCS may be obtained at the time of admission when these factors are present. This has led some investigators to use the best GCS for scoring purposes (Bion *et al.*, 1985; Jacobs *et al.*, 1988), and some to award higher or normal scores when in doubt (Chang *et al.*, 1988a). The GCS is a component of the APACHE II, MPM and the SAPS systems, and the variability which it introduces into the total scores is a cause of concern.

The use of scoring systems that are based on single sets of observations at admission or from the first 24 h of intensive care is unsatisfactory. It ignores treatment that may or may not have been applied before admission. In other words, a given score may indicate a graver prognosis in a patient admitted after aggressive resuscitative efforts than the same score in a patient admitted before optimum resuscitation has been completed. This so called 'lead time bias' has been documented (Dragsted *et al.*, 1989). Thus, even scores obtained at the time of admission to the ICU cannot be said to be treatment independent. Furthermore, the use of a score obtained early in an admission to predict mortality ignores the dynamic character of critical illness and implies that outcome is fixed from that time on. It would be unacceptable to attempt to base decisions relating to an individual on a single score. Consequently, a number of investigators have evaluated the use of daily scoring and have shown that this can improve predictive accuracy (Bion *et al.*, 1985, 1988; Chang *et al.*, 1988a,b; Lemeshow *et al.*, 1988). The APACHE III system will also use daily scoring.

Validation of the APACHE II system specifically excluded patients who had undergone coronary artery bypass surgery because their admission scores were high but their overall mortality extremely low. Similarly, APACHE II is a poor predictor of mortality in conditions which produce profound physiological disturbance but which are amenable to specific treatment, such as diabetic ketoacidosis. Thus, scoring systems tend to predict mortality accurately only in conditions where treatment is supportive. Furthermore, although it has been suggested that earlier scoring confers greater 'treatment-independence' on the resultant mortality prediction (Knaus *et al.*, 1985a), it is intuitively apparent that actual mortality is the result of the interaction between the patient's disease and the therapy administered. This raises the question of periodic revalidation of scoring systems in order to allow for improvements in therapy.

Therefore, while the role of scoring systems in the stratification of patients into risk groups is accepted, their proposed use for individual patient decisions remains controversial. As noted above, these decisions relate to patients who either do not require intensive care or who cannot benefit from it. Knaus and colleagues (1981a) noted that a substantial number of patients in a large teaching hospital were admitted to ICU for monitoring only, and that only 14% of these patients subsequently received one or more active treatments considered to be unique to the intensive care environment. A further study in 5790 patients from 13 hospitals was carried out (Wagner *et al.*, 1987). A total of 1941 patients required monitoring only. A predictive equation was estimated from data on 778 admissions and then validated in a further 1163 patients. Multivariate logistic regression was used to select variables predictive of active treatment in ICU and a decision criterion of 10% chance of treatment used to divide those with a 'low risk' from those with a 'high risk' of requiring treatment. The study showed that, of 1163 patients in the validation group who received only monitoring services on admission to ICU, 849 were predicted to have less than a 10% chance of requiring subsequent active treatment. Only 37 patients (4.3%) actually received such treatment. The authors concluded: 'For these patients, the potential requirement for ICU services may be low enough that the potential harm from ICU admission might outweigh the benefit' (Wagner *et al.*, 1987).

The decision to withdraw treatment must be based primarily on clinical assessment, although the use of a scoring system may provide some statistical support of the clinician's judgement. It must be made only after the most careful consideration not only of outcome in terms of life and death, but also quality of life and any wishes expressed by the patient prior to the present illness. These patients are, by definition, dependent on the supportive measures provided in the ICU and a prediction of death leading to withdrawal of treatment will inevitably result in death. Chang and colleagues (1986) reported a study in which they used the APACHE II system to predict mortality in 26 patients treated with total parenteral nutrition (TPN). Using a decision criterion of 0.6 on the day of admission, or a combined criterion of <0.6 on the day of admission and >0.3 on day of referral for TPN, they were able to predict the death of eight patients (specificity 100%, sensitivity 53%). They suggested that if TPN had been withheld from these patients, a financial saving could have been realized without prejudicing patient care (Chang *et al.*, 1986). A later study by Hopefl and colleagues (1989) using a decision criterion of 0.6 on the day of referral for TPN in 61 patients revealed a sensitivity of 27.6% and specificity of only 96.9% in predicting mortality (one of nine patients predicted to die, survived). Therefore on the basis of the decision criteria defined in Chang's study, nutrition might have been withheld from a patient who survived with the benefit of this therapy. However, it should be appreciated that calculation of risk in some cases may support the continuation of treatment in situations where clinical assessment suggests a grave prognosis (Chang et al., 1988b) and that the reliability of clinical assessment in making these decisions is difficult to quantify. Much further work is required before scoring systems may be used to assist in individual patient decisions and it seems likely that decision criteria of 0.9 or greater will have to be used.

Advances in the investigation of the critically ill may also be incorporated into future scoring systems. A group of 80 critically ill patients were divided into groups determined by the gastric intramucosal pH (measured by a tonometer; see below) at the time of admission (Doglio et al., 1991). Patients with a 'low' intramucosal pH had a group mortality of 65.4%, whereas those with a normal intramucosal pH had a mortality of 43.6%. The APACHE II scores for the two groups were not significantly different.

It is also important to remember that the mortality predictions by intensive care staff have been shown to be similar in accuracy to predictions based on the APACHE II score (Bion et al., 1988; Kruse et al., 1988) and that: 'Regardless of the number of patients studied, prognostic estimates are still only estimates' (Knaus et al., 1985a).

Monitoring in the intensive care unit

Monitoring is essential in the critically ill patient. It assists diagnosis, guides adjustment of therapy and allows early detection of deterioration in the patient's condition. The level of monitoring required for an individual patient is determined by the presenting condition and its predicted course, the existence of concurrent disease, and, in the case of invasive monitoring techniques, the risk : benefit ratio. In general, instrumental monitoring is indicated if it provides information which is not available from clinical observation, if it is likely to provide early warning of an unpredictable change or if it helps to quantify a predictable change.

Although it is convenient to classify monitoring techniques with respect to physiological systems, haemodynamic and respiratory monitoring should be considered in tandem, as oxygen transport to the cell is dependent on the functions of both the cardio-vascular and respiratory systems.

Haemodynamic monitoring

Electrocardiography

ECG monitoring provides information on heart rate and rhythm. Changes in the pattern of the ECG complex may indicate electrolyte disturbances or myocardial ischaemia. Detection of these changes requires regular observation by the nursing and medical staff, although devices are now available which detect changes in ECG pattern and indicate rhythm disturbances or onset of ischaemia.

Arterial pressure

Measurement of arterial pressure is essential. In some patients, intermittent non-invasive measurement is adequate. However, direct pressure monitoring is preferable in any patient whose condition is unstable, as rapid changes in arterial pressure are not detected by intermittent observations. In addition, continuous access to an artery permits regular measurement of arterial blood gases without the need to perform multiple arterial punctures.

The radial artery is used most commonly for arterial pressure monitoring, although some authorities believe that a larger artery, such as the brachial or femoral artery, is less likely to become occluded because of the higher flow rate of blood around the cannula. Femoral artery cannulation is indicated in the shocked patient, or if difficulty is experienced in inserting a radial artery cannula. Although it has been suggested that the femoral route is more likely to lead to infective complications (Band & Maki, 1979), the overall complication rates for femoral and radial routes are similar (Russell et al., 1983). The incidence of complications resulting from radial artery cannulation may be reduced if a parallel-sided Teflon cannula no larger than 20 gauge in adults, or 22 gauge in children, is used, and if multiple attempts at cannulation are avoided (Russell et al., 1983).

The information provided by an intra-arterial cannula may be inaccurate unless careful attention is paid to the damping of the transducer system. Overdamping may result from a kinked or partially occluded catheter, or the presence of air bubbles in the transducer tubing. An excessive length of tubing may result in underdamping, with overestimation of systolic and underestimation of diastolic pressure. Measurement of arterial pressure by cannulation of the dorsalis pedis artery is often subject to under-damping. The reading from the transducer system should be calibrated regularly by checking the arterial pressure with a cuff and mercury sphygmo-manometer.

There are several potential complications of direct arterial pressure measurement. Disconnection leads to haemorrhage, which may be lethal, especially in children, if it is not noticed and arrested promptly. The risk of haemorrhage is reduced if Luer locks are used at all connections and if the number of connections is kept to a minimum. Integral tubing systems containing a flushing device, transducer dome and connecting tubing are available which reduce the number of connections, and are cheaper than construction of a system from individual components. The cannula and connecting tubing should always be visible to the nursing staff, and should not be hidden underneath bandages or dressings. Excessive flushing of the cannula at high pressure can produce retrograde flow in the artery, with proximal embolization; this is a particular risk in children.

As with any procedure in which the skin is penetrated, arterial cannulation carries a risk of infection. Septic emboli may result also from an infected arterial cannula. Methods of minimizing the risk of infection are described later in this chapter.

The most feared complication of arterial cannulation is distal ischaemia resulting from arterial occlusion. Occlusion of the radial artery occurs in up to 50% of patients during or after long-term arterial cannulation; patency is re-established usually, but this may take up to 11 weeks (Bedford & Wollman, 1973). Clinical evidence of ischaemia is relatively uncommon (up to 4% during radial artery cannulation), but is not predicted accurately by Allen's test (Allen, 1929) to determine adequacy of the collateral circulation through the ulnar artery. Necrotic damage is rare provided that the cannula is removed promptly when distal ischaemia is recognized.

Central venous pressure

Measurement of central venous or right atrial pressure (CVP, RAP) gives an indication of the preload of the right ventricle. The RAP increases if the right ventricle fails because of overtransfusion, increased pulmonary vascular resistance or increased back pressure from the left ventricle, and decreases in the presence of hypovolaemia with normal ventricular function. Right ventricular failure alone is relatively uncommon in the ICU patient; it is usually secondary to acute pulmonary disease or left ventricular failure. The principal use of RAP measurement in the ICU is therefore assessment of the adequacy of the circulating volume.

The commonest sites for insertion of a central venous catheter are the subclavian vein, the internal jugular vein, the femoral vein and, less frequently now, the antecubital fossa. The internal jugular route is associated with the highest incidence of correct positioning of the catheter tip in the vena cava or right atrium (over 90%), although insertion into an arm vein has fewest early complications (Rosen *et al.*, 1981). The major complications of the four routes are summarized in Table 82.4.

Two complications are common to all routes of insertion. Infection, which may remain localized or may result in bacteraemia, can be reduced substantially by ensuring that a fully sterile technique is used; this is discussed more fully later. The tip of the catheter may not be in the correct position. Extra-

Table 82.4 Major complications of central venous catheterization

Arm veins
High incidence of incorrect placement (25–30%)
Thrombophlebitis — almost 100% at 48 h

Subclavian vein
Pneumothorax
Haemothorax
Hydrothorax
Subcutaneous emphysema
Brachial plexus palsy
Phrenic nerve paralysis
Subclavian artery puncture
Innominate vein puncture
Subclavian vein thrombosis
Knotted catheter
Air embolism

Internal jugular vein
Pneumothorax
Haemothorax
Hydrothorax
Carotid artery puncture
Thrombophlebitis
Thoracic duct puncture
Horner's syndrome
Tracheal tube cuff puncture
Vocal cord paralysis
Air embolism
Superior vena cava thrombosis
Aortic catheterization
Ventricular fibrillation

Femoral vein
Thrombophlebitis
Femoral and iliac vein thrombosis
Inferior vena cava thrombosis
Serious infection

vascular insertion may result in infusion of intravenous fluids into tissues, or more seriously, into the pleural cavity. The catheter tip may remain in a vein, but lie outside the thorax or in an anomalous intrathoracic vessel; this results in inaccurate measurements of pressure, and may cause vascular damage if hypertonic fluids are infused. It is essential to check the position of the tip after insertion by ensuring that venous blood can be aspirated freely, and by chest radiography; it may be necessary to inject a small volume of radio-opaque dye to highlight relatively radiolucent catheters.

Measurement of RAP or CVP can be undertaken with a water-filled manometer. The true zero reference point is the right atrium; the surface marking is the midaxillary line opposite the fourth costal cartilage. The normal range of values in the spontaneously breathing patient is $0-6\,cmH_2O$. The manubriosternal junction is used often as a more convenient zero reference point, but this is $5-10\,cm$ above the right atrium, depending on body build and the position of the patient, and the CVP value is correspondingly lower. If drugs are infused through the central venous line, administration ceases during the $30-45\,s$ during which the CVP measurement is made. It is preferable to use a multilumen catheter so that one lumen can be dedicated to measurement of CVP. In many units, CVP measurement is made continuously using a pressure transducer.

Trends in measurement are more important than the absolute value of RAP. There is considerable interindividual variation in the normal measurement, the zero reference point is not always consistent between patients and the use of positive-pressure ventilation increases RAP by an amount which varies with the inspiratory and expiratory pressures and the compliance of the lungs. A downward trend in RAP suggests that the circulating volume is decreasing (e.g. haemorrhage), whilst an upward trend suggests right ventricular failure. In the hypotensive patient with RAP within the normal range, the technique of a 'fluid challenge' is often used to help determine the volaemic status. Factors that influence RAP are summarized in Table 82.5.

Pulmonary artery pressures

A balloon-tipped, flow-guided catheter may be inserted by any of the routes appropriate for central venous catheterization. Because of their large diameter, pulmonary artery catheters are inserted through a wide-bore cannula following dilatation of the vein with a dilator advanced over a guide wire.

Table 82.5 Factors that influence right atrial (central venous) pressure

Blood volume
  Total
  Volume of blood on venous side
  Rate of transfusion or fluid administration
Left ventricular failure
Cor pulmonale
Venoconstriction
Vasopressor administration
Increased intrathoracic pressure
  Mechanical ventilation
  Mediastinal emphysema
  Pneumothorax
  Haemothorax
  Postoperative ileus
Pulmonary embolism
Air embolism
Pulmonary arterial hypertension
Superior vena cava obstruction
Pericardial tamponade
Constrictive pericarditis
Artefacts
  Blocked catheter
  Catheter tip in right ventricle

When the tip is in a central vein, a pressure transducer is connected to the saline-filled distal lumen and the balloon at the tip is inflated. With careful manipulation, the balloon follows the flow of blood through the right atrium and ventricle and into the main pulmonary artery; its progress is assessed by monitoring the pressure waveform (Fig. 82.1). As the catheter is advanced further, its tip enters a branch of the pulmonary artery with a diameter equal to that of the balloon; at this point, the balloon becomes wedged and the arterial pulsation disappears from the trace. When the balloon is deflated, the pulmonary arterial pressure (PAP) trace returns.

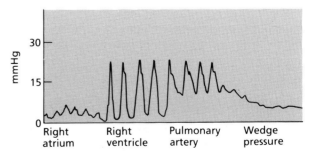

Fig. 82.1 Pressure waveform as a pulmonary artery catheter passes through right atrium, right ventricle and main pulmonary artery to become wedged in a small branch of the pulmonary artery.

Table 82.6 Complications of pulmonary artery catheterization

Ventricular arrhythmias
Valve erosions
Subacute bacterial endocarditis
Pulmonary emboli
Pulmonary infarction
Pulmonary artery rupture
Arteriovenous fistula
Knot formation in right ventricle
Infection

Most pulmonary artery catheters have at least three lumens. The distal lumen is used to record PAP and to obtain samples of mixed venous blood from the pulmonary artery. The proximal lumen, situated approximately 25 cm from the tip, should lie in the right atrium or superior vena cava when the catheter is positioned correctly; it may be used for infusions, injection of fluid for calculation of cardiac output, or for measuring CVP. The third lumen carries air to the balloon at the tip. Additional lumens may be incorporated to carry wires for a thermistor (see below) or for cardiac pacing.

The complications of pulmonary artery catheterization are summarized in Table 82.6. In addition, any of the complications of cannulation at the site of insertion may be encountered. The position of the catheter must be confirmed always by a chest X-ray. PAP is usually measured continuously, and the waveform displayed on an oscilloscope. When wedging occurs, the PAP trace disappears, to be replaced by a trace similar to that seen in the right atrium, and the pressure declines gradually as blood flows towards the left atrium. The pressure plateaus when pressure in the pulmonary artery branch equilibrates with left atrial pressure (LAP). The pressure measured in this way is not always identical to LAP, and is referred to as pulmonary capillary wedge pressure (PCWP) or pulmonary artery occlusion pressure (PAOP).

PCWP should be measured during end-expiration. It is influenced by positive end-expiratory pressure (PEEP), and on average, PCWP is increased by approximately 40% of the end-expiratory pressure. It should always be less than pulmonary artery diastolic pressure (PADP). Overinflation or eccentric inflation of the balloon, or the presence of mitral regurgitation or complete heart block, should be suspected if PCWP exceeds PADP. PCWP may reflect LAP inaccurately in severe left ventricular dysfunction, or if the tip of the catheter is wedged in the upper zones of the lung where pulmonary capillaries may become occluded during inspiration. The pressure *must* be measured

only intermittently, as occlusion of the branch of the pulmonary artery for more than 30–45 s may result in pulmonary infarction; the balloon must be deflated after each measurement has been made and the return of a PAP waveform confirmed. If the PAP trace assumes a 'wedged' pattern with the balloon deflated, the catheter has probably advanced so that the tip is wedged in a small branch of the artery. Its patency should be checked by aspirating blood, and if the waveform remains unchanged, the catheter should be withdrawn until a pulmonary arterial waveform is obtained.

The indications for pulmonary artery monitoring include clinical or anticipated left ventricular dysfunction, particularly in patients with ischaemic heart disease, and titration of therapy to optimize LAP when dissociation between left and right atrial pressures exists, e.g. pulmonary oedema, chronic pulmonary disease and ARDS. Normal values for PAP and PCWP are shown in Table 82.7; however, as with RAP, trends are often more useful than absolute values.

The risks of infection and valvular damage associated with pulmonary artery catheters increase with time, and the catheter should be removed after 48 h unless there are strong indications for its continued use.

Cardiac output

Measurement of cardiac output ($\dot{Q}_T$) may be useful in assessing oxygen delivery, cardiac performance, or the response of the cardiovascular system to treatment. However, all methods of measurement are prone to inaccuracy, and it is important to make other assessments of circulatory adequacy (see below) in conjunction with $\dot{Q}_T$ measurement.

Table 82.7 Normal pressures and oxygen saturations in cardiac chambers

	Pressure (mmHg)	Saturation (%)
Right atrium	0–7	77
Right ventricle	14–30/0–7	75
Pulmonary artery	14–30/5–12	75
Left atrium	4–10	97
Pulmonary capillary wedge pressure	4–10	75
Left ventricle	110–135/4–10	97
Aorta	110–135/60–80	96

Non-invasive techniques

Non-invasive techniques of $\dot{Q}_T$ measurement are available, but, despite manufacturers' claims, they are often inaccurate at measuring absolute values. However, they do reflect changes accurately and may be valuable in following a patient's clinical progress. Impedance cardiography detects voltage changes caused by the ejection of blood from the ventricles. Transcutaneous aortovelography uses ultrasound to detect the velocity of blood flow in the ascending aorta. Stroke volume and cardiac output may be estimated also after injection of technetium-99m-labelled albumin; however, this technique is expensive, and exposes the patient and staff to radioactivity.

Invasive techniques

Invasive techniques of measuring cardiac output are subject to error also, but at present are more reproducible than any of the non-invasive methods. All are based on the Fick principle. The direct Fick method requires measurements to be made of arterial and mixed venous oxygen contents (Cao_2, $C\bar{v}o_2$), and oxygen consumption ($\dot{V}o_2$); the latter is calculated by measuring expired minute volume and inspired and mean oxygen concentrations. $\dot{Q}_T$ is calculated from the formula:

$$Q_T = \frac{\dot{V}o_2}{Cao_2 - C\bar{v}o_2}$$

However, unless very expensive equipment and microprocessor calculation are used, this technique is time consuming, cumbersome and subject to error particularly in the artificially ventilated patient receiving a high fractional inspired oxygen concentration (F_Io_2).

Indicator dilution techniques compute $\dot{Q}_T$ by calculating the degree of dilution of a bolus of indicator after mixing with blood. Two indicators are in common use. Indocyanine green may be injected as a bolus into the right atrium or pulmonary artery. Blood is sampled from a peripheral artery, commonly the radial, and the average concentration of dye and its transit time are measured by sampling blood continuously through a densitometer. $\dot{Q}_T$ can be calculated from these data. This method is also rather cumbersome because of the need to draw blood continuously from the peripheral artery using a syringe pump, and because calibration of the densitometer is required for each patient. In addition, indocyanine green accumulates in the circulation

and limits the frequency with which measurements can be made.

The thermodilution technique is now the most commonly employed. A known volume of liquid at a known temperature (significantly different from the temperature of the patient) is injected into the right atrium, and the temperature of blood in the pulmonary artery measured using a pulmonary artery catheter with a thermistor at its tip. The 'dilution' of temperature difference is calculated, and cardiac output computed from the mean temperature dilution and the transit time of the temperature drop. The accuracy of the method improves if ice-cold liquid is used, especially in children, small adults or low output states. Errors are introduced by injecting the liquid slowly or irregularly. The mean of three measurements, each of which differs by no more than 10%, is usually calculated in order to minimize the errors of individual measurements. The method is easy to perform; the catheters are precalibrated and thermodilution cardiac output computers are easy to use. There is no problem with a shifting baseline. The major disadvantage is that large volumes of fluid are injected if measurements are made frequently. With both dye and thermodilution techniques, the accuracy depends on the shape of the dilution curve; this should be recorded, and calculations based on unsatisfactory curves should be rejected. Cardiac output varies with ventilation. Although reproducibility of cardiac output measurements is improved by injecting the indicator at the same point in the respiratory cycle, the true cardiac output is probably reflected more accurately by averaging values obtained after injection at intervals spread evenly throughout the respiratory cycle (Versprille, 1984).

Derived haemodynamic variables

A number of variables can be calculated after cardiac output and cardiovascular pressures have been measured. Table 82.8 indicates the necessary calculations and normal values of these variables. They are often of value in determining the optimum mode of therapy in the presence of hypotension or cardiac failure. Table 82.9 shows methods of calculating oxygen delivery.

Perfusion

The aim of cardiovascular support in the ICU is usually to obtain satisfactory perfusion of the tissues.

Table 82.8 Derived haemodynamic variables

Variable	Derivation	Normal value (70 kg)
Cardiac output (CO)	SV × heart rate	5 litres/min
Cardiac index (CI)	$\dfrac{CO}{Body\ surface\ area}$	$3.2\ litres \cdot min^{-1} \cdot m^{-2}$
Stroke volume (SV)	$\dfrac{CO}{HR} \times 1000$	80 ml
Stroke index (SI)	$\dfrac{SV}{Body\ surface\ area}$	$50\ ml/m^2$
Systemic vascular resistance (SVR)	$\dfrac{Mean\ arterial\ pressure - CVP}{CO} \times 80$	$1000-1200\ dynes \cdot s^{-1} \cdot cm^{-5}$
Pulmonary vascular resistance (PVR)	$\dfrac{Mean\ pulmonary\ artery - left\ atrial\ pressure}{CO} \times 80$	$60-120\ dynes \cdot s^{-1} \cdot cm^{-5}$
Left ventricular stroke work index (LVSWI)	$\dfrac{1.36\ (Mean\ arterial - left\ atrial\ pressure)}{100} \times SI$	$50-60\ g \cdot m \cdot m^{-2}$
Rate pressure product (RPP)	Systolic arterial pressure × heart rate	
Ejection fraction (EF)	$\dfrac{End\text{-}systolic - end\text{-}diastolic\ volumes}{End\text{-}diastolic\ volume}$	>0.6

Table 82.9 Oxygen delivery

Variable	Derivation	Normal value (70 kg)
Oxygen content (Co_2)	$Hb \times So_2 \times 1.34 + Po_2 \times 0.0225$	18−20 ml/dl
Oxygen delivery ($\dot{D}o_2$)	$CO \times Cao_2 \times 10$	850−1050 ml/min
Oxygen consumption (Vo_2)	$CO \times C(a-\bar{v})o_2$	180−250 ml/min
Oxygen extraction rate	$C(a-\bar{v})o_2/Cao_2$	20−30%

Hb, haemoglobin concentration (g/dl); CO, cardiac output (litres/min); Po_2, oxygen tension (kPa); So_2, fractional oxygen saturation; a, arterial; $\bar{v}$, mixed venous.

An assessment of the perfusion of all tissues may be obtained from the mixed venous oxygen saturation which is reduced in states leading to increased oxygen extraction (e.g. cardiogenic shock) and increased in states of reduced oxygen extraction (e.g. sepsis syndrome). However, there is an increasing awareness that not all tissues become ischaemic simultaneously and therefore there is a requirement for monitoring of individual organs. Urine output gives an impression of renal perfusion but is not reliable alone, because non-oliguric renal failure is a relatively common form of acute renal failure. The advent of *gastric tonometry* has provided a means of monitoring gastric mucosal oxygenation (Fiddian-Green *et al.*, 1982). It is based on the premise that ischaemia leads to a decrease in tissue pH. The tonometer resembles a nasogastric tube. At its tip is a gas-permeable silicone balloon connected by a narrow lumen in the wall of the tube to the proximal end of the tonometer. A small volume of saline is introduced into the balloon and allowed to equilibrate with the intragastric Pco_2. The saline is aspirated and its Pco_2 measured in a blood-gas analyser. An arterial blood sample drawn simultaneously is analysed for bicarbonate concentration. These values are substituted into a modified Henderson−Hasselblach equation in order to produce a value for the intramucosal pH (pH_i). This device has been shown to produce results that correlate with directly measured pH_i. The tonometer may be of great value in the management of the critically ill in view of the increasing awareness of the importance of splanchnic ischaemia in these patients (see below).

The difference between core temperature and the temperature of the large toe has in the past been related to outcome in critically ill patients (Henning *et al.*, 1979). However, a more recent study of 26 critically ill patients (Woods *et al.*, 1987) did not reveal any relationship between core/peripheral temperature gradient and cardiac output or systemic vascular resistance, and the authors counselled against the use of this measurement as an aid to therapeutic decision making.

The degree of cardiovascular monitoring, and the frequency with which observations are made, depend on the severity and nature of the illness. Indications for invasive monitoring are shown in Table 82.10.

Respiratory monitoring

Ventilatory volume and frequency

Gas volumes are usually measured directly, using one of the devices listed in Table 82.11. Monitoring of tidal or minute volume is relatively easy in the ventilated patient, and many ICU ventilators incorporate either a vane respirometer or pneumotachograph. In the patient who is breathing spontaneously without a tracheal tube, a closely fitting mask can be applied and connected to a respirometer, but continuous monitoring can be effected with an impedance or inductance plethysmograph. Ideally, tidal or minute volume should be monitored continuously in the patient undergoing mechanical ventilation so that the development of a large leak in the system, or significant changes in volumes from altered pulmonary compliance or resistance, can be detected rapidly. When this is not possible, measurements should be made at regular intervals, e.g. every 30–60 min. Respiratory frequency is displayed by a number of types of ventilator, or may be counted by nursing staff; it is important to count also the rate of spontaneous ventilation in patients receiving intermittent mandatory or mandatory minute ventilation.

Airway pressure

Changes in airway pressure may indicate a change in compliance, as may occur with the development of pulmonary oedema or pneumothorax, or changes in resistance, e.g. from bronchospasm. It is difficult to measure airway pressure accurately in the spontaneously breathing patient who is without a tracheal

Table 82.10 Indications for invasive cardiovascular monitoring

High-risk, preoperative patients (e.g. recent MI)
Combined acute cardiac and pulmonary disease
Multiple trauma
Pre-existing cardiorespiratory or renal disease
Multiple organ failure
Septic shock
Pulmonary embolism
Fat embolism

Table 82.11 Methods of measuring gas volumes in the ICU

Respirometer (e.g. Wright's)
Pneumotachograph
Heated wire
Vortex spirometer
Inductance plethysmograph

tube. During artificial ventilation, a short end-inspiratory pause permits monitoring of alveolar pressure, which is related to compliance; the difference between peak and pause pressures is influenced predominantly by airway resistance when constant flow ventilators are used. End-expiratory pressure should be monitored also in patients receiving PEEP or continuous positive airways pressure (CPAP). Airway pressure may be measured mechanically or electronically.

However, if expiratory time is insufficient (a situation most commonly encountered in patients with airways obstruction) then alveolar pressure may exceed proximal airway pressure at end-expiration. This phenomenon has been termed auto-PEEP (Pepe & Marini, 1982) and it can lead to progressive air-trapping in the alveoli. Its presence is revealed by an increase in tracheal pressure after end-expiration, measured with the inspiratory and expiratory ventilator limbs occluded.

Pressure/flow–volume loops

Using electronic monitoring techniques, pressure–volume or flow–volume loops can be displayed regularly. Pressure–volume loops are useful in detecting changes in compliance and resistance. The expiratory flow–volume pattern is useful in monitoring the resolution of bronchospasm in asthmatic patients.

Respiratory gas concentrations

The fractional inspired oxygen concentration is an important determinant of alveolar oxygen tension ($P_A o_2$). It should be monitored routinely during artificial ventilation so that adjustments can be made accurately as indicated by arterial blood-gas analysis, and in order to calculate $P_A o_2$ when calculations of alveolar–arterial oxygen tension gradient or intrapulmonary shunt are required. The fractional inspired oxygen concentration is measured usually by a polarographic or fuel cell or using a paramagnetic analyser. These devices have a response time which is too slow to record tidal variations at the airway, and are used only in the inspiratory limb to measure $F_I o_2$.

End-tidal carbon dioxide tension ($P_{ET} co_2$) is derived from end-tidal carbon dioxide concentration, which is measured most commonly using an infrared spectrometer. These devices have a rapid response time. End-tidal carbon dioxide pressure is related to $Pa co_2$, but in patients with pulmonary disease, the gradient between the two may be greater than the normal 0.7 kPa (5.25 mmHg). However, measurement of $P_{ET} co_2$ is useful in following trends in $Pa co_2$, and for calculation of physiological deadspace. Most infrared capnographs show an analogue or digital display of $P_{ET} co_2$, and many also display the expired carbon dioxide waveform. Computer analysis of this waveform has been used in critically ill patients to analyse pulmonary function (Fletcher *et al.*, 1981).

Mass spectrometry is used in some units to analyse respiratory gases. The mass spectrometer has an extremely fast response time, and can simultaneously measure the concentrations of carbon dioxide, oxygen, nitrogen and anaesthetic gases. Using a tracer gas-dilution technique, it is also possible to measure mixed expired concentrations of carbon dioxide and oxygen for calculation of oxygen consumption, carbon dioxide excretion and respiratory quotient.

Blood-gas analysis

Arterial oxygen and carbon dioxide tensions and pH are measured usually intermittently from samples of arterial blood drawn from an arterial puncture or indwelling cannula. Modern blood-gas analysers contain three electrodes and display Po_2, Pco_2 and pH within 1–2 min of inserting a small sample (usually less than 0.25 ml) of heparinized blood. The machines are self-calibrating and may be used by non-technical staff. However, errors may occur unless careful attention is paid to methods of sampling and storage.

Excessive heparin in the sampling syringe decreases pH and Pco_2, and results in large errors in calculated bicarbonate and base excess concentrations. When sampling from an indwelling cannula, the heparinized saline in the connecting tube must be aspirated and discarded before the sample is drawn. Bubbles or air in the syringe should be expelled immediately, or the gases dissolved in blood tend to equilibrate with gas in the bubbles. Storage of the sample for more than a few minutes results in oxygen consumption and carbon dioxide production, particularly by leucocytes; if analysis cannot be carried out immediately, the syringe should be capped and stored in ice-cold water. The syringe should be rotated gently immediately before injection into the analyser in order to ensure complete mixing of blood. The analysing electrodes are maintained at 37°C, and mathematical corrections are required to all three measurements if the patient's temperature is different.

Frequency of arterial blood-gas analysis is determined usually by the clinical condition of the patient. Mixed venous blood-gas analysis can be undertaken by sampling from a pulmonary artery catheter when calculation of intrapulmonary shunt is required.

Continuous monitoring of blood gases has been made possible by the development of intravascular catheters with inbuilt electrodes. All of these devices suffer from having a relatively slow response time. Although pH and Pco_2 electrodes are available, they are relatively unstable and require frequent calibration. Indwelling oxygen electrodes are more stable, and may be useful in monitoring $Pa o_2$ in the very sick patient. However, pulse oximetry is probably superior in most patients.

Oximetry

Oximeters estimate the oxygenation of haemoglobin by measuring either the reflectance or the transmission of light in the red and infrared ranges. Pulse oximeters are used widely in the ICU. Most of these are accurate in all but the severely vasoconstricted patient, and provide a continuous display of oxygen saturation derived from the absorption spectrum of the pulsatile component at the sampling site ($Sp o_2$). $Sp o_2$ is closely related to arterial oxygen saturation ($Sa o_2$), which is almost directly proportional to oxygen content in blood. Thus, it is in many ways a more useful measurement than $Pa o_2$ when arterial oxygenation is impaired. The technique is non-invasive, and its use permits continuous monitoring of arterial oxygenation. Continuous measurement of

Spo_2 may be of value in the patient in whom it is impossible to maintain a normal Pao_2 (e.g. severe ARDS), and in the spontaneously breathing patient with threatened respiratory failure. It may be useful also during such procedures as physiotherapy or tracheal suction, although there is a relatively slow response time when a finger probe is used.

Continuous measurement of mixed venous oxygen saturation ($S\bar{v}o_2$) can be achieved using a pulmonary artery catheter which incorporates three fibre-optic bundles. Light from light-emitting diodes is transmitted through two of the bundles to the tip of the catheter, and light reflected by pulmonary arterial blood is transmitted up the third bundle to a detector at the proximal end of the catheter. Once calibrated, these systems are accurate in the range of 25–95% saturation. Mixed venous oxygen saturation is influenced by cardiac output, arterial oxygenation and tissue oxygen consumption and reflects the average oxygenation of the tissues. The difference between Sao_2 and $S\bar{v}o_2$ indicates oxygen consumption if cardiac output is known. Values of $S\bar{v}o_2$ below 50% in critically ill patients, or failure of $S\bar{v}o_2$ to improve with therapy, are associated with a poor prognosis, whilst values over 65% indicate usually a satisfactory outcome (Kaznitz et al., 1976).

Central nervous system

Clinical examination of the CNS is the single best method of monitoring brain function. However, in the comatose patient, other means may be necessary.

Electroencephalogram

The rhythm, amplitude and waveform pattern of the EEG may be used to monitor patients with suspected CNS dysfunction. However, EEG interpretation requires skilled assistance. In addition, there is considerable variability in the normal EEG, and the relationship between clinical and EEG abnormalities is often poor. Conventional EEG monitoring can be performed only intermittently, and is subject to interference from other apparatus in the ICU. A variety of methods is available for processing the EEG signal to provide a continuous and more easily interpreted form of monitoring.

Frequency domain analysis

This technique displays the frequency distribution of the EEG. The compressed spectral array (Fig. 82.2) is an example of this form of monitoring. The

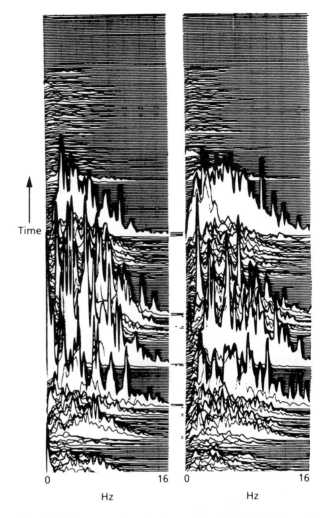

Fig. 82.2 Compressed spectral array, showing fitting followed by electrical silence in a patient with meningoencephalitis. (Redrawn from Willatts, 1985.)

amplitudes at each frequency are displayed as a series of 'hills' and 'valleys'. Monitoring can be carried out continuously, but interpretation is difficult in the comatose patient unless gross abnormalities are present.

Time domain analysis

The cerebral function monitor (CFM) displays the integrated electrical activity from the cerebral cortex as a trace of amplitude plotted against time (Fig. 82.3). Electrical activity increases in the presence of seizures, and decreases if cerebral ischaemia or hypoxia occur. Sedation with intravenous anaesthetic agents also decreases the amplitude of the trace.

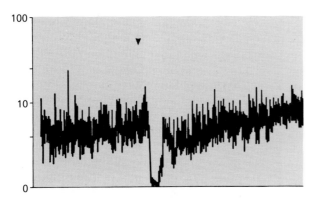

Fig. 82.3 Trace from a cerebral function monitor, showing interruption of the circulation at the arrow causing a transient absence of cerebral activity. (Redrawn from Willatts, 1985.)

Time and frequency domain analysis

The cerebral function analysing monitor (CFAM) displays the total electrical activity of the brain together with the percentage of that activity which falls in the α-, β-, γ- and δ-frequency bands. Its role in ICU has yet to be established.

Evoked potentials

Auditory, visual and somatosensory evoked potentials can be used to assess the integrity of pathways in the brainstem and cerebral cortex. Asymmetrical conduction or absent potentials are poor prognostic signs after cerebral trauma. Delayed conduction may occur in the presence of anaesthetic agents or oedema.

Intracranial pressure

Intracranial pressure (ICP) may increase and cerebral perfusion pressure (CPP) decrease in some categories of comatose patient, e.g. traumatic or metabolic coma. These patients often receive heavy sedation or are paralysed in order to provide artificial ventilation so that adequate oxygenation and a decrease in arterial carbon dioxide tension may be achieved. Consequently, it is virtually impossible to monitor neurological function clinically. The likelihood of permanent cerebral damage increases if ICP exceeds 3.3–4.0 kPa (25–30 mmHg), or if CPP is less than 8 kPa (60 mmHg). Continuous monitoring of ICP permits early therapeutic intervention if ICP starts to increase, and, intuitively, careful control of ICP should help to reduce the probability of secondary cerebral damage occurring. ICP is monitored most accurately using a fluid-filled catheter inserted into the lateral ventricle,

but this technique is associated with the highest incidence of infective complications. Measurement of pressure in the subarachnoid space can be achieved by insertion of a catheter through a conventional burrhole, or using a 'bolt' threaded into a smaller burrhole in the skull. Despite the anticipated advantages of ICP monitoring, there is little evidence to show that control of ICP improves outcome in patients with severe head trauma. However, computerized analyses of the ICP waveform and automated recognition of patterns of ICP change may be able in future to predict dangerous increases in ICP, and might be useful in improving prognosis.

Infection control

Hospital-acquired (nosocomial) infection complicates the course of at least 40% of patients admitted to ICU. It has been estimated that 150 000 deaths occur each year in the USA alone as a direct result of infections which were not present, and not incubating, in patients at the time of admission to hospital (Farber, 1987). The survivors spend a longer period of time in hospital and often require treatment with the most expensive antibiotics. ICU patients are particularly susceptible to infection for a number of reasons. The body's natural defences are breached by a tracheal tube, intravascular monitoring cannulae and urinary catheters; the immune system may be depressed by the severity of the patient's illness; infection may be transmitted from other patients after incubation in items of equipment or by staff; and antibiotics prescribed for infection by relatively susceptible microorganisms may permit superinfection by resistant bacteria.

Pneumonia

Nosocomial lower respiratory tract infections are the third most common type of hospital-acquired infection; only wound and urinary infections are more frequent. The overall mortality has been reported to be 30% (Farber, 1987), although the rate may be considerably higher in specific situations such as polymicrobial pneumonia (Celis *et al.*, 1988). The incidence of nosocomial pneumonia in ICU patients has been estimated at 9–15%. In a recent European multicentre study, 33% of patients admitted to ICU with no evidence of pulmonary infection developed pneumonia subsequently (Ruiz-Santana *et al.*, 1987). Unfortunately, sputum cultures for the diagnosis of pneumonia in hospitalized patients have a specificity of approximately 30%, and the true incidence of nosocomial pneumonia is extremely difficult to estimate using this technique. Celis and colleagues (1988) noted that clinically diagnosed nosocomial pneumonias in which no organism could be identified had a relatively benign prognosis and suggested that 60% of patients without a definitely identified microbial pathogen may have had lung infiltrates that were not pneumonic. This has implications for any study which assesses the incidence of pneumonia. However, 11 of 12 patients treated with an 'inappropriate antibiotic' subsequently died.

Blood cultures are relatively rarely positive in primary pneumonia (Crim, 1989) and thus interest currently centres on the bronchoscopic techniques of broncoalveolar lavage (BAL) and the protected brush catheter (PBC) for the diagnosis of nosocomial pneumonia. These techniques use special catheters introduced through a bronchoscope into a distal bronchus in the region suspected of being infected. The BAL technique involves the recovery and culture of a small volume of lavage fluid, while the PBC uses a special brush which is used to sample secretions from the distal airways. The brush is located within a protective sleeve during introduction and removal, thus preventing contamination of the sample. However, a review of the published investigations of these techniques criticized the methodology of most of the studies, and suggested that the definitive study of these techniques had yet to be performed (Cook et al., 1991). Nevertheless, a patient who has clinical signs of pneumonia and who has a negative PBC and/or BAL may require antibiotics for treatment of a non-pulmonary infection.

Causes

A number of factors may increase the risk of nosocomial pneumonia (Table 82.12). The most important of these are thoracic or thoracoabdominal surgery, and artificial ventilation, especially if continued for more than 72 h.

The most common causative organisms found in one large study are listed in Table 82.13. Most are Gram-negative bacilli, although the exact pattern varies in different hospitals and depends in part on the original complaint of the patient. *Klebsiella* and *Staphylococcus aureus* infections are more common in obstetric and paediatric patients, and *Haemophilus influenzae* in ICU patients who have suffered trauma. Viruses may be responsible for a proportion of cases of pneumonia in the ICU; these may be transmitted by staff, but are thought more often to be the result of reactivation of latent disease as a result of temporary

Table 82.12 Factors which increase risk of developing nosocomial pneumonia

Thoracoabdominal surgery
Mechanical ventilation
Thoracic surgery
Upper abdominal surgery
Smoking
Low serum albumin
Prolonged surgery (>3 h)
High ASA classification
Corticosteroids
Prolonged hospital stay (>40 days)
Other infection
Social class
? Age
? Male gender
? Obesity

Table 82.13 Causative organisms of hospital-acquired pneumonia in decreasing order of frequency. (From Ruiz-Santana et al., 1987)

Pseudomonas aeruginosa
Proteus mirabilis
Escherichia coli
Staphylococcus aureus
Serratia marcescens
Klebsiella pneumoniae
Other Gram-negative aerobes
Enterobacter spp.
Streptococcus pneumoniae
Haemophilus influenzae
Other *Pseudomonas* spp.
Other Gram-positive aerobes
Other *Serratia* spp.
Bacteroides fragilis
Bacteroides spp.
Other Gram-negative anaerobes
Fungi

immunosuppression. Patients with severe immunosuppression may develop infections with uncommon pathogens; this subject is dealt with in a separate section below.

There are three mechanisms by which organisms may infect the lower respiratory tract in the critically ill patient. There may be blood-borne spread. Infected material may be aspirated from the pharynx; this may contain upper respiratory tract flora, or may consist of gastrointestinal contents regurgitated from the stomach. Finally, there may be inhalation of droplets containing bacteria.

Normally, the lung is well protected against entry of foreign material. The laryngeal reflex is usually sufficiently strong to prevent aspiration of pharyngeal contents. The nose and nasopharynx filter out inhaled particles or droplets which exceed 3 μm in diameter, and those larger than 1 μm are deposited on the tracheal or bronchial mucosa, and removed by ciliary transport. The growth of microorganisms which reach the alveoli is inhibited by surfactant and complement, and removed by phagocytosis, which is stimulated by immunoglobulins and complement products.

These defence mechanisms are altered by disease, and may be influenced by treatment. The gag reflex is depressed in patients with neurological disease involving the cranial nerves, and in those who are semiconscious or debilitated; 70% of patients with depressed consciousness aspirate during sleep (Huxley et al., 1978). Aspiration is not prevented completely by the presence of a cuffed tracheal tube. Indeed up to 60% of ventilated patients regurgitate gastric contents to the pharynx and 30% aspirate past the tracheal tube cuff into the trachea (Ibanez et al., 1988; Nachtkamp et al., 1988). The normal bacterial flora of the nasopharynx inhibit the growth of more virulent strains; when antibiotics are administered, staphylococci and coliform bacilli proliferate. Elderly patients who have been hospitalized for some time have colonies of Klebsiella, Escherichia coli or Enterobacter in the oropharynx even if no antibiotics have been administered. The incidence of colonization is highest in those who have been in hospital longest, and those with respiratory infections or severe illness. It has been shown that over 80% of patients become colonized with one or more hospital-acquired potentially pathogenic microorganisms in the first 5 days of admission to an ICU (Stoutenbeek et al., 1984). Thus, aspiration of fluid from the oropharynx appears to be the source of many cases of respiratory infection.

The majority of bacteria which colonize the oropharynx originate in the gut. In patients with ileus, and those with high intraluminal pH, the gastric content is not sterile. Patients treated with antacids or H_2-receptor antagonists have a high gastric pH, and bacteria can be cultured from gastric aspirate. In several studies, the same organism has been cultured from tracheal and gastric aspirates in a large proportion of ICU patients with pneumonia (du Moulin et al., 1982).

Chronic lung disease and anaesthetic drugs inhibit ciliary movement. Alveolar defences are impaired by nutritional deficiency, pulmonary oedema or ARDS. Tracheal intubation allows droplets of any size to bypass the nasopharynx, and prevents ciliary transport of infected material. High inspired oxygen concentrations inhibit ciliary movement and surfactant production.

Any equipment used to deliver gases may act as a source of infection, particularly if it contains fluids. Nebulizers used during physiotherapy to loosen bronchial secretions, and those used for drug administration, are likely to become colonized with Pseudomonas organisms. Ventilator humidifiers may act as a breeding ground for bacteria unless maintained at an adequate temperature. The expiratory ventilator tubing becomes contaminated with secretions where bacteria multiply; some of this infected material may be reintroduced into the patient's bronchial tree if fluid in the expiratory limb is not collected in traps. The tip of the tracheal tube becomes contaminated almost always with infected secretions. The incidence of colonization with Gram-negative organisms is higher if the tracheal tube is left in place for more than 8 days. During tracheal suctioning, crusts of infected material may be dislodged into the bronchial tree.

Prevention

In patients about to undergo major elective surgery, smoking should be discontinued, pre-existing infection treated with appropriate antibiotic therapy and physiotherapy, and any congestive cardiac failure should be controlled. The risk of nosocomial pneumonia in the ICU may be minimized by using only sterile water in humidifiers, and by ensuring that they are maintained at an appropriate temperature. Water in the ventilator tubing becomes infected in both inspiratory and expiratory limbs, and must not be allowed to drain towards the tracheal tube. Bacteria may migrate along the inspiratory limb towards the humidifier. Because of this, it is normal practice to change humidifier water and ventilator tubing every 24 h, although there is some evidence that changing ventilator tubing only every 48 h does not increase the risk of contamination. The introduction of infection by droplet spread from the atmosphere may be minimized by placing bacterial filters on the air inlet port of air-entraining ventilators and humidifiers, and filtering gas at the expiratory port reduces contamination of the atmosphere by infected material from the expiratory limb. The use of a filter between the tracheal tube and the ventilator reduces contamination of the patient's lungs from the inspired gas, and of the expiratory limb from the patient's bronchial tree, and acts as a condenser humidifier. It has been suggested that this obviates the need for a water humidifier, and so eliminates the risk of humidifier contamination. However, there is some doubt as to whether these filters are efficient enough in the critically ill patient to prevent tracheal secretions from becoming thick and difficult to remove.

Inappropriate use of antibiotics should be avoided, as this may encourage the growth of resistant strains of bacteria in the lungs. Meticulous attention by staff to hand-washing is important in reducing the risk of cross-infection. The use of H_2-receptor antagonists may not be appropriate in patients with a high risk of developing nosocomial pneumonia. Chest physiotherapy is believed to reduce the risk, or at least the severity, of nosocomial pneumonia, although there are few data to confirm this. In the patient who is breathing spontaneously, adequate analgesia must be provided to permit deep breathing and coughing, but excessive sedation must be avoided. After abdominal surgery, there is a decrease in functional residual capacity (FRC), which may decline below closing capacity (CC). Atelectasis is likely to occur in this situation. Positive pressure breathing produced intermittently by pressure-cycled ventilation applied through a mouthpiece may help to reduce atelectasis. However, the use of CPAP increases FRC, and can be applied comfortably using a mask (Fig. 82.4). CPAP improves gas exchange and reduces nosocomial infection in patients who have undergone major abdominal or thoracic surgery and in those being weaned from intermittent positive-pressure ventilation (IPPV) (Feeley et al., 1975).

Selective decontamination of the gastrointestinal tract (SDD) in order to reduce the likelihood of aspiration into the lungs of infected gastrointestinal fluid has been extensively investigated in recent years. It is based on the concept that the majority of infections in the critically ill are endogenous and are caused by potentially pathogenic organisms (PPM) — predominantly Gram-negative aerobes — which have previously colonized the patient at the expense of the indigenous intestinal flora. These PPM may be present when the patient is admitted, and cause early infection (primary endogenous infection) or colonize the patient in the course of the admission causing later infection (secondary endogenous infection). Selective decontamination sets out to minimize gastrointestinal colonization, protect indigenous anaerobic bacterial populations and thus reduce infection. The technique involves intensive bacteriological surveillance coupled with routine application of antibiotic/antifungal paste to the buccal mucosa and administration of a liquid preparation containing the same agents via the nasogastric tube four times

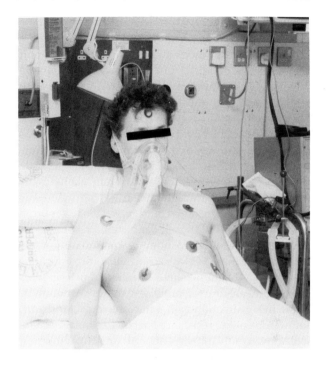

Fig. 82.4 A patient receiving continuous positive airway pressure (CPAP) by mask.

per day. An intravenous antibiotic is also administered from admission either for a fixed time period or until PPM are eliminated. It is therefore expensive in nursing time and bacteriological support services. The increased expenditure involved in prophylaxis may be offset to some extent by decreased antibiotic use in the treatment of later infections, but a detailed investigation of costs in one study failed to confirm this (van Dalen, 1991). The greatest decrease in infections with SDD has been in those of the lower respiratory tract. Very few trials have used the more sophisticated techniques detailed above to diagnose pneumonia. In three that did, two noted a decrease in infection rates but one recorded that this was not so in the subgroup of patients who remained in the ICU for more than 4 days. Unfortunately, the expected reductions in mortality and length of stay have not been realized in the general ICU population (Hammond et al., 1992). However, specific subgroups of patients may benefit from SDD (Ledingham et al., 1988). Although SDD promises much, it remains controversial and is still under investigation. The originators of this therapy find three indications for SDD — trauma, liver transplantation and the control of outbreaks of multiresistant microorganisms (van Sane et al., 1990). Antibiotic resistance has not been a significant problem to date.

Diagnosis and Treatment

Appropriate respiratory and cardiovascular support measures are required often in order to maintain adequate tissue oxygenation. Clearly, the patient's primary illness must be treated if possible. Nutritional support may be required also. Antibiotic therapy should be based ideally on sensitivity studies on bacteria cultured from the patient's lungs. However, this is often impractical, and leads to long delays in starting treatment. A Gram stain of the specimen may give an indication of the pathogenic organism. Chastre and colleagues (1988) reported that Gram stain of intracellular bacteria recovered by BAL might also be of help in determining early antibiotic treatment. Most nosocomial lung infections result from Gram-negative bacilli or *Staphylococcus aureus*. The choice of antibiotic therapy should be made in consultation with a microbiologist, and with knowledge of the resistance spectra of similar bacteria isolated recently in the ICU. At present, empirical therapy for Gram-negative bacilli consists often of an antipseudomonal penicillin and an aminoglycoside (although serum concentrations at the upper end of the therapeutic range are required because of poor penetration in the lung), or a third generation cephalosporin with an antipseudomonal penicillin or imipenem; a penicillinase-resistant penicillin should be used for staphylococcal infection.

When sensitivity studies have been undertaken, it may be necessary to change the antibiotic regimen.

Nosocomial bacteraemia

Approximately 5% of all nosocomial infections result in bacteraemia, and 25% of these are related to intravascular cannulae or catheters. The remainder are the result of infection acquired by other routes, e.g. secondary to nosocomial pneumonia or abdominal sepsis.

Table 82.14 lists the sites at which infection may be introduced when the integrity of the vascular system is breached by a cannula. The most common site of entry is the area of skin puncture. Contamination from this source is with the patient's own skin flora, such as *Staphylococcus epidermidis*, diphtheroids and some anaerobic organisms. However, the skin of patients who have been hospitalized for some days, and of those who have received antibiotic therapy, is often colonized with more virulent bacteria. Infection may be introduced also by hospital personnel during insertion of the cannula or subsequent dressing of the site. The hands of medical staff and nurses are

Table 82.14 Sites of introduction of infection to the bloodstream from intravascular devices

---

Intravenous fluids
    Contamination during manufacture
    Contamination during insertion of giving set
    Contamination introduced with additives
Injection ports
Stopcocks
Transducers
Flush solutions
Connections and Y-junctions
CVP manometers
Catheter insertion site
    Skin flora
    Contamination of operator's hands
    Contaminated or inadequate disinfectants

---

often contaminated with *Staphylococcus aureus* and Gram-negative bacilli.

Organisms gain access to the circulation by migrating along the cannula, and may then become attached to the fibrin sheath which forms around the intravascular portion of the cannula as a normal reaction to its presence. This sheath may then act as a medium for multiplication of bacteria, whilst also protecting the organisms from antibiotics.

Diagnosis

External signs of infection (erythema, swelling or pus) are present in less than 50% of subsequently proven, catheter-related infections, and the diagnosis is made often by process of exclusion when no other source of bacteraemia is found. Catheter-related sepsis should always be considered when appropriate antibiotics are unsuccessful in treating bacteraemia. Positive confirmation is made by culturing the tip of the catheter after its removal. Positive cultures may be obtained from a catheter tip which has been infected secondarily in patients with bacteraemia from another source. However, the number of colonies of bacteria cultured from the catheter tip is lower in these cases. A semiquantitative culture technique has been described (Maki *et al.*, 1977) which is claimed to identify if the catheter is the source of infection. However, this results in a high false-positive rate. A more recent rapid technique which involves slicing and Gram-staining the catheter tip appears to be more sensitive and specific (Cooper & Hopkins, 1985).

The most common organisms isolated from intravascular cannulae are *Staphylococcus aureus* and *Staphylococcus epidermidis*; although the latter is often thought of as a benign organism, it now appears to be a major pathogen (Ponce de Leon & Wenzel, 1984). *Enterococci, Klebsiella* and *E. coli* are also cultured commonly, and occasional reports have been made of infection of intravascular lines with *Candida*.

Relationship with type of catheter

Peripheral venous catheters are used most commonly throughout the hospital, and most ICU patients have at least one in place. Infection is more common if the cannula is inserted in an emergency, if an aseptic technique is not used, if a surgical cutdown is required, and if the cannula is left in position for more than 72 h. Daily dressing changes, the use of semipermeable dressings and local antibiotic ointment have been recommended, but there is no definite evidence that these reduce the risk of infection. In-line filters reduce the incidence of thrombophlebitis, but have not been proved to reduce infection.

Central venous catheters are often considered to present a higher risk of bacteraemia than peripheral cannulae, but the risk of infection per day of catheterization is lower. The incidence of infection is increased in the presence of distant infection (although blood-borne spread of infection to catheters is said to be rare) and, in the case of lines inserted in the jugular or subclavian veins, if a tracheostomy is in place. Infection is less common if a strict aseptic technique is used for insertion but postinsertion management is probably at least as important (Keohane *et al.*, 1983). Movement of the catheter increases the risk of infection, and it should be anchored well at its site of insertion. Silicone catheters are surrounded by a smaller fibrin sheath than plastic catheters, and are probably associated with a lower risk of infection.

Long-term central venous cannulae are used for intravenous nutrition or the administration of chemotherapy. The infection rate is extremely low if insertion is conducted aseptically and the catheter tunnelled subcutaneously so that the exit site in the skin is some distance from the site of venous puncture. The most common site of infection is the exit of the tunnel. Whilst this may be treated by systemic antibiotics, infection throughout the tunnel requires removal of the catheter. Catheters have been left in place successfully for as long as 2.5 years.

Pulmonary arterial catheters are associated with all the risks of central venous catheters, but in addition,

have a large puncture wound, are handled and manipulated usually to a considerable degree during insertion, are often left in place inside an introducing sheath which is filled with blood, and pass through the chambers of the heart resulting in damage to the endocardium. Endocardial lesions occur in over 50% of all patients in whom a pulmonary artery catheter has been inserted (Rowley *et al.*, 1984), and over 10% of these patients are likely to have infective endocarditis. It has been estimated that 3% of pulmonary artery catheters are a source of bacteraemia if left in place for longer than 72 h.

Arterial cannulae are associated with an increased risk of infection if left in place for more than 4 days. In one study, approximately 14% of arterial cannulae showed signs of local infection, and 4% were responsible for bacteraemia (Band & Maki, 1979). Although bacteraemia is the most serious complication, serious local skin infection may occur also; an abscess containing 30 ml has been reported at the site of a radial artery cannula, with minimal external signs of infection (Lindsay *et al.*, 1987).

There are no strict guidelines regarding the duration of catheter insertion beyond which the infection rate increases substantially. However, a recent prospective randomized study did not support routine changing of central or peripheral venous or intra-arterial catheters (Eyer *et al.*, 1990).

Prevention (Centers for Disease Control Working Group, 1981)

The operator's hands should be washed before insertion of any cannula. Soap and water is appropriate before insertion of a peripheral line, but an antiseptic should be used before insertion of any central line. Sterile gloves should be worn for insertion of any central line, and for insertion of any cannula requiring a cutdown. Veins in the arm or neck are preferable to veins in the leg or groin. The site should be prepared with iodine 1 or 2%, chlorhexidine or 70% alcohol; the solution should be in contact with the skin for at least 30 s before venepuncture is performed. The cannula should be secured firmly to the skin; if tape is used, it must not cover the puncture site. A topical antiseptic or antibiotic and sterile dressing should be applied. The date and time of insertion should be recorded.

The minimum number of connections between infusion bag and cannula should be made. Injection ports should be swabbed before use. Daily examination of catheter sites should be made, including palpation through the dressing to elicit tenderness. The intravenous administration set should be changed every 48 h. The entire administration system should be changed if there is any evidence of sepsis.

Disposable components should be used whenever possible. Those preassembled by the manufacturer are preferable. A closed flush system should be used. They should not be stored after preparation and flushing, although there is evidence that the risk of contamination is small over a 72-h storage period (Tenold *et al.*, 1987). Glucose solutions should never be used to flush intravascular pressure lines because of the increased risk of infection. Flush solutions should be changed every 24 h, and the administration and flushing set every 48 h. If any part of the system is contaminated with blood (except the tubing between catheter and sampling point), it is desirable to replace the contaminated sections. Three-way stopcocks should be used only if essential, and covered when not in use. The number of blood samples taken from indwelling lines should be kept to a minimum.

Sepsis syndrome

A recent study found that more than 50% of the critically ill patients investigated who fulfilled a specific definition of 'sepsis' did not have a demonstrable bacteraemia (Bone *et al.*, 1989). The similarity of the clinical pattern between the bacteraemic and non-bacteraemic patients suggests that some final common pathway might be involved and there is considerable evidence that the gut may play a role in this syndrome (Wilmore *et al.*, 1988). It has been known since the 1950s that haemorrhagic shock can result in a state of endotoxaemia and that this endotoxin derives from the gut. The 'leaky gut' hypothesis did not gain acceptance at the time, and has been 'rediscovered' recently. Animal models of haemorrhagic shock, gut ischaemia and burns have all demonstrated damage to the gut with resulting alteration in permeability of the mucosa to endotoxin and bacteria. Endotoxin infusion into the portal vein has been shown to produce a hypermetabolic state whereas systemic infusion does not (Arita *et al.*, 1988). Furthermore, endotoxin has been shown *in vitro* to stimulate Kuppfer cells to produce mediators which can produce the clinical picture of hypermetabolic sepsis and to alter cell−cell communication between hepatocytes, resulting in increased acute-phase protein production and decreased albumin production by these cells. Similar effects may result from bacterial translocation to the portal circulation. Thus, it seems that a number of insults may result in deterioration of gut function and consequent endotoxin and bacterial contamination of the circulation, possibly stimulating or perpetuating a state of hypermetabolic sepsis.

A burn model of sepsis showed a 50% loss of small bowel mucosal mass in the first 24 h after injury. This could be attenuated almost completely by immediate postburn enteral feeding (Dominioni *et al.*, 1984).

Although this process has not yet been proved to be of importance in humans, there is some evidence that similar processes occur. Rush and colleagues (1988) found that over 50% of trauma patients admitted with a systolic blood pressure of less than 10.6 kPa (80 mmHg) had positive blood cultures, whereas the incidence was 4% in those admitted with a systolic pressure greater than 14.6 kPa (110 mmHg). In addition, a preliminary study has shown a decreased incidence of infective complications in patients given total enteral nutrition within 12 h of injury compared to those given TPN started within the same period (Moore *et al.*, 1989).

Binding of endotoxin by polymixins and decreasing the load of Gram-negative organisms in the gut may be one of the mechanisms of action of selective decontamination. However, there is some evidence that SDD may increase translocation of Gram-positive organisms (Jackson *et al.*, 1990).

It is possible that the final common pathway of these insults is to produce intramucosal hypoxia. Although oxygenation of the mucosa is difficult to monitor, mucosal hypoxia will lead to a fall in intramucosal pH (pH_i). Manipulation of pH_i has been studied recently in a group of critically ill patients with improvement in outcome (see above).

'Gut failure' may be of central importance to the sepsis syndrome, multiple organ failure and death. It has been estimated that it may result in 100 000 deaths per year in the USA. Prevention and management of 'gut failure' warrants further investigation.

The immunosuppressed patient

The normal immunological defence mechanisms may be impaired by a number of diseases. Immunological depression may occur to some degree in many acute conditions, but specific depression of cellular immunity occurs in patients with Hodgkin's disease, some leukaemias and AIDS, and low levels of immunoglobulins are found in multiple myeloma. In addition, drug therapy may induce immunological depression. Steroids and chemotherapy for leukaemia, lymphoma and bone-marrow transplantation depress cellular immunity, and cytotoxic drugs used for some tumours result in impairment of both cellular and humoral immune mechanisms. Patients with a neutrophil count of less than 1×10^9 cells/litre appear to be most at risk. Immunocompromised patients are susceptible to any infection, although specific pathogens which are combated easily in the normal patient may result also in life-threatening illness. Infections are caused usually by organisms which have colonized the patient before the acute episode; in one study of patients with acute non-lymphocytic leukamia, almost 50% of these organisms were acquired within hospital (Schimpff et al., 1972).

Prevention of infection

Protective isolation

Simple isolation in an isolation room in which all staff wear a gown, mask and gloves, has not been found to reduce the risk of infection in the immuno-compromised patient (Nauseef & Maki, 1981). The use of filtered air, which removes virtually all particles greater than $0.3\,\mu$m in diameter, has been shown to reduce dramatically the number of airborne micro-organisms. However, neither protective 'bubbles' nor laminar airflow rooms supplied with filtered air have been shown to influence the incidence of infection in immunocompromised patients in most of the randomized trials which have been conducted, although there is some evidence to suggest that the infection rate, and particularly the incidence of pneumonia, is reduced in patients who remain isolated for more than 3 weeks (Yates & Holland, 1972). Patients undergoing bone-marrow grafting for aplastic anaemia or leukaemia have a reduced incidence of graft rejection if isolated in a laminar airflow environment.

Reduction of endogenous bacteria

The gastrointestinal tract is the major site of colonization with bacteria which may subsequently cause clinically important infection. Hospital food, particularly salads and vegetables, has a high content of pathogens. Immunocompromised patients do not require sterile food, but food with low bacterial counts should be available. Sterilization of the gastrointestinal tract with non-absorbable antibiotics (usually gentamicin, vancomycin and nystatin) is effective in suppressing gut flora, but has not been

proved conclusively to influence the incidence of infection; in addition, this regimen causes significant incidences of nausea, vomiting and diarrhoea. Selective suppression of gut flora with trimethoprim and sulphamethoxazole reduces the number of aerobic Gram-negative organisms in the gut, but has little effect on anaerobic bowel flora. This regimen has been shown to reduce the incidence of infections in immunocompromised patients with a variety of types of primary pathology. However, there is an increased risk of fungal infections, and little effect has been seen in the eventual outcome of the patients.

Topical antibiotic or antiseptic regimens have been suggested as a means of reducing skin flora. These involve usually bathing or showering daily in an antiseptic solution, with local antibiotic treatment of mouth and nose. However, it has proved to be virtually impossible to sterilize the skin completely, and the effect on infections remains unclear.

Specific prophylaxis

Viral infections are more common in immuno-compromised patients. Reactivation of latent herpes simplex occurs in up to 40% of patients, but the incidence can be reduced by the administration of acyclovir. The risks of contracting varicella zoster infection in children, and cytomegalovirus infection in all immunocompromised patients, may be reduced by administration of specific immunoglobulins. Trimethoprim/sulphamethoxazole treatment reduces the risk of Pneumocystis carinii infection, but is recommended only for patients in areas where infection with this protozoon is common because of fears that resistant strains may develop.

Granulocyte infusions have been shown to reduce the incidence of bacterial sepsis by 60% in patients with leukaemia (Strauss et al., 1981). However, overall infection rates and survival are not altered.

Prevention of spread of infection

There are three mechanisms (Table 82.15) by which infection may spread in the ICU. True airborne transmission in droplets of less than $10\,\mu$m in diameter, and transmission in larger droplets (i.e. greater than $10\,\mu$m) (which requires relatively close contact), have been implicated in spread of respiratory viral infections such as influenza, para-influenza, varicella, measles, rhinoviruses, rubella, echovirus and adenoviruses. Members of staff, rather than other patients, are usually the source. Paediatric patients are particularly susceptible. Aspergillus and other fungi may be

Table 82.15 Mechanisms of spread of infection and reservoirs in ICU

Contact	Airborne	Ingestion
Mattresses	Ventilators	Food
Bandages	Humidifiers	Enteral feeds
Stethoscopes	Nebulizers	Ice
Endoscopes	Air conditioning	
Bronchoscopes	False ceilings	
Thermometers	Building work	
Suction apparatus	Staff respiratory	
Pressure transducers	infections	
Contaminated disinfectants		
Sinks		
Toilets		
Flower vases		

present on dust particles in hospital, particularly during rebuilding programmes. *Pseudomonas* and staphylococci may be carried on droplets from infected linen. However, the major source is contaminated respiratory equipment, such as humidifiers and ventilators.

Indirect contact spread may occur if any item of equipment is contaminated by contact with an infected patient or staff member, and used subsequently without being sterilized. Stethoscopes are often contaminated with pathogens, especially *Staphylococcus aureus*, and should be cleaned regularly with 70% alcohol. Endoscopes are contaminated readily, and disinfection is difficult and time consuming. Bacteraemia following gastroduodenal endoscopy occurs in up to 8% of patients, and respiratory infection has been reported after use of contaminated bronchoscopes. Thermometers often harbour pathogenic organisms, despite the use of sheaths; perforation of plastic sheaths is common. Non-disposable items such as tracheal tubes, suction tubing or drains may also transmit infection, although most units now use only disposable items. Infection may also be spread by contact with the bed, mattress or bed linen.

Indirect spread may result also from contamination of staff. Medical and nursing staff may become contaminated after contact with another patient, or from another source in the unit. Sinks are a common source. *Pseudomonas* has been isolated from up to 59% of hospital sinks, and may contaminate staff either by direct contact or by large droplet spread during hand-washing. Heat traps are effective in reducing contamination of the waste pipe.

Many types of bacteria have been isolated from

water in flower vases. Nurses' hands may become contaminated after changing water in vases, or if spillage occurs. In most units, fresh flowers are not permitted for this reason. Contaminated water has been implicated in the transmission of intravascular infection; warm water baths for thawing fresh frozen plasma, and iced water baths for cooling syringes before thermodilution cardiac output measurements, can result in bacteraemia.

Isolation

Prevention of cross-infection from an infected patient requires that precautions must be taken which are appropriate to the nature of the infective organism, the source (e.g. respiratory tract, body secretions, skin) and the means of transmission. In many cases, adequate isolation may be achieved with the patient in the main area of the ward. However, an isolation room should be available for some categories of patient. This room should have a negative air pressure relative to the main unit, and the room should be vented directly to the outside of the building.

Isolation precautions may be considered as category-specific or disease-specific. Recommendations for category-specific isolation are summarized in Table 82.16, and examples of diseases requiring each category of isolation are shown in Table 82.17.

Antibiotic resistance

Resistance to antibiotics may occur by a number of mechanisms. Bacteria vary in the composition of the cell wall which surrounds the cell membrane; Gram-positive bacteria are relatively permeable to antibiotics, whereas Gram-negative organisms have a more complex wall which is less permeable. Many microorganisms synthesize enzymes which inactivate antibiotics. Beta-lactamases are a group of enzymes which can inactivate the β-lactam ring of a variety of antibiotics including most penicillins and cephalosporins. These enzymes may be excreted into the immediate surroundings of the bacteria, or may exist between the inner and outer cell membranes. They may be a normal constituent of the bacterium, or their production may be induced in the presence of an antibiotic. The capacity to produce the enzymes may be mediated by chromosomes or by plasmids; plasmid-mediated resistance may be transferred to other bacteria of the same, or occasionally of other, species. Some species of Gram-negative bacteria produce β-lactamases which are capable of inacti-

Table 82.16 Category-specific isolation requirements. (From Garner & Simmons, 1983)

Strict isolation
Private room, door kept closed
Mask, gown and gloves must be worn by all persons entering room
Hands must be washed after touching patient or contaminated articles
Contaminated articles, e.g. linen, must be discarded or bagged and labelled before being sent for decontamination

Contact isolation
Private room
Masks should be worn by those in close contact with patient
Gowns should be worn if soiling with infected material likely
Gloves should be worn if touching infected material
Hand-washing and disposal as for strict isolation

Respiratory isolation
Private room
Masks should be worn by those in close contact with patient
Hand-washing and disposal as for strict isolation

Tuberculous isolation
Private room with negative pressure, door closed
Masks should be worn if patient is coughing
Gowns should be worn if gross contamination likely
Hand-washing and disposal as for strict isolation

Enteric precautions
Private room if patient hygiene poor, or if incontinent
Gowns should be worn if soiling likely
Gloves should be worn when touching infected material
Hand-washing and disposal as for strict isolation

Drainage/secretion precautions
Gowns should be worn if soiling likely
Gloves should be worn when touching infected material
Hand-washing and disposal as for strict isolation

Blood/body fluid precautions
Private room if patient hygiene poor, or if incontinent
Gowns should be worn if soiling with blood or body fluids likely
Gloves should be worn if touching blood or body fluids
Hands must be washed immediately if contaminated with blood or body fluids, and always before touching another patient
Needlestick injuries should be avoided
Used needles should be placed immediately in a labelled, puncture-resistant container
Spilt blood should be cleaned immediately with sodium hypochlorite solution
Disposal as for strict isolation

Table 82.17 Category-specific isolation recommendations. (From Garner & Simmons, 1983)

Strict isolation
Varicella
Diphtheria
Viral haemorrhagic fevers (e.g. Lassa fever)
Pneumonic plague

Contact isolation
Multiply resistant, Gram-negative bacilli
Methicillin-resistant *Staphylococcus aureus*
Major wound sepsis
Group A *Streptococcus pneumoniae*
Rubella

Respiratory isolation
Measles
Meningococcal meningitis
Mumps
Pertussis

Tuberculous isolation
Active pulmonary tuberculosis
Laryngeal tuberculosis

Enteric precautions
Cholera
Enteroviral infections
Hepatitis A
Poliomyelitis
Salmonella enteritis

Drainage/secretion precautions
Minor abscess
Conjunctivitis
Minor infected decubitus ulcer
Minor wound infection

Blood/body fluid precautions
Acquired immunodeficiency syndrome
Hepatitis B
Hepatitis non-A, non-B
Malaria

vating the newer β-lactam antibiotics. Aminoglycoside-modifying enzymes are produced by some species of Gram-positive and Gram-negative bacteria, and account for most of the resistance which occurs to these antibiotics. Many of these enzymes are plasmid-mediated, and once induced in a hospital strain, resistance spreads rapidly. Chloramphenicol can be inactivated by a specific enzyme produced by some strains of *Haemophilus influenzae* and *Streptococcus pneumoniae*.

Alteration of the cellular target sites is perhaps the most serious method by which resistance can develop. Structural changes may occur in the penicillin-binding proteins, the normal target sites of penicillins of the cytoplasmic membrane. These changes reduce the affinity of the target sites for penicillin molecules, and render these antibiotics useless. This mechanism has been implicated in the development of resistance by enterococci, gonococci, *Haemophilus influenzae* and methicillin-resistant *Staphylococcus aureus*. Similar structural changes account for some types of resistance to other antibiotics, and are plasmid-mediated. There is therefore the possibility that this form of resistance could spread rapidly to many bacterial species.

The development of resistant strains of bacteria is related largely to the quantity of antibiotics administered. Almost 30% of hospitalized patients receive one or more antibiotics, and as many as 50% of these may be administered inappropriately. Areas of the hospital with the highest antibiotic usage, such as the ICU, have also the highest incidence of resistant strains (McGowan, 1983). A number of studies have shown that decreased use of an antibiotic to which resistance has developed leads to a decrease in the isolation of resistant strains.

Problem organisms

Staphylococcus aureus

This organism has produced a succession of phage types resistant to a variety of antibiotics. Previous resistant strains have disappeared without any apparent reason. The current resistant strain is not particularly virulent, but can cause postoperative sepsis, especially after vascular surgery. It is extremely resistant to almost all antibiotics, including gentamicin, methicillin and cloxacillin. Vancomycin is one of the few effective agents against this strain.

Staphylococcus epidermidis

The use of intravenous catheters and prosthetic surgery have resulted in this previously commensal organism becoming a serious pathogen. Most strains are resistant to the commonly used antibiotics.

Gram-negative bacteria

Although *Pseudomonas* species and *Klebsiella* are common causes of serious infection in the ICU, more unusual strains have started to emerge in patients treated with broad-spectrum antibiotics. These include *Enterobacter*, *Serratia* and *Acinetobacter*, which are often resistant to most antibiotics.

Infection control policy

Every hospital should have an infection control policy, which defines the criteria for isolation, gives guidance for the use of disinfectants and antiseptics in each department of the hospital, and for the decontamination and disinfection of equipment. However the implementation of these policies varies from unit to unit (Inglis *et al.*, 1992). The policy should be revised periodically by an infection control committee, which should be responsible in addition for education of staff, and implementation of the policy. It should give guidance also on local use of antibiotics. Control of antibiotic use varies, but in general, it is best if a hospital confines itself to the use of a single first-line drug in each of the following categories: aminoglycoside, second- or third-generation cephalosporin, broad-spectrum penicillin, antistaphylococcal penicillin, tetracycline. Toxicity and cost should be considered when selecting the first-line agents. Antibiotic prophylaxis for surgery should not be given for prolonged periods; in general, there is no advantage in continuing therapy for more than 24 h. By consultation with the microbiologists, it should be possible in most cases to select an appropriate empirical agent for treatment before culture and sensitivities have been obtained.

References

Allen E.V. (1929) Thromboangitis obliterans: methods of diagnosis of chronic occlusive arterial lesions distal to the wrist with illustrative cases. *American Journal of Medical Science* **178**, 237–44.

Arita H., Ogle C.K., Alexander J.W. & Warden G.D. (1988) Induction of hypermetabolism in guinea pigs by endotoxin infused through the portal vein. *Archives of Surgery* **123**, 1420–4.

Band J.D. & Maki D.G. (1979) Infections caused by arterial catheters used for hemodynamic monitoring. *American Journal of Medicine* **67**, 735–41.

Bedford R.F. & Wollman H. (1973) Complications of radial-artery cannulation: an objective prospective study in man. *Anesthesiology* **38**, 228–36.

Berenson R.A. (1984) *Intensive Care Units (ITUs): Clinical Outcomes, Costs and Decisionmaking (Health Technology Study 28).* Office of Technology Assessment, US Congress, OTA-HCS-28, Washington D.C.

Bion J.F., Edlin S.A., Ramsay G., McCabe S. & Ledingham I.M. (1985) Validation of a prognostic score in critically ill patients undergoing transport. *British Medical Journal* **291**, 432–4.

Bion J.F., Aitchison T.C., Edlin S.A. & Ledingham I.M. (1988) Sickness scoring and response to treatment as predictors of outcome from critical illness. *Intensive Care Medicine* **14**, 167–72.

Bone R.C., Fisher C.J. Jr, Clemmer T.P., Slotman G.J., Metz C.A.

& Balk R.A. (1989) Sepsis syndrome: a valid clinical entity. *Critical Care Medicine* **17**, 389–93.

Boyd C.R., Tolson M.A. & Copes W.S. (1987) Evaluating trauma care: the TRISS method. *Journal of Trauma* **27**, 370–8.

Celis R., Torres A., Gatell J.M., Almela M., Rodriguez-Roisin R. & Agusti-Vidal A. (1988) Nosocomial pneumonia. A multivariate analysis of risk and prognosis. *Chest* **93**, 318–24.

Centers for Disease Control Working Group (1981) *Guidelines for Prevention and Control of Nosocomial Infections.* VSDHS-PHS.

Champion H.R., Sacco W.J., Carnazzo A.J., Copes W. & Fouty W.J. (1981) Trauma score. *Critical Care Medicine* **9**, 672–6.

Chang R.W.S., Jacobs S. & Lee B. (1986) Use of APACHE II severity of disease classification to identify intensive-care-unit patients who would not benefit from total parenteral nutrition. *Lancet* i, 1483–7.

Chang R.W.S., Jacobs S. & Lee B. (1988a) Predicting outcome among intensive care unit patients using computerised trend analysis of daily APACHE II scores corrected for organ system failure. *Intensive Care Medicine* **14**, 558–66.

Chang R.W.S., Jacobs S., Lee B. & Pace N. (1988b) Predicting deaths among intensive care unit patients. *Critical Care Medicine* **16**, 34–42.

Chastre J., Fagon J.-Y., Soler P., Bornet M., Domart Y., Trouillet J.-L., Gibert C. & Hance A.J. (1988) Diagnosis of nosocomial bacterial pneumonia in intubated patients undergoing ventilation: comparison of the usefulness of broncho-alveolar lavage and the protected specimen brush. *American Journal of Medicine* **85**, 499–506.

Cook D.J., Fitzgerald J.M., Guyatt G.H. & Walter S. (1991) Evaluation of the protected brush catheter and broncho-alveolar lavage in the diagnosis of nosocomial pneumonia. *Intensive Care Medicine* **6**, 196–205.

Cooper G.L. & Hopkins C.C. (1985) Rapid diagnosis of intravascular catheter-associated infection by direct gram staining of catheter segments. *New England Journal of Medicine* **312**, 1142–7.

Crim C. (1989) The influence of respiratory failure on ITU patient outcome. *Problems in Critical Care* **3**, 616–30.

Cullen D.J. (1977) Results and costs of intensive care. *Anesthesiology* **47**, 203–16.

Cullen D.J. (1989) Reassessing critical care: illness, outcome, and cost. *Critical Care Medicine* **17**, 172S–3S.

Cullen D.J., Civetta J.M. & Briggs B.A. (1974) Therapeutic intervention scoring; method for quantitative comparison of patient care. *Critical Care Medicine* **2**, 57–62.

Deam R., Kimberley A.P.S., Anderson M. & Soni N. (1988) AIDS in ITUs: outcome. *Anaesthesia* **43**, 150–1.

Department of Health and Social Security (1970) *Intensive Therapy Unit.* Hospital Building Note (HBN) 27.

Doglio G.R., Pusajo J.F., Egurrola M.A., Bonfigli G.C., Parra C., Vetere L., Hernandez M.S., Fernandez S., Palizas F. & Gutierrez G. (1991) Gastric mucosal pH as a prognostic index of mortality in critically ill patients. *Critical Care Medicine* **19**, 1037–40.

Dominioni L., Trocki O., Mochizuki H., Fang C.H. & Alexander J.W. (1984) Prevention of severe postburn hypermetabolism and catabolism by immediate intragastric feeding. *Journal of Burn Care and Rehabilitation* **5**, 106–12.

Dragsted L., Jorgensen J., Jensen N.-H., Bonsing E., Jacobsen E.,

Knaus W.A. & Jesper Q. (1989) Interhospital comparisons of patient outcome from intensive care: I. Importance of lead-time bias. *Critical Care Medicine* **17**, 418–22.

Dudley H.A.F. (1987) Intensive care: a specialty or a branch of anaesthetics? *British Medical Journal* **294**, 459–60.

du Moulin G.C., Paterson D.G., Hedley-White J. & Lisbon A. (1982) Aspiration of gastric bacteria in antacid-treated patients: a frequent cause of postoperative colonisation of the airway. *Lancet* i, 242–5.

Durocher A., Ssulnier F., Beuscart R., Dievart F., Bart F., Deturck R. & Wattel F. (1988) A comparison of three severity score indexes in an evaluation of serious bacterial pneumonia. *Intensive Care Medicine* **14**, 39–41.

Elebute E.A. & Stoner H.B. (1983) The grading of sepsis. *British Journal of Surgery* **70**, 29–31.

Eyer S., Brummit C., Corssley K., Siegel R. & Cerra F. (1990) Catheter-related sepsis: prospective, randomized study of three methods of long-term catheter maintenance. *Critical Care Medicine* **18**, 1073–9.

Farber B.F. (1987) Nosocomial infections; an introduction. *Infection Control in Intensive Care* (Clinics in Critical Care Medicine 12) (Ed. Farber B.F.) pp. 1–7. Churchill Livingstone, New York.

Fedullo A.J. & Swinburne A.J. (1983) Relationship of patient age to cost and survival in a medical ITU. *Critical Care Medicine* **11**, 155–9.

Feeley T.W., Faumarez R., Klick J.M., McNabb T.G. & Skillman J.J. (1975) Positive end-expiratory pressure in weaning patients from controlled ventilation. A prospective randomized trial. *Lancet* ii, 725–8.

Fiddian-Green R.G., Pittenger G. & Whitehouse W.M. (1982) Back-diffusion of CO_2 and its influence on the intramural pH in gastric mucosa. *Journal of Surgical Research* **33**, 39–48.

Fletcher R., Jonson B., Cumming G. & Brew J. (1981) The concept of deadspace with special reference to the single breath test for carbon dioxide. *British Journal of Anaesthesia* **53**, 77–88.

Garner J.S. & Simmons B.P. (1983) Guideline for isolation precautions in hospitals. *Infection Control* **4**, 245–325.

Hammond J.M.J., Potgeiter P.D., Saunders G.L. & Forder A.A. (1992) Double-blind study of selective decontamination of the digestive tract in intensive care. *Lancet* **340**, 5–9.

Hanson G. (1985) Training doctors for intensive therapy. *Care of the Critically Ill* **1**, 4–5.

Henning R.J., Wiener F., Valdes S. & Weil M.H. (1979) Measurement of the temperature for assessing the severity of acute circulatory failure. *Surgery Gynecology and Obstetrics* **149**, 1–7.

Hopefl A.W., Taaffe C. & Herrmann V.M. (1989) Failure of APACHE II alone as a predictor of mortality in patients receiving total parenteral nutrition. *Critical Care Medicine* **17**, 414–17.

Huxley E.J., Viroslav J., Gray W.R. & Pierce A.K. (1978) Pharyngeal aspiration in normal adults and patients with depressed consciousness. *American Journal of Medicine* **64**, 564–8.

Ibanez J., Penafiel A., Raurich J.M., Marse P., Paternostro J.C. & Mata F. (1988) Gastroesophageal reflux and aspiration of gastric contents during nasogastric feeding, the effect of posture (abstr). *Intensive Care Medicine* **14** (Suppl. 2), 296.

Inglis T.J.J., Sproat L.J., Hawkey P.M. & Knappett P. (1992) Infection control in intensive care units: UK national survey. *British Journal of Anaesthesia* **68**, 216–20.

Intensive Care Society (1984) *Standards for Intensive Care Units*. Biomedica, London.

Jackson R.J., Smith S.D. & Rowe M.I. (1990) Selective bowel decontamination results in Gram-positive translocation. *Journal of Surgical Research* **48**, 444–7.

Jacobs S., Chang R.W.S., Lee B. & Lee B. (1988) Audit of intensive care: a 30 month experience using the APACHE II severity of disease classification system. *Intensive Care Medicine* **14**, 567–74.

Jacobs S., Chang R.W.S., Lee B. & Lee B. (1989) An analysis of the utilisation of an intensive care unit. *Intensive Care Medicine* **15**, 511–18.

Jennett B. (1984) Inappropriate use of intensive care. *British Medical Journal* **289**, 1709–11.

Kaznitz P., Druger G.L., Yorra F. & Simmonds D.H. (1976) Mixed venous oxygen tension and hyperlactemia. Survival in severe cardiopulmonary disease. *Journal of the American Medical Association* **236**, 570–4.

Keohane P.P., Jones B.J.M. & Attrill H. (1983) Effect of catheter tunnelling and a nutrition nurse on catheter sepsis during parenteral nutrition. *Lancet* **2**, 1388–90.

Kerr J.H., Coates D.P. & Gale L.B. (1985) Use of 'bollards' to improve patient access during intensive care. *Intensive Care Medicine* **11**, 33–8.

Knaus W. & Wagner D. (1989) Individual patient decisions. *Critical Care Medicine* **17**, 204S–9S.

Knaus W.A., Wagner D.P., Draper E.A., Lawrence D.E. & Zimmerman J.E. (1981a) The range of intensive care services today. *Journal of the American Medical Association* **246**, 2711–16.

Knaus W.A., Zimmerman J.E., Wagner D.P., Draper E.A. & Lawrence D. (1981b) APACHE — acute physiology and chronic health evaluation: a physiologically based classification system. *Critical Care Medicine* **9**, 591–7.

Knaus W.A., Draper E.A., Wagner D.P. & Zimmerman J.E. (1985a) APACHE II: a severity of disease classification system for acutely ill patients. *Critical Care Medicine* **13**, 818–29.

Knaus W.A., Draper E.A., Wagner D.P. & Zimmerman J.E. (1985b) Prognosis in acute organ failure. *Annals of Surgery* **202**, 685–93.

Kruse J.A., Thill-Baharozian M.C. & Carlson R.W. (1988) Comparison of clinical assessment with APACHE II for predicting mortality risk in patients admitted to a medical intensive care unit. *Journal of the American Medical Association* **260**, 1739–42.

Ledingham I.M. (Ed.) (1977) Care of the critically ill. In *Recent Advances in Intensive Therapy* pp. 1–7. Churchill Livingstone, Edinburgh.

Ledingham I.M., Alcock S.R., Eastaway A.T., McDonald J.C., McKay I.C. & Ramsay G. (1988) Triple regimen of selective decontamination of the digestive tract, systemic cefotaxime, and microbiological surveillance for prevention of acquired infection in intensive care. *Lancet* **i**, 785–90.

Le Gall J.R., Loirat P., Alperovitch A., Glaser P., Granthil C., Mathieu D., Mercier P., Thomas R. & Villers D. (1984) A simplified acute physiology score for ITU patients. *Critical Care Medicine* **12**, 975–7.

Lemeshow S., Teres D., Pastides H., Avrunin J.S. & Steingrub J.S. (1985) A method for predicting survival and mortality of ICU patients using objectively derived weights. *Critical Care Medicine* **13**, 519–25.

Lemeshow S., Teres D., Avrunin J.S. & Gage R.W. (1988) Refining intensive care unit outcome prediction by using changing probabilities of mortality. *Critical Care Medicine* **16**, 470–7.

Lindsay S.L., Kerridge R. & Collett B.J. (1987) Abscess following cannulation of the radial artery. *Anaesthesia* **42**, 654–7.

McGowan J.E. (1983) Antimicrobial resistance in hospital organisms and its relation to antibiotic use. *Reviews of Infectious Diseases* **5**, 1033–48.

Maki D.G., Weise C.E. & Sarafin H.W. (1977) A semiquantitative method for identifying intravenous-catheter-related infection. *New England Journal of Medicine* **296**, 1305–9.

Marrubini M.B. (1984) Classifications of coma. *Intensive Care Medicine* **10**, 217–26.

Moore E.E., Jones T.N. & Peterson V.M. (1989) TEN vs. TPN following major abdominal trauma — reduced septic morbidity. *Journal of Trauma* **29**, 916–23.

Murray J.F., Matthay M.A., Luce J.M. & Flick M.R. (1988) An expanded definition of the adult respiratory distress syndrome. *American Review of Respiratory Disease* **138**, 720–3.

Nachtkamp J., Bares R. & Winkeltau G. (1988) Keimbesiedlung des Magens unter medikamentöser Stresulcusprophylaxe-Ursache von broncho-pulmonalen Infektionen bei Beatmungspatienten? *Zeitschrift fur Gastroenterologie* **26**, 493.

Nauseef W.M. & Maki D.G. (1981) A study of the value of simple protective isolation in patients with granulocytopenia. *New England Journal of Medicine* **304**, 448–53.

Pepe P.E. & Marini J.J. (1982) Occult positive end-expiratory pressure in mechanically ventilated patients with airflow obstruction, the auto-PEEP effect. *American Review of Respiratory Disease* **126**, 166–70.

Ponce de Leon S. & Wenzel R.E. (1984) Hospital-acquired blood-stream infections with *Staphylococcus epidermidis*: review of 100 cases. *American Journal of Medicine* **77**, 639–44.

Ranson H.C., Rifkind K.M. & Roses D.F. (1974) Prognostic signs and the role of operative management in acute pancreatitis. *Surgery Gynecology and Obstetrics* **139**, 69–81.

Ranson J.H.C., Rifkind K.M. & Turner J.W. (1976) Prognostic signs and non-operative peritoneal lavage in acute pancreatitis. *Surgery Gynecology and Obstetrics* **143**, 209–19.

Ridley S., Biggam M. & Stone P. (1993) A cost–benefit analysis of intensive therapy. *Anaesthesia* **48**, 14–19.

Rosen M., Latto I.P. & Ng W. (1981) *Handbook of Percutaneous Central Venous Catheterisation*. W.B. Saunders, London.

Rowley K.M., Clubb S.K., Smith G.J.W. & Cabin H.S. (1984) Right sided infective endocarditis as a consequence of flow-directed pulmonary-artery catheterisation. A clinicopathological study of 55 autopsied patients. *New England Journal of Medicine* **311**, 1152–6.

Ruiz-Santana S., Jimenez A.G., Esteban A., Guerra L., Alvarez B., Corcia S., Gudin J., Martinez A., Quintana E., Armengol S., Gregori J., Arenzana A., Rosada L. & Sanmartin A. (1987) ITU pneumonias; a multi-institutional study. *Critical Care Medicine* **15**, 930–2.

Rush B.F., Sori A.J., Murphy T.F., Smith S., Flanagan J.J. & Machiedo G.W. (1988) Endotoxemia and bacteremia during hemorrhagic shock: the link between trauma and sepsis. *Annals of Surgery* **207**, 549–54.

Russell J.A., Joel M., Hudson R.J., Mangano D.T. & Schlobohm R.M. (1983) Prospective evaluation of radial and femoral artery catheterization sites in critically ill adults. *Critical Care Medicine* **11**, 936–9.

Rutledge R., Fakhry S.M., Rutherford E.J., Muakkassa F., Baker C.C., Koruda M. & Meyer A.A. (1991) Acute physiology and chronic health evaluation (APACHE II) score and outcome in the surgical intensive care unit: an analysis of multiple intervention and outcome variables in 1,238 patients. *Critical Care Medicine* **19**, 1048–53.

Schimpff S.C., Young V.M., Greene W.H., Vermeulen G.D., Moody M.R. & Wiernik P.H. (1972) Origin of infection in acute nonlymphocytic leukemia: significance of hospital acquisition of potential pathogens. *Annals of Internal Medicine* **77**, 707–14.

Shoemaker W.C. (1989) Methodologic assessment of outcome. *Critical Care Medicine* **17**, 169S.

Stevens L.E. (1983) Gauging the severity of surgical sepsis. *Archives of Surgery* **118**, 1190–2.

Stoddart J.C. (1986) A career post — with intensive therapy? *Anaesthesia* **41**, 1181–3.

Stoutenbeek C.P., van Saeme H.K.F., Miranda D.R. & Zandstra D.F. (1984) The effect of selective decontamination of the digestive tract on colonization and infection in multiple trauma patients. *Intensive Care Medicine* **10**, 185–92.

Strauss R.G., Connett J.E., Gale R.P., Bloomfield C.D., Herzig G.P., McCullough J., Maguire L.C., Winston D.J., Ho W., Stump D.C., Miller M.W. & Koepke J.A. (1981) A controlled trial of prophylactic granulocyte transfusions during initial induction chemotherapy for acute myelogenous leukemia. *New England Journal of Medicine* **305**, 597–603.

Teasdale G. & Jennett B. (1974) Assessment of coma and impaired consciousness. A practical scale. *Lancet* **ii**, 81–4.

Tenold R., Priano L., Kim K., Rourke B. & Marrone T. (1987) Infection potential of nondisposable pressure transducers prepared prior to use. *Critical Care Medicine* **15**, 582–3.

Teres D. (1989) Peer review, publication policy and APACHE.

Critical Care Medicine **17**, 169S–72S.

Teres D., Brown R.B. & Lemeshow S. (1982) Predicting mortality of intensive care patients. The importance of coma. *Critical Care Medicine* **10**, 86–95.

Teres D., Lemeshow S., Avrunin J.S. & Pastides H. (1987) Validation of the mortality prediction model for ICU patients. *Critical Care Medicine* **15**, 208–13.

van Dalen R. (1991) Selective decontamination in ICU patients: benefits and doubts. In *Update in Intensive Care and Emergency Medicine*, pp. 379–86. vol. 14 (Ed. Vincent J.L.) Springer-Verlag, Berlin.

van Saene J.K.F., Stoutenbeek C.P. & Gilbertson A.A. (1990) Review of available trials of selective decontamination of the digestive tract (SDD). *Infection* **18** (Suppl. 1), 5S–9S.

Versprille A. (1984) Thermodilution in mechanically ventilated patients. *Intensive Care Medicine* **10**, 213–15.

Wagner D.P., Knaus W.A. & Draper E.A. (1987) Identification of low-risk monitor admissions to medical-surgical ICUs. *Chest* **92**, 423–8.

Watt I. & Ledingham I.M. (1984) Mortality amongst multiple trauma patients admitted to an intensive therapy unit. *Anaesthesia* **39**, 973–81.

Willatts S.M. (1985) Physiology of the nervous system. In *Textbook of Anaesthesia* (Eds Smith G. & Aitkenhead A.R.) pp. 72–100. Churchill Livingstone, Edinburgh.

Wilmore D.W., Smith R.J. & O'Dwyer S.T. (1988) The gut: a central organ after surgical stress. *Surgery* **104**, 917–23.

Wilson L.M. (1972) The effect of outside deprivation in a windowless unit. *Archives of Internal Medicine* **130**, 225–6.

Woods I., Wilkins R.G., Edwards J.D., Martin P.D. & Faragher B. (1987) Danger of using core/peripheral temperature gradient as a guide to therapy in shock. *Critical Care Medicine* **15**, 850–2.

Yates J.W. & Holland J.F. (1972) A controlled study of isolation and controlled endogenous microbial suppression in acute myelocytic leukaemia patients. *Cancer* **32**, 1490–8.

Zimmerman J.E. (1989) *APACHE III Study Design: Analytic Plan for Evaluation of Severity and outcome.* Williams & Wilkins, Baltimore.

Drug Intoxication and Poisoning

L.F. PRESCOTT

Self-poisoning is one of the most common causes of acute medical admission to hospital. In the UK, the total number of admissions for self-poisoning approaches 150000 annually, but the true incidence is considerably higher, as not all patients are admitted or even referred to hospital. In adults and older children, self-poisoning is usually an intentional impulsive act which has been provoked by failure to cope with adverse social circumstances or breakdown in personal relationships. It is fashionable and it no longer carries the stigma of former times. It is indulged in more frequently by females than by males and the peak incidence is in the age range of 18–30 years. Self-poisoning must always be a game of toxicological roulette but the outcome is often not fatal. It would certainly not be so popular otherwise. The mortality in hospital patients is approximately 0.5% (Jacobsen *et al.*, 1984), with most fatalities occurring in elderly patients and in patients with serious underlying medical problems. The great majority of deaths from poisoning occur outside hospital and the total number in England and Wales is about 4000 per annum (Osselton *et al.*, 1984).

Epidemiology of acute poisoning

Classification of poisoning

Poisoning may be classified under the following main headings:

Intentional self-poisoning

This is the most common type in adults and older children, and the usual method is the taking of drugs in overdose. The adverse social and personal factors which lead up to the event include broken love affairs, separation, divorce, loneliness, homosexuality, debts, conflict with the law, court appearance,

alcoholism, drug abuse, poor housing, unemployment and disordered or inadequate personality. Some patients with intractable social problems, drug or alcohol abuse and inadequate personality poison themselves repeatedly over a period of months or years, despite all efforts at reform. They often carry a mind-boggling burden of psychotropic polypharmacy obtained by repeat prescription. Not only is this unlikely to help them, but potentially depressing drugs such as benzodiazepines and major tranquillizers may actually predispose to self-poisoning (Prescott & Highley, 1985). Reduction in the prescribing of anxiolytic-hypnotic drugs is associated with a reduced incidence of abuse and fatal poisoning (Melander *et al.*, 1991).

Children older than 8–10 years tend to copy their parents increasingly and take drugs in overdosage when they are unable to cope with pressures at home and at school. In addition, the abuse of drugs and solvents (glue sniffing) has become an increasing problem in school children, especially in boys. Self-poisoning in 12–15-year-olds is commoner during school term than in holidays (McGibben *et al.*, 1992). Intentional poisoning is being encountered with greater frequency now in elderly patients, and in this group, there is a higher incidence of serious complications and mortality (Klein-Schwartz & Oderda, 1991).

An important minority of patients have serious premeditated and persistent suicidal intent. Some of these suffer from genuine psychiatric illness such as schizophrenia and depression (as distinct from unhappiness, frustration or disappointment), and it is essential that a full psychosocial assessment is carried out in all cases on recovery so that such patients can be identified and treated. It is also important to remember that these patients may make further determined attempts on their life whilst under medical supervision. Other, less severely disturbed patients may require psychiatric follow-up and support also, and official guidance has been issued recently on the psychosocial assessment of self-poisoners (Department of Health and Social Security, 1984). Although described often as a 'suicide attempt' or 'suicide gesture', the intentional taking of drugs and poison is best referred to as 'self-poisoning', as this does not imply any motive. Most patients do not intend to kill themselves and seek only to escape from an intolerable situation.

Accidental poisoning

This is common in toddlers and very young children who eat almost anything that they can obtain. An incredible variety of substances and objects may be taken, including the whole range of domestic products together with plants (e.g. berries), nuts and bolts, batteries, fireworks and matches, etc. (Picaud et al., 1991). To these should be added drugs, most of which are now brightly coloured and as irresistible to an inquisitive youngster as Liquorice Allsorts. In 1984, more than 25 000 children were admitted to hospital in England with suspected accidental poisoning, but serious consequences are rare and the mortality is very low. In a survey of 2043 cases in children under 5 years of age, drugs were involved in 59%, household products in 37% and plants in 3% (Wiseman et al., 1987). Less than 5% of children taking household products suffer serious consequences (Craft et al., 1984). Hospital admission is often unnecessary (Sibert & Routledge, 1991).

Accidental poisoning is uncommon in adults and older children, and it occurs usually because of confusion over identity and labelling. All too often poisonous substances (e.g. paraquat concentrate) are decanted into beer or lemonade bottles without warning labels and left carelessly for an unsuspecting victim to drink. Accidental carbon monoxide poisoning may occur with incomplete combustion of carbon-containing fuels (e.g. a gas fire with a blocked flue) and inadequate ventilation. Other forms of accidental poisoning include toxicity caused by stings and bites (e.g. by adders), ingestion of contaminated food and the consumption of poisonous plants and fungi.

Non-accidental poisoning in children

In recent years it has been recognized that parents (usually the mother) may abuse their children by poisoning them with drugs deliberately (Dine & McGovern, 1982). In some cases, the objective may be to quieten the child, in others the circumstances resemble child battering with toxicological rather than physical assault, and in another group, drugs may be used to produce the equivalent of the syndrome of 'Munchausen by proxy'. Subacute and chronic intoxication produced by non-accidental poisoning may lead to extensive and expensive investigation before the true cause is recognized (Rogers et al., 1976).

Drug abuse and drugs 'for kicks'

Drug abuse is a very serious problem, and increasing numbers of young people are referred to hospital with complications (Horn et al., 1987). Overdosage may cause acute behavioural disturbances, coma and cardiorespiratory disasters. The drugs involved include hallucinogens and central stimulants such as lysergic acid diethylamide (LSD), anticholinergics, herbal cigarettes, 'magic mushrooms', cyclizine, sympathomimetics, amphetamines and cocaine, and depressants such as barbiturates, benzodiazepines, organic solvents (e.g. toluene and trichloroethane) and opioid analgesics. Inexperienced drug takers may become frightened by the effects produced by hallucinogens, whilst others become violent and uncontrollable. Mainlining abusers of 'street' opioids may overdose because they are ignorant of the strength and purity of what they inject, and multiple drug abuse is common. Some intravenous opioid abusers intend to kill themselves by overdosage knowing that they are condemned to a miserable and degrading existence from which there seems to be no other escape. Apart from the formidable list of medical complications of intravenous drug abuse, there is now the problem of acquired immunodeficiency syndrome (AIDS), and in some areas a substantial proportion of drug abusers already have positive tests for the human immunodeficiency virus (HIV) antigen (Brettle et al., 1987).

Therapeutic poisoning

This arises usually from the chronic excessive therapeutic use of cumulative drugs such as long-acting benzodiazepines, depot phenothiazines, diphenylhydantoin, phenobarbitone and salicylate. It is particularly likely to occur with drugs which have saturable dose-dependent kinetics within the therapeutic dose range, and diphenylhydantoin and salicylate may be cited as examples. The recognition of therapeutic poisoning is often delayed and the consequences may be serious. Thus, therapeutic salicylate intoxication carries a very high mortality, particularly in young and elderly patients (Anderson *et al.*, 1976). The liberal use of topical preparations may result in salicylate poisoning (Raschke *et al.*, 1991).

Occupational poisoning

This form of poisoning is less common with increasing recognition of hazards and legislation to ensure safer working conditions. However, patients may still be exposed inadvertently to toxic substances, and accidents may always occur. Inadequate ventilation may lead to poisoning with agents such as chlorine, oxides of nitrogen, hydrogen sulphide, carbon monoxide and metal fumes from welding. Established safety procedures are not always complied with and protective clothing may not be worn. The latter is particularly important with agents which are absorbed rapidly through the skin, e.g. organophosphate insecticides.

One unusual report of poisoning in the place of work referred to acute water intoxication caused by attempts to produce a dilute urine to avoid detection in screening for drug abuse (Klonoff & Jurow, 1991).

Homicidal poisoning

Homicide by poisoning is rare in the UK, but the possibility should always be kept in mind and investigated further if circumstances are in any way suspicious. Traditional poisons such as arsenic and cyanide have given way largely to more subtle agents and paraquat was fashionable at one time.

Agents used for self-poisoning

Most adults and older children poison themselves on impulse at a time of crisis, and they take usually whatever is immediately at hand. Drugs are taken by the great majority, and the remainder resort mostly to household products such as bleach, detergents and disinfectants. Patients with serious suicidal intent may deliberately choose traditionally dangerous poisons such as phenols ('Lysol'), cyanide, ethylene glycol (antifreeze) and paraquat. They may poison themselves also with carbon monoxide from a car exhaust.

Most self-poisoners have personal problems for which many have consulted their general practitioners during the preceding few weeks. They are often prescribed hypnotics, tranquillizers and antidepressants, and most patients who take overdoses repeatedly are being given these drugs long term. Not surprisingly, psychotropic drugs are involved in the majority of poisonings (more than 50%), and of these the ubiquitous benzodiazepines lead the field by a substantial margin. Analgesics (usually non-prescription products containing aspirin or paracetamol) are taken by approximately 30% of patients, mostly young women who have not been given prescribed drugs. The remaining patients take a wide range of miscellaneous drugs (Prescott & Highley, 1985). As many as 60% of patients may take more than one drug in overdosage and as prescribing fashions change gradually over time, so too do the drugs used for self-poisoning (Proudfoot & Park, 1978).

Alcohol

Most patients now take ethanol before they poison themselves. This is of considerable toxicological significance, as ethanol potentiates the toxicity of other CNS depressants, and the outcome may be rapidly fatal when it is taken in combination with particularly dangerous drugs such as barbiturates, D-propoxyphene ('Distalgesic') and chlormethiazole (McInnes, 1987). The consumption of ethanol by self-poisoners is related to age and sex. It is taken before an overdose by approximately 75% of males and more than 50% of females aged between 18 and 30 years.

Diagnosis of poisoning

Contrary to popular belief, many poisons and drugs taken in overdosage do not cause rapid loss of consciousness. However, overdosage must always be considered in the differential diagnosis of coma, and it is by far the most common cause in young-to-middle-aged adults.

The diagnosis of self-poisoning may be made almost always on clinical and circumstantial evidence, and laboratory confirmation is rarely necessary. Personal problems come to light usually with careful questioning of friends and relatives, there are often medicine bottles and containers at the scene and a 'suicide' note may be found. Although the clinical features of poisoning are often non-specific, the diagnosis can be made usually with reasonable certainty on the basis of the clinical state, circumstantial evidence and knowledge of the drugs available to the patient. Certain intoxications produce a characteristic clinical picture (Table 83.1).

Poisons information services

The range of toxic substances to which patients might

Table 83.1 Some characteristic clinical manifestations of poisoning

Common clinical manifestations	Drug or poison
Vomiting, deafness, tinnitus, hyperventilation, sweating, vasodilatation, tachycardia, mixed respiratory alkalosis (adults) and metabolic acidosis (young children)	Salicylates
Initial nausea and vomiting, delayed onset of liver tenderness, mild jaundice and biochemical evidence of acute hepatic necrosis. Hepatic and renal failure in severe untreated cases	Paracetamol
Coma, slow respiration, cyanosis, hypotension, pinpoint pupils	Opioid analgesics
Deep peaceful sleep, depressed reflexes, minimal cardiorespiratory depression	Benzodiazepines
Coma, muscle twitching, convulsions, cardiac arrhythmias (tachycardia, absent P-waves, QRS widening), dry mouth, dilated pupils, extensor plantar responses, urinary retention, agitation and delirium on recovery	Tricyclic antidepressants and other anticholinergics
Vomiting, restlessness, delirium, dilated pupils, tremor, hyperreflexia, convulsions, hyperventilation, tachycardia	Theophylline and sympathomimetics
Gross ataxia, dysarthria and nystagmus, stupor, dilated pupils	Diphenylhydantoin
Brief ataxia, muscle twitching, coma, convulsions (usually isolated)	Mefenamic acid
Coma, convulsions, bradycardia, conduction defects, hypotension, severe circulatory failure	Beta blockers
Confusion, deafness, tinnitus, cardiac arrhythmias, delayed onset blindness, fixed dilated pupils	Quinine
Vomiting, confusion, coma, hyperventilation (severe metabolic acidosis), circulatory failure, delayed blindness, fixed dilated pupils	Methanol
Vomiting, diarrhoea, colic, sweating, salivation, bronchospasm, pinpoint pupils, bradycardia, hypotension, muscle twitching, paralysis, respiratory failure, confusion, coma, convulsions	Cholinergics (organophosphates)

be exposed is enormous, and poisons information services have been established to assist doctors in the management of poisoning. The centres in the UK provide information concerning the composition and toxicity of a wide range of proprietary, domestic, industrial and agricultural products, the toxic principles of plant and animal poisons and the acute toxicity of drugs and medicines. Detailed information is available on the manifestations and management of poisoning. In the case of difficulty, advice should always be sought from the nearest centre. The Scottish Poisons Information Bureau has been converted to a computer viewdata system, and the database can be accessed by users with their own terminals throughout the UK (Proudfoot & Davidson, 1983).

Use of the laboratory

Specific antidotal therapy is available for very few commonly taken poisons. Management is not influenced usually by laboratory identification of drugs or knowledge of their concentrations in biological fluids. On the other hand, clinical biochemical investigation is essential for correct management of the serious complications of poisoning (Table 83.2). Careful monitoring of fluid, acid–base and electrolyte balance is required during forced alkaline diuresis, and laboratory assistance may be required to confirm the diagnosis and monitor treatment in patients with methaemoglobinaemia and poisoning with carbon monoxide and cholinesterase inhibitors. Laboratory identification is obviously important in medicolegal cases, and it is usually helpful in the confirmation of non-accidental poisoning in children (Flanagan et al., 1981).

The correct management of some poisonings does depend on emergency measurement of the plasma concentration of the agent in question (Table 83.3). In paracetamol poisoning for example, there are no reliable, early clinical indications of the severity of intoxication. Specific treatment with N-acetylcysteine must be started within 8–10 h to prevent severe

Table 83.2 Biochemical investigation in acute poisoning

Investigation	Relevant conditions
Arterial blood-gas analysis	Respiratory failure, metabolic acidosis (shock, severe poisoning with many agents including methanol, ethylene glycol, metformin, cyanide, salicylate and paracetamol)
Plasma electrolytes	Cardiac arrhythmias, haemolysis, renal failure, rhabdomyolysis, forced diuresis. Poisoning with potassium, saline emetics, salicylate, theophylline, sympathomimetics, digoxin, insulin, etc.
Plasma calcium	Cardiac arrhythmias, ethylene glycol and fluoride poisoning
Plasma urea and creatinine	Renal failure (shock, haemolysis, rhabdomyolysis, poisoning with salicylate, paracetamol, non-steroidal anti-inflammatory drugs, heavy metals, paraquat, chlorate, ethylene glycol, carbon tetrachloride, etc.)
Liver function tests	Hepatotoxicity — paracetamol, phenylbutazone halogenated hydrocarbons [e.g. carbon tetrachloride, paraquat, metals, *Amanita phalloides* (the death cap mushroom), etc.]
Prothrombin time ratio	Poisoning with paracetamol, anticoagulants and hepatotoxins, snake bites
Plasma glucose	Poisoning with hypoglycaemics, hepatotoxins, ethanol, salicylate
Plasma creatine phosphokinase and myoglobin	Muscle damage and rhabdomyolysis
Methaemoglobin	Poisoning with chlorate, nitrites, aromatic amines, phenols, drugs with oxidizing metabolites (sulphonamides, dapsone, phenazopyridine, etc.)
Carboxyhaemoglobin	Carbon monoxide poisoning
Plasma pseudocholinesterase	Organophosphate and carbamate poisoning

Table 83.3 Indications for emergency measurement of plasma concentrations of drugs and poisons

Drug or poison	Indication
Paracetamol	Treatment with N-acetylcysteine
Salicylate	Active removal, e.g. forced alkaline diuresis
Iron	Treatment with desferrioxamine
Lithium	Active removal
Phenobarbitone	Active removal
Digoxin	Treatment with antidigoxin Fab fragments
Methanol, ethylene glycol	Treatment with ethanol, active removal
Paraquat	Assessment of prognosis and risk of complications
Other drugs	Removal by haemodialysis or haemoperfusion (Table 83.7)

and sometimes fatal liver damage, and only a small minority of patients is at risk. Emergency estimation of the plasma paracetamol concentration is therefore necessary, and treatment is indicated in patients with concentrations above the treatment line shown in Fig. 83.1. Without treatment, 60% of such patients suffer severe liver damage (Prescott, 1983). Ideally, toxic substances should be indentified and quantitated before attempts to enhance their elimination by techniques such as haemodialysis, haemoperfusion or forced alkaline diuresis, and the efficacy of

treatment should be monitored by serial estimation of plasma concentrations. Unfortunately, most hospitals have a very limited repertoire of emergency toxicological analyses, and many drugs and poisons are not detected by comprehensive screening programmes (Wiley, 1991). However, the position is improving with technical advances and the growth of therapeutic drug monitoring.

Toxicological results should be interpreted with caution, and must considered always in relation to the clinical state of the patient. Some simple assays

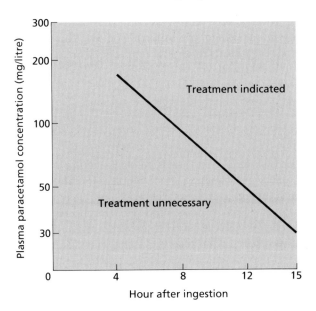

Fig. 83.1 Graph relating plasma paracetamol concentrations to the risk of liver damage after overdosage. Treatment with N-acetylcysteine is indicated in patients with values above the treatment line. Measurements made less than 4 h after ingestion cannot be interpreted.

necessarily used for emergency work are non-specific and subject to interference by other drugs and inactive metabolites. The relationship between drug concentrations and toxicity is complex. Patients often take multiple drugs in overdosage, ethanol is also often taken, and there is often great individual variation in response. Published lists of 'toxic', 'lethal' or 'potentially lethal' concentrations of drugs and poisons may be useful as a guide (Stead & Moffat, 1983), but they can be very misleading and are often inaccurate.

Drug pharmacokinetics are unpredictably abnormal in severely poisoned patients (Rosenberg *et al.*, 1981). Absorption may be slow or delayed, distribution may be restricted because of poor tissue perfusion, plasma protein binding is reduced at high concentrations and elimination is often impaired because of saturation of drug-metabolizing enzymes and reduced hepatic and renal blood flow. Hypothermia may also depress drug metabolism (Koren *et al.*, 1987). The time since ingestion must usually be taken into account in the interpretation of drug concentrations, and serial measurements are much more useful than a single estimation. It is essential to be aware of the units used by the laboratory for drug measurement. Unfortunately, although mass units have always been used in clinical toxicology, the recent unofficial introduction of molar units by many

laboratories has caused dangerous confusion. To make matters worse, drug concentrations measured in these new units cannot be related to conventional mass units unless the molecular weight is known (Prescott *et al.*, 1987).

Principles of management

Antidotes are available for very few commonly encountered poisons, and treatment is usually nonspecific and symptomatic. In such circumstances, management consists of emergency first aid and resuscitation, intensive care and supportive therapy, removal of unabsorbed drug and if appropriate, measures to enhance the elimination of the drug or poison. It is important to remember the possibility of delayed onset of toxicity following ingestion of slow-release and enteric coated dosage forms (Pierce *et al.*, 1991).

Emergency measures and resuscitation

The unconscious patient should be transported and nursed initially in the head-down semiprone position to minimize the risk of inhalation of gastric contents. The depth of coma is assessed most conveniently according to the Edinburgh coma scale (Table 83.4). The first priority is to establish a clear airway and to ensure that ventilation is adequate. If it is not, the lungs should be ventilated with oxygen and the trachea should be intubated if the conscious level permits. Reoxygenation often transforms the clinical state of an unconscious, seemingly moribund patient, and can rapidly restore an effective cardiac output and circulation. The adequacy of ventilation should be monitored by arterial blood-gas analysis. The combination of coma, cyanosis, slow respiration and pinpoint pupils is virtually diagnostic of poisoning with opioid analgesics, and a trial of intravenous naloxone in sufficient dosage (up to 2 mg) is mandatory. Potentially serious abnormalities such as metabolic acidosis, hyperkalaemia and hypoglycaemia may require correction as a matter of urgency.

Hypotension with peripheral circulatory failure is

Table 83.4 Assessment of depth of coma in poisoned patients (Edinburgh coma scale)

Grade 0	Fully conscious
Grade 1	Drowsy but responding to commands
Grade 2	Ready response to painful stimuli
Grade 3	Minimal response to maximal painful stimuli
Grade 4	No response to any stimulus

treated first by correction of hypoxia and acidosis, and by elevation of the foot of the bed. If adequate perfusion is not restored by these measures, the circulating volume should be increased by administration of a plasma expander (see Chapter 28). Cardiac arrhythmias are often improved or abolished by correction of hypoxia, acidosis and electrolyte imbalance. The temptation to give antiarrhythmic drugs must be resisted unless control of the rhythm disturbance is absolutely necessary. Many drugs and poisons can cause grand mal convulsions which, if repeated, should be controlled with intravenous diazepam.

The indications for other emergency measures depend on the agent involved and the severity of intoxication. Oxygen should be given in maximum concentration for carbon monoxide poisoning and transfer for hyperbaric oxygen therapy considered (Norkool & Kirkpatrick, 1985). Specific antidotal therapy may have to be given without delay, and examples include N-acetylcysteine for paracetamol poisoning, glucagon for severe beta-blocker intoxication, dicobalt edetate for cyanide poisoning and atropine with pralidoxime for organophosphate intoxication. Once the condition of the patient has been stabilized, decisions can be made about further management.

Removal of unabsorbed drug

Theoretically, unabsorbed drug in the stomach can be removed by gastric aspiration and lavage or by induction of emesis. In practice, neither procedure can be relied upon to empty the stomach, and most drugs and poisons seem to be absorbed surprisingly rapidly. Gastric lavage is performed normally in patients in Grade 3 or 4 coma, and in most other patients who are thought to have taken a potentially toxic dose of drug or poison within the preceding 4 h. This period is extended to 12 h with drugs which delay gastric emptying such as opioid analgesics, anticholinergics and salicylates. Gastric lavage is not carried out in unconscious patients unless an effective gag reflex is present or a tracheal tube is in place, and it is contraindicated in patients who have ingested corrosives or liquid hydrocarbons. Inhalation of the latter may cause a severe pneumonitis.

The patient is placed head-down on the left side on a trolley and a well-lubricated large-bore stomach tube (e.g. Jacques, 30 gauge) is passed. Suction must be available throughout the procedure. After siphoning out as much of the gastric contents as possible, the tube is connected to a large funnel with rubber tubing and successive volumes of 300 ml of warm tap-water poured into the stomach and removed by siphoning. When the return is clear, the tube is removed with its open end occluded.

In most cases, very little drug is removed by gastric lavage, but gratifyingly large amounts can occasionally be recovered. Its routine use has been questioned, and with the changing pattern of drugs taken in overdosage, it is probably unnecessary in at least 50% of patients (Blake et al., 1978). However, used with discrimination, gastric lavage retains an important place in the management of poisoning (Proudfoot, 1984). Complications of gastric lavage include inhalation of gastric contents and, very rarely, rupture of the oesophagus. It may also cause transient hypoxia, tachycardia, arrhythmias and ischaemic ECG changes (Thompson et al., 1987). It has even been suggested that gastric-emptying procedures may accelerate absorption by enhancing the passage of contents through the pylorus (Saetta et al., 1991).

Emesis is the preferred method of emptying the stomach in young children, and patients who refuse to submit to gastric lavage. Emetics obviously cannot be used in unconscious patients. Syrup of ipecacuanha is the fashionable emetic currently, and its active principle is emetine. In adults, a dose of 15 ml taken with 200 ml of water usually causes vomiting in 20 min. If there is no response, the dose may be repeated once. Serious complications of ipecac-induced emesis are extremely rare, but Mallory–Weiss oesophageal tears and fatal gastric rupture have been described (Knight & Doucet, 1987). Other emetics should not be used, as they can cause serious toxicity if retained. Saline emetics are often prepared with grossly excessive amounts of salt and can cause fatal hypernatraemia (Goulding & Volans, 1977).

Activated charcoal is a powerful absorbent which is often recommended as a means of reducing the absorption of ingested drugs and poisons. Unfortunately, it has little effect unless given within 1 h, and most patients arrive in hospital too late for it to be effective. There is no evidence that it limits drug absorption when administered after gastric lavage (Comstock et al., 1982). However, activated charcoal is safe and cheap. It is given as an aqueous suspension and the adult dose is 50–100 g.

Intensive supportive therapy

The primary objective of intensive supportive therapy is to maintain the vital functions to allow time for elimination of the poison and recovery. At the same time, potentially serious complications are anticipated and treated promptly if necessary.

Intensive supportive therapy is based on the principles of conservative intensive care. It includes such measures as the maintenance of respiration with assisted ventilation if necessary, regular removal of bronchial secretions, the use of humidified air or oxygen when the trachea has been intubated, regular chest physiotherapy, cardiovascular support, ECG monitoring, correction of hypo- and hyperthermia, close attention to fluid, acid–base and electrolyte balance, and conventional treatment of complications such as convulsions, pneumonia and renal failure. Central venous pressure monitoring and bladder catheterization may be required, but meddlesome medical interference should be kept to a minimum. Additional drugs should never be given unless they are necessary. Antibiotics are indicated only for demonstrable infection, and there is rarely, if ever, any need for the use of pressor agents. An exception is dopamine which is often effective in increasing renal blood flow and urine output in hypotensive patients with oliguria. Techniques for enhancing drug elimination should be employed only when justified by the clinical state and when they may be expected to be effective. Skilled nursing care is of great importance. In addition to regular observations and monitoring, this includes regular turning of the patient and removal of secretions, passive movements of the limbs, care of the skin, mouth and eyes and emptying of the bladder by fundal pressure.

Management of the complications of poisoning

Although recovery from self-poisoning is often rapid and uneventful, serious life-threatening toxicity may be caused by many poisons and commonly used drugs taken in large doses. The morbidity and outcome depend on the nature of the toxic agent(s), the dose absorbed, the rates of absorption and elimination, the duration of intoxication and many other factors including age, pre-existing disease, individual susceptibility, associated ingestion of ethanol and environmental temperature. Poisoning can cause serious adverse effects on virtually every organ system (Kulling & Persson, 1986). Coma is the most common complication, but it persists rarely for more than 24–36 h. It may be prolonged in poisoning with phenobarbitone and baclofen, and with long-acting benzodiazepines such as nitrazepam and flurazepam in elderly patients. Intoxication which is severe enough to produce Grade 4 coma is associated with a high incidence of morbidity and mortality (Arieff & Friedman, 1973).

Pulmonary complications

Pulmonary complications are common in unconscious poisoned patients and are important causes of morbidity and mortality (Jay et al., 1975). They include aspiration pneumonia, bronchial obstruction and collapse, infection, hypostatic pneumonia, and adult respiratory distress syndrome (ARDS). These are treated conventionally as described in Chapter 84.

Poisoned patients may develop pulmonary oedema of cardiac or non-cardiac origin. Cardiac pulmonary oedema is caused usually by the administration of excessive fluid, often in attempts to produce a forced diuresis in a severely poisoned patient. In this setting, myocardial and renal function are often impaired (Glauser et al., 1976). In addition, drugs such as salicylate and the non-steroidal anti-inflammatory drugs cause fluid retention. Cardiac pulmonary oedema should be treated with oxygen, fluid restriction, diuretics and if necessary, removal of excess fluid by haemodialysis.

Non-cardiac pulmonary oedema is a rather uncommon complication of severe poisoning with a variety of agents including opioid analgesics, salicylate, tricyclic antidepressants, diltiazem and quinine. Pulmonary capillary permeability is increased as a result of endothelial injury, and there is leakage of albumin-rich fluid into the interstitial and alveolar spaces. The pulmonary capillary wedge pressure is usually normal or low (Benowitz et al., 1979). A particularly acute form of pulmonary oedema may occur in drug addicts following the intravenous injection of opioid analgesics. More often, there is gradual development of interstitial oedema during the course of the intoxication. Inhalation of irritant gases such as chlorine, sulphur dioxide and oxides of nitrogen produces a chemical pneumonitis with associated pulmonary oedema. The treatment of non-cardiac pulmonary oedema consists of administration of oxygen, and if necessary, ventilation of the lungs with positive end-expiratory pressure (PEEP). Haemorrhagic pulmonary oedema occurs in severe, rapidly fatal paraquat poisoning and in less severe but ultimately fatal poisoning there is delayed onset of progressive proliferation of alveolar cells and pulmonary fibrosis. These changes resemble those of oxygen toxicity and are aggravated by oxygen.

Cerebral oedema

Cerebral oedema may occur in patients who have suffered hypoxic brain damage. It may also follow hypoglycaemia and other forms of metabolic brain damage such as may occur in poisoning with carbon monoxide, cyanide, methanol and salicylate. It also occurs in acute liver failure following paracetamol overdose. Cerebral oedema is aggravated by hypercapnia and by overhydration as may occur with misguided attempts at forced diuresis (Mühlendahl *et al.*, 1978). Treatment is directed towards correction of the underlying metabolic disorder and removal of excess fluid. Intracranial pressure may be reduced by administration of osmotic agents such as mannitol and if possible, hypocapnia should be induced by controlled hyperventilation. Dexamethasone is given often but its value in such circumstances is doubtful.

Convulsions and motor disorders

Many poisons and drugs taken in overdosage can cause grand mal convulsions: examples include mefenamic acid, tricyclic antidepressants, D-propoxyphene, theophylline, anticholinergics, antihistamines, monoamine-oxidase inhibitors, organophosphates, baclofen and salicylate. Isolated convulsions such as those produced by mefenamic acid do not require treatment, but repeated convulsions should be controlled with intravenous diazepam. If this fails, it may be necessary to paralyse the patient and ventilate the lungs.

Agents such as strychnine and α-chloralose may also cause extensor muscle spasms and opisthotonus provoked by tactile and auditory stimuli. The patient should be nursed in a dark, quiet room and sedated with diazepam. If the spasms cannot be controlled in this way, the patient should be paralysed.

A malignant neuroleptic hyperthermia syndrome characterized by coma, generalized muscle rigidity, tachycardia, hyperventilation and hyperpyrexia may occur in poisoning with monoamine–oxidase inhibitors and amphetamines, and with combinations of phenothiazines, butyrophenones and lithium. The sustained muscle activity may cause necrosis with myoglobinuria, hyperkalaemia and renal failure. The onset of this syndrome is usually delayed and muscle rigidity and hyperpyrexia can usually be brought under control rapidly with intravenous dantrolene (Harpe & Stoudemire, 1987). Dantrolene may also be useful for the control of muscle rigidity associated with severe theophylline poisoning (Parr & Willatts, 1991).

In normal therapeutic doses, the phenothiazines, butyrophenones and metoclopramide may cause bizarre acute dystonic reactions involving primarily the muscles of the head and neck. The onset is delayed usually for 12 h or more, most cases occur in young adults, and females are affected more often than males. These reactions are probably caused by inhibition of central dopamine receptors and resulting imbalance with the cholinergic system. They can be terminated rapidly with intravenous procyclidine or benztropine.

Hypothermia

Prolonged, deep, drug-induced coma may result in hypothermia, especially in elderly patients and when environmental temperatures are low and vasodilators such as ethanol have been taken. Mild hypothermia (down to about 33°C), is normally reversible rapidly and of little consequence. In more severe hypothermia, there is bradycardia, hypotension and slow respiration (this is not necessarily harmful, as the metabolic rate is correspondingly depressed). The results of arterial blood-gas analysis may appear less worrying if corrected for low temperature, but there is evidence that myocardial function is optimal at an uncorrected blood pH of 7.4 (Matthews *et al.*, 1984). After initial resuscitation, patients with severe hypothermia should be wrapped in a reflective 'space' blanket and nursed in a warm room with extra wool blankets. There is usually a rapid, spontaneous return to normal temperature, and this may be followed by an overshoot to 38°C or more. Atrial fibrillation with a slow ventricular rate may occur as the temperature rises, but it is usually self-limiting. Active rewarming is potentially dangerous as it causes peripheral vasodilatation with demands for increased cardiac output while the core temperature remains low. It is rarely, if ever, indicated in poisoned patients.

Hypotension

Some degree of hypotension is common in moderate to severe poisoning, and it is almost always present in patients in Grade 3 and 4 coma. It does not require treatment unless there is peripheral circulatory failure with cold extremities or the systolic pressure is less than approximately 10.6 kPa (80 mmHg). Several factors contribute to hypotension, depending on the drugs taken and the severity and stage of intoxication (Benowitz *et al.*, 1979). Many poisons and drugs taken in overdosage cause myocardial depression, and this is often aggravated by factors such as hypoxia and acidosis. In addition, CNS depressants and other drugs impair the autonomic reflex control of vascular tone causing vasodilatation, relative hypovolaemia and a decrease in the venous return to the heart. Hypovolaemia may result also from vascular injury with increased capillary permeability and loss of fluid into the tissues (Shubin & Weil, 1985). Arterial pressure and the circulation can often be improved dramatically by correction of hypoxia and acidosis, and by raising the foot of the bed to increase the venous return. If these measures fail, the blood volume should be increased by infusion of plasma expanders such as albumin solution, preferably with monitoring of the central venous or pulmonary capillary wedge pressure. Pressor agents are not normally recommended because the peripheral resistance may be raised already but dopamine infusion may produce a beneficial increase in cardiac output without decreasing renal blood flow.

Hypertension

Hypertension severe enough to warrant treatment may occasionally complicate overdosage with central stimulants. The administration of labetolol would be logical, and sublingual nifedipine has been used also (Gibson *et al.*, 1987).

Cardiotoxicity and arrhythmias

Many drugs and poisons can cause cardiac arrhythmias and conduction abnormalities. The mechanisms are complex and although the ECG may appear alarming (Fig. 83.2), most rhythm disturbances in poisoned patients are self-limiting. They often respond promptly to correction of hypoxia, acidosis and electrolyte balance. Tricyclic antidepressant overdosage is a common cause of worrying arrhythmias and these often respond to correction of hypoxia and

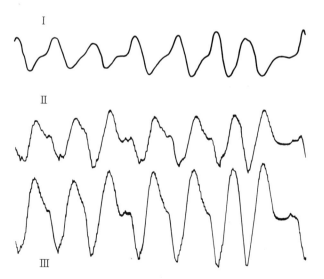

Fig. 83.2 Electrocardiogram (standard leads I, II and III) in a young woman with severe imipramine poisoning. Recovery was uneventful without the use of antiarrhythmic drugs. (Redrawn from Prescott, 1987.)

treatment of acidosis with sodium bicarbonate, or even administration of sodium chloride (Dziukas & Vohra, 1991; Hoegholm & Clementsen, 1991). The administration of cardiotoxic antiarrhythmic drugs to a patient with an already poisoned myocardium is fraught with danger. These drugs should only be given, and then with great caution, if the cardiac output is seriously compromised by the abnormal rhythm, or progression to a malignant arrhythmia is considered likely and simpler measures have failed. The chaotic cardiac rhythm in a patient with chloral hydrate intoxication shown in Fig. 83.3 was associated with a good cardiac output, and in this context there was no indication for treatment. However, chloral hydrate sensitizes the myocardium to catecholamines, and there is a risk of ventricular fibrillation. The multifocal ventricular ectopic activity was abolished safely with a very small intravenous dose of a β-adrenergic blocker. Pacing may be required occasionally for extreme bradycardia or atrioventricular conduction block.

Solvent abuse may cause chronic cardiotoxicity (McLeod *et al.*, 1987), and heart transplantation has been carried out in a glue sniffer for dilated cardiomyopathy associated with abuse of toluene (Wiseman & Banim, 1987). Myocardial infarction is an uncommon complication of poisoning. It may occur in carbon monoxide poisoning, and it has been described also in glue sniffers (Cunningham *et al.*, 1987) and abusers of cocaine and amphetamine (Carson *et al.*, 1987).

Renal failure

Renal function may be impaired in any poisoned patient with severe hypotension and persistent circulatory failure. In such circumstances it is important to avoid both under- and overhydration, and central venous pressure monitoring with hourly measurement of urine volume is essential for the correct control of fluid balance. Renal blood flow and urine output can be improved usually by infusion of low-dose dopamine (Henderson *et al.*, 1980), and these measures may prevent otherwise irreversible ischaemic renal failure.

Many drugs and poisons (Table 83.2) may cause proximal tubular necrosis and acute renal failure (Kulling & Persson, 1986). Acute drug-induced rhabdomyolysis is another cause of renal failure in poisoned patients (Hampel *et al.*, 1983; Forwell & Hallworth, 1986). In addition to fluid replacement, correction of acidosis and circulatory support as described above, and the use of antidotes and measures to enhance elimination if appropriate, little can be

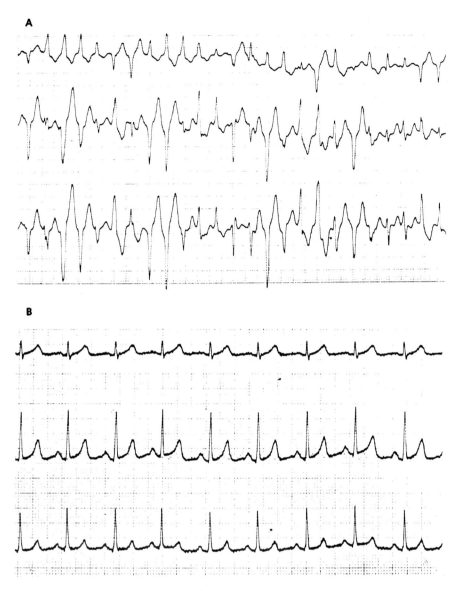

Fig. 83.3 Electrocardiograms in a patient with chloral hydrate intoxication. Gross multifocal ventricular ectopic activity (A) was abolished completely by the intravenous injection of 1 mg of practolol (B).

done to prevent renal failure in such circumstances. There is some evidence that early diuresis may limit nephrotoxic renal damage, but attempts to force a diuresis as renal failure is developing are hazardous and not to be undertaken lightly. Established acute renal failure is treated conventionally as described in Chapter 85.

Liver damage

Acute hepatic necrosis is a common complication of paracetamol overdosage, and it may occur also in poisoning with a number of other agents (Table 83.2). In addition, prolonged hypotension may cause ischaemic liver damage. Acute hepatic necrosis

induced by paracetamol can be prevented by the early administration of N-acetylcysteine (see below). Otherwise, severe liver damage and hepatic failure are managed as described in Chapter 61. Heroic measures such as liver transplantation are now feasible in some areas (O'Grady *et al.*, 1991).

Skin blisters, peripheral nerve injury and muscle damage

Poisoned patients who remain deeply unconscious and immobile with poor peripheral perfusion for many hours may develop erythema of the skin progressing to bullous blister formation at pressure points. These lesions are caused probably by local ischaemia. Similarly, prolonged pressure may cause ischaemic peripheral nerve injury and muscle necrosis. Injury to nerves often becomes apparent only on recovery of consciousness, and functional recovery may be delayed for weeks or months. Muscle damage is manifest by swelling, brawny induration, oedema and severe pain on passive movement when consciousness returns. The diagnosis of a compartmental syndrome may be facilitated by direct pressure measurement (Macey, 1987), and fasciotomy may be required to restore the blood supply, relieve pressure on nerves and prevent further muscle necrosis. More generalized muscle damage (rhabdomyolysis) is a less common complication of severe poisoning with a variety of agents including amphetamines, theophylline, opioid analgesics and isopropanol. Myoglobinuria is associated with gross elevation of plasma creatine phosphokinase activity, hyperkalaemia and oliguric renal failure (Forwell & Hallworth, 1986).

Behaviour disturbances

Agitation, restlessness, delirium and hallucinations may be caused by drug abuse and intoxication with a variety of agents, particularly those with a central anticholinergic action. Delirium may persist for several days after consciousness is regained after tricyclic antidepressant overdosage, and phenobarbitone intoxication may cause a prolonged period of disruptive disinhibited behaviour. Sedation may be required to prevent injury in a disturbed patient, but obvious causes of restlessness such as a distended bladder must first be excluded. The safest method, in the author's experience, is oral administration of diazepam in doses of 50–100 mg repeated hourly until the patient is asleep but easily roused. Prevention is always better than cure, but if oral therapy is not practicable, restraint may be necessary and diazepam should be given intravenously in small graded doses. A large total dose may be needed in an acutely disturbed patient and in such circumstances oral or intramuscular chlorpromazine has a potent synergistic effect.

Methods for enhancing drug elimination

The efficacy of regimens for enhancement of drug elimination from the body can be predicted to a large extent if the physico-chemical properties, disposition and pharmacokinetics of the substance are known (Prescott, 1974; De Broe et al., 1986). Nevertheless, these measures have often been employed indis-

criminately without clinical or toxicological justification, and in circumstances where only insignificant amounts of drug could be removed. The use of these techniques has been encouraged by numerous anecdotal reports of successful treatment in which survival of the patient is accepted as proof of efficacy. Unfortunately, it is not often possible to obtain proof of clinical benefit with such treatment in controlled clinical trials, but its use can be justified if rapid removal of a toxicologically significant fraction of the total body burden of the active drug can be demonstrated. Invasive and potentially dangerous methods for drug removal should be restricted to seriously poisoned patients who do not improve with conservative management and whose survival would otherwise be in doubt. Ideally, the toxic substance should be identified and its plasma concentrations monitored before, during and after the procedure.

Repeated oral activated charcoal

Repeated oral activated charcoal is effective in accelerating the removal of many drugs and poisons after absorption has occurred (Palatnick & Tenenbein, 1992). It is thought to act by irreversibly binding drug which diffuses from the circulation into the gut lumen under 'sink' conditions and the process has been referred to as gastrointestinal dialysis. Compounds which are excreted into the bile during enterohepatic circulation are bound also in the gut and their reabsorption is prevented.

Repeated oral charcoal is most effective with drugs which have a small volume of distribution, a small endogenous clearance and a long half-life (Table 83.5). It is the only means known of enhancing significantly the removal of drugs such as diphenylhydantoin and quinine, and with salicylate and phenobarbitone it is at least as effective as forced alkaline diuresis and haemodialysis (Fig. 83.4) (Hillman & Prescott, 1985; Boldy et al., 1986). Efficacy depends on keeping an adequate mass of charcoal moving down the intestine, and on the absorptive capacity of the preparation used. An initial dose of 100 g of charcoal is given as a

Table 83.5 Some drugs which can be removed effectively by repeated oral activated charcoal

Phenobarbitone	Diphenylhydantoin
Carbamazepine	Salicylate
Theophylline	Dapsone
Barbiturate hypnotics	Meprobamate
Digoxin	Digitoxin
Quinine	Cyclosporin

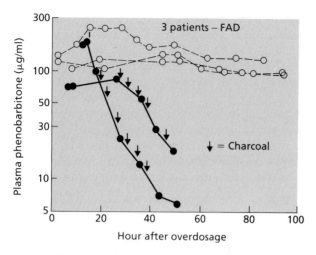

Fig. 83.4 Rapid removal of phenobarbitone by repeated oral activated charcoal in two patients (●——●). The charcoal was administered at the times indicated by the arrows. Plasma phenobarbitone concentrations are shown for comparison in three patients treated by forced alkaline diuresis (FAD) (○----○). (Redrawn from Prescott, 1987.)

slurry in 200 ml of water followed by 50 g every 4 h until recovery. In unconscious patients, the charcoal may be given by nasogastric tube, and the stomach contents should be aspirated before each dose is given. The major disadvantages are unpalatability and difficulty of administration in patients with nausea and vomiting. Complications of repeated administration of oral charcoal include fatal pulmonary aspiration (Menzies *et al.*, 1988) and intestinal pseudo-obstruction (Longdon & Henderson, 1992).

Forced diuresis

There are relatively few indications for forced diuresis. It can only increase the renal clearance of drugs which undergo tubular reabsorption, and it can only enhance usefully the overall elimination of drugs which are excreted unchanged in the urine to the extent of 30% or more. Diuresis alone has relatively little effect on drug elimination because at best the renal clearance is only proportional to the urine flow rate. In the case of drugs which are weak organic acids and bases with pKa values of 3.0–7.5 and 7.5–10.5 respectively, a much greater effect on clearance can be obtained by manipulation of the urine pH. The lipid solubility and hence tubular reabsorption of such acidic and basic drugs is decreased in alkaline and acid urine respectively, and their renal clearance is increased correspondingly. This relationship is logarithmic, and theoretically for each change of one

unit in urine pH, the renal clearance could change by a factor of 10. Urine pH is therefore much more important than urine flow rate (Fig. 83.5).

In practice, forced alkaline diuresis is restricted largely to poisoning with phenobarbitone and salicylate, although much of the effect in lowering plasma salicylate concentrations results from haemodilution rather than increased urinary excretion (Prescott *et al.*, 1982). Repeated oral activated charcoal is much more effective in removing phenobarbitone (Fig. 83.4), and simple alkalinization of the urine is as effective as forced alkaline diuresis for the removal of salicylate. Alkaline diuresis is effective in the treatment of intoxication with the selective weedkiller 2,4-dichlorophenoxyacetic acid (Prescott *et al.*, 1979) and it would be effective also in removing chlorpropamide (Neuvonen & Kärkkäinen, 1983). Forced acid diuresis is potentially much more hazardous than alkaline diuresis, and there are no proven indications for its use.

Before forced diuresis is undertaken, the state of hydration and electrolyte balance should be assessed together with cardiac and renal function. Regular monitoring is necessary during the procedure. A standard 'cocktail' containing sodium bicarbonate and potassium may be used for forced alkaline diuresis in salicylate poisoning (Lawson *et al.*, 1969) and a less aggressive regimen is used to produce alkaline urine at a rate of about 500 ml/h for pheno-

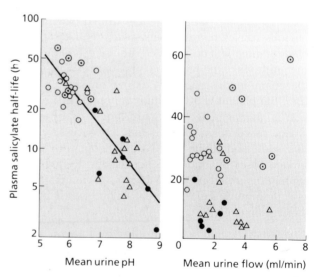

Fig. 83.5 Relationship between plasma salicylate half-life and urine pH and flow rate in patients with salicylate poisoning treated by forced alkaline diuresis (△), alkali alone (●), forced diuresis alone (■) and in control patients (○). There is a highly significant correlation with urine pH but not with flow rate. (Redrawn from Prescott *et al.*, 1982.)

barbitone poisoning (Vale & Meredith, 1981). Any form of forced diuresis is potentially dangerous. It is contraindicated in patients with cardiac and renal impairment, and great caution is needed in elderly patients. Complications include water intoxication, disturbances of acid–base and electrolyte balance, left ventricular failure with pulmonary oedema and cerebral oedema. Deaths have occurred as a result of unnecessary and inappropriate forced diuresis (Mühlendahl et al., 1978).

Haemodialysis, peritoneal dialysis and haemoperfusion

These regimens have been used extensively in attempts to enhance the elimination of drugs in poisoned patients. In many cases little clinical benefit could be expected on the basis of the pharmacokinetic characteristics of the drug, and when measured, the amounts removed have often been toxicologically insignificant. Nevertheless, haemodialysis and haemoperfusion may be very effective in appropriate circumstances (Fig. 83.6) (Pond, 1991). The conditions which must be met for the effective removal of toxic substances by haemodialysis and haemoperfusion are summarized in Table 83.6. Apart from the efficacy of removal of the drug from the blood by the device, the most important factors are the volume of drug distribution, the extent of binding to plasma proteins and the ratio of the extracorporeal to endogenous

Table 83.6 Characteristics necessary for effective removal of drugs by haemodialysis and haemoperfusion

Low molecular size and weight for good dialysance (haemodialysis)
Great affinity for and irreversible binding to adsorbent (haemoperfusion)
Small volume of distribution
Minimal binding to plasma proteins
Rapid transfer from peripheral tissues to the circulation
Extracorporeal clearance similar to or greater than endogenous clearance
Adequate extracorporeal blood flow

clearance. The maximum extracorporeal clearance cannot exceed the blood flow rate, and an adequate flow may be difficult to obtain in the most seriously poisoned patients. At the end of the day, the most important criteria are the survival of the patient and the amount of active drug removed relative to the total body burden.

Some drugs which can be removed reasonably effectively by haemoperfusion and haemodialysis are listed in Table 83.7. In general, haemoperfusion with coated charcoal or exchange resins is more effective than haemodialysis, although the latter may be preferred for simultaneous correction of acid–base and electrolyte balance (e.g. in salicylate poisoning). Haemodialysis is also the method of choice for

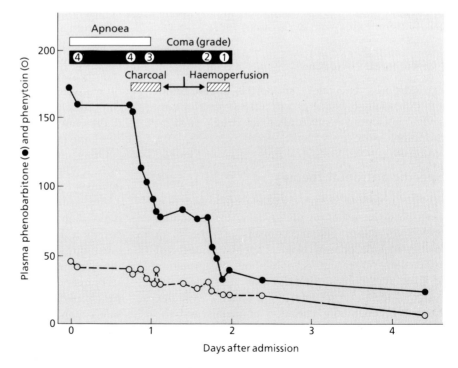

Fig. 83.6 Rapid removal of phenobarbitone by charcoal haemoperfusion in a 29-year-old woman in Grade 4 coma with prolonged apnoea requiring ventilation following overdosage of phenobarbitone, diphenylhydantoin, pentazocine and diazepam. Large doses of naloxone had no effect and she met the criteria for brain death. Adequate spontaneous respiration returned after the first haemoperfusion and consciousness was regained after the second. Note that haemoperfusion had no effect on the plasma concentrations of diphenylhydantoin. Drug concentrations are in mg/litre.

Table 83.7 Some drugs which can be removed effectively by haemodialysis and haemoperfusion

Phenobarbitone	Carbamazepine
Other barbiturates	Meprobamate
Salicylate	Theophylline
Dapsone	Most antibiotics
Lithium*	Chloral hydrate*
Methanol*	Ethylene glycol*

* Haemodialysis only.

removal of methanol, ethylene glycol and lithium. Peritoneal dialysis is much less effective and it is used rarely. It has the advantages that unlike the other methods it can be continued without interruption for long periods and does not require special facilities. The complications of haemodialysis and haemoperfusion include hypotension, haemorrhage, air embolism and removal of white blood cells and platelets. Peritoneal dialysis may be complicated by fluid and electrolyte abnormalities, perforation, peritonitis and adhesions.

Exchange transfusion and plasmapheresis

Drug removal by these regimens is very inefficient, and there is rarely, if ever, any indication for their use in poisoned patients. Even with drugs which have limited tissue distribution such as theophylline, the fraction removed by exchange transfusion is clinically insignificant (Wolff & Dreissen, 1983).

Extracorporeal circulation

Extracorporeal circulatory support is an important and potentially life-saving form of treatment for very severe poisoning with cardiotoxic drugs such as propranolol (McVey & Corke, 1991).

Specific antidotal therapy

Specific antidotes are not available often and they must be given usually without delay for maximum protective action. The mechanisms of reversal of toxicity include pharmacological agonist–antagonist interactions at receptors, inhibition of formation of toxic metabolites, provision of substrates and cofactors to stimulate detoxifying enzyme systems, enzyme regeneration, chelation of metals and the binding of toxins with specific antibodies. Some examples are listed in Table 83.8.

Agonist–antagonist interactions

Toxicity caused by block or stimulation of specific receptors may be reversed by administration of pharmacological agonists and antagonists respectively. The overall effect of combinations of competitive agonists and antagonists depends on their relative concentrations, their relative affinities for the receptor, and their intrinsic activities. The dose required to reverse toxicity therefore depends on the drugs involved and the severity of intoxication.

Naloxone has a very high affinity for opioid receptors but is virtually devoid of agonist activity. When given intravenously in adequate dosage it rapidly reverses coma, respiratory depression and hypotension in patients with opioid analgesic intoxication (Evans et al., 1973). The most common mistake is the use of too small a dose, and up to 2 mg may be required initially to obtain a response. Even larger doses are needed to counteract the effects of partial agonist–antagonists such as pentazocine, and the effects of buprenorphine cannot be reversed by naloxone in any reasonable dose. Naloxone has a relatively short duration of action and repeated doses may be necessary in poisoning with long-acting opioids such as methadone. The complete reversal of severe opioid analgesic intoxication with intravenous naloxone results in an abrupt return to full consciousness, with dilatation of the pupils, tremor, piloerection, hyperventilation and tachycardia. These latter effects are mediated probably by massive catecholamine release, and this may be relevant to the rare induction of serious ventricular arrhythmias by naloxone (Cuss et al., 1984). It is probably safer to give repeated incremental doses of 0.4 mg to allow a more gradual return to consciousness. The effects of naloxone cannot be regarded as specific, as it can partially reverse coma produced by other CNS depressants such as ethanol, benzodiazepines and clonidine (Kulig et al., 1982; Jeffreys & Volans, 1983).

Other examples of useful receptor interactions include those between adrenergic and cholinergic agonists and antagonists. Poisoning with β-adrenergic blockers can cause severe myocardial depression with virtual electromechanical dissociation. Isoprenaline is the pharmacological antagonist, but very large doses may be required, and safe titration in an emergency is impossible. Although recommended universally, atropine is useless in this situation. Prenalterol may have a wider margin of safety than isoprenaline and it has been used successfully in beta-blocker poisoning (Wallin & Hulting, 1983). However, the preferred treatment for severe

Table 83.8 Specific antidotal therapy

Drug or poison	Specific therapy	Mechanism of protection
Opioid analgesics	Naloxone	Pharmacological antagonism
Beta blockers	Isoprenaline Prenalterol Glucagon	Pharmacological antagonism
Sympathomimetics Theophylline	Beta blockers	Pharmacological antagonism
Phenothiazines Metoclopramide (acute dystonic reactions)	Anticholinergics (e.g. benztropine)	Pharmacological antagonism
Anticholinergics	Physostigmine	Pharmacological antagonism
Cholinesterase inhibitors	Atropine Pralidoxime	Pharmacological antagonism Enzyme regeneration
Benzodiazepines	Flumazenil	Pharmacological antagonism
Warfarin	Vitamin K Clotting factors	Pharmacological antagonism Replacement of factors
Ethylene glycol, methanol	Ethanol	Inhibition of metabolic activation
Paracetamol	N-acetylcysteine (methionine)	Stimulation of glutathione synthesis
Digoxin	Antidigoxin Fab	Binding and inactivation of digoxin in tissues
Iron	Desferrioxamine	Chelation
Lead	Calcium sodium edetate, D-penicillamine	Chelation
Other heavy metals	Dimercaprol D-penicillamine	Chelation
Cyanide	Dicobalt edetate Sodium nitrite Sodium thiosulphate	Chelation Methaemoglobin binds cyanide Provides sulphur for conversion to thiocyanate
Oxidizing agents	Methylene blue	Reversal of methaemoglobinaemia

poisoning with these drugs is glucagon. It activates cardiac adenyl cyclase by a mechanism independent of that mediated by catecholamines without causing excessive stimulation. In graded intravenous doses up to 10 mg it reverses myocardial depression effectively and restores an effective cardiac output (Illingworth, 1979).

Atropine blocks acetylcholine receptors and antagonizes the toxic effects of cholinergic agonists and cholinesterase inhibitors such as organophosphates. Again, very large doses may be needed. Conversely, anticholinesterases such as physostigmine have been used as antidotes for poisoning with tricyclic antidepressants and other anticholinergics. However, physostigmine is a potent non-specific central stimulant, and it has a very short duration of action which makes it difficult to use. Although it restores consciousness effectively, in mild to moderate poisoning with a variety of drugs, including the tricyclic antidepressants, it does not reverse the lethal cardiac toxicity produced by the latter. It causes convulsions and asystole has been reported (Pentel & Peterson, 1980). The use of physostigmine may have limited diagnostic value but its therapeutic benefit is minimal (Nilsson, 1982). It is not recommended. The availability of benzodiazepine antagonists such as flumazenil is of limited relevance to the treatment of overdosage with benzodiazepines as their acute toxicity is rarely serious or life threatening. Flumazenil may have a place as an aid to the diagnosis of unexplained coma (Höjer et al., 1990), but its alerting effect may precipitate convulsions in patients who have taken benzodiazepines in combination with other drugs such as tricyclic antidepressants (Burr et al., 1989).

Other antidotal therapy is based on receptor-mediated interactions involving parallel or opposing physiological systems. Thus, β-adrenergic blockers such as propranolol antagonize many of the effects attributed to excessive adenyl cyclase activity in theophylline toxicity, atropine may reverse brady-cardia in mild β-adrenergic blocker and digoxin poisoning, and other anticholinergics such as benz-tropine abolish acute dystonic reactions produced by central dopamine antagonists.

Inhibition of metabolic activation

Many agents cause toxicity through the formation of reactive intermediate metabolites by drug-metabolizing enzymes. There are many examples of prevention of this form of toxicity by inhibition of microsomal enzymes in experimental animals. However, the clinical application of this principle is very limited and extends only to the use of ethanol to inhibit the metabolism and reduce the toxicity of other alcohols. Given acutely to maintain a blood concentration of approximately 100 mg/100 ml, ethanol is a potent inhibitor of alcohol dehydrogenase and it reduces the rate of conversion of methanol and ethylene glycol to the highly toxic metabolites formate and glycolate which cause severe acidosis, blindness and encephalopathy (Jacobsen & McMartin, 1986).

Stimulation of detoxifying enzyme systems

The capacity of major routes of elimination is an important determinant of toxicity. Drug metabolizing enzymes may become saturated at high toxic concentrations, and the availability of substrates and cofactors may become a limiting factor. Endogenous protective mechanisms such as the conjugation of reactive nucleophilic metabolites with glutathione may fail if substrates for its synthesis become depleted. This is a critical factor in hepatotoxicity following overdosage with paracetamol.

The metabolic activation of paracetamol results in the formation of a minor reactive metabolite (N-acetyl-p-benzoquinoneimine) which is normally inactivated rapidly by conjugation with reduced glutathione. Following overdosage, glutathione is depleted rapidly and the excess metabolite damages liver cells causing necrosis (Mitchell et al., 1974). The availability of cysteine is rate limiting for glutathione synthesis. The administration of precursors such as

N-acetylcysteine stimulates glutathione synthesis and it is very effective in preventing liver damage if given intravenously within 8–10 h. Its protective action declines rapidly after this time, and it was thought not to be effective after 15 h (Prescott, 1983). However, recent reports suggest that the later administration of N-acetylcysteine may be of value and safe (Harrison et al., 1990). Oral methionine has been used also but its absorption and efficacy may be compromised because nausea and vomiting occur in most severely poisoned patients. Only a minority of patients are at risk of severe liver damage and N-acetylcysteine should be given only to those with plasma paracetamol concentrations above the treatment line shown in Fig. 83.1. However, treatment should be started immediately in patients admitted 8–15 h after the overdose, and it must not be withheld after 8 h whilst awaiting the laboratory result. N-acetylcysteine may be discontinued if the plasma paracetamol is found subsequently to be below the treatment line.

Glutathione protects against the toxicity of many other agents, including heavy metals and halogenated hydrocarbons such as chloroform. Thus, N-acetylcysteine is effective in preventing nephrotoxicity induced by mercuric chloride (Girardi & Elias, 1991). The toxicity of carbon tetrachloride is not glutathione dependent, and N-acetylcysteine does not prevent it from causing liver damage in humans (Ruprah et al., 1985).

Another example of the enhancement of detoxification is the use of sodium thiosulphate for cyanide poisoning. It provides sulphur which is rate limiting for the inactivation of cyanide through conversion to thiocyanate by the enzyme rhodanase.

Enzyme regeneration

Organophosphate compounds irreversibly phosphorylate the ester site of the cholinesterase receptor and cause severe cholinergic toxicity by inhibiting the hydrolysis of acetylcholine. Spontaneous recovery is very slow as it depends on resynthesis of the enzyme. Pralidoxime binds to the anionic site of the receptor and regenerates the enzyme by forming a stable complex with the organophosphate moiety. Poisoning with organophosphate is treated with large doses of atropine to block the acetylcholine receptors, and pralidoxime is given to regenerate the cholinesterase. Repeated doses may be necessary, and treatment is not effective if it is delayed for more than about 12 h (Lotti, 1991).

Chelation

Chelating agents form inert stable complexes with heavy metals and can reduce their toxicity if administered without delay. Currently available chelating agents include desferrioxamine (for iron), calcium disodium edetate (for lead) and thiols such as dimercaprol and D-penicillamine (for arsenic, antimony, bismuth, gold, mercury, lead and copper). Newer chelating agents such as 2,3-dimercaptosuccinic acid hold promise of greater efficacy and safety (Jones, 1991). Iron poisoning is relatively common, especially in children, but it does not often cause serious toxicity (Proudfoot et al., 1986). Treatment with desferrioxamine has been recommended in patients with serum iron concentrations above 8–10 mg/litre (145–180 μmol/litre), and vomiting and diarrhoea are useful predictors of severe poisoning with serum iron concentrations above 300 mg/litre (Lacouture et al., 1981). Prompt treatment with desferrioxamine may prevent the acute toxicity of severe iron poisoning but not late complications such as intestinal stricture (Henretig et al., 1983). Objective criteria have been proposed to allow discontinuation of desferrioxamine therapy in patients with iron poisoning (Yatscoff et al., 1991).

Cyanide inactivates cytochrome oxidases and is a very rapidly acting metabolic poison. It has a very high affinity for cobalt, and dicobalt edetate has now replaced sodium nitrite and thiosulphate for the treatment of cyanide poisoning.

Methaemoglobinaemia

Oxidizing agents cause methaemoglobinaemia in which the iron of haemoglobin is converted to the ferric form with loss of oxygen carrying capacity (Table 83.2). Methaemoglobinaemia can be recognized by slatey grey cyanosis which is unrelieved by oxygen and a characteristic chocolate-brown colour of the blood. Severe methaemoglobinaemia (exceeding 40%) causes symptomatic tissue hypoxia, and it can be reversed with intravenous methylene blue (Hall et al., 1986).

Immunotherapy

The use of antibodies to reverse toxicity is not new but there have been important recent developments, and the treatment of severe digoxin intoxication has been revolutionized by the introduction of digoxin-specific Fab antibody fragments. These fragments are less immunogenic than the complete IgG antibody and they have a much greater affinity for digoxin than binding sites in the myocardium and other tissues. Following their intravenous administration, there is a precipitous decrease in the plasma concentrations of free digoxin, and rapid reversal of life-threatening cardiac arrhythmias and hyperkalaemia (Smith et al., 1982; Hickey et al., 1991). The inactive complex with digoxin is partially degraded, and eventually excreted in the urine (Schaumann et al., 1986). The dose of Fab fragments is calculated according to the estimated body load of digoxin, but treatment is very expensive and it should be reserved for life-threatening intoxication. Digoxin-specific Fab antibody fragments bind other cardiac glycosides also such as digitoxin and lanatoside C. With recent developments in genetic engineering and DNA biotechnology, the potential exists for effective specific immunotherapy of intoxication with many other lethal poisons.

References

Anderson R.J., Potts D.E., Gabow P.A., Rumack B.H. & Schrier R.W. (1976) Unrecognized adult salicylate intoxication. Annals of Internal Medicine 85, 745–8.

Arieff A.I. & Friedman E.A. (1973) Coma following nonnarcotic drug overdosage: management of 208 adult patients. American Journal of the Medical Sciences 266, 405–26.

Benowitz N.L., Rosenberg J. & Becker C.E. (1979) Cardiopulmonary catastrophes in drug-overdosed patients. Medical Clinics of North America 63, 267–96.

Blake D.R., Bramble M.G. & Grimley Evans J. (1978) Is there excessive use of gastric lavage in the treatment of self-poisoning? Lancet ii, 1362–4.

Boldy D.A.R., Vale J.A. & Prescott L.F. (1986) Treatment of phenobarbitone poisoning with repeated oral administration of activated charcoal. Quarterly Journal of Medicine 235, 997–1002.

Brettle R.P., Bisset K., Burns S., Davidson J., Davidson S.J., Gray J.M.N., Inglis J.M., Lees J.S. & Mok J. (1987) Human immunodeficiency virus and drug misuse: the Edinburgh experience. British Medical Journal 295, 421–4.

Burr W., Sandham P. & Judd A. (1989) Death after flumazenil. British Medical Journal 298, 1713.

Carson P., Oldroyd K. & Phadke K. (1987) Myocardial infarction due to amphetamine. British Medical Journal 294, 1525–6.

Comstock E.G., Boisaubin E.V., Comstock B.S. & Faulkner T.P. (1982) Assessment of the efficacy of activated charcoal following gastric lavage in acute drug emergencies. Journal of Toxicology, Clinical Toxicology 19, 149–65.

Craft A.W., Lawson G.R., Williams H. & Sibert J.R. (1984) Accidental childhood poisoning with household products. British Medical Journal 288, 682.

Cunningham S.R., Dalzell G.W.N., McGirr P. & Khan M.H. (1987) Myocardial infarction and primary ventricular fibrillation after glue sniffing. British Medical Journal 294, 739–40.

Cuss F.M., Colaço C.B. & Baron J.H. (1984) Cardiac arrest after reversal of effects of opiates with naloxone. *British Medical Journal* **288**, 363–4.

De Broe M.E., Bismith C., De Groot G., Heath A., Okonek S., Ritz D.R., Verpooten G.A., Volans G.N. & Widdop B. (1986) Haemoperfusion: a useful therapy for a severely poisoned patient? *Human Toxicology* **5**, 11–14.

Department of Health and Social Security (1984) The management of deliberate self-harm. *Department of Health and Social Security Health Notice* HN(84)25.

Dine M.S. & McGovern M.E. (1982) Intentional poisoning of children — an overlooked category of child abuse: report of seven cases and review of the literature. *Pediatrics* **70**, 32–5.

Dziukas L.J. & Vohra J. (1991) Tricyclic antidepressant poisoning. *Medical Journal of Australia* **154**, 344–50.

Evans L.E.J., Roscoe P., Swainson C.P. & Prescott L.F. (1973) Treatment of drug overdosage with naloxone, a specific narcotic antagonist. *Lancet* **i**, 452–5.

Flanagan R.J., Huggett A., Saynor D.A., Raper S.M. & Volans G.N. (1981) Value of toxicological investigation in the diagnosis of acute drug poisoning in children. *Lancet* **ii**, 682–5.

Forwell M.A. & Hallworth M.J. (1986) Nontraumatic rhabdomyolysis and acute renal failure. *Scottish Medical Journal* **31**, 246–9.

Gibson R.G., Oliver J.A. & Leak D. (1987) Nifedipine therapy of phenylpropanolamine-induced hypertension. *American Heart Journal* **113**, 406–7.

Girardi G. & Elias M.M. (1991) Effectiveness of N-acetylcysteine in protecting against mercuric chloride-induced nephrotoxicity. *Toxicology* **67**, 155–64.

Glauser F.L., Smith W.R., Siefkin A. & Morton M.E. (1976) Renal hemodynamics in drug-overdosed patients. *American Journal of the Medical Sciences* **272**, 147–52.

Goulding R. & Volans G.N. (1977) Emergency treatment of common poisonings: emptying the stomach. *Proceedings of the Royal Society of Medicine* **70**, 766–70.

Hall A.H., Kulig K.W. & Rumack B.H. (1986) Drug- and chemical-induced methaemoglobinaemia: clinical features and management. *Medical Toxicology* **1**, 253–60.

Hampel G., Horstkotte H. & Rumpf K.W. (1983) Myoglobinuric renal failure due to drug-induced rhabdomyolysis. *Human Toxicology* **2**, 197–203.

Harpe C. & Stoudemire A. (1987) Aetiology and treatment of neuroleptic malignant syndrome. *Medical Toxicology* **2**, 166–76.

Harrison P.M., Keays R., Bray G.P., Alexander G.J.M. & Williams R. (1990) Improved outcome of paracetamol-induced fulminant hepatic failure by late administration of acetylcysteine. *Lancet* **335**, 1572–3.

Henderson I.S., Beattie T.J. & Kennedy A.C. (1980) Dopamine hydrochloride in oliguric states. *Lancet* **ii**, 827–9.

Henretig F.M., Karl S.R. & Weintraub W.H. (1983) Severe iron poisoning treated with enteral and intravenous desferrioxamine. *Annals of Emergency Medicine* **12**, 306–9.

Hickey A.R., Wenger T.L., Carpenter V.P., Tilson H.H., Hlatky M.A., Furberg C.D., Kirkpatrick C.H., Strauss H.C. & Smith T.W. (1991) Digoxin immune Fab therapy in the management of digitalis intoxication: safety and efficacy results of an observational surveillance study. *Journal of the American College of Cardiology* **17**, 590–8.

Hillman R.J. & Prescott L.F. (1985) Treatment of salicylate poisoning with repeated oral activated charcoal. *British Medical Journal* **291**, 1472.

Hoegholm A. & Clementsen P. (1991) Hypertonic sodium chloride in severe antidepressant overdosage. *Journal of Toxicology: Clinical Toxicology* **29**, 297–8.

Höjer J., Baehrendtz S., Matell G. & Gustafsson L.L. (1990) Diagnostic utility of flumazenil in coma with suspected poisoning: a double blind, randomized controlled study. *British Medical Journal* **301**, 1308–11.

Horn E.H., Henderson H.R. & Forrest J.A.H. (1987) Admissions of drug addicts to a general hospital: a retrospective study in the northern district of Glasgow. *Scottish Medical Journal* **32**, 41–5.

Illingworth R.N. (1979) Glucagon for beta-blocker poisoning. *Practitioner* **223**, 683–5.

Jacobsen D. & McMartin K.E. (1986) Methanol and ethylene glycol poisonings: mechanisms of toxicity, clinical course, diagnosis and treatment. *Medical Toxicology* **1**, 309–34.

Jacobsen D., Frederichsen P.S., Knutsen K.M., Sorum Y., Talseth T. & Odegaard O.R. (1984) Clinical course in acute self-poisonings: a prospective study of 1125 consecutively hospitalised adults. *Human Toxicology* **3**, 107–16.

Jay S.J., Johanson W.G. & Pierce A.K. (1975) Respiratory complications of overdose with sedative drugs. *American Review of Respiratory Disease* **112**, 591–8.

Jeffreys D.B. & Volans G.N. (1983) An investigation of the role of the specific opioid antagonist naloxone in clinical toxicology. *Human Toxicology* **2**, 227–31.

Jones M.M. (1991) New developments in therapeutic chelating agents as antidotes for metal poisoning. *CRC Critical Reviews in Toxicology* **21**, 209–33.

Klein-Schwartz W. & Oderda G.M. (1991) Poisoning in the elderly: epidemiological, clinical and management considerations. *Drugs and Ageing* **1**, 67–89.

Klonoff D.C. & Jurow A.H. (1991) Acute water intoxication as a complication of urine drug testing in the workplace. *Journal of the American Medical Association* **265**, 84–5.

Knight K.M. & Doucet H.J. (1987) Gastric rupture and death caused by ipecac syrup. *Southern Medical Journal* **80**, 786–7.

Koren G., Barker C., Goresky G., Bohn D., Kent G., Klein J., MacLeod S.M. & Biggar W.D. (1987) The influence of hypothermia on the disposition of fentanyl — human and animal studies. *European Journal of Clinical Pharmacology* **32**, 373–6.

Kulig K., Duffy J., Rumach B.H., Mauro R. & Gaylord M. (1982) Naloxone for treatment of clonidine overdose. *Journal of the American Medical Association* **247**, 1697.

Kulling P. & Persson H. (1986) Role of the intensive care unit in the management of the poisoned patient. *Medical Toxicology* **1**, 375–86.

Lacouture P.G., Wason S., Temple A.R., Wallace D.K. & Lovejoy F.H. (1981) Emergency assessment of severity in iron overdose by clinical and laboratory methods. *Journal of Pediatrics* **99**, 89–91.

Lawson A.A.H., Proudfoot A.T., Brown S.S., MacDonald R.H., Fraser A.G., Cameron J.C. & Matthew H. (1969) Forced diuresis in the treatment of acute salicylate poisoning in adults. *Quarterly Journal of Medicine* **38**, 31–48.

Longdon P. & Henderson A. (1992) Intestinal pseudo-obstruction following the use of enteral charcoal and sorbitol and mechanical ventilation with papaveretum sedation for theophylline poisoning. *Drug Safety* **7**, 74−7.

Lotti M. (1991) Treatment of acute organophosphate poisoning. *Medical Journal of Australia* **154**, 51−5.

Macey A.C. (1987) Compartmental syndromes in unconscious patients: a simple acid to diagnosis. *British Medical Journal* **294**, 1472−3.

McGibben L., Ballard C.G., Handy S. & Silveira W.R. (1992) School attendance as a factor in deliberate self-poisoning by 12−15 year old adolescents. *British Medical Journal* **304**, 28.

McInnes G.T. (1987) Chlormethiazole and alcohol: a lethal cocktail. *British Medical Journal* **294**, 592.

McLeod A.A., Marjot R., Monaghan M.J., Hugh-Jones P. & Jackson G. (1987) Chronic cardiac toxicity after inhalation of 1,1,1-trichloroethane. *British Medical Journal* **294**, 727−9.

McVey F.K. & Corke C.F. (1991) Extracorporeal circulation in the management of massive propranolol overdose. *Anaesthesia* **46**, 744−6.

Matthews A.J., Stead A.L. & Abbott T.R. (1984) Acid−base control during hypothermia. *Anaesthesia* **39**, 649−54.

Melander A., Henricson K., Stenberg B., Löwenhielm P., Malmvik J., Sternebring B., Kaij L. & Bergdahl U. (1991) Anxiolytic−hypnotic drugs: relationships between prescribing, abuse and suicide. *European Journal of Clinical Pharmacology* **41**, 525−9.

Menzies D.G., Busuttil A. & Prescott L.F. (1988) Fatal pulmonary aspiration of oral activated charcoal. *British Medical Journal* **297**, 459−60.

Mitchell J.R., Thorgiersson S.S., Potter W.Z., Jollow D.J. & Keiser H. (1974) Acetaminophen-induced hepatic injury. Protective role of glutathione in man and rationale for therapy. *Clinical Pharmacology and Therapeutics* **16**, 676−84.

Mühlendahl K.E., Krienke E.G. & Bunjes R. (1978) Fatal overtreatment of accidental childhood intoxication. *Journal of Pediatrics* **93**, 1003−4.

Neuvonen P.J. & Kärkkäinen S. (1983) Effects of charcoal, sodium bicarbonate, and ammonium chloride on chlorpropamide kinetics. *Clinical Pharmacology and Therapeutics* **33**, 386−93.

Nilsson E. (1982) Physostigmine treatment in various drug-induced intoxications. *Annals of Clinical Research* **14**, 165−72.

Norkool D.M. & Kirkpatrick J.N. (1985) Treatment of acute carbon monoxide poisoning with hyperbaric oxygen: a review of 155 cases. *Annals of Emergency Medicine* **14**, 1169−71.

O'Grady J.G., Wendon J., Tan K.C., Potter D., Cottam S., Cohen A.T., Gimson A.E.S. & Williams R. (1991) Liver transplantation after paracetamol overdose. *British Medical Journal* **303**, 221−3.

Osselton M.D., Blackmore R.C., King L.A. & Moffat A.C. (1984) Poisoning-associated deaths for England and Wales between 1973 and 1980. *Human Toxicology* **3**, 201−21.

Palatnick W. & Tenenbein M. (1992) Activated charcoal in the treatment of drug overdose. *Drug Safety* **7**, 3−7.

Parr M.J.A. & Willatts S.M. (1991) Fatal theophylline poisoning with rhabdomyolysis. A potential role for dantrolene treatment. *Anaesthesia* **46**, 557−9.

Pentel P. & Peterson C.D. (1980) Asystole complicating physostigmine treatment of tricyclic antidepressant overdose. *Annals of Emergency Medicine* **9**, 588−90.

Picaud J.C., Cochat P., Parchoux B., Berthier J.C., Gilly J.,

Chareyre S. & Larbre F. (1991) Acute renal failure in a child after chewing of match heads. *Nephron* **57**, 225−6.

Pierce R.P., Gazewood J. & Blake R.L. (1991) Salicylate poisoning from enteric-coated aspirin. Delayed absorption may complicate management. *Postgraduate Medicine* **89**, 61−4.

Pond S.M. (1991) Extracorporeal techniques in the treatment of poisoned patients. *Medical Journal of Australia* **154**, 617−22.

Prescott L.F. (1974) Limitations of haemodialysis and forced diuresis. In *The Poisoned Patient: the Role of the Laboratory*. pp. 269−82. Ciba Foundation Symposium 26. Associated Scientific Publishers, Amsterdam.

Prescott L.F. (1983) Paracetamol overdoses: pharmacological considerations and clinical management. *Drugs* **25**, 290−314.

Prescott L.F. (1987) Drug overdosage and poisoning. In *Drug Treatment* 3rd edn. (Ed. Speight T.M.) pp. 283−302. ADIS Press, Auckland.

Prescott L.F. & Highley M.S. (1985) Drugs prescribed for self-poisoners. *British Medical Journal* **290**, 1633−6.

Prescott L.F., Park J. & Darrien I. (1979) Treatment of severe 2,4-D and mecoprop intoxication with alkaline diuresis. *British Journal of Clinical Pharmacology* **7**, 111−16.

Prescott L.F., Balali-Mood M., Critchley J.A.J.H., Johnstone A.F. & Proudfoot A.T. (1982) Diuresis or urinary alkalinisation for salicylate poisoning? *British Medical Journal* **285**, 1383−6.

Prescott L.F., Proudfoot A.T., Widdop B., Volans G.N., Vale J.A., Whiting B., Griffin J.P. & Wells F.O. (1987) Who needs molar units for drugs? *Lancet* **1**, 1127−9.

Proudfoot A.T. (1984) Abandon gastric lavage in the accident and emergency department? *Archives of Emergency Medicine* **2**, 65−71.

Proudfoot A.T. & Davidson W.S.M. (1983) A viewdata system for poisons information. *British Medical Journal* **286**, 125−7.

Proudfoot A.T. & Park J. (1978) Changing pattern of drugs used for self-poisoning. *British Medical Journal* **1**, 90−3.

Proudfoot A.T., Simpson D. & Dyson E.H. (1986) Management of acute iron poisoning. *Medical Toxicology* **1**, 83−100.

Raschke R., Arnold-Capell P.A., Richeson R. & Curry S.C. (1991) Refractory hypoglycemia secondary to topical salicylate intoxication. *Archives of Internal Medicine* **151**, 591−3.

Rogers D., Tripp J., Bentovim A., Robinson A., Berry D. & Goulding R. (1976) Non-accidental poisoning: an extended syndrome of child abuse. *British Medical Journal* **1**, 793−6.

Rosenberg J., Benowitz N.L. & Pond S. (1981) Pharmacokinetics of drug overdose. *Clinical Pharmacokinetics* **6**, 161−92.

Ruprah M., Mant T.G.K. & Flanagan R.J. (1985) Acute carbon tetrachloride poisoning in 19 patients: implications and treatment. *Lancet* **1**, 1027−9.

Saetta J.P., March S., Gaunt M.E. & Quinton D.N. (1991) Gastric emptying procedures in the self-poisoned patient: Are we forcing gastric content beyond the pylorus. *Journal of the Royal Society of Medicine* **84**, 274−6.

Schaumann W., Kaufmann B., Neubert P. & Smolarz A. (1986) Kinetics of the Fab fragments of dioxin antibodies and of bound digoxin in patients with severe digoxin intoxication. *European Journal of Clinical Pharmacology* **30**, 527−33.

Shubin H. & Weil M.H. (1985) The mechanism of shock following suicidal doses of barbiturate, narcotics and tranquillizing drugs, with observations on the effects of treatment. *American Journal of Medicine* **38**, 853−63.

Sibert J.R. & Routledge P.A. (1991) Accidental poisoning in

children: can we admit fewer children with safety. *Archives of Disease in Childhood* **66**, 263−6.

Smith T.W., Butler V.P., Haber E., Fozzard H., Marcus F.I., Bremner W.F., Schulman I.C. & Phillips A. (1982) Treatment of life-threatening digitalis intoxication with digoxin-specific Fab anti-body fragments. *New England Journal of Medicine* **307**, 1357−62.

Stead A.H. & Moffat A.C. (1983) A collection of therapeutic, toxic and fatal blood drug concentrations in man. *Human Toxicology* **2**, 437−64.

Thompson A.M., Robins J.B. & Prescott L.F. (1987) Changes in cardiorespiratory function during gastric lavage for drug overdose. *Human Toxicology* **6**, 215−18.

Vale J.A. & Meredith T.J. (1981) Forced diuresis, dialysis and haemoperfusion. In *Poisoning Diagnosis and Treatment* (Eds Vale J.A. & Meredith T.J.) pp. 59−68. Update Books, London.

Wallin C.-J. & Hulting J. (1983) Massive metoprolol poisoning treated with prenalterol. *Acta Medica Scandinavica* **214**, 253−5.

Wiley J.F. (1991) Difficult diagnoses in toxicology: Poisons not detected by the comprehensive drug screen. *Pediatric Clinics of North America* **38**, 725−37.

Wiseman M.N. & Banim S. (1987) 'Glue sniffer's' heart? *British Medical Journal* **294**, 739.

Wiseman H.M., Guest K., Murray V.S.G. & Volans G.N. (1987) Accidental poisoning in childhood: a multicentre survey. 1. General epidemiology. *Human Toxicology* **6**, 293−301.

Wolff E.D. & Dreissen O.M.L. (1983) End kind met theofyllinevergiftiging. *Nederland Tijdschrift voor Geneeskunde* **121**, 896−9.

Yatscoff R.W., Wayne E.A. & Tenenbein M. (1991) An objective criterion for the cessation of deferoxamine therapy in the acutely iron poisoned patient. *Journal of Toxicology: Clinical Toxicology* **29**, 1−10.

Ventilatory Failure

D. ROYSTON

The view that the heart was the furnace where the 'fire of life' kept the blood boiling has long been relegated to antiquity. Current views on cell biology hold that each cell has its own set of furnaces — the mitochondria. These organelles are specialized towards supplying the cell with its energy needs by oxidation of organic substrates. The mitochondrion is equipped with a set of enzymes which degrade sugars to carbon dioxide, extracting hydrogen ions in the process which are, in time, combined with oxygen to produce water. This fundamental process of energy production by oxidation depends totally on an adequate and continuous supply of oxygen.

The respiratory system is the first part in the complex chain which, by securing effective continuous exchange of oxygen and carbon dioxide between air and blood, enables respiration to proceed at cellular level without interference.

If this exchange between air and blood becomes discontinuous or impaired because of failure of one or more of the normal mechanisms of transfer, respiratory failure occurs.

The purpose of this chapter is to outline certain concepts of the mechanism by which this happens and to discuss the management of this problem. It is worth highlighting that the majority of the modern multidisciplinary intensive therapy units were established on the basis of the ability of anaesthetists to take control efficiently of patients' breathing and thereby provide some support for the failing respiratory system. It is also important to underline that the concept of respiratory support units is comparatively new. Whilst major advances have and continue to be made, there are still yawning gaps in our knowledge.

Definition

Many attempts have been made to provide a univer-sally accepted definition for use by the clinician in all circumstances. As outlined above, the role of the respiratory system is to maintain gas exchange. The definition of failure of the system is based usually on measuring blood-gas tensions in the end-organ (arterial blood) and allocating levels of normality. If the tension of carbon dioxide in arterial blood exceeds 6.7 kPa (50 mmHg) or that of oxygen is less than 8.0 kPa (60 mmHg) while the patient is at rest, breathing air at sea level and when there is no primary metabolic alkalosis, this is defined as respiratory failure (Sykes, et al., 1976). Whilst this definition is extremely useful in terms of characterizing certain pathophysiological states, it does not necessarily define clinical management strategies. For example a $Paco_2$ of 6.7 kPa (50 mmHg) would not automatically lead to the institution of controlled ventilation in a patient with chronic obstructive airway disease and known carbon dioxide retention. In contrast, aggressive intervention may be instituted at a $Paco_2$ lower than 6.7 kPa (50 mmHg) in, for example, a young asthmatic who fails to respond adequately to medical management of an acute attack.

None the less, the definition of respiratory failure on blood-gas tension criteria remains the most accepted and will remain so until other more suitable methods are established.

Failure of respiration

It is axiomatic from the above that 'respiratory failure' at the tissue level determines the ability of an organism to survive. The partial failure of the lungs and respiratory system alone may be compensated for by other mechanisms aimed at improving oxygen availability, e.g. by improvements in the circulation or the gas transport capacity of the blood. For this reason, failure of the respiratory system alone is not considered in isolation but rather as part of an integrated interactive system. The concept of 'pulmonary failure' may then be discussed in two broad areas.

Failure of ventilation (ventilatory failure)

This may result from problems of mechanics or ventilatory control. In these conditions there is usually an increase in arterial blood carbon dioxide tension in addition to a reduction in oxygen tension.

Failure of tissue oxygenation (hypoxaemic failure)

This type of failure may have both pulmonary and extrapulmonary aetiology. The majority of such disorders are inflammatory in nature and/or are related to pathology of the pulmonary vasculature with alterations in ventilation and perfusion leading to an increase in shunting of venous blood. Causes unrelated to the lung include reductions in oxygen-carrying capacity of the blood. Examples of this latter form of hypoxaemic failure are the reduced haemoglobin associated with anaemia or the functional anaemia found in carbon monoxide poisoning.

Causes of respiratory failure

As an exhaustive list of causes of respiratory failure would be extremely long, this section deals with the more commonly occurring causes leading to ventilatory and hypoxaemic failure. Although this classification aids description, it is not intended to suggest that the two terms and types of failure cannot be interlinked and the patient may present with hypoxaemic failure and progress rapidly to ventilatory failure.

Ventilatory failure

This is defined by an increase in the arterial carbon dioxide tension. This represents the balance between carbon dioxide production and alveolar ventilation. Ventilatory failure therefore follows if:
1 There is a reduction in alveolar ventilation to an amount which does not allow adequate exchange of carbon dioxide with ambient air.
2 Ventilation cannot increase to compensate for an increased carbon dioxide production.
3 There is insufficient removal from inappropriate matching of pulmonary perfusion and ventilation.

It is usual and convenient to consider the various causes of ventilatory failure by defining the underlying lesion according to its anatomical site.
1 Central nervous system.

2 Neuromuscular.
3 Thoracic cage and pleura.
4 Lungs and airways.

Central nervous system

An increase in total ventilation accompanies emotional surges and is normal prior to energetic physical activity, e.g. in athletes immediately prior to a race. However, the majority of processes affecting the respiratory neuronal mechanism situated around the fourth ventricle produce depressed respiration.

The main causes of respiratory centre depression are:
1 Drugs.
2 Trauma.
3 Intracranial disease.
4 Hypoxia.
5 Hypercapnia.

The most common cause of respiratory centre depression is the administration of drugs, particularly those used to provide anaesthesia, analgesia and sedation. The mode of action to produce this depression varies between compounds. For example, the opioid analgesics do not affect tidal volume significantly but cause the internal cycling system in the respiratory centre to slow down or stop. The frequency of breathing is thus reduced until apnoea develops. In contrast, the barbiturates and volatile anaesthetics reduce the ventilation by decreasing tidal volume whilst having usually little effect on respiratory frequency.

It is important to remember that in the presence of other causes of CNS depression, such as hypoxaemia or trauma, the respiratory centre is more sensitive to the effects of sedative and analgesic agents.

Trauma to the brain may produce central depression either as a direct result of trauma itself or secondary to an increase in intracranial pressure; producing a reduction in cerebral perfusion pressure and cerebral blood flow. The most extreme example of the effects of trauma and raised intracranial pressure is coning of the medulla leading to apnoea.

Ventilatory depression consequent to the raised intracranial pressure from intracranial tumours is usually a preterminal event. However, there are several inflammatory diseases of the nervous system which may lead to reductions in ventilation. Encephalitis and bulbar involvement in ascending polyneuritis represent the most common examples of this type of lesion in the UK. More rarely, patients with poliomyelitis and tetanus may demonstrate also the same derangement in ventilatory control.

Finally, moderate hypoxaemia and hypercapnia act as stimulants to breathing, the former via peripheral chemoreceptors, the latter acting centrally. However, with severe hypoxia the pattern of respiration becomes irregular and of so-called Cheyne–Stokes pattern: apnoea follows if hypoxaemia is not relieved. Similarly, with acute elevations in the Pa_{CO_2} to values of $11-12\,kPa$ ($80-90\,mmHg$) there is an increasing tendency to depression of ventilation with a reduction in conscious level at levels above about $13\,kPa$ ($97.5\,mmHg$).

Neuromuscular

In this type of ventilatory failure, there is a normal central respiratory drive but the peripheral neural and muscular responses are abnormal.

There are four main causes of this problem:
1 Drugs and toxins.
2 Spinal cord dysfunction from trauma or infection.
3 Congenital or acquired muscle disease.
4 Myasthenia gravis.

As in the case of the central depression of ventilation, this type of ventilatory failure most commonly follows administration of drugs, particularly those used to provide neuromuscular block. Persistent respiratory inadequency after their withdrawal is invariably a result of overdosage, especially if these compounds are given in full dosage to patients with myasthenia gravis or Eaton–Lambert syndrome. Other causes of inadequate reversal include disorders of acid–base balance and electrolyte disorders, especially those affecting calcium homeostasis.

Two further causes of myoneuronal block now seen rarely are poisoning with organophosphorus insecticides and botulinus toxin. The former acts as an anticholinesterase producing an excess of acetylcholine at the motor end-plate and the latter acts by inducing a failure to release this neurotransmitter. Whilst the final effect of both toxins is to produce a flaccid paralysis, it may be that patients with organophosphorus poisoning have a period of time where there are excitatory phenomena and convulsions.

The most common inflammatory lesion in the UK affecting the spinal cord is acute polyneuritis (Guillain–Barré syndrome) which is usually a self-limiting and reversible condition of the lower motor neurone producing flaccid paralysis. Infections of the anterior horn cell with poliomyelitis virus are now extremely rare in the UK and USA but are still a considerable cause of morbidity and mortality in the world.

Patients with muscular dystrophies and myositis present occasionally with ventilatory failure. However, ventilatory failure in these conditions usually follows chest infection, acquired as a complication of treatment rather than to muscle weakness alone.

Patients with myasthenia gravis may present with ventilatory failure either as a consequence of their disease or as a complication of therapy. In addition, myasthenia gravis patients often require ventilatory support in the perioperative period after thymectomy.

Thoracic cage and pleura

This system is the force generator for respiration. Failure of the system leading to hypercapnic respiratory failure results from problems with either the muscles of inspiration or the 'mechanical' connection to provide adequate lung movement.

Inspiratory muscle fatigue (the patient getting 'tired') is probably the most common reason for instituting mechanical ventilatory support. It is also an area in which there is a comparative paucity of well-controlled clinical trials and research.

In addition to the more hereditary muscle diseases such as muscular dystrophy, the respiratory muscles may be compromised in many ways. Increased work of breathing, usually a consequence of an underlying lung problem, mechanical disadvantage, impaired nutritional status, shock, hypoxaemia and electrolyte deficiencies (especially potassium, magnesium and organic phosphates) are major factors which contribute to respiratory muscle fatigue and failure.

To allow the chest-wall muscles and mechanics to work at their best advantage, the thoracic cage should be both uniform and firm. If the thoracic cage is not uniform (for example, in patients with kyphoscoliosis) or has a flail segment (following thoracic trauma), ventilatory failure may develop rapidly. Interestingly, in patients suffering from ankylosing spondylitis with the stiff (or immobile) chest wall but with uniformity of shape, the incidence of ventilatory failure is low.

Lungs and airways

Ventilatory failure with hypercapnia is a late event in the majority of disease processes affecting the lungs and airways. The majority of patients have hypoxaemia as the primary abnormality.

Large airway disease

The pivotal mechanism by which ventilatory failure is produced in larger airways disease is by airway narrowing. As the flow resistance of an airway is inversely proportional to the fourth power of the radius, small changes in the lumen have profound effects on air flow rates and increase the work of breathing, leading eventually to inspiratory muscle fatigue. By far the most common cause of large-airway lumen obstruction is the presence of secretions.

Other less commonly seen but easily treated causes include upper airway obstruction after infection (epiglottis, laryngotracheitis, 'croup'), trauma (post-intubation) and tumour (either directly or via involvement of the recurrent laryngeal nerve).

Sleep apnoea syndrome

One final cause of ventilatory failure which does not at present fit comfortably into any single classification is the so called sleep apnoea—hypopnoea syndrome (SAHS). This was described originally as general alveolar hypoventilation (Fishman *et al.*, 1966) and is a syndrome of respiratory and cardiac failure in patients with normal lungs (Strohl *et al.*, 1986). Patients with this condition are usually obese (nearly always 30% greater than their ideal weight, sometimes three times heavier!), although it is not known if this is the cause or effect of the disease. During rapid eye movement (REM) sleep, the patients develop complete upper airway obstruction to air flow for periods lasting over 15 s. The desaturation of arterial blood which follows leads to arousal and relief of the obstruction. Daytime somnolence is a part of the syndrome.

The patients eventually develop crippling pulmonary hypertension with hypoxaemia, hypercapnia and right heart failure. The diagnosis of sleep apnoea syndrome is made by continuously monitoring respiration, oxygen saturation, electro-oculography (for eye movement) during sleep. Similar periods of pronounced episodic desaturation related to obstructive hypopnoea and apnoea have been recorded in the first 16 postoperative hours in patients given morphine for analgesia. These episodes are not seen in patients who had analgesia provided by local anaesthetic block (Catley *et al.*, 1985).

Therapy in SAHS is focused to relieve the upper airway obstruction (Hanly, 1992). This is usually achieved with nocturnal nasal [continuous positive airway pressure (CPAP)] devices. However, the com-pliance of the patient with this therapy is only about 80% (Hoffstein *et al.*, 1992). Some patients have surgical interventions such as pharyngoplasty, and more rarely today, tracheostomy. For further discussion of this subject, the reader is referred also to Chapter 1.

Lower airway obstruction

Lower airway narrowing is a predominant feature of the respiratory failure associated with several diseases, particularly:
1 Asthma.
2 Bronchiolitis.
3 Chronic obstructive lung disease.
The presence of intraluminal secretions has profound effects on airway calibre leading to increasing airway resistance (chronic bronchitis, asthma, bronchiolitis), although airway narrowing by either bronchiolar muscle spasm (asthma) or a lack of appropriate elastic recoil (emphysema) play a part also. Nevertheless, the predominant and primary effect of all these diseases is to produce a mismatching of ventilation and perfusion ($\dot{V}:\dot{Q}$) leading to arterial hypoxaemia; ventilatory failure is usually a late event in these patients.

Hypoxaemic respiratory failure

Hypoxaemia may develop as a consequence of:
1 Low inspired oxygen concentration.
2 Alveolar hypoventilation.
3 Increased $\dot{V}:\dot{Q}$ mismatching.
4 Increase in intrapulmonary shunting.
5 Limitation of diffusion across the alveolar capillary barrier.

The alveolar : arterial oxygen tension difference is normal in the first two causes and elevated in the latter three. Diffusion limitation once held as a major component and cause of hypoxaemia, is currently not believed to contribute to clinical respiratory failure.

The principle underlying lesion in hypoxaemic failure is abnormality of $\dot{V}:\dot{Q}$ matching in the lung. Table 84.1 shows several disease processes associated causally with the development of hypoxaemic failure from $\dot{V}:\dot{Q}$ mismatch. Although for convenience the diseases have been listed under vascular and alveolar unit causes of this defect, there are certain conditions which overlap these boundaries. For example, patients suffering from the so-called adult respiratory distress syndrome (ARDS) have pulmonary vascular abnormalities in addition to pulmonary oedema and alveolitis.

The predominant effect of most of these diseases is

Table 84.1 Disease processes associated with the development of hypoxaemia and respiratory failure

Alveolar Unit
Pneumonia
Bronchiectasis (especially in cystic fibrosis)
Inhalation
    Firesmoke
    Gastric contents
    Near drowning
Interstitial lung disease
    Idiopathic fibrosis
    Radiation and chemotherapy for malignant disease
Haemorrhage and contusion
    Immunological (Goodpasture syndrome)
    Traumatic
Opportunist infections (especially in the immune-compromised, e.g. transplants or AIDS)
    Aspergillus and other fungi
    Cytomegalovirus
    Pneumocystis carinii

Circulation
Cardiac pulmonary oedema
Pulmonary artery embolism
    Fat
    Thrombus
    Amniotic fluid
Pulmonary hypertension
    Primary (plexiform lesions)
    Secondary (Eisenmenger's syndrome)

to produce increased stiffness of the lung parenchyma and reduction in lung compliance necessitating increased work of breathing to maintain ventilation. Infiltration of the lung parenchyma with inflammatory cells, exudates and oedema fluid is thought to lead to stimulation of the J-receptor in the lung parenchyma. This leads to the sensation of shortness of breath which is usually the predominant and primary symptom in patients with such diseases.

There are two further pathological conditions where there is impaired tissue oxygenation, although the arterial Po_2 may not be reduced:
1 Limitation of oxygen delivery to the peripheral tissues so that aerobic metabolism cannot be maintained. Examples include severe anaemia, carbon monoxide poisoning and low cardiac output states.
2 Failure to extract oxygen at tissue level to allow its use for aerobic metabolism. The most obvious example of this is poisoning with cyanide. However, there is a recent body of evidence to suggest that in certain disease processes, associated with multi-system failure, improvements in delivery are not matched by increases in peripheral usage. The so-called supply dependence of oxygen consumption

had a large vogue and following in the late 1980s. However, this concept was based on calculations of tissue oxygen consumption by the reverse Fick method. Introduction of systems which directly measure oxygen consumption by calorimetry have shown that there is a consistent error and discrepancy between these direct measures and the reversed Fick calculation (Bizouarn *et al.*, 1992). The significance of this difference is still hotly debated. One suggestion is that as the Fick technique does not take into account pulmonary metabolism and oxygen consumption then this variable is measured by the differences in the results from the two techniques.

Principles of management of respiratory failure

These may be classified into two broad categories based on the aetiological subgroups.
1 Methods to improve gas transfer to alveoli.
2 Methods to improve tissue oxygenation.

Methods to improve gas transfer

These can be subdivided further into:
1 General methods to improve ventilation.
2 Specific methods based on treating certain known underlying disease processes especially airflow obstruction. Included in this section is a discussion of the management of the patient with chest trauma.

General management

Ventilatory failure with a high arterial carbon dioxide tension can be reversed only by altering those factors which affect this gas tension — carbon dioxide production and alveolar ventilation, $\dot{V}_A$.

Carbon dioxide production may be reduced using antipyretics such as aspirin or paracetamol, by surface cooling, using antibiotics in the presence of a proven infection and by the judicious use of sedatives to reduce excessive muscle activity from shivering or agitation.

Alveolar ventilation may be improved by restoring normal control of ventilation, overcoming lung restriction and, most importantly, by reducing airflow obstruction mainly by ensuring clearance of secretions. Tracheal intubation and mechanical support may be necessary if these measures fail.

Retained secretions increase airway resistance and thereby the work of breathing. Clearance of secretions may therefore produce a major reduction in the work of breathing.

Causes of retained secretions include:

1 Mucus hypersecretion as found in asthma or in bronchiectasis (e.g. cystic fibrosis).

2 Impaired ciliary function, most commonly from chronic inhalation of irritants such as tobacco smoke. However, there are many iatrogenic causes of decreased ciliary beat frequency. The most important are increases in inspired oxygen concentration and the administration of anaesthetics, opioids and sedatives.

3 Ineffective or absent cough may occur in patients with neuromuscular disease or following CNS or spinal trauma. Drug overdose either by intent or iatrogenic is a further potent cause of absent cough. Adequacy of cough to expel secretions requires the generation of an explosive expiratory flow. Inability to take a deep breath, weak abdominal muscles or unwillingness to contract them because of pain, and small airways collapse on forced expiration (as occurs in obstructive lung disease) all reduce cough efficiency significantly.

4 Alterations or abnormalities of mucus secretion may be important. The mucus secretions of the large airways are a complex mixture of mucopolysaccharides which act as a thyxotrope. Purulent sputum has different viscoelastic properties to non-purulent sputum. One factor known to modify the transport velocity of sputum is the degree of hydration. Experimental work has shown that mucus flow may be reduced by 25% in the presence of systemic dehydration.

5 Bronchoconstriction and airway collapse potentiate secretion retention. Airway collapse may lead also to plugging of airways with subsequent atelectasis of the distal segment thereby decreasing lung compliance to increased $\dot{V}:\dot{Q}$ inequalities.

Therapy to improve clearance of secretions

From the above outline of causes, a simple management plan to improve clearance should include:

1 *Adequate hydration*. This is attained by ensuring that humidification of the inspired gas is appropriate using either a nebulizer or hot-water device. Additionally, any systematic dehydration should be corrected. The viscoelastic properties of sputum may also be modified pharmacologically. In particular, *N*-acetyl cysteine and bromhexene have been suggested as therapies to reduce the 'stickiness' of sputum and aid its removal. Unfortunately, controlled clinical trials have not been in agreement regarding the value of these compounds (Wanner & Rao, 1980).

2 *Chest physiotherapy*. This is the mainstay of therapy to remove secretions by using techniques such as postural drainage, percussion and vibration when accompanied by cough to clear secretions. If the patient's ability to cough is inadequate, secretions may be expelled with the aid of artificial breaths and suctioning (bagging and sucking). This does not necessarily require tracheal intubation but may be performed using a T-piece and mask following insertion of a nasopharyngeal airway under local anaesthesia. Such techniques of physical therapy have been shown to be highly beneficial even with large quantities of tenacious secretions, as found in cystic fibrosis (Mortensen *et al.*, 1991).

There are several relative contraindications to chest physiotherapy which include:

(a) Raised intracranial pressure.

(b) Active or recent lung haemorrhage.

(c) Multiple rib fractures when percussion and vibration may lead to pneumothorax.

(d) Lung abscess and empyema unless it is possible to institute powerful tracheal and endobronchial suction in the case of rupture.

(e) Uncontrolled hypoxaemia when postural changes induce haemodynamic disturbances.

(f) Patients with severe shortness of breath, low cardiac output or cardiac arrhythmia should be treated with caution, as the physiotherapy itself is known to produce an increase in $\dot{V}:\dot{Q}$ mismatch during the procedure.

Finally, several patients with chronic sputum retention develop acute lobar atelectasis in the perioperative period probably because of mucus plugging. Bronchoscopy and removal of the plug under direct vision is often suggested as the therapy of choice. However, a prospective study of the use of fibreoptic bronchoscopy and physiotherapy in patients with acute lobar atelectasis showed no benefit of bronchoscopy compared with physiotherapy alone (Marini *et al.*, 1979).

Airflow obstruction may be relieved also by using an artificial airway which is used usually for four specific indications:

1 Prevention or reversal of upper airway obstruction, e.g. permanent tracheostomy in a patient with sleep apnoea syndrome or laryngeal tumours.

2 Protection against aspiration in patients with impairment of the level of consciousness from drugs or organic CNS disease.

3 Facilitating tracheobronchial toilet. A fine suction catheter via a nasopharyngeal airway passed into the trachea for suctioning at the time of chest physiotherapy is often of great benefit.

4 To allow mechanical ventilation. This is by far

the commonest indication for tracheal intubation whether by the oral or nasal route. When choosing the route for tracheal intubation, it is often worth considering the technique proposed to wean the patient from ventilation. There is, for example, little point in passing a 7-mm nasotracheal tube in a patient with chronic obstructive lung disease as the tube itself produces a resistance to airflow some four times higher than that of the patient's own airway. In this case it may be that an early tracheostomy with the insertion of a 12-mm tube (which has the same resistance to airflow as the patient) may be more useful.

Management of chest trauma

The management of chest injuries depends on the nature and site of the injury and the expertise and equipment available in the hospital concerned.

The history of the traumatic insult gives an insight into the potential injuries produced. The lesion in a crush injury depends on the direction of the force. Anterior−posterior trauma is more likely to lead to a flail segment, airway rupture and fracture of the spine. Lateral crushing tends to produce ipsilateral rib fractures and traumatic rupture of the spleen or liver.

With high-velocity (rapid deceleration) injuries, as found in road traffic accidents then the injury usually leaves the chest intact but with an anterior flail segment, possibly with a fracture of the sternum. In addition to the flail segment there may be an underlying aortic rupture, cardiac contusion, rupture of the diaphragm or a major airway. Extra to the chest injuries there is a high probability that the patient has maxillofacial, cervical and hepatic or splenic injuries.

Low-velocity injury is usually caused by a direct blow, as, for example, in pedestrians involved in road traffic accidents or in falls from a height. In this event there are usually rib fractures on the side of the injury with underlying pulmonary contusions. Laceration of the liver or spleen is likely if the lower five or six ribs are involved.

A simple visual examination of the patient reveals the presence of a flail segment. Subcutaneous emphysema and haemoptysis suggests that major airway rupture has occurred. Aortic dissection is most easily diagnosed with an ultrasound scan. Suspicion of such a problem is suggested on a chest radiograph if the mediastinal shadow is greater than 8 cm on a standard 100 cm anterior−posterior film, if there is shift to the right of the trachea or a depression

of the air bronchogram of the left main bronchus to less than an angle of 40° to the trachea. The chest radiograph also shows if there is air or fluid in the pleural space.

Diagnosis of cardiac contusion and injury is made by finding evidence of ischaemia or arrhythmia on the electrocardiogram. Additional evidence can be obtained by detecting elevated concentrations of creatinine phosphokinase in the plasma and by detecting abnormal wall motion with echocardiography (ECHO) or gated radionuclide scanning. Children with cardiac contusion rarely, if ever, develop ECHO abnormalities with cardiac injury (Ildstad et al., 1990).

The child with a chest injury is also less likely to present with rib fractures due to the relative suppleness of their ribs and therefore sometimes present considerable diagnostic difficulties.

It is useful to have a baseline arterial blood-gas estimation performed as early as possible on presentation of the patient into the hospital.

Management of the patient with blunt chest trauma depends on the extent of the injury. Air or fluid in the pleura should be drained with a tube thoracostomy and an under-water sealed drain. With early drainage and appropriate antibiotic cover, empyema requiring operative decortication is reported in about 1:14 patients with blunt chest injury (Helling et al., 1989).

The two principal problems for the patient are pain from fractures and respiratory difficulties due to a flail segment or underlying lung contusion. The pain leads to difficulties with coughing and deep breathing which in turn is associated with a greater chance of atelectasis and an increased risk for the development of a pulmonary infection.

Good analgesia and physiotherapy to maintain adequate ventilation is usually all that is necessary with a unilateral injury and stable blood-gas tensions with five or less fractured ribs. The best method of producing analgesia is still debated. In young patients, intramuscular opioid and other simpler analgesics are all that is usually required. In the older patient and particularly in elderly patients, a continuous local analgesic technique with either intrapleural local anaesthesia or an extradural technique should be considered. In patients more than 60 years of age, the use of extradural analgesia has been shown to have significant benefits to decrease mortality and the development of pulmonary infections in patients with blunt chest injury (Wisner, 1990).

Continuous extradural analgesia would also be the preferred method of analgesia in patients with multiple (i.e. >5) fractures and an unstable or flail segment. These patients also tend to have relatively poor arterial blood-gas values. To prevent deterioration of arterial oxygen tension with increasing atelectasis it is also valuable to apply CPAP, in addition to intensive physiotherapy. The use of regional analgesia and CPAP has been shown to be superior to the use of tracheal intubation and intermittent positive-pressure ventilation (IPPV) with a positive end-expiratory pressure (PEEP) in patients with multiple rib fractures. Bolliger and van Eeden showed in 1990 that patients treated with regional analgesia and CPAP had a three-fold reduction in the incidence of pulmonary infections and a two-fold reduction in the time in intensive care and hospital compared with patients treated by tracheal intubation and IPPV.

Patients with multiple bilateral fractures and significant deformity rarely have the chest injury as their sole lesion and usually require general anaesthesia for a separate reason. In this case it is conventional to maintain the patient with IPPV and PEEP until recovery from the non-pulmonary lesion.

Surgical management of chest trauma is best undertaken at a specialist centre. Before repair of an aortic rupture, it is necessary to perform angiography to confirm the site of the injury and to ensure that the lesion is not multiple. Cardiovascular instability is common after this procedure and if this occurs then urgent transfer to the operating theatre is needed.

The need for urgent thoracotomy following chest injury is associated with a mortality of about 80%. This high mortality was attributed universally to exsanguination (Devitt *et al.*, 1991). It is obvious that if such surgery becomes necessary then the usual precautions used when torrential bleeding is anticipated are used. In addition, if a major intrathoracic disruption is suspected, then it may be necessary to perform bronchoscopy and possibly intubation with a double-lumen tube to isolate the injury while the patient is awake.

Ventilatory support

Mechanical support

Mechanical ventilatory support is indicated when there is hypercapnia from CNS depression or neuromuscular disease. In addition, many centres would institute controlled hyperventilation in patients with cerebral trauma in order to produce hypocapnia, to aid the reduction of post-traumatic oedema.

As suggested earlier, the exact timing of institution of ventilatory support based on blood-gas tensions is more difficult to define in patients with pulmonary disease. It is usually based on additional clinical criteria such as patient age, chronicity of the underlying disease process and prospects for recovery from the disease.

Probably of equal controversy is the type of ventilator to use and the pattern of ventilation to select. Earlier ventilators were negative-pressure devices of the tank or cuirass type. Until recently, this mode of support has been reserved for patients with normal lungs with muscle weakness or neuromuscular dysfunction.

More modern ventilators apply intermittent positive pressure to the airway to facilitate gas transfer. The simplest such devices provide a near-sinusoidal waveform, and only the frequency of breathing and the volume of each breath can be altered independently. Attempts to overcome the many disadvantages and potential deleterious affects of such systems have taxed engineers and clinicians alike. Such systems as assisted mechanical ventilation (AMV) and (synchronized) intermittent mandatory ventilation [(S)IMV] have been developed. It is thought that AMV would spare the patient the energy cost of breathing by providing the inspiratory power from the machine. However, measurements in clinical practice suggest that some patients receiving mechanical assistance with AMV may continue to perform respiratory work at levels which stress the ventilatory reserve and as a consequence work levels during AMV may be comparable with the work of chest inflation during spontaneous ventilation (Marini *et al.*, 1986). Similarly, the use of (S)IMV has failed to show the major benefits ascribed originally to the method (Luce *et al.*, 1981).

High-frequency ventilation (HFV) using high-pressure jets or oscillators has been suggested as an advance in ventilatory support. However, in the presence of airflow limitation, the devices produce a highly predictable increase in resting-lung volume with increased likelihood of barotrauma. In patients with low lung compliance, there is a theoretical benefit for increased respiratory frequency compared to conventional IPPV. However, studies designed to investigate this theory have failed to show any significant benefit of HFV (Brichart *et al.*, 1986).

An increasing vocabulary has been developed to describe patterns and modes of ventilation. The microprocessor has allowed an increasingly complex series of instructions to be converted into gasflow generation. Despite this, there is a paucity or absence of well-controlled trials or comparisons between different patterns or styles of ventilation in relation to outcome and complications.

The optimum ventilator and pattern of ventilation which is applicable universally to patients with ventilatory failure remains unclear.

Pharmacological support of ventilation

Increased alveolar ventilation may be achieved in certain conditions using pharmacological support. Doxapram stimulates an increase in minute ventilation and aminophylline and isoprenaline can restore the force of contractility of the diaphragm (Aubier et al., 1981). However, there have been no controlled clinical trials to examine the application and efficiency of such support in acute (and chronic) ventilatory failure.

Specific therapy to relieve airflow obstruction with particular reference to asthma

There is considerable interest in the definition and concept of airflow limitation and its management. Historically, airflow limitation has been designated according to the response to a set dose of a known bronchodilator. Thus, patients suffered from either reversible disease, perceived as asthma in the young, atopic non-smoker with a family history, or irreversible disease, found in older, tobacco smokers often with bronchitis and emphysema.

The study by Eliasson and de Graff (1985), however, showed that airflow limitation (measured as the forced expiratory volume in 1 s, $FEV_{1.0}$) would not distinguish between those patients with 'asthma' and those with chronic obstructive airway disease (COAD). These authors questioned the practice of classifying patients with known airflow limitation as either asthmatic or COAD. Studies such as this together with reappraisals of the meaning of the term 'obstructive airway disease' (Fletcher & Pride, 1984) imply that the majority of patients with airflow obstruction (except those with fixed upper airway lesions) may benefit from a trial of bronchodilator therapy. Indeed, it has been argued cogently (Luce et al., 1984) that acute ventilatory failure in patients with COAD is manageable nearly always without mechanical ventilation if the patient is alert on admission. This point is amplified by a review suggesting that 94% of patients admitted with respiratory failure and with a history of COAD did not receive ventilatory support and left hospital (Rosen, 1986). In addition, these patients pose a special problem in regard to weaning from ventilatory support

and the primary goals of therapy must be to avoid mechanical support.

In cases where ventilatory support is felt to be justified, there is a reported mortality of approximately 25% of patients with COAD requiring more than 24 h ventilation, compared with the mortality of 80% in patients with multiple organ failure (Gillespie et al., 1986).

Recent surveys have shown the incidence and mortality from acute asthma is rising. This has led to the publication of guidelines for the diagnosis and management of acute severe asthmatic attacks from the National Institutes of Health in North America (National Asthma Program, 1991) and a joint group representing the National Asthma Campaign in the UK (Statement of the British Thoracic Society, Research Unit of the Royal College of Physicians of London, Kings Fund Centre and National Asthma Campaign, 1990). Both reports have similar recommendations but vary as to the precise pharmacological interventions to undertake. A severe, life-threatening asthma attack is defined as being present if:

1 The patient has increasing wheeze or breathlessness to prevent completion of a spoken sentence or to limit mobility, for example, getting out of a chair.
2 If the heart rate is more than 110 beats/min.
3 If the respiratory rate is more than 25 breaths/min.
4 If the peak expiratory flowrate is less than 40% of the predicted normal or best normally achieved or less than 200 litres/min if the best normally achieved is not known.
5 Pulsus paradoxus (a reduction in arterial pressure on inspiration) of more than 1.33 kPa (10 mmHg).

Imminently life-threatening features are a silent chest on auscultation, bradycardia, cyanosis and exhaustion, confusion or unconsciousness. These latter features are absolute indications to perform tracheal intubation and commence positive-pressure ventilation. Measurement of arterial blood-gas tensions should always be performed in any patient with acute severe asthma. The finding of a high hydrogen ion concentration and hypoxia [$Pao_2 < 8$ kPa (60 mmHg)] with a high inspired oxygen concentration or a normal or raised carbon dioxide tension in a breathless patient also suggests a very severe or life-threatening attack.

Other investigations to conduct are a chest radiograph to show if there is a second pathology such as a pneumothorax or lung collapse. An ECG may also show evidence of right-heart strain or failure. Measurement of haemoglobin concentrations, white cell count and plasma urea and electrolytes is useful in defining if infection is a problem and also the state of hydration of the patient.

The recommendations for therapy other than intubation are:

1 Give oxygen at as high a concentration as possible, usually 60%.

2 Administer high doses of a β_2-agonist by inhalation following nebulization of the drug with oxygen. In the UK the recommendation is salbutamol, 2.5–5 mg, or terbutaline, 5–10 mg. In the USA metaproterenol, 15 mg, or isoetharine, 5 mg, are also recommended.

3 Administer high-dose steroids. Hydrocortisone 200 mg, or methyl prednisolone, 80 mg i.v., and/or prednisolone, 30–60 mg, orally.

4 Parenteral bronchodilators. Both sets of guidelines recommend giving aminophylline at a rate of about $0.6 \, mg \cdot kg^{-1} \cdot h^{-1}$. The major point of discussion about administration of methyl xanthines is related to whether a loading dose of about 6 mg/kg should be given. If the patient is already taking methylxanthines then this added dose may lead to problems of toxicity, especially cardiac arrhythmias and tachycardia. Lower doses are more likely to be necessary in patients taking cimetadine, ciprofloxacin or erythromycin or who have impaired liver function. In contrast, smokers may need a higher dose. It is probable that treatment with methylxanthines will become less common as newer therapies are developed. These newer therapeutic interventions act by preventing the inflammatory aspects of acute asthma. None the less the phosphodiesterase inhibitors still play a part in current practice (Lam & Newhouse, 1990).

Other agents suggested for single-dose parenteral administration are β_2-agonists (salbutamol, 200 μg, or terbutaline, 250 μg) by the intravenous route or subcutaneously (adrenaline, 300 μg, or terbutaline, 250 μg). Salbutamol and terbutaline can be given as continuous infusions at dose rates between 3–20 μg/min. The dose depends on the response of the patient in terms of the increase in heart rate associated with the use of such drugs and the improvement in airflow.

All patients with acute severe asthma should be admitted to an intensive care unit for monitoring and management. The progression of acute asthma to respiratory arrest is not understood and many patients are thought to have died because the severity of the disease was not recognized and they were therefore undertreated (Molfino et al., 1991).

Monitoring should include measurement of peak expiratory flow rates about 30 min after starting therapy, before and after therapy with nebulized β_2-agonists usually four times a day. Arterial blood-gas tensions should be measured again within 2 h of starting treatment and also if the Pao_2 was less than 8 kPa (60 mmHg) or there was a normal or raised carbon dioxide tension. Many cases of hypercapnia resolve within 6 h of the start of an asthmatic attack (Mountain & Sahn, 1988). Heart rate and rhythm should be monitored continuously and if methyl xanthines are being given, the plasma concentrations should be measured every day to maintain the concentration between 56 and 111 μmol/litre.

Controversy still exists on the timing and also the need for institution of positive-pressure ventilation. The arguments in this area mirror those concerning the management of patients with chronic obstructive pulmonary disease. Authors from certain centres recommend the early institution of mechanical support in a high proportion of patients during acute exacerbations of their asthma (Cottam & Eason, 1991). In contrast other groups have reported a mortality rate of zero in patients managed without mechanical ventilation (Bramman & Kaemmerlen, 1990). This latter result was attributed, by the authors, to avoiding the deleterious effects of mechanical ventilation.

This zero mortality in patients with asthma and the 6% mortality in patients with other chronic obstructive disease processes treated without mechanical interventions (Rosen, 1986) suggests strongly that the institution of ventilatory support should be undertaken with some caution. However, as in all therapies, there is a middle-ground approach. Most clinicians would also agree that with worsening hypoxia or hypercapnia, if consciousness is impaired or frank respiratory arrest occurs then mechanical ventilation is required urgently.

Methods to improve tissue oxygenation

Classically, tissue hypoxaemia has been classified into four aetiological groups.

1 Hypoxic hypoxia.

2 Anaemic hypoxia.

3 Stagnant hypoxia.

4 Cytotoxic hypoxia.

In patients with respiratory failure, the problem is hypoxic hypoxia where arterial oxygen tension is abnormal as a result of a $\dot{V}:\dot{Q}$ mismatch in the lung. However, in the clinical situation where hypoxaemia is refractory to therapeutic intervention, it may be that therapy to improve oxygen transport (increasing the red cell mass) and availability (improving tissue blood flow) may have profoundly beneficial effects. As other variables can determine tissue oxygenation, the measurement of arterial blood tension of oxygen alone may be misleading. In some situations, monitoring cardiac output together with oxygen contents of arterial and mixed venous blood may be important.

Therapy to improve arterial blood oxygenation

Increasing inspired oxygen concentration

Administration of added oxygen is the most obvious first step in reversing or diminishing arterial hypoxaemia. Oxygen is administered often as first-line and potentially life-saving therapy although in theory administration of oxygen to patients with relatively fixed right–left shunting should be ineffective. However, it is important to note that giving added oxygen may not be without dangers. This is true in patients with chronic respiratory failure who present with an acute exacerbation. The hypoxic ventilatory drive diminishes greatly when the PaO_2 increases above 8.7 kPa (65 mmHg). In patients whose breathing is stimulated primarily by hypoxic drive, the administration of added oxygen may produce severe hypoventilation or apnoea.

Additionally high inspired oxygen tensions have other adverse and toxic effects which are discussed more fully in the section on oxygen toxicity. It is therefore important to define the goals of oxygen administration.

The curvilinear relationship between arterial oxygen tension and the saturation of haemoglobin is well known. Because of this relationship, an increase in PaO_2, of say 3 kPa (22.5 mmHg) has differing effects depending on the original PaO_2. If this were 6 kPa (45 mmHg), a 3 kPa (22.5 mmHg) increase raises saturation from 75–90%, equivalent to oxygen content increasing from 15 ml/dl to 18 ml/dl for a haemoglobin of 15 g/dl. However, a 3 kPa (22.5 mmHg) increase in PaO_2 from 10.7 kPa (80 mmHg) increases haemoglobin saturation by only 3%, a content increase of only about 0.5 ml/dl.

For this reason it is conventional to attempt to maintain PaO_2 at or just above 10 kPa (75 mmHg) in an attempt to balance the beneficial effects of added oxygen against its potentially deleterious effects.

Raising airway pressure

It has been known for some time that raising end-expiratory pressure [conventionally termed continuous positive airway pressure (CPAP) for spontaneous breathing and positive end-expiratory pressure (PEEP) for patients receiving assisted ventilation] can improve PaO_2. These techniques are used in addition to added inspired oxygen in conditions where there is diffuse, restrictive disease associated with a reduction in functional residual capacity (FRC). Classically, these disorders represent the pulmonary complications of anaesthesia, surgery and inadequately treated primary ventilatory failure. Whilst raising the airway pressure has beneficial effects, it can be deleterious and inappropriate, particularly in patients who already have abnormally high FRC, e.g. in obstructive airway disease, raising FRC further may have deleterious effects on gas exchange and simply increase the incidence and severity of barotrauma. Additionally, in patients with large physiological deadspace as a result of vascular occlusions, a further increase in this deadspace induced by PEEP/CPAP may result in alveolar hypoventilation and retention of carbon dioxide. The use of PEEP is relatively contraindicated in the presence of localized and unhomogeneous disease, especially if there is evidence of gas trapping.

Correctly used PEEP/CPAP can restore an abnormally low FRC towards normal. None the less, there is still a lack of agreement concerning the most appropriate means of determining the optimum timing, levels and outcome of the application of PEEP.

Before applying PEEP it is worth asking:
1 Is this manoeuvre likely to benefit the patient?
2 What level of raised airway pressure is optimal for this individual patient?
Therefore the goals of the therapy need to be defined. Application of PEEP in an attempt to allow an adequate PaO_2 at a safe F_IO_2 should be beneficial in patients with severe hypoxaemia from increased $\dot{V}:\dot{Q}$ mismatch, where the disease is diffuse and where there is a reduction in lung volumes.

Raising lung volumes above normal by raising airway pressure, increases both pleural and intrathoracic pressures throughout both the respiratory and the cardiac cycles. This leads to a reduction in cardiac output from decreased venous return to the right atrium. The amount of PEEP necessary to produce this effect is reduced markedly in patients with hypovolaemia, intrinsic cardiac dysfunction and especially in patients with raised pulmonary vascular resistance. The increase in venous pressure and reduction in arterial pressure induced by PEEP make this modality of therapy inappropriate also in patients with raised intracranial pressure.

Attempting to minimize shunt from $\dot{V}:\dot{Q}$ mismatch requires very high levels of PEEP, an approach which requires intensive and aggressive cardiovascular support. This approach produces the best Pao_2 for the lowest F_1o_2 and is appropriate when pulmonary oxygen toxicity may be a significant problem. However, some clinicians aim to maintain relatively low intravascular volumes. It is therefore more appropriate to apply PEEP to a level which has minimal effect on cardiac output whilst hopefully increasing haemoglobin saturation. The concept of optimum PEEP therefore depends on the objective of the therapy.

The application of PEEP and CPAP require usually the presence of a tracheal tube. However, techniques of applying CPAP by close-fitting mask have been described. This technique may be useful in such conditions as viral pneumonia or following inhalation of toxic smoke and fumes. However, the technique does require that the patient is fully conscious and co-operative and is able to remove the mask if vomiting occurs.

Other deleterious and beneficial effects of PEEP or CPAP are discussed more fully in the later section on ARDS.

Effects of position

In unilateral lung disease, a change in posture can have profound beneficial effects in returning $\dot{V}:\dot{Q}$ mismatch towards normality. Perfusion is increased to the dependent lung. Ventilation to the upper lung is greatest during controlled ventilation and to the lower lung during spontaneous breathing. In diffuse lung disease postural changes are also of great benefit with an increase in the Pao_2 in the prone position (Douglas et al., 1977; Langer et al., 1988).

Hyperbaric oxygenation

Hyperbaric oxygenation may have potential areas of benefit. However, its use in the management of acute respiratory failure has never been justified.

Therapy to improve tissue oxygenation

This may be classified into:
1 Increasing blood flow.
2 Increasing oxygen transport by haemoglobin or synthetic oxygen carriers.

Measurement of blood flow usually entails the use of a thermodilution cardiac output pulmonary artery catheter. The insertion of such a catheter is not routine in most patients with respiratory failure and their beneficial use in such situations is not known.

Increasing a reduced red cell mass may often have a beneficial effect on tissue oxygen delivery. For example, raising the total oxygen delivery to the tissues from 500 ml/min to 600 ml/min could be achieved by raising the haemoglobin concentration by 1.5 g/dl. This could probably be achieved more easily than raising the cardiac output from 5 litres/min to 6 litres/min or the Pao_2 from 8.0 kPa (60 mmHg) to 12 kPa (90 mmHg) to produce the same effect. Notwithstanding these obvious benefits of blood transfusion, there are worries related to the transmission of blood-borne diseases. The quest for synthetic substitutes for haemoglobin has been, and still continues to be, the subject of intensive research. At present, perfluorocarbon preparations (e.g. Fluosol DA) have significant toxic side-effects. However, newer less toxic substances are being prepared and these may lead to significant improvements in the future.

Adult respiratory distress syndrome

Background

The term ARDS is used to designate an episode of acute respiratory failure developing in association with a separate, usually non-pulmonary, medical or surgical illness. When recognized, the syndrome should be appreciated as simply a statement of an immediate clinical condition, which needs to be defined in terms of the responsible aetiological factors. Although this type of respiratory failure had been described in detail previously (Cameron, 1948), the war in Vietnam emphasized the occurrence of the condition and brought this type of respiratory failure to the notice of a global audience. The paper by Ashbaugh and colleagues in 1967 was the first to describe the problem in civilian practice. They described the sudden respiratory distress of 12 adult patients who had no evidence of either prior lung disease or heart failure. The disease was characterized by dyspnoea and reduced lung compliance. In addition, the patients exhibited low arterial oxygen tensions, refractory to increased inspired oxygen concentrations and diffuse infiltrates on chest radiography, which strongly suggested pulmonary oedema. This condition was termed acute respiratory distress in adults (Ashbaugh et al., 1967).

Later studies by the same group (Petty & Ashbaugh, 1971) centred on the observation that histological damage to the lung and reduced surfactant activity resembled that found in neonates with idiopathic respiratory distress syndrome. They coined the term adult respiratory distress syndrome (ARDS) to describe the clinical condition.

This condition still occurs and despite a vast amount of research, the pathophysiology of the condition is poorly understood. Even more striking is the fact that there is still no consensus as to the management of the condition and there is currently no specific targeted therapy of proven value. It is important to try to explain why there has been no apparent progress in clinical terms despite there being over 25 years since the first description of the condition. Three main areas will be critically appraised with regard to (i) defining the condition and its prevalence; (ii) the putative pathophysiology; and (iii) the causative mechanism(s) for this pathophysiology. In the second part of this section the aim is to discuss those aspects of care which may be important to reduce morbidity and mortality from this acute lung injury.

Definition, diagnosis and incidence

The obvious first step in understanding and managing a problem is to develop a definition of that problem. Unfortunately, and in common with defining respiratory failure, there had been no universally accepted definition of the condition. It is therefore clear that the true incidence of ARDS cannot be known accurately. The Task Force of the National Heart Lung and Blood Institute suggested that 150 000 cases of ARDS occurred each year in the USA alone and with a mortality of 80% (Murray, 1977). This incidence figure of some 0.6 cases : 1000 of the population per year has been challenged by a survey in one health service region of the UK (Webster et al., 1988). These UK figures suggest that the incidence is 10% of that suggested in the USA. This difference almost certainly reflects the problem associated with the definition of the condition. Acute lung injury follows a continuum from an acute oedematous picture through to a chronic fibrotic type of pattern. Certain centres may not diagnose ARDS till this fibrotic state is reached, others may exclude the chronic injury from their definition. An additional problem is related to the likelihood of ARDS developing as a consequence of a specific cause varies with that predisposition. The incidence and mortality for certain 'at-risk' populations is shown in Table 84.2. These data were obtained from prospective studies of ARDS in the USA (Pepe et al., 1982; Fowler et al., 1983). It must be emphasized that the criteria for the diagnosis of ARDS were extremely strict compared to the original definition (Ashbaugh et al., 1967). The patients had to fulfil the following five criteria for ARDS to be diagnosed.

1 Respiratory failure requiring mechanical ventilation.

2 Alveolar : arterial oxygen tension ratio of less than 0.3.

3 Static lung compliance of less than 50 ml/cmH$_2$O.

4 Bilateral diffuse infiltrates on the chest radiograph.

5 Pulmonary capillary wedge pressure (PCWP) of less than 2.4 kPa (18 mmHg).

These criteria do not differentiate between acute and chronic forms of the syndrome. Thus, it may be that the incidence of the syndrome has been underestimated because of this strict definition. It may be also that by using these criteria only the most ill patients fulfilled the authors strict definition of ARDS and this resulted in the increased mortality.

The effect of modifying the definition of ARDS is apparent when the criteria for diagnosing ARDS are more akin to the original described criteria (Ashbaugh et al., 1967) i.e.:

1 Diffuse infiltrates on the chest X-ray.

2 Respiratory failure requiring mechanical ventilation with an inspired oxygen of more than 40% (i.e. a greater than 20% shunt).

3 Absence of heart failure (i.e. low heart filling pressures).

Table 84.2 The percentage of patients who developed adult respiratory distress syndrome following a specific predisposing factor. Also included is the mortality in those patients who developed the condition. (Data from Pepe et al., 1982; Fowler et al., 1983)

Predisposition	Percentage of patients developing ARDS	Percentage of mortality in ARDS patients
Bacteraemia	30	78
Aspiration of gastric contents	36	94
Disseminated intravascular coagulation	22	50
Massive blood transfusion	5	45
Long-bone or pelvic fracture	5	0
Following cardiopulmonary bypass	2	50

Using these criteria nearly all patients having open-heart surgery could be diagnosed as having a form of ARDS in the immediate postoperative period. It is true also that simple cardiorespiratory support during the initial period of respiratory distress following open-heart surgery ensures that the mortality from this more loosely defined condition is essentially zero.

To overcome some of these problems, a new definition of acute lung injury has been suggested (Murray et al., 1988). The lung injury itself is scored for severity using four criteria.

1 Oxygenation ($Pao_2 : F_IO_2$ ratio).
2 Chest radiograph.
3 Static respiratory system compliance.
4 Amount of PEEP.

Table 84.3 Components and calculation of the lung injury score. The final value is obtained by dividing the number of components which have made up the score by the sum of these scores. Mild-to-moderate lung injury is defined as a score of 0.1–2.5. Severe lung injury (ARDS) is present when the lung injury score is >2.5

	Value	Score
1 *Chest radiography score*		
No alveolar shadowing	—	0
Alveolar shadowing in one segment	—	1
Alveolar shadowing in two segments	—	2
Alveolar shadowing in three segments	—	3
Alveolar shadowing in all segments	—	4
2 *Hypoxaemia score* ($Pao_2 : F_IO_2$)		
	>300	0
	225–299	1
	175–224	2
	100–174	3
	<100	4
3 *Respiratory system compliance*		
	>80 ml/cmH$_2$O	0
	60–79 ml/cmH$_2$O	1
	40–59 ml/cmH$_2$O	2
	20–39 ml/cmH$_2$O	3
	<19 ml/cmH$_2$O	4
4 *PEEP*		
	<5 cmH$_2$O	0
	6–8 cmH$_2$O	1
	9–11 cmH$_2$O	2
	12–14 cmH$_2$O	3
	>15 cmH$_2$O	4

Criteria and calculation of the severity index for respiratory failure is shown in Table 84.3.

In addition, any associated clinical disorders such as trauma, cardiopulmonary bypass or aspiration are considered as is a third element defining other organ systems which are impaired. The use of this system should allow a more quantitative assessment of pulmonary and non-pulmonary organ failure and hence a more accurate incidence of acute lung injury and the prognosis for recovery. These aspects have been reviewed by the group from San Francisco (Wiener-Kronisch et al., 1990).

Notwithstanding these problems of definition, there is little doubt that acute pulmonary failure as a consequence of a separate non-pulmonary cause is responsible for a high proportion of admissions to the intensive therapy unit. Patients with ARDS have been reported to account for approximately 1:15 patients requiring ventilation in a district general hospital (Searle, 1985).

Pathophysiology

The majority of the studies designed to identify and understand the mediators and modulators of this pulmonary injury have been performed in animals. The starting premise for such studies was that there was pulmonary capillary leak of protein-rich oedema fluid into the interstitium and airspaces.

In 1896 Starling defined the relationship between the forces which governed the rate of fluid flux across the capillary membrane. This relationship is stated simply as:

$$Q_{\text{fluid}} = K_f \times \Delta P$$

where Q_{fluid} is the net fluid flow, K_f is the fluid filtration coefficient (or index of the 'leakiness' of the barrier to that fluid) and ΔP is the driving pressure for that fluid across the capillary. The term ΔP comprises the difference between hydrostatic pressure (tending to force fluid out of the circulation) and colloid oncotic pressure (tending to draw fluid into the circulation).

The development of the balloon flotation catheter allowed indirect determination of left-heart filling pressures. It soon became obvious that patients with ARDS did not have increased intravascular pressures as the cause of the lung failure; the 'cause' must therefore result from changes in K_f, or leakiness of the lung. Further evidence to imply increased lung leak came from investigations in humans with ARDS who had mean oedema fluid to plasma protein concentration ratios which were statistically greater than those found in patients with cardiac oedema (Sprung et al., 1981). However, this was not found universally and there was overlap between the results of these protein ratios and the cardiac oedema and ARDS patients.

At the same time as the development of the theory of ARDS based on Starling forces, an animal model was described in which lung lymph was collected from the caudal mediastinal lymph node of the unanaesthetized sheep (Staub et al., 1975). Alteration in the rate of flow of this lymph, together with any changes in the concentration of the constituent proteins, can be ascribed to changes in driving pressure (cardiac oedema) or increased permeability/surface area of the alveolar capillary barrier (noncardiac permeability oedema).

Increased flows for high-protein lung lymph or frank pulmonary oedema, suggesting increased permeability of the alveolar capillary barrier, have been produced in this model by infusions of bacteria and endotoxin (simulating sepsis), fibrin degradation products (simulating disseminated intravascular coagulopathy, DIC) and microemboli (air or glass beads) (Rinaldo & Rogers, 1982). The ability to produce an ARDS-like syndrome in experimental animals with evidence of increased lung leakiness led to the concept of treatment based on mechanical ventilatory support together with manipulation of the Starling forces.

Over the past few years, several methods have been developed for use in humans which quantify lung solute and water leakiness using radiotracer techniques. Of these, the permeability surface area product for urea, clearance of aerosolized radio-labelled diethylene triamine pentacetate (DTPA) and the accumulation of radiolabelled protein in the lung have been used in patients who fulfilled the five strict criteria for ARDS outlined above. In these studies it was apparent that increased lung leakiness was not a universal finding. Using these methods, between 20 and 40% of patients with ARDS did not demonstrate an increase in solute flux outside the normal range (Royston et al., 1987; Rocker et al., 1989). These data suggest that the manipulation of Starling forces will meet with little success.

Extra to these observations are the data obtained from histological examination of biopsy specimens obtained before and after death from patients with ARDS in the American extracorporeal membrane oxygenator study. These samples revealed that the concept of ARDS being purely a capillary-leak syndrome causing non-cardiac, pulmonary oedema was oversimplified. The normal Type I epithelial cells

were lost rapidly and replaced with proliferating Type II cells, leading to a greatly thickened alveolar septa. The interstitial space became infiltrated with inflammatory cells and fibroblasts. There was rapid obliteration of alveolae, alveolar ducts and interstitium by fibrous tissue. The pulmonary vasculature became obliterated early in the development of this progressive response (Pratt et al., 1979). These histological features showed clearly that changes which occur over weeks or months in patients not receiving cardiopulmonary support could occur in days in patients receiving such support.

With this extremely complex series of events, it is not surprising that mechanical ventilatory support and manipulation of Starling forces has met with little success.

Cause

Because of the lack of a beneficial treatment there has been a great deal of effort directed to establishing the mediators and modulators of the acute oedematous lesion. A vast number of humoral and cellular mediators have been implicated. Table 84.4 shows a number of humoral mediators of capillary macromolecular leakage in hamsters (Svensjo & Grega, 1986). Extrapolation of data to human pulmonary injury is difficult as there are many discrepancies in the data. For example, histamine but not bradykinin will increase lung lymph flow in sheep. Similarly, the pulmonary effects of the leukotrienes LTC_4, D_4 and E_4 [the so-called slow-reacting substances of anaphylaxis (SRSA)] will depend on the species studied. Cat and rabbit lungs are relatively immune to the effects of infusions of these leukotrienes. Guinea pig and sheep lungs respond readily with increases in

Table 84.4 Humoral mediators shown to increase macromolecular transport across capillaries. Also shown to illustrate relative potency are molar concentrations of substance producing this effect

Mediator	Effective concentration (M)
ADP, adenosine, inosine	10^{-6}
Histamine, hydroxytryptamine	10^{-7}
Bradykinin, substance P	10^{-8}
Prostaglandin E_1, E_2, F_2	$<10^{-8}$
Leukotrienes C_4, D_4, E_4, B_4	$<10^{-9}$
C_3a C_5a	$<10^{-9}$
Platelet — activating factor	$<10^{-9}$
Fibrin — derived products	—
Free radicals	—
Immune complexes	—

both pulmonary vascular pressure and permeability (Malik *et al.*, 1985).

Of the formed elements of the blood, considerable interest has been focused on the role of the neutrophil in inducing the lung injury leading to ARDS. One commonly discussed hypothesis is that neutrophils are activated by complement conversion products and these activated white cells will induce lung microvascular injury. These activated neutrophils can do this by being sequestered in the lung where they release cytotoxic substances; released normally as part of the body's defences. Activated neutrophils release reactive oxygen species (ROS). These highly toxic species can degrade DNA and hyaluronic acid, peroxidize membrane lipids, destroy endothelial cells and increase capillary permeability. In addition, they inactivate α_1-antiproteinase rapidly, a crucially important defence mechanism against proteolytic enzymes. The neutrophil can also release proteases that destroy collagen, elastin and the adhesive glycoprotein, fibronectin. These proteases can also cleave fibrinogen, complement and Hageman factor (Factor XII) (Fig. 84.1).

Humans with severe ARDS have evidence of activated neutrophils in the circulation (Zimmerman *et al.*, 1983). There is also evidence in humans for a significant increase in oxidant and proteolytic activity in the lungs of patients with ARDS (Cochrane *et al.*, 1983; Brigham & Meyrick, 1984). However, these observations do not provide a universal explanation for the lung injury in ARDS.

Complement activation occurs as commonly in ill patients without pulmonary failure as in those with lung injury (Weinberg *et al.*, 1984). The necessary role of the white cell has also been questioned. In particular ARDS has been reported in patients without evidence of neutrophil involvement (Braude *et al.*, 1985).

The role of platelets in triggering or augmenting the original lung injury of ARDS has not been characterized as thoroughly. In the sheep, infusion of platelet microemboli does not produce increased lymph flow; nor does platelet depletion protect from the injury induced by microemboli infusions (Malik *et al.*, 1985). However, the platelet lifespan was reduced in patients with ARDS, and thrombocytopenia was a common finding in patients with sepsis and ARDS (Rinaldo & Rogers, 1982).

Finally, although an increased permeability of the alveolar capillary barrier is thought to be pivotal in the genesis of ARDS, it is not a universal clinical finding as discussed previously. This may, in part, be explained by the relationship to the Starling hypothesis of capillary leakage. The Starling hypothesis is based on the view of the capillary as a static system allowing passive diffusion. However, this mechanism cannot account for all macromolecule transport (Renken, 1985), and there is interest in the hypothesis of active membrane transport first suggested by Heidenheim in 1891 (Grega, 1986).

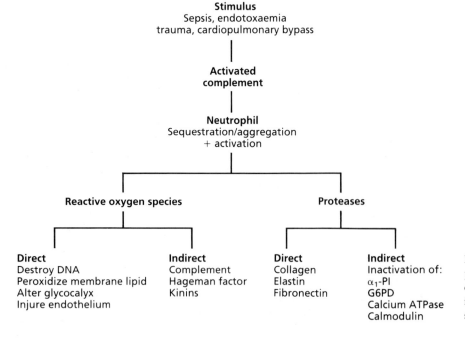

Fig. 84.1 Schematic outline of proposed mechanisms of cytotoxic effects of neutrophils leading to lung injury and adult respiratory distress syndrome.

Management of the patient

The principles of patient management for ARDS are to:
1 Improve oxygenation.
2 Reduce oedema formation.
3 Prevent secondary infection.
4 Reduce or prevent the potentially noxious sequelae of the initial lung injury or its therapy.

Improve oxygenation

Therapy designed to improve oxygenation is the same as for other forms of ventilatory failure. However, the lungs of patients with ARDS tend to have greatly reduced compliance as a consequence of:
1 Loss of surfactant with increased surface tension.
2 Loss of lung volume from obliteration of alveolated regions by oedema and cellular infiltrate.
3 Development of fibrotic response.
In addition, the $\dot{V}:\dot{Q}$ mismatch is usually greater than with other causes of respiratory failure. Because of these problems, the patient with ARDS is more likely to require very high inspired oxygen concentrations to maintain adequate arterial tensions and also to require a high inflation pressure to deliver an adequate tidal volume. The problems associated with breathing hyperoxic gas mixtures are discussed more fully later. The question to be answered is what is the optimum (or least detrimental) method of ventilatory support for the patient with ARDS?

What has been appreciated for some time in humans is that ventilation with very high peak airway pressures is associated with an increased incidence of barotrauma to the lung (pneumothorax, pneumomediastinum, etc.) (Hillman, 1985). Studies in animal models have shown also that periods of ventilation at high pressures for periods as short as 1 h can induce increases in lung water and protein escape into the lung (Dreyfuss et al., 1985). These physiological data augment the histological evidence of the same damaging effects of high inspiratory pressures obtained 10 years previously (Webb & Tierney, 1974). In an effort to reduce inspiratory pressures, there was a vogue to employ a faster rate of respiration with a low tidal volume, using either high-frequency jet or oscillating ventilation. Unfortunately, controlled trials of the use of high-frequency ventilation have failed to show any advantage over well-managed, conventional systems in adult patients with respiratory failure (Brichart et al., 1986). The majority of reports of the benefits of higher rates are largely anecdotal.

Equally controversial is the use of PEEP in preventing or treating ARDS.

Positive end-expiratory pressure

The arterial partial pressure of oxygen tends to have a direct relation to the FRC for a given inspired oxygen fraction. There is little doubt that the application of PEEP allows the reduction of F_IO_2 to a 'safer' concentration whilst maintaining arterial Pao_2. What is more controversial is the role of PEEP in 'treating' ARDS. The prime report of acute respiratory distress (Ashbaugh et al., 1967) suggested that PEEP was highly beneficial. However, prospective controlled trials in patients 'at risk' of developing ARDS have failed to show benefit in preventing the occurrence of the syndrome or reducing mortality in those who developed ARDS (Pepe et al., 1984). It is also not clear if the application of PEEP augments or produces injury. In humans, the occurrence of bronchiolar injury assessed by histology has been associated significantly with both the time of application and degree of PEEP (Slavin et al., 1982). In contrast, the application of $10\,cmH_2O$ PEEP prevented the injury to rat lungs induced by high peak airway pressures (Webb & Tierney, 1974). A further potentially beneficial effect of this level of PEEP was that protein leak into the lung was reduced in injured lungs (Nolop et al., 1987).

Alternative methods of respiratory support

The concept of ARDS as an 'inflammatory' pulmonary lesion has led to the logical premise that reducing the load on the system and allowing it to rest may aid recovery.

Two approaches have been suggested:
1 Dietary and thermal modifications to reduce tissue oxygen consumption and carbon dioxide production.
2 Extracorporeal support and gas exchange.

The use of diets including a greater ratio of lipid : carbohydrate to provide energy should reduce the load on the respiratory system by reducing the carbon dioxide production for each calorie of energy produced. There are no well-designed studies in humans to show that this is beneficial in patients with ARDS.

Cooling the patient should reduce the metabolic needs of the patient and reduce the need for ventilatory support. Again there are no well-controlled studies to show any benefit of this approach. However, what is well known is that hypothermia depresses the normal immune response thereby augmenting bacterial infections.

The use of extracorporeal respiratory support is a *tour de force*. Extracorporeal membrane oxygenation in end-stage ARDS was shown to be of no benefit, and was fraught with complications.

Partial support of respiration using venovenous bypass with a twin-membrane lung system has been used to aid removal of carbon dioxide: so-called extracorporeal carbon dioxide removal ($ECCO_2R$). During $ECCO_2R$, the lungs are inflated at a low frequency with 100% oxygen (Pesenti *et al.*, 1981). Although the group in Milan have reported great benefits with this technique, reports from other centres are largely anecdotal. The results from well-controlled trials of this therapy are awaited. The preliminary data from such a study have, thus far, failed to show any benefits of $ECCO_2R$ when compared to conventional ventilation which was altered so as to maintain a constant arterial blood pH (Morris *et al.*, 1992). This latter technique of ventilatory control allows a degree of 'passive hypercapnia'.

These disappointing preliminary data in adult patients contrast sharply with the results for the use of extracorporeal support in infants with severe respiratory distress. In this condition there have been several encouraging studies. These show a survival, currently reported as about 90%, but with a degree of residual pulmonary impairment, probably related to the underlying cause of the respiratory distress (Garg *et al.*, 1992).

Reduce oedema formation

Based on the putative pathophysiology of the underlying pulmonary injury and the Starling forces, there are four approaches to reducing the oedema formation in the lung.
1 Decrease the hydrostatic pressure.
2 Increase the colloid osmotic pressure.
3 Reduce the capillary leak.
4 Increase lymphatic drainage and fluid clearance.

Decrease hydrostatic pressure

This is the only treatment modality which has been shown to have benefit. By reducing capillary hydrostatic pressure the fluid flux from the capillary should be reduced. In addition, pulmonary hypertension is a frequent finding in patients with ARDS (Zapol & Snider, 1977) and reduction of pulmonary vascular resistance is associated with an improved outcome (Shoemaker *et al.*, 1985). Similar outcome studies have shown that there is a three-fold reduction in mortality in those patients in whom the pulmonary

capillary wedge pressure fell by over 25% compared with those with no reduction (Humphrey *et al.*, 1990).

However, at present neither the pulmonary artery dilator of choice nor the duration for its administration are known. Suggested agents include prostacyclins, prostaglandin E_1, nitrates, sodium nitroprusside and calcium-channel antagonists. There is some evidence to show that administration of a dilator of the pulmonary circulation may lead to right-heart ischaemia if the coronary perfusion pressure is not maintained (Priebe, 1992). For this reason, there has been a constant search for a specific dilator of the pulmonary circulation. In this respect there has been considerable interest in the use of inhaled nitric oxide (the putative endothelial derived relaxing factor) as such a specific pulmonary artery dilator. It remains to be seen if this line of therapy is either specific or beneficial in acute lung injury in adults.

Increase colloid osmotic pressure

In theory, increasing the intravascular colloid oncotic pressure should draw water from the interstitium and alveoli of the lung. However, in the face of a capillary leak the usual effect is for the administered substance to pass rapidly into the interstitium increasing the oedema and worsening the problem (Robin *et al.*, 1972). Studies in a number of animal models of ARDS have failed also to show any benefit of administering substances to increase oncotic pressure.

Reduce capillary leak

Simple mechanical cardiorespiratory support has failed to prevent the development of ARDS or to reduce the mortality from the syndrome. Because of this, there has been an explosion in research aimed at understanding the mechanism of the increase in capillary permeability and in providing pharmacological means of preventing or reducing that injury.

Based on studies performed in the sheep lung lymph model the use of steroids in treating patients with ARDS had a considerable vogue. However, prospective controlled studies have shown that steroids had no benefits in preventing ARDS (Weigelt *et al.*, 1985). Indeed, in this study, there was an increase in the incidence of ARDS in the treated group. More worrying was the finding that the steroid-treated group had a much higher incidence of sepsis. This finding was enhanced by a study in patients given steroids for neural trauma. They also developed sepsis and multisystem failure more frequently than non-steroid treated patients (De Maria *et al.*, 1985). Based on this evidence, the use of high-dose steroids to treat patients with ARDS can no longer be recommended routinely.

Considerable interest has been shown in three other areas.

1 Arachidonic acid metabolites and inhibitors of metabolism.

2 Oxidant free-radical scavengers.

3 Fibronectin and antiprotease augmentation.

The vast majority of evidence suggesting efficacy of these approaches has been performed in animal models of lung injury. When human studies have been performed, the results have been less dramatic. In particular the short-term administration of prostaglandin E_1 and the thromboxane antagonist, dazoxiben, have been shown to be of no benefit (Leeman *et al.*, 1985; Shoemaker & Appel, 1986). However, the administration of prostaglandin E_1 in a very high dosage of $30\,ng \cdot kg^{-1} \cdot min^{-1}$ for 30 days was reported to be associated with a two-fold improvement in survival in these treated patients (Holdcroft *et al.*, 1986).

A number of non-steroidal anti-inflammatory (NSAI) agents have been shown to have benefits in animal studies. Unfortunately, these data have been difficult to reproduce in humans. In addition the NSAI drugs are known to be associated with a number of potent toxic side-effects including an increased incidence of gastrointestinal bleeding and renal dysfunction.

Several lung injuries may be reduced by the administration of antioxidants and free-radical scavengers. In particular, the increased lung lymph flow following endotoxin administration in the sheep can be prevented by the prior administration of *N*-acetyl cysteine (normally used as a source of sulphydryl groups in paracetamol overdose). Unfortunately, this agent increased mortality in other oxidant stress injuries such as the administration of bleomycin (Patterson *et al.*, 1985). Moreover, increasing antioxidant protection to endotoxin-treated sheep by administering superoxide dismutase (SOD) increased the permeability injury (Traber *et al.*, 1985). These data suggest that it would be premature to design clinical trials of antioxidants and free-radical scavengers in ARDS.

Reversal of opsonic deficiencies by administration of cryoprecipitate which is rich in fibronectin has been claimed to be highly beneficial. However, controlled trials have failed to demonstrate clear differences in fibronectin concentrations between survivors and non-survivors in intensive therapy units. The benefit of giving antiproteinase compounds awaits human studies.

Overall, it is obvious that there is currently no specific therapy which reduces the permeability injury of ARDS from any cause.

Increased lymphatic drainage and fluid clearance

Data related to methods of increasing lung fluid clearance are sparse. Essentially, nothing is known of the factors which modify active lung lymph flow. There is, however, a body of evidence to suggest active transport plays a major role in lung fluid clearance, e.g. infusions of β-agonists increase lung liquid clearance in neonatal lambs. Airway instillation of amiloride (which inhibits sodium transport) slows fluid clearance in adult sheep (Staub, 1983). Obviously, a great deal more needs to be known of such active transport systems before controlled trials and guidelines for therapy can be instituted.

Prevention of complications

As there is no proven direct therapy for patients with ARDS, the outcome is dependent on natural healing and prevention of complications, particularly further lung injury manifest clinically as barotrauma or fibrosis. The incidence of severe barotrauma may be reduced, if not prevented, by measures to minimize airway pressures and lung volumes (Hillman, 1985). The ability to produce a nadir in mean airway pressure, while maintaining adequate alveolar ventilation, has been the focus of attention of a large body of expertise. This goal has, almost by default, led to an increase in methods of applying assisted ventilation. Each of these methods have their own acronym and supporters. None the less 'After 40 years of critical care mechanical ventilation support we still are searching for new and better techniques without generating any controlled data to establish the superiority of any method over another, in any patient group' (Räsänen, 1992).

Little is known of the intermediate messages that link the early capillary leak syndrome to the later disordered fibrotic response. As discussed previously, this fibrotic response can occur within $24-48\,h$ of clinical presentation with the syndrome. Biochemical agents aimed specifically at collagen synthesis have been studied in models of lung injury (Rinaldo & Rogers, 1982). However, there have been no controlled clinical trials of these compounds, and it is clear that some of these agents would have limited use in conditions where collagen turnover is high, for example, in healing wounds.

Prevention of infection

Prevention of infection and sepsis is of great importance. In a prospective study of outcome of patients with ARDS, the patients with sepsis had a significantly greater incidence of multiple organ failure and a far greater mortality (Bell *et al.*, 1983). This progression of disease occurred even in patients who were improving or had recovered from their respiratory failure. As endotoxin is thought to be the major trigger to developing organ failure, there is current interest in developing methods of preventing or reducing the effects of endotoxaemia.

Methods aimed at reducing the incidence of sepsis and endotoxaemia have been concentrated on modification of gut functions. This line of approach follows from the view that the gut is the only obvious source of bacteria and toxins. Methods have included selective bowel decontamination and more recently the use of agents which might divert blood flow to potentially ischaemic areas of the gut and splanchnic circulation.

Unfortunately, the early enthusiasm for gut decontamination has been tempered by the results of controlled trials. These show that the use of selective bowel decontamination was not associated with a reduction in sepsis or mortality and morbidity (Hammond *et al.*, 1992).

The alternative strategy is to give compounds which 'mop up' any circulating endotoxin. Administration of polyclonal antibodies against the core lipid of endotoxin reduced the mortality from sepsis (Ziegler *et al.*, 1982). Subsequently, a human monoclonal antibody against the core lipid of endotoxin has been developed. Early studies, in animals, showed that this antibody would prevent endotoxin-induced lung capillary leak (Feeley *et al.*, 1987). A further randomized controlled study has also shown that this antibody will reduce mortality in certain septic states in humans. There was significant efficacy in patients with blood cultures positive for Gram-negative organisms. There was no significant efficacy in patients with sepsis but with negative cultures (Ziegler *et al.*, 1991).

Sepsis and endotoxaemia are therefore still significant problems in the intensive care setting.

One further complication of therapy which may develop is that of oxygen toxicity. Discussion of this topic makes up the final section of this chapter.

Oxygen toxicity

Whilst oxygen is necessary for life, it is clear also that increased concentrations can be toxic and induce organ dysfunction. There are three major organs at risk of hyperoxic injury.
1 *Central nervous system.* Only affected under hyperbaric conditions.
2 *The lens of the eye in newborns.* High arterial partial pressures of oxygen are associated with neoangiogenesis of the posterior aspect of the lens. These new vessels allow the laying down of fibrous tissue, and this retrolental fibrous dysplasia leads to a reduced visual acuity and eventually to blindness.
3 *The lung.* The effects of normobaric hyperoxia in patients who rely on their hypoxic respiratory drive are well known. Similarly, it has been well demonstrated that breathing of 100% oxygen leads to instability of terminal ventilatory units and reversible absorption collapse (Winter & Smith, 1972). Breathing 100% oxygen at high atmospheric pressure, even for short periods, induces other changes in lung function in humans. In particular in these studies the volunteers developed substernal discomfort and significant reductions in airflow without changes in lung volume or diffusing capacity. One of the thirteen subjects had convulsions during the hyperbaric period as anticipated from the known toxic effects of hyperbaric oxygen on the CNS (Clark *et al.*, 1991).

In the next section the mechanisms of oxygen as an agent toxic to lung structure and function will be discussed.

Pathophysiology of pulmonary oxygen toxicity

The inhalation of high partial pressures of oxygen is known to be toxic to the lung of all mammals (Clark & Lambertson, 1971). The improved supportive care of patients with pulmonary failure and especially those with ARDS has resulted in prolonged survival, with the concomitant increase in the length of time the lung is exposed to high concentrations of inspired oxygen. The patient with respiratory failure has an added risk of an increase in lung injury, as the levels of oxygen partial pressures used in this situation are potentially toxic. Several questions thus require answers. How does oxygen induce this injury? How does the body normally protect itself from such injury? What are the effects of oxygen therapy on lung injury and repair? Are there means to prevent these deleterious effects?

How does oxygen induce tissue injury?

In recent years, a biochemical mechanism involving cellular production of partially reduced metabolites of oxygen (sometimes termed oxidant free radicals) has been proposed as the basis of oxygen toxicity. In brief, the two outer bonding electrons of molecular oxygen have parallel spins (Fig. 84.2). This configuration imparts a dipole to the molecule (this paramagnetic effect is used in clinical measurement) and also restricts the molecule into accepting further electrons one at a time — the so called Hund rule. This single-step transfer is essential for the controlled electron transport which is necessary for mitochondrial high-energy phosphate production.

Reduction of oxygen follows this single transfer system and is shown diagramatically in Fig. 84.3.

The compound $O_2^- \cdot$ is termed superoxide and is a free radical, i.e. a species capable of independent existence and which contains an unpaired electron in an outer orbital, signified usually by a dot. The molecular configurations of superoxide and peroxide radicals are shown in Fig. 84.2.

In life, the reaction is more complex as highlighted by the role of coenzyme Q (CoQ) in electron transport. The active site in CoQ is a semiquinone (Fig. 84.3) which has two oxygens capable of accepting electrons to produce a semiquinone free-radical (CoQ·), which is then protonated.

In the conditions where there is a hyperoxic state the semiquinone free radical is thought to react with molecular oxygen to produce superoxide according to the following:

$$CoQ + e^- \rightarrow CoQ^- \cdot + O_2 \rightarrow CoQ + O_2^- \cdot$$

Although superoxide and peroxide radicals are oxidizing agents, they are relatively unreactive. The danger lies in their ability to react or combine to form other species of considerable potency and reactive

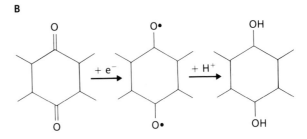

Fig. 84.3 (A) Molecular oxygen accepting an electron to pass through the stage of being a free radical prior to protonation. (B) The semiquinone moiety of coenzyme Q accepting an electron to produce a free radical intermediary prior to protonation. This free radical generation is absolutely essential for the cytochrome chain of ATP production.

capability, in particular hydroxyl radical (OH·) and singlet oxygen ($^1O_2$). Molecular configurations of these moieties are shown in Fig. 84.2.

Four cell and tissue components are at greatest risk from oxidant attack:

1 Sulphydryl-containing enzymes and proteins. Most importantly α_1-antiproteinase is inactivated rapidly. Glucose-6-phosphate dehydrogenase and enzymes of the citric acid cycle are also at risk.

2 Nucleic acids are damaged irreversibly by oxidants; a useful mode of action of a number of antitumour agents such as bleomycin. Cell death follows as intracellular components are not regenerated.

3 Collagen and glycoproteoglycan oxidation is thought to play a major part in the development of emphysema.

4 Peroxidation of polyunsaturated cell membrane lipids by oxidants leads to an increase in membrane permeability associated with a decreased fluidity.

Fig. 84.2 Configurations of oxygen and certain reactive oxidant species to show direction of spin and number of outer bonding electrons, the number of protons and electrons, the presence (Y) or absence (N) of a charge and the definition of the species as a free radical.

Outer bonding electron spin	↑↑	↑↓↓	↑↓↑↓	↑↓	↑↓	↑
Protons	16	16	16	16	16	9
Electrons	16	17	18	16	16	9
Charge	N	Y	Y	N	N	Y
Radical	N	N	N	N	N	Y
Species name	Ground state	Super oxide	Peroxide	Σg	Δg	Hydroxyl radical
					Singlet oxygen	

Protection from free-radical tissue injury

It is obvious that with such a potentially destructive ability the body has developed a system of anti-oxidant defences. These defences are based on two systems: an enzymatic system for aiding removal of superoxide and hydrogen peroxide (Fig. 84.4) and a system directed towards minimizing the effects of oxidant tissue injury by removing the secondary free radicals, usually lipids (designated ROO·) produced by the initial radical injury. Reduced glutathione can provide a source of protons from sulphydryl groups to protonate lipid radicals. The reduced glutathione is itself oxidized and the oxidized glutathione regenerated using energy-dependent processes (Fig. 84.5). Other compounds such as α-tocopherol (vitamin E), ascorbate (vitamin C), caeruloplasmin, etc. can act to reduce oxidant injury usually by accepting the free electron of the free-radical species (Halliwell & Gutteridge, 1985).

These antioxidant defences are found in high concentrations in metabolically active organs such as the liver and kidney. The lung is relatively poorly supplied with these defences and may therefore be at greater risk of hyperoxic injury.

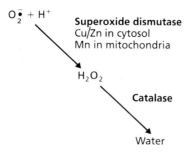

Fig. 84.4 Enzymatic conversion of the superoxide radical by way of hydrogen peroxide to water. Superoxide dismutase is found in the mitochondria (the manganese form) and in the cytosol as the copper/zinc form.

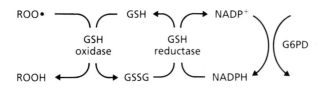

Fig. 84.5 Antioxidant protection using the tripeptide glutathione (GSH). Glutathione is oxidized during protonation of the lipid free radical (ROO·) to produce the non-reactive lipid hydroperoxide and oxidized glutathione (GSSG). The reduced glutathione is regenerated using energy from the pentose phosphate pathway.

What are the effects of hyperoxia on the lung and on lung injury?

Breathing 100% oxygen produces profound effects on the lung over a short time-period; within hours there is severe substernal pain, associated with cessation of mucociliary transport. Inflammation of the airways follows within 18 h. The vital capacity decreases after approximately 24 h following abnormalities of carbon monoxide diffusing capacity and the widening of the alveolar : arterial oxygen tension difference. Confirmation of lung toxicity in ventilated patients comes from a study in 10 patients who were diagnosed as brain-dead. Five patients ventilated with oxygen had oedematous, heavy lungs associated with increased alveolar : arterial oxygen tension differences, reduced compliance and increased dead-space : tidal volume ratios (Barber *et al.*, 1970). However, the patients in the study had received steroid therapy, which may have affected the outcome.

The majority of studies determining the effects of added oxygen on injured lungs have been performed in animals or *in vitro*. Oxygen promoted increased fibrosis in injured mouse lungs. Exposure of normal mouse lung to 70% oxygen for 24 h or 50% for 6 days produced no effects. However, the same dose/time product regimens produced extensive interstitial fibrosis when given to animals whose lungs were injured previously with butylated hydroxytoluene (Witsch *et al.*, 1981).

Potentiation of oxygen toxicity is induced by several pharmacological and physical interventions (Table 84.5). The role of steroids in augmenting or reducing oxygen toxicity to the lung depends on their time of administration. Pretreatment with dexamethasone augmented lung injury, and was associated with decline in lung antioxidant defences. However, when dexamethasone was administered at the end of the exposure to oxygen, the effect was protective (Koizumi *et al.*, 1985).

It is not known if there is toxic interaction between oxygen administration and any of the mass of anti-bacterial, vasoactive or inotropic agents used in critically ill patients.

It has been argued cogently (Rinaldo & Roger, 1982) that oxygen may increase or affect lung injury in a variety of different ways. Oxidants deactivate the lung antiprotease defences and induce alveolar macrophages to release neutrophil chemotoxins. Oxygen reduces the lung host defences by causing cessation of cilial action, by reducing alveolar macrophage migration and by increasing the adherence of

Table 84.5 Agents known to augment pulmonary toxicity in animals. (References can be found in Clark & Lambertson, 1971)

Agents which increase tissue metabolism
Thyroxine (or hyperthyroidism)
Adrenaline
Amphetamines
Hyperpyrexia

Exogenous agents
Paraquat
Nitrofurantoin
Disulfiram (Antabuse)
Ionizing radiation

Dietary deficiency
Selenium
Copper
Vitamin C
Vitamin E
Sulphur-containing amino acids

Gram-negative organisms to lower respiratory tract epithelium.

In the light of this array of potentially damaging effects, it is not surprising that the 'toxic threshold' for oxygen to the injured lung is unknown.

Prevention of oxygen toxicity

Augmenting the lung antioxidant defences has been studied as a means of reducing toxicity.

Administration of excess vitamins C or E has no effect. However, liposome-encapsulated enzymes, SOD and catalase had beneficial effects. Unfortunately, giving liposomes is associated with a depression of bacterial clearance and killing which may lead to an increased risk of sepsis (McDonald *et al.*, 1985).

Stimulation of production of enzymatic protective mechanisms may be achieved by increasing the concentration of inspired oxygen slowly, although this method has limited clinical usefulness.

A further approach is the administration of endotoxin. Paradoxically, this manoeuvre leads to protection from hyperoxic pulmonary injury in the rat. Originally, this protective effect was thought to be via increasing enzymatic antioxidants such as superoxide dismutase or catalase. More recent studies have failed to demonstrate increases in enzyme levels despite protection by endotoxin (Spence *et al.*, 1986).

There is a great interest currently in attempting to modify the endotoxin molecule to produce protective substances which have no inherent toxic action, so-called endotoroids.

Finally, there is evidence that instillation of erythrocytes into the lung will protect animals from oxygen toxicity, possibly by increasing lung glutathione content (Brigham, 1986).

We are left with the conclusion that oxygen is known to be a potent damaging agent to the lung. However, the significance of this to human disease is still far from clear.

References

Ashbaugh D.G., Bigelow D.B., Petty T.L. & Levine B.E. (1967) Acute respiratory distress in adults. *Lancet* **ii**, 319–23.

Aubier M., De Troyer A. & Sampson M. (1981) Aminophylline improves diaphragmatic contractility in man. *New England Journal of Medicine* **305**, 249–50.

Barber R.E., Lee J. & Hamilton W.K. (1970) Oxygen toxicity in man; a prospective study in patients with irreversible brain damage. *New England Journal of Medicine* **283**, 1478–84.

Bell R.C., Coalson J.J. & Smith J.D. (1983) Multiple organ failure and infection in adult respiratory distress syndrome. *Annals of Internal Medicine* **99**, 293–8.

Bizouarn P., Soulard D., Blanloeil Y., Guillet A. & Goarin Y. (1992) Oxygen consumption after cardiac surgery; a comparison between calculation by Fick's principle and measurement by indirect calorimetry. *Intensive Care Medicine* **18**, 206–9.

Bolliger C.T. & van Eeden S.F. (1990) Treatment of multiple rib fractures. Randomized controlled trial comparing ventilatory with non-ventilatory management. *Chest* **97**, 943–8.

Braman S. & Kaemmerlen J. (1990) Intensive care status asthmaticus: a ten year experience. *Journal of the American Medical Association* **264**, 366–8.

Braude S., Apperley J., Krausz T., Goldman J.M. & Royston D. (1985) Adult respiratory distress after allogeneic bone marrow transplantation; evidence for a neutrophil independent mechanism. *Lancet* **i**, 1239–42.

Brichart J.F., Rouby J.J. & Viars P. (1986) Intermittent positive pressure ventilation with either positive end-expiratory pressure or high frequency jet ventilation (HFJV), or HFJV alone in human acute respiratory failure. *Anesthesia and Analgesia* **65**, 1135–42.

Brigham K.L. (1986) Role of free radicals in lung injury. *Chest* **89**, 859–63.

Brigham K.L. & Meyrick B.O. (1984) Interactions of granulocytes with the lungs. *Circulation Research* **54**, 623–35.

Cameron G.R. (1948) Pulmonary oedema. *British Medical Journal* 965–72.

Catley D.M., Thornton C., Jordan C., Lehane J.R., Royston D. & Jones J.G. (1985) Pronounced episodic oxygen desaturation in the postoperative period; its association with ventilatory pattern and analgesic regimen. *Anesthesiology* **63**, 20–8.

Clark J.M. & Lambertson C.J. (1971) Pulmonary oxygen toxicity; a review. *Pharmacological Reviews* **23**, 37–134.

Clark J.M., Jackson R.M., Lambertson C.J., Geland R., Hiller W.D. & Unger M. (1991) Pulmonary function in men after oxygen breathing at 3 ATM for 3.5 hours. *Journal of Applied Physiology* **71**, 878–85.

Cochrane C.G., Spragg R. & Revak S.D. (1983) Pathogenesis of the adult respiratory distress syndrome; evidence of oxidant activity in brochoalveolar lavage fluid. *Journal of Clinical Investigation* **71**, 754–61.

Cottam S. & Eason J. (1991) The intensive care management of acute asthma. In *Anaesthesia Reviews* vol. 8 (Ed. Kaufman L.) pp. 71–8. Churchill Livingstone, London.

De Maria E.J., Reidman W., Kenney P.R., Armitage J.M. & Gann D.S. (1985) Septic complications of corticosteroid administration after central nervous system trauma. *Annals of Surgery* **202**, 248–52.

Devitt J.H., McLean R.F. & Koch J.P. (1991) Anesthetic management of acute blunt thoracic trauma. *Canadian Journal of Anaesthesia* **38**, 506–10.

Douglas W.W., Rehder K., Beynen F.M., Sesslet A.D. & Marsh M.H. (1977) Improved oxygenation in patients with acute respiratory failure; the prone position. *American Review of Respiratory Disease* **115**, 559–65.

Dreyfuss D., Basset G., Soler P. & Saumon G. (1985) Intermittent positive-pressure hyperventilation with high inflation pressures produces pulmonary microvascular injury in rats. *American Review of Respiratory Disease* **132**, 880–4.

Eliasson O. & de Graff A.C. (1985) The use of criteria for reversibility and obstruction to define patient groups for brochodilator trials. *American Review of Respiratory Disease* **132**, 858–64.

Feeley T.W., Minty B.D., Scudder C.M., Jones J.G., Royston D. & Teng N.H.H. (1987) The effect of human antiendotoxin monoclonal antibodies on endotoxin induced lung injury. *American Review of Respiratory Disease* **135**, 665–70.

Fishman A.P., Goldring R.M. & Turino G.M. (1966) General alveolar hypoventilation: a syndrome of respiratory and cardiac failure in patients with normal lungs. *Quarterly Journal of Medicine* **35**, 261–75.

Fletcher C.M. & Pride N.B. (1984) Definition of emphysema, chronic bronchitis, asthma and airflow obstruction; 35 years from the CIBA symposium. *Thorax* **39**, 81–5.

Fowler A.A., Hausmann R.F., Good J.T., Benson K.H., Baird M., Eherle D.G., Petty T.L. & Hyers T.M. (1983) Adult respiratory distress syndrome; risk with common predispositions. *Annals of Internal Medicine* **98**, 593–7.

Garg M., Kurzner S.I., Bautista D.B., Lew C.D., Ramos A.D., Platzker A.C.G. & Keens T.G. (1992) Pulmonary sequellae at six months following extracorporeal membrane oxygenation. *Chest* **101**, 1086–90.

Gillespie D.J., Marsh H.M.M., Divertie M. & Meadows J.A. (1986) Clinical outcome of respiratory failure in patients requiring prolonged (>24 hours) mechanical ventilation. *Chest* **90**, 364–9.

Grega G.J. (1986) Role of the endothelial cell in regulation of microvascular permeability to molecules. *Federation Proceedings* **45**, 75–95.

Halliwell B. & Gutteridge J.M.C. (1985) *Free Radicals in Biology and Medicine* p. 67. Clarendon Press, Oxford.

Hammond J.M., Potgeiter P.D., Saunders E.L. & Forder A.A. (1992) Double-blind study of selective decontamination of the digestive tract in intensive care. *Lancet* **ii**, 5–9.

Hanly P.J. (1992) Mechanisms and management of central sleep apnoea. *Lung* **70**, 1–17.

Helling T.S., Gyles N.R., Eisenstein C.L. & Soracco C.A. (1989) Complications following blunt and penetrating injuries in 216 victims of chest trauma requiring tube thoracostomy. *Journal of Trauma* **29**, 1367–70.

Hillman K. (1985) Pulmonary barotrauma. *Clinics in Anesthesiology* **3**, 877–98.

Hoffstein V., Viner S., Mateika S. & Conway J. (1992) Treatment of obstructive sleep apnoea with continuous positive airway pressure; patient compliance, perception of benefits and side effects. *American Review of Respiratory Disease* **145**, 841–5.

Holdcroft J.W., Vassar M.J. & Weber C.J. (1986) Prostaglandin E1 and survival in patients with the adult respiratory distress syndrome. *Annals of Surgery* **203**, 371–8.

Humphrey H., Hall J., Sznajder L., Silverstein M. & Wood L. (1990) Improved survival in ARDS patients associated with a reduction in pulmonary capillary wedge pressure. *Chest* **97**, 1176–80.

Ildstad S.T., Tollerud D.J., Weiss R.G., Cox J.A. & Martin L.W. (1990) Cardiac contusion in paediatric patients with blunt thoracic trauma. *Journal of Pediatric Surgery* **25**, 287–9.

Koizumi M., Frank L. & Massaro D. (1985) Oxygen toxicity in rats. Varied effects of dexamethasone treatment depending on duration of hyperoxia. *American Review of Respiratory Disease* **131**, 907–11.

Lam A. & Newhouse M. (1990) Management of asthma and chronic airflow limitation. *Chest* **98**, 44–52.

Langer M., Mascheroni D., Marcolin R. & Gattinoni L. (1988) The prone position in ARDS patients. *Chest* **94**, 103–7.

Leeman M., Boeynaems J.M., Degante J.P., Vincent J.L. & Kahn R.J. (1985) Administration of Dazoxiben, a selective thromboxane synthetase inhibitor in the adult respiratory distress syndrome. *Chest* **87**, 727–30.

Luce J.M., Pierson D.J. & Hudson D. (1981) Intermittent mandatory ventilation; a critical review. *Chest* **79**, 678–85.

Luce J.M., Tyler M.C. & Pierson D.J. (1984) *Intensive Respiratory Care* p. 195. W.B. Saunders, Philadelphia.

McDonald R.J., Berger E.M., White C.V., Freeman B.A. & Reine J.E. (1985) Effect of superoxide dismutase encapsulated in liposomes or conjugated with polyethylene glycol on neutrophil bactericidal activity *in vitro* and bacterial clearance *in vivo*. *American Review of Respiratory Disease* **131**, 633–7.

Malik A.B., Selig W.M. & Burhop K.E. (1985) Cellular and hormonal mediators of pulmonary oedema. *Lung* **163**, 193–219.

Marini J.J., Pierson D.J. & Hudson L.D. (1979) Acute lobar atelectasis; a prospective comparison of fibreoptic bronchoscopy and respiratory therapy. *American Review of Respiratory Disease* **119**, 971–8.

Marini J.J., Rodriguez J. & Lamb V. (1986) The inspiratory workload of patient initiated mechanical ventilation. *American Review of Respiratory Disease* **134**, 902–9.

Molfino N.A., Nannini L.J., Martelli A.N. & Slutsky A.S. (1991) Respiratory arrest in near fatal asthma. *New England Journal of Medicine* **324**, 285–8.

Morris A.H., Wallace C.J., Clemmer T.P., Orme J.F., Weaver L.K., Dean N.C., Menlove R. & East T. (1992) Final report: computerized protocol controlled clinical trial of new therapy which includes ECCO$_2$R for ARDS. *American Review of Respiratory Disease* **145** 184A.

Mortensen J., Falk M., Groth S. & Jensen C. (1991) The effect of postural drainage and positive end expiratory pressure physiotherapy on tracheobronchial clearance in cystic fibrosis. *Chest* **100**, 1350−7.

Mountain R. & Sahn S. (1988) Clinical features and outcomes in patients with acute asthma presenting with hypercapnia. *American Review of Respiratory Disease* **138**, 535−9.

Murray J.F. (1977) Mechanisms of acute respiratory failure. *American Review of Respiratory Disease* **115**, 1071−8.

Murray J.F., Matthay M.A., Luce J. & Flick M.R. (1988) An expanded definition of the adult respiratory distress syndrome. *American Review of Respiratory Disease* **138**, 720−72.

National Asthma Education Program (1991) Expert Panel Report. *Guidelines for the Diagnosis and Management of Asthma.* National Heart Lung and Blood Institute publication number 91−3042. National Institutes of Health, Bethesda, July 1991.

Nolop K.P., Braude S., Taylor K.M. & Royston D. (1987) Epithelial and endothelial solute flux after bypass in dogs; effect of positive end expiratory pressure. *Journal of Applied Physiology* **62**, 1244−9.

Patterson C.E., Butler J.A., Byrne F.D. & Rhodes M.E. (1985) Oxidant lung injury; intervention with sulphydryl reagents. *Lung* **163**, 23−32.

Pepe P.E., Potkin R.T. & Rens D.N. (1982) Clinical predictors of the adult respiratory distress syndrome. *American Journal of Surgery* **144**, 124−30.

Pepe P.E., Hudson L.D. & Carrico C.J. (1984) Early application of positive end expiratory pressure in patients at risk from the adult respiratory distress syndrome. *New England Journal of Medicine* **311**, 281−6.

Pesenti A.A., Pelizzola D., Muscheroni L., Uzriel E., Pirovano U., Fox L., Gattinoni L. & Kolobow T. (1981) Low frequency positive pressure ventilation with extracorporeal CO_2 removal (LFPPV−$ECCO_2$R) in acute respiratory failure (ARF): technique. *Transactions − American Society for Artificial Internal Organs* **27**, 263−6.

Petty T.L. & Ashbaugh D.G. (1971) The adult respiratory distress syndrome clinical features, factors influencing prognosis and principles of management. *Chest* **70**, 223−9.

Pratt P.C., Vollmen R.T., Shelburne J.D. & Crapo J.D. (1979) Pulmonary morphology in a multihospital collaborative extracorporeal membrane oxygenation project. *American Journal of Pathology* **95**, 191−214.

Priebe H.J. (1992) Myocardial ischemia during vasodilator therapy in a canine model of pulmonary hypertension and coronary insufficiency. *Anesthesiology* **76**, 781−91.

Räsänen J. (1992) IMPRV − synchronized APRV, or more? *Intensive Care Medicine* **18**, 65−6.

Renken E.M. (1985) Capillary transport of macromolecular pores and other endothelial pathways. *Journal of Applied Physiology* **58**, 315−25.

Rinaldo J.E. & Rogers R.M. (1982) Adult respiratory distress syndrome; changing concepts of lung injury and repair. *New England Journal of Medicine* **306**, 900−9.

Robin E.D., Carey L.C., Grenvik A., Glansen F. & Gandio R. (1972) Capillary leak syndrome with pulmonary oedema. *Archives of Internal Medicine* **130**, 66−71.

Rocker G.M., Wiseman M.S., Peason D. & Shale D.J. (1989) Diagnostic criteria for adult respiratory distress syndrome: time for reappraisal. *Lancet* i, 120−3.

Rosen R.L. (1986) Acute respiratory failure and chronic obstructive lung disease. *Medical Clinics of North America* **70**, 895−907.

Royston D., Braude S. & Nolop K.B. (1987) Clearance of aerosolised 99m TcDTPA does not predict outcome in patients with adult respiratory distress syndrome. *Thorax* **42**, 494−9.

Searle J.F. (1985) The outcome of mechanical ventilation; report of a five year study. *Annals of the Royal College of Surgeons* **67**, 187−9.

Shoemaker W.C. & Appel P.C. (1986) Effects of prostaglandin E1 in adult respiratory distress syndrome. *Survey* **99**, 275−82.

Shoemaker W.C., Bland R.D. & Appel P.L. (1985) Therapy of critically ill postoperative patients based on outcome prediction and prospective trials. *Surgical Clinics of North America* **65**, 811−33.

Slavin G., Nunn J.F., Crow J. & Dore C.J. (1982) Bronchiolectasis − a complication of artificial ventilation. *British Medical Journal* **285**, 931−4.

Spence T.H., Jenkinson S.G., Johnson K.H., Collins J.F. & Lawrence R.A. (1986) Effects of bacterial endotoxin on protecting copper-deficient rats from hyperoxia. *Journal of Applied Physiology* **61**, 982−7.

Sprung C.L., Rackow E.C., Fein A., Jacob A.L. & Isikoff S.K. (1981) The spectrum of pulmonary oedema; differentiation of cardiogenic, intermediate and non-cardiogenic forms of pulmonary oedema. *American Review of Respiratory Disease* **124**, 718−22.

Statement of the British Thoracic Society, Research Unit of the Royal College of Physicians of London, Kings Fund Centre, National Asthma Campaign (1990) Guidelines for the management of asthma in adults: II acute severe asthma. *British Medical Journal* **301**, 797−800.

Staub N.C. (1983) Alveolar flooding and clearance. *American Review of Respiratory Disease* **127**, 544−51.

Staub N.C., Bland R.D., Brigham K.L. & Woolverton C. (1975) Preparation of chronic lung lymph fistulas on sheep. *Journal of Surgical Research* **19**, 315−21.

Strohl K.P., Cherniak N.S. & Gotle B. (1986) The physiological basis of therapy for sleep apnoea. *American Review of Respiratory Disease* **134**, 791−802.

Svensjo E. & Grega G.J. (1986) Evidence for endothelial cell regulation of macromolecular permeability by post capillary venules. *Federation Proceedings* **45**, 89−95.

Sykes M.K., McNicol R. & Campbell E.J.M. (1976) Introduction. In *Respiratory Failure* 2nd edn, p. xi. Blackwell Scientific Publications, Oxford.

Traber D.L., Adams T., Sziebert L., Stein M. & Traber L. (1985) Potentiation of lung vascular responses to endotoxin by superoxide dismutase. *Journal of Applied Physiology* **58**, 1005−9.

Wanner A. & Rao A. (1980) Clinical indications for and effects of bland, mucolytic and microbial aerosols. *American Review of Respiratory Disease* **122** (Suppl.), 79−87.

Webb H.H. & Tierney D.F. (1974) Experimental pulmonary oedema due to intermittent positive pressure ventilation with high inflation pressures; protection by positive end expiratory pressure. *American Review of Respiratory Disease* **120**, 556−65.

Webster N.R., Cohen A.J. & Nunn J.F. (1988) Adult respiratory distress syndrome − how many cases in the UK? *Anaesthesia* **43**, 923−6.

Weigelt J.A., Norcross J.F., Bormon K.R. & Snyder U.K. (1985) Early steroid therapy for respiratory failure. *Archives of*

Surgery **120**, 536—40.

Weinberg P.F., Matthay M.A., Welsten R.O., Roskos K.V., Goldstein T.M. & Murray J.F. (1984) Biologically active products of complement and acute lung injury in patients with the sepsis syndrome. *American Review of Respiratory Disease* **130**, 791—6.

Wiener-Kronisch J.P., Gropper M.A. & Matthay M.A. (1990) The adult respiratory distress syndrome: definition and prognosis, pathogenesis and treatment. *British Journal of Anaesthesia* **65**, 107—29.

Winter P.M. & Smith G. (1972) The toxicity of oxygen. *Anesthesiology* **37**, 210—41.

Wisner D.H. (1990) A stepwise logistic regression analysis of factors affecting morbidity and mortality after thoracic trauma; effect of epidural analgesia. *Journal of Trauma* **30**, 799—804.

Witsch H.R., Haschek W.M., Klein M., Szanto A.J.P. & Hakkinen P.J. (1981) Potentiation of diffuse lung damage by oxygen; determining variables. *American Review of Respiratory Disease* **123**, 98—103.

Zapol W. & Snider M. (1977) Pulmonary hypertension in severe acute respiratory failure. *New England Journal of Medicine* **296**, 476—80.

Ziegler E.J., McCutchan J.A., Fierer J., Glansen M.P., Sadoff J.C., Douglas H. & Braude A.I. (1982) Treatment of gram negative bacteremia and shock with human antiserum to a mutant *Escherichia Coli*. *New England Journal of Medicine* **307**, 1225—30.

Ziegler E.J., Fisher C.J., Sprung C.L., Straube R.C., Sadhoff J.C., Foulke G.E., Wortel C.H., Fink M.P., Dellinger R.P., Teng N.H.H., Allen E., Berger H.J., Knatterud G.L., LoBuglio A.F. & Smith C.R. (1991) Treatment of gram negative bacteremia and septic shock with HA-1A human monoclonal antibody against endotoxin: a randomized double-blind placebo-controlled trial. *New England Journal of Medicine* **324**, 429—36.

Zimmerman G.A., Renzetti A.D. & Nill H.R. (1983) Functional and metabolic activity of granulocytes from patients with adult respiratory distress syndrome: evidence for activated neutrophils in the pulmonary circulation. *American Review of Respiratory Disease* **127**, 290—300.

Renal Failure

A. INNES AND G.R.D. CATTO

Acute renal failure, which may occur following trauma, infection or surgery, continues to carry a high mortality of approximately 50%. Its prevention and treatment present considerable challenges if mortality and morbidity are to be reduced. As patients with chronic renal failure now have a considerably longer life expectancy than 20 years ago, anaesthetists care for such patients in an increasing number of surgical procedures which may or may not be related to their initial renal disease. Renal transplantation has become an accepted form of treatment for patients with end-stage renal disease, enabling successful recipients to have a relatively normal quality of life. However, these patients present anaesthetists with particular problems because of the non-specific immunosuppressive therapy and consequent increased risk of opportunistic infections. All of these aspects of the management of patients with renal failure necessitate a combined approach to their care by surgeon, anaesthetist and nephrologist.

Chronic renal failure

The definition is arbitrary, with the onset of symptoms often poorly related to the degree of renal impairment, but chronic renal failure is usually considered to be present when the glomerular filtration rate (GFR) is less than 12−15 ml/min.

The incidence of chronic renal failure is higher in elderly patients. In all age groups it shows a marked racial difference. The overall incidence of patients developing advanced renal failure in a recent UK study was 148 per million (Feest *et al.*, 1990), increasing with advancing age. Chronic renal failure may result from any underlying renal disease but the most frequent causes are glomerulonephritis, hypertension, diabetes mellitus, interstitial nephropathy and polycystic disease.

Pathophysiology

When renal function starts to decline, the effects of progressive nephron loss are compensated by glomerular hyperfiltration in the remaining intact nephrons — at least in animals. This is achieved by increasing the glomerular capillary plasma flow and glomerular transcapillary hydrostatic pressure. Such adaptation may be the reason why patients remain relatively asymptomatic until approximately 80% of nephrons are destroyed. These vascular protective changes are, however, deleterious and the resulting hyperfiltration may damage the remaining nephrons and cause glomerulosclerosis — indeed this may be one mechanism by which renal function continues to deteriorate even after the initial damaging stimulus is no longer detectable as in many cases of chronic glomerulonephritis (Olsen *et al.*, 1982). Extrapolation to humans has been difficult and indeed some studies have contradicted this hypothesis (Williams *et al.*, 1988). Whatever the explanation, when serum creatinine concentration is greater than 200−400 μmol/litre, the GFR almost invariably declines gradually until end-stage renal failure results.

Nitrogen balance

Nitrogenous waste products of protein metabolism accumulate in chronic renal failure and cause increases in serum urea, creatinine and urate concentrations. These substances are important only because they are relatively simple to measure and not because they are particularly toxic; they may be regarded as representative of a large number of poorly characterized substances excreted normally by glomerular filtration. However, it is known that the factors responsible for the toxicity of uraemia have a molecular weight in the range 500−5000 — intermediate in size between small substances removed by dialysis such as urea and large non-dialysable proteins; they have been termed 'middle molecules' but have not been characterized further (Contreras et al., 1982).

Serum urea

As the GFR decreases, serum urea concentration does not increase proportionately — it increases above the upper limit of normal only when the filtration rate is reduced to less than 50% of its normal value. Thus, an individual with mild renal disease may have a GFR as measured by creatinine or ^{51}Cr-EDTA clearance of 80 ml/min and a normal serum urea concentration; with progression of the renal disease, the GFR may decline to 10 ml/min and serum urea may increase to 30 mmol/litre.

Serum urea concentrations are influenced not only by changes in GFR but also by: (i) the protein content of the diet; (ii) hypercatabolic states such as severe infection, trauma and surgery; and (iii) urinary flow rates — urea is a relatively small molecule which tends to diffuse out of the tubules back into the circulation during states of reduced urine flow. For all these reasons, urea provides a less satisfactory measure of GFR than serum creatinine concentrations.

Serum creatinine

In patients not gaining or losing muscle rapidly, creatinine is produced at a constant rate in proportion to the muscle mass, and is excreted largely by glomerular filtration; only a small proportion is excreted by tubular secretion. Serum creatinine concentration thus provides a useful method of assessing GFR. Because individuals vary widely in muscle mass, single measurements of serum creatinine concentration must be evaluated with care — a concentration of 125 μmol/litre may indicate a normal GFR in a healthy young man but suggests a marked decrease in GFR in a frail elderly woman. When in doubt, GFR should be measured by ^{51}Cr-EDTA or creatinine clearance techniques (Shemesh et al., 1985).

Serum urea and creatinine concentrations

When serum concentrations of both urea and creatinine are measured, additional diagnostic information may be available.

1 Serum urea and creatinine concentrations are elevated equally in established renal failure, both acute and chronic.

2 Serum creatinine may be raised out of proportion to urea because of:

    (a) Rhabdomyolysis, associated with elevation of muscle enzymes.

    (b) Long-term dialysis treatment as urea molecules are smaller and more readily dialysable than creatinine.

Occasionally, drugs such as aspirin or cotrimoxazole cause a similar but more minor effect by blocking the tubular secretion of creatinine.

3 Serum urea may be raised out of proportion to creatinine because of:

    (a) Salt and water depletion or diuretic therapy.

    (b) Dietary protein or gastrointestinal haemorrhage.

    (c) Hypercatabolic states resulting from surgery, trauma and infection or drugs such as corticosteroids and tetracyclines (except doxycycline) which has an antianabolic effect.

4 Serum urea concentration may be decreased out of proportion to creatinine in liver failure, low-protein diet, high fluid intake and pregnancy.

Sodium and water balance

As the GFR decreases, there is a compensatory increase in the fractional excretion of both sodium and water from each nephron. It is postulated that the decline in GFR leads to sodium retention and expansion of blood volume, stimulating volume receptors which decrease sodium reabsorption from the renal tubules.

Recently, atrionatriuretic peptides (ANP) have been discovered. Their formation is stimulated by atrial distention and causes a marked natriuresis, which may be responsible for the increased fractional excretion of sodium observed in chronic renal failure (Suda et al., 1988). ANP may have a physiological role in the regulation of fluid volume and arterial pressure in chronic renal failure and may be important in the adaptation of tubular function occurring with reduced nephron mass (Swainson & Craig, 1991).

In chronic renal failure, the kidney is less efficient in varying urinary sodium excretion. Eventually, nephrons lose their ability to dilute or concentrate urine and cannot excrete more than 200 mmol of sodium per day. As a result of the osmotic gradient created by excess sodium in body fluid, water is generally retained together with salt, and the serum sodium concentration remains normal. When sodium intake exceeds output, extracellular volume increases, hypertension develops, body weight tends to increase and features of cardiac failure may become apparent. As a result of the adaptive increase in fractional sodium excretion, clinical problems of oliguria, severe fluid overload and oedema are uncommon until chronic renal failure is advanced — although minor degrees of sodium retention contribute undoubtedly to the hypertension which affects 75% of patients with renal failure (Bricker, 1982).

Conversely, as such patients are unable to reduce urinary sodium excretion rapidly when intake is diminished, they are at risk of volume depletion, especially after surgery or during intercurrent infection, e.g. gastroenteritis. Clinically, they present with polyuria, anorexia, nausea and hypotension. Obligatory urinary sodium losses may cause a decrease in GFR perhaps producing 'acute-on-chronic' renal failure. In this situation, an intravenous infusion of saline is essential to restore extracellular fluid volume, renal perfusion and renal function.

Potassium balance

Potassium is filtered normally by the glomerulus and then reabsorbed almost completely in the proximal tubule and loop of Henle. As renal function declines, potassium homeostasis is maintained by increasing secretion at the distal tubule and decreasing fractional reabsorption. Faecal loss of potassium increases three- or four-fold as a further adaptive mechanism in chronic renal failure. However, animal studies have shown that despite these homeostatic changes, an acute potassium load is not tolerated well in uraemia (Linas et al., 1979).

These adaptive mechanisms help to maintain potassium balance until an advanced stage of renal failure — despite the reduction of GFR and the shift of potassium from intracellular to extracellular fluid which accompanies the development of acidosis. Moderate hyperkalaemia is noted usually when the GFR decreases to below 15 ml/min; as renal function deteriorates further, severe hyperkalaemia may occur — particularly if the patient becomes oliguric.

Acid–base balance

Mild metabolic acidosis develops when the GFR declines to 25% of normal and is therefore present at a relatively early stage of the disease. The compensatory mechanisms involved in acid–base balance are less efficient than those governing sodium, potassium and water homeostasis (Warnock, 1988). These mechanisms include:

1 Respiratory hyperventilation and loss of carbon dioxide:

$$HCO_3^- + H^+ \rightarrow H_2O + CO_2$$

2 Buffering by the alkaline skeletal calcium salts; calcium is leached from bone with increased urinary calcium excretion as hydrogen ions are buffered.
3 Secondary hyperparathyroidism, which increases the buffering capacity of an acute acid load by increasing the excretion of titratable acid and mobilizing extrarenal buffers.
4 Renal responses — increasing ammonia production ($NH_3 + H^+ \rightarrow NH_4^+$), enhanced reabsorption of bicarbonate, increased titratable acid excretion and increased distal tubular delivery of sodium and potassium for hydrogen ions.

In spite of these measures, there is a reduction in serum bicarbonate concentration, a decrease in P_{CO_2} and a decrease in arterial pH. Initially, the anion gap is normal, but as renal function deteriorates, the gap increases by retention of sulphate and phosphate. The anion gap is calculated by subtracting the sum of the serum bicarbonate and chloride concentrations from the serum sodium concentrations; normally the result obtained is within the range 10–16 mmol/litre.

The acidosis is exacerbated further by decreased ammonia secretion leading to decreased hydrogen ion excretion, although the urinary pH may remain low. Proximal tubular reabsorption of bicarbonate is also impaired. Clinically, acidosis is exacerbated if diarrhoea (bicarbonate loss), hypotension or a hypercatabolic state is present.

Haemopoietic and immune systems

When the creatinine concentration increases to over 300 μmol/litre, anaemia invariably develops. Thereafter, there is only a poor correlation between the degree of anaemia and the reduction in GFR. The aetiology of the anaemia is multifactorial. There is decreased production of erythropoietin, decreased bone-marrow activity and increased red cell fragility leading to decreased red cell half-life and microangiopathic haemolysis (the latter being an acquired abnormality of the red cell pentose phosphate pathway) (Fisher, 1980).

The haemoglobin concentration decreases to below 5 g/dl rarely. Compensatory mechanisms are again important; a shift in the oxyhaemoglobin dissociation curve to the right (from acidosis and the red cell 2,3-diphosphoglycerate concentration), releases more oxygen to the tissues and there is also an increase in cardiac output.

Clinical bleeding is a manifestation of renal failure and is multifactorial. Bleeding time is prolonged and platelets exhibit decreased adhesion (Remuzzi, 1988). Increased susceptibility to infection with impairment of both cellular and humoral immunity may also be noted. Neutrophil chemotaxis and antibody responses are reduced, and there is a decrease in the number of circulating lymphocytes.

Symptoms

Gastrointestinal system

Early morning nausea and vomiting with progressive anorexia are common features of chronic renal failure. Hiccups may be troublesome and the stomach-emptying time prolonged (often doubled in patients on dialysis) — of particular relevance in anaesthetic practice.

Neurological system

Neurological complications of uraemia can vary from minor mental changes to grand mal seizures, drowsiness and coma. Uraemic twitching, cramps and restless legs may occur also. The peripheral neuropathy of chronic renal failure is sensory in type initially, but may progress to a mixed sensory and motor pattern. It is almost invariably present electromyographically when the GFR is less than 10 ml/min. Myopathy and autonomic dysfunction may also occur, particularly in patients with end-stage disease. The cerebrospinal fluid (CSF) in uraemia often has an increased protein content but there are no changes in pressure, cell count or glucose concentration.

Respiratory system

The anaemia and acidosis of uraemia contribute to the dyspnoea of chronic renal failure. The so-called 'uraemic lung' is probably largely the result of pulmonary oedema caused by fluid overload and generally improves when the patient is dialysed adequately (Rocker et al., 1988). However, there are peculiar abnormalities associated with uraemia. Transfer factor and vital capacity are both reduced. Fibrosis can occur and calcification has been noted in alveolar septa. Pleural effusions present in 20% of patients may be either exudates or transudates — serous, serosanguinous, or even haemorrhagic in type.

Cardiovascular system

Fluid overload, hypertension and anaemia all contribute to the congestive failure which is common in chronic renal failure. Expansion of the extracellular fluid compartment causes hypertension in 90–95%

of patients. Hypertension is a result also of increased activity of the renin–angiotensin system and overactivity of the autonomic nervous system. Approximately 30% of patients have hyperreninaemia, and, although bilateral nephrectomy used to be advocated, it produced no improvement in 20% of cases. By further reducing erythropoietin, it inevitably exacerbated the anaemia.

Plasma catecholamine concentrations are also elevated. Autonomic neuropathy may occur particularly in dialysis patients and is often accompanied by marked hypotension, particularly postural, despite volume expansion. Pericarditis, a frequent late complication of uraemia, is present in 60% of untreated patients. Tamponade occurs in only 20% of patients with pericarditis.

Other cardiac manifestations include uraemic cardiomyopathy — although its existence as a distinct entity is disputed (Mall et al., 1990). Peripheral vascular disease is frequently present as a result of the increased incidence of hypertension and atherosclerosis in uraemia patients. Calcification of blood vessels is noted often on X-ray and complicates vascular surgical procedures.

Calcium and phosphate homeostasis

In conservatively treated chronic renal failure, a falling GFR leads to an increase in serum phosphate and a decrease in serum calcium concentrations. However, the ionized fraction of the serum calcium concentration is protected by the systemic acidosis and hence tetany is rare. These patients should not be given bicarbonate routinely in order to control the acidosis or Kussmaul's respiration as this may precipitate tetany and generalized convulsions.

Deficiency of the active form of vitamin D (1,25-dihydroxyvitamin D_3) normally produced by the renal tubular cells, leads to defective mineralization of bone and reduced calcium absorption from the gut. As serum calcium concentrations decrease, secretion of parathyroid hormone (PTH) is stimulated. The increased PTH tends to raise serum calcium concentrations and reduce serum phosphate concentrations initially through its effects on the kidney but later at the expense of increased bone resorption; when this happens, serum phosphate concentrations may increase considerably, as both calcium and phosphate are released from bone into the blood and the excess phosphate cannot be excreted in the urine because of the renal impairment. Eventually, the solubility product of calcium phosphate is exceeded and soft-tissue calcifications may develop. Although particularly noted in blood vessels and around joints (especially when the calcium–phosphate product exceeds 4 mmol/litre), it may occur at any site including lungs, myocardium and the bundle of His. With the continued stimulation of hypocalcaemia, the mass of the parathyroid glands becomes very large and a degree of autonomous (tertiary) hyperparathyroidism with hypercalcaemia may develop.

Renal bone disease is manifest by osteomalacia, osteosclerosis and osteoporosis. Osteitis fibrosa cystica and subperiosteal erosions of the phalanges, usually with an increase in serum alkaline phosphatase activity, are thought to be pathognomonic of parathyroid overactivity. Clinically, patients may complain of bone pain but fractures are unusual. Radiological changes themselves are now uncommon as most patients are treated before these become manifest. In addition, changes are insensitive and may be misleading (Malluche & Faugere, 1990).

Other endocrine effects

Chronic renal failure reduces the production of certain hormones and increases the effect of others by reducing their degradation and elimination. Erythropoietin and 1,25-dihydroxyvitamin D, as discussed previously, are reduced. The concentrations of many peptides are elevated — insulin (giving glucose intolerance), somatostatin, calcitonin, glucagon, vasopressin, growth hormone and gastrointestinal peptides. Peripheral insulin resistance may occur in non-diabetic patients. Moreover, as the kidney is an important site for insulin metabolism, insulin dosage may have to be decreased substantially in diabetic patients developing end-stage renal failure (DeFonzo & Alvestrand, 1980).

The clinical symptoms and signs of uraemia relate to the pathophysiological processes in chronic renal failure. These features are summarized in Table 85.1.

Conservative treatment of chronic renal failure

In this section, the treatment of chronic renal failure at the stage before the need for renal replacement therapy is discussed. When possible, any underlying cause should be treated. However, in practice this is confined usually to urinary obstruction, hypertension and drug-induced causes. Treatment is otherwise directed towards ameliorating the biochemical and toxic consequences of uraemia. Possible interventions in chronic renal failure have been reviewed by Curtis (1990).

Table 85.1 Clinical features of chronic renal failure

Dermatological	*Nervous system*
Pallor	Tremor
Pruritus	Convulsions
Purpura	Lethargy
	Malaise
Cardiovascular	Peripheral neuropathy
Hypertension	Autonomic neuropathy
Congestive cardiac failure	
Pericarditis	*Gastrointestinal*
Cardiomyopathy	Anorexia
	Nausea, vomiting
Respiratory	Hiccups
Infection	Ulcerations
'Uraemic lung'	Parotitis
Acidotic respiration	Mouth ulcers
Haemopoietic	*Endocrine and metabolic*
Anaemia	Renal bone disease
Platelet dysfunction	Hyperuricaemia
Bleeding tendency	Carbohydrate intolerance

Dietary measures

Protein

Dietary protein restriction has long been used in the symptomatic management of patients with chronic renal failure. There have been recent claims that such treatment may slow or halt the progression of renal disease. In animal studies, the survival rate of animals with chronic renal failure given a low-protein diet is increased. At present, the case for such diets in humans has not been firmly established, and although symptoms may be relieved, nutritional problems may ensue.

Restriction of protein to 20 g/day is possible with a Giordano–Giovanotti diet, nitrogen balance being maintained by supplements of essential amino acids. However, this regimen is very monotonous, leads to weight loss and is unacceptable to most patients. A 40-g protein diet is reasonably palatable and does not lead to nitrogen imbalance. Although there is strong evidence that protein restriction slows down the progression of chronic renal failure in animal models, firm evidence in humans is lacking. The most recent controlled trial, although flawed, offered little support that protein restriction retards the progression of renal failure (Locatelli et al., 1991). Until more definite evidence is available, it would appear prudent to confine protein restriction to patients with uraemic symptoms. Dietary advice of this type will help also to reduce the systemic acidosis but must provide a high calorific content, to prevent catabolism of skeletal muscle. All protein-restricted diets have a low calcium content and if maintained below 30 g/day, deficiencies of iron and zinc may occur also. The use of essential amino acids or ketoacid analogues as supplements to low-protein diets remains controversial. Most studies involving the use of essential amino acids have been short term and not long enough to assess any changes in GFR. There are no data which demonstrate an advantage of ketoacid analogue supplements and some evidence that severe muscle wasting can occur. When the facilities exist, it is preferable to commence patients on some form of renal replacement therapy (dialysis or transplantation) rather than persevere with such difficult conservative measures which, in any event, carry a poorer prognosis.

One problem in assessing the effects of low-protein diets lies in monitoring the nutritional status of patients with chronic renal failure. Weight is a poor indicator of nutritional status in advanced uraemia. Significant muscle wasting has been observed without any change in serum albumin or transferrin concentrations (El Nahas & Coles, 1986; Giovannetti, 1986).

Potassium

Restriction of potassium is usually necessary only in the late stages of the disease. The patient should be advised on a reduced potassium diet (40 mmol/day) and told which foods contain high concentrations of potassium.

Sodium

Sodium restriction is indicated for most patients with chronic renal failure who have evidence of salt and water retention and hypertension. The average Western diet contains approximately 100 mmol of sodium per day. Diets containing less than 20 mmol/day are unpalatable but an intake of 60 mmol/day can be achieved by avoiding salted foods such as salted crisps.

Thus, in patients with advanced chronic renal failure, a commonly prescribed diet would contain 40 g protein, 40 mmol potassium and 40 mmol sodium.

Renal osteodystrophy

Treatment consists of maintaining serum phosphate concentrations within normal limits by dietary means or by giving oral phosphate-binding agents if necessary (Maschio et al., 1980). Aluminium hydroxide,

the most effective of these drugs, is now known to cause aluminium toxicity — a severe form of fracturing bone disease and a type of progressive dementia. Oral calcium carbonate binds phosphate, buffers the acidosis and provides calcium supplements. It is given usually in a dose of 2 g/day together with calcitriol (1,25-dihydroxyvitamin D_3), 0.25 µg/day, or alfacalcidol (1α-hydroxyvitamin D_3), 0.25–0.5 µg/day, to patients with normo- or hypocalcaemia (Muirhead et al., 1982). Hypercalcaemic patients cannot be treated in this way and are subjected usually to parathyroidectomy and then given vitamin D replacement therapy. Fragments of excised parathyroid gland may be embedded in forearm muscles; this allows the patient to re-establish normal calcium homeostasis in the event of a future renal transplant or to have the gland excised easily should hyperparathyroidism develop again (Malluche & Faugere, 1990).

Acidosis

The metabolic acidosis of chronic renal failure is normally tolerated reasonably well by patients. However, it may contribute to other problems with potassium homeostasis and to dyspnoea and lethargy. If symptoms resulting from the acidosis become severe, this is usually an indication that dialysis is required. Before this, oral sodium bicarbonate therapy may be considered but its use is limited by the high sodium content which may lead to oedema and worsening of arterial pressure control and the increased risk of tetany as discussed earlier.

Anaemia

Because of the shift in the oxygen dissociation curve, anaemia is also tolerated well. A change from the characteristic normochromic, normocytic pattern should be investigated and any concomitant vitamin, folate or iron deficiency treated. The symptomatic improvement produced by blood transfusion is short lived and may suppress erythropoiesis further; transfusions are given to patients with chronic renal failure for the improvement in subsequent graft survival rates they produce. The use of recombinant human erythropoietin is considered subsequently.

Hypertension, salt and water balance

The salt and water overload that occurs in chronic renal failure responds usually to loop diuretics. There is a dose relationship with the falling GFR. Frusemide is the drug of choice in doses of 250–500 mg/day given in a single dose. Potassium-sparing diuretics should be avoided because of the risk of producing hyperkalaemia. Dietary sodium restriction should be instituted if there is evidence of salt and water excess — despite the potential danger of volume depletion leading to a decrease in renal perfusion. In practice, it is often useful to allow a small amount of peripheral oedema to remain towards the end of the day as a safeguard against excessive volume depletion.

Beta blockers are widely used to control arterial pressure, although they tend to reduce both renal blood flow and GFR. Atenolol and nadolol are excreted unchanged by the kidney and doses should be reduced in renal failure; metoprolol which is metabolized by the liver, may prove more useful in practice.

Methyldopa increases the GFR even in chronic renal failure but still requires dosage modification; unfortunately, its numerous side-effects limit its acceptability to patients. Captopril has led to further deterioration in renal function in patients with renal artery stenosis and pre-existing renal impairment (Hricik et al., 1983). Calcium antagonists appear to be safe drugs although some have been shown to interact with cyclosporin in transplant recipients.

Additional therapy

Pruritus is a common and extremely distressing symptom of uraemia. It can be difficult to control adequately, and scratching may provoke secondary infection. Occasionally, the itch results from deposition of phosphate salts in the skin. This may respond to correction of serum calcium and phosphate concentrations as discussed previously. Chlorpheniramine, or the less sedating terfenadine, may give some symptomatic relief.

Persistent nausea and vomiting is usually an indication that dialysis is necessary. Metoclopramide may give some temporary benefit.

The onset of peripheral neuropathy is a further indication for dialysis which usually produces an improvement. Continuous ambulatory peritoneal dialysis (CAPD) appears to be more effective in this regard. Should dialysis not result in an improvement, other causes of neuropathy must be sought; alcohol and nitrofurantoin are aetiological factors overlooked in uraemic patients.

Factors of particular relevance in anaesthesia

The complications of chronic renal failure pose special problems for anaesthetic practice. Anti-hypertensive therapy should be continued up to and including the day of anaesthesia and surgery. Cannulae should not be inserted into forearm veins, as these may be required later as vascular access for haemodialysis.

The compensatory mechanisms in uraemic anaemia generally permit adequate oxygenation of the tissues. However, preoxygenation for 5 min is recommended to improve the removal of nitrogen. Anaemia decreases the blood : gas partition coefficients of halothane and methoxyflurane and thus assists rapid induction when these agents are used. Rapid recovery from anaesthesia occurs also.

Intraoperative fluid and electrolyte balance should be monitored carefully. In chronic renal disease, adequate hydration and the administration of isotonic saline preoperatively may prevent the further deterioration in renal function often associated with major surgery. Serum potassium concentration should be measured and ECG monitoring is essential; ECG abnormalities associated with potassium excess are tall, peaked T-waves, loss of P-waves and widening of the QRS complex. Catabolic states, infection or increasing acidosis may all produce dangerous elevation of the serum potassium concentration. The metabolic acidosis is usually mild, but when severe, it has been suggested that hyperventilation be maintained during anaesthesia.

After induction of anaesthesia and a neuromuscular-blocking agent are given, tracheal intubation should be performed with cricoid pressure applied. The problem of delayed stomach emptying has been discussed previously. Reversal of muscle paralysis may be achieved with neostigmine, although its half-life is prolonged in renal failure. Pyridostigmine has been preferred because of the possibility of recurarization. If there is weak hand grip or poor head lift, ventilation of the lungs may be required until full reversal is obtained. Postoperatively, supplemental oxygen should be continued for at least 4—6 h (Deutsch et al., 1969).

Anaesthetic agents (See Chapter 62)

Acute renal failure

Acute renal failure has been defined as a sudden decrease in GFR sufficient to cause uraemia. Oliguria (less than 15 ml/h) is a usual feature, but non-oliguric acute renal failure may occur. In contrast to chronic renal failure, acute renal failure develops over days or weeks, rather than months or years, and some forms are reversible or potentially reversible. Often, however, the distinction between the two conditions is difficult and an acute deterioration in a patient with chronic renal impairment (acute-on-chronic) may occur.

The classification of acute renal failure into postrenal, prerenal and intrinsic renal failure is probably satisfactory for most purposes. The three groups and their specific management will be discussed separately. The treatment of the general sequelae of acute renal failure will be considered under intrinsic renal failure category.

The major causes of acute failure in each category are listed in Table 85.2.

Postrenal renal failure

The possibility of obstruction should always be considered as it is a potentially treatable condition. An obstructive lesion is suggested by a history of total anuria, haematuria, urinary infection or loin pain. Occasionally, partial obstruction may result in paradoxical polyuria as the back pressure of urine may impair the concentrating ability of the collecting ducts. A history of previous urological problems, such as urinary calculi, should be sought.

Rectal or pelvic examination may reveal a palpable bladder caused by outlet obstruction. Calculi or blood clots, if bilateral or occurring on the side of a solitary functioning kidney, may cause acute renal failure. Analgesic abuse may produce papillary necrosis leading to ureteric obstruction. Intermittent oliguria is a common feature of retroperitoneal fibrosis and, perhaps surprisingly, pain is often absent.

The possibility of an obstructive aetiology is supported by the absence of proteinuria or urinary casts. Real-time ultrasound may be used to confirm or exclude obstruction (more accurately, dilatation of the urinary tract) and has the advantages of being non-invasive and portable. Retrograde pyelography is now seldom indicated — the site of obstruction is defined usually by antegrade pyelography performed under local anaesthesia with ultrasound control.

Removal of the obstruction is the aim of treatment. Normal renal function may not return immediately, particularly if prerenal elements (e.g. dehydration or sepsis) are present, and supportive therapy including dialysis may be necessary.

Prerenal acute renal failure

Reduction in renal perfusion leads to the development of acute renal failure; common causes are listed in Table 85.2. Clinically, the signs of incipient shock

Table 85.2 Causes of acute renal failure

Postrenal
Calculi
Papillary necrosis
Tumour
Retroperitoneal fibrosis
Bladder dysfunction
Renal vein thrombosis

Prerenal
Haemorrhage
Cardiogenic shock
Cardiac surgery
Cardiac failure
Sepsis
Gastrointestinal loss
Burns
Urinary loss
Muscle damage
Hypercalcaemia
Hepatorenal syndrome

Intrinsic renal
Postischaemic acute tubular necrosis (ATN)
Nephrotoxins
   Antibiotics
   Analgesic
   Heavy metals
Myeloma protein
Acute glomerulonephritis
Acute interstitial nephritis
Polyarteritis nodosa
Acute pyelonephritis
Postpartum renal failure
Haemolytic uraemic syndrome
Acute cortical necrosis
Thrombotic thrombocytopenia purpura

may be found; reduced skin tissue turgor, oliguria, hypotension and tachycardia. These features may be obscured in patients undergoing artificial ventilation and in elderly and obese patients. Septicaemia may cause profound hypotension and marked vasodilatation mediated by bacterial toxins. In complex situations central venous or pulmonary wedge pressures should be monitored to allow circulating plasma volume to be restored to normal by adequate but not excessive fluid replacement. Failure to restore plasma volume will result in the development of intrinsic renal failure, and at that stage renal function will not return to normal with fluid replacement. The renal response to hypoperfusion is to produce a small volume of concentrated urine. Urinary sodium concentration is less than 20 mmol/litre, and urinary osmolality increased; the ratio of the osmolality in urine and plasma (U : P ratio) is greater than 1 : 1. The ratio of urinary urea : serum urea concentrations is greater than 10 : 1. Whilst these measurements may be useful clinically, they can be unreliable in the presence of sodium depletion, diuretic therapy and in patients with acute-on-chronic renal failure. The conditions of prerenal uraemia and established renal failure are two ends of a clinical spectrum and intermediate grades of disease may give confusing results. In these situations, calculation of the fractional excretion of sodium may be worthwhile (Miller *et al.*, 1978).

If the conditions producing renal hypoperfusion are not corrected, one type of intrinsic renal failure — acute tubular necrosis — may develop. In this situation, fluid replacement above the restoration of normal circulating volume results in fluid overload and pulmonary oedema.

Intrinsic renal failure

The major causes of acute renal failure from intrinsic renal lesions are given in Table 85.2. If untreated, prerenal uraemia progresses to produce a potentially reversible form of intrinsic renal failure, known as acute tubular necrosis (ATN). This form of renal lesion is both common and, because of its good prognosis, important clinically. It can be caused not only by ischaemia but also by nephrotoxins, e.g. following excessive doses of gentamicin, paracetamol or heavy metals. The kidneys become swollen, the cortex pale and the medulla dark and congested. Histologically, the glomeruli appear intact but tubular damage predominates. This may be patchy in post-ischaemic renal failure but it is widespread and confluent following nephrotoxic damage. In both situations, the proximal tubules are affected predominantly.

Pathophysiology

A number of pathophysiological mechanisms (Table 85.3) have been proposed. It should be noted that these are not mutually exclusive.

Table 85.3 Proposed pathophysiological mechanisms in acute renal failure

Tubular obstruction
Vascular alterations
Tubular-fluid back leak
Altered glomerular permeability
Tubuloglomerular feedback

Tubular obstruction

Abnormally high intratubular pressures are present early in acute renal failure; there is impaired sodium reabsorption and an inability to concentrate urine. Obstruction of the tubules by debris and swollen tubular cells may be a major factor, and it is possible that the high back pressure within the tubules prevent glomerular filtration.

Vascular alterations

Renal blood flow has been shown to be reduced both in humans and in animal models of acute renal failure. This may decrease glomerular capillary pressure to a level at which filtration ceases and causes ischaemia of the tubular cells.

Tubular-fluid back leak

The tubular epithelium loses its integrity and it has been proposed that glomerular filtrate may leak back through the damaged epithelium. Following open-heart surgery, a back leak of inulin of between 5 and 50% has been noted.

Altered glomerular permeability

This has been proposed and indeed, a diminished ultrafiltration coefficient has been observed in acute renal failure. The presence, however, of intact glomerular histology makes this a less likely mechanism in the pathogenesis of acute renal failure.

Tubuloglomerular feedback

Reduced sodium and/or chloride reabsorption results in increased salt within the distal tubule. This is detected by the cells of the macula densa which forms one side of the triangle containing the juxtaglomerular apparatus (the other sides being the afferent and efferent glomerular arterioles). The local renin–angiotensin system is activated and angiotensin II causes constriction of the afferent arteriole and a reduction in the GFR.

Diagnosis of intrinsic acute renal failure

A thorough history is essential. Previous episodes or a history of the nephrotic syndrome may suggest acute glomerulonephritis. Documented or possible exposure to occupational, environmental or iatrogenic nephrotoxins may be important.

On urinalysis, red-cell casts suggest strongly a diagnosis of acute glomerulonephritis. In acute pyelonephritis a positive urinary culture may be obtained. Evidence of a multisystem disorder or vasculitis may be apparent clinically.

Autoantibodies, antisteptolysin-O titres and complement levels may also aid the investigation of intrinsic disease. An eosinophilia may indicate an acute interstitial nephritis — induced generally by non-steroidal anti-inflammatory drugs or antibiotic therapy.

Abdominal ultrasound is valuable in determining renal size (and thus helping to identify the small shrunken kidneys of chronic renal failure) and in detecting the dilatation of the renal tract associated with obstructive nephropathy (Webb, 1990). Renal biopsy may be required to confirm a diagnosis, although in seriously ill patients severe hypertension or a coagulopathy may preclude such an invasive technique. It is useful to determine if glomerular disease is present — important if cases of crescentic nephritis presenting as acute or rapidly progressive renal failure are to be treated adequately; it is also of value in elucidating the histological features and hence the prognosis in those patients who were thought to have a form of ATN but whose renal function has failed to return after several weeks. Routine renal biopsy is not indicated in most cases of ATN (Madaio, 1990).

Complications

When oliguria persists despite correction of prerenal factors and there is no evidence of obstructive uropathy, intrinsic acute renal failure has almost certainly developed. Non-oliguric renal failure is increasingly seen and is encountered most often in patients with ATN secondary to burns or nephrotoxins. The prognosis is better and the hospital stay shorter than for the oliguric form.

Fluid balance

Prerenal uraemia may occasionally remain undiagnosed and therefore untreated in severely debilitated or unconscious patients. More commonly, however, fluid overload is present due either to injudicious fluid replacement or to the inappropriate use of large quantities of sodium bicarbonate in an attempt to correct the acidosis. Fluid overload can lead to hypertension, peripheral pulmonary and cerebral oedema.

Sodium balance

Hyponatraemia, is common in acute renal failure, and this may be dilutional due to fluid overload or may indicate true sodium loss (e.g. caused by vomiting or diarrhoea). Hypernatraemia is noted less frequently but may occur in situations of volume depletion when more water than salt is lost, or rarely, after excessive sodium infusion.

Potassium balance

Hyperkalaemia when not caused by foods, drinks, drugs and infusions containing potassium, most frequently results from leak of intracelullar potassium and is often associated with hypercatabolic states such as severe infection or trauma. Acidosis also exacerbates the hyperkalaemia by aiding the shift of potassium from the intracellular compartment. Electrocardiogram changes are common once the serum potassium increases above 6.5 mmol/litre and can ultimately lead to ventricular arrhythmias, cardiac arrest and death.

Acid–base balance

A metabolic acidosis is usual in acute renal failure and may exacerbate already existing hypotension and hyperkalaemia. Rarely, alkalosis can occur when gastrointestinal fluid losses are substantial. Respiratory acidosis may be present also if pulmonary infection, trauma or oedema are present.

Anaemia

Bleeding, haemodilution or haemoconcentration may all obscure the initial stages of acute renal failure. Subsequently, normochromic normocytic anaemia develops as in patients with chronic renal failure. A rapidly falling haemoglobin concentration may result from bleeding or disseminated intravascular coagulopathy.

Uraemia

The accumulation of uraemic toxins is noted particularly in hypercatabolic states, and the serum urea concentration may increase rapidly. An acute fibrinous pericarditis may occur with the danger of tamponade. Hiccups and gastrointestinal bleeding are common. If untreated, the patient's mental condition deteriorates rapidly from apathy and confusion to coma, convulsions and death.

Calcium balance

Hypocalcaemia is usual and accompanies the increase in serum phosphate concentrations caused by the decreased GFR. Plasma concentrations of 1,25-dihydroxyvitamin D_3 are reduced, and it is believed that the elevated phosphate concentrations cause precipitation of insoluble calcium phosphate complexes in soft tissues and exacerbate the tendency to hypocalcaemia. The precise mechanisms are only poorly understood. The systematic acidosis protects against tetany.

Infection

In addition to being a cause of acute renal failure, infection may occur as a complication of the disease itself. Chest, urinary and oral infections predominate and should be sought and treated actively.

Treatment

If practicable, treatment should be directed towards removal of the underlying cause or withdrawal of an offending nephrotoxin. When, as is usual, primary treatment of this type is not possible, the principal aim of management is to prevent death from uraemia or any other cause while the kidneys are recovering from ATN. When the acute renal failure results from a non-reversible renal lesion, the patient should receive the appropriate treatment and rehabilitation necessary to prepare for some form of renal replacement therapy — dialysis or transplantation.

Management

Conservative therapy may be all that is required for patients with mild disease who are not hypercatabolic or oliguric. Conversely, patients who are severely ill following trauma, sepsis or major surgery often require continuing supportive measures and dialysis.

Fluid balance must be monitored stringently by daily weighing of the patient, accurate fluid balance charts and central venous pressure (CVP) measurements when appropriate. Evidence of infection should be actively sought and treated with non-nephrotoxic antibiotic. Blood and urine cultures should be obtained from all patients presenting with acute renal failure. Physiotherapy is essential for patients undergoing artificial ventilation and those with severe chest infections. Prophylactic systemic antibodies are not recommended as they may produce superinfection of the mouth and gastrointestinal tract.

The verdict on the use of selective decontamination of the gastrointestinal tract is probably currently 'not proven' (Sanderson, 1989).

If a prerenal element is suspected, a fluid challenge with a test infusion of saline (1 litre in 1 h) may be helpful. If within 1–2 h the urine flow doubles, the infusion should be continued — provided that CVP remains below 8–10 cmH_2O. If a saline infusion proves ineffective and after ensuring that the patient is volume replete, treatment with frusemide may increase urinary output as it improves renal blood flow and induces a salt diuresis. Although it does not reduce the number of dialyses required, the overall mortality or the period of renal insufficiency, it may, in doses of 1–3 g/day, convert oliguric to non-oliguric renal failure.

Mannitol has been advocated in renal failure because of its effects of increasing renal perfusion and urine flow by inducing an osmotic diuresis. Intravenous mannitol will, however, cause a considerable increase in extracellular fluid volume by attracting water from the intracellular fluid. There is little evidence that it is effective in preventing the development of intrinsic acute renal failure and because of the risks of pulmonary oedema, cerebral dehydration and haemolysis should seldom be used.

When cardiac failure has caused renal hypoperfusion, CVP monitoring may be inadequate, as right-sided cardiac filling pressure may not reflect left-sided pressure. In this situation, a catheter should be inserted into the pulmonary artery so that the pulmonary capillary wedge pressure, and thus, indirectly, the left-sided filling pressure, may be monitored.

Fluid replacement may not abolish hypotension even though the circulating volume returns to normal. In this situation, dopamine and/or dobutamine are useful pressor agents. Both have renal vasodilatory effects at low dosage in addition to acting as cardiac inotropes at higher dosage. Unfortunately, as the dose of each increases, the renal vasodilatory effect becomes a pressor effect and may well result in a further impairment of renal perfusion. It is probably best to commence with dopamine at a dose of $2\,\mu g \cdot kg^{-1} \cdot min^{-1}$, increasing to a maximum of $10\,\mu g \cdot kg^{-1} \cdot min^{-1}$. If a generalized pressor effect is still required because of persistent hypotension, the addition of dobutamine at a dose of $2.5\,\mu g \cdot kg^{-1} \cdot min^{-1}$ may provide an adequate pressor effect while maintaining or improving renal perfusion (Henderson et al., 1980).

Hyperkalaemia, if mild, may be controlled by diet and by avoiding potassium supplements and potassium-sparing diuretics. If this is insufficient, ion-binding resins (e.g. calcium resonium, 15 g 6-hourly) given either orally or rectally are effective in 24–48 h. In situations of severe life-threatening hyperkalaemia, a combination of soluble insulin (10 units) and dextrose (50 g) given intravenously drives potassium into the intracellular compartment. Its effect is short lived and may have to be repeated. Intravenous salbutamol can also be used in urgent situations, either alone or in combination with glucose/insulin. Its use is not recommended, however, in patients with acute ischaemic heart disease (Lens et al., 1989). Calcium gluconate does not lower the serum potassium level, but appears to protect the myocardium from the deleterious effects of hyperkalaemia. The treatment of hyperkalaemia is summarized in Table 85.4.

It is important when investigating patients with acute renal failure to consider first those conditions which, if treated specifically, may be reversible. This applies to postrenal and prerenal factors in particular. Many patients may be so ill on admission that treatment, often including dialysis, must precede all but the most basic investigations. The incidence of gastrointestinal haemorrhage, which is a common problem in such acutely ill patients, has been decreased by the prophylactic use of H_2-antagonists (Priebe et al., 1980).

When immediate life-threatening problems have been tackled, the difficulties of maintaining adequate hydration whilst limiting excessive protein or potassium intake remain. Fluid balance is critically important. Overhydration overloads the cardiovascular system and predisposes to pulmonary oedema; underhydration with a reduction in the extracellular fluid volume delays the return of renal function. For most afebrile patients in temperate climates it is sufficient generally to supply 500 ml fluid daily in addition to the volume of urine excreted.

Dietary protein intake may have to be decreased but it is very important that a high-energy diet (at least 12 000 kJ or 3000 cal) be provided to prevent catabolism of endogenous proteins. When the facilities are available, it is preferable to begin dialysis early and to encourage adequate nutrition, if necessary by total parenteral nutrition, than to persist in prolonged conservative measures.

Dialysis is therefore normally required in acute renal failure to control hyperkalaemia, acidosis and fluid overload, and to relieve the symptoms and signs of uraemia. The current trend is to introduce dialysis early, as uraemic complications are reduced if the serum urea is maintained below 33 mmol/litre (Rainford, 1977).

Peritoneal dialysis, which requires no specialized facilities, may be sufficient in non-catabolic patients and is useful in small children, elderly patients and patients with bleeding problems. It is less efficient than haemodialysis in removing large amounts of fluid and cannot be used after abdominal surgery. Protein depletion and peritonitis can occur and respiration may be compromised in debilitated patients.

Haemodialysis is discussed in greater detail subsequently. It is more satisfactory for fluid removal (using ultrafiltration or haemofiltration) and more useful in correcting biochemical abnormalities rapidly. It requires specialized facilities and vascular access. It is more efficient in correcting serum biochemical abnormalities than peritoneal dialysis in hypercatabolic patients. Such patients may also need total parenteral nutrition — the large amounts of fluid which can be removed by ultrafiltration (or haemofiltration) may enable adequate nutrition to be provided.

Recovery from acute tubular necrosis

The prognosis in acute renal failure depends on the aetiology (Table 85.2). From some conditions, the prognosis is poor and patients may require long-term renal replacement therapy. Conversely, patients with ATN generally recover and the principal aim of management is to support the patient until recovery of some function occurs — usually within 6 weeks (Moran & Myers, 1985). Recovery is marked by a diuretic phase during which urinary output generally increases; rarely, a patient may pass 10 litres/day of

Table 85.4 Treatment of severe hyperkalaemia

Calcium gluconate (10%), 10–30 ml i.v. Sodium bicarbonate, 50–150 mmol i.v.	Immediate therapy to stabilize cell membrane and shift potassium into cells
Glucose, 50 g i.v. Soluble insulin 10 units i.v. Salbutamol, 0.5 mg i.v. over 15 min	Effective within 15–30 min in shifting potassium into cells
Cation exchange resins (Na^+ or Ca^{2+}) 30–60 g rectally or 30 g orally	Acts within 1–2 h and removes potassium from the body
Haemodialysis and peritoneal dialysis	Used only in renal failure and begins to remove potassium from the body within 15–30 min of starting treatment

dilute urine. This polyuria, which may require considerable fluid and potassium replacement, occurs partly as a result of the osmotic diuresis induced by the retained urea, creatinine, etc. and partly because the medullary hypotonicity, and hence renal concentrating ability, has been lost (Swann & Merrill, 1953).

Recovery of renal function as measured by a reduction in serum urea and creatinine concentration lags usually a few days behind the diuresis. Even when adequate renal function has returned, some impairment of GFR or tubular defects in urinary concentration or acidification may remain.

The overall mortality of acute renal failure from ATN has only improved slightly in the last 30 years and remains approximately 50%. However, there has been an improvement in mortality from traumatic and obstetric causes and also a decrease in the incidence of these cases. In medical conditions an increase in the average age of the patients treated and the more serious primary conditions precipitating acute renal failure have offset the considerable improvement in patient management and dialysis techniques (Turney et al., 1990).

Factors of particular relevance to anaesthesia

Overall, trauma and surgery predispose to over 50% of cases of acute renal failure. Anaesthetists caring for seriously ill and postsurgical patients in intensive therapy units are responsible for considerable numbers of patients with renal failure. Prerenal uraemia is usually the most common form, but this may progress to established acute renal failure, especially if appropriate treatment is not given rapidly. Close monitoring of urinary output, fluid intake, weight and CVP is necessary. Early correction of hypovolaemia and sepsis increases urinary output and decreases blood urea.

The prognosis is dependent primarily on the factors which precipitated acute renal failure initially and the prognosis of the underlying disease. The prognosis is worse in patients with oliguric acute renal failure compared with the non-oliguric form. Mortality from obstetric causes is very low and, indeed, the incidence of acute renal failure from such causes has fallen markedly in recent years.

In contrast, the mortality in patients with burns, trauma and sepsis remains very high (approximately 50%) and has not changed significantly in the past 20 years. Death is usually a result of gastrointestinal haemorrhage or sepsis. Jaundice at presentation indicates a poor prognosis. The unchanging prognosis in severely ill patients probably reflects the underlying condition and the degree to which acute renal failure, can be prevented in less ill patients. Patients with both ventilatory failure and acute renal failure have a particularly poor prognosis (Turney et al., 1990).

Renal replacement therapy

End-stage renal disease (ESRD) has been defined as the situation in which, despite conservative therapy, the patient with chronic renal failure dies without renal replacement therapy. It may be defined in terms of clinical and biochemical criteria. Renal replacement therapy includes both haemodialysis and CAPD, and transplantation.

The overall incidence of ESRD is unknown, and the incidence of new patients requiring treatment for ESRD is difficult to obtain. In the USA, a figure of 100 patients per million of the population per year is given. In the UK (in the age group 15−60 years) a figure of approximately 40 patients per million was claimed in 1986 (European Dialysis and Transplantation Association Registry, 1986). In 1988, 55.1 patients per million were accepted for renal replacement therapy. Most recent data suggest that in the UK 75−80 new patients per million population per year would be suitable for dialysis (Feest et al., 1990; McGeown, 1990). The reasons for these marked differences in national data depend partly on the great variation in the provision of facilities for treating patients with ESRD and partly on such medicopolitical considerations as a statutory right to treatment which pertains in some countries. Ideally, need for treatment should be determined solely on medical criteria and all patients with ESRD should be assessed by a nephrologist. The indications for dialysis are listed in Table 85.5.

Haemodialysis

Both haemodialysis and peritoneal dialysis are based on the ability of crystalloids but not colloids to diffuse down a concentration gradient through a semi-permeable membrane separating two solutions — blood and an ideal dialysis fluid — dialysate. For

Table 85.5 Indications for dialysis in ESRD

Uraemic symptoms
Peripheral neuropathy
Pericarditis
Acidosis
Hyperkalaemia

haemodialysis, the membrane is made usually of cellulose derivatives whilst in peritoneal dialysis the peritoneum itself serves as the membrane.

Haemodialysis requires the circulation of blood through an artificial kidney at 200 ml/min and therefore repeated access to the circulation is necessary. For short-term use, particularly in acute renal failure, percutaneous catheterization of central veins is the method of choice. This is achieved by cannulation of either the femoral or the subclavian vein. Subclavian cannulation may be used for longer-term dialysis (for several months) by tunnelling the cannula through a subcutaneous track to reduce the risk of infection.

An arteriovenous (Scribner) shunt was the first method of obtaining repeated access to the circulation although is used less frequently now (Quinton et al., 1960). A shunt is a moulded silastic tube: one limb is inserted into an artery, the other into a vein to provide blood flow from and to the patient. When not being used for dialysis, blood simply flows through the loop formed by joining arterial and venous limbs. If possible, the shunt should be inserted in the leg to preserve arm vessels for subsequent fistula construction if the patient should require long-term dialysis. The lifetime of a shunt is limited by clotting or infection.

These problems have led to the use of arteriovenous (Cimino) fistulas (Brescia et al., 1966). The formation of a fistula, however, must be regarded as an elective procedure as the arterialized venous drainage may not produce the distended veins suitable for repeated vascular access for several weeks. The forearm is the most suitable site. Once mature, the fistula can be used for dialysis either by inserting needles at two sites on the fistula for inflow and outflow, or by using a double-lumen cannula. Using specialized equipment, single-needle dialysis is possible also.

The use of an extracorporeal circulation requires anticoagulation. In patients on long-term dialysis, this is provided by a loading dose of heparin (3000–5000 IU) followed by a constant infusion of 1000–1500 IU/h. In ill patients, particularly those with clotting problems, minimal heparinization should be used to prevent bleeding problems. Minimal heparin therapy involves a loading dose of 1500 IU or less, and additional doses of 500 IU as necessary to maintain the clotting time in the range 15–20 min. Prostacycline has been used as an alternative to heparin in high-risk patients (Lindsay & Smith, 1989).

Modern haemodialysis machines provide equipment to generate dialysate from a concentrate and integrate blood and anticoagulant pumps with a system of alarms and monitors. They require a flow of suitably purified water of approximately 500 ml/min. Dialysers are available in a variety of models with different ultrafiltration and clearance capabilities. These have a surface area of semipermeable membrane of $1.0–1.2\,m^2$, although smaller areas are available for children and larger areas may be useful when increased efficiency is required.

Fluid removal is achieved by ultrafiltration. This involves transfer of water from the blood compartment to the dialysate by varying the suction pressure applied across the dialysis membrane.

Although haemodialysis removes fluid and toxins and corrects the biochemical abnormalities of uraemia, it does so intermittently and therefore, between dialyses, considerable dietary restrictions remain necessary. In adequately nourished patients, an intake of 0.75–1.0 g/kg body weight of protein with a calorie intake of approximately 2000 kcal is recommended. Both sodium and potassium intake has to be restricted, whilst any fluid restriction depends upon urine output and clinical status of the patient.

Complications

Failure to adhere to salt and water restrictions or a change in the ideal body weight causes fluid overload with weight gain, hypertension, peripheral and pulmonary oedema. Left ventricular hypertrophy is an important determinant of survival on dialysis (Silberberg et al., 1989). Hypertension is usually salt and water dependent and responds to ultrafiltration. This may, however, not be tolerated well, and antihypertensive therapy may remain necessary. Hypotension and cramps are common complications of haemodialysis. Hypotension may develop within minutes of starting dialysis and is related usually to myocardial insufficiency, inadequate response of peripheral blood vessels and poor filling of the vascular bed from the interstitial space. Other reasons invoked have been the use of acetate dialysis, autonomic neuropathy and hypoxaemia. The problem may be alleviated by using either bicarbonate in place of the conventional acetate buffer or sequential ultrafiltration and haemodialysis. Bicarbonate haemodialysis has been advocated for severely ill patients with acute renal failure, hypotension and impaired myocardial contractility.

Anaemia is almost invariable in dialysis patients; the exceptions are patients with polycystic kidneys who may have haemoglobin values in the normal range. In addition to the causes discussed earlier, there is a small amount of blood lost at each dialysis

(3–5 ml) although larger quantities can be lost occasionally as a result of membrane rupture, clotting of blood within the dialyser or haemorrhage from a fistula or shunt. It is necessary, therefore, to provide iron supplements to compensate for this loss and most units also give folic acid, although in adequately nourished patients this may be unnecessary.

The production of erythropoietin by recombinant DNA technology has led to its clinical use in the anaemia of chronic renal failure. Erythropoietin corrects the anaemia although it appears that aiming for a haemoglobin slightly less than the conventional normal range avoids many of the drug's side-effects. These include hyperkalaemia and vascular problems — hypertension and thrombosis of A–V fistulas (Casati et al., 1987). Despite these drawbacks, the routine use of erythropoietin in haemodialysis and CAPD patients represents a major advance in improving the lives of dialysis patients. Its use in acute renal failure and chronic renal failure (not requiring dialysis) remains to be fully determined.

Hyperlipidaemia, a common finding, may require further dietary restrictions. Renal osteodystrophy is a frequent feature in patients with ESRD and has been discussed previously. This may be high-turnover hyperparathyroid bone disease, an adynamic low-turnover type or a mixed picture. Treatment is based on the use of oral phosphate-binding agents and vitamin D (calcitriol). Vitamin D therapy may lead to hypercalcaemia, particularly when used with calcium-containing phosphate binders, and the serum calcium should be monitored frequently. Vitamin D analogues have been developed which do not appear to produce hypercalcaemia, although they have not reached clinical use yet.

In common with other trace materials, aluminium is not eliminated in renal failure, and toxicity can result from the use of aluminium-containing phosphate-binding agents and aluminium-rich dialysis water. Aluminium is deposited in the bones causing an osteodystrophy (Parkinson et al., 1979). Multiple fractures are common, particularly of the ribs. Histologically, the lesion resembles osteomalacia but serum alkaline phosphatase concentrations (and PTH) are normal. A characteristic encephalography may also occur. Water supplies should be treated by reverse osmosis to reduce the aluminium content of the dialysate. Desferrioxamine has been used to chelate aluminium from the tissues with subsequent removal by dialysis and has produced some clinical improvement in the encephalography and osteodystrophy. The desferrioxamine test may be a useful tool to assess aluminium toxicity (Milliner et al., 1984). Other phosphate-binding agents which do not contain an aluminium salt (usually calcium containing) can be used. Magnesium-containing antacids (though having a weaker binding effect) have been investigated. Hypermagnesaemia is prevented by using dialysate low in magnesium. Recently, a unique variety of amyloid deposit has been found in the tissues of long-term dialysis patients. The main clinical features are carpal tunnel syndrome, bone cysts, pathological fractures and scapulohumeral periarthritis (Fenves et al., 1986).

Acquired cystic disease of the kidneys has been described in dialysis patients who did not have any form of renal cystic disease as a cause of their renal failure (Rudge, 1986).

Hepatitis B, once a scourge of dialysis centres, is now an uncommon problem in the UK since screening blood donations and stringent aseptic techniques have been adopted widely. Within the UK, all staff and patients are screened regularly for HBsAg and positive patients are treated in a separate dialysis unit. Acquired immune deficiency syndrome (AIDS) is at present a relatively uncommon condition in long-term dialysis patients, but is likely to increase in the near future (Goldman et al., 1986). It is clearly a major problem among young drug addicts, many of whom may present with acute renal failure secondary to septicaemia.

Peritoneal dialysis

Peritoneal dialysis makes use of the peritoneum, the semipermeable membrane separating blood from the ideal fluid solution — the dialysate. Until recently, difficulty in obtaining repeated access to the peritoneal cavity and problems of malnutrition and peritonitis restricted this simple but relatively inefficient technique to the treatment of patients with non-hypercatabolic acute renal failure. The development, almost 20 years ago, of the permanent indwelling Tenckhoff catheter, made of flexible silastic and anchored to the anterior abdominal wall by dacron cuffs, allowed peritoneal dialysis to be used for the long-term treatment of patients with chronic renal failure.

Intermittent peritoneal dialysis, performed generally by an automated peritoneal dialysis machine, was used by some renal units but costs and technical problems limited its usefulness. It has now been largely replaced by CAPD, developed a decade ago. A combination of the two therapies, so-called continuous cycling peritoneal dialysis (CCPD), is used by some units to ease the burden of frequent exchange

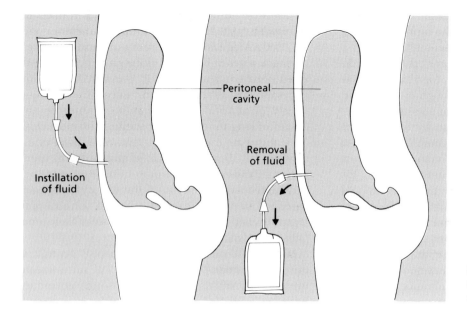

Fig. 85.1 The technique of continuous ambulatory peritoneal dialysis (CAPD).

with CAPD. Continuous ambulatory peritoneal dialysis is now used widely in the UK where 50% of children and 30% of adults are treated in this way. It has enabled units to increase the numbers of patients treated for ESRD (Morgan & Burden, 1986). Despite this growth in its use, its future is uncertain. With high failure rates, these large numbers of patients treated with CAPD need adequate back-up facilities for haemodialysis.

Nevertheless, once the catheter system is inserted, the technique for dialysis is simple and rapidly learned by patients (Fig. 85.1). Training is achieved in 7–10 days, it can be performed at home, no complicated equipment is necessary and no costly adaptations to the home are required.

Contraindications are usually relative. Intraperitoneal adhesions or abdominal stomas may both cause problems. Hernias should be repaired before CAPD is commenced. Inflammatory bowel disease and diverticular disease may be associated with the spread of bowel organisms. Difficulties either due to visual handicap, comprehension or arthritis may interfere with the aseptic technique. The advantages of CAPD to patients are several. There is better removal of middle molecular weight solutes, patients often feel better on CAPD and an improvement in peripheral neuropathy may be noted.

Haemoglobin concentrations are higher than in patients on haemodialysis, making patients more active physically and increasing their feeling of well-being. Fluid and dietary restrictions are less severe than with haemodialysis and an increased protein intake is required to counteract protein loss into the peritoneal cavity.

No vascular access is required, making this form of treatment useful in children (with a low vascular volume), diabetics and arteriopaths with poor peripheral vasculature. The haemodynamic fluctuations and their associated symptoms, noted on haemodialysis, are avoided. Growth rates in children may be better and control of osteodystrophy is equal to that achieved on haemodialysis. Blood glucose control in insulin-dependent diabetics is easily achieved generally, although insulin requirements are increased. Insulin may be added to the CAPD bags and is thus given intraperitoneally rather than subcutaneously.

Conversely, the technique has considerable disadvantages. There is a high technical failure and drop-out rate. Only 72% of those beginning CAPD in 1981 were still using the technique 10–12 months later. A recent study found only 40% of patients remained on CAPD 2 years later. Hyperglycaemia and hyperlipidaemia result from the use of necessarily hypertonic solutions with a high glucose content. This may pose problems in existing diabetics leading to poor control and increased insulin requirements and may worsen the hyperlipidaemia which occurs in many renal patients.

Some data suggest that there is long-term damage to the peritoneal membrane. There is a gradual reduction in the efficiency of dialysis with time, and by 2 years, 30% of patients have lost a substantial proportion of their ultrafiltration capacity

(Slingeneyer *et al.*, 1983). This is often the result of recurrent bacterial infections. The use of dialysis solutions containing acetate has also been implicated, although it has been reported as well when lactate-containing solutions are used. Occasionally 'resting' the membrane by using haemodialysis for a period allows recovery of function to take place.

Psychological and psychosocial problems may occur in patients and their relatives who feel unable to cope with the presence of the catheter, bag and tubing.

Peritonitis is a frequent complication of CAPD treatment. The incidence varies but is probably around one episode per 4–12 patient months. It arises usually from contamination of the dialysate when the bags are changed; less frequently, it may pass through the anterior abdominal wall down the catheter track or arise from the bowel. Peritonitis presents as a cloudy CAPD bag (caused by poly-morphonuclear leucocytes in the peritoneal effluent) with or without abdominal pain and fever. Approximately 50% of infective episodes are caused by Gram-positive cocci, usually *Staphylococcus epidermidis* and 20% by Gram-negative bacteria. A sterile peritonitis is usually a result of inadequate bacteriology or previous antibiotic therapy. Fungal peritonitis may occur, often following treatment of bacterial infection. Antifungal therapy is seldom effective and catheter removal may be essential. For bacterial infection, intraperitoneal antibiotics given with the dialysate are usually satisfactory. As Gram-positive cocci are almost always sensitive to vancomycin and Gram-negative bacteria to gentamicin, treatment with a combination of these antibiotics may be commenced while bacterial sensitivities are awaited. Drug concentrations should be monitored. Infections of the catheter exit site and track may occur. Antibiotic therapy is often ineffective and removal of the catheter may be required.

Subacute sclerosing peritonitis is a rare complication of CAPD. The small bowel becomes encapsulated in thickened fibrosed peritoneum. This causes loss of ultrafiltration and a subacute small-bowel obstruction. The cause is uncertain, although certain antiseptic solutions (Chlorhexidine) and acetate have been implicated. Surgical relief may be unsuccessful and mortality is high (Gandhi *et al.*, 1980).

There appears to be little difference in terms of cost between CAPD and haemodialysis when hospitalization, peritonitis, antibiotic therapy and loss of earnings are taken into consideration. Differences in survival rates between the two techniques are difficult to assess. Most studies comparing survival rates had noted, however, that those on CAPD have a higher prevalence of cardiovascular disease and diabetes, but corrected for such variables, patient survival appears similar on CAPD and haemodialysis (Gentil *et al.*, 1991).

Continuous ambulatory peritoneal dialysis, therefore, appears to be an acceptable form of treatment for certain groups of patients. Individuals with severe cardiovascular disease, children, diabetic patients, elderly patients and those who fear machines may all benefit from this form of therapy. In the absence of a successful transplant, haemodialysis probably continues to be the treatment of choice for most other categories of patient.

Transplantation

Renal transplantation is now the treatment of choice for most patients with ESRD. Initially successful only between identical twins, kidneys from unrelated cadaver donors and from living-related donors are now transplanted with increasing chances of success. This continuing improvement (with grafts from living-related donors having a graft survival rate at 1 year of 95% and from cadavers of 75–80%) is largely a result of advances in immunosuppressive therapy; patient survival at 1 year is about 95%.

When a living-related transplant is performed, anaesthesia is required for both donor and recipient. In some countries, when cadaver donors are used, the anaesthetist may be called upon to supervise ventilations and maintain cardiovascular stability.

Suitable cadaver donors are patients under 70 years of age, in whom a diagnosis of brain death has been made. Potential donors are excluded if sepsis or malignancy (apart from primary cerebral tumours) is present. Significant hypertension or a history of renal disease are also exclusions.

Transplantation must be based on the principles of ABO compatibility. Matching for HLA A, B and DR specificities has been shown to improve graft survival although some doubt about serological testing remains (Opelz *et al.*, 1991). In living-related donor transplantation, a single haplotype mismatch is suitable if a complete two-haplotype mismatch is not available.

For many years, blood transfusion of potential graft recipients was avoided to prevent sensitization of patients to Class I antigens (HLA A, B and C). Later it was observed that transplant recipients who had received pretransplant blood transfusions from third-party donors had improved graft survival. The reasons for this improvement or enhancement of graft survival are still not fully understood. More recent data suggest that although the 'transfusion effect' exists, other improvements have led to increased graft survival in untransfused patients (Opelz, 1987). Thus, the transfusion effect appears to have lost much of its influence on graft survival, a finding which has led to many units stopping elective transfusions (Innes et al., 1993).

Hyperacute rejection with rapid graft destruction within hours of transplantation was not an uncommon occurrence. It was caused by preformed cytotoxic antibodies present in recipient serum and directed to the graft and has fortunately become much less frequent following the introduction of the 'cross-match test'. Donor lymphocytes from spleen in lymph node are incubated with recipient serum in the presence of complement. A positive test in which the serum kills the donor cells indicates the presence of cytotoxic antibodies to donor tissue and precludes transplantation.

The surgical techniques are beyond the scope of this chapter. The anaesthetist is, however, responsible for patients with ESRD; these patients may be considered in terms of two subgroups. The recipient of a living-related donor transplant will be adequately prepared, optimally hydrated and recently dialysed. By contrast, the recipient of a cadaver transplant will have been notified at short notice and may require haemodialysis and preparation before theatre. Patients should not be volume depleted before surgery, and fluid losses during the transplant operation need to be replaced cautiously and potassium balance monitored in case the transplanted kidney does not function immediately.

Immunosuppression

Within the graft, donor cells possess surface antigens differing from those of the recipient. The more important of these are encoded by the genes of the HLA gene complex, the human major histocompatibility complex, located on the short arm of the sixth chromosome. Recognition of these antigens by the recipient initiates cellular and humoral responses leading to acute rejection. Current immunosuppressive regimens which vary considerably are used to prevent rejection occurring or are given as additional therapy to reverse acute rejection. The most commonly used regimens employ varying combinations of prednisolone, azathioprine and cyclosporin (Jones et al., 1988).

Cyclosporin, which inhibits lymphocyte proliferation mediated by interleukins I and II, results in a reversible impairment of T-cell-dependent immunity. Its use has resulted in graft survival figures for cadaver donor transplants now approaching those achieved in living-related transplants. It has led to a decrease in steroid dosage and the related serious effects. Unfortunately, however, cyclosporin therapy has significant but different side-effects, notably renal toxicity — acute toxicity is often difficult to distinguish from rejection and chronic toxicity is a complication in the longer term (Mihatsch et al., 1988). Important drug interactions occur in patients treated with cyclosporin notably with ketoconazole, erythromycin and diltiazem (Cockburn, 1986).

Since 1962, prednisolone has been used as an immunosuppressive agent in combination with azathioprine. Steroids are now given in relatively low doses of 20–30 mg prednisolone in daily or alternate day regimens (Morris et al., 1982). To treat episodes of acute rejection, higher doses of steroids (oral prednisolone, 200 mg daily, or intravenous methyl-prednisolone, 0.25–1 g daily) are used. Such treatment reverses episodes of acute rejection in 90% of cases but in 50% this reversal is only temporary; repeated immunological attack may prove unresponsive to further steroid therapy.

Antilymphocytic globulin, is obtained by immunizing animals with human lymphoid cells. It is associated with fever, thrombocytopenia, leukopenia and, rarely, anaphylactoid reactions. More recently, monoclonal antibodies directed to specific receptors on T-cell subsets have become available. The most extensively investigated is OKT3, which is now used both in prevention of acute rejection in high-risk patients but also in its treatment (Norman, 1988). Novel agents such as the macrolide immunosuppressant FK506 are currently being evaluated (MacLeod & Thomson, 1991).

Complications

Early complications of renal transplantation are related usually to failure of the graft to function. Delayed function may result from a degree of ATN in the graft whereas decreasing function may result from acute rejection, cyclosporin A nephrotoxicity or mechanical problems with the transplanted ureter. A later decline in renal function may result from chronic rejection, further ureteric problems, stenosis of the arterial anastomosis, urinary infection or recurrence of the original pathology (e.g. glomerulonephritis). A chronic rejection process is usually unresponsive to antirejection therapy.

Other long-term complications relate to the need

for persisting immunosuppressive therapy and have been reviewed by Braun (1990). Infection is a major cause of morbidity and mortality after transplantation. Bacterial chest infections are produced by common pathogens generally, such as pneumococci or *Haemophilus influenzae*. Tuberculosis may, however, be reactivated in immunosuppressed patients. 'Opportunistic infections' with fungae and protozoa may occur. Oral candidiasis usually responds readily to topical nystatin. Pulmonary infections may be caused by *Aspergillus*, *Histoplasma* and *Cryptococcus*, which may also produce a meningitis. *Pneumocystis carinii* presents usually as an undiagnosed pulmonary infiltrate in a febrile dyspnoeic patient. Diagnosis depends on lung biopsy and cotrimoxazole is the treatment of choice.

Cytomegalovirus is a common problem in some centres and presents usually with fever and leukopenia (Editorial, 1989). Herpes simplex and varicella zoster infection can occur but respond to therapy with the antiviral agent, acyclovir. Certain tumours (particularly lymphomas in cyclosporin-treated patients) have an increased incidence in transplant patients (Penn, 1990).

Despite the problems associated with transplantation, cadaver graft survival figures of over 80% have been obtained. Successful transplantation offers the patients with ESRD the best opportunity of achieving a normal lifestyle.

Haemofiltration

Haemofiltration differs from conventional haemodialysis in that no dialysate is used. It is used most frequently in the treatment of acute renal failure, but in some countries it is used also for long-term dialysis despite the expense involved. In haemofiltration, a 'high flux' membrane very permeable to water and solutes is used. Fluid and molecules of molecular weight 6000–12 000 in size are removed by convection. Twenty-five to 30 litres of ultrafiltrate can be removed at one 4-h session — the equivalent of a GFR of 17–20 ml/min for that day. The advantages over haemodialysis are less hypotension and hypoxia during treatment, better control of hypertension, improved control of plasma lipids, peripheral and autonomic neuropathy. One disadvantage is that to maintain volume homeostasis large quantities of crystalloid solution have to be reinfused such that the net removal of fluid may only be 2 litres per session. It may, however, be useful in patients with a tendency to hypotension on dialysis who have not benefited from a change to bicarbonate haemodialysis.

Continuous prolonged haemofiltration can be used in acute renal failure to remove fluid overload and will also permit parenteral feeding to be achieved without fluid restriction or overload. It is most useful in patients with multiorgan failure and cardiovascular instability. Several methods have evolved. Continuous arteriovenous haemofiltration can be achieved by the addition of continuous dialysis to this technique (CAVHD) (Stevens *et al.*, 1988). A further development, continuous venous–venous haemofiltration (CVVH), avoids the necessity for arterial access but requires a blood pump.

Drugs and the kidney

Many drugs are excreted at least partially by the kidney and dosage schedules require modification frequently in patients with chronic renal failure. Drugs which are excreted by non-renal routes may require dosage modification also as the volume of distribution, protein binding of the drug and the response of the target organ may all be altered in renal failure. In patients undergoing renal replacement therapy, either haemodialysis or peritoneal dialysis may complicate dosage regimens further as some drugs are removed by these routes. The particular problems of agents used in anaesthetic practice have been dealt with in Chapter 62. In this chapter, the general principles of drug modification in renal failure are discussed.

In uraemia, some drugs which are excreted normally by the kidney, may be metabolized or excreted by other organs, notably the liver and gastrointestinal tract. Conversely, drug accumulation may occur when normal hepatic pathways such as oxidation, conjugation and acetylation are affected adversely by the biochemical effects of uraemia. Chronic renal failure also affects the protein binding of certain drugs. Drugs which are anionic, including warfarin, frusemide, phenytoin, sulphonamides and salicylates are less protein bound in uraemic patients. Nonionic drugs, such as propranolol, morphine and diazepam are not affected in this manner by renal failure. In nephrotic patients, the reduction in plasma albumin concentration will also alter the binding of acidic drugs.

If more than 50% of a drug or its active metabolite undergoes renal excretion, the dosage usually requires to be modified when the GFR is less than 40–50 ml/min or the serum creatinine is greater than 200–250 µmol/litre. The loading dose of a particular drug should not be changed but thereafter the dosage can be modified by prolonging the interval between doses or by reducing subsequent doses. Recommended doses for patients with chronic renal failure are given in the *British National Formulary*.

References

Braun W.E. (1990) Longterm complications of renal transplantation. *Kidney International* 37, 1363−73.

Brescia M.J., Cimino J.E., Appel K. & Hurwich B.J. (1966) Chronic haemodialysis using venipuncture and a surgically created arteriovenous fistula. *New England Journal of Medicine* 275, 1089−92.

Bricker N.S. (1982) Sodium homeostasis in chronic renal disease. *Kidney International* 21, 886−97.

Casati S., Passerini P. & Campise M.R. (1987) Benefits and risks of protracted treatment with human recombinant erythropoietin in patients having haemodialysis. *British Medical Journal* 295, 1017−20.

Cockburn I. (1986) Cyclosporin A: a clinical evaluation of drug interactions. *Transplantation Proceedings* 18, 50−5.

Contreras P., Later R., Navarro J., Touraine J.L., Freyria A.M. & Traeger J. (1982) Molecules in the middle molecular weight range. *Nephron* 32, 193−201.

Curtis J.R. (1990) Interventions in chronic renal failure. *British Medical Journal* 301, 622−4.

DeFonzo R.A. & Alvestrand A. (1980) Glucose intolerance in uraemia: site and mechanism. *American Journal of Clinical Nutrition* 33, 1438−45.

Deutsch S., Bastron R.D., Pierce G.C. & Vandam L.D. (1969) The effects of anaesthesia with thiopentone, nitrous oxide, narcotics and neuromuscular blocking on renal function in normal man. *British Journal of Anaesthesia* 41, 807−14.

Editorial (1989) Cytomegalovirus infection in allograft recipients. *Lancet* i, 303−4.

El Nahas A.M. & Coles G.A. (1986) Dietary treatment of chronic renal failure: ten unanswered questions. *Lancet* i, 597−600.

European Dialysis and Transplantation Association Registry (1986) *Demography of Dialysis and Transplantation in Europe 1984* pp. 1−8.

Feest T.G., Mistry C.D., Grimes D.S. & Mallick N.P. (1990) Incidence of advanced chronic renal failure and the need for end stage renal replacement treatment. *British Medical Journal* 301, 897−900.

Fenves A.Z., Emmett M., White M.G., Greenway G. & Michaels D.B. (1986) Carpal tunnel syndrome with cystic bone lesions secondary to amyloidosis in chronic haemodialysis patients. *American Journal of Kidney Diseases* 7, 130−4.

Fisher J.W. (1980) Mechanism of the anaemia of chronic renal failure. *Nephron* 25, 106−11.

Gandhi V.C., Humayun H.M., Ing T.S., Daugirdas J.T., Jablokow V.R., Iwatsuki S., Geis P. & Hano J. (1980) Sclerotic thickening of the peritoneal membrane in maintenance peritoneal dialysis patients. *Archives of Internal Medicine* 140, 120−3.

Gentil M.A., Carriazo A., Pavon M.I., Rosado M., Castillo D., Ramos B., Algarra G.R., Tejuca F., Banasco V.P. & Milan J.A. (1991) Comparison of survival in continuous ambulatory peritoneal dialysis and hospital haemodialysis: a multicentric study. *Nephrology, Dialysis, Transplantation* 6, 444−51.

Giovannetti S. (1986) Answers to ten questions on the dietary treatment of chronic renal failure. *Lancet* ii, 1140−2.

Goldman M., Vanherweghem J.L., Liesnard C., Dolle N., Sprecher S., Thiry, L. & Toussaint C. (1986) Markers of AIDS-associated virus in a haemodialysis unit. *Nephrology, Dialysis, Transplantation* 1, 130.

Henderson I.S., Beattie T.J. & Kennedy A.C. (1980) Dopamine hydrochloride in oliguric states. *Lancet* ii, 827−8.

Hricik D.E., Browning P.J., Kopelman R., Goorno W.E., Madias N.E. & Dzau V.J. (1983) Captopril induced functional renal insufficiency in patients with bilateral renal artery stenosis or renal artery stenosis in a solitary kidney. *New England Journal of Medicine* 308, 373−6.

Innes A., Dennis M.J., Morgan A.G., Ryan J.J. & Burden R.P. (1993) Attitudes to elective pre-transplant blood transfusions in UK renal units. *Transplantation* 53, 934−5.

Jones R.M., Murie J.A., Allen R.D., Ting A. & Morris P.J. (1988) Triple therapy in cadaver renal transplantation. *British Journal of Surgery* 75, 4−8.

Lens X.M., Montoliu J., Cases A., Campastrol J.M. & Revert L. (1989) Treatment of hyperkalaemia in renal failure: salbutamol v. insulin. *Nephrology, Dialysis, Transplantation* 4, 228−32.

Linas S.L., Peterson L.N., Anderson R.J., Aisenbrey G.A., Simon F.R. & Berl T. (1979) Mechanisms of renal potassium conservation in the rat. *Kidney International* 15, 601−11.

Lindsay R.M. & Smith A.M. (1989) Practical use of anticoagulants. In *Replacement of Renal Function by Dialysis* (Ed. Maher J.F.) pp. 246−75. Kluwer, Dordrecht.

Locatelli F., Alberti D., Graziani G., Buccianti G., Redaelli B. & Giangrande A. (1991) Prospective, randomised multicentre trial of effect of protein restriction on progression of chronic renal insufficiency. *Lancet* 337, 1299−304.

McGeown M.G. (1990) Prevalence of advanced renal failure in Northern Ireland. *British Medical Journal* 301, 900−3.

MacLeod A.M. & Thomson A.W. (1991) FK 506: an immunosuppressant for the 1990s. *Lancet* 337, 25−7.

Madaio M.P. (1990) Renal biopsy. *Kidney International* 38, 529−43.

Mall G., Huther W., Schneider J., Lundin P. & Ritz E. (1990) Diffuse intermyocardiocytic fibrosis in uraemia patients. *Nephrology, Dialysis, Transplantation* 5, 39−44.

Malluche H. & Faugere M.-C. (1990) Renal bone disease 1990: an unmet challenge for the nephrologist. *Kidney International* 38, 193−211.

Maschio G., Tessitore M., D'Angelo A., Morachiello P., Previato G. & Fiaschi E. (1980) Early dietary phosphorus restriction and calcium supplementation in the prevention of renal osteodystrophy. *American Journal of Clinical Nutrition* 33, 1546−54.

Mihatsch M.J., Steiner K., Abeywickrama K.H., Landman J. & Thiel G. (1988) Risk factors for the development of chronic cyclosporin nephrotoxicity. *Clinical Nephrology* 29, 165−75.

Miller T.R., Anderson R.J., Linas S.L., Henrich W.L., Berns A.S., Gabow P.A. & Schrier R.W. (1978) Urinary diagnostic indices in acute renal failure. *Annals of Internal Medicine* 89, 47−50.

Milliner D.S., Nebeker H.G., Ott S.M., Andress D.L., Sherrard D.J., Alfrey A.C., Slatopolsky E.A. & Coburn J.W. (1984) Use of desferrioxamine infusion test in the diagnosis of aluminium related osteodystrophy. *Annals of Internal Medicine* **101**, 775–80.

Moran S.M. & Myers B.D. (1985) Pathophysiology of protracted acute renal failure in man. *Journal of Clinical Investigation* **76**, 1440–8.

Morgan A.G. & Burden R.P. (1986) Effect of continuous ambulatory peritoneal dialysis on a British renal unit. *British Medical Journal* **293**, 935–7.

Morris P.J., Chan L., French M.E. & Ting A. (1982) Low dose oral prednisolone in renal transplantation. *Lancet* **i**, 525–7.

Muirhead N., Adami S., Sandler L.M., Fraser R.A. Catto G.R.D., Edward N. & O'Riordan J.L.H. (1982) Long-term effects of 1,25-dihydroxyvitamin D_3 and 24,25-dihydroxyvitamin D_3 in renal osteodystrophy. *Quarterly Journal of Medicine* **51**, 427–44.

Norman D.J. (1988) An overview of the use of the monoclonal antibody OKT3 in renal transplantation. *Transplantation Proceedings* **20**, 1248–52.

Olsen J.L., Hostetter T.H., Rennke H.G., Brenner B.M. & Ventakatachlam M.A. (1982) Altered glomerular permselectivity and progressive sclerosis following extreme ablation of renal mass. *Kidney International* **22**, 112–26.

Opelz G. (1987) Improved kidney graft survival in non-transfused recipients. *Transplantation Proceedings* **19**, 147–52.

Opelz G., Mytilineos J., Scherer S. *et al.* (1991) Survival of DNA HLA-DR typed and matched cadaver kidney transplants. *Lancet* **338**, 461–3.

Parkinson I.S., Ward M.K., Feest T.G., Fawcett R.W.P. & Kerr D.N.S. (1979) Fracturing dialysis osteodystrophy and dialysis encephalopathy. *Lancet* **i**, 406–9.

Penn I. (1990) Cancers complicating organ transplantation. *New England Journal of Medicine* **323**, 1767–9.

Priebe H.J., Skillman J.J., Bushnell L.S., Long P.C. & Silen W. (1980) Antacid versus cimetidine in preventing acute gastrointestinal bleeding. *New England Journal of Medicine* **302**, 426–30.

Quinton E., Dillard D. & Scribner B.H. (1960) Cannulation of blood vessels for prolonged haemodialysis. *Transactions of the American Society of Artificial Internal Organs* **6**, 104–13.

Rainford D.J. (1977) The immediate care of acute renal failure.

Anaesthesia **32**, 277–81.

Remuzzi G. (1988) Bleeding in renal failure. *Lancet* **i**, 1205–8.

Rocker G.M., Morgan A.G. & Shale D.J. (1988) Pulmonary oedema and renal failure. *Nephrology, Dialysis, Transplantation* **3**, 244–6.

Rudge C.J. (1986) Acquired cystic disease of the kidney: serious or irrelevant. *British Medical Journal* **293**, 1186–7.

Sanderson P.J. (1989) Selective decontamination of the digestive tract. *British Medical Journal* **299**, 1413–14.

Shemesh O., Golbetz H., Kriss J.P. & Myers B.D. (1985) Limitations of creatinine as a filtration marker in glomerulopathic patients. *Kidney International* **28**, 830–8.

Silberberg J.S., Barre P.E., Prichard S.S. & Sniderman A.D. (1989) Impact of left ventricular hypertrophy on survival in end stage renal disease. *Kidney International* **36**, 286–90.

Slingeneyer A., Canaud B. & Mion C. (1983) Permanent loss of ultrafiltration capacity of the peritoneum in long term peritoneal dialysis: an epidemiological study. *Nephron* **33**, 133–8.

Stevens P.E., Riley B., Davies S.P., Gower P.E., Brown E.A. & Kox W. (1988) Continuous arteriovenous haemodialysis in critically ill patients. *Lancet* **ii**, 150–2.

Suda S., Weidman P., Saxenhofer H., Cottier C., Shaw S.G. & Ferrier C. (1988) Atrial natriuretic factor in mild to moderate chronic renal failure. *Hypertension* **11**, 483–90.

Swainson C.P. & Craig K.C. (1991) Effects of atrial natriuretic peptide (99–126) in chronic renal disease in man. *Nephrology, Dialysis, Transplantation* **6**, 336–41.

Swann R.C. & Merrill J.P. (1953) The clinical course of acute renal failure. *Medicine* **32**, 215–92.

Turney J.H., Marshall D.H., Brownjohn A.M., Ellis C.M. & Parsons F.M. (1990) The evolution of acute renal failure 1956–1988. *Quarterly Journal of Medicine* **74**, 83–104.

Warnock D.G. (1988) Uremic acidosis. *Kidney International* **34**, 278–87.

Webb J.A.W. (1990) Ultrasonography in the diagnosis of renal obstruction. *British Medical Journal* **301**, 944–6.

Williams P.S., Fass G. & Bone J.N. (1988) Renal pathology and proteinuria determine progression in untreated mild, moderate chronic renal failure. *Quarterly Journal of Medicine* **67**, 343–52.

Cardiovascular Failure

I. McA. LEDINGHAM, I. H. WRIGHT AND J. L. VINCENT

Cardiovascular failure may be defined as a pathological state in which the tissues are perfused insufficiently in relation to their metabolic needs. In the context of the intensive therapy unit (ITU), this condition may have a variety of causes and often demands prompt and aggressive intervention.

In order to understand and treat cardiovascular failure in the ITU, it is necessary to possess a good working knowledge of the relevant cardiovascular physiology, to understand the underlying physiological derangement caused by specific disease processes, to know the indications for, and the limitations and possible hazards of, available monitoring techniques, to be aware of the spectrum of treatment options and their rationale and to be able to set treatment goals which correlate with increased survival.

Applied physiology

Regulation of cardiac output (see also Chapter 12)

Stroke volume

Cardiac output is determined by the product of stroke volume and heart rate. Stroke volume is determined by the preload, contractility and afterload (Table 86.1).

Preload

Starling's law of the heart states that the force of contraction is a function of the length of the myocardial fibres prior to contraction: an increase in length (preload) produces a more forceful contraction. In the intact heart, preload is taken to be the volume of blood in the ventricle at the end of diastole: the end-diastolic volume (EDV). For any given EDV, the end-diastolic pressure (EDP) depends on the compliance of the ventricle: the less compliant (i.e. stiffer)

the ventricle, the higher the EDP for any EDV. It is possible to measure EDV using radionuclide imaging, and modern techniques using short half-life tracers such as ^{195}Au allow repeated estimations of EDV (Matthay & Berger, 1983). There are technical problems of separation of counts from the different chambers of the heart, and the technique is expensive, and not available widely. For these reasons, it is usual to measure EDP as an index of preload, although this involves certain assumptions which if unrecognized may be misleading.

The pressure−volume relationship is alinear (Fig. 86.1) such that at higher volumes, a further small increase in EDV causes a disproportionate increase in EDP. Compliance of the ventricle is not only determined by the elasticity of the myocardium but also by the geometry and wall thickness of the ventricle and ultimately, by the constricting effect of the intact pericardium (Belenkie et al., 1992; Calvin & Ascah, 1992). A single curve cannot describe ventricular compliance, and a family of parallel curves provides a more accurate illustration of changes in compliance. For example, a decrease in compliance associated with ischaemia or the use of some inotropic drugs shifts the curve upwards and to the left, and conversely an increase in compliance shifts the curve downwards and to the right (Fig. 86.1).

It can be seen, therefore, that a high EDP need not reflect a high EDV. However, although compliance may be altered acutely either by disease or treatment, it is still valid to investigate the relationship between EDP and EDV, and this can be achieved best by noting the response to a fluid challenge (see below). A rapid increase in EDP (or some other pressure taken as an indication of preload) in response to a bolus of fluid, indicates that the ventricular pressure−volume relationship lies on the steeply ascending portion of the compliance curve, and that further volume expansion should be considered carefully.

Many factors affect preload in the intact patient.

Table 86.1 Determinants of stroke volume

Factors affecting preload

Increase	Decrease
Fluid infusion*	Hypovolaemia
Venoconstriction	Venodilatation
Posture	Raised intrathoracic pressure
Leg elevation	Raised intrapericardial pressure
Muscle pump	Decreased ventricular compliance
	Loss of atrial transport

Factors affecting contractility

Increase	Decrease
Sympathetic stimulation	Ischaemia
Endogenous catecholamines	Hypoxia
Inotropes*	Severe sepsis
Improved myocardial oxygenation	Metabolic derangement
Tachycardia	Negatively inotropic drugs*

Factors affecting afterload

Increase	Decrease
High aortic impedance	Low aortic impedance
Arteriolar constriction	Arteriolar dilatation
	Vasodilating agents*
Increased ventricular radius	Decreased ventricular radius
	Intra-aortic balloon pump*

* Iatrogenic influence.

The venous return to the atrium is determined by the balance between circulating volume and venous capacitance, and the presence or absence of the skeletal 'muscle pump', and is reduced by a high intrathoracic or intrapericardial pressure [as a consequence of, for example, intermittent positive-pressure ventilation (IPPV) with or without positive end-expiratory pressure (PEEP), pericardial fibrosis or tamponade]. The loss of atrial transport during arrhythmias or ventricular pacing may reduce preload crucially, especially in a non-compliant ventricle, as may also atrioventricular valve dysfunction (Ganong, 1983). The preload is altered also by changes in myocardial contractility and afterload (see below).

Contractility

It is a useful concept to plot a graph with preload on the abscissa and some parameter of ventricular performance on the ordinate, such as stroke volume (end-diastolic volume — end-systolic volume) or more usually stroke work (mean arterial pressure × stroke volume) or even in the clinical setting, cardiac output. Such a graph is described as a ventricular function curve (VFC) (Fig. 86.2) and allows contractility to be deduced. If the afterload (see below) is held constant, increasing contractility produces a greater degree of work for any given preload. This is seen clinically with sympathetic nerve stimulation, release of catecholamines or exogenously administered inotropes. The VFC moves upward and to the

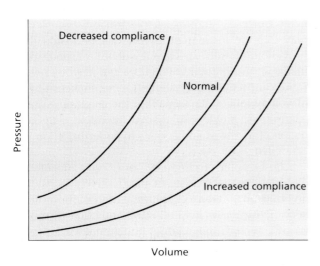

Fig. 86.1 Ventricular compliance curves (see text for details).

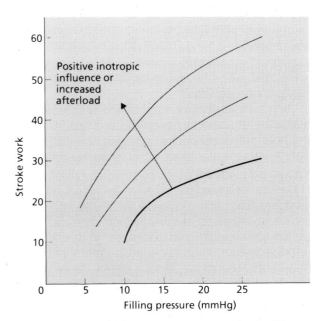

Fig. 86.2 Ventricular function curves (see text for details).

left. The converse applies with negatively inotropic influences such as hypoxia, ischaemia, metabolic and acid–base derangements and certain drugs (see below) (Braunwald *et al.*, 1977). The concept of the VFC is useful clinically, as exemplified by the technique of 'fluid challenge'. A bolus of colloid (of the order of 50–200 ml depending on the size and condition of the patient) is given over a short period of time, and this may be repeated. Variables reflecting preload and myocardial performance are measured [e.g. pulmonary capillary wedge pressure (PCWP) and cardiac output], and when further fluid challenges do not result in improvements in myocardial performance, the circulating volume should not be expanded further. The end-point of a series of fluid challenges is indicated usually by a rapid increase in filling pressures in response to a bolus of fluid (Vincent, 1991). This increase reflects the position of the ventricle on the steeply ascending part of the compliance curve (Fig. 86.1) and implies that further volume challenge produces only an increase in venous pressures with the attendant risk of systemic or pulmonary oedema.

Afterload

The tension in the ventricular wall during systole is taken to be the afterload on the ventricle, and is determined partly by the resistance against which the ventricle ejects blood, and partly by the physical characteristics of the ventricle (Braunwald *et al.*, 1977).

The outflow resistance is determined by the aortic impedance (rate of change of pressure divided by instantaneous aortic flow, i.e. a reflection of aortic compliance) and arteriolar run off. For any given stroke volume, if the aorta and major vessels are non-compliant (e.g. atherosclerotic) or the patient vasoconstricted, the pressure generated, and thus the afterload, are increased.

Ventricular wall tension is related to ventricular radius and intracavitary pressure by Laplace's law: $P = 2T/R$ (P = intracavitary pressure, T = wall tension, R = ventricular radius), i.e. for any given pressure, as the radius increases, so does the wall tension.

The clinical importance of afterload is that for any given preload and contractility, if the afterload increases, either the ventricular stroke work (and oxygen consumption) has to increase, or cardiac output decreases.

Heart rate

The denervated sinoatrial node depolarizes spontaneously at a rate of approximately 120 beats/min, and the predominant vagal tone acting on the heart slows this rate to 55–100 beats/min in the normal resting heart.

As the heart rate slows, diastole lengthens, which leads to increased ventricular filling, increased end-diastolic volume, and cardiac output is therefore maintained. At very low rates, e.g. less than 40 beats/min, it is not possible for the normal heart to increase stroke volume sufficiently to compensate, and the diseased heart copes even less well. This is especially so if the slow rate is nodal or ventricular in origin.

As the heart rate increases, diastole shortens, and diastolic stress relaxation produces a reduction in compliance (Covell & Ross, 1973). Diastolic filling is therefore compromised, and stroke volume and cardiac output tend to decrease. This effect is overcome at rates up to 180 beats/min by the intrinsic increase in contractility caused by an increased heart rate (the 'treppe' effect; Braunwald *et al.*, 1977) and the positive inotropic effect of sympathetic stimulation (which is usually the cause of the tachycardia) which leads to a relative shortening of systole. At very high rates (180 beats/min or greater), diastolic filling is so compromised that this compensation is ineffective, especially if atrial transport is lost as in many supraventricular arrhythmias, or if ventricular function is compromised by ventricular arrhythmias or myocardial depression (Ganong, 1983).

Determinants of myocardial metabolism
(Table 86.2)

The haemodynamic alterations in disease and ITU treatment have profound implications for myocardial metabolism. Direct measurement of adequacy of perfusion and oxygenation of the myocardium is difficult. Coronary sinus lactate or cardiac enzyme levels may indicate inadequate myocardial perfusion, but provide only retrospective evidence of poor perfusion and/or myocardial damage and may not reveal significant regional ischaemia. Acute changes in the ECG may reflect ischaemia, but the commonly used, continuous, single-lead display monitors only one region of the heart and serious hypoperfusion can be concealed.

Echo-Doppler techniques can now document dyskinetic/akinetic areas of progressively ischaemic myocardium. Transoesophageal techniques have been particularly helpful in cardiovascular monitoring although they cannot be maintained for long periods of time (Thomas & Weyman, 1991; Reichert *et al.*, 1992). Nor can they be readily used during such

Table 86.2 Determinants of myocardial oxygen metabolism

Oxygen supply
Arterial oxygen content
Coronary vessel calibre (the concentration of myocardial
    metabolic products and the P_{CO_2})
Coronary perfusion pressure (diastolic — LVEDP)
Coronary perfusion time (1/heart rate)

Oxygen demand
External work (mean arterial pressure × stroke volume)
    Preload
    Contractility
    Aortic compliance and arteriolar run-off
Internal work (during isovolumic contraction)
    Pressure generated
    Ventricular radius
Heart rate

critical periods as tracheal intubation or extubation.

A knowledge of the determinants of myocardial oxygen supply and demand allows prediction of the effects of alteration of haemodynamic parameters.

Myocardial oxygen supply

This is determined by arterial oxygen content (proportional to haemoglobin concentration × oxygen saturation) and coronary blood flow, which depends on coronary vessel calibre, perfusion pressure [diastolic pressure — left ventricular end-diastolic pressure (LVEDP)] and perfusion time (i.e. duration of diastole).

Inotropes, pressor agents, vasodilators and P_{CO_2} may affect coronary vessel calibre directly (except in rigid, atherosclerotic vessels). However, the predominant determinant of calibre is accumulation of local metabolites (in response to increased myocardial work) which causes vasodilatation and overrides the direct effects of vasoactive drugs.

The pressure in the left ventricle during systole is slightly greater than in the aorta, and subendocardial vessels are compressed by the increased wall tension during systole, so perfusion of the left ventricular muscle occurs predominantly during diastole (although the atria and right ventricle are perfused throughout the cardiac cycle). Perfusion pressure depends, therefore, on the differences between aortic diastolic pressure and LVEDP. As heart rate increases, diastole shortens, and perfusion time is therefore inversely proportional to heart rate.

Coronary blood flow is affected also by viscosity of blood, and may be decreased locally by atherosclerotic lesions.

Myocardial oxygen demand

Oxygen demand is proportional to the amount of work performed by the ventricle. Stroke work is calculated as the product of mean arterial pressure and stroke volume (although it should be noted that this is only an estimate of external work performed by the ventricle, and takes no account of internal work performed when the inflow valve is closed and the outflow valve has not yet opened). Factors which increase myocardial oxygen consumption are therefore increased ventricular wall tension, increased contractility, increased stroke volume and increased heart rate. 'Pressure' work raises oxygen consumption much more than 'volume' work, reflecting the internal work performed in increasing wall tension before the ejection phase (Sonnenblick & Skelton, 1971) and this demonstrates the importance of afterload as a prime determinant of myocardial oxygen consumption.

Maintenance of intravascular volume

There is a complex series of inter-relating mechanisms to maintain circulating volume and vascular capacity within the normal range, which in the short term are protective but may cause further problems eventually and indeed lead to the breakdown of cellular integrity. These mechanisms may be considered under the headings of neurohumoral and passive responses.

Neurohumoral response (Fig. 86.3)

Reduction in blood volume stimulates vascular mechanoreceptors in the great vessels of the chest leading to release of antidiuretic hormone (ADH). Baroreceptor stimulation increases heart rate and causes peripheral vasoconstriction, and activation of the renin–angiotensin–aldosterone axis leads to salt and water retention. Afferent stimuli integrated in the hypothalamus cause release of stress hormones from the anterior pituitary, chiefly adrenocorticotrophic hormone (ACTH) but also growth hormone and prolactin, and lead also to a massive outpouring of catecholamines from the adrenal medulla, in addition to direct sympathetic stimulation. The net result of these responses is to reduce vascular capacity by sympathetic nervous system and catecholamine-induced vasoconstriction, to increase circulating

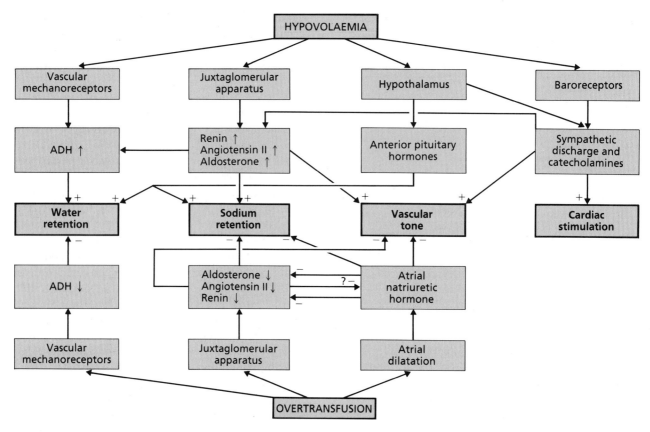

Fig. 86.3 The neurohumoral response to hypovolaemia and overtransfusion. ADH, antidiuretic hormone.

volume by causing salt and water retention and incidentally to mobilize energy reserves directly and as a result of insulin antagonism. Release of β-endorphin from the anterior pituitary and met-enkephalin from the adrenal medulla caused by these same stimuli tends to antagonize the actions of catecholamines (Watson *et al.*, 1984).

An increased blood volume partially reverses the response noted above and causes vasodilatation and diuresis, chiefly via reduced plasma ADH and renin concentrations. Atrial natriuretic hormone causes a natriuresis by increasing glomerular filtration rate, exerting an antirenin and antiangiotensin action, and directly relaxing vascular smooth muscle. Atrial distension is a key factor responsible for the release of atrial natriuretic hormone.

Passive response

The transfer of fluid between the intravascular and interstitial fluid compartments is governed by Starling's hypothesis that a net outward hydrostatic force is balanced by a slightly smaller inward oncotic force. Thus, there is a net outflow of fluid from the

intravascular compartment into the interstitial compartment under normal circumstances, and this returns to the circulation via the lymphatics.

The balance of these forces is altered in cardiovascular failure. In the early stages of shock, the effects of sympathetic stimulation result in constriction of the resistance vessels on both sides of the capillary bed. Precapillary resistance is increased (by arteriolar constriction) to a greater extent than postcapillary (venular) resistance. This reduces the intravascular pressure so that there is net transfer of fluid from the interstitial space to the intravascular space. Both the gel and the free fluid phases of the interstitium are involved (Haljamäe, 1984), and because the interstitial compartment contains approximately four times the volume of fluid compared with the intravascular compartment, there is considerable scope for autotransfusion to occur. However, as the shock process continues and in the absence of effective resuscitation, there is a marked change in vascular reactivity. The arteriolar constriction 'fades' much more rapidly than venular constriction, and the accumulation of local metabolites such as lactate has a greater vasodilatory effect on arterioles than venules. The result is an increased mean capillary pressure which causes net transfer of fluid initially into the interstitium and later into the cells. This process is exacerbated by the increase in capillary permeability induced by the release of various vasodilators in severe sepsis.

Metabolic response to cardiovascular failure

Hormonal and substrate variations (Table 86.3)

The initial metabolic response to injury is uniform, whatever the mechanism of the injury. Hyperglycaemia occurs early, and increased uptake of precursor substrates such as lactate, pyruvate and gluconeogenic amino acids cause increased hepatic glucose production (Wilmore et al., 1980). The hormones adrenaline and cortisol, released as part of the systemic response to injury, and glucagon, released by adrenaline, have a synergistic hyperglycaemic action (Heath, 1980). Plasma adrenaline concentrations increase rapidly, causing extensive muscle glycolysis, and the lactate produced is converted to glucose in the liver. Glucagon increases later, reaching a peak within 2 h, and stimulates hepatic glycogenolysis, gluconeogenesis and amino acid uptake. Cortisol, released rapidly and in proportion to the severity of the insult (Stoner et al., 1979), increases and prolongs the action of adrenaline and glucagon, and stimulates peripheral release of amino acids. Relative insensitivity to insulin occurs 2–7 days after injury; this is termed insulin resistance and potentiates the hyperglycaemia.

Table 86.3 Metabolic response to injury

Hormonal response	Substrate response
Increased adrenaline	*Carbohydrate*
Increased glucagon	Increased glycogenolysis
Increased cortisol	Increased peripheral glycolysis
	Increased hepatic gluconeogenesis
	Increased lactate and pyruvate
	Increased glucose (late fall in sepsis)
	Lipid
	Increased lipolysis
	Increased free fatty acids (down in severe injury)
	Protein
	Increased visceral protein turnover
	Negative nitrogen balance

Catecholamine-induced lipolysis leads to an increase in plasma free-fatty acid concentration initially, in concert with increasing severity of injury, but this correlation no longer holds in severe injury because of poor perfusion of fat depots, and reesterification stimulated by increasing lactate concentrations (Stoner et al., 1979).

Injury causes an increase in whole-body protein turnover, breakdown increasing more than synthesis (especially in severe injury or sepsis) resulting in a net negative nitrogen balance.

These metabolic changes are exaggerated in sepsis; lipolysis is prominent and there may be a marked lipaemia. Intracellular glucose oxidation and ketone body utilization are decreased in muscle, and there is therefore increased utilization of branched-chain amino acids. Hyperglycaemia with insulin resistance is superseded by hypoglycaemia, produced by depletion of glycogen stores, depressed gluconeogenesis (Wilmore et al., 1980) and increased tissue utilization of glucose, and hypoinsulinaemia from depressed pancreatic secretion associated with high plasma catecholamine concentrations.

Plasma lactate concentration correlates with severity of injury as shown by the Injury Severity Score (Stoner et al., 1979) or the mortality rate (Bakker et al., 1991). This may reflect hypoperfusion although endotoxin may increase lactate levels by altering the pyruvate dehydrogenase enzyme complex even in the absence of cellular hypoxia (Vary et al., 1988).

Cellular dysfunction

Failure of perfusion of the respiring tissues deprives the cells of oxygen and substrate, and causes inability to remove products of cellular metabolism. This damages the cell in three ways: altered cell volume regulation, altered energy metabolism and intracellular release of lysosomal enzymes. Anaerobic metabolism leads to a reduction in cellular adenosine triphosphate (ATP) content. This essential energy source for the ionic pump of the plasma membrane is broken down normally to adenosine diphosphate (ADP) and phosphate in the presence of ATPase. The absence of high-energy phosphate bonds leads to depression of pump function and cell swelling, the cells tending to approach Gibbs–Donnan equilibrium with an increase of intracellular sodium, calcium and water content and a loss of potassium and magnesium.

When oxygen tension decreases to below 0.1 kPa (0.75 mmHg) in the mitochondria (Nunn, 1977) electron transport stops immediately. Oxidative phosphorylation is uncoupled and ATP production ceases, and eventually structural changes appear in the outer and inner mitochondrial membranes. These mark the 'point of no return' (Trump *et al.*, 1976) beyond which the mitochondria and therefore the cells are damaged irreparably.

ATP deficiency and intracellular lactic acidosis alter calcium flow within the cell, and the excess intracellular calcium has been postulated as a major cause of irreversibility of damage in ischaemia (Jennings, 1976). The reduced intracellular pH causes alteration in lysosomal structure and function leading to release of hydrolases from the lysosomes. This seems to be a late effect however, and not a causative event in the sequence of cellular derangement (Trump *et al.*, 1976).

Aetiology of shock

The four classic clinical subdivisions of shock (Table 86.4) are discussed in this section. Their causes, the resulting primary physiological insults and compensatory reactions are described. The clinical pictures, and the effects on myocardial metabolism and

Table 86.4 Aetiology of shock

Hypovolaemic shock
Haemorrhage, oedema
Burns
Salt and water deficits
e.g. Addison's disease
Gastrointestinal fistulae
Diabetes insipidus
Cardiogenic shock
Primary myocardial failure
e.g. Ischaemia
Arrhythmias
Valvular damage
Cardiomyopathy
Secondary myocardial failure
e.g. Drugs
Hypoxia
Acute rise in afterload
Obstructive shock
Pulmonary embolism
Tamponade
Aortic dissection
Distributive shock
Sepsis
Anaphylaxis
Late stages of hypovolaemic shock

tissue perfusion follow logically from these descriptions, although the complexity of septic shock makes interpretation difficult.

Hypovolaemia

The effects of hypovolaemia vary with its nature, severity and duration, the patient's age and general health, and with the speed and adequacy of resuscitation. The causes of hypovolaemia are well known, have been reviewed recently (Ledingham & Ramsay, 1986) and are therefore not considered further. Whatever the cause, the primary physiological insult is a reduction in venous return which causes reduction in cardiac output and a reduction in major organ perfusion. In early and uncomplicated hypovolaemia, the intravascular space is replenished at the expense of the interstitial space. The neurohumoral response to hypovolaemia causes salt and water retention, sympathetic stimulation of the heart and peripheral vasoconstriction which tends to redistribute blood centrally, notably improving perfusion of the heart and the brain at the expense of skin, muscle and splanchnic circulation.

The cumulative effect of the primary insult and the compensatory mechanisms leads to the development of the typical clinical picture: clouding of consciousness, tachypnoea, pallor, hypotension, tachycardia, poor peripheral perfusion and oliguria.

Prompt and effective resuscitation reverses this picture. However, if the shock is prolonged or especially severe, secondary complications may arise as a consequence of reduced perfusion of the heart and other organs.

The effect of hypoperfusion on the heart is to reduce coronary perfusion pressure, and the compensatory tachycardia reduces the duration of coronary perfusion. In addition, arterial oxygen content is often reduced as a result of anaemia and hypoxia. Sympathetic stimulation increases heart rate and contractility, and peripheral vasoconstriction increases afterload. The net effect of these changes is to reduce myocardial oxygen supply and increase myocardial oxygen demand, which may cause myocardial failure, especially in elderly patients with pre-existing cardiac disease.

Prolonged ischaemia causes irreversible cellular dysfunction as noted above, but the susceptibility of different cells is variable. Astrocytes cease to function after seconds, whilst skeletal muscle functions anaerobically for 30 min, and hepatocytes for several hours. The effects of hypovolaemia may be complicated by absorption of endotoxin or translocation of bacteria from underperfused bowel (Haglund & Lundgren, 1978; Wardle, 1978). Ultimately therefore, a patient with hypovolaemic shock may manifest signs also of cardiogenic or septic shock as a preterminal event.

Cardiogenic shock

Cardiogenic shock results from pump failure, a mechanical dysfunction which is caused usually by myocardial infarction involving more than 40% of the ventricle. It may be especially severe where rupture of a papillary muscle or a ventricular septal defect interferes with normal forward flow of blood.

In the past, attention has focused on left ventricular dysfunction, but the important role of acute right ventricular dysfunction is increasingly recognized (Ducas & Prewitt, 1988). Right ventricular infarction is relatively rare as an isolated entity. Much more common is right ventricular dysfunction resulting from increase in right ventricular afterload, the right ventricle being unable to generate high intracavitary pressures (Matthay & Berger, 1983; Sibbald et al., 1986). Failure of the right ventricle causes distension of the systemic venous system which therefore sequesters a proportion of the intravascular volume, left ventricular preload decreases, and thus, cardiac output diminishes (Furey et al., 1984). Right ventricular dilatation may also occur in an attempt to maintain right ventricular output. The interventricular septum bulges into the left ventricle causing an acute decrease in left ventricular compliance and consequently in cardiac output (Sibbald & Driedger, 1983).

Even if right or left ventricular failure is the primary cause of the cardiogenic shock, failure is exacerbated by brady- or tachyarrhythmias.

The initial physiological derangement is therefore reduced cardiac output, with acutely decreased ventricular compliance resulting in high ventricular end-diastolic pressures in the face of normal or slightly increased end-diastolic volumes. Increased pulmonary and systemic venous pressures result in net outflow of fluid from the intravascular to the interstitial space, whilst the neurohumoral response tends to cause salt and water retention, peripheral vasoconstriction and increased sympathetic stimulation of the heart. There is usually a tachycardia but contractility may be little enhanced because of intrinsic myocardial dysfunction.

The clinical picture is similar to hypovolaemia with clouding of consciousness, tachypnoea and orthopnoea, hypotension, tachycardia, poor peripheral perfusion, an elevated jugular venous pressure and oliguria.

Pulmonary oedema may cause hypoxia, coronary perfusion pressure and time is reduced, and coronary vessel lesions decrease myocardial oxygen supply further. Tachycardia and peripheral vasoconstriction increase myocardial oxygen demand, and the worsening myocardial oxygen supply : demand ratio may lead to further deterioration of myocardial function and increase in the size of myocardial infarction, resulting in a downward spiral of clinical deterioration.

Hypoperfusion results in cellular dysfunction (see above) and the effects are liable to be worsened by critical stenotic lesions in major vessels (e.g. the carotid and renal arteries), such that ischaemia occurs at a higher mean pressure than would otherwise be the case. As major organ dysfunction supervenes the metabolic derangement, and hypoxia worsens, endotoxaemia may occur from gut hypoperfusion, and secondary myocardial depression exacerbates the physiological derangement.

Obstructive shock

In this form of shock, the primary defect is represented by an obstruction within the cardiovascular system, such as a large pulmonary embolism, the presence of pericardial tamponade or an aortic dissection.

Distributive shock

In distributive shock, cardiac output may be increased, but altered distribution of blood flow causes hypoperfusion of respiring tissues. The prime example of this type of shock is septic shock.

Sepsis may be defined as the systemic response to microorganisms of all types. In the past it was thought that the response to sepsis depended on the organism involved but more recent work has shown that the response is host determined and is not peculiar to a specific pathogenic microorganism (Wiles et al., 1980). A proportion of septic patients proceed to frank septic shock, displaying either unexplained systemic hypotension [exceeding 10.6 kPa (80 mmHg) systolic] or reduced systemic vascular resistance (exceeding $800 \, \mathrm{dyne \cdot s \cdot cm^{-5}}$) or unexplained metabolic acidosis. Such patients comprise 1% of the hospital population, or 100 000–300 000 cases per year in the USA, with a mortality rate of around 60% (Bakker et al., 1991).

The complex cellular and humoral mechanisms

which underlie the septic response are summarized elsewhere.

The pathophysiological dysfunction in sepsis has been well characterized and reflects the combined actions of various mediators on vascular tone, patency and permeability. In the past, hyperdynamic and hypodynamic responses to sepsis have been described (MacLean et al., 1967; Kwaan & Weil, 1969) and both forms of clinical presentation are common. However, it is increasingly accepted that the hypodynamic, low cardiac output, high systemic vascular resistance picture is a result of either inadequate volume resuscitation and/or intrinsic myocardial disease (Wiles et al., 1980). It is thought that the primary response to sepsis is a profound reduction in systemic vascular resistance which is maintained until the moment of death in the majority of non-survivors, presumably as a result of locally released mediators, and that this reduction is often refractory to exogenous vasopressors, even in large doses (Parker et al., 1984a). An apparent increase in capillary permeability leads to a net outflow of fluid from the intravascular to the interstitial space (Fleck et al., 1985), and this, in addition to the peripheral vasodilatation, causes a relative hypovolaemia. Pulmonary vascular resistance is increased, and the combination of raised pulmonary arterial pressure and leaking capillaries causes interstitial and often intra-alveolar oedema formation.

In addition, myocardial function is depressed by a number of factors, including myocardial oedema, hypoxia and metabolic derangement, right heart failure (consequent upon acute increases in pulmonary vascular resistance), coronary hypoperfusion and circulating substances. Providing there is adequate volume replacement, cardiac output is increased to supranormal levels as a result of increased preload associated with dilatation of the heart (Parker et al., 1984b). Despite this compensation, the reduction in systemic vascular resistance is so profound that the patient often remains hypotensive.

The role of cytokines in the development of sepsis-related myocardial depression has been increasingly recognized in recent years. Tumour necrosis factor (TNF), interleukin-1 (IL-1), platelet activating factor (PAF), arachidonic acid metabolites and even nitric oxide have all been implicated in this myocardial depression. Interestingly, the same mediators could be involved in the peripheral and the cardiac alterations of severe sepsis. This may explain why the non-survivors from septic shock have a more severe systemic vasodilatation and also a more profound myocardial depression (Vincent et al., 1992c).

The clinical picture in volume-repleted septic shock is one of variable confusion, tachypnoea associated with a characteristic 'white-out' pattern on the chest X-ray consistent with pulmonary oedema, warm, dilated extremities with tachycardia and bounding pulse, hypotension and oliguria.

The effect on the myocardial oxygen supply: demand ratio is marked. Supply decreases as a result of decreased arterial oxygen content and decreased coronary perfusion pressure and duration. The increase in heart rate produces an increased demand, and the tendency for afterload to decline as a result of peripheral vasodilatation is counter-balanced by an increase as ventricular radius enlarges.

Cellular dysfunction results from a number of factors in sepsis. In addition to hypotension, microvascular thrombi, direct endothelial damage, increased interstitial fluid and maldistribution of blood through the capillaries, result in failure of oxygenation of the respiring tissues. Serum lactate concentrations increase markedly, reflecting imbalance between oxygen supply and demand (Bakker et al., 1991).

Pathogenesis of cardiovascular failure

The preceding section dealt with the four types of shock and made clear distinctions between them. In fact, the situation is rarely so clear: hypovolaemia may be complicated by the manifestations of sepsis in prolonged shock, sepsis may be complicated by absolute or relative hypovolaemia, and hypotension may precipitate myocardial infarction leading to cardiogenic shock. Anaphylactic shock can combine features of hypovolaemic and distributive types of shock. It is more useful for immediate therapeutic purposes to assess the underlying mechanism of the cardiovascular failure in terms of physiological dysfunction. A short summary of myocardial failure is followed by a more complete account of peripheral circulatory failure, although it should be noted that the two often coexist.

Myocardial failure

Myocardial failure may precipitate or complicate an admission to the ITU, and may result either from primary myocardial dysfunction or secondary to other disease processes or treatment (Fig. 86.4).

Primary myocardial dysfunction

The incidence of coronary artery disease increases

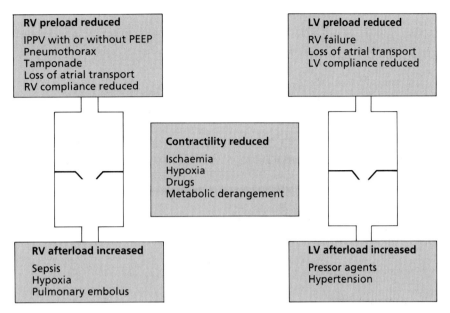

Fig. 86.4 The causes of secondary myocardial failure. RV, right ventricular; LV, left ventricular.

with increasing age, and cardiac ischaemia, with or without frank infarction, is a common finding in patients in the ITU, either causing the admission, or, as a result of adverse effects on the myocardial demand:supply ratio as detailed above, complicating other disease processes. Tachy- and brady-arrhythmias are often a cause of myocardial failure and may be difficult to treat. Rarer causes include cardiomyopathies, acute or chronic valvular dysfunction as a result of ischaemic, traumatic or infective damage, and blunt or penetrating myocardial trauma. Some of these causes are not obvious immediately in the context of a complex ITU patient, but they should be borne in mind and excluded if necessary.

Secondary myocardial dysfunction

This is probably more common in the general ITU than primary dysfunction. There may be global myocardial dysfunction or one or the other ventricle may be primarily affected.

Global dysfunction is seen in hypoxia (especially in patients with pre-existing coronary disease; Coetzee *et al.*, 1984), electrolyte imbalance (especially hypo-kalaemia) and metabolic derangement (especially acidosis). Negatively inotropic drugs such as sedative agents or beta blockers may be given therapeutically or taken in overdose. Sepsis or even hyperthermia alone may cause myocardial dysfunction.

Specific ventricular dysfunction is seen with acute changes in the preload or afterload occurring in either ventricle. For example, right ventricular preload may be reduced by a tension pneumothorax, or IPPV with or without PEEP (Fig. 86.5). Acute changes in right ventricular afterload have been discussed above, as has the inter-relationship between increased right ventricular afterload and left ventricular preload and compliance. Left ventricular afterload may be altered acutely by vasodilators or pressor agents, the effect on cardiac output depending on the balance between direct effects and changes secondary to altered myocardial perfusion.

Peripheral circulatory failure

Tissue perfusion may be inadequate as a result of disturbances in the peripheral circulation. These may result from an absolutely or relatively inadequate circulating volume, regional redistribution of blood flow, or microvascular changes including diversion of blood away from respiring tissues, intravascular thrombi and interstitial compartment expansion as a result of increases in vascular permeability.

Hypovolaemia is the most common cause of shock in a general hospital population (Ledingham *et al.*, 1974). There may be absolute hypovolaemia, as in loss of fluid from the body, transfer of fluid from the intravascular compartment to the interstitial or intracellular compartments, or to closed body cavities (e.g. pleural effusion, ascites), or relative hypovolaemia

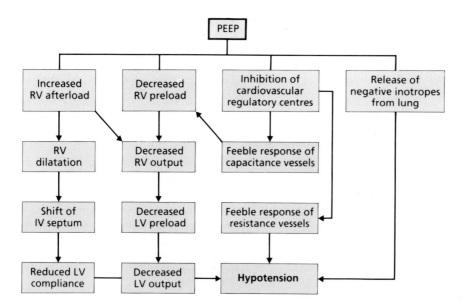

Fig. 86.5 The haemodynamic effects of PEEP. RV, right ventricular; IV, interventricular; LV, left ventricular.

produced by dilatation of blood vessels, often venous capacitance vessels.

During shock, there is autoregulation of blood flow to the brain and heart, and to a lesser extent the kidneys, mediated partly by an intrinsic property of the vascular smooth muscle and partly by accumulation of metabolites such as adenosine. However, if cardiac output reduces whilst blood flow to these organs is maintained, it implies that there is regional redistribution of blood flow such that muscle, skin and the splanchnic circulation are relatively deprived. Gilmour and colleagues (1980) showed that a 10% reduction in blood volume produced negligible alterations in arterial pressure and heart rate, but a 30% reduction in colon blood flow and oxygen availability, and Kram and colleagues (1986) showed that 30 ml/kg blood loss in a dog was associated with a linear reduction in intestinal oxygen saturation whilst renal oxygen saturation was maintained at significantly higher levels.

An important effect of this redistribution of blood flow may be a reduction in gut perfusion, which produces also a reduction in hepatic perfusion (because 80% of hepatic perfusion is via the portal vein). It has been proposed that the gut wall becomes permeable and allows release of gut organism-derived endotoxin into the circulation. Hepatocellular and reticuloendothelial function is reduced, and since 85% of the fixed macrophages are in the liver, clearance of particulate debris, bacteria and endotoxin is greatly impaired (Prytz et al., 1976). Evidence for this in humans remains to be provided.

Microcirculatory disturbances are difficult to quantify and treat, but become increasingly important in the late stages of cardiovascular failure, especially in sepsis. Vasoconstriction occurs partly as a response to circulating catecholamines and angiotensin II, and partly as a response to locally released mediators such as the prostaglandins, leukotrienes and thromboxanes.

Such alterations in vascular tone and increased capillary permeability cause fluid shifts which tend to expand the interstitial compartment, impairing delivery of oxygen and substrates to the respiring cells and removal of products of metabolism. Complement-mediated aggregation of white cells, aggregation of platelets and activation of the clotting cascade lead to intravascular thrombi formation in the microcirculation, impairing perfusion further. The reduced oxygen extraction in septic shock may be explained either by diversion of blood away from normally respiring tissue, by increased diffusion distances for oxygen from capillaries to cells, or by direct metabolic disturbances inhibiting cellular respiration.

Oxygen consumption is normally independent of oxygen delivery (Fig. 86.6). As oxygen delivery declines, capillary recruitment occurs, thereby reducing the mean distance between the respiring cells and the capillaries; oxygen extraction ratio is consequently increased. Below a critical level of total oxygen delivery, no further recruitment takes place and therefore consumption becomes supply dependent, with an increase in lactate. In sepsis, oxygen

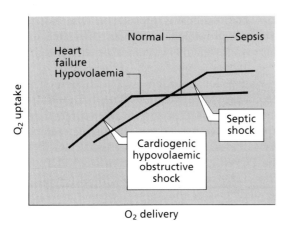

Fig. 86.6 Oxygen delivery—consumption relationships in normal patients and those with shock.

consumption is supply dependent over a much greater range, induced by reduced capillary reserve (Cain, 1986).

The above observations indicate why mixed venous oxygen measurement may be of limited value in the diagnosis and treatment of some complex forms of cardiovascular failure.

Monitoring

It is important to examine the critically ill patient regularly from top to toe. This has the dual function of stimulating a fresh assessment of each system on at least a daily basis, allowing early identification of new problems or deterioration of the existing complaint, and ensures also that the patient is treated as a whole.

A vast array of complex, invasive and expensive investigations and monitoring procedures has developed in the last two decades, but the temptation to monitor comprehensively every patient should be resisted. There is a risk:benefit ratio for every procedure, and in these days of increasing medical expenditure, costs cannot be ignored. Monitoring of cardiovascular failure may include invasive and non-invasive monitoring of haemodynamic parameters, and monitoring of the biochemical consequences of hypoperfusion.

Non-invasive haemodynamic measurement

These techniques are used most commonly in the general wards, but have a limited role in the ITU. The most commonly recorded parameters are pulse and arterial pressure measurement, and although these

may alter markedly in cardiovascular failure, they are not diagnostically or prognostically useful. Core/peripheral temperature gradient is a useful index of the adequacy of peripheral perfusion and may follow closely changes in cardiac output (Joly & Weil, 1969); it is not, however, synonymous with systemic vascular resistance (Woods et al., 1987). Similarly, hourly measurements of urine output reflect renal perfusion and intrarenal distribution of blood flow.

Transcutaneous measurement of oxygen tension has been evaluated, and correlates well with arterial oxygen tension providing the subject is haemodynamically stable (Fink et al., 1984). However, artefacts are introduced by the necessity to heat the skin to arterialize the circulation, and haemodynamic stability cannot be assumed in ITU patients. At best therefore, this device provides an early warning system: if transcutaneous oxygen tension declines, either arterial oxygen tension or tissue perfusion has decreased and further diagnostic steps are necessary. Transconjunctival oxygen tension ($TcjO_2$) may be measured also, using an unheated electrode which therefore avoids heating artefacts. On an experimental model, $TcjO_2$ was shown to be a substantially more effective measurement of the adequacy of resuscitation than mean arterial pressure (Abraham & Fink, 1986).

Oxygen saturation may be determined by pulse oximetry from the absorption of light in a finger tip or ear lobe, intermittent (i.e. arterial) absorption being electronically distinguished from constant (i.e. capillary and venous) absorption. It reflects accurately the arterial oxygen tension, but errors occur in low flow states, hypothermic and jaundiced patients. It is important also to appreciate that because of the alinearity of the oxygen dissociation curve above approximately 90% saturation, small changes in saturation reflect large changes in oxygen tension. Its main use is probably to identify acute hypoxic episodes associated with physiotherapy, suctioning and similar patient care manoeuvres (Taylor & Whitwam, 1986). Continuous monitoring of the ECG is useful, enabling changes in rhythm to be identified early, and frequent chest X-rays may record the causes or effects of myocardial and peripheral circulatory failure.

Two-dimensional echocardiography enables the physician to estimate ventricular function non-invasively including ventricular volumes and ejection fractions. Valvular function can also be estimated accurately. Transoesophageal techniques are particularly helpful in intubated patients, as they provide better visualization of the cardiac structures with minimal risk to the patient (Thomas & Weyman, 1991; Reichert et al., 1992).

Invasive haemodynamic measurement

Invasive monitoring is ubiquitous in the ITU, and often provides continuous measurement of physiological variables. Diagnosis becomes more exact, treatment is regulated more rigorously, and prognostic information may be derived. These benefits should be balanced by a recognition of the risks involved, the problems of interpretation of the data and the often large costs incurred.

Continuous intra-arterial pressure monitoring is employed frequently, and provides beat-to-beat display of changes in arterial pressure, in addition to allowing repeated blood sampling for blood gas and other estimations. There is a small incidence of thrombosis, and local infection can occur which may act as a focus for systemic spread.

Preload is determined most accurately by measurement of EDV, but for practical reasons, pressure monitoring is employed generally. The ideal would be to measure EDP directly, but again for practical reasons, 'upstream' pressures are used.

Insertion of a central venous catheter (via a central vein or threaded up the brachial vein) allows manometry of the right atrial pressure, which reflects right ventricular preload. However, the right-sided and left-sided filling pressures may differ. An understanding of the underlying physiological concepts, complications and data interpretation problems may allow rational selection of the optimum monitoring technique.

Using right atrial pressure as an indirect index of left ventricular EDP depends on normal physiology and a patent anatomical pathway between the two cardiac chambers, i.e. normal tricuspid valve, pulmonary vasculature, mitral valve and left ventricular compliance. If there is marked abnormality in any of these sites, left-sided pressures have to be monitored. Examples of indications for a pulmonary artery catheter therefore include conditions in which a marked disparity of ventricular function is expected, as after a large myocardial infarction, conditions where low-pressure or non-cardiogenic pulmonary oedema is likely, and conditions such as sepsis where more detailed physiological measurements are needed for diagnostic, therapeutic and prognostic purposes. A balloon-tipped, flow-directed pulmonary artery catheter may be inserted to measure pulmonary artery pressures, PCWP, cardiac output by thermodilution and mixed venous oxygen saturation

(Svo_2). The composite information may be used to construct a physiological profile, consisting of pulmonary and systemic vascular resistances, right and left ventricular stroke work, oxygen delivery (DO_2) and oxygen consumption (VO_2). Pulmonary artery catheters provide a wealth of data, but their use has not always been selective. Table 86.5 summarizes the complications associated with the use of a pulmonary artery catheter.

The PCWP is a valid reflection of LVEDP only if the tip of the catheter is in Zone III of the lung, the dependent part of the lung in which vascular pressures are always higher than the airway or alveolar pressure. In fact, this zone correlates with that part of the lung below the level of the left atrium.

In a non-compliant ventricle, the LVEDP is raised at a normal left ventricular end-diastolic volume (LVEDV) and is therefore less useful in assessing preload, especially as small changes in LVEDV cause large changes in LVEDP.

The transmural PCWP is equal to the measured value minus pleural pressure. In normal, spontaneously breathing subjects, pleural pressure approximates to zero and transmural pressures are the same as measured values. This does not apply in conditions where there may be large variations in pleural pressure such as in asthma or in association with IPPV especially if PEEP is applied. All intravascular pressures should be measured at end-expiration. When a high level of PEEP is applied, accurate measurements of PCWP can be obtained by transient disconnection of the ventilator system to obtain a nadir-PCWP (Pinsky et al., 1991). In patients with stiff lungs, low-level PEEP does not affect the measured value greatly.

Having assessed preload, contractility may be inferred from construction of a ventricular function curve as described previously. Afterload is assessed indirectly by calculating systemic vascular resistance which takes into account aortic impedance and arteriolar run-off.

Table 86.5 Complications of pulmonary artery catheterization

- Complicated venous insertion (bleeding, haemopneumothorax, nerve injury)
- Arrhythmias (ventricular tachycardia or fibrillation, A-V block etc.)
- Catheter knotting
- Pulmonary thrombosis or infarction
- Endothelial/endocardial damage
- Catheter-related infection
- Pulmonary artery rupture

The above apply to the systemic circulation, but in acute right heart failure, either primary or secondary to changes in the pulmonary circulation, the appropriate right-sided parameters should be obtained. Right atrial pressure assesses preload, contractility is assessed as before and pulmonary vascular resistance is an index of afterload (Ducas & Prewitt, 1988).

Pulmonary vascular resistance is a summation of the pre- and postcapillary resistances. The precapillary resistance provides the bulk of the resistance normally, in which case the pulmonary capillary pressure is equal to the PCWP. If, however, the postcapillary resistance is increased disproportionately as in histamine release or endotoxaemia for example (D'Orio *et al.*, 1986), pulmonary capillary pressure exceeds PCWP and pulmonary oedema may occur at normal or low PCWP (Editorial, 1986). The pulmonary capillary pressure may be determined from the point of inflection (Fig. 86.7) between the fast and slow components of the decreasing pressure profile after pulmonary artery occlusion (Cope *et al.*, 1986). This technique has not yet found wide clinical application.

A pulmonary artery catheter enables determination of Svo_2 either intermittently (from blood samples withdrawn from the pulmonary artery) or continuously (using fibre-optic filaments). Svo_2 varies directly with arterial oxygen saturation (Sao_2) and cardiac output (CO) and inversely with VO_2. Continuous measurement of arterial and mixed venous oxyhaemoglobin saturation using combined pulse and pulmonary artery oximetry has been shown to provide a rapid assessment of acute cardio-respiratory changes. A derived ventilation/perfusion index is a valuable indicator of gas exchange (Downs & Rasanen, 1987).

Oxygen extraction (O_2 extr.) can be easily calculated as follows:

$$O_2 \text{ extr.} = \frac{VO_2}{DO_2} = \frac{CO\,(Cao_2 - Cvo_2)}{CO \cdot Cao_2}$$

$$= \frac{Hb \cdot C \cdot Sao_2 - Hb \cdot C \cdot Svo_2}{Hb \cdot C \cdot Sao_2} = \frac{Sao_2 - Svo_2}{Sao_2}$$

C = oxygen-carrying capacity.
Cao_2 = arterial oxygen content.

A diagram representing cardiac index versus O_2 extr. can be useful to evaluate the relation between VO_2 and DO_2 in critically ill patients. It has the advantage over a VO_2–DO_2 diagram in that the values are obtained more simply and independently, thus avoiding the problem of mathematical coupling of data when the thermodilution cardiac output value is introduced in the calculation of both VO_2 and DO_2 (Silance *et al.*, 1993).

In Fig. 86.8, myocardial dysfunction is illustrated by a positioning of the haemodynamic data below a

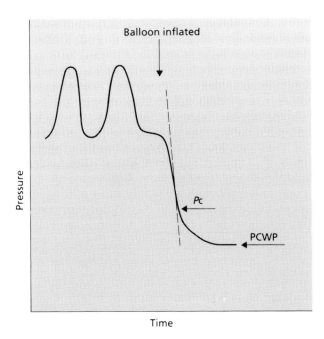

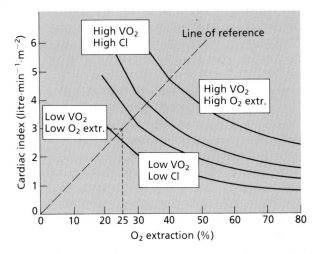

Fig. 86.7 Pressure tracing following inflation of pulmonary artery flotation catheter balloon: the point of inflection between the fast and slow components of the diminishing pressure profile indicates the pulmonary capillary pressure. Pc, pulmonary capillary pressure; PCWP, pulmonary capillary wedge pressure.

Fig. 86.8 Relation between cardiac index and oxygen extraction, in which oxygen consumption (VO_2) is represented by a series of curvilinear isopleths. The line passing through the origin and normal values for cardiac index (3 litre · min^{-1} · m^{-2}) and oxygen extraction (25%) represents a reference to physical exercise.

line of reference representing equal changes in cardiac index and O_2 extr.

Recent clinical studies measuring right ventricular volumes by the thermodilution technique during fluid challenge are encouraging (Reuse et al., 1990).

Biochemical monitoring

The function of the cardiovascular system is to provide sufficient perfusion such that the cells are provided adequately with oxygen and substrates and metabolic products are removed. Haemodynamic monitoring provides diagnostic information but does not usually reflect tissue perfusion directly, and this function is performed better using biochemical monitoring which measures substrate supplied to and metabolites derived from the respiring tissues.

Blood-gas analysis is the most common form of biochemical monitoring. The arterial oxygen tension may fall as a result of cardiovascular failure (e.g. as a result of pulmonary oedema) or may reveal the cause of secondary myocardial depression. Acid—base analysis (from pH, standard bicarbonate and base deficit values given by most blood-gas machines) may likewise show an acidosis as the result of poor tissue perfusion leading to anaerobic metabolism, or may reveal the cause of secondary myocardial depression. The hormonal and substrate changes in shock as detailed in a previous section have been characterized but unfortunately are of limited clinical value. For example, measurement of serum lactate, a product of anaerobic metabolism, has shown good correlation with outcome in shock, but the correlation is less valid in septic shock (Cowan et al., 1984; Bakker et al., 1991). Serial lactate measurements were better than a single estimation (Cowan et al., 1984).

A number of experimental and clinical studies have shown that the VO_2/DO_2 dependency phenomenon is associated with elevated blood lactate levels (Haupt et al., 1985; Kruse et al., 1990; Vincent et al., 1990a; Bakker & Vincent, 1991). However, the interpretation of blood lactate levels can be complicated by the fact that they reflect both production and elimination of lactate and the latter can be protracted, especially in patients with liver dysfunction.

Determination of gastric intramucosal pH (pHi) can be useful to assess the degree of gut hypoxia (Gutierrez et al., 1992). pHi measurements have been shown to be of prognostic value in critically ill patients (Gutierrez et al., 1992). Moreover, the combination of blood lactate levels and pHi may be useful in monitoring tissue hypoxia (Friedman & Vincent, 1993). However, the two parameters are not entirely independent as pHi is calculated from the local Pco_2 (from the modified gastric tube) and from the arterial bicarbonate concentration (Boyd et al., 1993).

Attempts to construct more complex biochemical 'profiles' have proved to be of value as a research tool but so far are not used routinely in clinical practice.

Knaus and colleagues (1985) have derived a scoring system (APACHE II) which ascribes a weighted value to derangements of haemodynamic + metabolic parameters from normal. When measured as a single value on admission to the ITU, a close correlation with outcome has been demonstrated. The difficulty is that overlap between different score bands makes it impossible to apply to the individual patient, although it is valuable as a research and audit tool. In addition, although the general relationship that increasing APACHE II score is associated with increasing mortality is true, the precise correlation varies with different categories of disease. Patients with haematological malignancy, for example, have a higher mortality for any particular APACHE II score than the average (Lloyd-Thomas et al., 1986).

Treatment

In considering treatment of cardiovascular failure in the ITU, indirect influences which contribute to myocardial dysfunction and peripheral circulatory failure should be identified and minimized.

Hypoxaemia should be regarded as a major priority and treated initially by increasing inspired oxygen concentration. Ultimately, IPPV with or without PEEP may be required, accepting that the latter may have deleterious effects on myocardial performance. There are occasions when intractable hypoxaemia dictates the use of IPPV with PEEP despite cardiovascular instability. A balance has to be struck between high levels of PEEP producing good oxygenation but less than optimal tissue perfusion, and low levels of PEEP producing good tissue perfusion but less than adequate oxygenation. In these circumstances, PEEP may be optimized by maximizing oxygen delivery (cardiac output × arterial oxygen content). The use of mechanical ventilation may be beneficial also by reducing the oxygen demand of the respiratory muscles (Aubier et al., 1982). In the presence of fever, oxygen requirement may also be reduced by the use of antipyretic medications. However, it must be appreciated that the febrile response may enhance the immune reaction to invading organisms. Oxygen consumption may need to be reduced. This can be achieved by increasing sedation and analgesia, with or without the use of relaxant drugs, although it should be borne in mind that such agents are often both negative inotropes and peripheral vasodilators.

Metabolic parameters should be restored to as near normal as possible. Electrolyte derangements (especially hypokalaemia) and acid–base abnormalities (especially acidosis) are both arrhythmogenic and negatively inotropic, and may impair the action of inotropic agents. However, the use of sodium bicarbonate to combat metabolic acidosis has been challenged and is no longer recommended in the treatment of acute circulatory failure. Dichloroacetate, a substance which maintains pyruvate dehydrogenase in an active state, can correct lactic acidosis but does not improve prognosis (Stacpoole *et al.*, 1992). These observations emphasize that correction of the cause of the acidosis should remain the ultimate goal of therapy.

Drugs taken in overdose or given therapeutically often have adverse effects on myocardial performance, the intracardiac conducting system and peripheral vascular tone. Unfortunately, a drug that is vital for treatment may have unwelcome side-effects, e.g. the arrhythmogenicity of many inotropic agents, but each drug given should be scrutinized carefully and its risk : benefit ratio assessed. The adverse effects of many drugs are not recognized easily. For example, etomidate was used by infusion as a sedative agent in the ITU before it was noted that it increased mortality (Ledingham & Watt, 1983).

Having dealt with indirect influences, treatment of cardiovascular failure *per se* is now considered (Fig. 86.9). In order to perfuse the respiring tissues, an adequate cardiac output is required, and this goal is achieved by ensuring optimal preload, heart rate, contractility and afterload. Cardiac output should be distributed appropriately between and within vital organs. Treatment is best considered, therefore, under these headings.

Optimization of preload

The effective circulating volume should be increased or decreased to optimize preload.

In increasing the circulating volume, two questions must be considered: what fluid to administer and how much? A controversy has raged for years between the proponents of crystalloids (such as normal saline or Hartmann's solution) and colloids, substances which remain in the intravascular space when transfused, e.g. modified gelatin solutions, hydroxyethyl starch (Macintyre *et al.*, 1985) or plasma protein derivatives (Vincent, 1991).

Proponents of crystalloids state that because of passive fluid shifts (see above) the whole of the

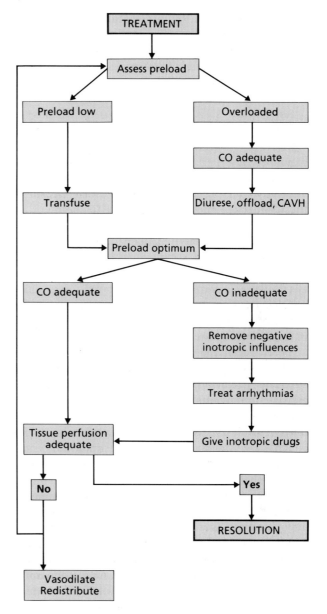

Fig. 86.9 Simplified treatment algorithm. CO, cardiac output; CAVH, continuous arteriovenous haemofiltration.

extracellular space (intravascular plus interstitial space) is depleted in hypovolaemia, and because crystalloids are distributed to both spaces (in a 3 : 1 interstitial : intravascular ratio), crystalloids are more appropriate (Virgilio *et al.*, 1979a). There is less likely to be a rapid increase in preload because 75% of the fluid is distributed to the interstitial space (Virgilio *et al.*, 1979b), and crystalloids are free from the risk of infection or anaphylaxis seen occasionally with colloids (Messmer, 1984). Crystalloids are also considerably cheaper.

Proponents of colloid state that it is more logical to replenish circulating volume with a substance that not only remains in the intravascular space, but by increasing plasma oncotic pressure may increase circulating volume further by aiding passive transfer of fluid from the interstitium: as a smaller volume is infused, resuscitation is more rapid (Shoemaker et al., 1981; Twigley & Hillman, 1985).

As in most such long-standing controversies, a choice, based on personal experience, is made. Where circulating volume needs to be replenished rapidly to restore tissue perfusion or where the interstitial space is already overloaded, colloid may be used with advantage. Because preload, which measures the adequacy of intravascular volume replacement, is measured readily, fine control of repletion with colloid is achieved easily. Maintenance fluid requirements are estimated according to less rigorous and exact parameters such as clinical judgement, plasma electrolyte concentrations and measured losses, and crystalloids are more appropriate, especially if deficits of the interstitial space are expected, as, for example, in losses from gastrointestinal fistulae.

More crucial than the particular choice of fluid used is the volume required for restoration of adequate perfusion. A balance has to be struck between an insufficient transfusion causing inadequate tissue perfusion and overloading causing cardiorespiratory embarrassment. In all critically ill patients a ventricular function curve should be constructed as described previously using the technique of fluid challenge. The sicker the patient, the more invasive the measurements tend to be: for example, a young, healthy trauma victim, who is obviously hypovolaemic, may reasonably have central venous pressure used as an index of preload and arterial pressure as an index of cardiac performance, whilst the elderly septic patient may require more frequently a pulmonary artery catheter and PCWP plotted against cardiac output. The principle remains the same, however, that repeated fluid challenges should be given until the preload increases and there is no further improvement in cardiac performance. Of course, contractility and afterload may vary during treatment, prompting continual reassessment of the optimum preload. Studies have been carried out to determine optimum filling pressures, e.g. Packman and Rackow (1983) suggested that the PCWP should not exceed 1.6 kPa (12 mmHg) in septic and hypovolaemic patients. However, they (and others in similar studies) arrived at this figure by a process of fluid challenge as outlined above, and it is preferable to treat each patient as an individual.

Some patients may become relatively fluid overloaded as a result of overenthusiastic replacement,

renal failure or myocardial failure, and such patients need a reduction in their effective circulating volume. This is accomplished most simply by the use of appropriate diuretic therapy, given as a bolus or by infusion, which reduces intravascular and interstitial fluid volumes, and exerts direct effects on cardiovascular haemodynamics (Brater & Chennavasin, 1984). Unfortunately, many patients in the ITU have impoverished renal function which, although not precluding this approach, makes it less feasible, especially if rapid reductions in circulating volume are necessary. In these circumstances, the use of vasodilators, especially venodilators such as isosorbide dinitrate or nitroglycerine may be used to reduce filling pressures rapidly whilst slower methods of fluid removal are instituted.

In the past, removal of fluid from a patient with renal impairment involved haemodialysis and ultrafiltration, a technique which often causes hypotension and is, by definition, intermittent. An alternative technique is continuous arteriovenous haemofiltration (CAVH) in which blood passes from a patient's artery over a dialysis membrane and is returned to a vein. Under the influence of the patient's own hydrostatic pressure, an ultrafiltrate of plasma is formed and extracellular fluid is therefore removed. Small volumes may be removed to allow, for example, intravenous feeding and drug administration, or up to 20 litres/day may be removed, and partially replaced by crystalloid fluids. By manipulation of the fluid intake and output in this way, a net loss of fluid can occur. This technique is inexpensive, does not require specially trained personnel and is tolerated very well haemodynamically. Coraim and colleagues (1986) demonstrated its efficacy in shocked patients [mean arterial pressure 6.6 kPa (50 mmHg)] and showed that cardiac index, VO_2 and Pao_2 increased.

Venovenous haemofiltration with pump assistance can also be used with greater safety and efficiency.

Optimization of heart rate

The effect of brady- and tachyarrhythmias has been discussed above; both may cause acute reductions in cardiac output. Arrhythmias in patients in the ITU are often secondary to hypoxia and/or metabolic disturbance, and are tolerated poorly by patients whose cardiovascular system is compromised from underlying illness. Hypotension, poor tissue perfusion and disturbances of gas exchange occur rapidly (Edwards & Kishen, 1986).

Most antiarrhythmic drugs are negative inotropes and vasodilators, and are often ineffective in critically ill patients. The first line of treatment is to correct as far as possible underlying physiological disorders. For example, in six carefully documented patients whose atrial fibrillation proved refractory to digoxin and DC cardioversion, correction of hypovolaemia was associated with prompt improvement in cardiac output and reversion to sinus rhythm (Edwards & Wilkins, 1987). Further treatment should be directed initially to optimizing heart rate rapidly. Brady-arrhythmias may require atropine, a chronotropic drug such as isoprenaline, or transvenous pacing. Supraventricular tachyarrhythmias may respond to amiodarone or verapamil given by infusion (Edwards

& Kishen, 1986). It should be noted that sinus tachycardia is often necessary to maintain adequate cardiac output, and attempts to slow such a rate with beta blockers, for example, may prove disastrous.

If the pragmatic approach outlined above is ineffective, a selection of conventional agents to meet individual requirements has been described (Rae & Hutton, 1986; Fig. 86.10).

Increasing contractility

Correction of preload or heart rate disturbances often leads to restoration of adequate tissue perfusion but

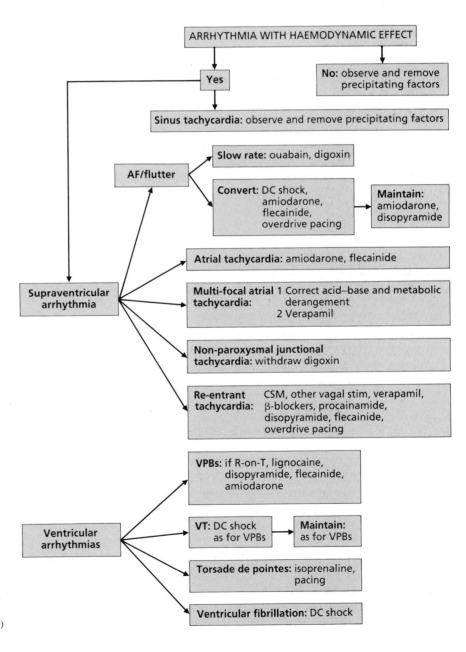

Fig. 86.10 Algorithm for the treatment of cardiac arrhythmias. CSM, carotid sinus massage; VPBs, ventricular premature beats. (Redrawn from Rae & Hutton, 1986.)

occasional recourse has to be made to augmentation of cardiac contractility.

Calcium salts are potent short-acting inotropes, and may be given as a bolus dose in an emergency to maintain tissue perfusion whilst other agents are diluted and administered. Calcium may be of value also in overcoming the negative inotropic effects of calcium antagonists such as verapamil.

The most common inotropic agents are the adrenergic agonists, which bind to specific receptors and exert their action via the second messenger, cyclic AMP. They are given usually by infusion via a central vein, and are used to improve myocardial performance for any given pre- and afterload, thus shifting the VFC upwards and to the left. They have also other direct and indirect actions which alter heart rate, afterload and myocardial oxygen supply and demand, and rational selection of a particular inotrope should take these actions into account.

Dopamine

In low doses ($0.5-3\,\mu g \cdot kg^{-1} \cdot min^{-1}$) dopamine (DA) has a specific action on DA_1-receptors in the renal and mesenteric vascular beds. In doses of $5-20\,\mu g \cdot$

$kg^{-1} \cdot min^{-1}$, its β_1 actions predominate, increasing the force of contraction and heart rate, and thus cardiac output (Fig. 86.11). In doses exceeding $20\,\mu g \cdot kg^{-1} \cdot min^{-1}$, α_1 actions are most obvious, and although arterial pressure is maintained by vasoconstriction, it may be at the expense of tissue perfusion. High doses may cause an increase in PCWP, pulmonary vascular congestion and arterial desaturation (Loeb et al., 1977), tachycardia and an increased incidence of ventricular ectopics (Leier et al., 1978).

With increasing dose, the increased contractility, heart rate and afterload increase myocardial oxygen demand, although supply is maintained by locally mediated coronary vasodilatation and high diastolic pressures. Stemple and colleagues (1976), using epicardial ST-mapping and coronary sinus lactate estimation, showed that DA worsened myocardial ischaemia after coronary occlusion.

In septic shock, there is no close relationship between dose of DA and haemodynamic effects; optimal response to DA administration should be assessed, therefore, by detailed and frequent haemodynamic measurement in individual patients (Edwards & Tweedle, 1986).

DA is often administered at low doses with the aim of exerting renal protective effects. However, there is no evidence that the use of low dose DA prevents the development of renal failure (Vincent, 1993).

Dobutamine

Dobutamine is given in a dose range of $0-40\,\mu g \cdot kg^{-1} \cdot min^{-1}$, and has both β_1 and β_2 actions. The β_1 actions increase the heart rate and force of contraction. Its β_2 actions tend to cause vasodilatation in skeletal muscle, which reduces afterload. It has only weak α activity and no effect on DA-receptors. In contrast to DA, PCWP often decreases with dobutamine infusions (Leier et al., 1978).

The net effect of these actions is that dobutamine increases cardiac output, whilst reducing right and left ventricular afterload, and the myocardial oxygen supply : demand ratio may be unchanged (Vatner et al., 1974b). Gillespie and colleagues (1975) could demonstrate no increase in cardiac enzymes in patients with evolving myocardial infarctions treated with dobutamine. It is therefore of special value in the treatment of myocardial failure; Shoemaker and colleagues (1986) demonstrated significant increases in DO_2 and VO_2 in critically ill surgical patients. The administration of limited doses of dobutamine to

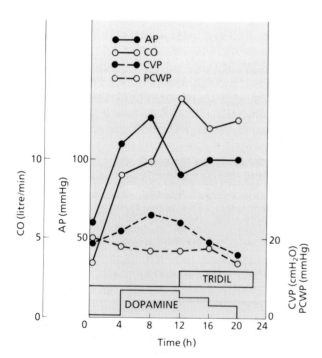

Fig. 86.11 An inotropic dose of dopamine increased arterial pressure (systolic) and cardiac output to adequate levels, but at the expense of unacceptably high filling pressures. The addition of a small dose of tridil (nitroglycerine) reduced the filling pressures, and although arterial pressure decreased, cardiac output increased.

increase DO_2 has been shown to be safe (Vincent et al., 1990b); DO_2 was increased in patients with altered tissue perfusion (Vincent et al., 1990a).

Adrenaline

Adrenaline is given in a dose range of $0.1-0.2\,\mu g \cdot kg^{-1} \cdot min^{-1}$, and has α, β_1 and β_2 actions. It is a potent and effective inotrope but in higher doses its α actions predominate and may reduce major organ blood flow critically (Stephenson et al., 1976). The use of adrenaline has been recommended in the treatment of septic shock (Bollaert et al., 1990). Its effect on contractility and afterload worsens the myocardial oxygen supply : demand ratio as would be expected. Having noted that, some patients with severe cardiovascular failure may need such a potent and effective inotrope, and the invariable increase in cardiac output may increase peripheral perfusion paradoxically despite the direct α effects.

Noradrenaline

Noradrenaline in doses of $0.01-0.1\,\mu g \cdot kg^{-1} \cdot min^{-1}$ is a pressor agent rather than an inotrope, with principally α-agonist actions. The vasoconstriction in the renal, mesenteric and peripheral vascular beds increases afterload vastly, often causing a reflex bradycardia, and although arterial pressure is increased, cardiac output often decreases. The vast increase in afterload worsens the oxygen supply : demand ratio usually, and vital organ perfusion is reduced (Vatner et al., 1974a). It is used mainly in an effort to overcome the profound reduction in systemic vascular resistance caused by sepsis, but, in addition to the drawbacks noted above, may be unable to overcome such locally mediated vasodilatation (Parker et al., 1984a); even when beneficial haemodynamic effects occur, changes in DO_2 and VO_2 are inconsistent (Meadows et al., 1988), and tissue oxygen extraction does not appear to improve significantly (Bakker & Vincent, 1993).

Isoprenaline

Isoprenaline acts on β_1- and β_2-receptors causing an increase in force of contraction, heart rate and peripheral and pulmonary vasodilatation. Cardiac output increases significantly, but at the expense of a greatly increased myocardial oxygen demand consequent upon the tachycardia, and a reduced supply consequent upon reduced diastolic pressures and its role in myocardial failure is therefore questionable.

Glucagon

The pancreatic polypeptide, glucagon, causes an increase in contractility and heart rate by stimulating adenyl cyclase which increases intracellular cyclic AMP concentrations. Nausea and vomiting, a dose-dependent side-effect, limits its use, but it may be useful in beta blocker overdose, since its action does not depend on drug receptor interaction.

Inodilating agents

All the above inotropes have an adverse effect on myocardial oxygen supply : demand ratio to a greater (noradrenaline) or lesser (dobutamine) extent. Combining an inotrope with a vasodilator (Fig. 86.11) to minimize this effect is useful and efforts have been made to synthesize agents which combine the attributes of both.

Phosphodiesterase (PDE) inhibitors such as amrinone, milrinone or enoximone exert positive inotropic effects by increasing the cyclic AMP content of the myocardium and exert strong vasodilating effects. Their use as sole agents has been limited by their inherent risk of decreasing blood pressure. The prolonged half-life of these compounds further complicates their administration in acute conditions. The combination of PDE inhibitors with adrenergic agents has been found effective in the management of severe heart failure and even cardiogenic shock (Vincent et al., 1988; Vincent et al., 1992d; Thuillez et al., 1993). The combination of PDE inhibitors with noradrenaline has been found to increase oxygen availability to the tissues in experimental septic shock (De Boelpaepe et al., 1989).

Dopexamine is a recently developed synthetic catecholamine which combines inotropic, vasodilating and dopaminergic properties. Its administration has been found useful in patients with cardiorespiratory failure (Vincent et al., 1989) and even in patients with septic shock (Colardyn et al., 1989). Dopexamine may exert beneficial effects by selectively improving the oxygen supply to the gut.

Whatever the theoretical risks in terms of myocardial perfusion, in practice inotropes are often necessary to ensure adequate peripheral perfusion. Inotropes should be discontinued as soon as possible by a slow weaning process, and in many instances volume loading is necessary as the inotrope is reduced, relating preload to myocardial performance as usual.

Afterload manipulation

Left sided

Vasodilators act on the systemic circulation and may reduce afterload predominantly by arteriolar dilatation (e.g. hydralazine) or may reduce pre- and afterload by arteriolar and venular dilatation (e.g. sodium nitroprusside). The result of this therapy is to increase cardiac index, stroke volume index and stroke work index whilst decreasing left ventricular filling pressures.

Hydralazine acts directly on arteriolar smooth muscle causing vasodilatation and a reduction in afterload. Arteriolar pressure may decrease but the myocardial oxygen supply:demand ratio improves, and cardiac output increases despite lower filling pressures as a result of the improvement in myocardial energetics (Mehta et al., 1978).

Sodium nitroprusside acts on both the arterial and venous sides of the circulation, and therefore lowers both preload and afterload by a direct action on vascular smooth muscle. Its dose should be titrated against effect and the doses should be limited to avoid the risk of cyanide toxicity (Robin & McCauley, 1992).

Its principal action is to reduce afterload, thus increasing cardiac output, and, providing diastolic pressure is not reduced too far, exerting a beneficial effect on the myocardial oxygen:supply ratio. Preload is reduced also, and if that decreases markedly, cardiac output decreases, although this effect may be offset by volume replacement with colloid.

Vasodilators tend to reduce preload, afterload and myocardial oxygen demand, but vital organ perfusion may decline as a result of systemic hypotension. Inotropes increase cardiac output and arterial pressure, but may increase preload and afterload, and increase myocardial oxygen demand.

The intra-aortic balloon pump (IABP) is a mechanical method of reducing left-sided afterload. A balloon is inserted via the femoral artery into the descending aorta; in synchrony with the pressure waveform or the ECG, the balloon is inflated during diastole, thus increasing coronary perfusion, and deflated during systole, reducing afterload. Myocardial oxygen supply is increased and demand reduced, this combination being especially useful in primary myocardial failure (Kern et al., 1993).

Right sided

As described previously, acute increases in right ventricular afterload reduce left ventricular preload.

The right ventricle dilates in an attempt to maintain output by the Starling mechanism, the interventricular septum bulges into the left ventricle and reduces left ventricular compliance, and cardiac output decreases (Sibbald & Driedger, 1983). In these circumstances, further volume challenge merely increases right ventricular dilatation, leading to a greater reduction in cardiac output. Therapy may be directed therefore towards lowering pulmonary vascular resistance. Although vasodilators such as hydralazine or nitrates are effective pulmonary vasodilators, they may also compromise systemic blood pressure. Prostanoids such as prostaglandin E1 may be preferred because they are primarily metabolized during their passage through the lungs (Vincent et al., 1992b). Dobutamine is an agent of choice in right ventricular failure because it improves ventricular contractility but has no significant effect on pulmonary artery or systemic pressure. In the presence of severe pulmonary hypertension a vasopressor may be required to restore right ventricular perfusion pressure (Priebe, 1992), provided coronary perfusion pressure is maintained (Prewitt & Ghignone, 1983).

Redistribution of blood flow

Manipulation of cardiac output is usually straightforward using the methods outlined above. There is no guarantee, however, that cellular oxygen availability will improve proportionally if the distribution of blood flow is simultaneously altered. Attempts have been made to manipulate the microcirculation.

As was mentioned before, the use of low dose dopamine has not been shown to improve renal function. The use of vasopressor agents has not been shown significantly to improve the oxygen extraction capabilities in septic shock (Bakker & Vincent, 1993).

The role of centrally and peripherally released endogenous opioid peptides in shock has become clearer. Consequently, naloxone and partial opioid agonists (such as meptazinol and nalbuphine) have been evaluated in several types of shock. Results of clinical trials have been equivocal and their routine use is not recommended currently (Hinds & Donaldson, 1988).

It is postulated that the microcirculatory disturbances of shock are mediated via locally released substances of which there are a large (and increasing) number. The microcirculatory changes are reversed readily if the cause of shock is eliminated promptly, and several pharmacological agents are known to attenuate or even reverse some of the adverse effects, for example ATP$-$MgCl$_2$ (Chaudry *et al.*, 1983), glucose$-$insulin$-$potassium (Bronsveld *et al.*, 1986), calcium-channel blockers (Hackel *et al.*, 1981) and steroids (Goldfarb & Glenn, 1983). None of these agents is of proven clinical value.

A number of inhibitors of eicosanoid synthesis have been evaluated in animal models with some success, but it has proved difficult to extrapolate these experimental findings to the clinical situation. It remains a promising area for future research, in which the precise role of eicosanoids in shock may be elucidated (Ball *et al.*, 1986).

Chernow and Roth (1986) reviewed the pharmacological manipulation of the peripheral vasculature in shock, emphasizing its unresponsiveness to exogenous catecholamines, probably because of release of local mediators and down-regulation of α-receptors.

Some immunotherapeutic modalities may exert beneficial haemodynamic effects. For instance, antibodies directed at TNF appear to improve myocardial contractility in experimental studies (Heard *et al.*, 1992) and in early clinical experiences (Vincent *et al.*, 1992a; Lanore *et al.*, 1993). The interleukin-1 receptor antagonist (IL-1 ra) also seems to improve cardiac function during septic shock in primates (Fischer *et al.*, 1992). Antagonists to PAF may also improve cardiac function (Anderson *et al.*, 1991). Nitric oxide (NO), which is released in greater amounts in severe sepsis, may contribute to the myocardial depression as well (Brady *et al.*, 1992).

Specific treatment

Although treatment is directed initially towards correcting physiological derangements, specific problems may require specific treatment. It may be impossible to treat the patient without first combating the initiating insult, e.g. in major haemorrhage, the source of bleeding should be identified and secured as a priority before or at the same time as resuscitation is proceeding. On the other hand, in septic shock where a septic focus must be drained, the surgical procedure is tolerated better following initial resuscitation in the ITU.

The choice of fluid for restoration of circulating volume in hypovolaemia has been covered previously, but controversy still surrounds the optimum haematocrit necessary to maximize oxygen delivery to the tissues. The greater oxygen carrying capacity as the haematocrit increases is counter-balanced by increased viscosity which reduces flow through smaller vessels. In the normal subject, a compromise is reached at a haemoglobin value of approximately 9$-$9.5 g/litre, but this may not hold for the severely ill and septic patient.

A major development in the treatment of myocardial infarction has been the administration of fibrinolytic agents.

The mainstay of the treatment of sepsis remains efficient surgical drainage (Meakins *et al.*, 1980), and laparotomies may have to be repeated if sepsis is to be eradicated effectively. Broad-spectrum antibiotics (guided where possible by positive bacteriology) have a lesser role to play. Episodes of infection in patients in the ITU are acquired often from endogenous sources such as the gut or oropharynx. The gut flora may be modified by non-absorbable antibiotics given enterally, such that Gram-negative aerobes are reduced in number while anaerobes remain to prevent overgrowth with resistant organisms. Studies (Ledingham *et al.*, 1988) have shown a reduced infection rate with such a regimen of selective decontamination of the digestive tract. However, a significant effect on outcome has not been conclusively demonstrated.

Conclusion

Throughout this chapter, emphasis has been placed on the physiology of the cardiovascular system: how it alters in disease, how to assess the physiological derangement and how to manipulate the cardiovascular system in the light of such knowledge.

A sound understanding of the relevant cardiovascular physiology is essential, as it is imperative to diagnose, monitor and treat the underlying physiological derangement before it worsens.

Before using invasive monitoring procedures, a risk:benefit assessment should be considered. This entails objective evaluation of the severity of the illness using a measure such as the APACHE II score, and using clinical experience to identify those patients at risk of further deterioration. Having assessed the disordered physiology, rational treatment may then be applied. The question remains as to what end-point should be sought when deciding on treatment. The ultimate goal is obviously survival of the patient but it remains difficult to define interim treatment goals. Those parameters measured most commonly, such as arterial pressure, pulse rate and filling pressures, are of no predictive value, and returning them to within a range of normal values does not increase survival. Of greater practical value, a spectrum of parameters should be repeatedly evaluated. It is salutary to note that some of these parameters, such as cardiac filling pressures, cardiac output, DO$_2$ and VO$_2$ represent increases of the values into the supraphysiological range. These observations are consistent with the recently acquired understanding of the relationship between oxygen supply and demand at the microcirculatory level. In the case of septic shock, the flow-dependent oxygen consumption is pathological and a higher than normal oxygen supply may be required to achieve optimal oxygen availability and elimination of lactic acidosis (Astiz et al., 1987).

Cardiovascular failure remains a condition in which mortality is high and the improvement in intensive care over the last 20 years has not improved survival greatly in the individual case. Advances in future must include enhanced understanding of the disordered physiology, realistic treatment goals and the ability to manipulate the circulation at the microvascular level.

References

Abraham E. & Fink S. (1986) Cardiorespiratory and conjunctival oxygen tension monitoring during resuscitation from haemorrhage. *Critical Care Medicine* **14**, 1004–9.

Anderson B.O., Bensard D.D. & Harken A.H. (1991) The role of platelet activating factor and its antagonists in shock, sepsis and multiple organ failure. *Surgery, Gynecology and Obstetrics* **172**, 415–24.

Astiz M.E., Rackow E.C., Falk J.L., Kaufman B.S. & Weil M.H. (1987) Oxygen delivery inpatients with hyperdynamic septic shock. *Critical Care Medicine* **15**, 26–8.

Aubier M., Viires N., Syllie G., Mozes R. & Roussos C. (1982) Respiratory muscle contribution to lactic acidosis in low cardiac output. *American Review of Respiratory Diseases* **126**, 648–52.

Bakker J. & Vincent J.-L. (1991) The oxygen supply dependency phenomenon is associated with increased blood lactate levels. *Journal of Critical Care* **6**, 152–9.

Bakker J. & Vincent J.-L. (1993) The effects of norepinephrine and dobutamine on oxygen transport and consumption in a dog model of endotoxic shock. *Critical Care Medicine* **21**, 425–32.

Bakker J., Coffernils M., Leon M., Gris P. & Vincent J.-L. (1991) Blood lactate levels are superior to oxygen derived variables in predicting outcome in human septic shock. *Chest* **99**, 956–62.

Ball H.A., Cook J.A., Wise W.C. & Halushka P.V. (1986) Role of thromboxane, prostaglandins, and leukotrienes in endotoxic and septic shock. *Intensive Care Medicine* **12**, 116–26.

Belenkie I., Dani R., Smith E.R. & Tyberg J.V. (1992) The importance of pericardial constraint in experimental pulmonary embolism and volume loading. *American Heart Journal* **123**, 733–42.

Bollaert P.E., Bauer P., Audibert G., Lambert H. & Larcan A. (1990) Effects of epinephrine on hemodynamics and oxygen metabolism in dopamine resistant shock. *Chest* **98**, 949–53.

Boyd O., Mackay C.J., Lamb G., Bland J.M., Grounds R.M. & Bennett E.D. (1993) Comparison of clinical information gained from routine blood-gas analysis and from gastric tonometry for intramural pH. *Lancet* **34**, 142–6.

Brady A.J., Poole-Wilson P.A., Harding S.Z. & Warren J.B. (1992) Nitric oxide production within cardiac myocytes reduces their contractility in endotoxaemia. *American Journal of Physiology* **32**, H1936–6.

Brater D.C. & Chennavasin P. (1984) Prolonged haemodynamic effect of furosemide in congestive heart failure. *American Heart Journal* **108**, 1031–2.

Braunwald E., Ross J. & Sonnenblick E.H. (1977) Mechanisms of contraction of the normal and failing heart. *New England Journal of Medicine* **277**, 910–20.

Bronsveld W., van Lambalgen A.A., van den Bos G.C., Thijs L.G. & Koopmans P.A.R. (1986) Regional blood flow and metabolism in canine endotoxin shock before, during and after infusion of glucose–insulin–potassium. *Circulatory Shock* **18**, 31–42.

Cain S.M. (1986) Assessment of tissue oxygenation. *Critical Care Clinics* **2**, 537–50.

Calvin J.E. & Ascah K. (1992) Impact of leftward septal shift and potential role of ischemia in its production during experimental right ventricular pressure overload. *Journal of Critical Care* **7**, 106–17.

Chaudry I.H., Ohkawa M., Clemens M.G. & Baue A.E. (1983) Alterations in electron transport and cellular metabolism with shock and trauma. In *Molecular and Cellular Aspects of Shock and Trauma* (Eds Lefer A.F. & Schumer W.) pp. 67–88. Liss, New York.

Chernow B. & Roth B.L. (1986) Pharmacologic manipulation of the peripheral vasculature in shock: clinical and experimental approaches. *Circulatory Shock* **18**, 141–55.

Coetzee A., Foex P., Holland D., Ryder A. & Jones L. (1984) Effect of hypoxia on the normal and ischaemic myocardium. *Critical Care Medicine* **14**, 1027–31.

Colardyn F.C., Vandenbogaerde J.F., Vogelaers D.P. & Verbeke J.H. (1989) Use of dopexamine hydrochloride in patients with septic shock. *Critical Care Medicine* **17**, 999–1003.

Cope D.K., Allison R.C., Parmentier J.L., Miller J.N. & Taylor A.E. (1986) Measurement of effective pulmonary capillary pressure using the pressure profile after pulmonary artery occlusion. *Critical Care Medicine* **14**, 16–22.

Coraim F.J., Coraim H.P., Ebermann R. & Stellwag F.M. (1986) Acute respiratory failure after cardiac surgery: clinical experience of continuous arteriovenous haemofiltration. *Critical Care Medicine* **14**, 714–18.

Covell J.W. & Ross J. (1973) Nature and significance of alterations in myocardial compliance. *American Journal of Cardiology* **32**, 449–55.

Cowan B.N., Burns H.J.G., Boyle P. & Ledingham I.McA. (1984) The relative prognostic value of lactate and haemodynamic measurements in early shock. *Anaesthesia* **39**, 750–5.

D'Orio V., Halleux J., Rodriguez L.M., Wahlen C. & Marcelle R. (1986) Effects of E. coli endotoxin on pulmonary vascular resistance in intact dogs. *Critical Care Medicine* **14**, 802–6.

De Boelpaepe C., Vincent J.-L., Contempre B., Luypaert P., Schwartz D., Coussart E. & Cantraine F. (1989) Combination of norepinephrine and amrinone in the treatment of endotoxin shock. *Journal of Critical Care* **4**, 202–7.

Downs J.B. & Rasanen J. (1987) Dual oximetry in assessment of cardiopulmonary function. In *Update in Intensive Care and*

Emergency Medicine (Ed. Vincent J.-L.) pp. 342–8. Springer Verlag, Berlin.

Ducas J. & Prewitt R.M. (1988) Right ventricular dysfunction, detection and treatment. In *Recent Advances in Critical Care Medicine* 3 (Ed. Ledingham I.McA.) pp. 109–18. Churchill Livingstone, Edinburgh.

Editorial (1986) Pulmonary capillary pressure? *Critical Care Medicine* **14**, 76–7.

Edwards J.D. & Kishen R. (1986) Significance and management of intractable supraventricular arrhythmias in critically ill patients. *Critical Care Medicine* **14**, 280–2.

Edwards J.D. & Tweedle D.E. (1986) Haemodynamic response to dopamine in severe human septic shock. *British Journal of Surgery* **73**, 503.

Edwards J.D. & Wilkins R.G. (1987) Atrial fibrillation precipitated by acute hypovolaemia. *British Medical Journal* **294**, 283–4.

Fink S., Ray W., McCartney S., Ehrlich H. & Shoemaker W.C. (1984) Oxygen transport and utilization in hyperoxia and hypoxia: relation of conjunctival and transcutaneous oxygen tensions to haemodynamic and oxygen transport variables. *Critical Care Medicine* **12**, 943–8.

Fischer E., Marano M.A., Van Zee K.J., Rock C.S., Hawes A.S., Thompson W.A., DeForge L., Kenney J.S., Remick D.G. & Bloedow D.C. (1992) Interleukin-1 receptor blockade improves survival and hemodynamic performance in *Escherichia coli* septic shock, but fails to alter host responses to sublethal endotoxemia. *Journal of Clinical Investigation* **89**, 1551–7.

Fleck A., Hawker F., Wallace P.G.M., Raines G., Trotter J., Ledingham I.McA. & Calman K.C. (1985) Increased vascular permeability. A major cause of hypoalbuminaemia in disease and injury. *Lancet* **I**, 781–4.

Friedman P.J. & Vincent J.-L. (1993) Comparison of blood lactate levels and pHi in septic patients. *American Review of Respiratory Diseases* **147**, 623A.

Furey S.A., Zieske H.A. & Levy M.N. (1984) The essential function of the right ventricle. *American Heart Journal* **107**, 404–10.

Ganong W.F. (1983) *Review of Medical Physiology* 11th edn., pp. 414–506. Lange Medical Publications, California.

Gillespie T.A., Roberts R., Ambos H.D. & Sobel B.E. (1975) Salutory effects of dobutamine on haemodynamics without exacerbation of arrhythmia or myocardial injury. *Circulation* **52** (Suppl. II), 76.

Gilmour D.G., Aitkenhead A.R., Hothersall A.P. & Ledingham I.McA. (1980) The effect of hypovolaemia on colon blood flow in the dog. *British Journal of Surgery* **67**, 82–4.

Goldfarb R.D. & Glenn T.M. (1983) Regulation of lysosomal membrane stabilization via cyclic nucleotides and prostaglandins: the effects of steroids and indomethacin. In *Molecular and Cellular Aspects of Shock and Trauma* (Eds Lefel A.M. & Schumer W.) pp. 147–66. Liss, New York.

Gutierrez G., Palizas F., Doglio G., Wainsztein N., Gallesio A., Pacin J., Dubin A., Schiavi E., Jorge M., Pusajo J., Klein F., San Roman E., Dorfman B., Shottlender J. & Giniger R. (1992) Gastric intramucosal pH as a therapeutic index of tissue oxygenation in critical patients. *Lancet* **339**, 195–9.

Hackel D.B., Mikat E.M., Reimer K. & Whalen G. (1981) Effect of verapamil on heart and circulation in haemorrhagic shock

in dogs. *American Journal of Physiology* **241**, H12–17.

Haglund U. & Lundgren O. (1978) Intestinal ischaemia and shock factors. *Federation Proceedings* **37**, 2729–33.

Haljamäe H. (1984) Interstitial fluid response. In *Clinical Surgery International*, vol. 9. Shock and Related Problems. (Ed. Shires G.T.) pp. 44–60. Churchill Livingstone, New York.

Haupt M.T., Gilbert E.M. & Carlson R.W. (1985) Fluid loading increases oxygen consumption in septic patients with lactic acidosis. *American Review of Respiratory Disease* **131**, 912–16.

Heard S.O., Perkins M.W. & Fink M.P. (1992) Tumor necrosis factor-alpha causes myocardial depression in guinea pigs. *Critical Care Medicine* **20**, 523–7.

Heath D.F. (1980) Carbohydrate metabolism after injury. The development and maintenance of hyperglycaemia. In *Advances in Physiological Science*, vol. 26. Homeostastis in Injury and Shock. (Eds Biro Z.S., Kovách A.G.B., Spitzer J.J. & Stoner H.B.) pp. 63–70. Pergamon, Oxford.

Hinds C.J. & Donaldson M.J.S. (1988) Endogenous opioid peptides. In *Recent Advances in Critical Care Medicine* 3 (Ed. Ledingham I.McA.). Churchill Livingstone, Edinburgh.

Jennings R.B. (1976) Relationship of acute ischaemia to functional defects and irreversibility. *Circulation* **52** (Suppl. I), 26–9.

Joly H.R. & Weil M.H. (1969) Temperature of the great toe as an indication of the severity of shock. *Circulation* **39**, 131–8.

Kern M.J., Aguirre F.V., Tatineni S., Penick D., Serota H., Donohue T. & Walter K. (1993) Enhanced coronary blood flow velocity during intraaortic balloon counterpulsation in critically ill patients. *Journal of the American College of Cardiology* **21**, 359–68.

Knaus W.A., Draper E.A., Wagner D.P. & Zimmerman J.E. (1985) APACHE II: a severity of disease classification system. *Critical Care Medicine* **13**, 818–29.

Kram H.B., Appel P.L., Fleming A.W. & Shoemaker W.C. (1986) Assessment of intestinal and renal perfusion using surface oximetry. *Critical Care Medicine* **14**, 707–13.

Kruse J.A., Haupt M.T., Puri V.K. & Carlson R.W. (1990) Lactate levels as predictors of the relationship between oxygen delivery and consumption in ARDS. *Chest* **98**, 959–62.

Kwaan H.M. & Weil M.H. (1969) Differences in the mechanism of shock caused by bacterial infections. *Surgery, Gynecology and Obstetrics* **128**, 37–45.

Lanore J.J., Dhainaut J.F., Fisher C.J., Opal S.M., Zimmerman J., Nightingale R., Stephens S., Schein R.L., Panacek E.R., Vincent J.-L., Foulke G.E., Warren E.L., Garrard C., Park G., Bodmer M.W., Cohen J., Van der Linden G., Sadoff J.C. & Pochard F. (1993) Effects of an anti-TNF IgG monoclonal antibody on left ventricular performance in septic patients. *American Review of Respiratory Disease* **147**, 202A.

Ledingham I.McA. & Ramsay G. (1986) Hypovolaemic shock. *British Journal of Anaesthesia* **58**, 169–89.

Ledingham I.McA. & Watt I. (1983) Influence of sedation on mortality in critically ill multiple trauma patients. *Lancet* **i**, 1270.

Ledingham I.McA., McArdle C.S., Fisher W.D. & Madden M. (1974) The incidence of shock syndrome in a general hospital. *Postgraduate Medical Journal* **50**, 420–4.

Ledingham I.McA., Alcock S.R., Eastaway A.T., McDonald I.C., McKay I.C. & Ramsay G. (1988) Triple regimen of selective decontamination of the digestive tract, systemic cefotaxime, and microbiological surveillance for prevention of acquired infection in intensive care. *Lancet* **I**, 785–90.

Leier C.V., Heban P.T., Huss P., Bush C.A. & Lewis R.P. (1978) Comparative systemic and regional haemodynamic effects of dopamine and dobutamine in patients with cardiomyopathic heart failure. *Circulation* **58**, 466–75.

Lloyd-Thomas A.R., Wright I.H. & Hinds C.J. (1986) Intensive therapy for life-threatening medical complications of malignancy. *Intensive Care Medicine* **12** (Suppl.), 249.

Loeb H.S., Bredakis J. & Gunnar R.M. (1977) Superiority of dobutamine over dopamine for augmentation of cardiac output in patients with chronic low output cardiac failure. *Circulation* **55**, 375–81.

Macintyre E., Mackie I.J., Ho D., Tinker J., Bullen C. & Machin S.J. (1985) The haemostatic effect of hydroxyethyl starch (HES) used as a volume expander. *Intensive Care Medicine* **II**, 300–3.

MacLean L.D., Mulligan W.G., McLean A.P.H. & Duff J.H. (1967) Patterns of septic shock in man — a detailed study of 56 patients. *Annals of Surgery* **166**, 543–62.

Matthay R.A. & Berger H.J. (1983) Noninvasive assessment of right and left ventricular function in acute and chronic respiratory failure. *Critical Care Medicine* **11**, 329–38.

Meadows D., Edwards J.D., Wilkins R.G. & Nightingale P. (1988) Reversal of intractable septic shock with norepinephrine therapy. *Critical Care Medicine* **16**, 663–6.

Meakins J.L., Wicklund B., Forse R.A. & McLean A.P.H. (1980) The surgical intensive care unit: current concepts in infection. *Surgical Clinics of North America* **60**, 117–32.

Mehta J., Pepine C.J. & Conti C.R. (1978) Haemodynamic effects of hydralazine and glyceryl trinitrate paste in heart failure. *British Heart Journal* **40**, 845–50.

Messmer K. (1984) Blood substitutes in shock therapy. In *Clinical Surgery International*, vol. 9. Shock and Related Problems. (Ed. Shires G.T. III) pp. 192–205. Churchill Livingstone, Edinburgh.

Nunn J.F. (1977) *Applied Respiratory Physiology* 2nd edn. Butterworths, London.

Packman M.I. & Rackow E.C. (1983) Optimum left heart filling pressure during fluid resuscitation of patients with hypovolaemic and septic shock. *Critical Care Medicine* **11**, 165–9.

Parker M.M., Shelhamer J.H., Bacharach S.L., Green M.V., Natanson C., Frederick T.M., Damske B.A. & Parillo J.E. (1984a) Profound but reversible myocardial depression in patients with septic shock. *Annals of Internal Medicine* **100**, 483–90.

Parker M.M., Shelhamer J.H., Natanson C., Masur H. & Parillo J.E. (1984b) Serial haemodynamic patterns in survivors and non-survivors of septic shock in humans. *Critical Care Medicine* **12**, 311.

Pinsky M.R., Vincent J.-L. & De Smet J.M. (1991) Estimating left ventricular filling pressure during positive end-expiratory pressure in humans. *American Review of Respiratory Disease* **143**, 25–31.

Prewitt R.M. & Ghignone M. (1983) Treatment of right ventricular dysfunction in acute respiratory failure. *Critical Care Medicine* **11**, 346–52.

Priebe H.J. (1992) Myocardial ischemia during vasodilator therapy in a canine model of pulmonary hypertension and coronary insufficiency. *Anaesthesiology* **76**, 781–91.

Prytz H., Holst-Chrustensen B., Korner B. & Liehr H. (1976) Portal venous and systemic endotoxaemia in patients without liver disease and systemic endotoxaemia in patients with cirrhosis. *Scandinavian Journal of Gastroenterology* **11**, 857–63.

Rae A.P. & Hutton I. (1986) Cardiogenic shock and the haemodynamic effects of arrhythmias. *British Journal of Anaesthesia* **58**, 151–68.

Reichert C.L., Visser C.A., Koolen J.J., Van den Brink R.B., Van Wezel H.B., Myne N.G. & Dunning A.J. (1992) Transesophageal echocardiography in hypotensive patients after cardiac operations. *Journal of Thoracic and Cardiovascular Surgery* **104**, 321–6.

Reuse C., Vincent J.-L. & Pinsky M.R. (1990) Measurements of right ventricular volumes during fluid challenge. *Chest* **98**, 1450–4.

Robin E.D. & McCauley R. (1992) Nitroprusside-related cyanide poisoning. Time (long past due) for urgent, effective interventions. *Chest* **102**, 1842–5.

Shoemaker W.C., Schluchter M., Hopkins J.A., Appel P.L., Schwartz S. & Chang P. (1981) Fluid therapy in emergency resuscitation: clinical evaluation of colloid and crystalloid regimens. *Critical Care Medicine* **9**, 367–8.

Shoemaker W.C., Appel P. & Kram H.B. (1986) Haemodynamic and oxygen transport effects of dobutamine in critically ill general surgical patients. *Critical Care Medicine* **14**, 1032–7.

Sibbald W.J. & Driedger A.A. (1983) Right ventricular function in acute disease states: physiologic considerations. *Critical Care Medicine* **11**, 339–45.

Sibbald W.J., Driedger A.A., Cunningham D.G. & Cheung H. (1986) Right and left ventricular performance in acute hypoxemic respiratory failure. *Critical Care Medicine* **14**, 852–7.

Silance P.G., Simon C. & Vincent J.-L. (1993) The relation between cardiac index and oxygen extraction in acutely ill patients. *Chest* (In press).

Sonnenblick E.H. & Skelton C.L. (1971) Myocardial energetics: basic principles and clinical implications. *New England Journal of Medicine* **285**, 688–75.

Stacpoole P.W., Wright E.C., Baumgartner T.G., Bersin R.M., Buchalter S., Curry S.H., Duncan C.A., Harman E.M., Henderson G.N., Jenkinson S., Lachin J.M., Lorenz A., Schneider S.H., Siegel J.M., Summer W.R., Thompson D., Wolfe C.L. & Zorovich B. (1992) A controlled clinical trial of dichloroacetate for treatment of lactic acidosis in adults. *New England Journal of Medicine* **327**, 1564–9.

Stemple D., Griffin J.C., Kernoff R.S. & Harrison D.C. (1976) Metabolic and electrophysiologic effects of nitroprusside and dopamine in experimental acute myocardial infarction. *Clinical Research* **24**, 141A.

Stephenson L.W., Blackstone E.H. & Kouchoukos N.T. (1976) Dopamine vs. epinephrine in patients following cardiac surgery. *Surgery Forum* **27**, 272–5.

Stoner H.B., Frayn K.M., Barton R.N., Threlfall C.J. & Little R.A. (1979) The relationship between plasma substrates and hormones and the severity of injury in 277 recently injured patients. *Clinical Science* **56**, 563–73.

Taylor M.B. & Whitwam J.G. (1986) The current status of pulse oximetry: clinical value of continuous noninvasive oxygen saturation. *Anaesthesia* **41**, 943–9.

Thomas J.D. & Weyman A.E. (1991) Echocardiographic Doppler evaluation of left ventricular diastolic function. *Circulation* **84**, 977–90.

Thuillez C., Richard C., Teboul J.L., Annane D., Bellissant E.,

Auzepy P. & Guidicelli J.F. (1993) Arterial hemodynamics and cardiac effects of enoximone, dobutamine, and their combination in severe heart failure. *American Heart Journal* **125**, 799–808.

Trump B.F., Mergner W.J., Kahng M.W. & Saladino A.J. (1976) Studies on the subcellular pathophysiology of ischaemia. *Circulation* **53** (Suppl. I), 17–25.

Twigley A.J. & Hillman K.M. (1985) The end of the crystalloid era? *Anaesthesia* **40**, 860–71.

Vary T.C., Siegel J.H. & Rivkind A. (1988) Clinical and therapeutic significance of metabolic patterns of lactic acidosis. *Perspectives in Critical Care* **1**, 85–132.

Vatner S.F., Higgins C.B. & Braunwald E. (1974a) Effects of norepinephrine on coronary circulation and left ventricular dynamics in the conscious dog. *Circulation Research* **34**, 812–23.

Vatner S.F., McRitchie R.J. & Braunwald E. (1974b) Effects of dobutamine on left ventricular performance, coronary dynamics and distribution of cardiac output in conscious dogs. *Journal of Clinical Investigation* **53**, 1265–73.

Vincent J.-L. (1991) Fluids for resuscitation. *British Journal of Anaesthesia* **61**, 185–93.

Vincent J.-L. (1993) Renal effects of dopamine: may our dream ever come true? *Critical Care Medicine* (In press).

Vincent J.-L., Carlier E., Berré J., Armistead C.W., Kahn R.J., Coussaert E. & Cantraine F. (1988) Administration of enoximone in cardiogenic shock. *American Journal of Cardiology* **62**, 419–23.

Vincent J.-L., Reuse C. & Kahn R.J. (1989) Administration of dopexamine, a new adrenergic agent, in cardiorespiratory failure. *Chest* **96**, 1233–6.

Vincent J.-L., Roman A., DeBacker D. & Kahn R.J. (1990a) Oxygen uptake/supply dependency: effects of short-term dobutamine infusion. *American Review of Respiratory Diseases* **142**, 2–8.

Vincent J.-L., Roman A. & Kahn R.J. (1990b) Dobutamine administration in septic shock: addition to a standard protocol. *Critical Care Medicine* **18**, 689–93.

Vincent J.-L., Bakker J., Marécaux G., Schandene L., Kahn R.J. & Dupont E. (1992a) Anti-TNF antibodies administration increases myocardial contractility in septic shock patients.

Chest **101**, 810–15.

Vincent J.-L., Carlier E., Pinsky M.R., Goldstein J., Naeije R., Lejeune P., Brimioulle S., Leclerc J.L., Kahn R.J. & Primo G. (1992b) Prostaglandin E1 infusion for right ventricular failure after cardiac transplantation. *Journal of Thoracic and Cardiovascular Surgery* **103**, 33–9.

Vincent J.-L., Gris P., Coffernils M., Leon M., Pinsky M.R., Reuse C. & Kahn R.J. (1992c) Myocardial depression and decreased vascular tone characterize fatal course from septic shock. *Surgery* **111**, 660–7.

Vincent J.-L., Leon M., Berré J., Melot C. & Kahn R.J., (1992d) Addition of enoximone to adrenergic agents in the management of severe heart failure. *Critical Care Medicine* **20**, 1102–6.

Virgilio R.W., Rice C.L., Smith D.E., James D.R., Zarins C.K., Hobelmann C.F. & Peters R.M. (1979a) Crystalloid vs. colloid resuscitation: is one better? *Surgery* **85**, 129–39.

Virgilio R.W., Smith D.E. & Zarins C.K. (1979b) Balanced electrolyte solutions: experimental and clinical studies. *Critical Care Medicine* **7**, 98–106.

Wardle E.N. (1978) A review of endotoxin and its absorption from the gut. In *Antigen Absorption by the Gut* (Ed. Hemmings W.A.) pp. 183–8. Medical and Technical Publishing, Lancaster.

Watson J.K., Varley J.G., Hinds C.J., Bouloux P., Tomlin S. & Rees L.H. (1984) Adrenal vein and systemic levels of catecholamines and metenkephalin like immunoreactivity in canine endotoxic shock; effects of naloxone administration. *Circulatory Shock* **13**, 47.

Wiles J.B., Cerra F.B., Siegel J.H. & Border J.R. (1980) The systemic septic response: does the organism matter? *Critical Care Medicine* **8**, 55–60.

Wilmore D.W., Goodwin C.W., Aulick L.H., Powanda M.C., Mason A.D. & Pruitt B.A. (1980) Effect of injury and infection on visceral metabolism and circulation. *Annals of Surgery* **192**, 491–500.

Woods I., Wilkins R.G., Edwards J.D., Martin P.D. & Faragher E.B. (1987) The danger of using peripheral/core temperature gradient as a guide to therapy in shock. *Critical Care Medicine* **15**, 850–2.

Nutrition

S.M. WILLATTS

Nutritional disturbances are extremely common in patients requiring intensive therapy and such disturbances have far-reaching consequences. The critically ill develop a marked stress response to trauma with disturbances of carbohydrate, fat and protein metabolism. Oxygen consumption is increased, fluid overload is common and susceptibility to sepsis is high.

The effects of malnutrition are legion. The topic is discussed by Cahill (1970), although Studley (1936) first noticed the adverse effect of a reduction in body weight. Acute weight loss in excess of 20% is associated with a postoperative mortality of 33% compared with 3.5% in those who have not lost weight. Malnutrition is generally held to lead to progressive weakness and other well known effects listed in Table 87.1, although the efficacy of peri-operative parenteral nutrition in reducing mortality and morbidity has been continuously questioned (Biebuyck, 1981; Veterans Affairs Total Parenteral Nutrition Cooperative Study Group, 1991). The ability to respond to infection is attributed in part to a group of proteins, leucocyte endogenous mediators, which are reduced in malnutrition and restored by increased protein intake.

It has been estimated that 40–50% of medical and surgical patients exhibit protein energy malnutrition at some time during their hospital stay (Bistrian et al., 1974). Unfortunately, we do not have a simple nutritional index of sufficient predictive power to define that group of patients who need feeding (Baker et al., 1982). Whilst malnutrition is clearly widespread in hospitalized patients and many of its effects are evident and at least partially preventable, associated disturbances in drug disposition (Pantuck et al., 1984; Vessell & Biebuyck, 1984), neurotransmitter release (Pardridge, 1983) and conscious level (Glaeser et al., 1983) are more difficult to manage.

The volume of nutritional support is often limited by salt and water retention produced by increased aldosterone and antidiuretic hormone (ADH) secretion whilst complications of overzealous nutritional replacement can be severe, ranging from respiratory failure to hyperosmolar states. An understanding of basic metabolism and energy requirements is therefore very important. It is illogical to infuse nutritional substances without knowledge of energy requirements and metabolic measurement of the consequences (Biebuyck, 1983).

A national survey undertaken in 1988 (Payne-James et al., 1991) reviewed current practice for management of nutritional depletion. Despite advances in enteral and parenteral nutritional support, wide variation was found in delivery of clinical nutritional support with very little use of nutritional advisory teams. With the cost of parenteral nutrition approaching £100/day it is essential that studies are set up to show the benefit of this compared with enteral nutrition which, additionally, may maintain intestinal mucosal integrity.

The energy substrates

Carbohydrate

Under normal circumstances of adequate nutrition, carbohydrate is almost always ingested in excess of requirements but blood glucose concentration is maintained at 4–8 mmol/litre. Carbohydrate is absorbed from the gut as hexoses (glucose, fructose, galactose) and reaches the liver in the portal circulation where the major uptake occurs. Some glucose bypasses the liver and is metabolized in other tissues, especially muscle where it is used to replenish glycogen stores. The arrival of glucose at the liver has two major effects.

1 Inhibition of endogenous glucose production.
2 Phosphorylation of glucose to glucose-6-phosphate,

Table 87.1 Effects of malnutrition. (Redrawn from Irvin, 1978)

Progressive weakness
Reduced vital capacity, respiratory rate, minute volume
Increased risk of respiratory infection
Difficulty in weaning from ventilatory support
Reduced cardiac output, myocardial contractility and
    compliance
Reduced tensile strength of skin, increased wound dehiscence
Breakdown of anastomoses
Reduced plasma proteins, susceptibility to salt and water
    overload
Reduced host resistance

which is converted into glycogen or metabolized first to pyruvate via the Embden—Myerhof pathway and thence to acetyl co-enzyme A (CoA) and fatty acids.

There are several mechanisms whereby ingested carbohydrate is stored, either as carbohydrate or lipid, for use during fasting. However, the human body has only limited reserves of energy substrates, and hepatic glycogen is depleted rapidly in starvation (Table 87.2).

In the normal human body, the CNS is dependent entirely on glucose except in the starved state. Red blood cells and the adrenal medulla are entirely glucose dependent. Glucose is the main substrate, therefore, for oxidative metabolism, and the only one for anaerobic metabolic. Oxidative metabolism continues *in vivo* with a small mitochondrial Po_2 0.067 kPa (0.5 mmHg), producing 38 moles of adenosine triphosphate (ATP) from 1 mole of glucose. Whilst adequate ingested carbohydrate is essential to maintain a normal blood glucose, there are dangers of hyperglycaemia which, if persistent, causes increased polyol accumulation in tissues, hyperlacta-taemia, hormone imbalance and glycosylation of tissue proteins including haemoglobin. In this respect, an increase in the proportion or absolute amount of starchy foods may be of benefit to both carbohydrate and fat metabolism because of its reduced hyperglycaemic response.

Regulation of carbohydrate metabolism

Mechanisms of regulation of carbohydrate metabolism are summarized in Table 87.3.

In the fed state, insulin secretion increases in response to carbohydrate and protein feeding. The effect of insulin is to increase phosphorylation of glucose, to activate glycogen synthetase and allow rapid disposal of glucose into glycogen stores. Insulin also increases glycolysis and pyruvate dehydrogenase activity with an increase in acetyl CoA carboxylase which therefore directs glucose towards fatty acid (FA) (implying non-esterified fatty acid) synthesis (Table 87.4).

Table 87.3 Mechanisms of regulation of carbohydrate metabolism

Endocrine	Non-hormonal
Anabolic	*Glucose infusion*
Insulin	Inhibits hepatic glucose output
Catabolic	*Glucose—FA—KB cycle*
Glucagon	Increased circulating FAs and KBs
Cortisol	inhibit glucose oxidation in heart
Catecholamines	and muscle
Growth hormone	

Table 87.4 Effects of insulin

Stimulates
Glucose phosphorylation
Glycogen synthetase
Pyruvate dehydrogenase
Acetyl CoA carboxylase, directing glucose towards fat
    synthesis

Inhibits
Glycogenolysis
Gluconeogenesis
Lipolysis
Proteolysis

Table 87.2 Nutritional reserves of a 70-kg man

	kg	Duration	kcal
Carbohydrate (mainly liver glycogen)	0.2	6—12 h	800
Fat	12—15	20—25 days	109 000—136 000
Protein (mainly muscle)	4—6	10—12 days	16 000—24 000

The net effect of insulin secretion, therefore, is to increase glucose transport into muscle and fat, to inhibit lipolysis and proteolysis and thus to reduce gluconeogenic precursors. In starvation, plasma insulin concentrations are low and act mainly to inhibit catabolism.

Catabolic hormones

Most of the hormonal effects on glucose metabolism are mediated by endocrine receptors found in all cells. Hormones may affect the action of each other by altering the affinity or the number of receptors for other hormones. Both cortisol and growth hormone alter insulin receptors, and insulin can 'down-regulate' its own receptors which is important in insulin resistance of stress states. Carbohydrate metabolism, therefore, depends on the balance between circulating insulin and catabolic hormones (Table 87.5).

In the fed situation, insulin predominates; if the subject is fasted, there is a predominance of catabolic hormones. In circumstances where the stress response is activated, despite the fed state, a surge of catabolic hormones occurs.

Fat

Lipids make a large contribution to energy stores and they may be stored as compact water-insoluble droplets in adipose tissue. Triacylglycerol (TAG) is the current term for the combination of three FAs with glycerol, termed previously neutral fat or triglyceride. Triacylglycerol has a very high calorie content (9.3 kcal/g). Ketone bodies (KBs) are produced from lipids especially during starvation when they may reduce the requirements for glucose and minimize gluconeogenesis from amino acids. After 4 days of fasting, triacylglycerol, non-esterified FA and KB

Table 87.5 Catabolic hormones

Glucagon
Maximal effects between feeding
Stimulates glycogenolysis (short term)
Stimulates hepatic uptake of amino acid

Cortisol
Enhances peripheral proteolysis
Increases FA release for gluconeogenesis

Catecholamines
Enhance glycogenolysis
Increase lactate output

Growth hormone
Short term increases glucose transport to muscle
Longer term impairs glucose uptake, increasing use of
    alternative substrates

constitute approximately 85% of the potential energy available in plasma (Table 87.6).

Fat exists in the body in a great variety of forms: the main ones are summarized in Table 87.7.

Metabolism of lipids and ketone bodies

Ingested lipid is hydrolysed in the duodenum to glycerol and FAs. These latter are absorbed by epithelial cells and resynthesized into TAG which is incorporated into chylomicrons (CMs) and apoproteins A and B, and pass eventually into the thoracic duct and then the circulation. Some TAG is taken up by the liver where essential. FAs are possibly removed. Some is taken up by the heart and muscle but most goes to adipose tissue. Non-esterified FAs are very important fuels of respiration with half-lives in the circulation of 2–3 min.

The liver converts FAs into TAG and very low-density lipoproteins (VLDLs) or oxidizes FAs to KBs. Adipose tissue stores TAG and controls its release as FAs. Lipoproteins are confined to the intravascular

Table 87.6 Fuels in circulation

| Substrate | Overnight fast | | Four-day fast | |
	Concentration (µmol/ml)	Available energy (%)	Concentration (µmol/ml)	Available energy (%)
FAs	0.42	9	1.15	20
TAG	1.0	65	1.0	54
Glucose	4.7	25	3.6	16
Lactate	0.5	<1	0.5	<1
KBs	0.03	<1	2.9	9

Table 87.7 Fats in the body

Triacylglycerol (TAG)	8–100 nm, soluble in aqueous media, carried in plasma as micelles with lipoproteins, found in liver and intestine
Chylomicrons (CMs)	100–1000 nm, produced by intestine and liver from dietary fat, removed rapidly from plasma
Lipoproteins	Structure aids carriage and delivery TAG to target tissues
Very low density lipoproteins (VLDLs)	30–80 nm, produced from TAG in liver, secreted into plasma, an important energy source
Low-density lipoproteins	25–30 nm, cholesterol enriched, correlation with atherosclerosis
High-density lipoproteins	8–20 nm, esterify cholesterol, mediate exchange of apoproteins, inverse correlation with atherosclerosis
Apoproteins	Synthesized in liver and intestine, used in assembly of VLDLs and CMs, activate enzymes, interact with specific cell-wall receptors, mark residual fat particles for removal by reticuloendothelial system
Fatty acids (FAs)	Non-esterified FAs transported in plasma bound to albumin, at pH 7.4 carboxyl group almost completely dissociated
Ketone bodies (KBs)	β-hydroxybutyrate and acetoacetate are lipid derived and relatively polar

space. Metabolism of CMs depends on hydrolysis in the circulation to FAs and glycerol. Glucose cannot be synthesized directly from FAs but glycerol is a gluconeogenic precursor and FAs can be converted into ketone bodies. Hydrolysis of TAG is catalysed by lipoprotein lipase which is found on the luminal surface of capillaries in adipose tissue, heart and skeletal muscle. Fatty acids can then cross capillary membranes where they can be used by most tissues except the CNS for oxidation and TAG synthesis as a local energy reserve. In heart muscle, FAs are preferred to glucose and when both are present, glucose uptake and oxidation are reduced greatly. Synthesis of TAG requires glucose as the precursor of glycerol-3-phosphate. During starvation, insulin secretion is reduced thereby reducing glucose uptake and TAG synthesis. Lack of glucose favours lipolysis and release of FAs. Lipolysis is stimulated by catecholamines, cortisol and thyroxine.

The concentration of KBs is increased during starvation, diabetes, uraemia, a high-fat diet, exercise, infancy and the perinatal period. All tissues except the liver have the ability to oxidize KBs. The plasma concentration depends on the balance between hepatic synthesis and peripheral utilization. Oxidation of KBs reduces the demand for glucose, the necessity for gluconeogenesis and degradation of protein, and in starvation the concentration of insulin, an antilipolytic hormone, decreases. Infants and children have more active KBs transport systems and a greater capacity to extract KBs from blood. This

mechanism may be important particularly in children who can become hypoglycaemic (and hyperketonaemic) after a very short fast. The influence of hormones on fat metabolism is summarized in Table 87.8.

Brown fat is found in cervical, interscapular, axillary, intrathoracic and perirenal depots and is responsible for buffering changes in food intake. Catecholamine stimulation of brown fat increases the supply of FAs for mitochondrial oxidation. The calorigenic effect of catecholamines may result from their effect of mobilizing free FAs. Heat is dissipated by uncoupling of mitochondrial oxidative processes and

Table 87.8 The influence of hormones on fat metabolism

Insulin
Promotes esterification of fatty acids (FAs)
Inhibits lipolysis
Stimulates glucose entry into fat cells (glycerol-3-phosphate)
Stimulates intracellular lipase
Reduced supply of FAs to liver inhibits ketone-body (KB)
   formation

Glucagon
Stimulates lipolysis, possibly only when insulin level is low
Stimulates gluconeogenesis
Inhibits glycolysis and FA synthesis

Cortisol, growth hormones, catecholamines, thyroid hormones together and separately mobilize FAs from adipose tissue. All these effects reversed by insulin.

heat production proceeds at maximal level. Central control mechanisms for this activity lie in the hypothalamus (Himms-Hagen, 1984).

Grossly obese patients have apparently defective thermogenesis in the mitochondria of brown fat. Exposure of anaesthetized, paralysed patients to a cold environment induces non-shivering thermogenesis, which is greater in lean subjects, with accompanying increased oxygen consumption. Obese patients have higher expenditure during normal life. Self-recorded energy intake tends to be underestimated in the obese (Prentice et al., 1986).

Fasting

During fasting, glucose must be produced at 180 g every 24 h. This is effected by glycogenolysis and gluconeogenesis. These two processes occur in the liver where phosphorylase is activated to produce glucose-6-phosphate from which free glucose is liberated. The substrates for gluconeogenesis are lactate, pyruvate, glycerol and the glucogenic amino acids (AAs); alanine, glutamine and glycine. Lactate provides approximately 50% of the precursor pool. Under normal circumstances, the liver can remove up to 400 g of lactate daily from the circulation, but if hypoxia intervenes, liver blood flow and function are impaired and this capacity is reduced. Glycerol provides 5–10% of the gluconeogenic precursor pool. The liver metabolizes normally 80–90% of available glycerol which in the fasting state is converted to glucose. The remainder of new glucose is derived from AAs, especially alanine which is formed by transamination of pyruvate in peripheral tissues.

As glycogen reserves are limited, most glucose is derived from gluconeogenesis, and protein breakdown occurs to provide the AAs. This process is limited by keto-adaptation. The CNS may use KBs as oxidative fuels in conditions of starvation, such that the total glucose requirement of the CNS decreases by 50% after approximately 5 weeks of starvation. During starvation, overall energy needs of the body are reduced, energy expenditure diminishes by up to 35%, ketoacids are substituted for glucose as brain fuel and the pool of free FAs increases.

Short-term starvation consumes glycogen stores, and proteolysis and lipolysis begin. As proteolysis proceeds, there is a reduction in muscle mass and muscle weakness and respiratory complications develop with an increased incidence of infection resulting occasionally in death. The greatest losses of nitrogen after trauma occur in well-fed young men. After long-term starvation, nitrogen losses in the urine are low because of protein-sparing mechanisms which come into play. These include enhanced KB production and their utilization by the CNS. In total starvation, the basal metabolic rate (BMR) declines by 20% after 3 weeks and 40% by 6 months. However, when the stress response is activated postoperatively, insulin concentrations increase, lipolysis is inhibited and metabolism is more dependent on glucose again. In the fasting state, the heart can metabolize FAs as a primary energy substrate. In the presence of a high concentration of glucose and insulin, myocardial stores of glycogen can be increased, which is valuable (should the heart suddenly become hypoxic) to provide substrate for anaerobic metabolism.

Adult volunteers electively starved for 10 days develop negative potassium, phosphate, magnesium and nitrogen balance. If they are subsequently fed, they develop equilibrium or positive nitrogen and electrolyte balance but with a decrease in muscle membrane potential (Legaspi et al., 1988). Thus, restoration of lean tissue protein and cellular function does not occur at a rate which might be inferred from positive nitrogen balance. A persistent defect of cellular function is evident after starvation but short periods (10 days) of parenteral nutrition are insufficient to restore skeletal muscle integrity. Nitrogen retained is distributed between lean body mass and the humoral protein compartment and thus is not necessarily an indication of improved muscle mass, and this could not be demonstrated in the elemental balance techniques used in this study.

Protein turnover

Protein synthesis and degradation are under independent control. Muscle plays a key role in uptake of AAs after a meal and in release of AAs during fasting. Protein synthesis decreases by 50% during starvation. During periods of rapid growth, protein synthesis increases but this is associated also with increased protein degradation. In animals, starvation leads to loss of pulmonary surfactant and reduced acetyl CoA carboxylase activity and FA synthesis.

Loss of weight in the first few days after surgery is likely to result from water loss, but after 10–14 days is produced by loss of protein and fat. Kinney and Hessov (1981) calculate that the protein contribution to this weight loss could amount to 10–14% over a 3-week period. In a very ill catabolic patient with sepsis, up to 22% of the resting energy expenditure (REE) is derived from protein.

Stress response to trauma

Surgery or trauma activates a typical metabolic and hormonal response which may be mediated by pain or some other neural mechanism (Fig. 87.1) and may be accompanied by immunosuppression (Bardosi & Tekeres, 1985).

Cuthbertson and Tilstone (1969) described an 'ebb' and a 'flow' phase. Loss of nitrogen (N_2), potassium (K) and sodium (Na) from the body are greatest during the flow phase and changes recede if the patient recovers and anabolism begins. Arnold and Little (1991) discuss the evidence for the purported reduction in cardiac output during the ebb phase. There is increasing evidence of immediate increase in catecholamines and insulin counterregulatory hormones. During the flow phase there is certainly increased cardiac output and metabolic rate, enhancement of substrate utilization and increased release of FAs which are the preferred substrate for oxidation. In sepsis, changes are similar to those of the flow phase and where tissue injury has occurred, the reduction in oxygen consumption is not reversed by restoration of tissue oxygen delivery. After injury, blood flow to adipose tissue falls significantly and this, coupled with reduction in plasma albumin for FA binding, may significantly reduce FA utilization. Impaired tissue perfusion also increases lactate which enhances re-esterification of FAs to triacylglycerol.

A wound is in effect an extra organ demanding a significant fraction of the cardiac output. Cells involved in repair consume preferentially a large amount of glucose by anaerobic glycolysis: lactate is then converted back to glucose aerobically in the liver (at metabolic cost). Glucose turnover rate is increased after injury. Hepatic gluconeogenesis in the flow phase cannot be inhibited by infusion of large amounts of dextrose. The net loss of protein is shared by the whole body except the CNS.

In rats, division of afferent fibres from the site of injury suppresses development of the neuroendocrine response. Extensive extradural analgesia (Engquist et al., 1977) to block both somatic and sympathetic afferent activity, centrally acting morphine, fentanyl, alfentanil and high spinal-cord lesions suppress the response which can also be modified by pre-existing fear and anxiety. There is some evidence for a humoral pathway, which would not be modified by the above measures. Prostaglandins, bacterial endotoxin and other pyrogens have been postulated as 'wound hormones'. Interleukin-1 is the most investigated wound hormone which increases lysosomal protein degradation, an action which is mediated by prostaglandin E_2 (Baracos et al., 1983) although other peptides are involved also.

Endocrine changes

The hypothalamus acts as a final common pathway for the neuroendocrine response which involves secretion of pituitary hormones and sympathetic activity (Table 87.9).

Most hormones increase in proportion to the severity of the surgery although the adrenocorticotrophic hormone (ACTH) is a poor index of the severity of injury and the growth hormone (GH) response may vary with age.

Insulin secretion is depressed during surgery (Allison et al., 1969), presumably by increased concentrations of noradrenaline (Nakao & Miyata, 1977). Insulin concentrations can be increased by alpha block, but suppression is short-lived in uncomplicated surgery (Aarimaa et al., 1978), returning to

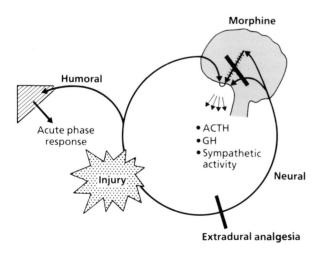

Fig. 87.1 Neuroendocrine response to stress. (Redrawn from Elliott & Alberti, 1983.)

Table 87.9 Hormones involved in the endocrine response to surgery

Neuroendocrine response	Systemic response
Adrenocorticotrophic hormone	Insulin
Vasopressin	Cortisol
Growth hormone	Glucagon
Thyroid-stimulating hormone	Thyroxine, triiodothyronine
Adrenaline	Aldosterone
Noradrenaline	Angiotensin

normal in about 7 days. Plasma glucose concentration and β-adrenergic activity increase. There is evidence also of tissue resistance to insulin (Thomas et al., 1979). Early hyperglycaemia (6–18h) is probably the result of adrenal medullary output rather than sympathetic nervous discharge. Studies in non-septic patients with musculoskeletal injury (Frayne et al., 1984) showed high plasma concentrations of insulin for the prevailing glucose concentration with peak urinary nitrogen excretion corresponding with maximum insulin concentration. As noted above, early after injury fat oxidation is high and later oxidation of carbohydrate increases relative to the concentrations of glucose and insulin.

The increase in plasma cortisol concentration is rapid, occurring within a few hours and is proportional to the severity of surgery (Stoner et al., 1979). Cortisol is termed the permissive hormone as it has little effect on glucose production, but acts by stimulating peripheral release of AAs as substrates for gluconeogenesis. The increase in glucagon is related also to the severity of injury and reaches a peak 18–48h after injury. Increased glucagon is thought to be caused by increased catecholamines (Porte & Robertson, 1975). Gluconeogenesis, glycogenolysis and AA uptake are stimulated in the liver (Woolfe et al., 1979).

Changes in thyroid hormones are variable (Goode et al., 1981) but extradural analgesia which suppresses cortisol has no effect on thyroid hormones (Brandt et al., 1976). Changes may be secondary to increased oxygen consumption after surgery. GH has only a minor effect, a normal metabolic response to trauma occurring in hypophysectomized patients receiving steroid replacement.

These hormonal effects stimulate mostly glucose production and catabolic processes, the so-called 'catabolic drive'. In normal male volunteers triple-hormone infusion of cortisol, glucagon and adrenaline produces significant hypermetabolism with a peripheral leucocytosis; a significant metabolic response to trauma (Bessey et al., 1984).

There is an increased demand for glucose after surgery to provide energy for wound repair. Whilst glycogenolysis continues, stimulated by catecholamines and glucagon, there is also an increase in lactate and pyruvate release from muscle. Pyruvate is taken up by the liver as a gluconeogenic substrate.

In severe injury, whole-body protein turnover increases but breakdown increases more than synthesis (Birkhahn et al., 1980). There is very little evidence for the assumption that the nitrogen loss in injury is produced by muscle breakdown (Rennie &

Harrison, 1984), although new isotope techniques may resolve this. Measurement of whole-body protein breakdown and 3-methyl histidine excretion in fasting shows a reduction in 3-methyl histidine excretion by total parenteral nutrition (TPN). However, increased non-muscle tissue breakdown is probably common in depleted patients (Lowry et al., 1985). There is a complex interaction between nutritional state and the degree of injury in severe trauma, burns and sepsis, and protein breakdown is relatively resistant to nutritional modification with marked unresponsiveness of protein metabolism to the normal anabolic effects of insulin. Catecholamine infusions used in these circumstances further increase glycogenolysis and hepatic gluconeogenesis and worsen insulin resistance.

Fat breakdown increases the release of glycerol and FAs which may be taken up by the muscles and used directly as an energy source or by the liver for conversion into KBs. Adrenaline and glucocorticoids stimulate adipose tissue lipolysis whilst glucagon speeds intrahepatic conversion of FAs and KBs. Isotope-tracing studies show increased fat cycling after injury which contributes to the increased metabolic rate. Propranolol infusion can reduce fat cycling in burned patients (Woolf et al., 1987).

In severe stress raised plasma lipid concentrations are partly a result of the action of tumour necrosis factor (TNF), which inhibits lipoprotein lipase.

One of the most prominent features of the stress response is therefore hyperglycaemia; both glucose oxidation and turnover are increased and the primary disturbance is one of increased hepatic output of glucose (Wilmore et al., 1980).

Severe metabolic derangements occur in the septic state with increased glucose utilization (Ryan, 1976) and often inappropriately low insulin concentrations, which correlate with cardiovascular decompensation, reduced cortisol (Sibbald et al., 1977) and reduced GH both of which are associated with a high mortality. Recovery is associated with return of a normal reciprocal relationship between insulin and glucagon.

Total-body oxygen consumption is increased. This may result from the hypermetabolism of infection (Gump et al., 1970a,b), or be catecholamine-induced after injury or following administration of excess glucose during TPN (Askanazi et al., 1980). This is discussed further below.

Effect of anaesthetic agents

Some aspects of the stress response to trauma may be modified by anaesthetic agents with the potential to improve postoperative nitrogen balance. In dogs receiving phentolamine and propranolol during a standard operation, urinary nitrogen losses, glutamine flux and muscle glutamine were not reduced by hormonal block but hindquarter nitrogen flux was diminished. Thus, hormonal block inhibits net skeletal muscle catabolism without altering whole-body nitrogen loss (Hulton et al., 1985).

Intrathecal diamorphine delays the hyperglycaemic response to colonic surgery and reduces cortisol compared with intravenous opioids. Extradural analgesia with local analgesic drugs and, to a lesser extent, opioids can improve nitrogen balance in the first 5 post-operative days and suppress plasma glucose and FA concentrations. Although midazolam obtunds catecholamine secretion during stress in animals through a central γ-aminobutyric acid (GABA) interaction, there is no blunting of the glycaemic response to surgery in humans (Dawson & Sear, 1986). Most anaesthetic techniques modify the response to surgery only for the duration of their intervention and pain relief per se may have little effect (Hjortso et al., 1985).

Malnutrition

The effects of malnutrition

A reduction in protein and calorie intake reduces protein turnover, synthesis and breakdown (Reeds & James, 1983). During repletion there are both increased synthesis and increased breakdown, but the former predominates with net accumulation of protein. Starvation occurring in the previously well-nourished patient increases plasma concentrations of branched-chain amino acids (BCAAs) and glycine and reduces plasma alanine. Specific plasma amino acid patterns are found in sepsis and hepatic failure, but these do not reflect necessarily the AA concentration of the muscle or the total pool of free AAs. Severe malnutrition is accompanied by profound disturbance of immune function (Shizgal, 1981).

Nutritional assessment (Table 87.10)

Most patients requiring intensive therapy show some evidence of malnutrition (Boles et al., 1984), although the aim in general is identification of patients with marginal malnutrition who might benefit from nutritional intervention to reduce postoperative mortality and morbidity.

It is difficult to determine ideal body weight in very ill patients and loss of body components is the final stage of malnutrition. Most other methods of assessment have their limitations, and plasma concentrations of visceral proteins are affected by conditions other than malnutrition such as dehydration and sepsis (Jeejeebhoy et al., 1982). 3-Methylhistidine was thought originally to be a valuable indication of muscle breakdown, but there is doubt regarding its

Table 87.10 Clinical and laboratory values and malnutrition

Parameter and standard	Degree of malnutrition		
	Mild	Moderate	Severe
Weight loss (of usual)	<10%	10−20%	>20%
Weight (of ideal)	80−90%	70−79%	<70%
Anthropometric measurements			
Triceps skin fold (of standard)	80−90%	60−79%	<60%
Arm muscle circumference (of standard)	80−90%	60−79%	<40%
Creatinine − height index (of standard)	60−80%	40−59%	<40%
Biochemical measurements			
Serum albumin (3.5−5.0 g/dl)	3.0−3.4	2.9−2.1	<2.1
Serum transferrin (175−300 mg/dl)	150−175	100−150	<100
Thyroxin-binding prealbumin (28−35 mg/dl)	25.2−28	23−25.2	<23
Retinol-binding protein (3−6 mg/dl)	2.7−3	2.4−2.7	<2.4
Immune competence			
Total lymphocytes (1500−5000/mm³)	1200−1500	800−1200	<800
Delayed cutaneous hypersensitivity	Reactive	Relative anergy	Non-reactive

These may be supplemented by dynamometry, measurement of 3-methylhistidine, creatinine excretion index and tests for muscle fatigue.

specificity (Rennie & Millward, 1983). It is, therefore, still difficult to identify at-risk patients. Daly and colleagues (1979) use two of the following three parameters:

1 Unintentional weight loss greater than 10%.
2 Albumin less than 35 g/litre.
3 A negative reaction to five skin antigens.

Plasma proteins vary with liver disease, septicaemia and other protein-losing states, so albumin is a non-specific measure of malnutrition. In 440 patients with gastric cancer, preoperative nutritional assessment was found beneficial for the prediction of postoperative complications with a close relationship between nutritional status and immunocompetence, lung complications and infection. Serum albumin and prealbumin reliably predicted nutritional status preoperatively and albumin, prealbumin and total lymphocyte count predicted postoperative complications (Yamanaka et al., 1989). However, in critically ill patients, visceral proteins better reflect severity of illness and prognosis than nutritional status or adequacy of nutritional support (Boosalis et al., 1989).

Pettigrew and Hill (1986) found that anthropometric measurements did not identify patients who subsequently had complications after operation but that decreased plasma proteins did, probably because they were reduced by preoperative sepsis rather than nutritional status. Even hand grip (an index of muscle function) is affected by factors other than nutrition (e.g. 35% reduction in acute sepsis, 50% after administration of sedative drugs) (Elia et al., 1984).

A prognostic nutritional index has been developed by Buzby and colleagues (1980) which uses albumin, prealbumin and delayed skin hypersensitivity and skin-fold thickness. This has been used to indicate when patients would benefit from preoperative parenteral nutrition before major gastrointestinal surgery (Smith & Hartemink, 1988).

An approach to assessing the benefit of TPN is that of Chang and colleagues (1986) who attempted to identify those patients admitted to an intensive therapy unit who would not benefit from TPN by using APACHE II scoring (Knaus et al., 1985). One problem with such an approach is the possibility of withholding TPN inappropriately thereby ensuring mortality.

Reliability of assessment

Forse and Shizgal (1980) evaluated the reliability of nutritional assessment by comparing the various parameters with simultaneous body composition measurements. Correlations were poor, the best being weight : height ratio. Many of the parameters are useful for epidemiological studies but not for individual nutritional assessment. Nutritional indices have poor discriminant value for individual prediction of survival (Apelgren et al., 1982).

Klidjian and colleagues (1980) found hand-grip dynamometry to be a useful screening test for detecting malnutrition. Loss of muscle power does predict those patients likely to show serious postoperative morbidity. Measurements of muscle fatigue were investigated by Jeejeebhoy (1985), who obtained a force frequency curve for adductor pollicis which correlates with that obtained from the diaphragm. Development of fatigue is a consistent finding in malnutrition and one which is not abnormal in nonspecific situations such as sepsis, administration of steroids, anaesthesia or moderate trauma.

The abnormalities of muscle contraction reported in malnourished patients are reviewed by Newman (1986). They include:

1 Excessively high force generation at low versus high stimulating frequencies.
2 Slow relaxation.
3 Increased fatiguability.

Moreover, measurements of fatigue are reversible with refeeding at a time when other indices of body composition remain abnormal (Russel et al., 1983). Brough and colleagues (1986) found that the ratio of force of contraction of the adductor pollicis at 10 Hz and 20 Hz gave the best combination of sensitivity (87%) and specificity (82%). After TPN, abnormal muscle function tests returned to normal before changes were detectable in anthropometric variables or plasma albumin concentration. However, these abnormal tests have been improved significantly by a regimen of glucose—potassium loading in preoperative malnourished patients (Chan et al., 1986).

It is unfortunately true that although an increase in body weight and nitrogen over months of observation is seen in patients receiving home nutrition, this is not the case in acutely ill patients receiving shortterm (<40 days) TPN in hospital. Despite apparent adequate intake of nitrogen and energy, little or no increase in total body nitrogen occurs although improved outcome can be demonstrated. These periods of nutrition are too short to alter body composition and therefore emphasis must be on muscle function and other outcome criteria (Jeejeebhoy, 1988).

However nutritional depletion is assessed, and loss of muscle power is at present the best guide, all patients require adequate nutrition administered ideally by the enteral route, but if this is not possible then parentally. Early enteral feeding is thought to reduce secretion of catabolic hormones and return immune responsiveness more rapidly.

Feeding

Some attempt should be made to evaluate the degree of existing malnutrition (see above). The American Society of Anesthesiologists (ASA) classification may be helpful (Table 87.11).

Alternatively, three patient categories may be defined: normal, depleted and hypercatabolic. Many authors stress the deficiencies in current methods used to define malnutrition (Baker et al., 1982) and that whilst a definitive single test of malnutrition is not available, clinical evaluation may be sufficient. It may be argued that all tests of malnutrition return to normal with resolution of the disease process regardless of the adequacy of nutritional therapy, but some continuous assessment of nutritional status should be made.

The diet should be as complete as possible (Elwyn et al., 1980), bearing in mind existing depletion (Table 87.12). Energy needs are based as far as possible on expenditure rather than intake. BMR or REE is the largest component of energy expenditure, hence the value of calculating other components as multiples of this. Irrespective of height, the BMR per kg body weight varies inversely with body weight. The basis for estimating protein requirement remains the nitrogen balance, which presents difficulties as it is extremely sensitive to energy intake. Resting metabolic rate of normal-weight and obese individuals is higher on a high-carbohydrate diet than on an isocaloric high-fat diet. The lower limit of intake for some nutrients is often defined by nutrient balance, measuring intake and excretion of nutrients. An estimate of variability of requirements is then added to the requirement to provide a safety margin. The upper limit of nutritional intakes appropriate to health are more difficult to define. There is obviously

Table 87.11 The American Society of Anesthesiologist's nutritional classification

Class I	Excludes patients with malnutrition
Class II	Those under 10% weight loss, partial starvation
Class III	Hypermetabolic, requiring vigorous nutritional support
Class IV	Complex, extreme catabolism, sepsis, multiple pathologies

Table 87.12 Recommended allowances of nutritional substances

Nutritional substance	Daily allowances to adults (per kg body weight)
Water	30 ml
Energy	30 kcal (0.13 MJ)
Amino acid nitrogen	90 mg (0.7 g amino acids)
Glucose	2 g
Fat	2 g
Sodium	1–1.4 mmol
Potassium	0.7–0.9 mmol
Calcium	0.11 mmol
Magnesium	0.04 mmol
Iron	1 μmol
Manganese	0.6 μmol
Zinc	0.3 μmol
Copper	0.07 μmol
Chlorine	1.3–1.9 mmol
Phosphorus	0.15 mmol
Fluorine	0.7 μmol
Iodine	0.015 μmol
Thiamine	0.02 mg
Riboflavine	0.03 mg
Nicotinamide	0.2 mg
Pyridoxine	0.03 mg
Folic acid	3 μg
Cyanocobalamin	0.03 μg
Pantothenic acid	0.2 mg
Biotin	5 μg
Ascorbic acid	0.5 mg
Retinol	10 μg
Ergocalciferol or cholecalciferol	0.04 mg
Phytylmenaquinone	2 μg
α-Tocopherol	1.5 mg

a wide range of intake. Published requirements relate to normal individuals, whereas considerable variation may occur in acute illness. Recommendations for electrolyte, vitamin and trace-element content of a TPN regimen are given below.

Wherever possible, the gastrointestinal tract should be used for feeding, as metabolic effects of nutrients given by this route are probably better than by the intravenous route (Yeung et al., 1979); visceral protein synthesis may improve, and it is associated with far fewer complications than the intravenous route.

Advantages of feeding enterally centre on maintenance of mucosal barrier function, prevention of bacterial translocation and portal endotoxaemia (Li et al., 1989; Maynard & Bihari, 1991). Translocation precedes septic shock, hypermetabolism and multiple organ failure (MOF) (Meakins & Marshall, 1989). Many TPN regimens lack glutamine and ketone bodies which are 'gut-specific' nutrients maintaining mucosal integrity whereas enteral nutrition post-operatively has been shown to reduce septic complications compared with TPN (Moore *et al.*, 1991). Impaired gut function has far-reaching consequences. In animals, protein malnutrition results in severe ileal atrophy but protein malnutrition by itself does not promote bacterial translocation from the gut to systemic organs but rather renders the subject more susceptible to endotoxin-induced bacterial translocation and less able to clear translocating bacteria than when normally nourished. Alverdy and colleagues in 1988 showed that parenteral nutrition promotes bacterial translocation from the gut by increasing caecal bacterial count and impairing intestinal defences.

Any event that results in sepsis and endotoxaemia initiates the 'interorgan glutamine cycle'. Translocated bacteria or endotoxin stimulate hepatic and pulmonary macrophages to release monokines such as interleukin-1 (IL-1) and TNF. The principal function of the interorgan glutamine cycle is to mobilize glutamine stores to repair 'injured' gut mucosa, generate substrate for renal ammonia production and support lymphocyte proliferation. If the gut is not repaired, a long-term catabolic state ensues. The advantages of glutamine supplements to enteral nutrition and to TPN include decreased bacterial translocation and restoration of secretory IgA (Burke *et al.*, 1989) and nitrogen-sparing equivalent to that produced by GH (Stehle *et al.*, 1989) without significant toxicity (Herskowitz & Souba, 1990).

Enteral nutrition

Palatability is important where these feeds are used without a nasogastric tube. Administration is ideally by fine-bore nasogastric tube, but these carry a risk of displacement and pulmonary aspiration of feeds. The presence of a tracheal tube, impaired cough reflex and the impossibility of retrograde withdrawal of feed, combined with the ready acceptability of these tubes, predispose to such pulmonary aspiration (Boscoe & Rosin, 1984). Fine-bore tubes may deliver 3–5 litres of nutrient solution in 24h without a pump.

Where gastric emptying is impaired but the intestine is functional otherwise, jejunostomy is invaluable. It is a very simple procedure and either wide- or fine-bore tubes may be used. Enteral feeding may take the form of nutritional supplementation, complete oral diets or elemental diets.

Pump-assisted enteral feeding to ensure a better-regulated delivery of the feed is indicated in a few patients with persistent diarrhoea and may obviate the need for TPN (Jones *et al.*, 1980). Whilst continuous feeding may be more comfortable for the patient and easier for nursing staff, it is metabolically less efficient than bolus feeding. An undiluted hypertonic feed gives rise to better nitrogen balance for similar side-effects compared with an isotonic feed (Keohane *et al.*, 1984). Starter regimens may also be abandoned when elemental diets are administered nasogastrically over 24h (Rees *et al.*, 1985).

Recent intestinal perfusion studies suggest that small peptides are absorbed faster from the small intestine than equivalent AAs. There is some evidence that antacids in combination with enteral feeds precipitate, forming plugs which may lead to oesophageal obstruction. Similarly, Osmolite suspension solidifies at low pH (below 4) and had caused complete lower-oesophageal obstruction, which was very difficult to remove (Myo *et al.*, 1986). The trace-element content of commercial enteral feeds may show a large discrepancy between levels stated by the manufacturers and those actually measured by analysis (Bunker & Clayton, 1983). Elemental diets consisting of free FAs, glucose, minerals and vitamins may result in essential FA deficiency with prolonged use, probably because of the low (1.3%) fat content. Table 87.13 shows some of the enteral products currently available.

The place of enteral feeding in hypermetabolic surgical patients has been reviewed by Cerra and colleagues (1989). Delivering enteral nutrition by total estimated calorie need may not produce an optimal nutritional result. Formulae with low non-protein calorie:nitrogen ratio give a better nutritional result. An approach similar to TPN, focusing on the metabolic needs of the patient rather than a target volume, should be the optimal end-point.

Very early enteral nutrition in burned patients resulted in earlier onset of positive nitrogen balance and reduced urinary catecholamine excretion and plasma glucagon in a study by Chiarelli and colleagues (1990). Very early enteral nutrition was safe, well tolerated and improved both control of the metabolic state and the clinical course.

Diarrhoea may be a troublesome problem believed by Brinson and Pitts (1989) to be related to hypoalbuminaemia which is common in critically ill patients and results in oedema of the gastrointestinal tract with protein exudation especially with enteral feeding. Peptide-based diets may then improve nitrogen absorption and increase plasma albumin. Medium-chain triglycerides may confer a similar

Table 87.13 Solutions for enteral nutrition

Product	Presentation features			Protein (g)	Fat (g)	CHO (g)	Energy (kcal)	Osmolality (mosmol/litre)
				Nutrients/amount for approx. 2000 kcal				
Whole protein/high-energy feeds								
Ensure Plus	250 ml	can	Can be taken orally	78	62.5	250	1875	473
	500 ml	bottle		95.8	75	300	2250	473
Clinutren 1.5	250 ml	can	Can be taken orally	75	84.5	212.5	1875	328
Fortison energy plus	500 ml	bottle		75	97.5	268.5	2250	320
Fresubin 750	500 ml	bottle	60% MCT fat	112.5	90	255	2250	300
Clinifeed extra	500 ml	dripac		99.7	77.7	225	1995	280
Whole protein/isocaloric feeds								
Ensure	250 ml	can	Can be taken orally	70	70	276	2000	380
Osmolite	250 ml	can	50% MCT fat	84	70	268	2000	241
	500 ml	bottle						
Clinutren 1	250 ml	can	Can be taken orally	80	76	254	2000	300
Suppliment	250 ml	can	High protein	125	66	226	2000	298
Fortison	500 ml	bottle		80	80	240	2000	260
Fresubin	500 ml	bottle	Can be taken orally	76	68	256	2000	300
Liquisorb	500 ml	bottle		80	80	236	2000	270
Liquisorbon MCT	500 ml	bottle	77% MCT fat	100	65	246	2000	230
Clinifeed favour	500 ml	dripac		75	78	250	2000	217
Modified protein feeds								
Peptamen	500 ml	can	70% MCT peptide based	80	78	254	2000	220
Pepti 2000 LF liquid	500 ml	bottle	Low-fat peptide based	80	20	376	2000	<400
Fresubin OPD	500 ml	bottle	Peptide based	90	52	300	2000	400
Peptisorb	500 ml	bottle	Low-fat peptide based	75	22.2	375	2000	340
Reabilan	500 ml	dripac	Peptide based	63	78	264	2000	300
Elemental 028	100 g	pack	Amino-acid based	50	33.2	352.5	1820	684
Whole protein/varied nutrient content (disease specific) feeds								
Jevity	500 ml	bottle	For long-term use, add fibre	82	70	268	2000	254
Pulmocare	500 ml	bottle	55% energy from fat	93	138	157.5	2000	385
Two-can HN	237 ml	can	Specialist use only	84	91	217	2000	533
Pre-Fortison	500 ml	bottle	Starter regimen only	40	40	120	1000	130
Fortison soya	500 ml	bottle	Milk free	80	80	240	2000	260
Fortison low sodium	500 ml	bottle	11 mmol Na/litre	80	80	240	2000	220
Fortison, low protein low mineral	500 ml	bottle	Renal failure	24	102	246	2000	175
Fresubin Plus F	500 ml	bottle	Added fibre	76	68	256	2000	250 350

MCT, medium-chain triglycerides; CHO, carbohydrates. A selection of sip feeds is available based on the above products such as Ensure, Ensure Plus, Fortimel, Fortisip, Fresubin, Fresubin plus fibre and Provide. The reader is referred to the current edition of MIMS for information on the frequently changing price and composition of these feeds.

advantage. Fibre-supplemented diets may also reduce the incidence of diarrhoea and short-chain fatty acids produced by bacterial metabolism of soluble fibre also stimulate mucosal growth, which helps to maintain integrity.

Total parenteral nutrition

Indications for TPN include: hypercatabolism (multiple trauma, burns, septicaemia), pyloric stenosis, pancreatitis, cardiac surgery, gastro-intestinal cutaneous fistulae, inflammatory bowel disease, severe intra-abdominal sepsis after surgery, cancer surgery, cachexia.

If the gastrointestinal tract is functioning, oral or nasogastric supplements or full feeding is the nutritional method of choice. Many of the conditions requiring preoperative TPN, however, need continued feeding into the postoperative period.

Pancreatitis

Where pancreatitis is prolonged, TPN keeps patients alive until pseudocysts can be drained surgically and oral nutrition commenced (Goodgame & Fischer, 1977). However, if the duodenum is bypassed, jejunal feeding is a possibility.

Fistulae

In the presence of gastrointestinal cutaneous fistulae, TPN increases the spontaneous closure rate and reduces mortality (Sitges-Serra et al., 1982). The output of the fistula probably decreases more rapidly with TPN compared with enteral nutrition. Long-term TPN results in closure of gastrointestinal fistulae in 70–80% of cases. There is preliminary evidence that somatostatin facilitates closure of persistent fistulae where TPN alone has failed (Di Costanzo et al., 1982), although this is still contentious.

Inflammatory bowel disease

In the presence of inflammatory bowel disease there may be fewer postoperative complications and less extensive surgery may be required when preoperative TPN is used, and where disease extends beyond the superficial mucosal cells (Rombeau et al., 1982). The benefits of TPN depend on the site of the disease. Where this is in the colon, intravenous feeding has little effect on the disease, but there are some advantages of TPN in acute exacerbations of Crohn's disease of the small gut (Dickinson et al., 1980). 'Resting the gut' by the use of TPN, although it may maintain positive nitrogen balance, has an adverse effect on the gut, producing profound disuse atrophy (Williamson, 1983).

TPN was used by Main and colleagues (1981) for 9 weeks to sustain pregnancy in a patient with Crohn's disease. Despite evidence of placental insufficiency at 36 weeks, the baby was normal.

Cardiac cachexia

Cardiac cachexia probably requires a prolonged period of preoperative nutritional support if postoperative mortality is to be improved.

In patients with congestive cardiac failure, nasogastric feeding at $1.4-1.8 \times$ measured REE provided nutrition without increasing oxygen consumption or worsening cardiac failure (Heymsfield & Casper, 1989).

Cancer

Many patients with cancer, especially those with gastrointestinal malignancies, are malnourished. Nutrition in the cancer patient has been reviewed by Dickerson (1984). Some patients show elevated REE, disturbances of carbohydrate metabolism and a failure to adapt to reduced food intake which is characteristic of cachexia. There is no firm evidence that preoperative TPN in cancer patients is of benefit. It may not prolong life although it may improve the quality of life, place patients in a satisfactory condition for specific antitumour therapy and reduce major postoperative complications although there is the concern that TPN stimulates tumour growth (Popp et al., 1983).

Reviewing the effects of artificial nutrition on the nutritional status of cancer patients Bozzetti (1989) concluded that no nutritional variable worsened in cancer patients receiving either enteral or TPN. Nutritional support alone probably has a small part to play in a limited number of patients with advanced cancer who are dying primarily from malnutrition. Artificial nutrition also has a permissive role in treatment where oncological treatment could not be delivered because of poor nutritional status. A statement from the American College of Physicians (1989) said that parenteral nutrition was associated with net HARM; no condition could be defined where such treatment appeared to be of benefit. Therefore the routine use of TPN should be strongly discouraged although it is still possible that the severely malnourished might benefit.

Perioperative patients

The employment of parenteral nutrition in the perioperative period is extremely controversial (Mullen et al., 1980). It is clear that intestinal mucosal integrity depends upon food in the gut and blood flow to it (Bristol & Williamson, 1988). Surgery or trauma result in breakdown of muscle and redistribution of AAs to the liver for manufacture of visceral proteins and gluconeogenesis. Visceral protein concentrations can be maintained in serum by provision of >1.2 g · $kg^{-1} \cdot day^{-1}$ of AA i.v., which increases protein production by the liver (Tulikoura, 1988; Carli et al., 1990). Some evidence of benefit is provided by Young and colleagues (1989) who used intravenous nutrition perioperatively in patients with gastrointestinal-tract malignancy who had a liver biopsy at operation. These workers found a significant increase in protein synthesis by the liver even after 3 days of intravenous feeding. At this time, plasma levels of fibronectin and IgA had also increased but an increase in pre-albumin, IgM and C3 complement only increased significantly in those fed for 7 days. By the seventh postoperative day, however, plasma proteins had decreased to the same extent as those of patients who had not received perioperative intravenous nutrition.

Muller and colleagues (1982) examined the influence of 10 days preoperative TPN in patients with gastrointestinal cancer. They found fewer major complications and reduced mortality in the TPN group compared with controls fed a regular ward diet. They attributed this to improvement of humoral and cellular immunocompetence and to protein status in the TPN group whilst deterioration occurred in the control group. The design of this study has been criticized; treated and control groups were matched badly, malnutrition ill-defined and no distinction was made between the malnourished and those with normal nutrition or between patients with tumours at different sites. In a study of patients with gastric or oesophageal carcinoma, there was no reduction in the incidence of anastomotic leakage. Neither was there death in patients receiving TPN preoperatively, except in those with a low albumin concentration who had reduced incidence of wound infection and who would be expected to have poor healing and immunocompromise (Geefuysen et al., 1971).

This controversy has led to the publication of a position paper by the American College of Physicians in 1987 stating that:

1 Perioperative use of parenteral nutrition is recommended for severely malnourished patients having major surgery, such as intra-abdominal or non-cardiac intrathoracic surgery.

2 Postoperative use of parenteral nutrition is recommended for selected groups of moderately malnourished and previously well-nourished patients having surgery that usually results in prolonged periods (>10 days) of inadequate nutritional intake, although some of these patients could be fed via a jejunostomy.

3 Postoperative use of parenteral nutrition is recommended for previously well-nourished patients who develop postoperative complications expected to result in prolonged periods (>10 days) of inadequate intake. They also recommended further clinical trials to show the effectiveness of TPN in these patients.

There is some evidence (Bellatone et al., 1988; Fan et al., 1989) that whilst preoperative parenteral nutrition may benefit certain patients, its routine use cannot be advocated. They studied patients before oesophageal surgery and found that although body weight and nitrogen balance improved, there was no reduction in morbidity and mortality compared with patients who were not fed. The highest postoperative complication rate was found in those patients who gained weight but whose plasma albumin decreased (extracellular fluid expansion). Pulmonary infection and anastomotic leak are the principal causes of postoperative morbidity after oesophageal surgery and these are known to be related to malnutrition. Although intensive nutritional support can improve respiratory muscle strength, reverse immune deficiency and increase serum carrier proteins the clinical evidence for benefit from preoperative feeding is at best inconsistent and remains controversial. Starker and colleagues (1986), seeking appropriate criteria for effective TPN, found that patients who failed to increase serum albumin after one week of TPN had a high morbidity and mortality. Their data suggest that TPN should not be given for a fixed time but instead the patient's response should be the indication for proceeding with elective surgery.

Similarly, there is no support for the routine use of elective TPN in the postoperative period. Woolfson and Smith (1989) could not identify perioperatively a group of patients who might possibly benefit by such feeding and this conclusion was endorsed by the large study of perioperative parenteral nutrition (395 patients) undertaken by the Veterans Affairs TPN study group (1991) who found no benefit from the routine use of TPN unless the patient was severely malnourished, which returns to the problem of how such patients can be identified preoperatively.

Other indications

Nasogastric nutritional supplementation may accelerate growth and reduce the incidence and severity of complications in growth-retarded children with sickle-cell disease (Heyman et al., 1985). Nutritional support improves antibody response to influenza virus vaccine in elderly patients (Chandra & Puri, 1985). Very thin patients with fractured neck of femur and a poor oral intake benefited from overnight supplementation by nasogastric tube in addition to daily normal ward diet. This manoeuvre reduced rehabilitation time and hospital stay without reducing voluntary oral food intake during the day (Bastow et al., 1983).

Renal disease

Impending renal failure should not be a reason for withholding TPN. Instead, early artificial renal support should be provided to control the metabolic state and allow room for feeding. Whereas acute renal failure used to be treated with various modifications of the Giordano–Giovanetti diet consisting of essential L-AAs and glucose with vitamins, improved survival and recovery of renal function has been demonstrated by the use of TPN (Abel et al., 1973; Abel, 1983; Feinstein, 1987).

The effect of intravenous AA solutions after elective surgery has been found to reduce the protein breakdown that develops in control patients (Shizgal, 1981). This effect is a result of AAs themselves (Greenberg et al., 1976). Some authorities recommended use of AA solutions in those patients who require nutritional support but may be expected to return to oral intake after a few days or in traumatized patients who may fail to absorb from the gastrointestinal tract for some time. Others believe that this nitrogen sparing is no better than infusing an isocaloric amount of carbohydrate. Where nutrient intake must be limited, 10 g nitrogen and 1000 kcal total energy intake daily may provide optimal sparing of body cell mass. The minimal nitrogen requirement in normal people receiving adequate non-protein energy to achieve zero nitrogen balance is 0.1 g/kg daily.

Assessment of requirements for total parenteral nutrition

A variety of techniques exist for investigating substrate metabolism in patients. These include indirect calorimetry (Dauncey et al., 1978), substrate-load tests, measurements of arteriovenous differences (Fick principle) and isotope infusions (Royle et al., 1981; Rennie, 1985).

The measurement of gas exchange, although seldom available clinically, can be useful for evaluation of the nutritional needs of hospitalized patients. If the resting respiratory quotient (RQ) is known, together with nitrogen excretion, the proportion of calorie requirements to nitrogen can be calculated.

Kinney and Hessov (1981) developed a closed system with a rigid transparent head canopy and neck seal for determination of the metabolic state in septic, injured and nutritionally depleted patients but it cannot be adapted readily to the patient with mechanically ventilated lungs. A fully automated instrument for measurement of oxygen consumption, carbon dioxide production and RQ in ventilated patients has been used for routine clinical evaluation of nutritional needs.

In critically ill sedated patients with artificially ventilated lungs, total energy expenditure is only approximately 5% above REE, although this may increase to 18% during stressful procedures with a commensurate increase in carbon dioxide production (Weissman et al., 1986). Mann and colleagues (1985) pointed out that predicted metabolic requirements based on ideal body weight (1.75 REE) averaged 59% greater than metabolic expenditure measured by indirect calorimetry.

The recent development of the Siemens–Elema Servo Ventilator 900 series with attached carbon dioxide and oxygen analysers has been shown by Damask and colleagues (1982) to be accurate enough under a variety of conditions for continuous measurement of oxygen consumption and carbon dioxide production. However, such a system is clearly prone to error because of leakage. Measurement of energy requirements must be expressed as a function of body size. Measurement of total body energy expenditure in healthy subjects at rest represents the BMR of total cell mass of the body, which varies with age, sex and existing pathology. Body cell mass (BCM) is difficult to derive but correlates best with isotope measurements of potassium. Certain physiological states such as lactation seem to enhance metabolic efficiency (Illingworth et al., 1986). In malnutrition, there is a loss of protein and BCM fluid with water retention which expands extracellular volume. Smoking seems to increase total 24-h energy expenditure by 10% without change in physical activity and mean BMR. This is associated with increased urinary excretion of noradrenaline and the effect is probably mediated therefore by the sympathetic nervous system (Hofsteller et al., 1986). It may be that a reduction in energy expenditure occurs on stopping smoking with subsequent weight gain although other adaptive influences on body weight and variation in calorie intake have not been explored.

Our views of energy supply to patients requiring TPN have been modified greatly by the measurements made by Macfie (1984) who found the REE in uncomplicated convalescents to be only 10% greater than the preoperative state. More recent techniques using water double-labelled with deuterium and oxygen-18 and improved instrumentation give accurate energy expenditure in normal mobile individuals. In patients with multiple injuries, REE increases by 10–30% over 2 weeks which correlates with a period of nitrogen excretion. The highest levels of nitrogen excretion are associated often with fever. The effect of various conditions on REE has been described by Elia and colleagues (1984) (Fig. 87.2).

The thermic effects of parenteral nutrition in septic and non-septic patients have been studied by Arnold and colleagues (1989). Whilst baseline oxygen consumption is higher in septic patients, both groups showed a similar (25%) increase in consumption during feeding and at least part of this response was sympathetically mediated.

In depleted and normal adults, nitrogen balance may be increased by increasing either nitrogen or energy intake, but depleted patients can only achieve a positive nitrogen balance at zero energy balance (Elwyn *et al.*, 1979). Attempts to estimate nitrogen losses have hinged upon measurement of urinary urea:

Urine 24 h urea (mmol) × 0.035

+ Measured proteinuria
(divide by 6.25 to convert to g N$_2$)

+ Blood urea change in mmol/litre
× body weight (kg) × 0.017

However, the variability of non-urea nitrogenous components in the urine may make this an unreliable measure upon which to judge the nitrogen input requirement for a stressed postoperative patient (Loder *et al.*, 1989).

Where REE can be measured and repletion is required, the patient may be given 1.25–1.75 of daily REE for calorie requirements. Normal REE is approximately 115.5 kJ (27.5 kcal)/kg daily.

A nomogram is available for rapid estimation of metabolic requirements of patients with tracheal tubes *in situ* (Smith *et al.*, 1984). This involves indirect calorimetry measuring mixed expired carbon dioxide tension, assuming an RQ of 0.8 and a leak-free circuit and that each litre of oxygen consumed by the body produces 4.83 kcal at RQ 0.8.

Despite the limited evidence of reduced mortality and morbidity nutritional support is used widely for patients in ITUs (Woolfson, 1983). The aim is to give all nutrients required by the body in the appropriate proportion. A major dilemma at present is what is the most suitable energy substrate for which patient, the glucose versus fat controversy. The value of protein-sparing regimens in the postoperative period or specific AA therapy in various disease processes is unconfirmed.

Jeevanandam and colleagues (1990) studied patients after accidental trauma who were receiving TPN by indirect calorimetry. Five days of TPN, providing calories to match the measured basal REE and nitrogen to replace initial urinary losses, shifted RQ from 0.74 to 0.81, improved but could not reverse negative N$_2$ balance, reduced net fat oxidation, increased carbohydrate and protein oxidation and

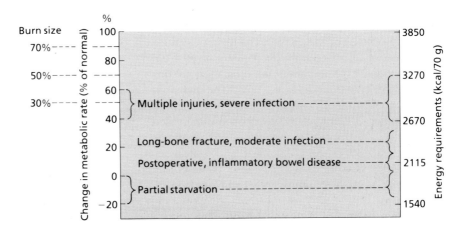

Fig. 87.2 Effects of various diseases on metabolic rate.

increased daily adrenaline and noradrenaline excretion rates. This also achieved positive energy balance. Thus, in patients who are catabolic after trauma positive energy balance can be achieved provided energy intake matches basal expenditure, plus 7–10% for activity. To prevent further loss of lean body mass a minimum of 350 mg/kg N_2 is needed.

Minimal technical detail of parenteral nutrition is given here except where it is relevant to the complications.

Disturbances of water and electrolytes and severe hypoalbuminaemia should be corrected prior to starting TPN. Analgesia should be adequate and where it is considered appropriate the stress response obtunded. Peripheral vein infusion is possible if isotonic nutrients are used, but usually this method cannot provide for the requirements of the critically ill. The author prefers a central line placed by the infraclavicular approach to the subclavian vein but internal jugular vein cannulation is associated with the highest rate of correct placement. LaSala and colleagues (1983) describe cannulation of the inferior vena cava via the saphenous system, tunnelling to mid-thigh level. Whichever route is used, the catheter should be inert and flexible, the best currently being silicone coated or polyethylene.

Administration of parenteral nutrition requires a volumetric infusion pump.

Glucose or fat as energy substrate

Glucose is the most advantageous sugar for TPN although others may induce less hyperglycaemia. Most of the early work on the use of glucose as a calorie source was undertaken in the USA where at the time all fat emulsions were banned. Dudrick and colleagues (1969) showed that normal growth and nutrition could be maintained with glucose as the major calorie source. In Europe, Wretlind successfully introduced Intralipid as an energy substrate at an early stage (Hallberg et al., 1966). The main objections to the use of fat in critically ill patients arose from earlier evidence of impaired fat utilization in this group of patients (Parodis et al., 1977). The increased insulin concentrations suppress fat mobilization. Later studies in humans, however, show increased fat clearance especially in hypermetabolic patients (Long et al., 1977), and Askanazi and colleagues (1981, 1982) have shown that these patients can oxidize fat in spite of intravenous glucose administration.

Nitrogen balance is influenced by the amount of nitrogen in the diet, the metabolic rate and the quantity and source of non-protein energy. Elwyn (1980) and others believe that glucose and fat are equally effective in maintaining positive nitrogen balance. The relative advantages of each of these substrates depends in part on the patients. Where protein intake is low or absent, fat administration has no effect on nitrogen excretion but carbohydrate administration reduces nitrogen loss. One hundred grams of carbohydrate are sufficient to replace gluconeogenesis from endogenous protein. When diet is adequate, isocaloric amounts of fat or glucose have equal nitrogen retention ability, although adaptation to the utilization of fat takes several days (Jeejeebhoy et al., 1976). In catabolic patients, carbohydrate is the main protein-sparing substrate (Long et al., 1977), although 80% of energy requirements are derived from endogenous fat. Ketosis does not develop and endogenous protein continues to be broken down for gluconeogenesis. Under these circumstances, infused fat spares endogenous fat stores but not muscle protein. Addition of insulin to the glucose infusion improves protein sparing and nitrogen balance although hypoalbuminaemia may result (Woolfson et al., 1979). A further advantage is that insulin enhances sodium-pump activity.

Administration of glucose in excess of an optimal $4 \, mg \cdot kg^{-1} \cdot min^{-1}$, however, is harmful as it leads to increased carbon dioxide production and fat deposition in the liver (Burke et al., 1979). Energy cannot be lost from a biological system, so that where carbohydrate is given in excess of requirements, approximately 20% increases REE and 80% is converted to fat with RQ increasing to 7–9 (Elwyn et al., 1981). This is associated with an increase in plasma noradrenaline concentration suggesting that increased sympathetic activity is the cause of the increased REE (Nordenstrom et al., 1981). Sympathetic-induced thermogenesis constitutes a further stress to the hypercatabolic-injured patient. Increased carbon dioxide production may lead to respiratory distress or failure in patients with compromised lung function. Oxygen consumption increases, particularly in hypercatabolic patients, and waste oxidation of FA occurs. This topic has been reviewed by Robin and colleagues (1981) and Askanazi and colleagues (1982).

On balance, a mixed energy source which combines the advantages of each and obviates the disadvantages is recommended. An energy source of 50% Intralipid, 50% glucose is suitable for the majority of patients requiring TPN. Catabolic patients require at least 60% glucose. The hormonal profile of insulin suppression and elevation of the counteracting hormones glucagon, catecholamines and cortisol forms a strong theoretical basis for use of fat emulsion in the seriously ill population. This is further discussed below. Administration of highly concentrated glucose solutions required for TPN results in local venous complications and systemic problems due to hyperglycaemia and the hypertonic solution.

Intralipid is the most widely used fat source in this country. The particle size of this emulsion is in the same range as CMs but its structure differs as it contains no apoproteins or cholesterol. It is probably metabolized similarly to CMs or VLDLs by lipoprotein lipase and is removed by the reticuloendothelial system (RES).

No significant changes were detected in respiratory mechanics, oxygen consumption, carbon dioxide production, REE, liver function or nitrogen balance following the addition of 550 kcal lipid emulsion to glucose calories sufficient for energy requirements (Abbott *et al.*, 1984).

Lipid emulsions in neonates and some adults can reduce Pao_2 and diffusing capacity. Fat has been shown to accumulate in the lungs of preterm infants fed Intralipid in less than the recommended maximum dose (Levene *et al.*, 1980). Intralipid may enhance the risk of bacterial sepsis. The serum of some acutely ill patients agglutinates Intralipid. This reaction is thought to be produced by C-reactive protein in the presence of calcium ions. At postmortem, such patients showed evidence of microemboli which could have been a result of this agglutination. In rabbits with oleic acid-damaged lungs, Intralipid infusion increased pulmonary production of vasodilating prostaglandins and hypoxaemia. This effect is thought to be due to inhibition of pulmonary hypoxic vasoconstriction and the resultant increase in intrapulmonary right–left shunt.

In injured adult patients, an alternative lipid, Lipofundin, did not produce any change in alveolar–arterial oxygen gradient. Lipofundin contains medium-chain triglycerides and when given to severely ill, malnourished patients receiving controlled mechanical ventilation of the lungs, it does not change arterial oxygen or carbon dioxide tensions, platelet or white cell count and does not activate complement.

Critically ill patients may have reduced intracellular carnitine content which might impair oxidation of long-chain FA. Further investigation is required to determine if carnitine should be added to the regimen or medium-chain FA substituted. Patients with carnitine deficiency are largely dependent on glucose for energy production. In septic patients, however, little advantage could be demonstrated for medium-chain triglycerides (Bach *et al.*, 1988) although structured lipids may be more promising.

Amino acid solutions

TPN regimens require crystalline L-AA solutions as a nitrogen source. There is considerable controversy regarding the value of specific AAs in the synthetic crystalline AA mixtures available commercially, particularly those which contain high concentrations of glycine. Jackson and Golden (1980) suggest that glycine is catabolized to free ammonia rather than contributing useful nitrogen for transamination reactions. The limits of glycine turnover of 200 mg/kg daily are exceeded easily in some high-nitrogen solutions available. *Drug and Therapeutics Bulletin* (1980) suggests the recosting of AA solutions excluding glycine. Amino-acid solutions must contain sufficient concentrations of all essential AA. The optimal non-essential AA content of the diet is unknown but egg protein is taken as the standard (51% essential AAs).

There is a relationship between nitrogen intake and balance (Fig. 87.3) up to a certain point beyond which no further effect is seen, and this relationship holds whatever the amount of energy supplied, although a more positive nitrogen balance may be achieved by supplying energy in excess of metabolic

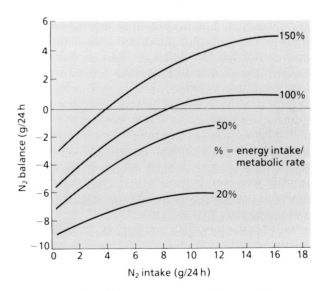

Fig. 87.3 Relationship between nitrogen balance and energy intake.

requirements together with adequate nitrogen intake (Woolfson *et al.*, 1979).

Urinary nitrogen excretion in starvation depends also on the preceding nitrogen intake. Starved patients have a greater capacity for nitrogen retention than normal patients. Very few patients can tolerate more than 20 g nitrogen i.v. daily as such levels saturate the hepatic metabolic pathways resulting in deamination of AAs and increased urea production. Amino acid infusions increase minute ventilation, oxygen consumption and the response to hypoxia and hypercapnia. Increased ventilatory drive produced by increased protein intake may result in dyspnoea with increased rate and work of breathing (Burki, 1980).

Branched-chain amino acids

In patients with cirrhosis, infusion of BCAAs may be beneficial (Vinnars, 1982), inducing a more positive nitrogen balance in the postoperative period than would a complete AA mixture. Patients with alcoholic hepatitis given 70–85 g of BCAA daily had an improvement in ascites, encephalopathy, plasma bilirubin and albumin compared with controls who were not given this supplement. Where this therapy was continued for 4 weeks, mortality rate decreased. In liver disease, aromatic AAs are not metabolized effectively and act as precursors for false neurotransmitters such as octopamine. BCAA concentrations are low in encephalopathic patients. Therapy to reduce gut uptake of glutamine or its conversion to ammonia may be useful.

BCAAs have certain unique characteristics including uptake into muscle rather than liver where they provide a nitrogenous source for glutamine. They may exert a specific regulatory effect on the rate of protein degradation and synthesis in muscle and liver (Skeie *et al.*, 1990).

Glutamine

Whole-body AA metabolism may be controlled by a carrier for glutamine isolated recently in rat muscle (Rennie *et al.*, 1986). These workers demonstrated a link between the size of the muscle glutamine pool and the rate of glutamine synthesis.

After injury or hypercatabolism there is marked reduction in intramuscular glutamine and a direct correlation between glutamine and protein synthesis. *In vitro* glutamine has been shown to have a positive effect on protein anabolic processes and it is now clear that it is essential for mucosal maintenance and especially important for gut-barrier function. Supplementation of parenteral nutrition with the dipeptide L-alanyl-L-glutamine after elective resection of the large gut improved nitrogen balance (Stehle *et al.*, 1989) and maintained intramuscular glutamine concentration close to the preoperative value. In rats, Burke and colleagues (1989) found that glutamine supplemented TPN protected against bacterial translocation from the gut; an effect which may be mediated by the secretory IgA immune system. In patients with burns, the decrease in plasma glutamine which lasts for at least 21 days may contribute to impaired immune function by decreasing both proliferation of lymphocytes and phagocytosis by macrophages (Parry-Billings *et al.*, 1990).

Nitrogen balance

Several means of improving nitrogen balance have been attempted. Remobilization is the best of these (Booth & Gollnick, 1983). However, malnutrition produces an increase in intracellular calcium, and exercise, including physiotherapy, may further increase intracellular calcium and produce more ultrastructural damage unless accompanied by adequate nutritional repletion (Jeejeebhoy, 1985).

There is evidence in elderly patients that prevention of heat loss during and after surgery causes a significant decrease in muscle-protein degradation and nitrogen loss as measured by 3-methyl histidine excretion and urea nitrogen loss (Carli & Itiaba, 1986).

Leucine has some stimulatory effect on protein synthesis *in vitro*, and BCAAs were found by Cerra and colleagues (1983) to increase nitrogen retention in postoperative and multiple trauma patients. Freund and Fischer (1985) also reported improved nitrogen balance in severely catabolic intensive-therapy patients with use of BCAA. Some visceral proteins improved, and insulin requirements decreased.

A metabolite of leucine, α-ketoisocaproate, can reduce negative nitrogen balance and 3-methylhistidine excretion (Sapir *et al.*, 1983), although the usefulness of this latter parameter has been questioned (see above). This nitrogen sparing may be related to:

1 The increased ketosis, as KBs inhibit oxidation of BCAAs in muscle and their concentration is increased.
2 Decreased protein degradation, as plasma prealbumin and retinol-binding protein were lower.
3 An effect on liver protein turnover.

The effect is unlikely to be a result of change in carbohydrate metabolism.

Prostaglandins are concerned with intracellular protein metabolism; it may therefore prove possible to reduce muscle protein breakdown with inhibitors of prostaglandin synthesis such as indomethacin (Rennie, 1984). Naftidrofuryl (Byrnes et al., 1981; Jackson et al., 1984), anabolic steroids, somatomedin and possibly proteinase inhibitors (Stracher, 1982) may also find a role in improving nitrogen balance. GH may be particularly valuable in elderly patients (Frayne et al., 1984) and a further approach is administration of β-adrenergic agonists which increase muscle mass (Arnold & Little, 1991).

Complications of total parenteral nutrition

The complications associated with TPN may be summarized: infective, metabolic, biochemical deficiencies, disorders of water, sodium and acid−base balance, jaundice, hypoalbuminaemia and technical complications. Many of these may occur also during enteral feeding.

Infection

Infection is a serious hazard of TPN, especially in the presence of invasive catheters, steroids and antibiotic-resistant, opportunistic organisms, and ranges from infusion phlebitis to suppurative mediastinitis and septicaemia. There is some evidence that surveillance cultures can identify those patients at high risk of infection, although this is controversial and stricter criteria for culture are required. The distinction between true infection and contamination is difficult (Collins et al., 1986). Catheter-associated infection may be reduced by the introduction of a 'control-of-infection team' giving proper education, advice and care. Filtration of the fluids may further reduce infection. Techniques and evaluation of tunnelling have been reviewed by Peters (1982). Keohane and colleagues (1983) believe that tunnelling can reduce sepsis where nursing care is less than optimal, although these findings have been criticized on the basis of diagnosis of sepsis.

Broviac and Hickman catheters are useful for long-term TPN because of the low incidence of catheter blockage by fibrin and lipid. These catheters have a Dacron cuff at the catheter exit site. Fibrous tissue grows into this with fixation of the catheter. Indwelling intravascular catheters such as the Hickman readily become colonized with organisms giving rise to a positive blood culture usually with Gram-positive organisms. This is especially so in the immuno-compromised patient, and whilst these organisms give rise to fever, they may produce no other clinical sequelae (Donnelly et al., 1985). Further confirmation and evaluation of this situation is required.

Some strains of coagulase-negative staphylococci seem able to survive cidal concentrations of certain antibiotics whilst adherent to polyvinyl chloride (PVC) catheters (Sheth et al., 1985).

Hyperglycaemia

Insulin therapy is required, ideally by continuous infusion using a dynamic scale. Insulin requirements vary throughout the day; the 'dawn phenomenon' of requirements increasing towards dawn is likely to be caused by a surge of GH at that time (Campell et al., 1985). Haemodynamic effects of infusion of hyper-osmolar glucose include expansion of blood volume, increase in stroke volume and reduction in pulmonary vascular resistance and wedge pressure.

Metabolic bone disease

Severe bone pain may occur with marked disability in the presence of normal calcium, phosphate, 25-hydroxyvitamin D_3 and parathyroid hormone. Bone biopsy may show osteomalacia, and hypercalciuria may occur, both of which resolve on discontinuing TPN. Hypercalcaemia may be precipitated by oliguria. The possibility remains that this is produced by administration of excessive phosphate (Allam et al., 1981).

Deficiencies

Deficiency of any and every dietary component has been described; only a few important ones are included here. Diuretics, aminoglycosides and amphoteracin B increase requirements for potassium and magnesium and patients receiving antineoplastic drugs such as cisplatin may have very high magnesium needs.

Zinc deficiency

This may be overt or subclinical, and results partly from the low concentration of zinc in some TPN solutions and partly from the formation of zinc−AA complexes with histidine and cysteine which are excreted in the urine. The effects are delayed wound healing and susceptibility to infection, diarrhoea, scaly rash and alopecia (Mozzillo et al., 1982). Zinc requirement is increased by diarrhoea and high fistula outputs (zinc concentration 12–17 mg/litre).

Phosphate depletion

This is common in postoperative patients especially if little blood has been transfused with phosphate in the anticoagulant solution. Hypophosphataemia is associated with diaphragmatic weakness and pulmonary insufficiency (Aubier et al., 1985) and CNS dysfunction resembling Guillain–Barré syndrome. In animals, acute hypophosphataemia occurring after weight loss and nutritional depletion produces rhabdomyolysis. Analysis of peripheral muscle shows accumulation of salt and water, loss of potassium and magnesium and severe phosphate loss with accumulation of calcium. Profound hypophosphataemia can mimic Wernicke's encephalopathy in alcoholics and simulate the clinical signs of brainstem death. Hypophosphataemic collapse has occurred with plasma phosphate 0.32 mmol/litre after marathon running but appears to be transient (Dale et al., 1986).

Current replacement solutions are reviewed by Kingston and colleagues (1985), iatrogenic hyperphosphataemia may occur (Chernow et al., 1981; Lamiell et al., 1990) accompanied by hypocalcaemia and hypomagnesaemia; hence, the importance of biochemical monitoring. Deficiency of magnesium alone is not uncommon.

Fatty acid depletion

Unless a fat emulsion is included in the regimen, essential FA deficiency is likely. This is most common in infants and presents as scaly dermatitis, alopecia, hepatomegaly, diminished skin pigmentation and fatty liver. Linoleic acid cannot be synthesized, and it is therefore recommended that 5–10% of calorie intake should be in the form of this essential FA. Stewart and Hensley (1981) describe four cases of acute polymyopathy associated with TPN which responded to discontinuation of the feeding regimen or intravenous lipid supplementation. In these cases, the aetiology was thought to be essential FA deficiency. Recent evidence has shown beneficial effects of polyunsaturated FAs found in fish (Phillipson et al., 1985). A diet rich in these FAs increased the eicosapentaenoic acid content of neutrophils and monocytes and inhibited 5-lipo-oxygenase pathways of arachidonic acid metabolism and leukotriene B_4-mediated inflammatory reactions (Lee et al., 1985). Dietary fish oils rich in Ω-3-FAs reduced plasma

lipid levels in normal patients and in those with hypertriglyceridaemia. The negative association between fish consumption and mortality from coronary heart disease is still controversial. However Ω-3-FAs are found in high concentration in purslane, a vegetable often used in soups and salads in Greece and Lebanon where such mortality is low. Fish oil contains the polyunsaturated FA eicosapentaenoate, and biosynthesis of thromboxanes (A_3) and prostacyclins (PGI_2) from this rather than the usual arachidonate may help to reduce the risk of atherosclerosis (Knapp et al., 1986). Fish oil may also reduce mild systolic hypertension (Norris et al., 1986). It seems likely that modification of fat solutions will take place in future.

Taurine deficiency

TPN does not contain taurine normally, and lack of this AA results in low blood concentrations and retinal dysfunction in children, which is reversed by adding taurine (Geggel et al., 1985).

Vitamin E deficiency

Vitamin E deficiency presenting as spinocerebellar syndromes may occur.

Intrahepatic cholestasis

This is not uncommon and may be related to intestinal overgrowth of anaerobic bacteria. The raised serum transaminase concentrations may be prevented by metronidazole (Capron et al., 1983).

Thrombosis and embolism

Subclavian vein thrombosis occurs in an estimated 5–35% of catheters used for TPN. Heparin and filtration may reduce the incidence of phlebitis in peripheral infusions, therefore inclusion of heparin in the TPN solution is logical (Falchuk et al., 1985). A dose of 1000 units/litre is recommended. This has the added advantage of activating lipoprotein lipase and enhancing fat clearance by speeding the hydrolysis of TAG. In patients receiving TPN, levels of antithrombin III are reduced. Intralipid has been incriminated in blockage of Hickman and Broviac catheters when mixed with all other nutrients for a prolonged period. This remains to be confirmed.

Catheter embolus is a serious complication which can occur even with tunnelled lines. Major complications such as cardiac perforation, pulmonary thrombosis and arrhythmia are likely if catheter emboli are not removed. Transvenous, non-surgical retrieval techniques are described. Paradoxical air embolus has been described associated with a cracked filter attached to a central TPN feeding catheter. Cardiac tamponade produced by a central catheter is a potentially fatal complication.

Air embolus may be prevented by use of certain intravenous filters, although these do reduce the flow rate and cannot be used with fat emulsions.

Mortality and home parenteral nutrition was considered in 1989 by Stokes and Irving. Fourteen of the 50 deaths in 228 patients recorded in the UK home parenteral nutrition register have died, not of their disease but from a cause attributable to administration of the home parenteral nutrition; septicaemia, subclavian thrombosis or hepatic failure.

Total parenteral nutrition in respiratory failure

The effects of TPN on oxygen consumption and carbon dioxide production have been discussed already. Diaphragmatic muscle fatigue occurs in malnutrition with onset of ventilatory failure (Rochester & Arora, 1983). The aim of feeding in respiratory failure is to improve respiratory muscle function and sensitivity to hypoxic drive. TPN may allow earlier weaning (Bassili & Dietal, 1981). Ventilator-dependent patients who respond to nutritional support by increasing protein synthesis are more likely to wean from mechanical ventilation than those who do not (Larca & Greenbaum, 1982). Early in ventilatory failure, intercostal muscles may be depleted of high-energy phosphates with increase in lactate, whilst skeletal muscle values remain normal. Phosphate-binding antacids worsen the situation. Acute respiratory acidosis depresses glycolytic activity with an increase in plasma phosphate which is excreted subsequently in the urine. When pH is restored, hypophosphataemia occurs as phosphate shifts from blood into cells when glycolytic activity increases.

There are two theoretical nutritional alternatives for patients with impending respiratory failure (Iapichino, 1989). The first is to supply energy at a rate below REE to minimize diet-induced thermogenesis. The second is to give a full calorie load of 1.2–1.5 × REE with a high-fat formula resulting in a lower RQ thereby reducing carbon dioxide for excretion. Exogenous lipid mainly replaces body fat stores that are continuously mobilized to meet energy expenditure. In patients with shock lung and increased catabolism, it is important not to increase carbon dioxide production, oxygen consumption,

ventilation or airway pressure. Then 1000–1300 kcal should be supplied as glucose with insulin if necessary and AAs, shifting the balance to enteral feeding as soon as possible, at a calorie load close to REE.

Sepsis

In the hypermetabolic phase of sepsis, in the absence of feeding, there is an increase in lipid metabolism that accounts for most of the oxidative substrate utilization. Adrenergic stimulation is at least partially responsible for increased mobilization of free FAs from adipose tissue. This leads to increased hepatic uptake of FAs thereby increasing the production and output of TAG. The rate of ketogenesis is impaired in severe sepsis when the influence of cytokines on metabolism increases. In severe shock release of FAs from adipose tissue falls as a result of blood flow limitation. In the presence of increased secretion of TNF and IL-1 from macrophages the capacity of extrahepatic tissues to clear FAs may be reduced due to suppression of lipoprotein lipase. The current consensus is not that fat should be avoided but that plasma-lipid concentrations should be carefully monitored.

Glucose recycling is enhanced in sepsis and is unrelated to eicosanoid production but experimentally TNF increases glucose metabolism. Immune tissues are stimulated under the influence of cytokines resulting in increased glucose utilization and lactate production. The combined changes in lipid and carbohydrate metabolism enable the body to rely on FA oxidation as a prime source of energy but to still supply tissues with special needs for glycolytic substrates (Cerra et al., 1988; Spitzer et al., 1988).

Total parenteral nutrition and drug administration

Antitumour drugs may have an effect on specific nutrients. 5-Fluorouracil, perhaps in combination with other drugs, may produce thiamine deficiency. There is some evidence that this drug is tolerated better in patients receiving TPN.

A reduction in dietary protein is known to depress renal plasma flow and creatinine clearance. In normal subjects given oxypurinol, renal clearance of the drug was reduced by 64% after changing from a high- to a low-protein diet. This was produced by a large increase in net renal tubular reabsorption (Berlinger et al., 1985).

The effect of TPN regimens on oxidative drug metabolism has been investigated by Vesell and Biebuyck (1984). It is known that diet can influence drug metabolism markedly (Pantuck *et al.*, 1979). In a study of volunteers, a change from intravenous dextrose to AAs resulted in an increase in antipyrine metabolism. Patients receiving TPN may have a variety of other disturbances of organ blood flow and drug interaction to complicate the issue. Therefore it is wise to be cautious with administration of drugs to patients receiving TPN.

Planning the regimen

Macfie (1986) proposed that the cost of TPN may be reduced without compromising efficiency if we first ask: Is TPN really necessary? What are the patient's actual requirements? What is the best way to administer them? and, Have we discussed it with the pharmacist?

There is little to choose between currently available TPN solutions, and it is not the intention to give a specific regimen here. It is better for the prescriber to be familiar with a few regimens and understand the principles involved.

Some centres prefer a standard feeding regimen (Harper *et al.*, 1983) which is very cost-effective and in this context, nutrition teams are valuable. However, most patients, and especially the critically ill, benefit from an individually planned regimen (Kirkpatrick *et al.*, 1981). Computer programs exist which can be used at the bedside to predict individual nutritional requirements, facilitating appropriate treatment and often producing financial savings compared with administration of a standard feeding regimen to all patients (Colley *et al.*, 1985).

The factors determining design of an optimal regimen are considered elsewhere (Willatts, 1984). Although carbohydrate infusion has a progressive nitrogen-sparing effect, and nitrogen balance is related directly to calorie intake (Elwyn *et al.*, 1979), the increased negative nitrogen balance associated with severe surgical stress cannot be prevented completely (Radcliffe *et al.*, 1980).

The ideal non-protein calorie : nitrogen ratio varies from 300 : 1 in starvation to 150 : 1 in hypercatabolic patients (Peters & Fischer, 1980). A scheme of optimal requirements is presented in Table 87.14.

Where fluid intake is restricted, a reasonable approach is to give as much protein as possible with a mixed-fuel energy supply (Echenique *et al.*, 1982) as glucose alone is inclined to lead to more fluid retention than other energy substrates (Yeung *et al.*, 1979; Macfie *et al.*, 1981). Insulin is given by a separate infusion at a rate determined by regular blood glucose estimation.

Table 87.14 Optimal calorie : nitrogen requirements. (Redrawn from Woolfson, 1979)

	Starving	Catabolic	Hyper-catabolic
Nitrogen (g/24 h) requirements for equilibrium	7.5	14	25
kcal (total including protein)	2000	3000	4000
Non-protein calorie : nitrogen ratio	250	200	135

Ethanol is no longer included in TPN regimens as a result of adverse metabolic effects which include hypoglycaemia, increased blood concentrations of lactate, 3-hydroxybutyrate and free FAs, and reduced GH.

The introduction of a 3-litre bag for infusion of a mixture of 24-h nutritional requirement has proved popular. There seems to be no deterioration of AAs and glucose in this system nor changes in concentration of major electrolytes for up to 72 h if the bags are refrigerated.

Vitamins and trace elements are less stable. Calcium may be precipitated if magnesium is low or pH high. If Intralipid is included in these mixtures, it causes a significant reduction in drop size of up to 40% depending on the concentration of the Intralipid or divalent cations, the amino acid solution and the presence of certain vitamin additives. Catheter occlusion with lipid material is reported with the use of ethylvinyl acetate bags containing Intralipid and other nutrients, and there is a risk of leaching of plasticizers from PVC containers by fat emulsions.

The stability of parenterovite is limited in the presence of light to 6 h. A variety of solutions is available to supplement TPN. Addamel and Addi-trace contain trace elements with electrolytes, Addi-phos contains sodium, potassium and phosphate whereas Solivito and Vitlipid contain water- and fat-soluble vitamins, respectively.

Solivito contains insufficient folic acid so that supplementation (15 mg weekly) is required. Hyper-vitaminosis A may occur with exfoliative dermatitis and ectopic calcium deposition. The thiamine content of Solivito seems inadequate to prevent deficiency (Anderson & Charles, 1985).

Recommended values for trace elements bear little relationship to clinical demands in the critically ill. Requirements are higher than in health. Table 87.15

Table 87.15 Electrolyte, vitamin and trace-element recommendations for patients receiving total parenteral nutrition

	Average patient	
Sodium	100–120 mmol/day (50–60 mmol/day in elderly and/or cardiopulmonary disease)	↑ with gastrointestinal losses
Potassium	80–120 mmol/day	↓ with renal failure
Magnesium	12–15 mmol/day	↑ with gastrointestinal losses
Phosphorus	14–16 mmol/day	↓ with renal failure
Calcium	6.8–10 mmol/day	
Vitamin A	2500 IU/day	
Vitamin D	400 IU/day	
Vitamin E	50 IU/day (α-Tocopherol)	
Vitamin K	10 mg/week	
Thiamine	5 mg/day	
Riboflavin	5 mg/day	
Niacin	50 mg/day	
Pantothenic acid	15 mg/day	
Pyridoxine	5 mg/day	
Folic acid	5 mg/day	
Vitamin B_{12}	12 μg/day	
Vitamin C	300–500 mg/day	
Biotin	60 μg/day	

Iron	Men: 1 mg/day
	Women:
	   Premenopausal 2 mg/day
	   Postmenopausal 1 mg/day	

Zinc	1 mg/day 2.5 mg/day when infusing amino acids +12 mg/litre of small intestinal fluid loss +17 mg/litre of stool loss	
Copper	0.3 mg/day 0.5 mg/day with diarrhoea None with abnormal liver function	
Chromium	10–20 μg/day	
Selenium	120 μg/day	
Iodine	120 μg/day	
Manganese*	0.2–0.8 mg/day None with abnormal liver function	

* No deficiency during TPN administration has been described in humans.

gives electrolyte, vitamin and trace element recommendations for patients receiving TPN (Lemoyne & Jeejeebhoy, 1986).

If surgery is required in a patient receiving TPN, great care must be taken with the lines, to reduce the risk of sepsis. Different intravenous lines should be established for the perioperative period. The importance of perioperative maintenance of glucose homeostasis cannot be overemphasized.

Home parenteral nutrition is commonplace in the USA and practised by several centres in the UK. A register of cases has been set up and the service is likely to develop in a similar way to home dialysis. The main indications in the UK and Ireland are

Crohn's disease, mesenteric vascular disease and extensive small-bowel resection (Mughal & Irving, 1986). A dedicated unit with strict protocols is essential for success.

As malnutrition is corrected by feeding, the rate of restoration of BCM falls to zero at normal nutritional state. At this point, nitrogen balance never exceeds zero unless the individual is 'body building'.

Rational prescription of TPN in the critically ill must take into account multisystem dysfunction encountered in these circumstances. Knowledge of metabolic derangements in severe illness and attention to detail are outstandingly important (Wilmore, 1989).

References

Aarimaa M., Gyvalahati E., Viikari J. & Ovaska J. (1978) Insulin, growth hormone and catecholamines as regulators of energy metabolism in the course of surgery. *Acta Chirurgica Scandinavica* **144**, 411–22.

Abbott W.C., Grakauskas A.M., Bistrian B.R., Rose R. & Blackburn G.L. (1984) Metabolic and respiratory effects of continuous and discontinuous lipid infusions. *Archives of Surgery* **119**, 1367–71.

Abel R.M. (1983) Nutritional support in the patient with acute renal failure. *Journal of the American College of Nutrition* **2**, 33–44.

Abel R.M., Beck C.H., Abbott W.M., Ryan J.A., Barnett G.O. & Fischer J.E. (1973) Improved survival from acute renal failure after treatment with intravenous essential L-amino acids and glucose. *New England Journal of Medicine* **288**, 695–9.

Allam B.F., Dryburgh F.J. & Shenkin A. (1981) Metabolic bone disease during parenteral nutrition. *Lancet* **i**, 385.

Allison S.P., Tomlin P.J. & Chamberlain M.J. (1969) Some effects of anaesthesia and surgery on carbohydrate and fat metabolism. *British Journal of Anaesthesia* **41**, 588–93.

Alverdy J.C., Aoys E. & Moss G.S. (1988) Total parenteral nutrition promotes bacterial translocation from the gut. *Surgery* **104**, 185–90.

American College of Physicians, Health and Public Policy Committee. Perioperative Parenteral Nutrition (Position Paper 1987). *Annals of Internal Medicine* **107**, 252–3.

American College of Physicians (1989) Parenteral nutrition in patients receiving cancer chemotherapy. *Annals of Internal Medicine* **110**, 734–6.

Anderson S.H. & Charles T.J. (1985) Parenteral nutrition. *British Medical Journal* **291**, 1723–4.

Apelgren K.N., Rombeau J.L., Twomey P.L. & Miller R.A. (1982) Comparison of nutritional indices and outcome in critically ill patients. *Critical Care Medicine* **10**, 305–7.

Arnold J. & Little R.A. (1991) Stress and metabolic response to trauma in critical illness. *Current Anaesthesia and Critical Care* **2**, 139–48.

Arnold J., Shipley K.A., Scott N.A., Little R.A. & Irving M.H. (1989) Thermic effects of parenteral nutrition in septic and non-septic individuals. *American Journal of Clinical Nutrition* **50**, 853–60.

Askanazi J., Carpentier Y.A., Elwyn D.H., Nordenstrom J., Jeejeevandam M., Rosenbaum S.H., Gump F.E. & Kinney J.M. (1980) Influence of total parenteral nutrition on fuel utilisation in injury and sepsis. *Annals of Surgery* **191**, 40–6.

Askanazi J., Nordenstrom J., Rosenbaum S.M., Elwyn D.H., Carpentier Y.A. & Kinney J.M. (1981) Nutrition for the patient with respiratory failure. *Anesthesiology* **54**, 373–7.

Askanazi J., Weissman C., Rosenbaum S.H., Hyman A.I., Milic-Emili J. & Kinney J.M. (1982) Nutrition and the respiratory system. *Critical Care Medical* **10**, 163–72.

Aubier M., Murciano D., Lecoguic Y., Vures N., Jaqueas Y., Squara P. & Pariente R. (1985) Effect of hypophosphataemia on diaphragmatic contractility in patients with acute respiratory failure. *New England Journal of Medicine* **313**, 420–4.

Bach A.C., Guiraud M., Gibault F.P., Schirardin H. & Frey A. (1988) Medium chain triglycerides in septic patients on total parenteral nutrition. *Clinical Nutrition* **9**, 157–64.

Baker J.P., Detsky A.S., Wesson D.E., Wolman S.J., Stewart S., Whitewell J., Langer B. & Jeejeebhoy K.N. (1982) Nutritional assessment. A comparison of clinical judgement and objective measurements. *New England Journal of Medicine* **306**, 969–72.

Baracos V., Rodemann P., Dinarello C.A. & Goldberg A.L. (1983) Stimulation of muscle protein degradation and prostaglandin E2 release by leucocyte pyrogen (Interleukin-1). *New England Journal of Medicine* **308**, 553–8.

Bardosi L. & Tekeres M. (1985) Impaired metabolic activity of phagocytic cells after anaesthesia and surgery. *British Journal of Anaesthesia* **57**, 520–3.

Bassili H.R. & Dietal M. (1981) Effect of nutritional support on weaning patients off mechanical ventilators. *Journal of Parenteral and Enteral Nutrition* **5**, 161–3.

Bastow M.D., Raowlongs J. & Allison S.P. (1983) Benefits of supplementary tube feeding after fractured neck of femur: a randomised controlled trial. *British Medical Journal* **287**, 1589–92.

Bellatone R., Doglietto G.B., Bossola M., Pacelli F., Negro F., Sofo L. & Crucitti F. (1988) Preoperative parenteral nutrition in the high risk surgical patient. *Journal of Parenteral and Enteral Nutrition* **12**, 195–7.

Berlinger W.G., Park G.D. & Spector R. (1985) The effect of dietary protein on the clearance of allopurinol and oxypurinol. *New England Journal of Medicine* **313**, 771–6.

Bessey P.Q., Watters J.M., Aoki T.T. & Wilmore D.W. (1984) Combined hormonal infusion simulates the metabolic response to injury. *Annals of Surgery* **200**, 264–81.

Biebuyck J.L. (1981) Total parenteral nutrition in the perioperative period – a time for caution? *Anesthesiology* **54**, 360–3.

Biebuyck J.L. (1983) Nutritional aspects of anaesthesia. *Clinics in Anaesthesiology*. W.B. Saunders, London.

Birkhahn R.H., Long C.L., Fitkin D., Dyger J.W. & Blakemore W.S. (1980) Effects of major skeletal trauma on whole body protein turnover in man measured by L-14C-leucine. *Surgery* **88**, 294–9.

Bistrian B.R., Blackburn G.L., Hallowell E. & Heddle R. (1974) Protein status of general surgical patients. *Journal of the American Medical Association* **230**, 858–60.

Boles J.M., Garre M.A., Youinou P.Y., Mialon P., Menez J.F., Jouquan J., Moissec P.J., Pennec Y. & Lemenn G. (1984) Nutritional status in intensive care patients; evaluation in 84 unselected patients. *Critical Care Medicine* **11**, 87–90.

Boosalis M.G., Ott L., Levine A.S., Slag M.F., Morley J.E., Young B. & McClain C.J. (1989) Relationship of visceral proteins to nutritional status in chronic and acute stress. *Critical Care Medicine* **17**, 741–7.

Booth F.W. & Gollnick P.D. (1983) Effects of disuse on the structure and function of skeletal muscle. *Medicine and Science in Sports Exercise* **15**, 415–20.

Boscoe M.J. & Rosin M.D. (1984) Fine bone enteral feeding and pulmonary aspiration. *British Medical Journal* **289**, 1421–2.

Bozzetti F. (1989) Effects of artificial nutrition on the nutritional status of cancer patients. *Journal of Parenteral and Enteral Nutrition* **13**, 406–20.

Brandt M.R., Kehlet H., Skovsted L. & Hansen J.M. (1976) Rapid increase in plasma tri-iodothyronine during surgery and epidural anaesthesia independent of afferent neurogenic stimuli and of cortisol. *Lancet* **ii**, 1333–6.

Brinson R.R. & Pitts W.M. (1989) Enteral nutrition in the critically ill patient: role of hypoalbuminaemia. *Critical Care Medicine* **17**, 367–70.

Bristol J.B. & Williamson R.C.N. (1988) Nutrition, operations and intestinal adaptation. *Journal of Parenteral and Enteral Nutrition* **12**, 299–309.

Brough W., Horne E., Blount A., Irving M. & Jeejeebhoy K.N. (1986) Effects of nutrient intake, surgery, sepsis and long term administration of steroids on muscle function. *British Medical Journal* **293**, 983–8.

Bunker V.W. & Clayton B.E. (1983) Trace element content of commercial enteral feeds. *Lancet* **ii**, 426–8.

Burke J.F., Wolfe R.R., Mullany C.J., Mathews D.E. & Bier D.M. (1979) Glucose requirements following burn injury. Parameters of optimal glucose infusion and possible hepatic and respiratory abnormalities following excessive glucose intake. *Annals of Surgery* **190**, 274–85.

Burke D.J., Alverdy J.C., Aoys E. & Moss G.S. (1989) Glutamine-supplemented total parenteral nutrition improves gut immune function. *Archives of Surgery* **124**, 1396–9.

Burki N.K. (1980) Dyspnoea in chronic airway obstruction. *Chest* **78** (Suppl.), 298–302.

Buzby G.P., Mullen J.I. & Matthews D.C. (1980) Prognostic nutritional index in gastrointestinal surgery. *American Journal of Surgery* **139**, 160–7.

Byrnes H.G.J., Galloway D.J. & Ledingham I.McA. (1981) Effect of naftidrofuryl on the metabolic response to surgery. *British Medical Journal* **283**, 7–8.

Cahill G.F. Jr. (1970) Starvation in man. *New England Journal of Medicine* **282**, 668–75.

Campbell P.J., Bolli G.B., Cryer P.E. & Gerich J.E. (1985) Pathogenesis of the dawn phenomenon in patients with insulin dependent diabetes mellitus. *New England Journal of Medicine* **312**, 1473–9.

Capron J.-P., Gineston J.-L., Herve M.-A. & Braillon A. (1983) Metronidazole in prevention of cholestasis associated with parenteral nutrition. *Lancet* **i**, 446–7.

Carli F. & Itiaba K. (1986) Effect of heat conservation during and after major abdominal surgery on muscle breakdown in elderly patients. *British Journal of Anaesthesia* **58**, 502–7.

Carli F., Webster J., Ramachandra V., Pearson M., Read M., Ford G.C., McArthur S., Preedy V.R. & Halliday D. (1990) Aspects of protein metabolism after elective surgery in patients receiving constant nutritional support. *Clinical Science* **78**, 621–8.

Cerra F.B., Mazuski J., Teasley K., Nuwer N., Lysne J., Shronts E. & Konstantinides F. (1983) Nitrogen retention in critically ill patients is proportional to the branched chain amino acid load. *Critical Care Medicine* **11**, 775–8.

Cerra F.B., Alden P.A., Negro F., Billiar T., Svingen B.A., Licari J., Johnson S.B. & Holman R.T. (1988) Sepsis and endogenous lipid metabolism. *Journal of Parenteral and Enteral Nutrition* **12**, 63S–8S.

Cerra F.B., Shronts E.P., Raup S. & Konstantinides N. (1989) Enteral nutrition in hypermetabolic surgical patients. *Critical Care Medicine* **17**, 619–22.

Chan S.T.F., McLaughlin S.J., Ponting G.A., Biglin J. & Dudley H.A.F. (1986) Muscle power after glucose-potassium loading in undernourished patients. *British Medical Journal* **293**, 1055–6.

Chandra R.K. & Puri S. (1985) Nutritional support improves antibody response to influenza virus vaccine in the elderly. *British Medical Journal* **291**, 705–6.

Chang R.W.S., Jacobs S. & Lee B. (1986) Use of Apache II severity of disease classification to identify intensive care unit patients who would not benefit from total parenteral nutrition. *Lancet* **I**, 1483–7.

Chernow B., Rainey T.G., Georges L.P. & O'Brian J.T. (1981) Iatrogenic hyperphosphatemia: a metabolic consideration in critical care medicine. *Critical Care Medicine* **9**, 772–4.

Chiarelli A., Enzi G., Casadei A., Baggio B., Valerio A. & Mazzoleni F. (1990) Very early nutrition supplementation in burned patients. *American Journal of Clinical Nutrition* **51**, 1035–9.

Colley C.M., Fleck A. & Howard J.P. (1985) Pocket computers; a new aid to nutritional support. *British Medical Journal* **290**, 1403–6.

Collins R.N., Braun P.A., Zinner S.H. & Kass E.H. (1986) Risk of local and systemic infection with polyethylene intravenous catheters: a prospective study of 1213 catheterisations. *New England Journal of Medicine* **279**, 340–3.

Cuthbertson D.P. & Tilstone W.J. (1969) Metabolism during the post-injury period. *Advances in Clinical Chemistry* **12**, 1–55.

Dale D., Fleetwood J.A., Inkster J.S. & Sainsbury J.R.C. (1986) Profound hypophosphataemia in patients collapsing after a 'fun run'. *British Medical Journal* **292**, 447–8.

Daly J.M., Dudrick S.J. & Copeland E.M. III (1979) Evaluation of nutritional indices and prognostic indicators in the cancer patient. *Cancer* **43**, 925–31.

Damask M.C., Weissman C., Askanazi J., Hyman A.I., Rosenbaum S.H. & Kinney J.M. (1982) A systematic method for validation of gas exchange measurements. *Anesthesiology* **57**, 213–18.

Dauncey M.J., Murgatroyd P.R. & Cole T.J. (1978) A human calorimeter for the direct and indirect measurement of 24 hour energy expenditure. *British Journal of Nutrition* **39**, 587–90.

Dawson D. & Sear J.W. (1986) Influence of induction of anaesthesia with midazolam on the neuroendocrine response to surgery. *Anaesthesia* **41**, 268–71.

Di Costanzo J., Cano N. & Martin J. (1982) Somatostatin in persistent gastrointestinal fistula treated by total parenteral nutrition. *Lancet* **ii**, 338–9.

Dickerson J.W.T. (1984) Nutrition in the cancer patient. *Journal of the Royal Society of Medicine* **77**, 309–15.

Dickinson R.J., Ashton M.G., Axon A.T.R., Smith R.C., Yeung C.K. & Hill G.K. (1980) Controlled trial of intravenous hyperalimentation and total bowel rest as an adjunct to the routine therapy of acute colitis. *Gastroenterology* **79**, 1199–204.

Donnelly J.P., Cohen J., Marcus R. & Guest J. (1985) Bacteraemia and Hickman catheters. *Lancet* **2**, 48.

Drug and Therapeutics Bulletin (1980) **18**, 77–88.

Dudrick S.J., Wilmore D.W., Vars H.M. & Rhoads J.E. (1969) Can intravenous feeding as the sole means of nutrition, support growth in a child and restore weight loss in an adult? *Annals of Surgery* **169**, 974.

Echenique M.M., Bistrian B.R. & Blackburn G.L. (1982) Theory and techniques of nutritional support in the ICU. *Critical Care Medicine* **10**, 546–9.

Elia M., Martin S. & Neale G. (1984) Effect of non-nutritional factors on muscle function tests. *Archives of Emergency Medicine* **1**, 175–8.

Elliott M.J. & Alberti K.G.M.M. (1983) The hormonal and metabolic response to surgery and trauma. In *New Aspects of Clinical Nutrition* (Eds Kleinberger G. & Deutsch E.) pp. 247–70. Karger, Basel.

Elwyn D.H. (1980) Nutritional requirements of adult surgical patients. *Critical Care Medicine* **8**, 9–20.

Elwyn D.H., Gump F.E., Munro H.M., Iles M. & Kinney J.M. (1979) Changes in nitrogen balance of depleted patients with increasing infusions of glucose. *Journal of Clinical Nutrition* **32**, 1597–611.

Elwyn D.H., Kinney J.M., Gump F.E., Askanzi J., Rosenbaum M.H. & Carpentier Y.A. (1980) Some metabolic effects of fat infusions in depleted patients. *Metabolism* **29**, 125–32.

Elwyn D.H., Kinney J.M. & Askanazi J. (1981) Energy expenditure in surgical patients. *Surgical Clinics of North America* **61**, 545–56.

Engquist A., Brandt M.R., Fernandes A. & Kehlet H. (1977) The blocking effect of epidural analgesia on the adrenocortical and hyperglycaemia responses to surgery. *Acta Anaesthesiologica Scandinavica* **21**, 330–3.

Falchuk K.H., Peterson L. & McNeil B.J. (1985) Microparticulate induced phlebitis: its prevention by in-line filtration. *New England Journal of Medicine* **312**, 78–82.

Fan S.T., Lau W.Y., Wong K.K. & Chan Y.P.M. (1989) Preoperative parenteral nutrition in patients with oesophageal cancer: a prospective, randomised clinical trial. *Clinical Nutrition* **8**, 23–7.

Feinstein E.I. (1987) Nutrition in acute renal failure. *Advances in Experimental Medical Biology* **212**, 297–301.

Forse R.A. & Shizgal H.M. (1980) The assessment of malnutrition. *Surgery* **88**, 17–24.

Frayne K.N., Little R.A., Stoner H.B. & Galasko C.S.B. (1984) Metabolic control in non-septic patients with musculo skeletal injuries. *Injury: The British Journal of Accident Surgery* **16**, 73–9.

Freund H.R. & Fischer J.E. (1985) The use of branched chain amino acids in injury and sepsis. In *Proceedings of the 4th World Congress on Intensive and Critical Care Medicine* pp. 177–80. King & Winth Publishing Co., London.

Geefuysen J., Rosen E.V., Katz J., Ipp T. & Metz J. (1971) Impaired cellular immunity in Kwashiorkor with improvement after therapy. *British Medical Journal* **iv**, 527–9.

Geggel H.S., Ament M.E., Heckenlively J.R., Martin D.A. & Kopple J.D. (1985) Nutritional requirements for taurine in patients receiving long term parenteral nutrition. *New England Journal of Medicine* **312**, 142–6.

Glaeser B.S., Maher T.J. & Wurtman R.J. (1983) Changes in brain levels of acidic, basic and neutral amino acids after consumption of single meals containing various proportions of protein. *Journal of Neurochemistry* **41**, 1001.

Goode A.W., Herring A.N., Orr J.S., Ratcliffe W.A. & Dudley H.A.F. (1981) The effect of surgery with carbohydrate infusion on circulating tri-iodothyronine and reverse tri-iodothyronine. *Annals of the Royal College of Surgeons* **63**, 168–72.

Goodgame J.T. & Fischer J.E. (1977) Parenteral nutrition in the treatment of acute pancreatitis: effect on complications and mortality. *Annals of Surgery* **186**, 651–8.

Greenberg G.R., Marliss E.B., Anderson G.H., Langer B., Spence W., Tovee E.B. & Jeejeebhoy K.N. (1976) Protein sparing therapy in post-operative patients. *New England Journal of Medicine* **294**, 1141–6.

Gump F.E., Kinney J.M. & Price J.B. (1970a) Energy metabolism in surgical patients; oxygen consumption and blood flow. *Journal of Surgical Research* **10**, 613–27.

Gump F.E., Price J.B. & Kinney J.M. (1970b) Whole body and splanchnic blood flow and oxygen consumption measurements in patients with intraperitoneal infection. *Annals of Surgery* **171**, 321.

Hallberg D., Schubert O. & Wretland A. (1966) Experimental and clinical studies with fat emulsion for intravenous nutrition. *Nutrition Dieta* **8**, 245–55.

Harper P.H., Royle G.T., Michell A., Greenall M.J., Grant A., Winsley B., Atkins S.M., Todd E.M. & Kettlewell M.G.W. (1983) Total parenteral nutrition: value of standard regimen. *British Medical Journal* **286**, 1323–7.

Herskowitz K., Souba W.W. (1990) Intestinal glutamine metabolism during critical illness; a surgical perspective. *Nutrition* **6**, 199–206.

Heyman M.B., Vichinsky E., Katz R., Gaffield B., Hurst D., Castillo R., Chiu D., Kleman K., Ammann A.J., Thaler M.M. & Lubin B. (1985) Growth retardation in sickle cell disease treated by nutritional support. *Lancet* **1**, 903–6.

Heymsfield S.B. & Casper K. (1989) Congestive heart failure: clinical management by use of continuous nasogastric feeding. *American Journal of Clinical Nutrition* **50**, 539–44.

Himms-Hagen J. (1984) Thermogenesis in brown adipose tissue as an energy buffer: implications for obesity. *New England Journal of Medicine* **311**, 1549–58.

Hjortso N.-C., Christensen N.J., Andersen J. & Kehlet H. (1985) Effects of the extradural administration of local anaesthetic agents and morphine on the urinary excretion of cortisol, catecholamines and nitrogen following abdominal surgery. *British Journal of Anaesthesia* **57**, 400–6.

Hofsteller A., Schutz Y., Jequier E. & Wahren J. (1986) Increased 24 hour energy expenditure in cigarette smokers. *New England Journal of Medicine* **314**, 79–82.

Hulton N., Johnson D.J., Smith R.J. & Wilmore D.W. (1985) Hormonal blockade modifies post-trauma protein catabolism. *Journal of Surgical Research* **39**, 310–15.

Iapichino G. (1989) Nutrition in respiratory failure. *Intensive Care Medicine* **15**, 483–5.

Illingworth P.J., Jung R.T., Howie P.W., Leslie P. & Isles T.E. (1986) Diminution of energy expenditure during lactation. *British Medical Journal* **292**, 437–41.

Irvin T.T. (1978) Effects of malnutrition and hyperalimentation on wound healing. *Surgery, Gynecology and Obstetrics* **146**, 33–7.

Jackson A.A. & Golden M.H.N. (1980) N15 glycine metabolism in normal man: the metabolic beta-amino nitrogen pool. *Clinical Science* **58**, 517–22.

Jackson J.M., Khawaja H.T., Weaver P.C., Talbot S.T. & Lee H.A. (1984) Naftidrofuryl on the metabolic response to surgery. *British Medical Journal* **289**, 581–4.

Jeejeebhoy K.N. (1985) Changes in body consumption and muscle function and effect of nutritional support. *Proceedings of 4th World Congress on Intensive and Critical Care Medicine* pp. 161–4. King & Winth Publishing Co., London.

Jeejeebhoy K.N. (1988) Bulk or bounce — the object of

nutritional support. *Journal of Parenteral and Enteral Nutrition* **12**, 539–49.

Jeejeebhoy K.N., Anderson G.H., Nakhooda A.F., Greenberg G.R., Sanderson I. & Marliss E.B. (1976) Metabolic studies in total parenteral nutrition. *Journal of Clinical Investigation* **57**, 125.

Jeejeebhoy K.N., Baker J.P., Wolman S.L., Wesson D.E., Langer B., Harrison J.E. & McNeill K.G. (1982) Critical evaluation of the role of clinical assessment and body composition studies in patients with malnutrition and after total parenteral nutrition. *American Journal of Clinical Nutrition* **35**, 1117–27.

Jeevanandam M., Young D.H., Schiller W.R. (1990) Influence of parenteral nutrition on rates of net substrate oxidation in severe trauma patients. *Critical Care Medicine* **18**, 467–73.

Jones B.J.M., Payne S. & Silk D.B.A. (1980) Indications for pump-assisted enteral feeding. *Lancet* **i**, 1057–8.

Keohane P.P., Jones B.J.M., Attrill H., Cribb A., Northover J., Frost P. & Silk D.B.A. (1983) Effect of catheter tunnelling and a nutrition nurse on catheter sepsis during parenteral nutrition. *Lancet* **ii**, 1388–90.

Keohane P.P., Attrill H., Love M., Frost P. & Silk D.B.A. (1984) Relation between osmolality of diet and gastrointestinal side effects in enteral nutrition. *British Medical Journal* **288**, 678–80.

Kingston M.R., Al-Siba'i M.B. & Siba M. (1985) Treatment of severe hypophosphatemia. *Critical Care Medicine* **13**, 16–18.

Kinney J.M. & Hessov I.B. (1981) Protein energy malnutrition. In *Nutrition and the Surgical Patient* (Ed. Hill G.L.) pp. 12–25. Churchill Livingstone, Edinburgh.

Kirkpatrick J.R., Dahn M.S. & Lewis L. (1981) Selective versus standard hyperalimentation, a randomised prospective study. *American Journal of Surgery* **141**, 116–19.

Klidjian A.M., Foster K.J., Kammerling R.M., Cooper A. & Karran S.J. (1980) Relation of anthropometric and dynamometric variables to serious postoperative complications. *British Medical Journal* **281**, 899–901.

Knapp H.R., Reilly I.A.G., Alessandrini P. & Fitzgerald G.A. (1986) *In vivo* indices of platelet and vascular function during fish oil administration in patients with atherosclerosis. *New England Journal of Medicine* **314**, 937–42.

Knaus W.A., Draper E.A., Wagner D.P. & Zimmerman J.E. (1985) APACHE II: a severity of disease classification system. *Critical Care Medicine* **13**, 818–29.

Lamiell J.J., Ducey J.P., Freese-Kepczyk J., Musio F. & Hansberry K.L. (1990) Essential amino acid-induced adult hyperammonemic encephalopathy and hypophosphatemia. *Critical Care Medicine* **18**, 451–2.

Larca I. & Greenbaum D.M. (1982) Effectiveness of intensive nutritional regimes in patients who fail to wean from mechanical ventilation. *Critical Care Medicine* **10**, 297–300.

LaSala P.A., Starker P.M. & Askanazi J. (1983) The saphenous system for long-term parenteral nutrition. *Critical Care Medicine* **11**, 378–80.

Lee T.H., Hoover R.L., Williams J.D., Sperling R.I., Revalese J. III, Spur B.W., Robinson D.R., Corey E.J., Lems R.A. & Austen K.F. (1985) Effect of dietary enrichment with eicosapentaenoic and docosahexanenoic acids on *in vitro* neutrophil and monocyte leukotriene generation and neutrophil function. *New England Journal of Medicine* **312**, 1217–24.

Legaspi A., Roberts J.P., Horowitz G.D., Albert J.D., Tracey K.J., Shires T. & Lowry S.F.(1988) Effect of starvation and total parenteral nutrition on electrolyte homeostasis in normal man. *Journal of Parenteral and Enteral Nutrition* **12**, 109–15.

Lemoyne M. & Jeejeebhoy K.N. (1986) Total parenteral nutrition in the critically ill patient. *Chest* **89**, 568–75.

Levene M.I., Wigglesworth J.S. & Desai R. (1980) Pulmonary fat accumulation in the pre-term infant. *Lancet* **ii**, 815–19.

Li M., Specian R.D., Berg R.D. & Deitch E. (1989) Effects of protein malnutrition and endotoxin on the intestinal mucosal barrier to the translocation of indigenous flora in mice. *Journal of Parenteral and Enteral Nutrition* **13**, 572–8.

Loder P.B., Kee A.J., Horsburgh R., Jones M. & Smith R.C. (1989) Validity of urinary urea nitrogen as a measure of total urinary nitrogen in adult patients requiring parenteral nutrition. *Critical Care Medicine* **17**, 309–12.

Long J.M., Wilmore D.W., Mason A.D. & Pruitt B.A. (1977) Effect of carbohydrate and fat intake on nitrogen excretion during total intravenous feeding. *Annals of Surgery* **185**, 417–20.

Lowry S.F., Horowitz G.D., Jeevanandam M., Legaspi A. & Brennan M.F. (1985) Whole body protein breakdown and 3-methylhistidine excretion during brief fasting, starvation and intravenous repletion in man. *Annals of Surgery* **202**, 21–7.

MacFie J. (1984) Energy requirements of surgical patients during intravenous nutrition. *Annals of the Royal College of Surgeons of England* **66**, 39–42.

MacFie J. (1986) Towards cheaper intravenous nutrition. *British Medical Journal* **292**, 107–10.

MacFie J., Smith R.C. & Hill G.L. (1981) Glucose or fat as non-protein energy source? A controlled clinical trial in gastroenterologic patients receiving intravenous nutrition. *Gastroenterology* **80**, 103–7.

Main A.N.H., Shenkin A., Black W.P. & Russell R.I. (1981) Intravenous feeding to sustain pregnancy in patient with Crohn's disease. *British Medical Journal* **283**, 1221–2.

Mann S., Westenstow D.R. & Houtchens B.A. (1985) Measured and predicted calorie expenditure in the acutely ill. *Critical Care Medicine* **13**, 173–7.

Maynard N.D. & Bihari D.J. (1991) Post-operative feeding. *British Medical Journal* **303**, 1007–8.

Meakins J.L. & Marshall J.C. (1989) The gut as the motor of multiple system organ failure. In *Splanchnic Ischaemia and Multiple Organ Failure* (Eds Marston A., Bulkley G., Fiddian-Green R.G. & Haglund U.) pp. 349–63. Edward Arnold, London, Melbourne, Auckland.

Moore F., Feliciano D., Andrassy R., McCardle A.H., Booth F., Morgenstein T. *et al.* (1991) Enteral feeding reduces postoperative septic complications. *Journal of Enteral and Parenteral Nutrition* **15** (Suppl.), 22S, 32S.

Mozzillo N., Ayala F. & Federici G. (1982) Zinc deficiency syndrome in patient on long term total parenteral nutrition. *Lancet* **i**, 744.

Mughal M. & Irvin M. (1986) Home parenteral nutrition in the United Kingdom and Ireland. *Lancet* **2**, 383–7.

Mullen J.L., Busby G.P., Matthews D.C., Small R.F. & Risarto E.G. (1980) Reduction of operative mortality by combined preoperative and postoperative nutritional support. *British Journal of Surgery* **66**, 893–6.

Muller J.M., Dienst C., Brenner U. & Pichlmaier H. (1982) Preoperative parenteral nutrition in patients with gastro-intestinal carcinoma. *Lancet* i, 68–71.

Myo A., Nichols P., Rosin M., Bryant G.D.R. & Peterson L.M. (1986) An unusual oesophageal obstruction during naso-gastric feeding. *British Medical Journal* 293, 596–7.

Nakao I.K. & Miyata M. (1977) The influence of phentolamine, an alpha-adrenergic blocking agent, on insulin secretion during surgery. *European Journal of Clinical Investigation* 7, 41–5.

Newman D.J. (1986) Nutritional status and skeletal muscle activity. *British Journal of Parenteral Therapy* 7, 93–6.

Nordenstrom J., Jeevanandam M., Elwyn D.H., Carpentier Y.A., Askanazi J., Robin A. & Kinney J.M. (1981) Increasing glucose intake during total parenteral nutrition increases norepinephrine excretion in trauma and sepsis. *Clinical Physiology* 1, 525–84.

Norris P.G., Jones C.J.-H. & Weston M.J. (1986) Effect of dietary supplementation with fish oil on systolic blood pressure in mild essential hypertension. *British Medical Journal* 293, 104–6.

Pantuck E.J., Pantuck C.B., Garland W.A., Min B.H. & Conney A.H. (1979) Stimulatory effects of brussel sprouts and cabbage on human drug metabolism. *Clinical Pharmacology and Therapeutics* 25, 88–95.

Pantuck E.J., Pantuck C.B., Weissman C., Askanazi J. & Conney A.H. (1984) Effects of parenteral nutrition regimes on oxidative drug metabolism. *Anesthesiology* 60, 534–6.

Pardridge W.M. (1983) Brain metabolism: a perspective from the blood brain barrier. *Physiological Reviews* 63, 1481.

Parodis C., Spanies A.H., Calder M. & Shizgal H.M. (1977) Total parenteral nutrition with lipid. *American Journal of Surgery* 135, 164–8.

Parry-Billings M., Evans J., Calder P.C. & Newsholme E.A. (1990) Does glutamine contribute to immunosuppression after major burns? *Lancet* 336, 523–5.

Payne-James J., de Gara C., Grimble G., Rees R., Bray J., Rana S., Cribb R., Frost P. & Silk D. (1991) Nutritional support in hospitals in the United Kingdom National Survey 1988. *Health Trends* 23, 9–13.

Peters J.L. (1982) The evolution of tunnelling techniques for central venous catheters. *British Journal of Parenteral Therapy* 3, 21–30.

Peters C.P. & Fischer J.E. (1980) Studies in calorie to nitrogen ratio for total parenteral nutrition. *Surgery, Gynecology and Obstetrics* 151, 1–8.

Pettigrew R.A. & Hill G.L. (1986) Indicators of surgical risk and clinical judgement. *British Journal of Surgery* 73, 47–51.

Phillipson B.E., Rothrock D.W., Coonor W.E., Harris W.S. & Illingworth D.R. (1985) Reduction of plasma lipids, lipo-proteins and apoproteins by dietary fish oils in patients with hypertriglyceridemia. *New England Journal of Medicine* 312, 1210–16.

Popp M.B., Wagner S. & Brito O.J. (1983) Host and tumour responses to increasing levels of intravenous nutritional support. *Surgery* 94, 300–8.

Porte D. & Robertson R.P. (1975) Control of insulin secretion by catecholamines, stress and the sympathetic nervous system. *Federation Proceedings* 32, 1792.

Prentice A.M., Black A.E., Coward W.A., Davies H.L., Goldberg G.R., Murgatroyd P.R., Ashford J., Sawyer M. & Whitehead D.G. (1986) High level of energy expenditure in obese women. *British Medical Journal* 292, 983–7.

Radcliffe A., Johnson A. & Dudley H.A.F. (1980) The effect of different calorific doses of carbohydrate on nitrogen excretion after surgery. *British Journal of Surgery* 67, 462–3.

Reeds P.J. & James W.P.T. (1983) Protein turnover. *Lancet* i, 571–4.

Rees R.G.P., Keohane P.P., Grimble G.K., Frost P.G., Atrill & Silk D.B. (1985) Tolerance of elemental diet administered without starter regimen. *British Medical Journal* 290, 1869–70.

Rennie M.J. (1984) The role of prostaglandins in the control of lean tissue mass. *British Journal of Parenteral Therapy* 5, 51–5.

Rennie M.J. (1985) The doubly labelled water method. *British Journal of Parenteral Therapy* 6, 90–4.

Rennie M.J. & Harrison R. (1984) Effects of injury, disease and malnutrition on protein metabolism in man. *Lancet* 1, 323–5.

Rennie M.J. & Millward D.J. (1983) 3-Methylhistidine excretion and the urinary 3-methylhistidine/creatine ratio are poor indicators of skeletal muscle protein breakdown. *Clinical Science* 65, 217–25.

Rennie M.J., Babji P., Taylor P.M., Hindal H.S., Jepson M.M., MacLellan P., Uatt D.W. & Millward D.J. (1986) Characteristics of a glutamine carrier in skeletal muscle have important consequences for nitrogen loss in injury, infection and chronic disease. *Lancet* 2, 1008–12.

Robin A.P., Askanazi J., Cooperman A., Carpentier Y.A., Elwyn D.H. & Kinney J.M. (1981) Influence of hypercalorie glucose infusions on fuel economy in surgical patients. *Critical Care Medicine* 9, 680–6.

Rochester D.F. & Arora N.S. (1983) Respiratory muscle failure. *Medical Clinics of North America* 67, 573–97.

Rombeau J.L., Barot R.L., Williamson C.E. & Mullen J.L. (1982) Preoperative total parenteral nutrition and surgical outcome in patients with inflammatory bowel disease. *American Journal of Surgery* 143, 139–43.

Royle G.T., Wolfe R.R. & Burke J.F. (1981) Techniques of investigating substrate metabolism in man. *Annals of the Royal College of Surgeons of England* 63, 413–19.

Russel D.M., Leiter L.A., Whitwell J., Marliss E.B. & Jeejeebhoy K.N. (1983) Skeletal muscle function during hypocalorie diets and fasting: a comparison with standard nutritional assessment parameters. *American Journal of Clinical Nutrition* 37, 133–8.

Ryan N.T. (1976) Metabolic adaptations for energy production during trauma and sepsis. *Surgical Clinics of North America* 56, 1073.

Sapir D.G., Stewart P.M., Walser M., Moreadith C., Moyer E.D., Imbembo A.L., Rosenstein M.B. & Munoz S. (1983) Effects of alpha ketoisocaproate and of leucine on nitrogen metabolism in post-operative patients. *Lancet* i, 1010–14.

Sheth N.K., Franson T.R. & Sohnle P.G. (1985) Influence of bacterial adherence to intravascular catheters on *in vitro* antibiotic sensitivity. *Lancet* 2, 1266–8.

Shizgal H.M. (1981) Nutrition and the immune function. *Surgery Annual* 12, 15–29.

Sibbald W.J., Short A., Cohen M.P. & Wilson R.F. (1977) Variations in adrenocortical responsiveness during severe bacterial infections. *Annals of Surgery* 186, 29–33.

Sitges-Serra A., Jaurrieta E. & Sitges-Creus A. (1982) Management of postoperative enterocutaneous fistulas: the roles of parenteral nutrition and surgery. *British Journal of Surgery* **69**, 147–50.

Skeie B., Kvetan V., Gil K.M., Rothkopf M.M., Newsholme E.A., Askanazi J. (1990) Branch chain amino acids: their metabolism and clinical utility. *Critical Care Medicine* **18**, 549–71.

Smith R.C. & Hartemink R. (1988) Improvement of nutritional measures during preoperative parenteral nutrition in patients selected by the prognostic nutritional index: a randomised controlled trial. *Journal of Parenteral and Enteral Nutrition* **12**, 587–91.

Smith H.S., Kennedy D.J. & Park G.R. (1984) A nomogram for rapid measurement of metabolic requirements of intubated patients. *Intensive Care Medicine* **10**, 147–8.

Spitzer J.J., Bagby G.J., Meszaros K. & Lang C.H. (1988) Alterations in lipid and carbohydrate metabolism in sepsis. *Journal of Parenteral and Enteral Nutrition* **12**, 53S–8S.

Starker P.M., LaSala P.A., Askanazi J., Todd G., Henzle T.W. & Kinney J.M. (1986) The influence of total parenteral nutrition upon morbidity and mortality. *Surgery, Gynecology and Obstetrics* **162**, 569–74.

Stehle P., Zander J., Mertes N., Albers S., Puchstein Ch., Lawin P. & Furst P. (1989) Effect of parenteral glutamine peptide supplements on muscle glutamine loss and nitrogen balance after major surgery. *Lancet* **1**, 231–3.

Stewart P.M. & Hensley W.J. (1981) Acute polymyopathy during total parenteral nutrition. *British Medical Journal* **283**, 1578.

Stokes M.A. & Irving M.H. (1989) Mortality in patients on home parenteral nutrition. *Journal of Parenteral and Enteral Nutrition* **13**, 172–5.

Stoner H.B., Frayne K.N., Barton R.N., Thretfall C.I. & Little R.A. (1979) The relationship between plasma substrates and hormones and the severity of injury in 277 recently injured patients. *Clinical Science* **56**, 563–73.

Stracher A. (1982) Proteinase inhibitors and muscle degradation. *Muscle and Nerve* **5**, 494.

Studley H.O. (1936) Percentage of weight loss. A basic indicator of surgical risk in patients with chronic peptic ulcer. *Journal of the American Medical Association* **106**, 458–60.

Thomas R., Aihawa N. & Burke J.F. (1979) Insulin resistance in peripheral tissues after burn injury. *Surgery* **86**, 742.

Tulikoura I. (1988) Maintenance of visceral protein levels in the serum during post-operative parenteral nutrition. *Journal of Parenteral and Enteral Nutrition* **12**, 597–601.

Vessell E.S. & Biebuyck J.F. (1984) New approaches to assessment of drug disposition in the surgical patient. *Anesthesiology* **60**, 529–32.

Veterans Affairs Total Parenteral Nutrition Cooperative Study Group (1991) Perioperative total parenteral nutrition in surgical patients. *New England Journal of Medicine* **325**, 525–32.

Vinnars E. (1982) Surgical trauma: conventional or special amino-acid solutions for parenteral nutrition. In *New Aspects of Clinical Nutrition* (Eds Kleinberger G. & Deutsch E.) pp. 422–7. Karger, Basel.

Weissman C., Kemper M., Elwyn D.H., Askanazi J., Hyman A.I. & Kinney J.M. (1986) The energy expenditure of the mechanically ventilated critically ill patient. An analysis. *Chest* **89**, 254–9.

Willatts S.M. (1984) Design of an optimal parenteral nutrition regimen. *British Journal of Parenteral Therapy* **5**, 117–23.

Williamson R.C.N. (1983) Effect of nutrition on the gut. *British Journal of Parenteral Therapy* **4**, 35–8.

Wilmore D.W. (1989) The practice of clinical nutrition: how to prepare for the future. *Journal of Parenteral and Enteral Nutrition* **13**, 337–43.

Wilmore D.W., Goodwin C.W., Aulick L.H., Powanda M.C., Mason A.D. & Pruitt B.A. (1980) Effect of injury on infection metabolism and circulation. *Annals of Surgery* **192**, 492–504.

Woolf R.R., Herndon D.N., Jahoor F., Miyoshi H. & Wolfe M. (1987) Effect of severe burn injury on substrate cycling by glucose and fatty acids. *New England Journal of Medicine* **317**, 403–7.

Woolfe B.M., Culebras J.M., Aoki T.T., O'Connor N.E., Finley R.J., Kaczowka A. & Moore F.D. (1979) The effects of glucagon on protein metabolism in normal man. *Surgery* **86**, 248.

Woolfson A.M.J. (1979) Metabolic considerations in nutritional support. *Research and Clinical Forums* **1**, 35–47.

Woolfson A.M.J. (1983) Artificial nutrition in hospital. *British Medical Journal* **287**, 1004–6.

Woolfson A.M.J. & Smith J.A.R. (1989) Elective nutritional support after major surgery: a prospective randomised trial. *Clinical Nutrition* **8**, 15–21.

Woolfson A.M.J., Heatley R.V. & Allison S.P. (1979) Insulin to inhibit protein catabolism after injury. *New England Journal of Medicine* **300**, 14–17.

Yamanaka H., Nishi M., Kanemaki T., Hosoda N., Hioki K. & Yamamoto M. (1989) Preoperative nutritional assessment to predict post-operative complication in gastric cancer patients. *Journal of Parenteral and Enteral Nutrition* **13**, 286–91.

Yeung C.K., Smith R.C. & Hill G.L. (1979) Effect of an elemental diet on body composition. *Gastroenterology* **77**, 652–7.

Young G.A., Chem C., Zeiderman M.R., Thompson M., McMahon M.J. (1989) Influence of preoperative nutrition upon hepatic protein synthesis and plasma proteins and amino acids. *Journal of Parenteral and Enteral Nutrition* **13**, 596–602.

Neurological Disease

L. LOH

Although there are several neurological diseases which may require intensive care management, the clinical problems which they present are often similar and generally fall into two main groups.

1 Patients in coma or with disorders of consciousness needing special nursing care, monitoring and protection of the airways.

2 Patients with impending or established ventilatory failure requiring close observation and perhaps artificial ventilation. Ventilatory failure may be an acute or chronic condition and may be central, arising from damage to the neural control of breathing, or peripheral as a result of respiratory muscle weakness.

Before specific neurological disorders are discussed, some preliminary comments are necessary on the anatomy of coma and the neural control of respiration. It is hoped that this may help in the assessment and management of disorders similar to those few illustrated in this chapter.

Coma

Consciousness is a state of awareness, both of self and the environment and this is demonstrated usually by voluntary and purposeful behaviour and speech in response to both internal and external stimuli. Coma is a sleep-like state in which the subject lies with eyes closed but it is distinguished from sleep as the subject cannot be roused by strong external stimulation. Coma is the converse of consciousness and may be defined in its simplest terms as an absence of awareness of self and environment.

The causes of coma generally involve either widespread dysfunction of both the cerebral hemispheres, as occurs in metabolic brain disease and hypoxic brain damage, or localized disruption of the ascending reticular activating system (ARAS) in the upper midbrain by external compression or an intrinsic lesion of the brainstem (Plum & Posner, 1980). It is important to stress the key role of the ARAS in the maintenance of consciousness.

The ARAS is composed of a diffuse core of neurones extending from the medulla to the upper midbrain. The main ascending pathway is the central tegmental tract which receives afferent signals from all areas of the brainstem and thalamus and projects to all areas of the cerebral cortex. A lesion of the upper midbrain which disconnects the ARAS from the cortex produces a state of coma; in experimental preparations it may be shown that such a lesion causes an EEG pattern similar to that of coma, whereas stimulation of this area may produce an awake-looking EEG (Bremer, 1937; Moruzzi & Magoun, 1949). A functioning ARAS is essential for awareness and presumably anaesthetics act primarily on the ARAS to produce unconsciousness.

The ARAS is very closely related anatomically to the brainstem nuclei. Brainstem death is essentially death of the ARAS and recognized indirectly by the cessation of function of the cranial nerve nuclei with which the ARAS is intimately connected.

Coma is not a disease in itself but the expression of an underlying disorder of the nervous system. Table 88.1 classifies the causes of coma into three main groups.

Causes

1 *Diseases which involve a widespread disorder of both cerebral hemispheres but where the brainstem function remains intact and there are no signs of focal neural damage.* With intoxication, metabolic disturbance or hypothermia, there is usually extensive reduction of neuronal activity and cerebral metabolic rate. Epilepsy produces unconsciousness if it has spread to both hemispheres or has involved the diencephalon and interrupted transmission from the ARAS. In this group of disorders the computerized tomography

Table 88.1 Causes of coma

Disorders of cortical function with no focal signs
Intoxications
Alcohol, barbiturates, opioids, etc.
Metabolic disturbances
Anoxia, uraemia, hepatic coma, hypo- and hyperglycaemia
Severe systemic infection
Pneumonia, typhoid, malaria, septicaemia
Cerebral ischaemia
Epilepsy
Hypo- and hyperthermia
Hypertensive encephalopathy
Concussion

Diseases with meningeal irritation
Subarachnoid haemorrhage, ruptured aneurysm,
   arteriovenous malformation, trauma
Acute bacterial meningitis
Aseptic meningitis, viral meningitis

Diseases causing focal brainstem or lateralizing cerebral signs
Brain haemorrhage
Brain infarction
Brain abscess
Brain tumour
Encephalitis
Cerebral thrombophlebitis

(CT) scan is often normal and so is the cerebrospinal fluid (CSF). Often the patients pass through various 'states of altered consciousness' with drowsiness, confusion and stupor, both as the disease develops and also during recovery. Sometimes the disease progresses to involve midbrain and more caudal structures either by direct extension of the disease process or through cerebral swelling causing tentorial herniation and brainstem compression. The clinical picture then changes to one with focal brainstem signs, and coma is likely to be compounded by disruption of the ARAS.

2 *Disorders with signs of meningeal irritation either from blood in the CSF or meningeal inflammation usually of bacterial origin.* The CSF is abnormal, containing blood or an excess of white cells, and there are signs of meningism such as neck stiffness and photophobia, headache and vomiting, before coma develops. There may or may not be focal neurological signs, and the CT scan may be helpful in the diagnosis.

3 *Diseases which demonstrate focal brainstem signs or lateralizing cerebral signs as a result of lesions which arise supra- or infratentorially and cause disruption of the ARAS by compression or destruction of the brainstem.* Supratentorial lesions arise frequently from one hemisphere and produce lateral compression of the brainstem, and there is a progression of signs which indicate, not necessarily with any great precision, the rostral-to-caudal involvement of the brainstem. These signs also indicate approximately the prognosis and response to treatment.

Of the many focal brainstem signs, probably the most useful clinically are those concerning the pupillary response, eye movements (oculocephalic and oculovestibular responses), motor responses to painful stimuli (extensor or flexor) and the pattern of respiration.

Pupillary responses

Pupil size and reactivity is determined not only by light falling on the retina but also the continuity of the parasympathetic (constrictor) and sympathetic (dilator) pathways to the pupil. The parasympathetic fibres are carried by the third nerve. The sympathetic pathway is tortuous from the hypothalamus down the brainstem to the first thoracic segment of the spinal cord. From there, sympathetic fibres pass out into the stellate ganglion and back via the carotid arteries or the fifth nerve and reach the orbit via the nasocilliary branch of V as the long ciliary nerves to the dilator muscles of the pupil.

Pupil size is determined by the balance between parasympathetic and sympathetic activity. If the third nerve is compressed, parasympathetic fibres are interrupted and the pupil becomes dilated and unreactive. If the sympathetic fibres from the hypothalamus and onwards are interrupted unilaterally, the pupil constricts, but may still show some reaction to light (Horner's syndrome). Bilateral pupillary constriction may occur if the descending sympathetic pathway is interrupted in the diencephalon and pontine tegmental region of the upper midbrain. If both parasympathetic and sympathetic supplies are interrupted by midbrain and pontine compression, the pupils are mid-dilated and unreactive. The fixed dilated pupils of acute cerebral ischaemia are thought to be the result of circulating hormonal factors induced by ischaemia.

Eye movements

In the awake state, eye movements are controlled by voluntary or behavioural cortical responses, and if the head is turned rapidly from side to side, the eye movement response is variable depending on what the subject is observing. In the unconscious state, this behavioural factor is abolished and turning the head from side to side reveals the basic reflex movements determined by the vestibular apparatus. These are the oculocephalic (or 'dolls eye') movements. Similarly, in the unconscious state, cooling or warming the tympanic membrane and the fluid in the semicircular canals produces reflex tonic deviation of the eyes, as demonstrated by the oculovestibular or caloric tests. These reflexes depend on the integrity of the vestibular nuclei in the pontine–medullary region and also on the III, IV and VI nerve nuclei which control eye movements. Absence of these reflex eye movements indicate severe brainstem injury.

Damage to the nuclei concerned with eye movements and their connecting tracts may also produce divergent or convergent squints or asymmetrical eye movements (internuclear ophthalmoplegia) indicative of localized brainstem damage.

Motor responses

Comatose subjects, although not aware, may still respond reflexly to a painful stimulus, and reflex withdrawal of a limb (a flexion response) to a painful stimulus is seen frequently in disorders involving just the cerebral hemispheres. However, if the lesion spreads to involve the diencephalon, the pattern of response may change to that of flexion of the upper limb and extension of the lower limb. This is often termed the decorticate response and is in effect a bilateral spastic hemiplegia. Further disruption of the upper midbrain gives rise to an extensor response in both upper and lower limbs which is termed the decerebrate response. Pontine–medullary involvement produces no motor response (flaccid response) and holds a grave prognosis.

Provided the subject is not under the influence of drugs which alter the brainstem responses, and having taken into account also the nature of the primary lesion, the above clinical signs may be used to assess the depth of coma, determine the site of the lesion, chart the progress of the disease and arrive at a prognosis. In a clinical setting, the picture is often not as definite as might be supposed from the above description and additional information may be derived from the study of the breathing pattern. In order to understand this, some knowledge of the anatomical organization of the neural control of breathing is necessary.

The neural control of breathing

Even after many years of investigation, the neural mechanisms which control breathing are still fairly obscure and the respiratory centres are regarded by the majority of anaesthetists as vague collections of neurones situated in the 'black box' of the pontine and medullary regions of the brainstem. Local trauma and disease of the brainstem and certain drugs acting on the brainstem have an effect on 'ventilation', which is the final result of the output of the breathing mechanism, but seldom are careful observations made of those changes in the pattern of breathing which may reflect the particular part of the system which is at fault.

An important point often forgotten is that there are two independent respiratory control mechanisms (Newsom-Davis, 1985). One relates to the voluntary control of breathing and may be termed the behavioural system. The other, the metabolic or automatic system, is devoid of conscious control and responds to metabolic and other afferent stimuli. It is of clinical importance to appreciate that there are these two systems when interpreting the various patterns of breathing seen in neurological disorders.

The behavioural system

Voluntary movements are subserved by the corticospinal tracts, the signals arising in the motor cortex and passing down the fibres of the internal capsule to decussate in the pons and thence, via corticospinal tracts in the lateral part of the spinal cord, to synapse with the anterior horn cells of the motor neurones supplying voluntary muscle. Voluntary control of breathing movements uses these same corticospinal pathways (Fig. 88.1). In general, it overrides the respiratory drive from the metabolic system. It should be noted that the respiratory function tests requiring voluntary manoeuvres, e.g. vital capacity, peak expiratory flow, maximum breathing capacity and voluntary cough, are only tests of the behavioural system and do not provide information on the integrity of the metabolic system.

The metabolic system

Groups of neurones forming longitudinal columns of cells in the medulla, concentrated in the regions of nucleus tractus solitarii (NTS) just beneath the floor of the fourth ventricle, and also nucleus retro-ambigualis (NRA) deeper in the medulla, cross in the medulla and project down the anterolateral part of the spinal cord to synapse with the anterior horn cells of respiratory muscles, probably via an internuncial neurone. The neurones of NTS and NRA

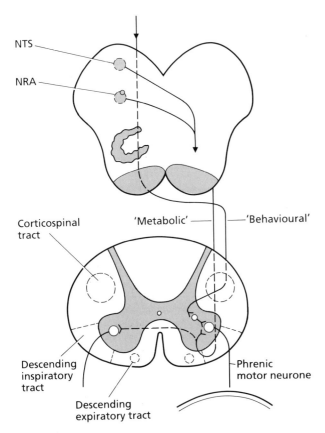

Fig. 88.1 Diagrammatic section through the medulla and midcervical cord showing the pathway of the corticospinal tract of the 'behavioural' system and the medullary nuclei and projections of the descending inspiratory and expiratory tracts of the 'metabolic' system. NTS, nucleus tractus solitarii; NRA, nucleus retroambigualis. (Redrawn from Loh, 1986.)

project to both inspiratory and expiratory muscles, although those of NTS are largely inspiratory to the diaphragm. They also receive projections from various other neurones in the pons and medulla.

The generation of a rhythmical pattern of breathing is a highly complex interaction between the pontine and medullary respiratory nuclei and has not been defined clearly in experimental animals, let alone in humans. There is probably a pontine rhythm generator which inhibits tonic inspiratory and expiratory medullary neurone activity, which are themselves mutually inhibitory (Sears *et al.*, 1982). These neurones may form the fundamental basis of a rhythmic breathing pattern which is modulated further by central and peripheral chemoreceptor drives, afferents from the lungs and chest-wall receptors and muscle spindles, in addition to pharyngeal, laryngeal and tracheal receptors. Body temperature and the general level of activity in the reticular activating system also modify the firing thresholds of

neurones, not only centrally, but also at the spinal level.

Figure 88.2 illustrates the breathing pattern of a male patient who has had the corticospinal tracts interrupted as a result of infarction of the ventral pontine region. He was unable to move voluntarily any muscle innervated below the level of the lesion and, although completely aware, was able to communicate only with eye movements — an example of the 'locked-in syndrome'. The breathing pattern is extremely regular, showing the metabolic system driving respiration in isolation, uninfluenced by the behavioural system. When asked to take a deep breath or stop breathing, the patient was unable to do either, and yet he could augment his breathing reflexly following an increase in inspired carbon dioxide.

Figure 88.3 shows the irregular breathing pattern of a man who had a tumour invading the floor of the fourth ventricle with destruction of NTS bilaterally. He was unable to sleep because he feared, quite correctly, that he would stop breathing if he did not voluntarily drive his breathing. He required artificial ventilation in order that he could sleep. The irregular pattern of breathing correlates with changes in EEG when lower-voltage activity, indicating short lapses in attention, is associated with slow respiration. This is an example of disruption of the metabolic system of respiratory control, a true 'Ondine's curse'. The patient could perform various voluntary respiratory manoeuvres but, when drowsy, would hypoventilate and show a slow irregular pattern of respiration with apnoeic periods.

Patients with a defect in the metabolic system may appear normal in the awake state, and may be able to perform satisfactorily various voluntary respiratory tests, but, if left alone, they may hypoventilate severely and even succumb, as a result of the failure by medical staff to recognize the abnormality in the metabolic system. Patients with medullary lesions should be observed very carefully for signs of hypoventilation, apnoeic episodes or slow irregular respiration, a situation not unlike an overdose of fentanyl, which is, in effect, a pharmacological disruption of the metabolic or automatic control system, with preservation of the behavioural mechanism.

The efferent and afferent neurones of the glossopharyngeal and vagal nuclei are situated close to NTS and NRA, and any lesion affecting one is likely to affect the other. Thus, patients who have loss of sensation of the pharynx and trachea or difficulty with swallowing, or who develop hiccup resulting from damage to the medulla, are likely in addition

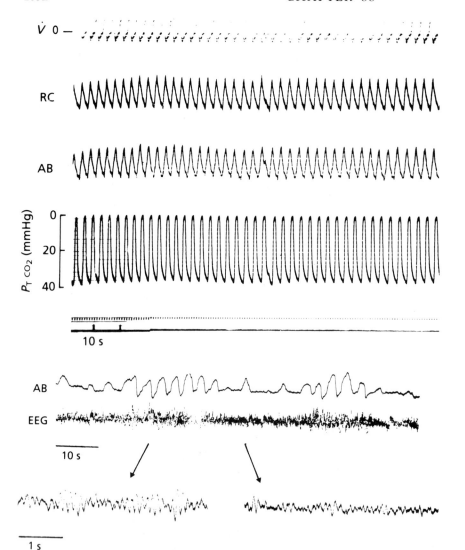

Fig. 88.2 Breathing pattern of a patient with 'locked-in' syndrome. V, airflow by pneumotachograph; RC, rib cage anteroposterior movement by magnetometers; AB, abdominal anteroposterior movement by magnetometers. Note the very regular pattern of breathing. In midtrace, the patient was asked to stop breathing, but no voluntary control was possible, the breathing being driven by the metabolic system in isolation. (Redrawn from Loh, 1986.)

Fig. 88.3 Irregular breathing pattern in a patient with disruption of the metabolic control system of breathing. AB, abdominal anteroposterior movement by magnetometer; EEG, simultaneous electroencephalogram. Below: expanded portions of EEG. Note low-voltage activity associated with slow respiratory rate. (Redrawn from Loh, 1986.)

to have respiratory disturbances of the metabolic system.

The descending tracts of NTS and NRA, which carry the respiratory drive to the anterior horn cells of respiratory muscles, lie in the anterolateral part of the cord in what may be termed the reticulospinal tracts (Nathan, 1963). When a high cervical cordotomy is performed for pain relief, a unilateral lesion of the spinothalamic tracts also frequently cuts the descending reticulospinal tract, giving rise to a temporary disturbance of automatic breathing. Bilateral lesions lead to death from total failure of the metabolic system, an irremediable Ondine's curse. Similar high-cervical lesions from other causes have the same effects.

Whilst tests of the behavioural system involve tests of voluntary function, tests of a metabolic system should include observation of the breathing pattern during quiet breathing or sleep. Frequent sighs, hiccups, slow irregular breathing and apnoeic periods are indicative of disturbance of the metabolic system. Specific tests of ventilatory response to hypoxia and carbon dioxide may be useful, although difficult to interpret.

The management of a deficiency of the metabolic system depends on the prognosis, but tracheostomy with artificial ventilation, especially during sleep, are necessary in the first instance. If the patient has a reasonable prognosis, this type of central respiratory failure is one of the few indications for phrenic nerve pacing (Glen *et al.*, 1972).

Disturbances of respiratory pattern

During normal quiet breathing in the awake subject, the pattern of breathing is reasonably regular, but the variations in tidal volume and inspiratory and expiratory time are greater than during slow-wave sleep, because the thinking individual alters his or her pattern of breathing when reading, listening or thinking. During sleep, breathing is more regular and less variable except during rapid eye movement (REM) sleep when possibly dreaming may influence breathing patterns. Several disturbances of the normal pattern of breathing have been described which are related to the part of the respiratory control mechanism which is at fault.

Cortical disturbances

Cheyne—Stokes respiration is a characteristic pattern of breathing occurring in patients with cortical damage or ischaemia and a slow circulation time. It is seen in the presence of an intact respiratory control mechanism. Breathing increases progressively in depth to a peak and then wanes, the cycle often ending with a period of apnoea before commencing again. The pattern of change is smooth and regular. Cherniack and Longobardo (1973) suggested that cortical damage reduced a central inhibition of carbon dioxide sensitivity and that the combination of an increase in carbon dioxide sensitivity and a slow circulation, causing unusual delays between blood-gas exchange in the lungs and the sensing of such changes by the chemoreceptors, caused a type of instability in the control mechanism which gave rise to the Cheyne—Stokes respiratory pattern.

Afferent stimulation from lung and chest wall

Tachypnoea which is a regular and persistent increase of breath frequency, is almost always the result of lung complications such as pneumothorax, pulmonary oedema, lobar collapse or consolidation. Again, the neural control mechanism is intact but the afferent discharge from the lungs and chest-wall receptors is altered by disease to produce a shortening of inspiration and a decrease in tidal volume and an increase in respiratory rate.

Midbrain and pontine lesions

Cluster breathing describes an abrupt increase in respiratory frequency for short periods which is quite unlike Cheyne—Stokes respiration. It is seen in patients with encephalitis and brainstem lesions and probably results from a disturbance of rhythm generation by a pontine tegmental lesion.

Apneustic breathing, when there is an involuntary breath-hold in inspiration and *ratchet breathing*, when inspiration occurs in a series of steps, have also been described in pontine lesions.

Neurogenic hyperventilation is again a manifestation of a pontine lesion, occasionally following head injury. The hyperventilation is difficult to control. In order to minimize respiratory work and prevent severe respiratory alkalosis, muscle paralysis and controlled ventilation may be necessary.

Medullary lesions

Irregular breathing with apnoeic periods is seen in lesions of NTS and NRA as illustrated in the case above, or when the descending reticulospinal pathway is interrupted. The subject may be reluctant to sleep, and careful examination may reveal damage to other cranial nerves arising from the medulla.

Hiccups may result from lesions in the region of NTS which remove an inhibitory influence which normally suppresses hiccups (Newsom-Davis, 1970). This periodic, massive inspiratory discharge is usually followed closely by glottic closure to produce the 'hic'. However, in patients in whom the trachea is intubated, limitation of inspiration by glottic closure cannot occur and the inspiratory activity produces large tidal volumes and gross hyperventilation. It appears that hypocapnia perpetuates the situation. Hiccups may sometimes be improved by carbon dioxide rebreathing. Strong vagal stimulation may also inhibit hiccups on occasion. It is important that hiccups in the patient with an intubated trachea are recognized and not mistaken for some other form of hyperventilation. It may be detected by the regular periodicity of inspiration, often interspersed with a few normal breaths.

Epilepsy

This is an intermittent derangement of the nervous system where sudden disorderly discharges of cerebral neurones produces disturbance in sensation, alterations in psychic function, convulsive movements and often loss of consciousness. Such an episode is often termed a seizure and is a manifestation of disease of the nervous system. Seizures may be idiopathic, when the nature of the original disease is unknown, or secondary to a known cause.

Seizures may take several forms which can be allocated into generalized or partial or focal seizures. Grand mal seizures are the most dramatic of the generalized seizures. They may sometimes start with an aura or may occur unexpectedly. There is first a tonic phase with generalized muscle spasm, loss of consciousness, incontinence, absent respiration and the pupils are usually dilated and unreactive. This then passes on to a clonic phase when a mild generalized trembling gives way to violent, rhythmic muscular contractions. Cyanosis, sweating, biting of the tongue and frothing of the lips are part of the picture. After 1—2 min the episode subsides, respiration resumes and for a minute the subject remains in a deep coma. The subject then regains consciousness but may remain drowsy for some hours. During the intense electrical activity there is an increase in local cerebral oxygen consumption and the possibility of severe local hypoxia and permanent neuronal damage is always present, although cardiac output and cerebral blood flow are increased during the episode in compensation.

There are numerous precipitating factors which result in epileptic episodes and some of these are outlined in Table 88.2 and the common anticonvulsants used in the treatment of grand mal seizures is shown in Table 88.3.

Table 88.2 Secondary causes of epilepsy

Cerebral trauma
Head injury
Postneurosurgical

Intracranial mass
Tumour
Abscess

Primary disease of the brain
Viral encephalitis
Parasitic disease
Creutzfeld—Jakob disease
Bacterial meningitis

Hypoxic encephalopathy
Cardiac arrest
Carbon monoxide poisoning

Complications of acute illness
Water intoxication
Hypertensive encephalopathy
Hyperglycaemia
Uraemia

Withdrawal of drugs
Alcohol
Addictive drugs
Anticonvulsants

Table 88.3 Some details of common anticonvulsants

Anticonvulsant	Daily adult dosage (mg)	Half-life (h)	Effective blood concentration (μg/ml)
Phenobarbitone	60—200	96	15—35
Phenytoin	200—400	24	10—20
Carbamazepine	600—1200	12	6—10
Sodium valproate	1000—2500	8	5—100

Status epilepticus

This occurs when recurrent generalized seizures occur sufficiently frequently that there is no recovery of consciousness. Approximately 8—10% of grand mal seizures result in status epilepticus and there is a 10% mortality in status epilepticus. This condition is therefore not benign, and prolonged convulsions also carry a high risk of permanent neurological damage. It is important to suppress the seizure activity as soon as possible. The first line of treatment should be to relieve any hypoxia by administering oxygen.

The intravenous route of administration of anticonvulsants is preferred, since the absorption from the oral route may not be practical and absorption via the intramuscular route is slow and unreliable. With some drugs, the rectal route is satisfactory, especially with children.

Table 88.4 shows the approximate intravenous loading doses of a number of anticonvulsants which may be used to gain rapid control of the seizures. These doses are approximate only and are derived mainly from the pharmaceutical data sheets. Many different dose regimens can be found in the literature and it is generally accepted that dose should be titrated according to response.

The benzodiazepines are usually the drugs of first choice. Diazepam is probably the most widely used because it acts rapidly, has a short duration of action and can be continued as repeated boluses or as an infusion. Clonazepam may be successful where diazepam has failed, especially in complex seizures. Because of their alinear elimination kinetics, prolonged high dosage may lead to prolonged recovery. Lorazepam may have an advantage because of its longer duration of action. However, the benzodiazepines are effective in less than 40% of patients in status and other agents must also be considered.

The barbiturates are potent anticonvulsants. Phenobarbitone has a prolonged action and may be

Table 88.4 Dosages of drugs used in the acute suppression of seizures in status epilepticus

Drug	Intravenous bolus	Maintenance
Diazepam	Adult 10–20 mg Child 0.2–0.3 mg/kg	Repeat bolus or infuse max. $0.3\,mg \cdot kg^{-1} \cdot h^{-1}$
Clonazepam	Adult 1–2 mg Child 0.05 mg/kg	
Lorazepam	Adult 0.1 mg/kg Child 0.05 mg/kg	Infusion not recommended
Phenobarbitone	Adult 10 mg/kg Child 5 mg/kg	Repeat half-dose in 12 h
Thiopentone	Adult 100 mg boluses until seizure control Child 3–5 mg/kg	Infusion $1–5\,mg \cdot kg^{-1} \cdot h^{-1}$
Phenytoin	Adult max. 15 mg/kg Slow $<1\,mg \cdot kg^{-1} \cdot min^{-1}$ Child 5 mg/kg	Repeat half-dose in 6–12 h
Chlormethiazole	Adult 5–15 ml/min Child $0.01\,ml \cdot kg^{-1} \cdot min^{-1}$	Infusion 0.5–1 ml/min
Paraldehyde	Adult 10 ml Child 0.1–0.15 ml/kg	Repeat in 2–4 h

effective without major sedation or respiratory depression. Thiopentone is the second most popular drug used in the acute management of status epilepticus since it seldom fails to control the seizures. But it is frequently necessary to intubate and control ventilation before and during treatment. Prolonged infusion can lead to slow recovery.

Chlormethiazole is also an effective anticonvulsant. Frequently, it is successful where diazepam has failed and at a dose which does not produce respiratory depression. The drug does have some disadvantages. It may cause thrombophlebitis and should be infused into a central vein. Infused as a 0.8% solution, it can pose a significant fluid load. Chlormethiazole may be absorbed by plastic tubing and the reaction with the plastic may liberate pyrogens which cause a pyrexia (Lingam et al., 1980). Nevertheless, chlormethiazole remains a useful drug.

Intravenous phenytoin can also be used to suppress convulsions in status epilepticus. However, the drug is usually prepared in propylene glycol which may induce acute cardiac failure. Phenytoin should be infused slowly (not faster than $1\,mg \cdot kg^{-1} \cdot min^{-1}$) with continuous monitoring of ECG and blood pressure. Its advantage is that it produces minimal sedation or respiratory depression.

Paraldehyde has been used as an anticonvulsant with success for many years. It may be administered slowly intravenously as a 4% solution or diluted in saline. It should not be delivered using plastic equipment and it has an unpleasant, lingering odour. For these reasons its use has declined.

When control of status epilepticus is achieved, it is essential to increase the maintenance anticonvulsant therapy with drugs such as phenytoin, phenobarbitone and sodium valproate. Plasma levels of these drugs should be checked to ensure that therapeutic concentrations are attained. There is little indication for muscle paralysis as this masks seizure activity which in turn may be causing local cerebral damage.

It is useful to monitor EEG to determine if seizure activity has been suppressed satisfactorily. The raw EEG signal is useful if it can be interpreted satisfactorily, but some intensive therapy units (ITUs) may find some form of cerebral function monitoring more useful. As a general rule, in severe status epilepticus, it is best to maintain suppression of seizures for approximately 24 h before starting to discontinue treatment, and if high doses of anticonvulsants are used, this period of elimination may be several days. A slow reduction of anticonvulsant over this period may be necessary with stepwise increases again if seizure activity recurs. It is wise to check the plasma concentrations of anticonvulsant frequently as drug interactions may alter these levels dramatically during the dynamic phases of control of seizures and the withdrawal of medication.

It is also essential to treat the precipitating cause of the convulsion and to arrange adequate supervision of the medical, physical and mental welfare of the patient after discharge from the ITU.

Herpes simplex encephalitis

Herpes simplex encephalitis is usually caused by the Type 1 virus and is the most common of the acute viral encephalitides in the UK. In about 50% of cases it is fatal, and those who survive are often severely damaged. The presentation is similar to other forms of acute viral encephalitis often starting with fever and headache and progressing to confusion, stupor and finally coma. The virus spreads possibly from the branches of the fifth nerve and fifth nerve ganglion to involve characteristically the temporal lobes and early temporal lobe seizures with gustatory and olfactory hallucinations and bizarre behaviour is sometimes observed.

In the CSF there is an increase in lymphocytes and sometimes red cells and the protein is raised. The intracranial pressure is raised as a result of the marked haemorrhagic necrosis and oedema found characteristically in the inferior and medial parts of the frontal and temporal lobes. It is the distribution of the lesion round the temporal lobes which enables a reasonably confident diagnosis to be made on CT scan. However, the virus is seldom isolated from CSF and confirmation of the diagnosis can be made only through brain biopsy using a fluorescent antibody technique or viral culture. Viral titres in blood are raised at a later stage and are not helpful in the initial diagnosis.

Oedema of the brain tissue increases intracranial pressure, and if tentorial herniation occurs, coma ensues, then further brainstem compression results in respiratory arrest. This carries a grave prognosis.

Treatment is directed towards early elimination of the virus before the onset of brainstem compression. Acyclovir is the antiviral agent of choice and is administered as a slow intravenous infusion over 1 h. The recommended dose is 10 mg/kg every 8 h for 10 days. Corticosteroids, osmotic diuretics and renal loop diuretics are used to reduce cerebral oedema and prevent tentorial herniation. Early decisions are required on the need to control ventilation and seizures. The mortality and morbidity is increased considerably once brainstem disturbances have developed.

Acute inflammatory polyradiculoneuropathy or Guillain–Barré syndrome

The Guillain–Barré syndrome, noted first by Landry in 1859 and subsequently by Guillain, Barré and Strohl in 1916, may best be described as an acute inflammatory polyradiculoneuropathy (AIP) (Hughes, 1978), with a prevalence of approximately 1.5 : 100 000 of the population. It may affect individuals at any age, but the peak incidence is in the fifth decade (Lesser et al., 1973). The disease is characterized by a progressive motor weakness, usually symmetrical, with areflexia and also some sensory symptoms (Asbury et al., 1978). In approximately 60% of patients, the onset of motor weakness is preceded by a mild non-specific viral infection, commonly of the upper respiratory tract. In approximately 30% of patients, high titres of antibody to cytomegalovirus have been found (Dowling et al., 1977), but several other viruses have been implicated, as have inoculations, mycoplasma, bacterial infections and pre-existing illness such as Hodgkin's disease and lymphoma. The motor weakness may progress rapidly over a few days, or the deterioration may occur more gradually, and in 90% of patients the weakness is maximum by 4 weeks. The weakness develops usually in the limbs, but may progress to involve the respiratory muscles and cranial nerves.

Sensory changes are typically paraesthesiae of the glove and stocking type. In addition, there is frequently autonomic dysfunction. The pathological changes are predominantly lymphocyte infiltration of the peripheral nerves up to the spinal roots, resulting in segmental demyelination. In severe cases, there is also secondary axonal degeneration. There is marked slowing or block of nerve conduction as a result of demyelination and denervation; muscle fibrillation indicates axonal degeneration. An increase in CSF protein concentration is seen usually by the second week, but only a few cells are present. The disorder should be distinguished from porphyria, lead neuropathy, volatile solvent abuse, toxic neuropathy (e.g. from organophosphorus compounds), poliomyelitis, botulism and diphtheria.

As AIP is likely to be the result of a sensitivity reaction to Schwann cell myelin or other peripheral nerve protein, various forms of immunosuppressive treatment have been tried. On the whole, steroids are not felt to be beneficial. There is some evidence of delayed recovery and a higher incidence of complication following steroid treatment (Hughes et al., 1978). Early use of plasma exchange may be useful in limiting the deterioration and demyelination (Editorial, 1984; Greenwood *et al.*, 1984; Osterman *et al.*, 1984). After studying 245 patients, the Guillain–Barré Syndrome Study Group (1985) came to the conclusion that plasma exchange was beneficial in inducing a quicker recovery and shortening hospital stay if introduced within 7 days of onset of symptoms.

Recently, intravenous immunoglobulin has been used instead of plasma exchange in the early stages of AIP (Van de Meche *et al.*, 1992). The dosage of $0.4\,g \cdot kg^{-1} \cdot day^{-1}$ was given on 5 consecutive days. Others have given a single dose of $2\,g/kg$. Both regimens are reported to be at least as effective as plasma exchange and may be safer and more easily available.

AIP is very variable in severity and is self-limiting. The signs of recovery of neuronal function are seen usually within 4 weeks of the onset of symptoms. The majority of patients make a full recovery over several months to 1 year, but approximately 10% are left with residual disability; mortality is approximately 10%. The prognosis, therefore, is good, and the aim of management is to prevent complications and thus keep the patient in good condition whilst awaiting spontaneous recovery.

Management

The main life-threatening problem in AIP is acute respiratory failure resulting from respiratory muscle weakness. This is likely to occur within the first 2 weeks of the illness and there is usually a progressive deterioration of respiratory muscle power over a few days. Vital capacity is a reasonable clinical test of respiratory muscle power, and if this shows a progressive decrease to less than 1 litre in an adult, it is likely that artificial ventilation is required.

A decreasing vital capacity together with bulbar weakness (with difficulty in swallowing and coughing) is a very dangerous combination as such patients may be precipitated into acute respiratory failure by the aspiration of small quantities of saliva. Under these circumstances, it is best to intubate the trachea, and perhaps the best guides to the need for tracheal intubation are if the patient begins to look anxious and is restless, and if the respiratory rate increases and the accessory muscles of respiration are being used. Arterial blood-gas tensions are not helpful in making an early decision to intubate the trachea.

The function of the diaphragm may be an important determinant of the need for tracheal intubation and ventilation, as it is the prime muscle of inspiration. Severe weakness or total paralysis of the diaphragm may be recognized by observation of the anterior abdominal wall during quiet respiration in the supine posture, when paradoxical inward movement of the upper abdominal wall occurs during inspiration. Such patients are likely to be distressed by the supine position and prefer to sit upright, and it is these patients who are most likely to require tracheal intubation and ventilation. It is also likely that satisfactory respiration will occur only after some diaphragm function has returned.

When tracheal intubation is necessary, early tracheostomy should be considered as it usually takes at least 2, and often several, weeks before extubation can take place satisfactorily. Patients accept artificial ventilation easily and there is no need for sedation or paralysis. The management of ventilation and care of the tracheostomy is straightforward and are not discussed further.

Vital capacity is a reasonable guide to recovery of respiratory muscle function. A vital capacity of 1–1.5 litres is often required before satisfactory spontaneous respiration can occur, and this is commonly when abdominal paradoxical movement disappears, signifying the return of diaphragm activity. It is probably unwise to decannulate the tracheostomy until it has been well established that bulbar function is adequate and the return of a satisfactory gag reflex and swallowing have been demonstrated. In some patients it is wise to change to an uncuffed silver tracheostomy tube with speaking attachment as an intermediate step before decannulation.

Autonomic disturbances

Second to respiratory failure, the most common cause of death in AIP is cardiac arrhythmia (Lichtenfield, 1971). Arrhythmias are associated frequently with autonomic abnormalities. Sinus tachycardia and persistent fluctuating hypertension are observed frequently early in the disease. Bradycardia and hypotension also occur, particularly following vagal stimulation from tracheal suction. Prolonged episodes of hypotension may occur with pallor and bouts of excessive sweating as a result of parasympathetic overactivity. Bladder and bowel function are seldom affected, although catheterization of the bladder may be needed for other reasons. Paralytic ileus lasting a few days, with failure to absorb feeds, may also be the result of autonomic dysfunction. Postural hypotension should be suspected, particularly when patients are being mobilized during the recovery phase of the illness.

Several studies have recorded sudden death in patients with autonomic disturbances, and our policy is currently to attempt to stabilize the cardiovascular system by partial beta block with propranolol to prevent tachycardia and hypertension, and also to give atropine, 0.6 mg three to four times a day, to avoid episodes of bradycardia during tracheal toilet and physiotherapy. Marked hypertension may be treated with a hypotensive drugs such as hydralazine. If episodes of marked bradycardia are noted, the insertion of a transvenous pacemaker should be considered.

Patients with profound muscle weakness are at risk from deep vein thrombosis and pulmonary embolus. Good nursing care, physiotherapy and hydration may help to prevent this complication. However, we prescribe routinely a subcutaneous heparin regimen (5000 IU twice daily).

Many patients complain of pain, which may last several days. It is often severe and persistent and felt usually in the back or calves. This pain is not relieved easily by analgesics and it may be most distressing.

The aim of management is to prevent complications and permit the natural recovery process to take place. Medical interference is secondary to good nursing care and physiotherapy. Attention must be paid to adequate nutrition and the prevention of muscle wasting. One of the most distressing problems is the inability of patients to communicate. Patients may be unable to signal with their hands or write, and in some cases the facial weakness is such that they cannot even signal with their eyes. Frequent reassurance is required. Television, radio and cassette tapes help to occupy the time and provide mental stimulation. Most important is the attitude and atmosphere created by the nursing staff and also the physiotherapy and occupational therapy staff who are involved throughout.

The milestones to recovery are return of respiratory muscle function and spontaneous breathing, recovery of speech, oral intake of food, decannulation of the tracheostomy, sitting up and supporting first the head and then torso, standing and walking with aid, and finally, walking unaided.

Myasthenia gravis

In recent years it has become clear that myasthenia gravis (MG) is an autoimmune disease (Newsom-Davis, 1982). In the majority (85%) of individuals with the disease, it is possible to demonstrate an antibody in the IgG fraction which, through complement-mediated lysis, causes an increase in the rate of breakdown of acetylcholine receptors (AchR) on the postjunctional membrane of the neuromuscular junction (NMJ). This antibody, the antiAchR antibody, eventually depletes the NMJ of acetylcholine receptors, giving rise to a characteristic fatiguable muscle weakness. The weakness may affect some muscle groups more than others, so that some patients complain only of ptosis and diplopia, others may have proximal limb weakness and the most severely affected may develop bulbar and respiratory muscle weakness which may require intensive care management.

The diagnosis is suggested on the history of muscle weakness which is worsened by exercise and improved by rest. An improvement in muscle power following the administration of an anticholinesterase drug such as edrophonium and a characteristic decrement of the electromyograph (EMG) on repetitive stimulation of peripheral nerves add weight to the diagnosis, but MG is confirmed by the demonstration of the anti-AchR antibody in the patient's plasma, although the disease cannot be excluded if no antibody is detected.

The prevalence of MG is approximately 1 : 20 000 of the population and affects all age groups. There is a female preponderance, particularly in the group younger than 40 years of age. Compston and colleagues (1980) showed an increased frequency of certain human leucocyte antigens in non-thymoma patients, indicating that genetic factors probably have a role in the aetiology of the disease. This has been confirmed by Kerzin-Storrar and colleagues (1988). Occasionally, MG is associated with other autoimmune disorders such as rheumatoid arthritis, thyrotoxicosis and pernicious anaemia.

Thymoma occurs in approximately 10% of patients with MG and, although usually benign, the tumour may show malignant change and locally invade important mediastinal structures such as phrenic nerve and aorta.

Other forms of myasthenia

There are some rarer disorders of neuromuscular transmission which should be distinguished from the usual acquired form of MG. Neonatal myasthenia occurs in one in eight babies born of mothers with MG and results from placental transfer of anti-AchR antibody from the mother (Morel et al., 1988). In the baby, this causes a transient muscle weakness which responds to anticholinesterases and which lasts usually for only 4–6 weeks. Following this, the baby is normal. A congenital form of myasthenia has been described, in which the abnormality is in the acetylcholine receptor itself, and no immunological abnormality is found; these patients do not respond to immunosuppression.

The Lambert–Eaton myasthenic syndrome is an immunological disorder which produces a presynaptic defect in the release of acetylcholine from the nerve terminal. It is frequently associated with an oat-cell carcinoma of the bronchus, although in some cases no malignancy is found. Muscle power is improved transiently with exercise and the neurophysiological characteristics are different from those of myasthenia gravis. No antibody has been identified yet, but the condition may be improved with plasma exchange and immunosuppression. Freeze-fracture electron microscopy indicated that there is a disorganization of calcium channels on the presynaptic membrane which may affect the liberation of the quanta of acetylcholine (Fukuoka et al., 1987).

Treatment of myasthenia gravis

Anticholinesterase drugs

These drugs delay the breakdown of acetylcholine by cholinesterase at the NMJ and therefore presumably allow the more efficient transfer of acetylcholine to the depleted acetycholine receptors on the postjunctional membrane. They produce symptomatic improvement, but do not alter the underlying pathology. In fact, there is some evidence that prolonged, high-dose anticholinesterase drugs may themselves produce undesirable changes at the NMJ. Too much anticholinesterase produces a cholinergic muscle weakness in addition to excessive salivation, colic, diarrhoea and other symptoms of parasympathetic overactivity. It is best to keep the patient suboptimally dosed, i.e. slightly myasthenic, rather than run the risk of cholinergic problems. Pyridostigmine bromide is the drug of choice, 30–120 mg 3-hourly, taken by mouth in tablet form or as an elixir via nasogastric tube. Atropine may be given to reduce the parasympathetic side-effects, but if the side-effects are troublesome, reduction in anticholinesterase therapy would be wise since the patient may be cholinergic, and alternative methods of management should be considered. Edrophonium (Tensilon) may be used as a test of the myasthenic or cholinergic state. After prior treatment with atropine, 0.3–0.6 mg i.v., usually not more than 5 mg of edrophonium i.v. is required to produce a satisfactory response. If the patient is myasthenic then, within 30 s, there should

be a marked improvement in muscle power which lasts for 2–3 min. The useful bedside tests of improved muscle power are loss of ptosis, recovery of facial muscle power, speech and voice, increased arm or leg outstretched time and improvement in vital capacity. If the improvement is marked, it would be reasonable to increase anticholinesterase therapy. However, if the response is marginal, one should contemplate a reduction in medication, bearing in mind that not all muscle groups behave equally and that some muscles may show a cholinergic response at the same time as others are myasthenic.

Thymectomy

Thymectomy alone produces an improvement in myasthenia gravis in approximately 60–70% of patients. The precise role of the thymus gland in MG is not clear, but it may be that some antigenic stimulus in the gland perpetuates the anti-AchR antibody production (Whiting et al., 1986). It has been demonstrated that, over a period of months, anti-AchR antibody concentrations decrease following thymectomy. Thymectomy is the treatment of choice in patients younger than 50 years, when the thymus usually shows hyperplasia. Thymectomy is indicated in cases of thymoma.

The thymus gland is removed most satisfactorily through a median sternotomy incision. The hazards of thymectomy are reduced considerably if patients come to operation in a good clinical state. Prior treatment with steroids or plasma exchange may improve the preoperative situation. The postoperative management is simplified by maintaining complete control of the airway with nasotracheal intubation for the first day or so after operation. Anticholinesterases are often discontinued before operation and reintroduced when indicated, usually at a lower dose, but guided by clinical state and testing with edrophonium. If comfortable, patients are allowed to breathe spontaneously through the nasotracheal tube, but at the first sign of respiratory distress, artificial ventilation is instituted easily. Extubation occurs when vital capacity is satisfactory and it is judged that respiratory assistance is unlikely to be required.

Immunosuppression

Immunosuppression with steroids may produce a remission of symptoms in approximately 80% of patients. This may be achieved using an alternate day regimen of prednisolone, starting at a low dose of 10 mg and slowly increasing over a period of weeks up to a maximum of 120 mg on alternate days. Thereafter, the dose may be reduced very slowly to a minimum dose which maintains the improvement. If steroids are introduced too rapidly at high dose, temporary deterioration in muscle power can occur which may require intubation and ventilation for a few days, but in this way, remission can be attained sooner. Thus, it may be justified to use a high-dose steroid regimen in those patients already in a poor clinical state and requiring artificial ventilation. Azathioprine may also be used for immunosuppression with a starting dose of 2.5 mg/kg body weight. Improvement is slow and may take up to 1 year, but the side-effects are probably less than with steroids. Regular checks of haematology and liver function are required.

Quite frequently, steroids and azathioprine are used in combination; steroids being used to produce a more rapid improvement and azathioprine for long-term immunosuppression. It seems that immunosuppression needs to be continued indefinitely. Because of the side-effects of steroids and azathioprine, there is a reluctance to use these drugs in the younger age group, especially in women of childbearing age. Thymectomy is still the treatment of choice in this younger age group because, if thymectomy alone produces a good remission, the problems of immunosuppression can be avoided.

Plasma exchange

Plasma exchange can reduce very effectively the anti-AchR antibody concentrations in blood and produce a remission of MG within a few days by allowing the effective regeneration of acetylcholine receptors. A series of approximately five daily exchanges removing approximately 50 ml/kg body weight of plasma each time can produce a marked clinical improvement, but it is relatively short-lived, lasting only 3–4 weeks. As the technique is very costly, it should be reserved for patients with severe disease who are awaiting the benefits of immunosuppression.

Immune globulin

Similar to the case of AIP, high-dose intravenous immunoglobulin (HDIVIg) in a dose of $0.4 \, \text{g} \cdot \text{kg}^{-1} \cdot \text{day}^{-1}$ for 5 days has been used in the treatment of MG. Improvement occurs in a few days and may last months (Cosi et al., 1991). In some individuals a transient weakness has been observed before improvement. The reason for the improvement in MG with HDIVIg is unclear. It is thought that immunoglobulin may interfere with the anti-AchR antibody binding to the AchR or may prevent complement activation. Possibly the benefit may be due to an anti-idiotypic effect. Further studies are required to determine the value of HDIVIg alone or in combination with other forms of immunosuppression in MG.

Intensive therapy unit problems

To the anaesthetist the most significant fact regarding MG is the severe reduction in the number of acetylcholine receptors, which implies that these patients are exceptionally sensitive to non-depolarizing muscle relaxants, but from the point of view of the intensive care specialist, the main problems are those of acute respiratory failure. Respiratory failure results usually from either a myasthenic or cholinergic crisis, but may be steroid-induced or the result of thymectomy. The majority are cholinergic crises.

Myasthenic crisis

This occurs in patients with severe myasthenia who suddenly deteriorate as a result of an acute infection or stress of some other type and in whom the anticholinesterase requirements increase. However, recovery may not be achieved by an increase in anticholinesterase alone. It is also necessary to deal with the precipitating factor (such as infection). The safest course is to ensure an adequate airway by tracheal intubation and to ventilate the lungs until an improvement is achieved. Plasma exchange may be performed for a rapid improvement and the opportunity to introduce more effective immunosuppression should be considered.

Cholinergic crisis

This occurs frequently from overdose with anticholinesterase drugs. The situation commonly arises following a myasthenic crisis in which only partial improvement with anticholinesterases occurs and more drug is administered progressively. This results in a cholinergic weakness which is not recognized as such. Eventually, the patient develops respiratory and bulbar muscle weakness, excessive salivation and abdominal cramps. Dangerous and acute respiratory failure may rapidly follow aspiration of secretions. Intubation and ventilation should be performed early and the anticholinesterase drugs withdrawn. In time, the patient returns to a myasthenic state and anticholinesterases may be reintroduced, and the process of weaning from the ventilator started. It is unwise to expedite tracheal extubation early, and, in general, patients should be able to breathe without assistance for at least 24 h before extubation. As with myasthenic crisis, plasma exchange and more effective immunosuppression should be considered.

It is worth noting that myasthenic patients may be made weaker by antibiotics of the aminoglycoside group such as streptomycin, gentamicin and neomycin, which reduce release of acetylcholine at the nerve terminal. Similarly, procainamide causes a reduction in release of acetylcholine, and quinine and quinidine reduce the speed of excitation along a muscle fibre, also making myasthenics weaker. In addition, a low serum potassium concentration should be avoided, since this potentiates muscle weakness.

Chronic neuromuscular respiratory failure

There are several neuromuscular disorders, the result of either neuronal damage such as poliomyelitis, or primary muscle disease as in the various myopathies and muscular dystrophies, which cause respiratory muscle weakness. Sometimes, the muscle weakness is such that a state of chronic respiratory failure develops in which the lungs are relatively normal, but the bellows function of the chest wall is impaired. If the condition is allowed to progress unrecognized, the patient may present in an ITU with unexplained respiratory failure. Occasionally, such patients are admitted having failed to breathe after anaesthesia or as difficult weaning problems, and some are admitted in congestive heart failure from chronic pulmonary hypertension. These neuromuscular problems may be diagnosed also as outpatients, provided one is attuned to the characteristic history. Patients often complain of breathlessness on exercise and often on assuming the supine posture, so that they sleep either propped up or in the lateral posture. A common feature is hypersomnolence with excessive sleepiness during the day, and yet disturbed sleep at night with frequent arousal and sometimes with nightmares. They are often difficult to rouse in the morning and wake up with a headache which clears shortly after getting up. These are symptoms of marked nocturnal hypoventilation with severe hypoxia and hypercapnia. On examination, there is evidence of neuromuscular weakness frequently affecting the shoulder girdle and neck muscles in addition to other muscle groups. In the majority of patients who suffer from this problem, there is evidence of marked diaphragm weakness (Newsom-Davis et al., 1976).

As mentioned earlier, weakness of the diaphragm may be seen best in the supine posture during quiet breathing, when the upper anterior abdominal wall moves paradoxically inwards during inspiration (Loh et al., 1977). This paradoxical movement is the result of the diaphragm failing to develop sufficient tension to prevent the abdominal contents moving up into the chest in the face of the more negative intrapleural pressure generated during inspiration. Awake, resting blood-gas tensions reveal hypoxia and hypercapnia which may be corrected to a degree by voluntary hyperventilation, and there is normally an increased bicarbonate concentration, indicating long-standing respiratory acidosis.

Lung function tests may reveal a reduced vital capacity, which may decrease further in the supine position. Ventilatory responses to hypoxia and hypercapnia are blunted, and exercise tolerance is poor. Pulmonary hypertension is a feature and signs of congestive heart failure may be present. One of the problems in making a correct diagnosis is that the patients often appear relatively normal when upright and awake, and the problem reveals itself only during sleep. During sleep, the patient is at a gross disadvantage, both from a mechanical point of view because of the recumbent posture and from the respiratory drive to the breathing muscles.

In the upright posture patients with weakness of the diaphragm may use abdominal muscle contraction to drive the abdominal contents up into the chest at end-expiration and then augment the inspiratory tidal volume by relaxing the abdominal muscles and allowing passive descent of the diaphragm and abdominal contents out of the chest in early inspiration. This mechanism is largely lost in the horizontal position. In addition, in the supine position the inspiratory muscles tend to be shorter and the mechanical advantage of extending the spine in the upright position is lost.

During sleep, the central drive to the breathing muscles is normally directed largely to the diaphragm and if this muscle is non-functional, hypoventilation is to be expected. Also because the ventilatory responses to hypoxia and hypercapnia are obtunded, there is a change in the threshold for arousal, and severe hypoxia and hypercapnia are allowed to persist. For these reasons, patients with diaphragm weakness are at risk during sleep and the correct diagnosis can be made only with certainty by observing what happens during sleep and making the relevant measurements.

When the diagnosis has been made, appropriate treatment may be attempted in the way of assisted ventilation during sleep with the aim of permanent use by the patient at home. This type of management should be undertaken by respiratory specialists and may be initiated in an ITU. The aims of treatment are to:

1 Prevent hypoxia and hypercapnia during sleep.
2 Reduce pulmonary hypertension.
3 Allow satisfactory sleep.
4 Rest fatigued respiratory muscles.

The results of satisfactory treatment are:

1 Abolition of hypersomnolence.
2 Reversal of congestive heart failure.
3 Induction of more normal blood-gas tensions.
4 Improved quality of life.
5 Prolonged survival.

Treatment

Nocturnal assisted ventilation

There are several ways of augmenting respiration during sleep. Rocking beds, which tip the patient head-up and then head-down regularly, assist ventilation by moving the abdominal contents in and out of the thorax, causing the diaphragm to act passively as a piston. Not all patients can tolerate the motion and, in some, ventilation is inadequate.

Positive-pressure ventilation via a tracheostomy or negative-pressure ventilation with a cuirass-type device are used more commonly for long-term home ventilation (Dunkin, 1983; Shneerson, 1991).

Positive-pressure ventilation via tracheostomy

Positive-pressure ventilation via a tracheostomy is suitable particularly for the severely disabled patient who might find difficulty using a negative-pressure device, for patients for whom there is minimal assistance at night, and if there is need for a tracheostomy to overcome the problem of upper airways obstruction during sleep or laryngeal incompetence. Small, reliable, relatively inexpensive, positive-pressure ventilators suitable for home use are available. If an uncuffed tracheostomy tube is used, the leakage of air into the pharynx during the inspiratory phase may not be tolerated well. However, with perseverance this problem can usually be overcome.

Negative-pressure respiration

Negative-pressure respiration is suitable provided the patient has a competent larynx, is able to breathe reasonably well on his/her own and is not entirely dependent on the device, and has adequate help at home. The advantage of negative-pressure devices is that tracheostomy may be avoided. Unfortunately, most of the devices are cumbersome, some may not be very efficient at ventilating and they may encourage upper airway obstruction during sleep.

Most of the apparatus available for home ventilation is of ancient design and, because of the small demand, commercial companies are reluctant to invest finance in the research and development of such apparatus. Specially tailored cuirass shells are available. It is possible to provide a patient with such equipment and a respiratory pump for approximately £4000.

Nasal intermittent positive-pressure ventilation

More recently, it has been demonstrated that intermittent positive-pressure ventilation delivered via a nasal mask is a realistic proposition for domiciliary ventilation (Ellis et al., 1987; Heckmatt et al., 1990). This method has the advantage of being simple and easy to apply, efficient in ventilation, overcomes the problems of upper airway obstruction and avoids tracheostomy (Branthwaite, 1991). The possible problems of aspiration of oral secretions into the trachea or distension of the abdomen by ventilating gas seldom arise and leakage of ventilating gas out of the mouth during sleep and pressure sores from the nasal mask are the main problems. These can be overcome usually with adjustment of the ventilation pressures, the use of a chin strap and care in fitting the mask. This method of assisted ventilation has now superseded negative-pressure respiration.

In order to pursue this type of therapy, one requires adequate medical expertise, adequate finance, good engineering back-up and interested and understanding nursing staff, so that the patient feels confident relying on the support of the hospital.

Many of the neuromuscular disorders which may be helped by assisted ventilation are only very slowly progressive, and often the condition affects young adults who have dependants. It can be extremely worthwhile and rewarding to assist these patients to lead happier, more productive and longer lives (Loh, 1983).

References

Asbury A.K., Arnason B.G.W., Karp H.R. & McFarlin D.E. (1978) Criteria for diagnosis of Guillain–Barré syndrome. *Annals of Neurology* **3**, 565–6.

Branthwaite M.A. (1991) Non-invasive and domiciliary ventilation: positive pressure techniques. *Thorax* **46**, 208–12.

Bremer R. (1937) L'activité cérébrale au cours du sommeil et de la narcose: contribution a l'étude de mechanisme de sommeil. *Bulletin de l'Academie Royale de Medicine de Belgique* **2**, 68—86.

Cherniack N.S. & Longobardo G.S. (1973) Cheyne—Stokes breathing. *New England Journal of Medicine* **288**, 952—7.

Compston D.A.S., Vincent A., Newsom-Davis J. & Batchelor J.R. (1980) Clinical, pathological, HLA antigen and immunological evidence for disease heterogeneity in myasthenia gravis. *Brain* **103**, 579—601.

Cosi V., Lombardi M., Piccolo G. & Erbetta A. (1991) Treatment of myasthenia gravis with high dose intravenous immunoglobulin. *Acta Neurologica Scandinavica* **84**, 81—4.

Dowling P.C., Mendonna J.P. & Cook S.D. (1977) Cytomegalovirus complement fixation antibody in Guillain—Barré syndrome. *Neurology* **27**, 1153—6.

Dunkin L.J. (1983) Home ventilatory assistance. *Anaesthesia* **38**, 644—9.

Editorial (1984) Plasma exchange in Guillain—Barré syndrome. *Lancet* **2**, 1312—13.

Ellis E.R., Bye P.T.P., Bruderer J.W. & Sullivan C.E. (1987) Treatment of respiratory failure during sleep in patients with neuromuscular disease. Positive-pressure ventilation through a nose mask. *American Review of Respiratory Disease* **135**, 148—52.

Fukuoka T., Engel A.G., Lang B., Newsom-Davis J., Prior C. & Wray D.W. (1987) Lambert—Eaton myasthenic syndrome: I. Early morphological effects of IgG on the presynaptic membrane active zones. *Annals of Neurology* **22**, 193—9.

Glen W.W.L., Holcomb W.G., McLaughlin A.J., O'Hare J.M., Hogan J.F. & Yasuda R. (1972) Total ventilatory support in a quadriplegic patient with radio frequency electrophrenic respiration. *New England Journal of Medicine* **286**, 513—16.

Greenwood R.J., Newsom-Davis J., Hughes R.A., Aslan S., Bowden A.W., Chadwick D.W., Gordon N.S., McLellan D.L., Millac P., Stott R.B. & Armitage P. (1984) Controlled trial of plasma exchange in acute inflammatory polyradiculopathy. *Lancet* **I**, 877—9.

Guillain—Barré Syndrome Study Group (1985) Plasmapheresis and acute Guillain—Barré syndrome. *Neurology* **35**, 5—104.

Heckmatt J.Z., Loh L. & Dubowitz V. (1990) Night-time nasal ventilation in neuromuscular disease. *Lancet* **335**, 579—82.

Hughes R.A. (1978) Acute inflammatory polyneuropathy. *British Journal of Hospital Medicine* **20**, 688—93.

Hughes R.A., Newsom-Davis J., Perkin G.D. & Pierce J.M. (1978) Controlled trial prednisolone in acute polyneuropathy. *Lancet* **ii**, 750—3.

Kerzin-Storrar L., Metcalfe R.A., Dyer P.A., Kowalska G., Ferguson I. & Harris R. (1988) Genetic factors in myasthenia gravis: a family study. *Neurology* **38**, 38—42.

Lesser R.P., Hauser W.A., Kurland L.T. & Mulder D.W. (1973) Epidemiologic features of the Guillain—Barré syndrome. Experience in Olmsted County, Minnesota. *Neurology* **23**, 1269—72.

Lichtenfield P. (1971) Autonomic dysfunction in the Guillain—Barré syndrome. *American Journal of Medicine* **50**, 772—80.

Lingam S., Bertwistle H., Elliston H.E. & Wilson J. (1980) Problems with intravenous chlormethiazole (Heminevrin) in status epilepticus. *British Medical Journal* **I**, 155—6.

Loh L. (1983) Editorial — home ventilation. *Anaesthesia* **38**, 621—2.

Loh L. (1986) Neurological and neuromuscular disease. *British Journal of Anaesthesia* **58**, 190—200.

Loh L., Goldman M. & Newsom-Davis J. (1977) The assessment of diaphragm function. *Medicine* **56**, 165—9.

Morel E., Eymard B., Vernet-der-Garabedian B., Pannier C., Dulac O. & Bach J.F. (1988) Neonatal myasthenia gravis, a new clinical and immunological appraisal on 30 cases. *Neurology* **38**, 138—42.

Moruzzi G. & Magoun H.W. (1949) Brainstem reticular formation and activation of the EEG. *Electroencephalography and Clinical Neurophysiology* **I**, 455—73.

Nathan P.W. (1963) The descending inspiratory pathway in man. *Journal of Neurology, Neurosurgery and Psychiatry* **26**, 487—99.

Newsom-Davis J. (1970) An experimental study of hiccup. *Brain* **93**, 851—72.

Newsom-Davis J. (1982) Myasthenia. In *Advanced Medicine*, vol. 18 (Ed. Sarner M.) p. 149—59. Pitman, London.

Newsom-Davis J. (1985) The neuronal control of respiratory function. In *Neurosurgery: The Scientific Basis of Clinical Practice* (Eds Crockard H.A., Hayward R.D. & Hoff J.) p. 200—11. Blackwell Scientific Publications, Oxford.

Newsom-Davis J., Goldman M., Loh L. & Cassan M. (1976) Diaphragm function and alveolar hypoventilation. *Quarterly Journal of Medicine* **45**, 87—100.

Osterman P.O., Fagius J., Lundemo G., Philstedt P., Pirskanen R., Siden A. & Safwenberg J. (1984) Beneficial effects of plasma exchange in acute inflammatory polyradiculoneuropathy. *Lancet* **2**, 1296—8.

Plum F. & Posner J.B. (1980) *The Diagnosis of Stupor and Coma* 3rd edn, pp. 11—14. F.A. Davis Company, Philadelphia.

Sears T.A., Berger A.J. & Philipson E.A. (1982) Reciprocal tonic activation of inspiratory and expiratory motorneurones by chemical drives. *Nature* **299**, 728—30.

Shneerson J. (1991) Non-invasive and domiciliary ventilation: negative pressure techniques. *Thorax* **46**, 131—5.

van de Meche F.G.A., Schmitz P.I.M. & the Dutch Guillain—Barré Study Group. (1992) A randomized trial comparing intravenous immune globulin and plasma exchange in Guillain—Barré syndrome. *New England Journal of Medicine* **326**, 1123—9.

Whiting P.J., Vincent A. & Newsom-Davis J. (1986) Myasthenia gravis: monoclonal antihuman acetylcholine receptor antibodies used to analyse specificities and responses to treatment. *Neurology* **36**, 612—17.

Head Injury

W. FITCH

Head injury is common but the overall incidence is not known with any degree of precision. For example, estimates of the frequency of trauma to the head in the USA vary from 180–673 : 100 000 of the population per annum. Each year, in the UK, 1 : 50 persons sustains an injury to the head of sufficient severity to require hospital attendance. In all probability, however, many others seek no medical advice unless complications develop. Fortunately, the majority of the injuries are minor: only 20–25% of those attending accident and emergency departments require admission to hospital. Nevertheless, the number of patients *admitted* to hospital as a consequence of an injury to the head has increased progressively (at least in Scotland) since the early 1960s. Of those admitted, most (approximately 60%) have comparatively trivial injuries, remain in hospital for less than 2 days and recover completely from their injury — with or without specific treatment.

At the other end of the spectrum, the *mortality* from head injury, although decreasing, is still substantial (9 : 100 000 deaths of the population of the UK in 1981). Head injury accounts for approximately 1% of all deaths in Western Europe (including the UK), 25% of all deaths from trauma and almost 50% of those associated with road traffic accidents. There are no national statistics on the mortality from head injury in the USA. However, annual death rates of 24–32 : 100 000 of the population have been reported in studies of selected geographical regions.

The frequency of head injury is greatest in young males (motor vehicle accidents, violence) and elderly people (falls). Not surprisingly, the proportion of deaths from head injury is much greater in young males than in females of equivalent age or in the general population. Head injury accounts for 15% of all fatalities in males between the ages of 15 and 40 years.

Sixty percent of all deaths from head injury occur *before* admission to hospital — 40% at the scene of the accident and 20% during transport to the nearest accident and emergency department, or before formal admission to the primary receiving unit. Even in hospital, the prognosis of the severely head-injured patient is poor: 30–50% dying despite a better understanding of the pathophysiology of head injury on the part of the clinician and the institution of apparently appropriate treatment.

This chapter considers principally the management of those patients with moderate to severe head injury (Glasgow coma score 13–3, p. 1869) who reach hospital alive. In such patients, the primary injury has been of insufficient severity to cause death at the time of the initial accident or in the period preceding admission to hospital. In theory at least, death should be preventable in such patients, as the sequelae of the secondary injury may be controlled by appropriate therapeutic interventions. This should not be taken to indicate that recovery is assured. The extent of the primary brain damage may be such that full recovery is 'out of the question': the patient remains severely disabled or vegetative. Nevertheless, it is this group of patients in whom good management may improve outcome materially and in whom inappropriate or inadequate treatment may decrease the chance of making a 'good' recovery. This chapter highlights certain fundamental *principles* relevant to the management of such patients, establishes a number of *priorities* in their management and, finally, details some current considerations on the *practicalities* of management.

Principles relevant to management

Brain damage never occurs in isolation

Although it is usual to place the emphasis on the damage to the brain *per se* as being the determinant of death or disability, injury to the *brain* never occurs in isolation. Although it is true that many of the most minor injuries require no more than the debridement and suturing of lacerations of the scalp, trauma of sufficient severity to injure the brain itself must, inevitably, damage other structures. Injury is inflicted on the scalp, skull and dura, perhaps on the spine and spinal cord and, especially in accidents involving motor vehicles, on the trunk, limbs and abdomen (30–40% of head-injured patients admitted to hospital have another significant injury elsewhere in the body). Such additional injuries may have devastating consequences as far as the traumatized brain is concerned. For example, a decrease in cerebral perfusion to critical values may be associated with haemorrhage from a ruptured spleen and the consequent decrease in systemic arterial pressure. Because arterial hypotension is a comparatively unusual feature of head injury *per se*, its presence should alert the clinician to the possibility of occult blood loss. If the dura is torn, meningitis may follow a depressed skull fracture or fracture of the anterior fossa and lead to severe disability — or even death — in a patient who should have recovered fully from a relatively trivial injury.

Brain damage may be primary or secondary

Primary brain damage

Following a severe insult to the brain — ischaemic, haemorrhagic or traumatic — a certain population of neurones is damaged irremediably. Function cannot be regained no matter how immediate or skilled the treatment. This primary injury is the result of the physical forces applied to the skull and the brain at the moment of the initial insult.

It is customary to characterize primary brain damage as being either focal (localized) or diffuse. Focal damage is the result of direct injury to the brain (as when associated with a depressed fracture or penetrating wound) or of the movement of the brain in relation to the skull. As a consequence of acceleration/deceleration forces, there may be obvious local bruising or more severe damage to the surface of the bain (contusions) localized to those areas of brain which have come into contact with the irregular bony prominences on the interior surface of the skull. If severe, contusions may be associated with actual lacerations of the cortex and haemorrhage from ruptured blood vessels.

Less obvious, but more significant, are small neuronal lesions which are scattered diffusely throughout the brain. These are the result of the movement of one part of the brain in relation to another part of the brain. For example, the degree of acceleration (or deceleration) imparted to the cortical mantle by a given force differs from that affecting the deeper structures such as white matter or corpus callosum. This results in a 'shearing' injury which stretches and tears nerve fibres (and blood vessels), particularly in the white matter. This form of primary brain damage is now recognized widely and has been referred to by a variety of names; 'diffuse degeneration of white matter', 'shearing injury', 'diffuse white matter shearing injury', 'inner cerebral trauma'. Histological studies show evidence of diffuse damage to the axons of the nerve cells: hence, the current preference for the term 'diffuse axonal injury'.

Unless it is severe and widespread (under which circumstance, of course, the patient may not reach hospital alive) primary *focal* damage to supratentorial structures does not, of itself, affect consciousness (Rafferty & Fitch, 1992). The initial severity of a head injury is determined by the number and extent of the *diffuse* lesions. If few in number and limited in extent, the patient is 'concussed': when they are more numerous and widespread, coma is irreversible.

Secondary brain damage

Clearly, if the patient reaches hospital alive, it may be assumed that the primary mechanical insult has been of insufficient severity to cause death. Likewise, if the patient has had a 'lucid interval' or has 'talked coherently', it can be accepted that the primary brain damage *per se* has not been severe enough to cause prolonged (or irreversible) unconsciousness. Thus, if death, or coma, occur later, it can be argued with some justification that the deterioration in neurological function must have resulted from a second series of events which, although initiated possibly at the time of the primary insult, have progressed to cause secondary brain damage. Secondary brain damage, therefore, occurs some time *after* the primary injury. Essentially, it is the result of cerebral ischaemia/hypoxia and is the sequel to the development of certain *intracranial* complications (haematoma, infection, cerebral oedema, brain shift and herniation, seizures) and/or the presence of one or more *extracranial* (systemic) factors (hypoxia, hypercapnia, anaemia, decrease in arterial pressure, pyrexia, coughing, straining, inappropriate anaesthesia).

At present, there is no treatment for primary brain damage. The role of the definitive management of the head-injured patient is to detect and treat (or better still prevent) secondary brain damage and so permit the greatest possible recovery of neuronal function consistent with the extent of the primary impact damage.

Secondary brain damage is preventable

Because secondary brain damage becomes evident after the initial insult, all the factors responsible for this second injury are potentially treatable. In theory, secondary brain damage is preventable. However, the clinical realities of the situation are less encouraging (Rose et al., 1977; Jennett & Carlin, 1978; Gentleman & Jennett, 1981). For example, these workers found that, after admission to hospital, one or more potentially avoidable factors were present in 74% of a group of patients who subsequently died having been sufficiently conscious to talk coherently some time after admission. In 54% of these patients it was concluded that one avoidable factor had contributed significantly to their eventual demise. Of those avoidable incidents which certainly contributed to mortality, 70% were intracranial and 30% extracranial (Table 89.1). Space does not permit a consideration of each factor individually: however, it is worth highlighting three.

Airway obstruction

Although airway obstruction was common, only approximately 1:4 of the incidents was regarded as having contributed definitely to the eventual death

Table 89.1 Avoidable incidents (as percentage of total preventable incidents) in a group of 166 patients who died after head injury. (Data from Jennett & Carlin, 1978)

Avoidable factors	Certain effect (%)	Total (%)
Intracranial		
Delay in treating haematoma	48	36
Inadequate control of epilepsy	8	10
Meningitis	7	4
Other	7	7
Total	70	57
Extracranial		
Airway obstruction	9	15
Hypotension	8	14
Other	13	14
Total	30	43

of the patient. What is of interest, however, was the finding that 50% of the incidents of airway obstruction occurred during the movement or transport of the patient *within* the hospital, or during transfer *between* hospitals. For example, in one cohort of comatose patients, being transferred from a primary receiving unit to the regional neurosurgical centre, it was found that 55% did not have a nasogastric tube in place, 36% had no form of artificial airway whatsoever and 61% had been transported lying supine on a non-tilting stretcher. These findings, which were obtained in 1980, can now be compared with the results of a more recent, but similar, investigation (Gentleman & Jennett, 1990). The comparison shows that there have been modest improvements in the care of the unconscious patient during transfer: more had a medical escort, fewer were hypoxaemic [$Pao_2 <$ 9.3 kPa (70 mmHg)] on arrival at the neurosurgical unit, and the trachea was intubated in a larger percentage of patients. Nevertheless, even in this more recent series, up to one-third of these comatose patients had no mechanical airway support, 10% had inadequately managed extracranial injuries and, of particular importance, 7% were considered to be significantly hypotensive on arrival.

Systemic arterial hypotension

The frequency of arterial hypotension [defined as a systolic arterial pressure of less than 12 kPa (90 mmHg)] is always underestimated. Decreases (or increases) in arterial pressure can be recognized only during those periods in which arterial pressure is measured accurately and recorded conscientiously. However, the significance of even minor decreases in arterial pressure is not in doubt (Table 89.2). When present, the combination of arterial hypotension and hypoxaemia was lethal in 100% of the patients studied by Gentleman and Jennett (1981).

Table 89.2 Effect of hypoxia and arterial hypotension on outcome after head injury. (Data from Gentleman & Jennett, 1981)

	No.	Dead (%)	Good recovery (%)
Hypotension alone	12	75	8
Hypoxia alone	29	59	17
Hypoxia or hypotension	46	67	13
Hypoxia and hypotension	5	100	0
Neither factor	104	34	34

Intracranial haematoma

The development of an intracranial haematoma may rapidly convert a relatively minor injury into a life-threatening emergency. Therefore, a high degree of suspicion is required by all those dealing with the head-injured patient. Although computerized tomographic (CT) scanning has proved to be a reliable, and usually non-invasive, means of diagnosing haematoma, not all hospitals are so equipped. Even in those hospitals with the facilities for CT scanning, it may be difficult to obtain repeated scans — particularly in the patient with multiple trauma receiving mechanical ventilation, cardiovascular support, etc. Moreover, several studies have shown that the availability of CT scanning does not, of itself, improve outcome because ideally, the haematoma must be detected *before* secondary brain damage occurs.

Neurological deterioration should be predicted and prevented

Delay in recognition (and hence in eventual evacuation) of an intracranial haematoma occurs because it is usual to become suspicious only when the patient's level of responsiveness has begun to deteriorate. However, it is recognized now that this policy of 'wait and see' implies that definitive action is taken too late: secondary brain damage is well established. In an attempt to pre-empt the development of secondary brain damage, a series of guidelines (Appendix 1) have been drawn up which should enable the clinician to manage the patient appropriately *before* neurological deterioration has become evident clinically. For example, the likelihood of a patient having a haematoma — even though he/she has not (as yet) shown signs of deteriorating neurological function — may be deduced from simple criteria (Teasdale & Galbraith, 1981) and suitable guidelines devised (Table 89.3).

Priorities in management

Resuscitation

If one accepts the principles outlined previously it is obvious that the patient with a moderate to severe head injury must receive — from the moment of injury if possible — appropriate care and aggressive resuscitation. It was noted above that 60% of all deaths from head injury occur before the patient is admitted to hospital. Although the majority of these

Table 89.3 Criteria for the transfer of patients with head injuries to the Institute of Neurological Sciences, Glasgow. (Data from Teasdale, 1982)

Indications
Deterioration in neurological status
Skull fracture, unless alert, orientated and asymptomatic
Focal neurological signs
Any impairment of consciousness greater than confusion
Confusion that persists for 6 h after injury

Contraindications
Major multiple injuries until resuscitated
Patients over 70 years of age in coma from time of injury
Patients of any age who are flaccid, with no motor response and apnoeic

patients die from overwhelming primary brain damage sustained at the time of the initial insult, there is a body of opinion which believes that more active treatment sooner might improve outcome in specific instances. Certainly, because the events precipitating secondary brain damage are triggered by the impact, one could argue logically that clinical management should begin at this time also. This view is supported by the results of a study in San Diego in which it was demonstrated that, after the introduction of 'advanced paramedic services', there was a significant decrease (25 to 14%) in the number of patients with uncontrollable intracranial hypertension [an intracranial pressure greater than 5.32 kPa (40 mmHg) despite standard aggressive therapy] on arrival at the hospital.

Wherever resuscitation is initiated, it should follow the classic pattern: airway, breathing, circulation. An adequate airway is essential: more patients die of hypoxia than from extradural haematoma. If necessary, the trachea should be intubated to secure the airway. The point at issue is not 'Does this patient require intubation of the trachea?' but 'Does this patient *not* require intubation of the trachea?' (in patients with protective reflexes it may be adequate to make use of the lateral position and an oropharyngeal airway). Intubation of the trachea does not require necessarily the administration of drugs or the institution of artificial ventilation. However, the head-injured patient must not be allowed to strain or cough on the tracheal tube and many advise that the patient be given thiopentone (even if unconscious) and/or neuromuscular-blocking drugs before intubation to ensure that he/she does not. Nasotracheal intubation is not indicated usually at this stage and is contraindicated if there is any suspicion that the patient may have a fracture of the base of the skull.

As far as the actual technique of intubation is concerned, one should assume that, until proven otherwise, there is a fracture of the cervical spine and take appropriate precautions. Ideally, the presence of a fracture/fracture−dislocation of the cervical spine should be determined before intubation is attempted. However, injuries to the cervical spine occur much less frequently than hypoxia. Thus, the decision to intubate the trachea, when clinically appropriate, should not be delayed unnecessarily. However, the maintenance of cervical alignment during any manipulation of the head and neck is vital. Some diagnostic hints as to the possibility of neck injury in an unconscious patient are given in Table 89.4.

Supplementary oxygen is always necessary, even if ventilation and colour appear adequate on clinical examination. Any improvement (or otherwise) in oxygenation can be assessed readily by the measurement of arterial oxygen tension which should be maintained at greater than 9.3 kPa (70 mmHg). If this value cannot be achieved with spontaneous ventilation (plus appropriate oxygen therapy) one should consider the use of artificial ventilation.

Pre-eminently, the adequacy of breathing must be assessed objectively (blood-gas analysis) and any evidence of underventilation treated. The indications for the urgent institution of artificial ventilation in the accident and emergency department are:

1 Pao_2 less than 9.3 kPa (70 mmHg) with air, or 13.3 kPa (100 mmHg) with an F_Io_2 of 0.4.

2 Underventilation [$Paco_2$ greater than 6.0 kPa (45 mmHg)] in association with spontaneous ventilation.

3 Hyperventilation [$Paco_2$ less than 3.5 kPa (25 mmHg)] in association with spontaneous respiration. (Note that not all units accept this criterion as an indication for the urgent institution of artificial ventilation.) (See Table 89.9 for additional indications for the use of artificial ventilation in the head-injured patient.)

Table 89.4 Neck injury in the unconscious patient

Diagnostic hints
Flaccid areflexia, especially with flaccid rectal sphincter
Diaphragmatic breathing
Patient can flex but not extend forearms
Patient grimaces to pain above the clavicle, but not to pain
   below clavicle
Hypotension without evidence of shock
Priapism
Scalp lacerations/bruising, particularly on forehead
Widening of posterior pharyngeal wall

The frequency of associated injuries in the patient with head injury has been emphasized previously: an intercostal drain (or drains) should be inserted if there is radiological evidence (or clinical suspicion) of the presence of a pneumothorax or haemothorax, before artificial ventilation is instituted.

The haemodynamic status of the patient is of great importance and must be monitored accurately and frequently. Intravenous access should be secured, and cannulation of a central vein is advantageous [measurement of central venous pressure (CVP), infusion of fluids, infusion of mannitol] and is recommended in the patient with multiple trauma. However, cannulation of the basilic, median cephalic or subclavian vein is to be preferred to cannulation of the internal jugular vein in the head-injured patient. As far as possible, hypovolaemia should be corrected and arterial pressure restored to the 'normal' for that individual using physiological saline, colloids and/or blood as appropriate. Occult blood loss is dangerous and the control of intrathoracic or intra-abdominal haemorrhage must take precedence over the more definitive management of the head injury. If there is any doubt, diagnostic pleural tap or peritoneal lavage should be considered.

At this point, certain other aspects of the early management of the patient with a head injury should be considered, although they are not specifically part of the initial resuscitation.

1 Mannitol (1 g/kg) should be administered normally, if required, once the advice of a neurosurgeon has been obtained. However, its administration is urgent if an intracranial haematoma is found on CT scanning and/or if there is clinical evidence of a dilating pupil or progressive deterioration in conscious level.

2 Convulsions should be controlled by the intravenous administration of an anticonvulsant (Table 89.5). Ventilatory support may be required if respiratory depression occurs in association with the administration of a barbiturate or benzodiazepine. Clearly, convulsive motor activity should not be controlled by the use of a neuromuscular-blocking drug alone.

3 It has now been shown that steroids are of no value in the management of the head injury itself (Dearden *et al.*, 1986). Thus, they should be given only if there is a separate indication for their use.

4 Pain is not only unpleasant for the patient: it also increases cerebral blood volume and intracranial pressure. Analgesia (morphine, up to 0.1 mg/kg; papaveretum, up to 0.2 mg/kg; fentanyl, up to 3 μg/kg) should not be withheld just because the patient

Table 89.5 Drugs (and doses) suitable for the management of seizures in the head-injured patient

Phenytoin
Slow intravenous injection (up to $1 \, mg \cdot kg^{-1} \cdot min^{-1}$)
Maximum loading dose: adults, 15 mg/kg; children, 5 mg/kg

Phenobarbitone
Slow intravenous injection (up to $1 \, mg \cdot kg^{-1} \cdot min^{-1}$)
Maximum loading dose 4 mg/kg

Thiopentone
Slow intravenous injection 2.5% (25 mg/ml) (up to $5 \, mg \cdot kg^{-1} \cdot min^{-1}$)
Maximum loading dose 20 mg/kg

Chlormethiazole
Intravenous infusion 0.8% (8 mg/ml) (up to 7 ml/min)
Maximum loading dose 10 mg/kg

has a head injury. Indeed, they may do more than relieve pain; they may also suppress acute increases in systemic arterial pressure and surges in intracranial pressure.

Assessment

The definitive neurological assessment of any patient with a head injury, i.e. the initial assessment of the severity of the brain damage, must be undertaken *after* the institution of appropriate resuscitative measures, and once time has been allowed for any improvement in the patient's general condition to become manifest. Attempts to assess the severity of the head injury before correction of hypoxaemia or replacement of blood loss lead to erroneous conclusions and may militate against the rational choice of the most appropriate definitive management. For example, fixed and dilated pupils and/or apnoea at the moment of entry to hospital may be the result of an obstructed airway, or arterial hypotension or drugs rather than head injury itself. Likewise, measures to select those head-injured patients in whom prognosis is hopeless before the effects of resuscitation have become evident could lead to the loss of a number of patients who would otherwise recover.

The most effective way to assess the integrity of central and peripheral neurological function has been and continues to be the *clinical* neurological examination. This requires that the patient *responds* to auditory, visual and tactile stimuli in a defined way. Until 1965, the neurological examination of the *comatose* (unresponsive) patient was limited to those aspects of the traditional neurological examination

which could be carried out — pupillary response to light, assessment of tendon reflexes and plantar response. In general terms, these provided little useful information. Once the role of the brainstem in the genesis of coma had become accepted, various measures were introduced by which the function of the brainstem could be assessed at the bedside. Subsequently, a number of 'coma' charts and 'coma' scales were designed and evaluated. The most widely used of these, the Glasgow coma scale (Table 89.6), is based on the assessment of three separate sets of function: eye opening, best verbal response and best motor response. Simple addition of the values on the right in Table 89.6 provides a coma 'score'. This is most useful as a means of classifying the severity of the brain damage: minor 14–15, moderate 9–13, severe 3–8. Use of the Glasgow coma scale alone does not ensure assessment of lower brainstem reflexes nor of changes in physiological variables such as heart rate, arterial pressure, or respiratory rate or pattern. Nevertheless, numerous studies have shown that it can serve as an adequate indicator of changing neurological state. However, in the individual patient, more information on overall neurological function may be obtained by the additional assessment of other physiological variables (arterial pressure, intracranial pressure).

What is assessed and how it is assessed varies from patient to patient. At one extreme there is the conscious patient who can talk, give an account of

Table 89.6 Glasgow coma scale. Numbers on the right may be added (one number for each index of neurological function) to produce the Glasgow coma score

Eye opening	
Spontaneous	4
To speech	3
To pain	2
None	1
Best verbal response	
Orientated	5
Confused	4
Inappropriate words	3
Incomprehensible sounds	2
None	1
Best motor response	
Obey commands	6
Localize pain	5
Normal flexion to pain	4
Abnormal flexion to pain	3
Extension to pain	2
None	1

his/her injury and respond verbally to the various facets of the clinical examination of his/her neurological function. At the other extreme is the head-injured patient in an intensive care environment in whom the lungs are ventilated mechanically (either as an elective procedure or as a sequel to respiratory insufficiency) and who may be receiving neuro-muscular-blocking drugs, hypnotics or opioids to permit compliance with artificial ventilation. In this latter group, the majority (or possibly all) of the *clinical* features relied upon normally to monitor neurological status are lost. Although it is customary to allow such patients to 'lighten' intermittently so that a neurological assessment may be obtained, this is not satisfactory, and it must be accepted that the ability of the clinician to detect changes in neuro-logical state is impaired. Despite this, there should be no hesitation in administering anticonvulsants, analgesics or neuromuscular-blocking drugs, when indicated, as most of the initial decisions in regard to treatment are based on the findings of the CT scan and/or measurements of intracranial pressure. Before concluding the initial assessment of the patient, it is important to exclude other causes of depression of consciousness (diabetes, alcohol, hypothermia, epilepsy, cerebrovascular accident, drugs, hypoxia).

The initial neurological assesment of the head-injured patient (at the correct point in time) is of fundamental importance. It acts as a baseline on which progress (or deterioration) can be judged, prognosis can be predicted and treatment can be evaluated. *Repeated* neurological assessment is the cornerstone of the management of this group of patients. Because this is so, this brief account should be augmented by a review of more comprehensive texts (Teasdale, 1976; Jennett & Teasdale, 1981; Teasdale, 1985; Miller, 1987).

Diagnosis

Definitive management of the patient with a head injury requires a definitive diagnosis. Nowadays, this is obtained almost exclusively by CT scanning which should be performed as soon as possible when the patient's cardiovascular and respiratory variables have been stabilized and when injury to the spine has been excluded (for indications for CT scanning see Appendix 2). An anaesthetic may be required, especially if the patient is restless, to abolish move-ment artifacts and so optimize the acquisition of reliable information. If so, a technique of anaesthesia described in Chapter 41 should be employed. If CT scanning is unavailable, the search for a diagnosis should be pursued by the use of ultrasound, angio-graphy and, possibly, burr hole exploration — *if equipment and expertise are available*. A good-quality CT scan shows the location and extent of focal lesions but shows little in patients with diffuse axonal injury. Patients who have a focal lesion with evidence of midline displacement require surgery and, normally, go directly to the operating theatre. In situations in which surgery is not indicated, it is usual to transfer the patient to an intensive therapy unit (ITU) either in the centre to which the patient has been referred, or in the primary receiving unit.

The performance of CT scanning (and, indeed, of other radiological investigations; skull, cervical spine, chest, abdomen, pelvis, limbs and any other area of clinical suspicion) requires that the patient be moved either within the accident and emergency department or the primary receiving unit or between hospitals. Clearly, this is a time of increased risk as far as the patient is concerned although, of course, the infor-mation sought is crucial to any further management. It is important that the basic care of the patient (supplementary oxygen, intravenous fluids, control of pain, monitoring of arterial pressure and neuro-logical function, etc.) be established before, and con-tinued throughout, such manoeuvres. As an aside, it is worth noting that one of the purposes of the continuous monitoring of intracranial pressure is to aid in the definition of those occasions when a radio-logical study is indicated and so decrease the number of unnecessary movements undertaken by an indi-vidual patient.

Maintenance of cerebral perfusion

Evidence of cerebral ischaemia is present in more than 90% of patients who die following a head injury and, when present in a patient who survives, is associated with a poorer outcome. The fact that ischaemia is present implies that the delivery of substrate to the brain was inadequate to meet its metabolic requirements.

The supply of oxygen to the brain is dependent on the amount of blood reaching brain tissue (cerebral blood flow) and the amount of oxygen carried per unit of blood (arterial oxygen content). Thus, the delivery of oxygen may be optimized by ensuring an adequate flow of fully oxygenated blood to the brain (ideally, to the most threatened regions). In the head-injured patient, cerebral blood flow (especially the blood flow to the damaged or potentially ischaemic regions) is dependent largely on systemic arterial pressure. Thus, it is mandatory that arterial pressure to be controlled adequately. However, care is necessary to prevent arterial pressure increasing significantly above the patients' preinjury value. As parts of the cerebral vasculature cannot constrict in response to such increases in arterial pressure (Chapter 41), there is a high probability of marked swelling of the brain and, consequently, of increases in intracranial pressure. Many devices are now available which permit non-invasive monitoring of arterial pressure from the arm, leg or finger, and one of these may suffice in the majority of patients with a pure head injury. In the patient with multiple trauma, however, there are advantages in monitoring arterial pressure directly.

Mean cerebral perfusion pressure is equal to mean arterial pressure minus mean intracranial pressure, therefore any increase in intracranial pressure decreases perfusion of the brain and increases the likelihood of ischaemic damage (unless arterial pressure increases concomitantly). Although the decision to institute measurement of intracranial pressure is made normally by the neurosurgeon, it is relevant to note that one of the cardinal indications for the use of the technique is the patient with a head injury undergoing artificial ventilation of the lungs.

The importance of considering values of arterial pressure *and* intracranial pressure when making therapeutic decisions cannot be overemphasized. In the patient with a head injury a marked increase in arterial pressure is frequently a sequel to a shift of brain and/or an increase in intracranial pressure. The correct management in this situation is to decrease intracranial pressure (see Chapter 41). Any decrease in arterial pressure alone increases the likelihood of cerebral ischaemia.

Practicalities of management

This section considers the practical clinical management of the head-injured patient in an ITU. It is assumed that the patient's cardiovascular system is stable, and the remit of this chapter is to consider those modalities of management relevant to the head injury *per se* (management of other aspects of multiple trauma is detailed in Chapter 46).

Currently, the intensive care of such patients involves a 'package' of measures designed to maximize the delivery of oxygen to the brain and, hence, prevent, or ameliorate, the effects of secondary brain damage.

Basic care of the head-injured patient

Good general care of the patient is vital. This includes nursing the patient with a 20–30° head-up tilt, regular changes of position and physiotherapy. Although it has been argued that the use of the physiotherapy and the frequency of tracheal suction should be limited because of the associated surges in intracranial pressure, the prevention of a chest infection (and of pressure sores) is of greater importance. In any case, if required, the acute increases in intracranial pressure associated with physiotherapy and other stimulating procedures can be obtunded by the prior administration of etomidate, 2–6 mg, thiopentone, 100–200 mg, γ-hydroxybutyric acid, 1 g, or propofol, 100 mg. The eyes should be protected and examined regularly for corneal abrasions/ulceration. Analgesics should be given as required to provide continuing relief of pain.

The optimum body temperature for the head-injured patient is 35°C. On no account should the patient be allowed to become pyrexial: tepid sponging, fanning and chlorpromazine, 0.1–0.2 mg/kg, may be helpful. Although routine prophylactic antibiotics should not be used (unless there is evidence of a fracture of the base of the skull) infection requires energetic and, preferably, specific therapy.

An anticonvulsant (for example, phenytoin, 15 mg/kg, in divided doses in day 1, 10 mg/kg in divided doses on day 2, thereafter 5 mg/kg) should be given prophylactically to all patients with an intracerebral haematoma or history of multiple post-traumatic seizures. If phenytoin is used, blood concentrations should be monitored from day 3 (therapeutic range 40–80 μmol/litre).

It is likely that a gastric tube will have been inserted at the accident and emergency department in order to decompress the stomach. Unless contraindicated, nasogastric drainage should be maintained until enteral feeding is commenced (usually around 48–72 h after the injury). Parenteral nutrition should be considered if enteral feeding is contraindicated or fails. It is customary to give ranitidine (50 mg 8-hourly) in an attempt to prevent ulceration of and bleeding from the mucosa of the stomach.

Fluid balance and electrolyte concentrations should be monitored, particularly as trauma to the brain may disturb physiological regulating mechanisms and lead to diabetes insipidus, the inappropriate secretion of antidiuretic hormone, water overload/retention (the most common cause of low serum sodium concentration in head injury) and water depletion (increased serum sodium concentration).

Diagnosis of these various problems requires measurement of urine volume, serum concentrations of sodium, potassium and urea, urinary content of sodium and potassium and serum, and urine osmolality.

Recent studies have highlighted the detrimental effects of increases in blood glucose concentration on neurological function after ischaemia (Fitch, 1988). Hence, it is necessary to monitor blood glucose concentrations repeatedly and maintain these within the physiological range (hypoglycaemia has, of course, been known for some time to cause brain damage).

In adults, hourly fluid input should equal the previous hour's output of urine +30 ml (to replace insensible losses) up to a maximum input of 150 ml/h. Customarily, it has been recommended that dextrose 5% in saline 0.45% (with 20 mmol potassium chloride per 500 ml) be used initially, and that appropriate adjustments to the nature of the fluid(s) and the additives be made in the light of the results of the biochemical investigations. Concern over the role of hyperglycaemia in the augmentation of ischaemic damage has prompted several groups of workers to argue that 'glucose-containing solutions be avoided in patients undergoing operations that may have a significant risk of intraoperative ischaemia'.

A reasonable compromise would be the use of colloid (salt-poor if indicated) to maintain circulating blood volume and cardiac filling pressure, saline 0.9% solution whilst monitoring repeatedly the serum sodium concentration, and dextrose 5% solution only as required to maintain normal blood glucose concentrations.

Specific treatment in the management of the head-injured patient

Specific treatment in the context of head injury aims to maximize the delivery of oxygen to the brain by optimizing the oxygen content of arterial blood and balancing cerebral metabolic demands and cerebral perfusion. This chapter has emphasized the importance of the former and the means by which the optimal carriage of oxygen may be realized (supplementary oxygen, correction of anaemia, management of chest injury, prevention of the aspiration of gastric contents, artificial ventilation). The latter can be achieved either by suppressing cerebral metabolism and so decreasing the demand for oxygen or by improving the supply. Although theoretically attractive, the use of barbiturates to decrease electively metabolic requirements of the damaged brain has not survived detailed prospective investigation

(Schwartz et al., 1984; Ward et al., 1985). Likewise, the elective use of hypothermia to temperatures of 32–33°C, as a means of decreasing cerebral metabolism deliberately, has fallen into disuse. Nevertheless, there are good theoretical arguments for attempting to achieve and maintain a core temperature of 35°C. This can be obtained often by controlling the heat generated by muscle activity and allowing the patient to 'find his/her own value of temperature' in relation to the environment. However, current interest centres on the means by which cerebral perfusion may be increased. It is evident from the arguments put forward above that this may be achieved by increasing systemic arterial pressure, by decreasing intracranial pressure, or by a combination of both. In practice, this implies normalization of systemic arterial pressure (correction of blood loss, optimization of cardiac filling pressures and myocardial performance, relief of pain) and control of intracranial hypertension.

Management of increases in intracranial pressure

Before discussing the specific modalities which may be employed to control intracranial pressure, it is important to consider two general points. First, it would seem logical intuitively to accept that a high intracranial pressure must be bad for the patient and, hence, any attempt to decrease it, beneficial. This presupposes that the increase in intracranial pressure is an aetiological *mechanism* in the development of cerebral ischaemia. The other side of this particular 'coin' is that the change in intracranial pressure is a *measure* of the damage to the brain with the proviso that one should treat, if possible, the cause of the brain swelling and not the measurement of its severity. Second, it must be stressed that, although we are about to consider the means by which increases in intracranial pressure may be attenuated or decreased, the ideal management would be to prevent any increase *ab initio*.

With a patient lying supine, the normal range of intracranial pressure is 0–2 kPa (0–15 mmHg) (Chapter 41). In those units which treat increases in intracranial pressure aggressively, specific therapy is introduced when intracranial pressure (measured with the zero reference at the external auditory meatus) exceeds 3.3 kPa (25 mmHg) for more than 5 min, *provided* there is no obvious, easily remediable cause (hypoxaemia, hypercapnia, pyrexia, compression of the jugular veins, 'fighting the ventilator', seizure activity).

The next stage in management is to validate the

measurement and then to select, as appropriate, one or more of the three measures (Miller, 1985) which are known to be effective in most patients and which carry a low risk of worsening the patient's condition (Table 89.7): hyperventilation, drainage of cerebrospinal fluid (CSF), administration of mannitol 20% solution.

In general terms, any increase in intracranial pressure can be considered as being due to vascular or non-vascular, factors. The vascular causes include active cerebral artery vasodilatation, passive arterial distension due to a combination of an increase in arterial pressure and an impairment of autoregulation, and venous engorgement due to an obstruction to the outflow of cerebral venous blood. The non-vascular causes include all forms of oedema and those factors which increase the outflow resistance of the cerebrospinal fluid pathways. The primary purpose behind any attempt to determine the cause of the increase in intracranial pressure in any individual patient is to ensure, whenever possible, that treatment is 'targeted' appropriately — in the belief that tackling the defined cause will be more successful and less detrimental, than treatment by trial and error. If the increase in intracranial pressure is due primarily to non-vascular factors, the most appropriate means of management are likely to be osmotherapy for cerebral oedema, and CSF drainage if there is an obstruction to the CSF pathways.

Broadly speaking, it can be proposed that hyperventilation (possibly plus the administration of hypnotic agents) ought to be considered when the increase in intracranial pressure is due to vascular causes (Dearden & Miller, 1989). As an aside, there is now evidence to suggest that the use of controlled arterial hypertension may be of value in decreasing intracranial pressure — as long as autoregulation is intact (Plets, 1989).

Mannitol 20% (0.5 g/kg) over 15–20 min is the drug used most commonly for the rapid control of intracranial hypertension. Usually, an infusion of mannitol is required early in the management of the patient in order to control intracranial pressure initially. Thereafter, it may not be necessary to give mannitol on more than one further occasion, provided controlled hyperventilation is continued. However, if necessary, the above dose may be repeated 4-hourly: indeed, a 'closed-loop' system is in use in at least one unit. Mannitol has very few disadvantages but may produce acidosis and renal failure if the plasma osmolality exceeds 320 mosmol/litre. Although the use of loop diuretics in the treatment of intracranial hypertension is controversial, frusemide, 0.4–0.6 mg/kg, in addition to the mannitol (frusemide given 15 min after the start of the mannitol) is often beneficial. Central venous pressure should be measured during and following the administration of mannitol as arterial hypotension may occur as a result of a decrease in circulating blood volume.

Drainage of CSF may be a useful means of decreasing intracranial pressure, although it is less effective if the ventricles are small (as in patients with diffuse axonal injury). To prevent the collapse of the ventricles in other patients, the CSF should be drained against a positive pressure [approximately 3 kPa (22 mmHg)].

In many units, controlled ventilation is the most widely practised specific measure in the management of the head-injured patient because, in theory at least, it helps to maximize the oxygen content of blood and control intracranial pressure (McDowall, 1985).

Advocates of the elective use of controlled ventilation decrease $Paco_2$ to 3.5–4 kPa (26–30 mmHg) in all patients liable to develop intracranial hypertension. More pronounced hyperventilation [$Paco_2$ 2.6 kPa (20 mmHg)] may be employed in the treatment of an increasing intracranial pressure. By inducing hypocapnia (Table 89.8), hyperventilation produces cerebral vasoconstriction, a decrease in cerebral blood volume and a decrease in intracranial pressure. Because it is important that the head-injured patient

Table 89.7 Proven methods of controlling increases in intracranial pressure. (Data from Miller, 1985)

Treatment	Limitations	Risks
Hyperventilation	Blood vessels must be responsive to changes in Pco_2	Vasoconstriction may produce brain ischaemia (although structural damage has never been shown to occur)
CSF drainage	From ventricular catheter only	Leakage of CSF may interfere with intracranial pressure recording. Haemorrhage in tract of cannula through brain
Mannitol	Serum osmolality must be less than 320 mosmol/litre	Fluid and electrolyte disturbance and renal failure

CSF, cerebrospinal fluid.

Table 89.8 Advantages and disadvantages of induced hypocapnia in the management of the head-injured patient

Advantages
Induces vasoconstriction in cerebral blood vessels responsive to effects of carbon dioxide: decreases cerebral blood flow, cerebral blood volume and intracranial pressure

May increase the perfusion to potentially ischaemic areas (inverse steal)

Improves autoregulation: protects against the effects of transient changes in arterial pressure

Helps to correct acidosis of brain tissue

Disadvantages
None — if patient is normovolaemic and if $Paco_2$ is not allowed to decrease below 2.7 kPa (20 mmHg)

Table 89.9 Indications for the use of artificial ventilation in the management of the head-injured patient. Note that the decision to introduce artificial ventilation as an elective procedure (i.e. not urgently) should be taken once the patient has been resuscitated and stabilized

Inadequate spontaneous breathing
$Pao_2 < 9.3$ kPa (70 mmHg) with F_1o_2 0.21
$Pao_2 < 13.3$ kPa (100 mmHg) with F_1o_2 0.40
$Paco_2 > 6.0$ kPa (45 mmHg)

Poor neurological function
No response to pain (Glasgow coma score 3)
Spontaneous extensor posturing (Glasgow coma score 4)
Repeated convulsions
Spontaneous hyperventilation: $Paco_2 < 3.5$ kPa (25 mmHg)
Intracranial pressure 3.5 kPa (25 mmHg) for more than 5 min (no obviously remediable cause)
After intracranial surgery (for 12–24 h)

Associated pathology
Chest injury
Prolonged surgery
Inhalation of gastric contents

does not cough, strain or 'fight the ventilator', neuro-muscular block and sedation if indicated should be used to aid compliance with mechanical ventilation. If possible, the tidal volume should be adjusted so as to produce an inflation pressure of 20 cmH$_2$O or less. Ideally, Pao_2 should be greater than 16 kPa (120 mmHg): certainly, it should not be allowed to decrease to less than 8 kPa (60 mmHg). If adequate oxygenation proves difficult to achieve, even after an increase in F_1o_2 to greater than 0.5–0.6, positive end-expiratory pressure (PEEP) may be employed. How-ever, a maximum value of +6 cmH$_2$O should not be exceeded (in the uncomplicated head injury), and cerebral perfusion pressure should be monitored closely.

The duration of mechanical ventilation is usually determined electively as 48–72 h in the first instance. It would then be customary to permit the return of neuromuscular transmission and assess the patient neurologically. If the indications for artificial venti-lation in the ITU (Table 89.9) remain, or if intracranial pressure increases again, hyperventilation is main-tained for a further 24–48 h — provided intracranial pressure decreases.

Monitoring the head-injured patient

Monitoring of the basic neurological, haemodynamic and respiratory status of the head-injured patient, and of the changes in the various indices, is a means of guiding the clinician so that appropriate thera-peutic steps may be taken. The various modalities of monitoring relevant to the management of the head-injured patient have been alluded to previously and are summarized in Table 89.10. Classically, it has

been customary to consider these as being inde-pendent, rather than interdependent, variables. As a result, considerable weight has been placed on the analysis of the changes in *isolated* physiological indices when, very probably, more clinically useful information could have been obtained through an appreciation of the simultaneous changes in a *series* of variables (Fitch *et al.*, 1993). Of particular value in this context has been the more widespread use of cannulation of the jugular bulb and the measurement and evaluation of the changes in the saturation of jugular venous blood, and the resultant ability to calculate the cerebral arteriovenous difference for oxygen (Robertson *et al.*, 1989; Andrews *et al.*, 1991). The results of the more widespread clinical appli-cation of diffuse near-infrared transmission spec-troscopy (McCormick *et al.*, 1991) (a means by which the cytochrome redox state of cerebral tissue may be measured non-invasively) are awaited with interest.

The goals of medical treatment in the head-injured patient are to preserve neurological function and promote physical and social rehabilitation. In this chapter we have considered only those aspects related to the acute phase of the illness. However, it must not be forgotten that this is but the beginning of a long and often difficult process of recovery. Although the primary objectives of treatment to the patient with a head-injury are to preserve neurological function and promote physical and social rehabilitation, the damage to the brain may be, or may become, such that function is destroyed and any capacity for

Table 89.10 Possible modalities of monitoring in the patient with a head injury. Note that the selected techniques of monitoring would be supplemented routinely with repeated assessments of fluid balance, serum electrolyte concentrations, urine and serum osmolalities

	Routinely	Frequently	Occasionally
Cerebral function	Neurological examination Coma scale/score Blood glucose concentration Temperature		EEG Evoked potentials CFM/CFAM Infrared spectroscopy
Cerebral perfusion	Arterial pressure/ICP Heart rate ECG $Paco_2$	CVP Expired CO_2 concentration TCD $S_{jv} o_2/A-jv\, Do_2$	CBF PCWP
Oxygen carriage	Haemoglobin concentration F_Io_2 $Paco_2$ Respiratory rate Expired minute volume	Sao_2 Pulse oximetry	Oxygen content

ICP, intracranial pressure; CVP, central venous pressure; TCD, transcranial Doppler blood flow velocity; CBF, cerebral blood flow; PCWP, pulmonary capillary wedge pressure.

recovery lost. A proportion of these patients become brain dead and may serve as a source of organ donation. The criteria for diagnosis of brain death are given in Appendix 3.

Appendix 1

Guidelines in regard to the initial management of an adult patient with a head injury
(Group of Neurosurgeons, 1984)

Criteria for X-ray examination of skull after a recent head injury (the presence of one or more of the following indicates a need for a skull X-ray):
1 Loss of consciousness or amnesia at any time.
2 Symptoms or signs of neurological deficit.
3 Cerebrospinal fluid or blood from nose or ear.
4 Suspected penetrating injury, scalp bruising or swelling.
5 Laceration of scalp.

Criteria for admission to hospital after a recent head injury (one or more of the following):
1 Confusion or any other depression of the level of consciousness at the time of examination (as measured by the Glasgow coma scale).
2 Fracture of the skull.
3 Neurological symptoms or signs, headache or vomiting.
4 Difficulty in the neurological assessment of the patient because of, e.g. alcohol, epilepsy, age (the very young).
5 Other associated medical conditions: diabetes mellitus, haemophilia, patient receiving anticoagulant therapy.
6 Social problems: in particular the lack of a responsible adult to supervise the patient.

NB: post-traumatic amnesia with full recovery is not itself an indication for admission to hospital. Relatives or friends of patients sent home should receive written instructions on possible complications and what to do (e.g. return to hospital).

Criteria for consultation with a regional neurosurgical unit (one or more of the following) (see also Table 89.3):
1 Coma continuing after resuscitation.
2 Neurological deterioration after admission.
3 Depressed skull fracture.
4 Linear fracture of the skull in combination with either:
  (a) Confusion or other depression of the level of consciousness.
  (b) Focal neurological signs, or
  (c) seizures.
5 Suspected open injury of the vault or the base of the skull.
6 Confusion or other neurological disturbances persisting for more than 12 h even if there is no fracture of the skull.

NB: although the above guidelines may be helpful, clinical judgement is always necessary.

Appendix 2

Guidelines for CT scanning in patients with head injury

Immediate CT scan

1 Patients in coma (Glasgow coma score 8 or less). (Chance of having an intracranial haematoma is greater than 40%.)
2 Patients in whom level of consciousness is depressed (Glasgow coma score 9–13) and who have a skull fracture. (Chance of haematoma or other significant intracranial lesion is around 20%.)
3 Patients who show neurological deterioration to coma (Glasgow coma score 8 or less).

Urgent CT scan (within 6 h)

1 Patients who are drowsy and/or disorientated (Glasgow coma score 14–15) and have a skull fracture. (Chance of haematoma 15%.)
2 Patients with abnormal neurological signs plus skull fracture. (Chance of haematoma 15%.)
3 Patients with depression of consciousness (Glasgow coma score 9–13) plus focal neurological deficit, irrespective of presence of skull fracture.
4 Patients with unexplained increase in intracranial pressure.

CT scan within 24 h

1 Patients who show neurological deterioration (by 2 or more points on Glasgow coma score).
2 Patients with confusion or severe headache, persisting for more than 48 h, but no skull fracture.

CT scan before surgery

Patients with multiple injuries which require surgery and general anaesthesia and who have a Glasgow coma score of 15. In such patients, it is important to exclude intracranial haematoma positively. However, scan should be undertaken only if airway is secure and haemodynamic status satisfactory. If not, surgery should be undertaken first and the scan performed afterwards.

Appendix 3

Diagnosis of brain death

Statement issued by the Honorary Secretary of the Conference of Medical Royal Colleges and their Faculties in the UK (1976)

Criteria for considering diagnosis of brain death (all of the following should co-exist):
1 The patient is deeply comatose.
  (a) There should be no suspicion that this state is due to depressant drugs.
  (b) Primary hypothermia as a cause of coma should have been excluded.
  (c) Metabolic and endocrine disturbances which can cause coma should have been excluded.
2 The patient is being maintained on a ventilator because spontaneous respiration had previously become inadequate or had ceased altogether.
  Relaxants (neuromuscular-blocking agents) and other drugs should have been excluded as a cause of respiratory inadequacy or failure.
3 There should be no doubt that the patient's condition is due to irremediable structural brain damage. The diagnosis should have been established fully.

Criteria for confirming brain death (all brainstem reflexes should be absent):
1 The pupils are fixed in diameter and do not respond to sharp changes in the intensity of incident light.
2 There is no corneal reflex.
3 The vestibulo-ocular reflexes are absent. These are absent when no eye movement occurs during or after the slow injection of 20 ml of ice-cold water into each external auditory meatus in turn, clear access to the tympanic membrane having been established by direct inspection. This test may be contraindicated on one or other side because of local trauma.
4 No motor responses within the cranial nerve distribution can be elicited by adequate stimulation of any somatic area.
5 There is no gag reflex or reflex to bronchial stimulation by a suction catheter passed down the trachea.
6 No respiratory movements occur when the patient is disconnected from the mechanical ventilator for long enough to ensure that the arterial carbon dioxide tension rises above the threshold for stimulating respiration, i.e. the Pa_{CO_2} must normally reach 6.7 kPa (50 mmHg). This is achieved best by measuring the blood gases; if this facility is available, the patient should be disconnected when the Pa_{CO_2} reaches 5.3–6.0 kPa (40–45 mmHg) after administration of

5% carbon dioxide in oxygen through the ventilator.

If blood-gas analysis is not available to measure the $Paco_2$ and Pao_2, the alternative procedure is to supply the ventilator with pure oxygen for 10 min (preoxygenation), then with 5% carbon dioxide in oxygen for 5 min, and to disconnect the ventilator for 10 min whilst delivering oxygen at 6 litres/min by catheter into the trachea.

Other considerations

1 Repetition of testing. It is customary to repeat the tests to ensure that there has been no observer error.

2 The interval between tests depends on the progress of the patient and might be as long as 24 h.

3 Integrity of spinal reflexes. Reflexes of spinal origin may persist or return after an initial absence in brain-dead patients.

4 Confirmatory investigations. It is now accepted widely that electroencephalography is not necessary for diagnosing brain death.

5 Body temperature. The body temperature in these patients may be low because of depression of central temperature regulation by drugs or by brainstem damage, and it is recommended that it should be not less than 35°C before the diagnostic tests are carried out. A low-reading thermometer should be used.

6 Specialist opinion and status of doctors concerned. Experienced clinicians in ITUs, acute medical wards, and accident and emergency departments should not normally require specialist advice. Only when the primary diagnosis is in doubt is it necessary to consult with a neurologist or neurosurgeon. The decision to withdraw artificial support should be made after all the criteria presented above have been fulfilled and can be made by any one of the following combinations of doctors:

(a) A consultant who is in charge of the case and one other doctor.

(b) In the absence of a consultant, his deputy who should have been registered for 5 years or more and who should have had adequate experience in the care of such cases, and one other doctor.

References

Andrews P.J.D., Dearden N.M. & Miller J.D. (1991) Jugular bulb cannulation: description of a cannulation technique and validation of a new continuous monitor. *British Journal of Anaesthesia* **67**, 553–8.

Dearden N.M. & Miller J.D. (1989) Paired comparison of hypnotic and osmotic therapy in the reduction of intracranial hypertension after severe head injury. In *Intracranial Pressure* (Eds Hoff J.T. & Betz A.L.) pp. 474–81. Springer-Verlag, Berlin, Heidelberg.

Dearden N.M., Gibson J.S., Gibson R.M., McDowall D.G. & Cameron M.M. (1986) Effects of high-dose dexamethasone on outcome from severe head injury. *Journal of Neurosurgery* **64**, 81–8.

Fitch W. (1988) Hyperglycaemia and ischaemic brain damage. In *Anaesthesia Review*, number 5 (Ed. Kaufman L.) pp. 119–30. Churchill Livingstone, Edinburgh.

Fitch W., Rafferty C., Stewart L. & Bullock R. (1993) Multimodality monitoring in the intensive care unit: studies in patients with a head injury. *Journal of Clinical Monitoring* **9**, 131.

Gentleman D. & Jennett B. (1981) Hazards of inter-hospital transfer of comatose head-injured patients. *Lancet* **ii**, 853–5.

Gentleman D. & Jennett B. (1990) Audit of transfer of unconscious head-injured patients to a neurosurgical unit. *Lancet* **335**, 330–4.

Group of Neurosurgeons (1984) Guidelines for initial management after head injury in adults. *British Medical Journal* **288**, 983–5.

Jennett B. & Carlin J. (1978) Preventable mortality and morbidity after head-injury. *Injury* **10**, 31–9.

Jennett B. & Teasdale G. (1981) Assessment of impaired consciousness. In *Management of Head Injuries. Contemporary Neurology*, number 20, pp. 77–93. F.A. Davis, Philadelphia.

McCormick P.W., Stewart M., Goetting M.G., Dujovny M., Lewis G. & Ausman J.I. (1991) Non-invasive cerebral optical spectroscopy for monitoring cerebral oxygen delivery and haemodynamics. *Critical Care Medicine* **19**, 89–97.

McDowall D.G. (1985) Artificial ventilation in the management of the head-injured patient. In *Head Injury and the Anaesthetist* (Eds Fitch W. & Barker J.) pp. 149–63. Elsevier, Amsterdam.

Miller J.D. (1985) Head injury and brain ischaemia — implications for therapy. *British Journal of Anaesthesia* **57**, 120–30.

Miller J.D. (1987) Neurological evaluation of the unconscious patient. In *Intensive Care and Monitoring of the Neurosurgical Patient* (Ed. Landolt A.M.) pp. 1–14. Karger, Basel.

Plets C. (1989) Arterial hypertension in neurosurgical emergencies. *American Journal of Cardiology* **63**, 40C–2C.

Rafferty C. & Fitch W. (1992) Consciousness and unconsciousness: definitions and differential diagnosis. In *Anaesthesia Review*, number 9 (Ed. Kaufman L.) pp. 158–72. Churchill Livingstone, Edinburgh.

Robertson C.S., Narayan R.K., Gokaslan Z.L., Pahwa R., Grossman R.G., Caram P. & Allen E. (1989) Cerebral arteriovenous oxygen difference as an estimate of cerebral blood flow in comatose patients. *Journal of Neurosurgery* **70**, 222–30.

Rose J., Valtonen S. & Jennett B. (1977) Avoidable factors contributing to death after head injury. *British Medical Journal* **ii**, 615–18.

Schwartz M.L., Tator C.H., Rowed D.W., Reid S.R. & Meguro K. (1984) The University of Toronto Head Injury Study: a prospective, randomised comparison of pentobarbital and mannitol. *Canadian Journal of Neurological Sciences* **11**, 434–40.

Teasdale G. (1976) Assessment of head injuries. *British Journal of Anaesthesia* **48**, 761−6.

Teasdale G. (1982) Management of head injuries. *The Practitioner* **226**, 1667−73.

Teasdale G. (1985) The clinical assessment of the head-injured patient. In *Head Injury and the Anaesthetist* (Eds Fitch W. & Barker J.) pp. 83−101. Elsevier, Amsterdam.

Teasdale G. & Galbraith S. (1981) Acute traumatic intracranial haematomas. In *Progress in Neurological Surgery* (Eds Krayenbyhl H., Maspes P.E. & Sweet W.H.) pp. 252−90. Karger, Basel.

Ward J.D., Baker D.P., Miller D., Choi S.C., Marmarou A., Wood C., Newton P.G. & Keenan R. (1985) Failure of prophylactic barbiturate coma in the treatment of severe head injury. *Journal of Neurosurgery* **62**, 383−8.

Acquired Haemostatic Failure

G. DOLAN AND C.D. FORBES

Disorders of blood coagulation may be congenital or acquired, and a detailed history and thorough clinical examination may often distinguish between the two. Although the majority of haemostatic problems which become manifest for the first time in adult life are acquired, it must be remembered that not all patients with a congenital coagulation disorder have a family history, and those with milder forms may not present until challenged by trauma or surgery, e.g. mild haemophilia, Christmas disease or von Willebrand's disease.

Acquired haemostatic failure is the result of a disease process affecting the haemostatic mechanism through one of the following mechanisms:

1 Disorders of synthesis of coagulation factors, e.g. malabsorption states, oral anticoagulants.

2 Increased loss of coagulation factors and platelets through consumption or blood loss, e.g. disseminated intravascular coagulation, cardiopulmonary bypass.

3 Through the production of substances which interfere with the function of coagulation factors, e.g. acquired inhibitors or drugs, or which interfere with platelet function, e.g. fibrinogen degradation products, drugs. Often, a combination of these mechanisms operate.

Clinical history

1 Specific questions about any family history should be asked.

2 The patient should be questioned on any previous haemorrhagic episodes:

(a) Any tendency to easy bruising or prolonged bleeding?

(b) Any haemorrhagic problems after operations, particularly tonsillectomy or dental extractions?

(c) Any episodes of gastrointestinal or genitourinary bleeding including menorrhagia and obstetric blood loss?

3 Systematic enquiry to uncover symptoms of underlying systemic disease such as neoplasms, connective tissue diseases or liver disease should be made.

4 A detailed drug history with specific reference to anticoagulants and antiplatelet drugs should be taken.

Clinical examination

A detailed clinical examination noting the following should be made:

1 Main sites of bleeding, including extent and distribution of skin lesions, mucous membrane bleeding, gastrointestinal bleeding, haematuria, haemoptysis and haemarthroses.

2 Any bleeding from wound sites or venepuncture sites should be noted.

3 If excessive bleeding is noted during surgery, a thorough search for a local bleeding point should be made to distinguish a primary surgical problem from diffuse bleeding.

4 Any evidence of systemic disease such as stigmata of liver disease, evidence of weight loss, abdominal masses, lymphadenopathy, splenomegaly suggestive of neoplasia or skin rashes and joint abnormalities which may suggest connective tissue disease.

5 There may be evidence also of sequelae of previous bleeding, e.g. neurological signs from cerebral bleeds, joint deformity from haemarthroses and other physical signs suggestive of nerve entrapment from haematoma. After completing the initial clinical assessment, the following basic screening investigations should be undertaken.

(a) Full blood count including platelet count and examination of blood film.

(b) Serum urea and creatinine measurements to assess renal function.

(c) Liver function tests.

(d) Further assessment of any abnormality noted

during clinical assessment, e.g. by radiological screening, antinuclear antibody testing or erythrocyte sedimentation rate (ESR) estimation.

Coagulation screen

The screening tests employed commonly in the investigation of coagulation disorders are the prothrombin time (PT), partial thromboplastin time (PTT) and the thrombin clotting time (TCT). These tests are designed to help localize any abnormality in the coagulation pathway into either the extrinsic pathway, intrinsic pathway or common pathway (Fig. 90.1).

Prothrombin time

This involves adding a source of thromboplastin (animal brain usually) and calcium to plasma thus activating Factor VII which activates Factor X. The cascade process continues with Xa and Va converting prothrombin to thrombin which in turn converts fibrinogen to fibrin. Thus, the PT bypasses the intrinsic pathway and is abnormal only with deficiencies of Factors VII, X, V, prothrombin or fibrinogen or if a coagulation inhibitor is present.

Partial thromboplastin time
(or kaolin cephalin clotting time)

In this test, the contact Factors XII and XI are activated by kaolin, and phospholipid accelerates the reactions involving VIII and V. Thus, factor X is activated and is followed by formation of thrombin and fibrin. From the diagram it may be seen that the only factor not involved in this pathway is VII and thus this test gives prolonged times with deficiencies of XII, XI, IX, X, V, prothrombin or fibrinogen or by inhibitors (e.g. heparin).

Thrombin clotting time

This involves adding a source of thrombin to plasma, thus bypassing the extrinsic, intrinsic pathways and common pathways to the level of conversion of fibrinogen to fibrin. The TCT is prolonged with deficiency of fibrinogen or by inhibitors of the fibrinogen to fibrin conversion, e.g. heparin or fibrin degradation products (FDPs).

Information obtained from these tests may help to localize a particular defect into one of the pathways and this may be followed by specific factor assays or inhibitor screens.

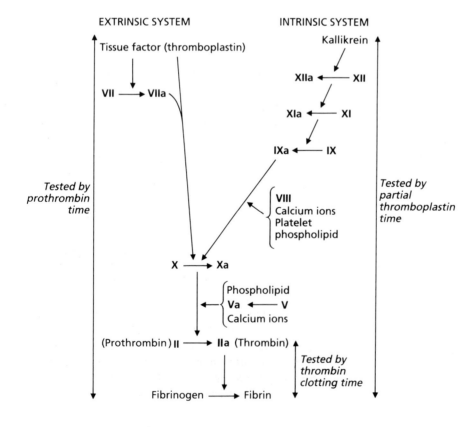

Fig. 90.1 The coagulation system. The addition of the letter 'a' indicates the active form of the coagulation factor.

Classification of acquired haemostatic disorders

Classifications of the acquired haemostatic disorders is complex as, in most instances, several mechanisms are involved. The following discussion is based on the more common situations seen in clinical practice.

Acquired haemostatic disorders:

1 Disseminated intravascular coagulation (DIC).
2 Primary fibrinolytic bleeding.
3 Haemostatic abnormalities associated with vitamin K deficiency.
4 Haemostatic failure associated with liver disease.
5 Haemostatic problems with anticoagulant drugs.
6 Acquired inhibitors of coagulation.
7 Haemostatic defects associated with renal disease.
8 Haemostatic defects associated with massive transfusion.
9 Haemostatic defects associated with cardiopulmonary bypass.
10 Psychogenic bleeding.

Disseminated intravascular coagulation

The haemostatic system is a dynamic one in which, under normal circumstances, there is a balance between intravascular coagulation and fibrinolysis. In DIC, a 'triggering' event occurs which disturbs this balance and leads to activation of the coagulation system with widespread deposition of fibrin and platelets and secondary activation of the fibrinolytic system.

DIC is not a disease or diagnosis in itself but occurs as part of the clinical picture of many diseases.

Pathogenesis

The initial event in the pathogenesis of DIC is activation of the coagulation sequence which may occur through three main triggering events (Muller-Berghaus, 1977).

Release of thromboplastin

This causes activation of the extrinsic system and is a major component of DIC seen in tissue injury (including placental damage) (Page et al., 1951), infection via the action of endotoxins (Cline et al., 1968; Rivers et al., 1975), released from leucocytes and also in disseminated malignancy (Gralnick & Abrell, 1973).

Direct activation of prothrombin and factor X

This is the probable mechanism in DIC seen after some cases of envenomation (Reid, 1984).

Damage of vascular endothelium

Widespread vascular damage occurs in a variety of circumstances which result in activation of Factor XII (Hageman factor) and activation of the intrinsic system (Wilmer et al., 1968). Exposed vascular endothelium also releases tissue thromboplastin and initiates platelet aggregation (Walsh, 1972).

Whatever the mechanism of activation of the coagulation sequence, the result is formation of thrombin. Once thrombin release has occurred, the pathophysiology follows a common pathway (Fig. 90.2).

Circulating thrombin cleaves fibrinopeptides from fibrinogen leaving behind fibrin monomers in the circulation. Most of these polymerize into fibrin in the microvascular circulation leading to microvascular and macrovascular thrombosis. The deposited fibrin in the microcirculation leads also to trapping of platelets and thrombocytopenia (Lasch et al., 1967; Owen et al., 1973).

Meanwhile, plasmin cleaves fibrinogen and fibrin into FDPs. These FDPs complex with fibrin monomers before they can polymerize, thus producing stable fibrin monomers which cannot polymerize (Fletcher et al., 1966; Bang & Chang, 1974; Jakobsen et al., 1974). FDPs have also a high affinity for platelet membranes, and coat the surfaces of platelets to produce significant platelet dysfunction. Thus, in addition to a quantitative deficiency of platelets, there is also a qualitative one (Kopec et al., 1968; Niewiarowski et al., 1972). Plasmin, in addition to degrading fibrin and fibrinogen, also degrades Factors V, VIII, IX and XI, contributing to deficiencies of these factors (Donaldson, 1960; Sharp, 1964; Pechet, 1965). Plasmin also activates the C1 and C3 complement sequence leading to red cell and platelet lysis, increased vascular permeability and shock. The liberation of kinins also contributes to shock (Schreiber & Austen, 1973; Kaplan et al., 1976).

Clinical aspects

DIC may manifest as a catastrophic illness with major haemorrhagic and thrombotic problems or as a chronic form with few clinical problems but which may progress to the acute form.

In the severely ill patient with DIC, general but non-specific signs of fever, hypotension, acidosis, hypoxia and proteinuria may be found. Often, it is not clear to what extent these signs result from the underlying clinical problem rather than to DIC.

More specific signs of coagulation upset such as

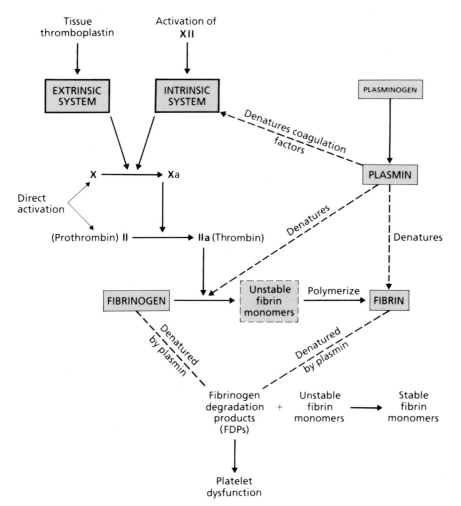

Fig. 90.2 Mechanisms involved in the pathogenesis of DIC.

petechiae and purpura, haemorrhagic bullae, central cyanosis and occasionally frank gangrene may be found.

Any pattern of haemorrhage may be seen but bleeding from several sites is common, especially from wound and venepuncture sites. Haemorrhage into any organ may occur, leading to organ dysfunction. Organ damage may also occur through microvascular and macrovascular thromboses which result in the high incidence of cardiac, pulmonary, renal and CNS dysfunction from ischaemia.

A microangiopathic haemolytic anaemia may result from fragmentation of red cells caused by the fibrin network within the microvasculature (Fig. 90.3).

Disorders associated with DIC

1 Infection.
2 Obstetric complications.
3 Neoplasia.

4 Shock.
5 Hepatic disease.
6 Intravascular haemolysis.
7 Vasculitis.
8 Snake venom.
9 Burns.
10 Extracorporeal circulation.
11 Metabolic diseases, e.g. severe diabetes mellitus hyperlipoproteinaemia.

Infection

Bacterial

Meningococcal septicaemia is the infection classically associated with DIC (McGehee *et al.*, 1967). Endotoxin from Gram-negative organisms can activate Factor XII directly, induce platelet aggregation, cause endothelial sloughing and initiate release of granulocyte procoagulant enzymes (McKay & Shapiro, 1958; Cline

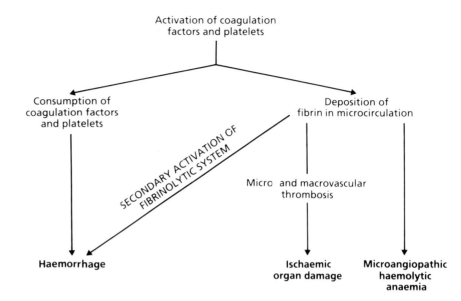

Fig. 90.3 Clinical manifestations of DIC.

et al., 1968). Studies on the mucopolysaccharide coating of Gram-positive organisms have shown similar properties (Cronberg *et al.*, 1973). Many other generalized bacterial infections are associated with DIC.

Viral

Many acute viraemias have been associated with DIC. Those implicated most commonly are varicella, hepatitis and cytomegalovirus. The mechanism is thought to involve antibody−antigen activation of XII, platelet release and endothelial sloughing (McKay & Margaretten, 1967; Wilmer *et al.*, 1968).

Others

Fungal infections, e.g. aspergillosis and candidiasis, rickettsial infections (Lasch *et al.*, 1967) and protozoan infections, e.g. malaria and schistosomiasis (Owen *et al.*, 1973; Bang & Chang, 1974) have all been associated with DIC.

Obstetric complications

Pregnancy may be considered to be a hypercoagulable state with increased concentrations of coagulation factors, depression of the fibrinolytic system and reduced reticuloendothelial clearance of activated coagulation factors all making the mother particularly susceptible to DIC (Kleiner *et al.*, 1970; Muller-Berghaus, 1977; Talbert & Blatt, 1979). Obstetric problems have long been associated with DIC, and in experimental models, DIC appears to be particularly severe in pregnant animals (Muller-Berghaus, 1977).

Placental abruption

Hypofibrinogenaemia is reported to occur in 25% of abruptions, usually within 8 h (Dieckman, 1936; Pritchard & Brekken, 1967). The full-blown picture of acute DIC with haemorrhage and thrombosis is much rarer, presumably from early delivery in such cases. From experimental work in animals, it seems likely that the mechanism involved is thromboplastins reaching the maternal circulation (Schneider, 1951; Cline *et al.*, 1968)

Amniotic fluid embolus

It has been shown that through damage to the uterus and tears in the membranes, amniotic fluid gains access to the maternal circulation (Morgan, 1979; Rushton & Dowson, 1982). The coagulation abnormalities which may follow are ascribed to the thromboplastic activity of amniotic fluid (Courtney & Allington, 1972; Yaffe *et al.*, 1977). Severe DIC may develop with hypofibrinogenaemia, reduced concentration of coagulation factors, thrombocytopenia and enhanced fibrinolysis (Bonnar, 1981). If the patient survives the initial cardiopulmonary collapse associated with embolism of amniotic fluid and fibrin thrombus in the pulmonary circulation, uncontrollable uterine haemorrhage may occur (Wiener & Reid, 1950).

Dead fetus syndrome

Evidence of DIC has been demonstrated in women in whom the fetus has died *in utero*, irrespective of the cause of death. It is thought that the triggering mechanism is the release of necrotic fetal tissues and enzymes acting as thromboplastins (Merskey *et al.*, 1966; Merskey *et al.*, 1967). If a woman retains a dead fetus *in utero* for more than 5 weeks, the incidence of DIC is approximately 30–40% (Pritchard, 1959, 1973), although in modern obstetric practice, this occurs rarely.

Abortion

Septic abortion, now a rarity because of legislative changes and availability of antibiotics, was once a relatively common cause of DIC. A combination of endotoxins and infected uterine tissue acting as thromboplastins being the likely 'triggering' agents (Rubenberg *et al.*, 1967).

Evidence of mild DIC has been shown to occur in some abortions using hypertonic saline and urea. Although there are usually no clinical problems, occasional reports of acute DIC have been made (Spivak *et al.*, 1972; MacKenzie *et al.*, 1975).

Evidence of DIC occurring in late dilatation and evacuation techniques, in addition to use of prostaglandin and oxytocin, has also been published (Davis & Liu, 1972; Grundy & Graven, 1976; Savage, 1982).

Pre-eclampsia and eclampsia

Patients with severe pre-eclampsia and eclampsia have changes consistent with low-grade DIC (Howie *et al.*, 1976; Edgar *et al.*, 1977; Douglas *et al.*, 1982). Thrombocytopenia and decreased titres of clotting factors are present more commonly than elevation of soluble fibrin and FDPs. The exact mechanism of activation of coagulation is not known (Howie *et al.*, 1975).

Neoplasia

Low-grade DIC has long been associated with neoplastic disease, especially disseminated malignancy (Bick, 1978; Goldsmith, 1984). This, however, rarely constitutes a clinical problem unless surgery is contemplated. Nevertheless, the low-grade nature may progress to an acute fulminating process when the disease progresses or with added stress such as infection. The pathogenesis is complex and is thought to involve the synthesis and release of thromboplastins and proteolytic enzymes which may activate coagulation factors and components accelerating the fibrinolytic pathway (Pitney, 1971; Mersky, 1973; Semararo & Donati, 1981). Acute promyelocytic leu-

kaemia, prostatic carcinoma and carcinoma of lung, pancreas and ovary have the strongest associations with DIC.

Shock

Many cases of shock are associated with DIC, especially if produced by trauma (Attar *et al.*, 1966; Hardaway, 1966). It is thought that the main aetiological factor is widespread vascular damage from endotoxin, immune complexes, hypoxia or acidosis. The observations that in shock, thrombocytopenia is common and fibrinogen concentrations are often raised, had led to the postulation that platelet aggregation and microthrombus formation are major 'triggering events' (Hardaway, 1967).

Hepatic disease

DIC is one of the several processes involved in the haemostatic failure associated with liver disease. This is discussed later (p. 1890).

Intravascular haemolysis

Haemolysed red cells have been recognized as a stimulus for DIC since early experimental work began (Krevans *et al.*, 1957). Severe DIC with marked hypofibrinogenaemia and thrombocytopenia has followed haemolytic reactions such as transfusion of incompatible blood (Muirhead, 1951; Langdell & Hedgpeth, 1959; Culpepper, 1975) and near drowning in fresh water (Mannucci *et al.*, 1969). Some workers have postulated that shock accompanying such haemolytic reactions is an important part of the pathogenesis (Crosby & Stefanini, 1952; Willoughby *et al.*, 1972).

Vasculitis

Collagen vascular diseases, haemolytic–uraemic syndrome and thrombotic thrombocytopenia purpura (Moskowitz syndrome) are among the vasculitic processes associated with DIC.

The haemolytic–uraemic syndrome is a disease of childhood in which renal impairment, thrombocytopenia and haemolytic anaemia occur (Brain, 1969; Lieberman, 1972; Willoughby *et al.*, 1972). The aetiological agent is uncertain but is probably of an infective nature. It has been suggested that damage to the vascular endothelium is responsible, possibly causing failure of prostacyclin relase (Remuzzi *et al.*, 1978).

Thrombotic thrombocytopenic purpura is a rare and fatal disorder of adults in which there is acute impairment of the CNS associated with microangiopathic haemolytic anaemia, renal impairment and a degree of DIC (Pisciotta & Goltschall, 1980). The aetiological agent has not been identified and is thought to cause widespread vascular damage (Grain & Chardry, 1981). Treatment is empirical and usually unsuccessful.

Snake venom

Disturbance of the haemostatic system is a well-recognized effect of the venom of members of the Viperidae family. Most of these venoms are strongly procoagulant and may result in defibrination; in addition, increased fibrinolytic activity and thrombocytopenia produced by vascular damage may occur (Warrell *et al.*, 1977; Lee, 1979; Reid, 1984).

Although encountered rarely in a clinical situation in the Western world, intravascular coagulation following snake bite is a more significant cause of morbidity and mortality from acquired haemostatic failure in a worldwide setting.

Laboratory diagnosis

In establishing the presence of DIC, one is aiming to demonstrate evidence of activation of the coagulation system and also of increased fibrinolytic activity. It is, however, important to realize that not all cases of DIC demonstrate the classical coagulation abnormalities.

Investigations may be classified into those that may be performed quickly and those that may provide additional information but which are either not practical or not required immediately (Table 90.1).

Additional tests

Reptilase time

This test is based on the fact that the venom of certain snakes act directly on fibrinogen to form fibrin. This action is not affected by heparin and the reptilase test may be a useful way of determining the contribution of heparin to an abnormal coagulation screen from a subject with multifactorial bleeding. The results are, however, less reliable if the level of FDPs is very high.

Ethanol gelation test (EGT) and the protamine sulphate precipitin test

Both tests detect the presence of fibrin monomer complexes in the blood. The results are non-specific, as fibrin monomer complexes are found also in trauma and infection.

Other abnormalities described in DIC have been reported widely and some of these are included in Table 90.2. Most of these investigations are time consuming, many are provided only in specialist centres and in the majority of cases yield little additional information.

Treatment

Much controversy exists concerning some aspects of the treatment of DIC, and many reports based on anecdotal observations or reports on small numbers

Table 90.1 First-line coagulation investigations in DIC

Investigation	Abnormality	Comment
Haemoglobin estimation	↓	Bleeding ± haemolysis
Platelet count	↓	May be normal in chronic DIC
Prothrombin time	↑	Markedly prolonged in acute DIC May be less so or normal in chronic DIC
Partial thromboplastin time	↑	May be markedly prolonged in acute DIC, less so in chronic DIC
Thrombin clotting time	↑	May be normal, depending on level of fibrinogen
Fibrinogen concentration	↓	May be normal or even increased in some circumstances
Fibrinogen degradation products	↑	Usually increased

↑ Prolonged or increased; ↓ shortened or decreased.

Table 90.2 Some of the abnormalities described in DIC

Assay of Factor V and VIII	Concentrations usually decreased
Factor VIII : C and VIII : RAg	There is often a discrepancy between these values with Factor VIII : C being relatively lower
Euglobulin lysis time	This may be shortened reflecting enhanced fibrinolysis
Fibrinopeptide A Fibrinopeptide B	Levels are elevated and are a sensitive reflection of thrombin generation
B β15–42 fragments	Provide confirmatory evidence of fibrinolysis
Platelet aggregation studies	Almost always abnormal but as there is no classical abnormality in DIC, these are of little diagnostic value
Beta-thromboglobulin (BTG)	Evidence of platelet activation and release of granules
Antithrombin III levels	Low plasma concentration is a common finding in DIC but is also found in many stressful situations. May be of value in monitoring therapy (see later section)

of patients are found in the literature. There are no reports on large controlled clinical trials.

The one point on which there is little disagreement is that the main aim should be to eradicate the underlying cause, as this is the only likely way in which resolution can occur (Cash, 1977; Brozovic, 1981; Preston, 1982; Collen, 1983; Nyman, 1985). Thus, in patients in whom there is evidence of infection, appropriate antibiotics should be administered immediately and in obstetric cases such as abruption, dead fetus syndrome and pre-eclampsia, evacuation of the uterus should be undertaken as soon as is feasible (Sharp *et al.*, 1958; Kleiner *et al.*, 1970; Bailton & Letsky, 1985).

With this single most important point in mind, other steps in management may be classified into:

1 Support of the patient.
2 Replacement therapy.
3 Controlling the haemostatic process.

Support of the patient

Patients with acute DIC are often critically ill, either because of the underlying condition or because of the complications of DIC, and these patients are often to be found in an intensive therapy unit (ITU). The presence of DIC may make management very difficult, e.g. haemorrhage and shock may necessitate transfusion of large volumes of fluid which may be made less feasible if there is impaired cardiac function as a result of ischaemia. Insertion of a central venous or/and arterial catheters which are often required in such patients is made hazardous by the haemorrhagic tendency.

Adequate oxygenation may be difficult to achieve

because of adult respiratory distress syndrome (ARDS) which has a strong but unclear association with DIC, and even if adequate arterial oxygenation is achieved, micro- and macrovascular thromboses may prevent adequate tissue oxygenation.

Attention to acid–base balance is also important because of the increased risk of thrombosis associated with acidosis (Beller, 1971; Bell, 1980).

Replacement therapy (see Chapter 27)

The authors recommend that despite abnormal results of coagulation screens, replacement of coagulation factors by blood products is not indicated unless uncontrolled bleeding occurs and the precipitating cause cannot be dealt with quickly (Bick *et al.*, 1976; Collen, 1983). The transfused factors and platelets may be of only temporary benefit if the consumption process is on-going and the balance of the haemostatic system may be further upset by adding 'fuel to the fire' (Preston, 1982; Prentice, 1985).

When heavy bleeding does occur, transfusion of blood and the following blood products may be useful:

Platelets

Transfusions of platelets are given usually if the platelet count is below 30×10^9/litre. It may be helpful to recheck the platelet count 1 h after transfusion to confirm that an increment has been achieved, as in some cases transfused platelets are consumed quickly and further therapy is likely to be useless unless the coagulation process is controlled.

Even when the platelet count remains above this

value, there is likely to be significant platelet dysfunction as the concentration of FDPs is high and transfused platelets are also likely to be affected in this circumstance (Kopec *et al.*, 1968; Niewiarowski *et al.*, 1972).

Fresh frozen plasma

Fresh frozen plasma (FFP) contains all the non-cellular coagulation factors including fibrinogen at a concentration which is less than that of normal plasma. FFP is useful as replacement therapy and also as a plasma expander. However, as the volumes required to maintain adequate levels of coagulation factors can be large, the practical applications are limited because of the risk of circulatory overload.

Cryoprecipitate

Cryoprecipitate provides a more concentrated source of fibrinogen and also of factor VIII. The actual concentrations vary (see Chapter 29). Cryoprecipitate is more useful in situations where hypofibrinogenaemia is marked. The volume of cryoprecipitate required for any given situation should be determined by measuring serum fibrinogen concentrations after transfusion, aiming for a plasma level within the normal range.

Stopping the coagulation process

Inhibitors of coagulation are used in some cases of DIC in the hope that the coagulation process can be halted, thus abolishing the stimulus to compensatory fibrinolysis and allowing resolution of the DIC process.

Heparin

The rationale for using heparin in DIC is that it augments the role of antithrombin III in inhibiting Factor Xa and thrombin, thus counteracting the acceleration of blood coagulation produced by thromboplastin release and thrombin formation in the circulation.

However, the use of heparin remains controversial (Brodsky & Siegel, 1970; Corrigan & Jordan, 1970; Deykin, 1970; Lawrence, 1971; Colman *et al.*, 1972) because of the lack of consistent response, lack of controlled clinical trials (Prentice, 1976) and the risk that heparin merely adds to the bleeding risk (Klein & Bell, 1974; Mant & King, 1979). Although used enthusiastically by earlier clinicians, its use is not

standard practice nowadays, and at present the decision as to whether or not to use heparin should be based on each individual case and on what the most likely triggering event is. Its use should be confined to those patients with no fresh wounds or raw surfaces from which haemorrhage may occur. Amniotic fluid embolus, some cases of shock including septicaemia, some cases of neoplasia and in patients in whom thrombosis is a major feature are conditions in which heparin may be less hazardous.

One recommended regimen is a bolus of 5000 units and 1000 units/h as a continuous infusion (Prentice, 1985) and serial measurements of fibrinogen and platelet count should be made to assess efficacy (Wilmer *et al.*, 1968; Gralnick & Abrell, 1973; Reid, 1984).

Antithrombin III

Considerable interest in using antithrombin III as a replacement therapy in DIC has been aroused following reports of successful treatment in small groups of patients.

Antithrombin concentrations are usually low in DIC and it is thought that by increasing these by infusion, deceleration of the coagulation process may be brought about by inhibition of Xa.

The attraction of this form of therapy is that it does not carry the same risk of bleeding as with heparin, and it is likely that it will be employed more as supplies become more available, although controlled clinical trials are required to justify widespread use (Schipper *et al.*, 1978; Laursen *et al.*, 1981; Blauhut *et al.*, 1982; Hellegren *et al.*, 1984).

Antiplatelet agents

Antiplatelet agents, e.g. prostacyclin, have aroused some interest which has been encouraged by occasional reports of successful treatment in haemolytic–uraemic syndrome and thrombotic thrombocytopenic purpura, and it may be that in cases where platelet aggregation is thought to be the main triggering event this would be useful.

Primary fibrinolytic bleeding

In DIC, increased fibrinolysis occurs secondary to increased intravascular coagulation. In some circumstances, fibrinolysis is increased by activation of plasminogen without evidence of intravascular coagulation (Fig. 90.4).

Primary fibrinolysis has been described in

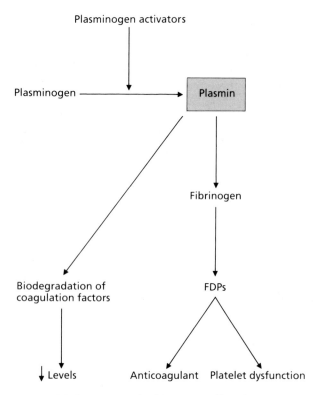

Fig. 90.4 Mechanisms involved in primary fibrinolysis.

association with neoplastic disease (Davidson *et al.*, 1969), and some tumours are thought to produce plasminogen activator.

Conditions in which primary fibrinolysis may be found

1 Carcinoma of prostrate (Tagnon *et al.*, 1952).
2 Carcinoma of pancreas (Ratnoff, 1952).
3 Acute leukaemias (Pisciotta & Schultz, 1955).
4 Systemic lupus erythematosus (SLE) (Zwicka *et al.*, 1961).
5 Hepatic cirrhosis (Grossi *et al.*, 1961; Fletcher *et al.*, 1964).

   Laboratory tests of coagulation may be very similar to those seen in DIC, and although a low platelet count is not usual in primary fibrinolysis, it may occur as a complication of the underlying disorder, e.g. cirrhosis, leukaemia. Time-consuming and elaborate tests measuring concentrations of coagulation factors and assessing fibrinolysis and its products may be required to distinguish between the two.

   This is of some clinical relevance in that if there is strong evidence of primary fibrinolysis, fibrinolytic inhibitors such as ε-amino-caproic acid (EACA) and tranexamic acid (cylocapron) may be of considerable benefit in controlling haemorrhage.

EACA acts as a competitive or non-competitive inhibitor of plasminogen, depending on the concentration. It is usually given orally at a dose of 3 g 6-hourly. Tranexamic acid has a similar action and may be given orally or intravenously. The use of these drugs may be hazardous in DIC, as unlysable thrombus may form in vessels or, in the presence of haematuria, unlysable fibrin clot may obstruct the urinary tract.

Haemostatic abnormalities associated with vitamin K deficiency

The vitamin K-dependent clotting Factors II, VII, IX and X undergo γ-carboxylation to form γ-carboxy-glutamic acid residue forms in order to develop calcium-binding properties which are essential for their normal activity (Hemker *et al.*, 1963; Nelsestuen *et al.*, 1974). Vitamin K acts as a cofactor in this carboxylation reaction (Fig. 90.5).

   Vitamin K is not synthesized by the body but is obtained from green vegetables and vitamin K-producing intestinal bacteria, and, being lipid soluble, requires the presence of bile salts in the small intestine for its absorption (Udall, 1956; Shearer *et al.*, 1980).

   Deficiencies of active vitamin K dependent clotting factors occur in the following circumstances.
1 Reduced availability of vitamin K, e.g. reduced dietary intake or use of antibiotics interfering with intestinal supply.
2 Malabsorption of vitamin K as in complete biliary obstruction or intestinal disease.
3 Failure of utilization as in common anticoagulant therapy or hepatic disease.
4 Very rarely, congenital deficiency from enzyme deficiency.

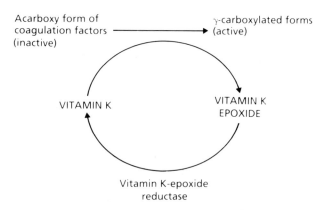

Fig. 90.5 Activation of vitamin K-dependent coagulation factors.

The following discussion considers the most common clinical examples:

Haemorrhagic disease of the newborn

The levels of the vitamin K-dependent clotting factors are decreased in the neonate and availability of vitamin K is low because human milk is a poor dietary source and the intestine has not yet been colonized by bacteria (Foley *et al.*, 1977; Donaldson, 1984).

This may cause a haemorrhagic tendency with bleeding from the umbilicus, gastrointestinal tract or intracranial bleeding. The bleeding problem can be corrected by parenteral administration of vitamin K, 1 mg 8-hourly, until coagulation returns to normal (Lucey & Dolan, 1958; Donaldson, 1984).

Malabsorption states

Malabsorption of vitamin K may result from:

Intestinal disease. Vitamin K deficiency may be part of a malabsorption syndrome with wide-ranging clinical features, e.g. coeliac disease, inflammatory bowel disease, intestinal surgery.

Biliary disease. In obstructive jaundice, there is a lack of bile salts in the small intestine and consequent malabsorption of vitamin K.

Inadequate intake. Patients with a poor diet for a long period of time may become deficient in vitamin K though this is rare and is usually accompanied by either surgery or prolonged use of broad spectrum antibiotics.

Coumarin-like anticoagulants

These drugs, the most commonly used being warfarin, antagonize the action of vitamin K thus blocking the β-carboxylation of the vitamin K-dependent clotting factors (see later section) (Muller-Berghaus, 1977).

Hepatic disease

The titres of vitamin K-dependent clotting factors are reduced in parenchymal liver disease, and utilization of vitamin K in carboxylation reaction is also defective (Goodnight *et al.*, 1971; Lechner, 1972).

Clinical features

There may be no bleeding problems despite an abnormal coagulation screen, or there may be multiple bruises and bleeding from mucous membranes, gastrointestinal, genitourinary tract or any other pattern of bleeding.

Of more immediate relevance is the need to treat any deficiency if surgery is contemplated, e.g. relief of biliary obstruction or intestinal surgery, or before liver biopsy.

Laboratory features

The defect in coagulation from vitamin K deficiency affects both the extrinsic and intrinsic pathways but does not cause a prolongation of TCT nor does it affect the platelet count (Table 90.3).

Treatment

If no bleeding occurs, parenteral vitamin K, 10 mg, should be given. This increases the concentrations of clotting factors and corrects the PT within 4–6 h.

If the patient is bleeding heavily and more rapid correction is required, transfusion of FFP or factor concentrates may be required. Vitamin K is required also for the γ-carboxylation of Protein C and Protein S which both inhibit the active forms of V and VIII. The activity of both these decrease in vitamin K deficiency leading to a potential thrombotic state which may be important when considering the action of coumarins.

Haemostatic failure associated with liver disease

The liver is thought to be the main site of synthesis of fibrinogen, Factors II, VII, IX, X, V, XI, XII, XIII in addition to plasminogen, antithrombin III and inhibitors of fibrinolysis. It follows that hepatocellular

Table 90.3 Coagulation test abnormalities in vitamin K deficiency

Investigation	Abnormality
Prothrombin time	↑
Partial thromboplastin time	↑
Thrombin clotting time	Normal
Fibrinogen	Normal
Platelet count	Normal

↑ Prolonged.

disease may cause a significant haemostatic defect which may involve several mechanisms (Ratnoff, 1963; Walls & Lavarsky, 1971; Roberts & Lederbaum, 1972; Duckert, 1973; Bloom, 1977; Shaw *et al.*, 1979; Flute, 1982).

Failure of synthesis of coagulation factors

Vitamin K-dependent clotting factor

As mentioned in the previous section, low titres of II, VII, IX and X are found as a result of decreased synthesis of protein precursors (Goodnight *et al.*, 1971; Lechner, 1972). This may be associated with vitamin K deficiency and there may also be defective utilization of vitamin K (Mann, 1952; Spector & Corn, 1967; Blanchard *et al.*, 1981).

Factor V deficiency

As with vitamin K-dependent clotting factors, low titres of V are found in a wide range of acute and chronic liver disorders (Owren, 1949; Rapaport *et al.*, 1960; Giddings *et al.*, 1975; Cederblad *et al.*, 1976) but not in obstructive jaundice, primary biliary cirrhosis or metastatic liver disease (Quick *et al.*, 1935; Owren, 1949; Rapaport *et al.*, 1960). Factor V contributes to the prolonged PT and PTT but its contribution to the bleeding tendency is perhaps less important, as patients with congenital factor V deficiency have lower concentrations of Factor V usually and have only a mild bleeding tendency.

In addition, defective synthesis, increased consumption in intravascular coagulation and plasmin degradation may occur.

Other factors

Deficiencies of XI, XII and XIII have been demonstrated in acute and chronic hepatic disorders but it is not thought that these are significant clinically (Hathaway & Alsever, 1970; Lechner *et al.*, 1977; Saito *et al.*, 1978).

Fibrinogen (Factor I)

The normal concentration of fibrinogen in plasma is 1.5–4.0 g/litre. This is synthesized by the liver and the concentration varies with stress (Miller *et al.*, 1951; Miller & Bale, 1954; Ratnoff, 1980a).

Plasma fibrinogen concentrations are not usually decreased in liver disease and are often normal or increased although the increase in fibrinogen in response to stress may be impaired in cirrhosis (Ratnoff, 1954; Volwiler *et al.*, 1955; Bergstorm *et al.*, 1960; von Felten *et al.*, 1969; Green *et al.*, 1977; Lipinski *et al.*, 1977; Higuchi *et al.*, 1980). Severe hypofibrinogenaemia is found usually as a near terminal phenomenon as in fulminant hepatitis when it may be a result of decreased synthesis, increased consumption in DIC, increased fibrinolysis or loss in massive haemorrhage.

Acquired dysfibrinogenaemia may be present at an early stage of a wide range of hepatic disorders including cirrhosis, hepatic carcinoma, severe acute hepatitis and chronic aggressive hepatitis but is reported to be rare in metastatic liver disease (Ham & Curtis, 1938; Hallen & Nilsson, 1964; Horder, 1969; Grun *et al.*, 1974; Hillenbrand *et al.*, 1974; Rubin *et al.*, 1978). The pathogenesis of this acquired defect is not clear but the end-result is reduced aggregation of fibrin monomers. This phenomenon may contribute to a bleeding tendency, although patients with congenital dysfibrinogenaemia tend to have a mild bleeding tendency.

Disseminated intravascular coagulation

In liver disease, several factors may be present which may encourage DIC. These include:
1 Reduced hepatic or reticuloendothelial clearance of activated coagulation factors (Ratnoff, 1991).
2 Decreased clearance of plasminogen activator (Murray-Lyon *et al.*, 1972; Ratnoff, 1991).
3 Decreased titres of antithrombin III (Damus & Wallace, 1975).
4 Decreased synthesis of fibrinolytic system inhibitors (Aoki & Yamanaka, 1978).

The triggering event may be necrotic hepatocytes acting as thromboplastins (Verstraete *et al.*, 1974), endotoxins (Wardle, 1974) or some other factor.

Intravascular infusion of ascitic fluid as occurs in systems such as the Le Veen shunt is also known to cause DIC (Lerner *et al.*, 1978; Harmon *et al.*, 1979).

Despite the great interest in the role of DIC in liver disease, firm laboratory support for the presence of DIC is not found in many patients with acute or chronic liver disease (Gralnick & Abrell, 1973; Rivers *et al.*, 1975; Reid, 1984). Assessment is made more difficult because reduced titres of coagulation factors and thrombocytopenia may already be present in liver disease (Ratnoff, 1991).

Disorders of platelets

Thrombocytopenia is common in liver disease, and

although the concentration is rarely low enough to cause spontaneous haemorrhage, bleeding from local lesions, e.g. varices or erosions, may be made worse and surgical procedures made more hazardous (Lasch *et al.*, 1967; Walsh, 1972; Owen *et al.*, 1973; Bang & Chang, 1974).

Causes of thrombocytopenia include:

1 Splenic sequestration from portal hypertension (Tocantins, 1948; Aster, 1966).

2 Decreased production because of concurrent folic acid deficiency in alcoholics (Jandl & Lear, 1956).

3 Decreased production through marrow suppression by alcohol (Larkin & Watson-Williams, 1984).

In addition to the quantitative defect in platelets described, various qualitative defects have been reported, although the clinical significance is not clear (Thomas *et al.*, 1967; Ballard & Marcus, 1976; Rubin *et al.*, 1977).

The coagulation screen may become abnormal before any other liver function test result, as in paracetamol poisoning where the PT is used to detect early liver damage.

PT is also the minimum investigation that should be undertaken prior to liver biopsy. If the PT is more than 1.5 times the control value, bleeding problems are likely after biopsy (Table 90.4).

Treatment

Vitamin K_1 should be administered, as deficiency may represent part of the defect. Ten mg each day for 3 days should be tried, although this is often only partially successful.

Management of patients with a haemostatic defect is aimed at supporting them until resolution of the underlying disease process. However, such patients have often a source of bleeding which may be aggravated by a haemostatic defect such as oesophageal varices, gastric erosions, peptic ulcers or require liver biopsy or surgery. In such circumstances, transfusion of FFP may be useful, although this may have to be repeated to maintain haemostasis.

Platelet transfusions may be beneficial because of thrombocytopenia and a qualitative defect, but the benefit may be short-lived if there is hypersplenism.

A prolonged TCT may indicate a qualitative or quantitative defect in fibrinogen and cryoprecipitate transfusion may be given.

If the patient is gravely ill, bleeding and cannot tolerate large volumes of fluid as may occur in advanced liver failure, activated prothrombin complex (contains Factors II, IX and X concentrate) may be given, although the risk of precipitating DIC is high.

Haemostatic problems with anticoagulant drugs

Heparin

There are several ways in which heparin can influence the coagulation system. The most important of these is its potentiation of the inhibition of Factors XIIa, XIa, IXa, Xa and thrombin by the plasma cofactor antithrombin III (Fig. 90.6).

Heparin is used widely in the prophylaxis and treatment of venous thromboembolism and is used also in extracorporeal circulations.

The main side-effect of heparin is bleeding, the risk of which is dependent on the following:

Table 90.4 Coagulation test abnormalities in liver disease

Investigation	Abnormality	Cause
Prothrombin time	↑	Reduced synthesis of factors Defective utilization of vitamin K
Partial thromboplastin time	↑	Consumption in DIC Plasmin degradation
Thrombin clotting time	↑	Dysfibrinogenaemia Hypofibrinogenaemia
Fibrinogen	May be low in advanced liver disease	Consumption in DIC
Platelets	↓	Splenic sequestration Decreased production

↑ Prolonged; ↓ decreased.

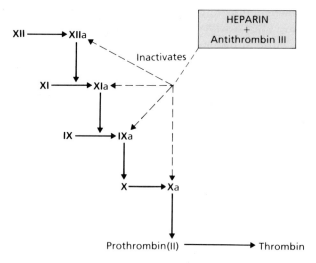

Fig. 90.6 The increased rate of inactivation of activated coagulation factors by the interaction of heparin and antithrombin III.

Dose

When low doses of heparin are used, as in prophylaxis of venous thrombosis, the risk of bleeding is low unless some other risk factor is present. The risk of bleeding is higher with increased anticoagulant effect (American Heart Association, 1973; Norman & Provan, 1977; Wilson & Lampman, 1979).

Route of administration

The risk of bleeding is lowest with subcutaneous administration, and incidence of bleeding is higher when intravenous intermittent administration is used compared with intravenous continuous infusion. This may be related also to the total dose delivered (Salzman *et al.*, 1975; Glazier & Cravell, 1976; Mant *et al.*, 1977; Wilson & Lampman, 1979).

Patient's characteristics

1 Risk of bleeding is increased in elderly patients, especially women (Jick *et al.*, 1968; O'Sullivan *et al.*, 1968; Viweg *et al.*, 1970; Glazier & Cravell, 1976; Wilson & Lampman, 1979).
2 Risk is increased if there is recent trauma or surgery (Salzman *et al.*, 1975; Wilson & Lampman, 1979).
3 Risk is increased if there is any other haemostatic defect (Pitney *et al.*, 1970).
4 Risk is increased if antiplatelet drugs are administered (Pitney *et al.*, 1970).
5 As heparin is metabolized by both the liver and

kidneys, any decrease in function may lead to prolonged half-life (Pitney *et al.*, 1970).

To reduce the risk of bleeding, the effect of heparin should be monitored carefully.

Monitoring therapy

In the past, the whole-blood clotting time was used as the method of monitoring heparin. Nowadays, measuring the activated partial thromboplastin time (APTT) or heparin level by protamine titration are the preferred methods.

Using the APTT method, the result is often expressed as a ratio compared to a control sample. The therapeutic range should be 1.5—2.0.

If the protamine titration method is used, the heparin concentration should be 0.3—0.5 units/ml (Hirsch, 1986).

Treatment of bleeding

If any invasive procedure is contemplated on a patient who is heparinized fully by infusion, heparin should be discontinued for 1—2 h before and after the procedure. As the half-life of heparin is 60 min, this should be sufficient to allow the coagulation system to return to normal. Also, if bleeding occurs during heparin administration and is mild and controlled easily, all that is required is to discontinue the heparin or reduce the dose.

With more severe bleeding, however, heparin should be neutralized by slow intravenous injection of protamine sulphate depending on the dose and time of administration of heparin. If protamine is given within minutes of an intravenous bolus of heparin, protamine sulphate, 1 mg/100 units heparin, should be given; if 30 min after, protamine sulphate, 0.5 mg/100 units heparin, should be given; if 2 h after, protamine sulphate, 0.25 mg/100 units heparin, should be given.

Protamine has anticoagulant properties *in vitro* (Ollendorff, 1962) but it is unlikely that enough would be administered in error to produce any clinical problem.

In the rare case of bleeding occurring after subcutaneous administration of heparin (usually associated with some other risk factor), repeated doses of protamine may be required, as heparin continues to be absorbed for 8—12 h afterwards. In this circumstance, 50% of the calculated dose of protamine should be given and repeated 3-hourly.

If bleeding persists or is marked, a coagulation screen including PT, APTT, TCT, reptilase time and platelet count should be measured, as there may be another cause for bleeding.

Thrombocytopenia is a well-recognized complication of heparin therapy and two distinct patterns may be seen. The more common form has been reported to occur in up to 30% of patients receiving heparin and causes a mild, reversible thrombocytopenia which is rarely of any clinical significance. The much rarer but potentially devastating antibody-mediated thrombocytopenia causes a marked drop in the platelet count and may be accompanied by arterial thrombosis due to aggregation of circulating platelets (Kelton & Levine, 1986). Bleeding problems are less common despite the sometimes marked thrombocytopenia.

It is therefore essential that patients on heparin therapy should have platelet counts checked, particularly between 6 and 12 days after starting treatment. If severe or progressive thrombocytopenia is found, heparin should be stopped and alternative forms of anticoagulation introduced.

Warfarin and related drugs

These drugs are derived from hydroxycoumarin and have a similar structure to vitamin K. Their anticoagulant action is complex and involves interfering with the cyclic interconversion of vitamin K and its 2,3-epoxide vitamin K form (Fig. 90.7).

The net result is that coagulation Factors II, VII, IX and X are not carboxylated and therefore not activated. The most widely used of these drugs is warfarin whose absorption, metabolism, excretion and bioavailability varies widely between individuals and is influenced greatly by drug therapy, disease and diet.

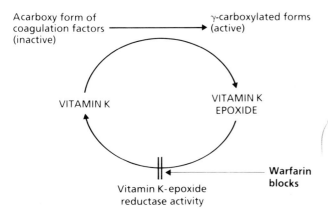

Fig. 90.7 Site of activation of warfarin.

Its main uses are in the treatment and prophylaxis of venous thromboembolism, valvular and arterial thromboses and vascular disease.

Bleeding is the main risk during warfarin therapy and may result from overdose, potentiation by other drugs, change in patient's clinical condition such as liver disease or habits, e.g. increased alcohol intake. Bleeding may be aggravated also in a pre-existing lesion such as peptic ulcer disease, even though the level of anticoagulation is well within the therapeutic range.

Monitoring

Warfarin therapy is monitored by measuring the PT, comparing the result to an international standard and expressing the result as a ratio, the international normalized ratio (INR). Previous methods were British comparative ratios (BCR) and Thrombotest.

The therapeutic range for INR is 2.0–4.5, depending on the clinical indication (British Society of Haematology, 1990).

Treatment of bleeding

When bleeding occurs, restoration of plasma levels of the vitamin-K dependent factors may be achieved by intravenous infusion of concentrates containing II, VII, IX and X. Alternatively, in non-urgent situations, intravenous vitamin K_1 may be used, though this may take up to 6 h to be effective. However, one has to take into account the possible risk of transmission of disease using blood products and the possible overcorrection of anticoagulation by vitamin K_1 which makes reintroduction of treatment very difficult for several days.

In patients who have a very long PT, reflected by an INR above the therapeutic range and who do not bleed, it is usually safe to stop warfarin for 24–48 h and restart at a lower dose. If the INR is above 7.0, one would consider giving 0.5–1 mg of vitamin K_1 orally or intravenously.

If bleeding occurs but is not life-threatening and the patients need to remain on anticoagulants, e.g. those patients with prosthetic heart valves, FFP should be given. This produces haemostatic levels of the vitamin K-dependent factors but this may have to be repeated.

In those who bleed and who do not require to remain on anticoagulants, vitamin K_1, 10 mg, should be given intravenously. This is effective within 8 h, and FFP may be required to secure haemostasis in the intervening period. Patients who have taken a massive overdose of warfarin may require repeated injections.

Those patients who cannot tolerate the fluid load of FFP may be given activated prothrombin complexes. This produces haemostatic levels of II, IX and X but carries a risk of causing thrombosis and carries also a risk of DIC.

Thrombolytic drugs

At present, the main thrombolytic drugs in clinical use are streptokinase, prepared from β-haemolytic streptococci, urokinase prepared from cultures of human fetal kidney cells and tissue-type plasminogen activator (t-PA) which is produced by recombinant DNA technology.

Streptokinase forms an active complex with plasminogen and this in turn converts plasminogen to plasmin (Kaplan *et al.*, 1978) (Fig. 90.8). Urokinase and t-PA activate plasminogen in a more direct manner. As streptokinase is antigenic, a loading dose of around 250 000 units is usually required to neutralize naturally occurring antibodies. This is followed by continuous intravenous infusion of 100 000 units/h to achieve a systemic thrombolytic state. Treatment with streptokinase is continued for 3—7 days during which time, antibodies will develop to the drug and limit its effectiveness. In recent years, however, especially in acute arterial ischaemia, e.g. myocardial infarction, much larger doses are given in a shorter period of time to promote maximal thrombolysis as quickly as possible. Both streptokinase and urokinase are relatively non-specific thrombolytic agents and produce a greater systemic effect on coagulation parameters than t-PA which is more clot specific. There is at present no consensus view as to how to monitor thrombolytic therapy, as there is poor correlation between laboratory parameters of systemic fibrinolysis, and the incidence of bleeding or thrombus resolution (Marder *et al.*, 1977; Marder, 1979).

As may be seen from Table 90.5, shortened whole-blood or euglobulin clot lysis time occurs, and reduction in plasma fibrinogen and coagulation factors (V and VIII) leads to prolongation of the PT, PTT and TCT. Elevated concentrations of FDPs may also contribute to these abnormalities. Reduced plasminogen and antiplasmin concentrations are also the result of enhanced fibrinolysis.

Table 90.5 Coagulation changes found during thrombolytic therapy with streptokinase and urokinase

Investigation	Result
Prothrombin time	↑
Partial thromboplastin time	↑
Thrombin clotting time	↑
Plasma fibrinogen	↓
Fibrin degradation products	↑
Euglobulin lysis time	Shortened
Whole-blood clot lysis time	Shortened
Plasminogen concentrations	↓
Antiplasmin concentrations	↓

↑ Prolonged or increased; ↓ decreased.

Bleeding problems

Patients should be selected carefully for thrombolytic therapy and should have a strong clinical indication for its use (e.g. pulmonary embolism) and should have no lesion from which bleeding may occur (e.g. recent operation, peptic ulcer).

The most common form of bleeding seen during therapy is oozing from venepuncture site or other small wound site. This may be controlled using local pressure. If more severe bleeding occurs or bleeding into any organ is suspected, therapy is stopped immediately and the patient is given transfusion of blood. Transfusion of cryoprecipitate, as a source of fibrinogen and FFP as a source of coagulation factors and antiplasmin may be required. If this is not effective, intravenous administration of antifibrinolytic agents such as EACA or tranexamic acid reverses the fibrinolytic state more rapidly. However, this is rarely required.

The efficacy and safety of the newer thrombolytic agents such as tissue-type plasminogen activator (t-PA), acylated streptokinase—plasminogen complex and single-chain urokinase-type plasminogen activator or prourokinase (scuPA) are *still* being evaluated in world-wide trials.

Antiplatelet agents

The most commonly used drug therapeutically is aspirin. The major effect of this drug is irreversible

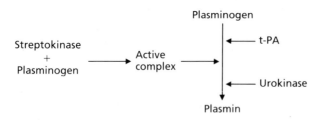

Fig. 90.8 Plasminogen activation by thrombolytic drugs.

acetylation of platelet cyclo-oxygenase with inhibition of synthesis of thromboxane A_2. This impairs platelet aggregation and in turn impairs haemostasis (Roth & Majevus, 1975; O'Grady et al., 1980).

As acetylation is irreversible, this defect remains for the duration of platelet lifespan, approximately 7–11 days. With otherwise normal haemostasis, however, the clinical risk of bleeding is small, and even with wounds, prolonged oozing is the only usual problem.

However, where there is another defect of haemostasis, e.g. heparin therapy, haemophilia or thrombocytopenia, bleeding may be severe, and treatment for the underlying disorder in addition to platelet transfusions may be required.

Prostacyclin infusions prevent platelets adhering to endothelial surfaces and may cause bleeding through this effect. If serious bleeding does occur, stopping the infusion should be sufficient, as prostacyclin has a very short half-life.

Acquired inhibitors of coagulation

Autoantibodies against coagulation factors may arise in patients with a congenital deficiency who have been treated with factor concentrates or may arise in individuals who have had no previous haemorrhagic problems (Shapiro, 1975; Green & Lechner, 1981).

Several specific inhibitors have been described, the most common and most clinically important being Factor VIII inhibitors.

Factor VIII inhibitors

Five to ten percent of patients with haemophilia A develop factor VIII inhibitors (Shapiro, 1975). These inhibitors are usually IgG or IgM antibodies and are more frequently seen in severe haemophiliacs. They also tend to persist. Haemophiliacs with inhibitors can be divided into:

1 *High responders.* In these patients, the inhibitor concentration is high and Factor VIII treatment tends to be unsuccessful and may produce an amnesic response. The titre may diminish if Factor VIII therapy is withheld but recurs after subsequent rechallenge.

2 *Low responders.* The concentrations of inhibitor is low and does not tend to increase after exposure to Factor VIII. These patients may be treated with high doses of Factor VIII.

Low responders may be managed successfully through operations or injuries using high doses of Factor VIII and rechecking the plasma concentration regularly. However, high responders are a considerable problem, and high-dose Factor VIII is rarely enough to ensure haemostasis. Other options for these patients include plasmapheresis, high purity porcine Factor VIII or prothrombin complex concentrates.

Factor VIII inhibitors have also been described in non-haemophiliac patients with a variety of clinical problems and in whom the pathogenesis is not clear:

1 Postpartum women (Voke & Letsky, 1977; Reece et al., 1982).
2 Drug reactions (particularly ampicillin and penicillin) (Allain et al., 1981; Green & Lechner, 1981).
3 Autoimmune disorders, e.g. SLE, rheumatoid arthritis (Shapiro, 1975; Green & Lechner, 1981).
4 Neoplastic disease, particularly lymphoproliferative disorders (Green & Lechner, 1981).
5 Apparently normal individuals (Shapiro, 1975; Allain et al., 1981; Green & Lechner, 1981).

In almost all of these cases, the inhibitor is discovered during investigation of haemorrhagic problems. The cause is variable and the inhibition may disappear spontaneously or with immunosuppressive treatment. If bleeding occurs, treatment with Factor VIII concentrate or prothrombin complex concentrates may be successful (Voke & Letsky, 1977; Green & Lechner, 1981; Spero et al., 1981).

Laboratory diagnosis

If a Factor VIII inhibitor is present, the PTT is prolonged and the clotting activity of Factor VIII (VIII : C) is low. When normal plasma is added to the plasma of a patient with an VIII inhibitor, these tests do not correct whereas in a patient with a pure deficiency state, they do correct. Further specialized assays can then measure the titre of the inhibitor (Table 90.6).

Lupus anticoagulant

Lupus anticoagulants are inhibitors which are directed against phospholipids and inhibit the interaction between the complex of (Xa, V, phospholipid and calcium ions) and prothrombin.

Lupus anticoagulant may be found in SLE, other autoimmune disorders and some haematological malignancies, but often no underlying disease state can be found (Schleider et al., 1976; Shapiro & Thiagarjan, 1982).

In laboratory screening tests, the most common finding is a prolonged PTT which is not corrected by addition of normal plasma. However, despite this prolongation of the PTT, bleeding is a rare event

Table 90.6 Features of other acquired inhibitors

Inhibitors	Coagulation abnormality	Features
IX	Partial thromboplastin time ↑	1–3% of patients with haemophilia B Acquired inhibitor in non-haemophiliac very rare
von Willebrand	Partial thromboplastin time ↑ Platelet dysfunction	Rare in patients with vW treated with cryoprecipitate Very rare in non-affected individuals
V	Prothrombin time ↑ Partial thromboplastin time ↑	Rare, usually occurs in previously normal individuals following surgery or antibiotics Usually mild bleeding problems
XII XI	Partial thromboplastin time ↑	Rare, may occur together Few bleeding problems
XIII	Unstable fibrin clot	Rare but may cause persistent and severe bleeding
Inhibitors directed at fibrinogen	May have: Prothrombin time ↑ Partial thromboplastin time ↑ Thrombin clotting time ↑	Rare Usually only mild bleeding tendency

↑ Prolonged.

unless some other haemostatic defect is present. The more common associated defects are thrombocytopenia and hypoprothrombinaemia.

Thrombotic events and recurrent abortions in pregnant patients are the more common clinical problems and these cases may be treated with immunosuppressants and anticoagulants (Carreras *et al.*, 1981; Scott, 1981; Shapiro & Thiagarjan, 1982).

Haemostatic defects associated with renal disease

Acute and chronic renal failure may be associated with haemostatic abnormalities which cause bleeding such as epistaxes and excess bruising, although occasionally more serious haemorrhage occurs. Even though clinical problems with bleeding are usually trivial, the problem assumes more importance when the patient with renal failure is faced with an operation or when an ill patient develops renal failure and needs a biopsy for proper assessment.

The most important haemostatic defect in renal failure is acquired platelet abnormalities (Rabiner, 1972b). Other potential problems are coagulation factor deficiencies and DIC.

Platelet abnormalities

Thrombocytopenia is a well-recognized finding in renal failure and may occur through several mechanisms.

1 Uraemia may lead to depression of megakaryocyte production, thus causing decreased platelet production.

2 Thrombocytopenia may occur as a prominent feature of the underlying condition causing renal failure, e.g. thrombotic thrombocytopenic purpura, haemolytic–uraemic syndrome, pre-eclamptic toxaemia. In these examples, much attention has been directed to the role of prostacyclin in pathogenesis.

3 Consumption of platelets may occur if DIC supervenes when septicaemia or some other problem develops.

Thrombocytopenia may develop with the use of heparin in dialysis.

Although thrombocytopenia is a well-recognized finding in renal failure, platelet count is a poor predictor of the risk of bleeding in these patients, and serious haemorrhage may occur with normal platelet counts (Rabiner, 1972a).

The major haemostatic defect associated with renal failure is abnormality of platelet function. Most *in vitro* tests of platelet function are abnormal (Remuzzi, 1988; George & Shattil, 1991). The bleeding time is commonly prolonged and there may be bleeding problems of varying severity. Prolonged bleeding times in uraemic patients may be temporarily corrected by:

1 Dialysis (Remuzzi, 1988).

2 Correction of anaemia (George & Shattil, 1991).

3 Cryoprecipitate (Remuzzi, 1988).

4 DDAVP infusion (Remuzzi, 1988).

Coagulation factors

Coagulation factor deficiency is uncommon in renal disease, indeed the plasma concentration of some factors, e.g. Factor VIII, are commonly increased.

As with any ill patient, especially if food intake is reduced and long-term antibiotics have been administered, vitamin K deficiency may occur with the corresponding coagulation abnormalities.

In advanced renal disease, hepatic impairment may occur and associated coagulopathy may develop.

Isolated deficiencies of Factor IX and XII have been reported in the nephrotic syndrome. The pathogenesis is not clear but appears to be related to proteinuria (Castaldi, 1984).

Disseminated intravascular coagulation

Evidence of localized DIC occurring in some cases of glomerular injury have been reported, and acute DIC may occur if some other factor such as septicaemia occurs. It has also been reported during rejection of renal transplant.

Laboratory diagnosis

A full blood and platelet count should be taken as well as a coagulation screen when any bleeding occurs or if an invasive procedure is contemplated. Appropriate tests should be undertaken if the patient has been exposed to heparin.

Platelet function tests are commonly abnormal, although these are performed rarely, as the bleeding time is the best indicator of the risk of haemorrhage.

Treatment

There are several approaches to the management of bleeding problems in uraemic patients but are often only temporarily effective. Dialysis may improve platelet function as may correction of anaemia either by transfusion of red cells or treatment with erythropoeitin. The packed cell volume should be kept above 30%. Cryoprecipitate and infusion of desmopressin acetate (DDAVP) may produce a rapid shortening of the bleeding time (Remuzzi, 1988) and may be sufficient to support haemostatic function during surgical procedures (Mannucci et al., 1983).

Vitamin K and blood products such as FFP and cryoprecipitate may be administered if there is evidence from coagulation studies that they are indicated, though patients with oliguria or anuria may not be able to tolerate the volumes unless dialysis or ultrafiltration techniques are used.

Heparin should be neutralized after dialysis.

Haemostatic defects associated with massive transfusion

Patients who require large transfusions of stored blood, as in severe trauma, may develop haemostatic abnormalities because of loss of coagulation factors and platelets by haemorrhage and replacement by fluids containing greatly reduced concentrations (Miller et al., 1971; Counts et al., 1979).

Stored blood contains reduced concentrations of Factors V, VIII and XI and virtually no platelets (Collins, 1976) (see Chapter 29).

The amount of stored blood transfused before haemostatic abnormalities become apparent is variable. Some abnormality is usual after transfusion of 10 litres but as little as 2.5 litres may cause significant problems if there is underlying disease, e.g. liver failure.

In addition to dilution, the other component contributing to the haemostatic defect is DIC (Collins, 1976). Patients who require massive transfusion may have experienced episodes of hypovolaemic shock which predisposes to DIC (Attar et al., 1966; Hardaway, 1966).

Thrombocytopenia is a frequent occurrence in massive transfusion, and although rarely falling below 50×10^9/litre, may cause serious surgical bleeding. If DIC occurs, profound thrombocytopenia with heavy bleeding may occur (Miller et al., 1971; Counts et al., 1979). Platelet function defects have also been noted.

Laboratory diagnosis

Standard coagulation screen, full blood count and platelet count are required. Hypofibrinogenaemia

Table 90.7 Coagulation test abnormalities which may be found through haemodilution in massive transfusion

Investigation	Result
Prothrombin time	↑
Partial thromboplastin time	↑
Thrombin clotting time	Normal
Platelet count	↓
Fibrinogen	Normal
Fibrin degradation products	Normal

↑ Prolonged; ↓ decreased.

and resultant long TCT time does not occur in massive transfusion *per se*, as fibrinogen concentration is not reduced in stored blood. This may help distinguish this coagulation abnormality from that of DIC.

Replacement therapy consisting of platelets and FFP is indicated if bleeding occurs, and prophylactic transfusions of both during blood transfusion are often given where blood loss is expected to be very high (Table 90.7).

Haemostatic defects associated with cardiopulmonary bypass

Much information has been gathered on abnormalities of the haemostatic system associated with cardiopulmonary bypass (CPB). Despite this, the clinical significance of many of the individual abnormalities is not certain, and the complex interrelationships involved in CPB are not understood completely (Ionescu *et al.*, 1981).

The more common abnormalities are described below.

Platelet abnormalities

Thrombocytopenia

This is a well-recognized finding following CPB (de Leval *et al.*, 1981), although there is a lower reported incidence in later studies probably reflecting differences in surgical and pumping techniques (Bick *et al.*, 1975; Bick, 1976).

There is a relationship between bypass time and the degree of thrombocytopenia, but a poor correlation between degree of thrombocytopenia and incidence of actual CPB haemorrhage (Kevy *et al.*, 1966; Porter & Silver, 1968; Signori *et al.*, 1969).

The aetiology of thrombocytopenia is not clear, although it is probable that damage to platelets during blood flow through the pump system is involved (Bick, 1985).

Platelet function defects

It has been shown that significant platelet function defect is induced in virtually all patients undergoing CPB (Bick, 1991).

A wide range of abnormalities of *in vitro* tests of platelet function have been reported. The actual aetiology is not certain although it seems likely that platelet membrane damage from contact with artificial surfaces or the action of shear forces in the pumping system plays a major role (Bick & Fekete, 1979; Edmunds *et al.*, 1982).

Platelet function defects are regarded as the most significant haemostatic abnormality associated with some CPB systems, particularly those using bubble or membrane oxygenator systems (Longmore *et al.*, 1981).

The major change in platelets occurs immediately following contact with artificial surfaces of the extracorporeal circuit and oxygenator. There is inhibition of platelets during bypass and this persists for some hours after cessation of the procedure. It is not clear if restoration of platelet function after CPB results from recovery of previously inhibited platelets or from formation of new platelets.

The potential haemorrhagic risk is increased if the patient has taken drugs which interfere with platelet function, e.g. aspirin (Bunting & Moncada, 1980).

Prostacyclin (Woods *et al.*, 1978) and heparin (Kalter *et al.*, 1979; Harker *et al.*, 1980) given during bypass have been shown to be effective in preserving platelet function and number.

Coagulation factor abnormalities

Decreased concentrations of coagulation factors may be found during CPB (Kalter *et al.*, 1979; Bick, 1991). Again, the aetiology is not certain, although decreased concentrations of II, V, VII, VIII, IX and X have been attributed to dilution and adsorption onto artificial surfaces (Harker *et al.*, 1980).

Decreased concentrations of fibrinogen and other coagulation factors have also been reported as being a result of increased fibrinolysis (O'Neill *et al.*, 1966; Porter & Silver, 1968; Bick *et al.*, 1975).

There is no clear relationship between these reported abnormalities and the incidence of bleeding.

In theory, excess heparin or inadequate neutralization may cause haemorrhage following bypass but it is reported rarely as the cause of bleeding after CPB. This may reflect greater experience in the use of heparin with CPB (Bick, 1985).

DIC was once considered a relatively common occurrence in CPB. The diagnosis, however, was difficult to establish in the presence of primary hyperfibrinolysis and heparin. More recent opinion suggests that DIC is in fact uncommon in CPB unless there is some other triggering factor such as sepsis present (Bick, 1991).

Increased fibrinolysis

Fibrinolytic activity is decreased usually during and after surgery (Tsitouris *et al.*, 1961; Lackner & Javid, 1973) except in CPB where it is shown to be increased frequently. It has been reported that a primary hyper-

Table 90.8 Patterns of abnormal coagulation tests which may be seen in cardiopulmonary bypass

| Test | Coagulation problem | | | | |
	Thrombocytopenia	Platelet dysfunction	DIC	Excess heparin	Primary hyperfibrinolysis
Platelet count	↓	Normal	↓	Normal	Normal
Prothrombin time	Normal	Normal	↑	↑	Normal
Partial thromboplastin time	Normal	Normal	↑	↑	May be ↑
Thrombin clotting time	Normal	Normal	↑	↑	↑
Fibrinogen	Normal	Normal	↓	Normal	May be ↓
Fibrin degradation products	Normal	Normal	↑	Normal	↑
Reptilase time (or equivalent)	—	—	↑	Normal	↑
Other relevant	—	Bleeding time	—	Protamine neutralization	Plasmin plasminogen studies

↑ Prolonged; ↓ shortened or decreased.

fibrinolytic state occurs in the majority of patients undergoing CPB (Bick, 1985).

The activation of the fibrinolytic system probably occurs in the pump/oxygenator systems.

The clinical significance of this increased fibrinolytic state is not clear. Controlled studies comparing patients in whom antifibrinolytic agents were used empirically with those in whom they were not given, show no difference in incidence of CPB haemorrhage (Tice & Worth, 1968; Verska et al., 1972). Some studies showed an increased incidence of bleeding with their use (Gomes & McGoon, 1970).

Other factors

Other factors known to be associated with increased risk of CPB haemorrhage (although the mechanisms involved are incompletely understood) include: long perfusion times (Bick, 1985), prior ingestion of coumarins (Verska et al., 1972), cyanotic congenital heart disease (Signori et al., 1969; Gomes & McGoon, 1970), hypothermic perfusions (O'Neill et al., 1966; Tice & Worth, 1968) and preoperative use of antiplatelet drugs (Bick & Fekete, 1979).

Investigation

A standard full blood count with platelet count and blood film should be taken. A coagulation screen consisting of PT, PTT, TCT and fibrinogen concentration should be performed.

In addition, if the TCT is prolonged, a reptilase time or heparin assay should be undertaken to exclude coagulation screen abnormalities caused by heparin.

Increased FDPs may be found in association with primary hyperfibrinolysis or DIC.

Many coagulation laboratories do not have the facilities for measuring components of the fibrinolytic system such as plasminogen or plasmin, but if available, these investigations may help to decide whether antifibrinolytic agents are indicated.

Table 90.8 summarizes patterns of abnormalities which may be found in association with CPB.

Treatment

Transfusion of platelets, cryoprecipitate and FFP may be required as an emergency in patients who are bleeding excessively after CPB. One should have ensured that heparin neutralization has been adequate before this step.

It is important to send samples to the laboratory for coagulation screen before transfusion of these blood products as the results may decide the strategy to be adopted, should haemorrhage continue.

Platelet concentrates should be given, even if there is a normal platelet count because of the likely platelet dysfunction present. FFP may be indicated to correct deficiencies occurring after adsorption of coagulation factors or dilution with stored blood and other fluids. Cryoprecipitate may be used as a source of fibrinogen if this is decreased from fibrinolysis.

Antifibrinolytic agents are indicated rarely and should be used only if there is clear evidence of primary hyperfibrinolysis without DIC and if previous measures have failed to control haemorrhage. Under these circumstances EACA, 5–10 g, should be slowly infused intravenously and followed by 1–2 g hourly until bleeding ceases (Bick, 1976).

Psychogenic bleeding

Rarely, a patient may present with a self-induced haemorrhagic state, and it is often only after exclusion of other potential causes that the diagnosis is made (Ratnoff, 1980b).

Warfarin ingestion and occasionally heparin administration in patients who have access to them, e.g. health workers have been reported. In these instances the usual patterns with coagulation results and the diagnosis is clinical with assay of specific drugs (Agle et al., 1970; Forbes et al., 1974; O'Reilly & Aggeler, 1976).

Patients suffering from hysterical states are also reported to have haemorrhagic events, although these are almost always minor and do not cause bleeding problems during surgery.

Conclusion

The anaesthetist deals with patients in a wide variety of clinical settings, including pre- and postoperative general surgical patients, cardiothoracic surgery, intensive care and obstetric practice, and this chapter has attempted to cover the more likely acquired haemostatic disorders that may be encountered in these situations.

Consultation with the haematologist or other specialist with an interest in coagulation is of great importance in planning investigation and management of patients with a haemostatic defect, as they are usually aware of the full resources of the local laboratory.

Most of the discussions in this chapter are up to date at the time of going to press but it is likely that future developments may significantly alter our thinking on some problems, e.g. pathogenesis and treatment of DIC.

References

Agle D.P., Ratnoff O.D. & Spring G.K. (1970) The anticoagulant malingerer, psychiatric studies on 3 patients. *Annals of Internal Medicine* **73**, 67–72.

Allain J.P., Gaillandre A. & Frommel D. (1981) Acquired haemophilia: functional study of antibodies to factor VIII. *Thrombosis and Haemostasis* **45**, 285–9.

American Heart Association (1973) The Urokinase Pulmonary Embolism Trial. A National Co-operative Study. Monograph No. 39. *Circulation* **47** (Suppl. 2), 11–108.

Aoki N. & Yamanaka T. (1978) The alpha 2-plasmin inhibitor levels in liver diseases. *Clinica Chimica Acta* **84**, 99–105.

Aster R.H. (1966) Pooling of platelets in the spleen: role of the pathogenesis of hypersplenic thrombocytopenia. *Journal of Clinical Investigation* **45**, 645–57.

Attar S., Mansberger A.R., Irani B., Kirby W., Masaitis C. & Cowley R.A. (1966) Coagulation changes in clinical shock II. Effect of septic shock on clotting times and fibrinogen in humans. *Annals of Surgery* **164**, 41–50.

Bailton F.E. & Letsky E.A. (1985) Obstetric haemorrhage: causes and management. In *Haematological Disorders in Pregnancy. Clinics in Haematology* (Ed. Letsky) pp. 683–728. W.B. Saunders, Philadelphia.

Ballard H.S. & Marcus A.J. (1976) Platelet aggregation in portal cirrhosis. *Archives of Internal Medicine* **136**, 316–19.

Bang N.U. & Chang M. (1974) Soluble fibrin complexes. *Seminars in Thrombosis and Hemostasis* **1**, 91–128.

Bell W.R. (1980) Disseminated intravascular coagulation. *Johns Hopkins Medical Journal* **146**, 289–99.

Beller F.K. (1971) Experimental animal models for the production of disseminated intravascular coagulation. In *Thrombosis and Bleeding Disorders* (Eds Bang N.U., Beller F.K., Deutsch E. & Mammen E.F.) p. 514. Academic Press, New York.

Bergstorm K., Blomback B. & Kleen G. (1960) Studies on the plasma fibrinolytic activity in a case of liver cirrhosis. *Acta Medica Scandinavica* **168**, 291–305.

Bick R.L. (1976) Alteration of hemostasis associated with cardiopulmonary bypass: pathophysiology, prevention, diagnosis and management. *Seminars in Thrombosis and Hemostasis* **3**, 59–82.

Bick R.L. (1978) Alterations of hemostasis associated with malignancy: etiology, pathophysiology, diagnosis and managment. *Seminars in Thrombosis and Hemostasis* **5**, 1–26.

Bick R.L. (1985) Hemostasis defects associated with cardiac surgery, prosthetic devices and other extracorporeal circuits. *Seminars in Thrombosis and Hemostasis* **11**, 249–80.

Bick R.L. (1991) Alterations of hemostasis associated with surgery, cardiopulmonary bypass surgery and prosthetic devices. In *Disorders of Hemostasis* (Eds Ratnoff O.D. & Forbes C.D.) pp. 382–422. Grune & Stratton, London.

Bick R.L. & Fekete L.F. (1979) Cardiopulmonary bypass haemorrhage. Aggravation by pre-op ingestion of anti-platelet agents. *Vascular Surgery* **13**, 277.

Bick R.L., Schmalhorst W.R., Crawford L., Holtermann M. & Arbegast N.R. (1975) The haemorrhagic diathesis created by cardiopulmonary by pass. *American Journal of Clinical Pathology* **63**, 588.

Bick R.L., Schmalhorst W.R. & Fekete L.F. (1976) Disseminated intravascular coagulation and blood component therapy. *Transfusion* **16**, 361–5.

Blanchard R.A., Furie B.C., Jorgensen M., Kruger S.F. & Furie B. (1981) Acquired Vitamin K dependent carboxylation deficiency in liver disease. *New England Journal of Medicine* **305**, 242–8.

Blauhut B., Necek S., Vinazzer H. & Bergman H. (1982) Substitution therapy with an anti-thrombin III concentrate in shock and DIC. *Thrombosis Research* **27**, 271–8.

Bloom A.L. (1977) Intravascular coagulation in the liver. *British Journal of Haematology* **30**, 1–7.

Bonnar J. (1981) Haemostasis and coagulation disorders in pregnancy. In *Haemostasis and Thrombosis* (Eds Bloom A.L. & Thomas D.P.) p. 454. Churchill Livingstone, New York.

Brain M.C. (1969) The haemolytic uraemic syndrome. *Seminars in Hematology* **6**, 162–80.

British Society for Haematology (1990) *Guidelines on Oral Anticoagulation*. BSCH Haemostasis and Thrombosis Task Force.

Brodsky I. & Siegel N.H. (1970) The diagnosis and treatment of disseminated intravascular coagulation. *Medical Clinics of North America* **54**, 555–65.

Brozovic M. (1981) Acquired disorders of blood coagulation. In *Haemostasis and Thrombosis* (Eds Bloom A.L. & Thomas D.P.) pp. 411–38. Churchill Livingstone, Edinburgh.

Bunting S. & Moncada S. (1980) Prostacyclin, by preventing platelet activation, prolongs activated clotting time in blood and platelet rich plasma and potentiates the anticoagulant effect of heparin. *British Journal of Pharmacology* **69**, 268–9.

Carreras L.O., Vermylen J., Spitz B. & Assche A. (1981) 'Lupus' anticoagulant and inhibition of prostacyclin formation in patients with repeated abortion, intrauterine growth retardation and intrauterine death. *British Journal of Obstetrics and Gynecology* **88**, 890–4.

Cash J.D. (1977) Disseminated intravascular coagulation. In *Recent Advances in Blood Coagulation* (Ed. Polle L.) p. 293. Churchill Livingstone, Edinburgh.

Castaldi P.A. (1984) Haemostasis and the kidney. In *Disorders of Haemostasis* (Eds Ratnoff O. & Forbes C.D.) pp. 473–84. Grune & Stratton, London.

Cederblad G., Korstan-Bengstein K. & Olsson R. (1976) Observation of increased levels of blood coagulation factors and other plasma proteins in cholestatic liver disease. *Scandinavian Journal of Gastroenterology* **11**, 391–6.

Cline M.J., Melman K.L., Davis W.C. & Williams H.E. (1968) Mechanism of endotoxin interaction with human leucocytes. *British Journal of Haematology* **15**, 539–47.

Collen D. (1983) Treatment of DIC. *Bibliotheca Haematologica* **49**, 295–305.

Collins J.A. (1976) Massive blood transfusion. *Clinics in Haematology* **5**, 201–21.

Colman R.W., Robbay S.J. & Minna J.D. (1972) Disseminated intravascular coagulation (DIC): an approach. *American Journal of Medicine* **52**, 679–89.

Corrigan J.J. & Jordan C.M. (1970) Heparin therapy in septicaemia with disseminated intravascular coagulation. *New England Journal of Medicine* **283**, 778–82.

Counts R.B., Haisch C., Simon T.L., Maxwell N., Heinbach D.M. & Carrico C.J. (1979) Haemostasis in massively transfused trauma patients. *Annals of Surgery* **190**, 91–9.

Courtney L.D. & Allington M. (1972) Effect of amniotic fluid on blood coagulation. *British Journal of Haematology* **22**, 353–5.

Cronberg S., Skansberg P. & Nivenius-Larsson K. (1973) Disseminated intravascular coagulation in septicaemia caused by beta haemolytic streptococci. *Thrombosis Research* **3**, 405–11.

Crosby W.H. & Stefanini M. (1952) Pathogenesis of the plasma transfusion reaction with especial reference to the blood coagulation system. *Journal of Laboratory and Clinical Medicine* **40**, 374–86.

Culpepper R.M. (1975) Bleeding diathesis in fresh water drowning. *Annals of Internal Medicine* **83**, 675.

Damus P.S. & Wallace G.A. (1975) Immunologic measurement of antithrombin III — heparin co-factor and 2 macroglobulin in disseminated intravascular coagulation and hepatic failure coagulopathy. *Thrombosis Research* **6**, 27–38.

Davidson J.F., McNicol G.P., Frank G.L., Anderson T.J. & Douglas A.S. (1969) A plasminogen activator-producing tumour. *British Medical Journal* **1**, 88–91.

Davis G. & Liu D.T. (1972) Mid-trimester abortion. *Lancet* **ii**, 1026.

de Leval M.R., Hill J.D. & Mielke C.H. (1981) Haematological aspects of extracorporeal circulation. In *Techniques in Extracorporeal Circulation* 2nd edn (Ed. Ionescu M.D.) p. 345. Butterworths, London.

Deykin D. (1970) The clinical challenge of disseminated intravascular coagulation. *New England Journal of Medicine* **283**, 636–44.

Dieckman W.J. (1936) Blood chemistry and renal function in abruptio placentae. *American Journal of Obstetrics and Gynecology* **31**, 734–5.

Donaldson V.H. (1960) Effect of plasmin *in vitro* on clotting factors in plasma. *Journal of Laboratory and Clinical Medicine* **56**, 644–51.

Donaldson V.H. (1984) Haemorrhagic disorders of neonates. In *Disorders of Haemostasis* (Eds Ratnoff O.D. & Forbes C.D.) p. 409. Grune & Stratton, London.

Douglas J.T., Shah M., Lowe G.D.O., Belch J.J.F., Forbes C.D. & Prentice C.R.M. (1982) Plasma fibrinopeptide A and β thromboglobulin in pre-eclampsia and pregnancy hypertension. *Thrombosis and Haemostasis* **47**, 54–5.

Duckert F. (1973) Behaviour of antithrombin III in liver disease. *Scandinavian Journal of Gastroenterology* **8** (Suppl. 19), 109–12.

Edgar W., McKillop C., Howie P.W. & Prentice C.R.M. (1977) Composition of soluble fibrin complexes in pre-eclampsia. *Thrombosis Research* **10**, 567–74.

Edmunds L.H. Jr., Ellison N., Colman R.W., Niewiarowski S., Rao A.K., Addonizio V.P., Stephenson L.W. & Edie R.N. (1982) Platelet function during cardiac operation. Comparison of membrane and bubble oxygenators. *Journal of Thoracic and Cardiovascular Surgery* **83**, 805–12.

Fletcher A.P., Biederman O., Moore D., Alkjaersig N. & Sherry S. (1964) Abnormal plasminogen–plasmin system activity (fibrinolysis) in patients with hepatic cirrhosis: its cause and consequences. *Journal of Clinical Investigation* **43**, 681–95.

Fletcher A.P., Alkjaersig N. & Fishers (1966) The proteolysis of fibrinogen by plasmin: the identification of thrombin-clottable fibrinogen derivatives which polymerize abnormally. *Journal of Laboratory and Clinical Medicine* **68**, 780–802.

Flute P.T. (1982) Acquired disorders of blood coagulation. In *Blood and its Disorders* 2nd edn (Eds Hardisty R.M. & Weatherall D.J.) p. 1161–89. Blackwell Scientific Publications, Oxford.

Foley M.E., Clayton J.K. & McNicol G.P. (1977) Haemostatic mechanisms in maternal, umbilical vein and umbilical artery blood at time of delivery. *British Journal of Obstetrics and Gynaecology* **84**, 81–7.

Forbes C.D., Prentice C.R.M. & Sclare A.B. (1974) Surreptitious ingestion of Warfarin. *British Journal of Psychiatry* **125**, 245–7.

George J.N. & Shattil S.S. (1991) The clinical importance of acquired abnormalities of platelet function. *New England Journal of Medicine* **324**, 27–39.

Giddings J.C., Shaw E., Tuddenham E.G.D. & Bloom A.L. (1975) The synthesis of factor V in tissue culture and isolated organ perfusion. *Thrombosis et Diathesis Haemorrhagia* **34**, 321.

Glazier R.L. & Cravell E.B. (1976) Randomized prospective trial of continuous v intermittent heparin therapy. *Journal of the American Medical Association* **236**, 1365–7.

Goldsmith G.H. (1984) Haemostatic disorders associated with neoplasia. In *Disorders of Haemostasis* (Eds Ratnoff O.D. & Forbes C.D.) pp. 351–66. Grune & Stratton, New York.

Gomes M.M. & McGoon D. (1970) Bleeding patterns after open heart surgery. *Journal of Thoracic and Cardiovascular Surgery* **60**, 87–97.

Goodnight S.H., Feinstein D.I., Osterud B. & Rapaport S.I. (1971) Factor VII antibody-neutralization material in hereditary and acquired factor VII deficiency. *Blood* **38**, 1–8.

Grain S.M. & Chardry A.N. (1981) Thrombotic thrombocytopenic purpura. A reappraisal. *Journal of the American Medical Association* **246**, 1243–6.

Gralnick H.R. & Abrell E. (1973) Studies on the procoagulant and fibrinolytic activity of promyelocytes in acute promyelocytic leukaemia. *British Journal of Haematology* **24**, 89–99.

Green D. & Lechner K. (1981) A survey of 215 non-hemophilic patients with inhibitors to Factor VIII. *Thrombosis and Haemostasis* **45**, 200–3.

Green G., Thomson J.M., Dymock I.W. & Poller L. (1977) Abnormal fibrin polymerization in liver disease. *British Journal of Haematology* **34**, 427–39.

Grossi C.E., Moreno A.H. & Rousselot L.M. (1961) Studies on spontaneous fibrinolytic activity in patients with cirrhosis of the liver and its inhibition by epsilon aminocapioic acid. *Annals of Surgery* **153**, 383–93.

Grun M., Liehr H., Brunswig D. & Thiel H. (1974) Regulation of fibrinogen synthesis in portal hypertension. *Thrombosis et Diathesis Haemorrhagia* **32**, 292–305.

Grundy M.F.B. & Graven E.R. (1976) Consumption coagulopathy after intra-amniotic urea. *British Medical Journal* **2**, 677–8.

Hallen A. & Nilsson I.M. (1964) Coagulation studies in liver disease. *Thrombosis et Diathesis Haemorrhagia* **11**, 51–63.

Ham T.H. & Curtis F.C. (1938) Plasma fibrinogen response in man. Influence of the nutritional state, induced hyperpyrexia, infectious disease and liver damage. *Medicine* **17**, 413–45.

Hardaway R.M. (1966) *Syndrome of Disseminated Intravascular Coagulation with Special Reference to Shock and Haemorrhage.*

Charles C. Thomas, Springfield.

Hardaway R.M. (1967) Disseminated intravascular coagulation in experimental and clinical shock. *American Journal of Cardiology* **20**, 161–73.

Harker L.A., Malpass T.W., Branson H.E., Hessel I.I. & Slichter S.J. (1980) Mechanism of abnormal bleeding in patients undergoing cardiopulmonary bypass: acquired transient platelet dysfunction associated with selective and granule release. *Blood* **56**, 824–34.

Harmon D.C., Dermirjian Z., Ellman L. & Fischer J.E. (1979) DIC with peritovenous shunt. *Annals of Internal Medicine* **90**, 774–6.

Hathaway W.E. & Alsever J. (1970) The relation of 'Fletcher factor' to factor XI and XII. *British Journal of Haematology* **18**, 161–9.

Hellegren M., Javelin L., Hagnevik K. *et al.* (1984) Antithrombin III concentrate as adjuvant in DIC treatment. A pilot study in 9 severely ill patients. *Thrombosis Research* **35**, 459–66.

Hemker H.C., Veltkamp J.J., Hensen A. (1963) Nature of pre-thrombinaemia in Vitamin K deficiency. *Nature* **200**, 589–90.

Higuchi A., Sakuruda R. & Miyazaki T. (1980) Acquired dys-fibrinogenaemia associated with liver disease. *Proceedings of the 18th Congress of the International Society of Haematology* p. 247.

Hillenbrand P., Parboo S.P., Jedrychowski A. & Sherlock S. (1974) Significance of intravascular coagulation and fibrinolysis in acute hepatic failure. *Gut* **15**, 83–8.

Hirsch J. (1986) Mechanisms of action and monitoring of anticoagulants. *Seminars in Thrombosis and Haemostasis* **12**, number 1.

Horder M.H. (1969) Consumption coagulopathy in liver cirrhosis. *Thromboses et Diathesis Haemorrhagia* **36** (Suppl.), 313.

Howie P.W., Prentice C.R.M. & Forbes C.D. (1975) Failure of heparin therapy to affect the clinical cause of severe pre-eclampsia. *British Journal of Obstetrics and Gynaecology* **82**, 711–17.

Howie P.W., Purdie D.W., Begg C.B. & Prentice C.R.M. (1976) Use of coagulation tests to predict the clinical progress of pre-eclampsia. *Lancet* **ii**, 323–5.

Ionescu M.I., Tandon A.P. & Roesler M.F. (1981) Blood loss following extracorporeal circulation for heart valve surgery. In *Techniques in Extracorporeal Circulation* 2nd edn (Ed. Ionescu M.I.) p. 345. Butterworths, London.

Jakobsen E., Ly B. & Kieulf P. (1974) Incorporation of fibrinogen with soluble fibrin complexes. *Thrombosis Research* **4**, 499–507.

Jandl J.H. & Lear A.A. (1956) The metabolism of folic acid in cirrhosis. *Annals of Internal Medicine* **45**, 1027–44.

Jick H., Slone D., Borda I.T. & Shapiro S. (1968) Efficacy and toxicity of heparin in relation to age and sex. *New England Journal of Medicine* **279**, 284–6.

Kalter R.D., Saul C.M., Wetstein L., Soriano C. & Reiss R.F. (1979) Cardiopulmonary bypass. Associated haemostatic abnormalities. *Journal of Thoracic and Cardiovascular Surgery* **77**, 427–35.

Kaplan A., Meier H. & Mandle R. (1976) The Hageman factor dependent coagulation pathways of coagulation, fibrinolysis and kinin generation. *Seminars in Thrombosis and Hemostasis* **3**, 1–26.

Kaplan A.P., Castellino F.J., Collen D., Wiman B. & Taylor F.B. (1978) Molecular mechanisms of fibrinolysis in man. *Throm-*

bosis and Haemostasis **39**, 263–83.

Kelton J.G. & Levine M.N. (1986) Heparin-induced thrombocytopenia. *Seminars in Thrombosis and Hemostasis* **12**, 59–62.

Kevy S.V., Glickman R.M. & Bernhard W.F. (1966) The pathogenesis and control of the hemorrhagic defect in open heart surgery. *Surgery, Gynecology and Obstetrics* **123**, 313–18.

Klein H.G. & Bell W.R. (1974) Disseminated intravascular coagulation during heparin therapy. *Annal of Internal Medicine* **80**, 477–81.

Kleiner G.J., Merskey C., Johnson A.J. & Markus W.B. (1970) Defibrination in normal and abnormal parturition. *British Journal of Haematology* **19**, 159–78.

Kopec M., Wegrzynowiczy Z. & Budzyski A. (1968) Interaction of fibrinogen degradation products with platelets. *Experimental Biology and Medicine* **3**, 73–80.

Krevans J.R., Jackson D.P., Cowley C.L. & Hartmann R.C. (1957) The nature of the haemorrhagic disorder accompanying haemolytic transfusion reactions in man. *Blood* **12**, 834–43.

Lackner H., Javid J.P. (1973) The clinical significance of the plasminogen level. *American Journal of Clinical Pathology* **60**, 175–81.

Langdell R.D. & Hedgpeth E.M. Jr. (1959) A study of the role of haemolysis in the haemostatic defects of transfusion reactions. *Thrombosis et Diathesis Haemorrhagia* **3**, 566–71.

Larkin E.C. & Watson-Williams E.J. (1984) Alcohol and the blood. *Medical Clinics of North America* **68**, 105–20.

Lasch H.G., Heene D.L., Huth K. & Sandritter W. (1967) Pathophysiology, clinical manifestations and therapy of consumption coagulopathy. *American Journal of Cardiology* **20**, 381–91.

Laursen B., Mortensen J.Z., Frost L. & Hansen K.B. (1981) Disseminated intravascular coagulation in hepatic failure treated with antithrombin III. *Thrombosis Research* **22**, 701–4.

Lawrence L. (1971) Lack of significant protection afforded by heparin during endotoxin shock. *American Journal of Physiology* **220**, 901–5.

Lechner K. (1972) Immune reactive factor IX in acquired factor IX deficiency. *Thrombosis et Diathesis Haemorrhagia* **27**, 19–24.

Lechner K., Niessner H. & Thaler E. (1977) Coagulation abnormalities in liver disease. *Seminars in Thrombosis and Hemostasis* **4**, 40–5.

Lee C.Y. (1979) *Snake Venoms*, vol. 52. Springer-Verlag, New York.

Lerner R.G., Nelson J.C., Corines P. & del Guercio L.R.M. (1978) DIC — complication of peritovenous shunts. *Journal of the American Medical Association* **240**, 2064–6.

Lieberman E. (1972) Haemolytic-uraemic syndrome. *Journal of Paediatrics* **80**, 1–16.

Lipinski B., Lipinska I. & Nova A. (1977) Abnormal fibrinogen heterogeneity and fibrinolytic activity in advanced liver disease. *Journal of Laboratory and Clinical Medicine* **90**, 187–94.

Longmore D.B., Bennett J.G., Hoyle P.M., Smith M.A., Gregory A., Osivand T. & Jones W.A. (1981) Prostacyclin administration during cardiopulmonary bypass in man. *Lancet* **i**, 800–4.

Lucey J.F. & Dolan R.G. (1958) Injections of a Vitamin K compound in mothers and hyperbilirubinaemia in the newborn. *Paediatrics* **221**, 605–6.

McGehee W.G., Rapaport S.I. & Hjort P.F. (1967) Intravascular coagulation in fulminant meningococcaemia. *Annals of Internal Medicine*, **67**, 250–6.

McKay D.G. & Margaretten W. (1967) Disseminated intravascular coagulation in virus diseases. *Archives of Internal Medicine* **120**, 129–52.

McKay D.G. & Shapiro S.S. (1958) Alterations in the blood coagulation system induced by bacterial endotoxin. 1: *in vitro* (generalized Schwartzman reaction). *Journal of Experimental Medicine* **107**, 353–67.

MacKenzie I.Z., Sayers L., Bonnar J. & Hillier K. (1975) Coagulation changes during second trimester abortion induced by intra-amniotic prostaglandin E_2 and hypertonic solutions. *Lancet* **ii**, 1066–9.

Mann J.D. (1952) Plasmin prothrombin in viral hepatitis and hepatic cirrhosis. Evaluation of the two stage method in 75 cases. *Gastroenterology* **21**, 263–70.

Mannucci P.M., Lobina G.F., Caocci L. & Dioguardi N. (1969) Effect on blood coagulation of massive intravascular haemolysis. *Blood* **33**, 207–12.

Mannucci M.M., Remuzzi G., Pusineri F., Lombardi R., Valsecchi C., Mecca G. & Zimmerman T.S. (1983) Desamino-8-D-Arginine vasopressin shortens the bleeding time in uremia. *New England Journal of Medicine* **308**, 8–12.

Mant M.J. & King E.G. (1979) Severe, acute disseminated intravascular coagulation. *American Journal of Medicine* **67**, 557–63.

Mant M.J., O'Brien B.D., Thong K.L., Hammond G.W., Birtwhistle R.V. & Grace M.G. (1977) Haemorrhagic complications of heparin therapy. *Lancet* **i**, 1133–5.

Marder V.J. (1979) Use of Thrombolytic agents: choice of patients, drug administration, laboratory monitoring. *Annals of Internal Medicine* **90**, 802–8.

Marder V.J., Soulen R.L. & Artichartalcon V. (1977) Quantitative venographic assessment of deep vein thrombosis in the evaluation of streptokinase and heparin therapy. *Journal of Laboratory of Clinical Medicine* **89**, 1018–29.

Merskey C. (1973) Defibrination syndrome or . . .? *Blood* **41**, 599–603.

Merskey C., Kleiner G.J. & Johnson A.J. (1966) Quantitative estimation of split products of fibrinogen in human series: relation to diagnosis and treatment. *Blood* **28**, 1–18.

Merskey C., Johnson A.J., Kleiner G.J. & Wohl H. (1967) The defibrination syndrome. Clinical features and laboratory diagnosis. *British Journal of Haematology* **13**, 528–9.

Miller L.L. & Bale W.F. (1954) Synthesis of all plasma protein functions except gamma globulins by the liver. The use of zone electrophoresis and lysine C^{14} to define the plasma proteins synthesized by the isolated perfused liver. *Journal of Experimental Medicine* **99**, 125–32.

Miller L.L., Bly G.G., Watson M.L. & Bale M.F. (1951) The dominant role of the liver in plasma protein synthesis. A direct study of the isolated perfused rat liver with the aid of lysine. *Journal of Experimental Medicine* **94**, 431–53.

Miller R.D., Robbins T.O., Tong M.J. & Barton S.L. (1971) Coagulation defects associated with massive blood transfusion. *Annals of Surgery* **174**, 794–801.

Morgan M. (1979) Amniotic fluid embolism. *Anaesthesia* **34**, 20–32.

Muirhead E.E. (1951) Incompatible blood transfusions with the emphasis on acute renal failure. *Surgery, Gynecology and*

Obstetrics **42**, 734–46.

Muller-Berghaus G. (1977) Pathophysiology of generalized intravascular coagulation. *Seminars in Thrombosis and Hemostasis* **3**, 209–46.

Murray-Lyon, Minchin Clarke H.G.M., McPherson K. & Williams R. (1972) Quantitative immunoelectrophoresis of serum proteins in cryptogenic cirrhosis, alcoholic cirrhosis and active chronic hepatitis. *Clinica Chimica Acta* **39**, 215–20.

Nelsestuen G.L., Zytkovicz T.H. & Havard J.B. (1974) Mode of action of Vitamin K, identification of carboxyglutamic acid as component of prothrombin. *Journal of Biological Chemistry* **249**, 6347–50.

Niewiarowski S., Regoeczi E., Stewart G., Senyi A.F. & Mustard J.F. (1972) Platelet interactions with polymerizing fibrin. *Journal of Clinical Investigation* **51**, 685–700.

Norman C.S. & Provan J.L. (1977) Control and complications of intermittent heparin therapy. *Surgery, Gynecology and Obstetrics* **145**, 338–42.

Nyman D. (1985) Discussion and definition of DIC and its treatment. *Scandinavian Journal of Clinical and Laboratory Investigation* **45** (Suppl. 178), 31–3.

O'Grady J., Bunting S. & Moncada S. (1980) Antithrombotic drugs in relation to prostaglandin metabolism. *Clinics in Haematology* **9**, 535–55.

Ollendorff P. (1962) The nature of the anticoagulant effect of heparin, protamine, polybrene and toludene blue. *Scandinavian Journal of Clinical and Laboratory Investigation* **14**, 267–76.

O'Neill J.A., Ende N., Collins J.S. & Collins H.A. (1966) A quantitative determination of perfusion fibrinolysis. *Journal of Thoracic and Cardiovascular Surgery* **51**, 777–82.

O'Reilly R.A. & Aggeler P.M. (1976) Covert anticoagulant ingestion: study of 25 patients and review of world literature. *Medicine* **55**, 389–99.

O'Sullivan E.F., Hirsh J., McCarthy R.A. & De Gruchy G.C. (1968) Heparin in the treatment of venous thrombo embolic disease. Administration, control and results. *Medical Journal of Australia* **2**, 153–9.

Owen C.A., Bawie E.J.W & Cooper H.A. (1973) Turnover of fibrinogen and platelets in dogs undergoing induced intravascular coagulation. *Thrombosis Research* **2**, 251–60.

Owren P.A. (1949) Diagnostic and prognostic significance of plasma prothrombin and factor V levels in parenchymatous hepatitis and obstructive jaundice. *Scandinavian Journal of Clinical and Laboratory Investigation* **1**, 131–40.

Page E.W., Fulton L.D. & Glendening M.B. (1951) The cause of the blood coagulation defect following abruptio placentae. *American Journal of Obstetrics and Gynecology* **61**, 1116–21.

Pechet L. (1965) Fibrinolysis. *New England Journal of Medicine* **273**, 966–73.

Pisciotta A.V. & Goltschall J.L. (1980) Clinical features of thrombotic thrombocytopenic purpura. *Seminars in Thrombosis and Hemostasis* **6**, 330–40.

Pisciotta A.V. & Schultz E.J. (1955) Fibrinolytic purpura in acute leukaemia. *American Journal of Medicine* **19**, 824–8.

Pitney W.R. (1971) Disseminated intravascular coagulation. *Seminars in Haematology* **8**, 65–82.

Pitney W.R., Pettit J.E. & Armstrong L. (1970) Control of heparin therapy. *British Medical Journal* **4**, 139–41.

Porter J.M. & Silver D. (1968) Alterations in fibrinolysis and coagulation associated with cardiopulmonary bypass. *Journal*

of Thoracic and Cardiovascular Surgery **56**, 869–78.

Prentice C.R.M. (1976) Heparin and disseminated intravascular coagulation. In *Heparin: Clinical Chemistry and Usage* (Eds Kakkar W. & Thomas D.P.) pp. 219–22. Academic Press, London.

Prentice C.R.M. (1985) Acquired coagulation disorders. In *Clinics in Haematology: Coagulation Disorders* pp. 413–42. W.B. Saunders, Philadelphia.

Preston F.E. (1982) Disseminated intravascular coagulation. *British Journal of Hospital Medicine* **28**, 129–320.

Pritchard J.A. (1959) Fetal death *in utero*. *Obstetrics and Gynaecology* **14**, 573–80.

Pritchard J.A. (1973) Haematological problems associated with delivery, placental abruption, retained dead fetus and amniotic fluid embolism. *Clinics in Haematology* **2**, 563–86.

Pritchard J.A. & Brekken A.L. (1967) Clinical and laboratory studies on severe abruptio placentae. *American Journal of Obstetrics and Gynecology* **97**, 681–95.

Quick A.J., Stanley-Brown M. & Bancroft F.W. (1935) A study of the coagulation defect in haemophilia and in jaundice. *American Journal of the Medical Sciences* **190**, 501–11.

Rabiner S.F. (1972a) Uraemic Bleeding. *Progress in Hemostasis and Thrombosis* **1**, 233.

Rabiner S.F. (1972b) The effect of dialysis on platelet function of patients in renal failure. *Annals of the New York Academy of Sciences* **201**, 234–42.

Rapaport S.I., Ames S.B., Mikkelsen S. & Goodman J.R. (1960) Plasma clotting factors in chronic hepatocellular disease. *New England Journal of Medicine* **263**, 278–82.

Ratnoff O.D. (1952) Studies as a proteolytic enzyme in human plasma VII. A fatal haemorrhagic state associated with excessive proteolytic activity in a patient undergoing surgery for carcinoma of head of pancreas. *Journal of Clinical Investigation* **31**, 521–8.

Ratnoff O.D. (1954) An accelerative property of plasma for the coagulation of fibrinogen by thrombin. *Journal of Clinical Investigation* **33**, 1175–82.

Ratnoff O.D. (1963) Haemostatic mechanisms in liver disease. *Medical Clinics of North America* **47**, 721–36.

Ratnoff O.D. (1980a) Why do people bleed? In *Blood, Pure and Eloquent* (Ed. Wintrobe M.M.) p. 600. McGraw Hill, New York.

Ratnoff O.D. (1980b) The psychogenic purpuras: a review of autoerythrocyte sensitization, autosensitization to DNA, 'hysterical' and factitial bleeding, and the religious stigmata. *Seminars in Hematology* **17**, 192–213.

Ratnoff O.D. (1991) Haemostatic defects in liver and biliary tract disease and disorders of vitamin K metabolism. In *Disorders of Haemostasis* (Eds Ratnoff O.D. & Forbes C.D.) pp. 459–79. Grune & Stratton, New York.

Reece E.A., Fox H.E. & Rapaport F. (1982) Factor VIII inhibitor: a cause of severe post partum haemorrhage. *American Journal of Obstetrics and Gynecology* **144**, 985–7.

Reid A.H. (1984) Clinical Haemostatic Disorders Caused by Venoms. In *Disorders of Haemostasis* (Eds Ratnoff O. & Forbes C.D.) pp. 511–26. Grune & Stratton, New York.

Remuzzi G. (1988) Bleeding in renal failure. *Lancet* **1**, 1205–8.

Remuzzi G., Marchesi D., Mecca G., Misiani R., Livio M., de Gactano G. & Donati M.B. (1978) Haemolytic−uraemic syndrome: deficiency of plasma factors regulating prostacyclin activity? *Lancet* **ii**, 871–2.

Rivers R.P.A., Hathaway W.E. & Weston W.L. (1975) Endotoxin induced coagulant activity of human monocytes. *British Journal of Haematology* **30**, 311–16.

Roberts H.R. & Lederbaum A.I. (1972) The liver and blood coagulation: physiology and pathology. *Gastroenterology* **63**, 297–320.

Roth G.J. & Majevus P.W. (1975) The mechanism of the effect of aspirin on human platelets. 1. Acetylation of a particular fraction protein. *Journal of Clinical Investigation* **56**, 624–32.

Rubenberg M.J., Baker L.R., McBride J.A., Sevitt L.H. & Brain M.C. (1967) Intravascular coagulation in a case of C1 perfringeus septicaemia. *British Medical Journal* **4**, 271–4.

Rubin M.H., Weston M.L., Bullock G., Roberts J., Langley P.G., White Y.S. & Williams R. (1977) Abnormal platelet function and ultrastructure in fulminant hepatic failure. *Quarterly Journal of Medicine* **46**, 339–52.

Rubin R.N., Kies M.S. & Posch J.J. (1978) Coagulation profiles with metastatic liver disease. *Blood* **52** (Suppl. 1), 193.

Rushton D.I. & Dowson I.M.P. (1982) The maternal autopsy. *Journal of Clinical Pathology* **35**, 909–12.

Saito H., Poon M.-C., Vicic W., Goldsmith G.H. & Menitove J.E. (1978) Human plasma prekallikrein (Fletcher factor) clotting activity and antigen in health and disease. *Journal of Laboratory and Clinical Medicine* **92**, 84–95.

Salzman E.W., Deykin D., Shapiro R.M. & Rosenberg R. (1975) Management of heparin therapy, controlled prospective trial. *New England Journal of Medicine* **292**, 1046–50.

Savage W. (1982) Abortion, methods and sequelae. *British Journal of Hospital Medicine* **27**, 364–84.

Schipper H.G., Kahle L.H., Jenkins C.S.P. *et al.* (1978) Antithrombin III transfusion in disseminated intravascular coagulation. *Lancet* **ii**, 854–6.

Schleider M.A., Nackman R.L., Jaffe E.A. & Coleman M. (1976) A clinical study of the lupus anticoagulant. *Blood* **48**, 499–509.

Schneider C.L. (1951) 'Fibrin embolism' (disseminated intravascular coagulation) with defibrination as one of the end results during placental abruption. *Surgery, Gynecology and Obstetrics* **92**, 27–34.

Schreiber A.D. & Austen K.F. (1973) Inter-relationships of the fibrinolytic, coagulation, kinin generation and complement systems. *Series Haematologica* **6**, 593–600.

Scott J.S. (1981) Connective tissue diseases antibodies and pregnancy. *American Journal of Reproductive Immunology* **6**, 19–24.

Semeraro N. & Donati M.B. (1981) Pathways of blood clotting initiation by cancer cells. In *Malignancy and the Haemostatic System* (Eds Donati M.B., Davidson J.F. & Garattini S.) pp. 65–81. Raven Press, New York.

Shapiro S.S. (1975) Acquired inhibitors to the blood coagulation factors. *Seminars in Thrombosis and Hemostasis* **1**, 336–85.

Shapiro S.S. & Thiagarjan P. (1982) Lupus anticoagulants. In *Progress in Haemostasis and Thrombosis*, vol. 6 (Ed. Spaed T.) p. 263. Grune & Stratton, New York.

Sharp A.A. (1964) Pathological fibrinolysis. *British Medical Bulletin* **20**, 240–5.

Sharp A.A., Howie B., Biggs R. & Methuen D.T. (1958) Defibrination syndrome in pregnancy (value of various diagnostic tests). *Lancet* **ii**, 1309–12.

Shaw E., Giddings J.C., Peake I.R. & Bloom A.L. (1979) Synthesis of procoagulant factor VIII, factor VIII related antigen and other coagulation factors by the isolated perfused rat liver. *British Journal of Haematology* **41**, 585–91.

Shearer M.J., Allan V., Haroon Y. & Barlchan P. (1980) Nutritional aspects of Vitamin K in the human. In *Vitamin K Metabolism and Vitamin K Department Proteins* p. 317. University Park Press, Baltimore.

Signori E.E., Penner J.A. & Kahn D.R. (1969) Coagulation defects and bleeding in open heart surgery. *Annals of Thoracic Surgery* **8**, 521–9.

Spector I. & Corn M. (1967) Laboratory tests of haemostasis. The relation to haemorrhage in liver disease. *Archives of Internal Medicine* **119**, 577–82.

Spero J.A., Lewis J.H. & Hasiba U. (1981) Corticosteroid therapy for acquired factor VIII:C inhibitors. *British Journal of Haematology* **48**, 635–42.

Spivak J.L., Springler D.B. & Bell W.R. (1972) Defibrination after intra-amniotic injection of hypertonic saline. *New England Journal of Medicine* **287**, 321–3.

Tagnon H.J., Whitmore W.F. & Schulman N.R. (1952) Fibrinolysis in metastatic carcinoma of prostate. *Cancer* **5**, 9–12.

Talbert I.M. & Blatt P.M. (1979) Disseminated intravascular coagulation in obstetrics. *Clinical Obstetrics and Gynaecology* **22**, 889–90.

Thomas D.P., Ream V.J. & Stuart R.K. (1967) Platelet aggregation in patients with Laennec's cirrhosis of the liver. *New England Journal of Medicine* **276**, 1344–8.

Tice D.A. & Worth M.H. (1968) Recognition and treatment of post-operative bleeding associated with open heart surgery. *Annals of the New York Academy of Science* **146**, 745–53.

Tocantins L.M. (1948) The haemorrhagic tendency in congestive splenomegaly: its mechanism and management. *Journal of the American Medical Association* **136**, 616–25.

Tsitouris G., Bellet S., Eilberg R., Feinberg L. & Sandberg H. (1961) Effects of major surgery on plasmin–plasminogen systems. *Archives of Internal Medicine* **108**, 98–104.

Udall J.A. (1956) Human sources of absorption of Vitamin K in relation to anticoagulation stability. *Journal of the American Medical Association* **194**, 127–9.

Verska J.J., Lonser E.R. & Brewer L.A. (1972) Predisposing factors and management of hemorrhage following open heart surgery. *Journal of Cardiovascular Surgery* **13**, 361–8.

Verstraete M., Vermylen J. & Collen D. (1974) Intravascular coagulation in liver disease. *Annual Review of Medicine* **25**, 447.

Viweg W.V.R., Pistcatelli R.L., Hauser J.J. & Proulx R.A. (1970) Complications of intravenous administration of heparin in elderly women. *Journal of the American Medical Association* **213**, 1303–10.

Voke J. & Letsky E. (1977) Pregnancy and antibody to factor VIII. *Journal of Clinical Pathology* **30**, 928–32.

Volwiler W., Goldsworthy P.D., MacMartin P., Wood P.A., MacKay I.R. & Freemont-Smith K. (1955) Biosynthetic determination with radioactive sulphur of turnover rates of various plasma proteins in normal and cirrhotic man. *Journal of Clinical Investigation* **34**, 1126–46.

von Felten A., Straub P.W. & Frick P.D. (1969) Dysfibrinogenaemia in a patient with primary haematoma. First observation of an acquired abnormality of fibrin monomer aggregation. *New England Journal of Medicine* **280**, 405–9.

Walls W.B. & Lavarsky M.S. (1971) The haemostatic defect of liver disease. *Gastroenterology* **60**, 108–11.

Walsh P.N. (1972) Evidence for an alternative pathway in intrinsic coagulation not requiring Factor XII. *British Journal of Haematology* **22**, 393–405.

Wardle E.N. (1974) Fibrinogen in liver disease. *Archives of Surgery* **109**, 741–6.

Warrell D.A., Davidson N. McD., Greenwood B.M., Ormerod L.D., Pope H.M., Watkins B.J. & Prentice C.R.M. (1977) Poisoning by bites of the saw scaled or carpet viper (*Echis carinatus*) in Nigeria. *Quarterly Journal of Medicine* **46**, 33–62.

Wiener A.E. & Reid D.E. (1950) Pathogenesis of amniotic fluid embolism III. Coagulant activity of amniotic fluid. *New England Journal of Medicine* **243**, 597–8.

Willoughby M.L.N., Murphy A.V., McMorris S. & Jewel F.G. (1972) Coagulation studies in haemolytic uraemic syndrome. *Archives of Diseases of Children* **47**, 766–71.

Wilmer G.D., Nossel H.D. & Le Roy E.C. (1968) Activation of Hageman Factor by Collagen. *Journal of Clinical Investigation* **47**, 2608–15.

Wilson J.R. & Lampman J. (1979) Heparin therapy: a randomized prospective study. *American Heart Journal* **97**, 155–8.

Woods H.F., Ash G., Weston M.J., Bunting S., Moncada S. & Yane J.R. (1978) Prostacyclin can replace heparin in hemodialysis in dogs. *Lancet* **ii**, 1075–7.

Yaffe H., Eldor A., Hornshslein E. & Sadovsky E. (1977) Thromboplastin activity in amniotic fluid during pregnancy. *Obstetrics and Gynaecology* **50**, 454–6.

Zwicka H., Kopec M., Latallo Z. & Kowalski E. (1961) Anticoagulant circulant vessemblant a l'antithrombin IV au cairs d'un lupus erythemateux dissemine. *Thrombosis et Diathesis Haemorrhagia* **6**, 63–72.

The Burned Patient

D.A.B. TURNER

Although the first written documentation describing the treatment of thermal injury dates back almost four millenia (Bryan, 1931), it is only in the last half of this century, with the refinement of fluid resuscitation techniques, the introduction of effective antimicrobial agents and the development of specialized burns units that any significant improvement in survival has occurred (Thomsen, 1977). In the last two decades, the realization that invasive infection and protein–calorie malnutrition are major factors contributing to delayed mortality has resulted in increasing enthusiasm for prompt excision and grafting of the burn wound using either autografts and/or cultured or artificial skin together with the early use of enteral or parenteral nutrition. These strategies would appear to improve outcome further, especially in patients with extensive injury (Demling, 1983a,b; Alexander, 1985).

In England and Wales, over 10 000 patients per annum sustain burns severe enough to warrant hospitalization, and of these, over 600 die as a result of their injuries. The overall mortality is related to the percentage of the body surface affected, the age of the patient and their premorbid physical status (Bull, 1971; Zawacki et al., 1979). Inhalation injury has a negative prognostic impact, being an important cause of death in patients with otherwise survivable cutaneous burns (Clarke et al., 1986).

Many complex physiological and metabolic adjustments accompany thermal injury and a clinical approach should be based logically on a thorough understanding of these associated pathophysiological events. Although thermal injury usually involves variable destruction of the skin and its appendages, severe burns are associated with alterations in virtually every organ system.

Pathophysiology of the burn injury

Cutaneous response

The skin is the largest organ of the body, constituting 15% of total body weight. It is usually the most severely affected organ in thermal injury and its destruction represents a breach in the body's protective shield allowing both uncontrolled evaporative water loss and bacterial colonization. Whilst the average insensible water loss through intact skin amounts to $15\,ml \cdot m^{-2} \cdot h^{-1}$ (700–1000 ml/day), loss through areas of full thickness burn may reach $200\,ml \cdot m^{-2} \cdot h^{-1}$. This is accompanied by loss of the latent heat of vaporization which approximates to 500 calories of heat for the evaporation of 1 litre of water. Thus, energy expenditure must be increased to maintain body temperature (Harrison et al., 1964). Bacterial proliferation of skin commensals occurs soon after cutaneous injury, and most wounds are colonized by Gram-negative organisms by the fifth day after burning.

Human skin can tolerate temperatures up to 40°C for relatively long periods of time without apparent injury. However, temperatures above this level result in a logarithmic increase in the degree of tissue destruction which is dependent on both the temperature and the duration of exposure to the heat source (Moritz & Henriques, 1947). Histologically, the area of tissue injury consists of three concentric zones. A central 'zone of coagulation' characterized by irreversible coagulation necrosis is surrounded by a 'zone of stasis' in which cells are potentially recoverable if the deleterious effects of infection and desiccation can be prevented. Peripherally is a 'zone of hyperaemia' in which there is minimal tissue destruction and in which spontaneous healing may be expected (Jackson, 1983).

Vascular response

The extent and severity of damage to local vasculature is variable and ranges from total destruction of superficial capillaries with widespread endothelial swelling and disruption to partial occlusion of vessels with thrombus.

The liberation from burned tissue of a multitude of vasoactive substances such as histamine, 5-hydroxytryptamine and bradykinin, results in a profound transcapillary fluid exchange which, at least initially, may be generalized and extend beyond the area of injury. Plasma-like fluid is sequestered in the extravascular space resulting in oedema formation in the burn wound. The magnitude of the oedema caused by this increased microvascular permeability is compounded by a generalized cell membrane defect that results in intracellular swelling (Baxter, 1974). A complication of the albumin loss is a decrease in plasma colloid osmotic pressure which promotes further extravascular fluid retention (Demling et al., 1984). In addition, blood viscosity is increased as a result of haemoconcentration secondary to this fluid loss.

The overall effect of these derangements on the systemic circulation is a profound loss of intravascular volume which is proportional to the extent of burn injury. The result of this decrease in intravascular volume is an initial decrease in cardiac output and thus tissue perfusion. As in most cases of hypovolaemic shock, the maintenance of cerebral and myocardial perfusion is obtained at the expense of the kidneys, liver and small intestine but the resulting state of uneven tissue perfusion may be corrected by early, aggressive and adequate volume resuscitation. The functional integrity of the capillary is re-established gradually over the ensuing 48–72 h; lymphatic drainage and the restoration of oncotic pressure gradients encourage re-entry of sequestered fluid into the intravascular space and the progressive reduction in intravascular volume slows. Red cell mass is decreased also following thermal injury (Muir, 1961). Red blood cells are destroyed directly by heat, but this is compounded by stasis and a reduced red blood cell half-life consequent upon increased fragility. The magnitude of loss of red cell mass is related to the size of full-thickness burn, and deficits of up to 40% may occur in severe injury.

Metabolic response

Extensive burns are associated with a rapid increase in metabolic rate which is greater than that seen with any other form of trauma or sepsis (Cope et al., 1953;

Moncrief, 1973). This increase reaches a peak only a few days postburn and persists until effective wound closure has occurred. Oxygen consumption studies have demonstrated that the basal metabolic rate (BMR) of $35-40$ cal $\cdot$ m^{-2} body surface area (BSA) $\cdot$ h^{-1} may double in patients whose burn affects more than 50% of their body surface and, in general, the degree of hypermetabolism is proportional to the size of the burn. This endocrine response to burn injury is characterized by protein catabolism, nitrogen wasting, hyperthermia, hyperglycaemia and increased carbon dioxide production and oxygen utilization (Kien et al., 1978). Although this was attributed originally to the need to generate more heat because of the large evaporative water losses from the burn wound, evidence exists which suggests that thermal injury triggers greatly increased activity of the sympathetic nervous system and the hypothalamic–pituitary–adrenal axis. This results in persistently increased levels of circulating catecholamines, glucocorticoids and glucagon (Wilmore et al., 1974). It is thought that these hormones are directly responsible for the runaway catabolism and that their effects may be compounded by any need to generate heat to maintain body temperature (Zawacki et al., 1970; Neely et al., 1974).

Immediate care of the burn victim

An evaluation of the extent and severity of the injury is conducted simultaneously with the institution of volume resuscitation (Brown & Ward, 1984).

Initial evaluation

The priorities of treatment that are well established for any trauma patient apply equally to the burn victim, and attention to the burn wound should not take precedence over the assessment and treatment of life-threatening problems such as cardiovascular collapse or upper airway obstruction. A primary survey should be conducted to ensure the patency of the patient's airway, the adequacy of ventilation and the ability of the cardiovascular system to maintain acceptable cerebral and coronary perfusion.

Burn size

A visual inspection delineates those areas of the body involved, and a rapid assessment of the appropriate percentage of the body surface area affected (excluding non-blistering erythematous areas) should be performed. The 'rule of nine' is a widely accepted method for this purpose (Lund & Browder, 1944). This rule is based on the fact that various regions of the body represent 9% of the BSA or a multiple thereof (Fig. 91.1). For smaller areas, a good guide is that the area covered by the patient's hand and fingers represents approximately 1% of their body surface. In general, if the total percentage BSA involved exceeds 15% in an adult or 10% in a child, then volume resuscitation should be instituted as a matter of urgency.

Burn depth

The assessment of burn depth (Fig. 91.2) is more prone to error but should be attempted as it has important therapeutic and prognostic implications. Although burn wounds have been classified conventionally into three 'degrees' of depth, the imprecision and subjectivity of this method (particularly with

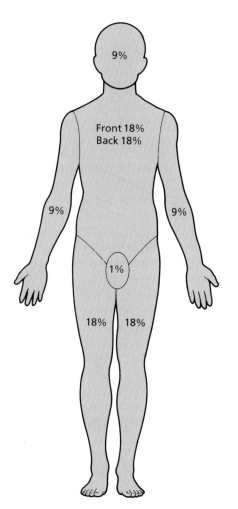

Fig. 91.1 'Rule of nine'.

Table 91.1 Classification of burn depth

Erythema	Damage is limited to epidermis resulting in a non-blistered erythematous area
	Minimal oedema
	Painful
	Heal spontaneously in 48–72 h
Partial thickness, superficial	Destruction of *outer* layers of dermis is also present, but hair follicles, sebaceous and sweat glands are spared
	Typically, vesicle formation occurs and erythema blanches with pressure
	Heals in 7–10 days if infection does not supervene
Partial thickness, deep	Only the deepest dermal appendages are spared
	Skin is blistered, oedematous and usually white
	Painless
	Hair can be pulled out easily
Full thickness	All epithelial elements and the full thickness of the dermis are destroyed
	The area is anaesthetic, dry and either charred or white

regard to second-degree injury) has led to the adoption of a simplified classification based on the depth of tissue destruction (Fig. 91.1 and Table 91.1).

When erythema is present, the protective barrier of the skin is maintained, there is minimal fluid loss or chance of infection and it is therefore not included in the burn-size calculations when estimating fluid requirements. Superficial, partial-thickness burns may be expected to heal in 7–10 days provided infection is prevented, but deep, partial-thickness burns require 4 weeks for epithelial regeneration to occur from the few remaining glands and hair follicles. In the case of full-thickness burns, healing may occur by wound contraction, and this requires skin grafting for definitive closure. Deep, partial-thickness burns may be converted to full-thickness by either infection or desiccation, and are treated often as full thickness.

Fluid resuscitation

Although the necessity for fluid resuscitation in patients with burns exceeding 15–20% BSA is not

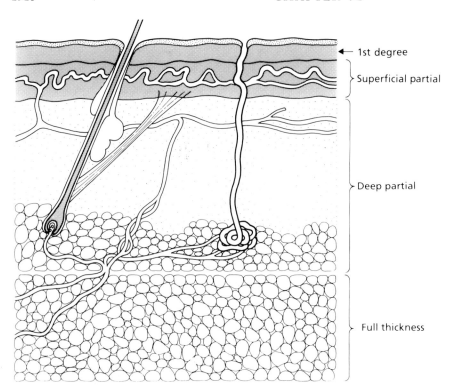

Fig. 91.2 Estimation of depth of burn.

questioned, the actual composition and rate of fluid administration remains the subject of controversy (Monafo *et al.*, 1973; Arturson, 1985; Demling, 1985). Over the years, numerous formulae have been advocated and most involve multiplying the product of percentage BSA involved and body weight by some constant 'factor'. This calculation determines the quantity of fluid to be infused during the first 24 h postburn. These formulae vary, depending on the value of this constant factor, and on the inclusion or exclusion of colloid-containing solution. Because of the marked increase in capillary microcirculatory permeability that occurs in burned tissue, most fluid resuscitation schemes produce some degree of burn tissue oedema. However, in patients with extensive burn injury, oedema occurs often in non-burned soft tissue. This appears to be attributable to the hypoproteinaemia consequent upon albumin loss in areas of injury rather than to some diffuse alteration in capillary protein permeability as was thought previously (Demling, 1985).

It is also difficult, in the absence of inhalation, to demonstrate any significant alteration in pulmonary capillary permeability. A number of studies have failed to demonstrate any early increase in extravascular lung water during controlled fluid administration after major burn injury (Tranbaugh *et al.*,

1980). This evidence would suggest that colloid infusion might minimize oedema in non-burned tissue and maintain plasma volume better than crystalloid solutions. This has resulted in the inclusion of colloid in the resuscitation regimens in many centres. The tendency, especially in North America, to avoid the use of colloid during the initial 24 h is based on the supposition that any colloid given during this period is of little benefit in maintaining plasma albumin concentration (and, therefore, osmotic gradients) because it leaks out into the extravascular space and further encourages extravascular fluid retention. Although there is some logic in this argument, it should be emphasized that definitive studies demonstrating the superiority of one resuscitation regimen over another are lacking, and it is *early* and aggressive fluid resuscitation that is of paramount importance. Regardless of the regimen used, the goal is to maintain an effective plasma volume and optimize vital and non-vital organ perfusion in the face of massive loss of protein and fluid from the circulation.

Two commonly used 'formulae' are presented in Table 91.2. The Mount Vernon formula popularized by Muir and Barclay in the 1950s (Muir *et al.*, 1987) is popular in the UK and relies heavily on the infusion of plasma protein fraction. The Brooke and Modified

Table 91.2 Fluid replacement formulae

Muir and Barclay	$0.5\,\text{ml}\cdot\text{kg}^{-1}\cdot\%$ BSA burn of colloid (as plasma protein fraction) is given every 4 h for the initial 12 h postburn and then every 6 h for the succeeding 12 h period
Brooke	$0.5\,\text{ml}\cdot\text{kg}^{-1}\cdot\%$ BSA burn of colloid *plus* $1.5\,\text{ml}\cdot\text{kg}^{-1}\cdot\%$ BSA burn of crystalloid (to a maximum limit of 50% BSA) *plus* 2 litres of water as dextrose 5% is the *total volume* given over the first 24-h period
	50% is given over the initial 8 h and 25% in the second and third 8-h periods

Time zero is the time of injury. All calculations are based from the time of injury.

Brooke (excludes colloid in the first 24 h) formulae are popular in North America and favour a more balanced regimen.

The two most common errors made in the resuscitation of the burn victim are *delay* in initiating resuscitation and failure to *vary* from the calculated requirements when signs of vital organ perfusion are not achieved. It cannot be overstated that all formulae are only guidelines for planning fluid therapy and may need to be adjusted frequently depending on clinical response (Aikawa *et al.*, 1982).

Monitoring resuscitation

The response to resuscitation should be assessed frequently using conventional clinical criteria (mental status, vital signs, capillary refill, urine output, central venous pressure) and laboratory data (packed cell volume, electrolytes, osmolalities). An adequate urine output ($0.5-1\,\text{ml}\cdot\text{kg}^{-1}\cdot\text{h}^{-1}$) is the most useful single guide to the adequacy of volume replacement (Settle, 1974). If urine output decreases below $0.5\,\text{ml}\cdot\text{kg}^{-1}\cdot\text{h}^{-1}$, the rate of fluid administration may need to be increased. If urine output exceeds $1.5\,\text{ml}\cdot\text{kg}^{-1}\cdot\text{h}^{-1}$, the patient should be re-evaluated to ascertain that fluid requirements have not been overestimated. The indications for the use of central venous or pulmonary artery flotation catheters are the same as for any trauma victim, and the burn injury itself does not contraindicate their use. Any patient who remains oliguric despite a fluid challenge requires an immediate haemodynamic assessment. This would require some assessment of right ventricular or left ventricular filling pressure (Aikawa *et al.*, 1978). The need for

transfusion of blood should be assessed at intervals, and most patients with extensive injury require transfusion if packed cell volume drops below 30%. In the context of severe burns, reliance on clinical judgement, vital signs and urine output results in inadequate resuscitation (Dries *et al.*, 1991).

From the practical standpoint, vascular access may present difficult problems in the burn patient. Nonburned areas are preferred for all peripheral and central insertion sites because of the risk of infection (as well as the problem of securing lines to eschar). However, line placement through burned tissue is allowable if the catheter is needed and no suitable non-burned site is available. As a rule, 'cutdowns' should be avoided because of the prohibitively high infection rates associated with their use.

Inhalation injury

Once the primary survey has been completed and volume resuscitation is in progress, the possibility of inhalation injury must be considered because effective treatment may depend on early recognition.

Three separate entities may be encountered with inhalation injury (Fein *et al.*, 1976; Trunkey, 1978); notably, direct thermal injury to the upper airway, carbon monoxide poisoning and smoke inhalation. Inhalation injury is more likely if the conflagration occurred in a closed space. Although each pattern of injury may occur in isolation, it is not uncommon for two or all three to exist in combination. The reader is referred to an excellent review of the pathophysiology of inhalation injury (Traber *et al.*, 1988).

Direct thermal injury

The clinical spectrum of direct heat injury ranges from asymptomatic supraglottic oedema to life-threatening upper airway obstruction. The upper airway possesses considerable heat-exchanging ability so that if hot air is inhaled, most of the heat energy is dissipated in the nose, pharynx and upper airway (Moritz *et al.*, 1945). This results in progressive mucosal oedema which is limited usually to the mouth, tongue and hypopharyngeal region. Heat injury below the level of the cords is rare but does occur if superheated steam is inhaled. The speed of onset, severity and duration of the oedema varies, but is usually maximal within the first 24 h. As mucosal burns are rarely full thickness, the oedema may be expected to subside in 3–5 days.

Suspicion of direct thermal injury should be aroused by any patient involved in a closed-space fire who has evidence of facial burns, particularly oedema of the lips, which is associated invariably with underlying pharyngeal oedema. If there is any clinical suggestion of upper airway obstruction, the presence of hypopharyngeal oedema should be assumed and the patient observed closely for evidence of increasing upper airway obstruction (Wanner & Cutchavaree, 1973). This allows complete obstruction to be pre-empted by tracheal intubation.

As fluid resuscitation might be expected to exacerbate oedema (and worsen airway obstruction), many authorities recommend an aggressive approach to diagnosis which involves direct visualization of the upper airway in any patient in whom direct thermal trauma is suspected. This may be achieved using a fibre-optic endoscope over which a nasotracheal tube may be passed should supraglottic oedema be present. As clinical experience with these instruments grows, it is likely that there will be an increasing tendency to perform early examination and intubation.

Carbon monoxide poisoning

Carbon monoxide (CO) is a colourless, odourless gas produced by the incomplete combustion of many carbon-containing materials. The primary hazard with CO lies with its propensity to tie up oxygen binding sites in the haemoglobin molecule (Douglas *et al.*, 1912). Although both gases bind to the α-chain, haemoglobin has an affinity for CO that is 230–270 times greater than its affinity for oxygen. Thus, CO fills oxygen binding sites at very low partial pressures. For example, a Paco of 0.133 kPa (1 mmHg) may result in a carboxyhaemoglobin saturation of over 40%. In addition, the rate of dissociation of CO from haemoglobin is slow, and high levels of carboxyhaemoglobin cause a leftward shift of the oxygen dissociation curve. Thus, the major concern with CO poisoning is tissue hypoxia, particularly cerebral and myocardial hypoxia.

Although the symptoms of CO poisoning tend to be vague, they do correlate with the carboxyhaemoglobin level to some extent (Table 91.3). The classical description of cherry red facial discoloration is helpful but by no means always present, and the diagnosis depends on a history of smoke or exhaust fume exposure in a closed space coupled with a direct measurement of CO saturation by CO-oximetry. A pitfall in the diagnosis of CO poisoning is to assume that a patient who is centrally pink with a normal arterial oxygen tension (Pao$_2$) is not hypoxic. Arterial

Table 91.3 Signs and symptoms of carbon monoxide poisoning

Percentage carboxyhaemoglobin	Clinical manifestations
0–10	None
10–20	Slight headache Angina may occur in patients with ischaemic heart disease
20–30	Throbbing headache Dyspnoea Dilatation of cutaneous blood vessels
30–40	*Above* plus nausea and vomiting Impairment of mental processes
40–50	Tachypnoea Tachycardia Syncope
60–70	Cardiovascular collapse and death

oxygen partial pressure may be normal in the presence of CO poisoning, and if oxygen saturation is derived (as it is on many blood-gas machines), instead of directly measured spectrophotometrically, the result may be misleading.

The treatment of CO poisoning involves facilitating the elimination of gas via the lungs. The rate of dissociation of CO from its oxygen binding sites is slow because there is usually only a small gradient in partial pressure at the alveolar interface. Alveolar CO partial pressure ($P_A$co) should approach zero and if Paco is 0.266 kPa (2 mmHg) there is a gradient of only 0.266 kPa (2 mmHg) available to displace CO from the haemoglobin molecule. However, as CO competes with oxygen for the same sites in the α-chain, increasing Pao$_2$ increases competition for the sites already occupied by CO. It has been demonstrated that the half-life of carboxyhaemoglobin is 5 h breathing room air (F_1o$_2$ 0.21), but this may be reduced to under 1 h by breathing 100% oxygen (F_1o$_2$ 1). Thus, increasing Pao$_2$ is the single most useful manoeuvre to enhance CO elimination. Patients with suspected CO poisoning and/or those in whom a spectrophotometrically measured carboxyhaemoglobin level exceeds 20% should be given 100% oxygen by nonrebreathing mask if this is practicable. If the patient is obtunded sufficiently, tracheal intubation protects the airway and allows titrated oxygen therapy. This should be continued until carboxyhaemoglobin levels are below 15–20%. Also absolute rest and ECG monitoring would seem appropriate. Patients who survive the initial period are at risk from delayed

Table 91.4 Delayed complications of carbon monoxide poisoning

Erythematous, bullous skin lesions
Rhabdomyolysis, myoglobinaemia, acute renal failure
Cerebral oedema (48 h to 2 weeks postinsult)
Demyelination/anoxic leukoencephalopathy manifesting as
    persistent neuropsychiatric symptoms

complications (Table 91.4) which are treated on standard lines. Permanent disability is not unusual (Smith & Brandon, 1973).

Smoke inhalation

The composition of smoke depends on the composition of the material that is burning. It consists usually of irritant carbon particles (ash) suspended in a mixture of gases and vapours, the chemical components of which cause airway irritability, airway obstruction (by damage to the tracheobronchial mucosa) and, occasionally, damage to the alveolar air–blood interface. The heat-induced decomposition of manufactured petrochemical byproducts, such as plastics and synthetic fibres, produces a bewildering spectrum of toxic fumes and gases (Table 91.5).

Despite this, it is unusual for smoke inhalation to constitute the predominant aspect of inhalation injury, probably because most victims succumb to CO poisoning before a sufficient 'smoke dose' has been inhaled. In addition, conscious victims may be able to escape from smoke especially if it contains some of the more pungent, soluble toxic gases such as chlorine, ammonia or sulphur dioxide. Some of the less pungent, insoluble, toxic gases and vapours, however, are recognized less easily and therefore

Table 91.5 Toxic products of combustion

Substance/material	Toxic product
Polyvinyl chloride (PVC)	Hydrochloric acid, phosgene, chlorine
Wood, cotton, paper	Acrolein, acetaldehyde, formaldehyde, acetic and formic acid
Polyurethane	Isocyanate, hydrogen cyanide
Nylon	Ammonia, hydrocyanic acid
Acrylics	Acrolein, carbon monoxide

tolerated for longer periods of time. These gases are more likely to be associated with lower airway injury (nitrogen dioxide, phosgene). Acrolein is an aldehyde produced during the combustion of wood, cotton, acrylics and some plastics. It produces intense irritation and inflammation of mucous membranes and pulmonary oedema. It has been incriminated frequently as a cause of mortality in house fires (Zikria et al., 1972). The combustion of polyvinylchloride (PVC), another common household material, results in the production of phosgene and chlorine. These gases, on contact with moist mucous membranes result in the formation of hydrochloric acid. Likewise, the thermal decomposition of nitrogen-containing polymers (polyurethane, nylon) result in the formation of hydrogen sulphide which, in addition to being a systemic poison, is hydrolysed to hydrocyanic acid. This causes an intense inflammatory reaction and cyanide toxicity.

Treatment of inhalation injury

Treatment of inhalation injury is mainly supportive. All patients need oxygen and this should be given in as high a concentration as possible until a carboxyhaemoglobin level has excluded CO poisoning. Early nasotracheal intubation may pre-empt complete airway obstruction in patients with supraglottic oedema. Patients who have been exposed to smoke or toxic fumes require meticulous respiratory care to prevent lethal complications. The importance of intensive physiotherapy and tracheobronchial toilet with efficient humidification of inspired gases cannot be overstated, and the fibre-optic bronchoscope is a useful aid to remove sloughed mucosa (Moylan et al., 1975). Minitracheostomy may be useful if this is a recurrent problem.

The use of continuous positive airway pressure (CPAP) or positive end-expiratory pressure (PEEP) in patients with alveolar injury who are hypoxaemic with poorly compliant lungs is logical but as airflow limitation with gas trapping is common after smoke inhalation, this modality of treatment should be applied with circumspection (Venus et al., 1981).

Definitive care of the burn victim

The primary goal of this stage of care is surgical closure of the burn wound, before invasive bacterial infection supervenes. Bacterial infection of burned tissues delays healing and may possibly destroy remaining epithelial cells and convert a partial-thickness burn into a full-thickness burn. It is also likely to prevent successful skin grafting. Bacterial invasion of underlying tissues may result in fulminating septicaemia. Prevention of burn-wound infection is, therefore, of paramount importance. Wound closure is accomplished definitively by surgery, but requires adequate metabolic support and meticulous nursing care to prevent burn wound contamination.

Prevention of infection

Any large, open wound that contains devitalized tissue represents an ideal culture medium for bacterial colonization. The burn wound itself, followed by the lungs are the most common sites for serious infection to occur. Whilst virulent strains of *Pseudomonas* and methicillin-resistant *Staphylococcus aureus* (MRSA) are being incriminated increasingly, it appears that diminished host resistance is a more important factor in determining the severity of burn-wound infection than the virulence of the causative organisms. The burn victim is in a state of immuno-compromise (Alexander *et al.*, 1978) and alterations in both the cellular and humoral components of the immune response have been identified. Impaired phagocyte function, reduced neutrophil chemotaxis and abnormalities in macrophage activity have all been demonstrated (Davies *et al.*, 1980). Derangements in lymphocyte function have also been reported. T-suppressor lymphocytes, which normally inhibit T-cell stimulation of antibody production are found in increased numbers in burn victims, and this may represent an indication of the risk of sepsis (McIrvine *et al.*, 1982). Reduced concentrations of both γ-globulin and the opsonic protein, fibronectin, occur also but the clinical significance of this is uncertain.

Protection of the patient against bacterial cross-infection involves strict attention to detail in all aspects of nursing care. More recently, many burns units have employed single-room isolation and barrier nursing techniques. The purpose of these units is to prevent bacterial contamination of the patient from staff and equipment, and from cross-contamination from other patients. In its simplest form, patients are placed in a single cubicle with reverse flow ventilation and strict barrier nursing, but more sophisticated laminar airflow units such as the bacteria-controlled nursing unit (BCNU) exist, which may reduce the chance of infection further. This provides a small (1.8 × 3 m) area which, through the use of clear, plastic walls and a continuous down-flow of filtered, bacteria-free air provides a non-contaminated environment (Burke *et al.*, 1977). With this unit, temperature and humidity may also be controlled.

Systemic antibiotics are unable to penetrate surface eschar, and control of bacterial growth over the burn wound is accomplished using topical antibiotics which continue to be the mainstay of wound-infection control. Numerous topical preparations are available and each has its inherent advantages and disadvantages (Moncrief, 1979).

Silver nitrate solution (0.5%) is a bacteriostatic agent effective against a broad spectrum of organisms. It is applied in the form of saturated mesh gauze which serves the dual purpose of reducing bacterial growth and minimizing evaporative water loss. Application is painless and, although little systemic absorption occurs, leaching of sodium from the burn wound in addition to reduced evaporative loss may result in hyponatraemia. Dressings are saturated with the solution every 2 h and the dressing changed once or twice a day.

Silver sulphadiazine cream (Flamazine) is also painless on application and is unable to penetrate eschar. It has broad antibacterial activity and side-effects are rare.

Mafenide acetate (Sulphamyalon cream) is a sulphonamide preparation that can penetrate surface eschar and control bacterial growth at the interface between eschar and granulation tissue. Proliferation of organisms at this site may progress to burn-wound invasion and infection in non-burned viable tissue. Application to partial-thickness burns is painful and it needs to be applied once or twice a day. Mafenide inhibits carbonic anhydrase activity leading to bicarbonaturia and metabolic acidosis. This is rarely a serious problem but has led to its use on an alternate-day basis with one of the other preparations.

Surgical approaches

The conventional surgical approach involves the use of topical antibiotics combined with repeated cleansing and debridement of the burn wound which, in time, either heals or allows skin grafting to be performed.

This form of conservative treatment is suitable for partial-thickness injuries. In cases where the differentiation between partial-thickness and full-thickness burns cannot be made with any degree of certainty, this conservative approach is warranted (to prevent infection and desiccation of the wound) until the distinction can be made (usually 14−21 days). The treatment of choice for full-thickness injury is removal of slough and early grafting. Indeed, in the presence of extensive injury when the conservative approach is both uncomfortable for the patient and involves the inherent danger of preserving an open wound in an immunocompromised host, there is increasing enthusiasm for prompt excision of the burn wound followed by immediate wound closure, especially for full-thickness and deep, partial-thickness burns (Burke et al., 1974). In one prospective study (Herndon et al., 1989) patients with >30% burns had their mortality reduced from 45% to 9% with early excision and grafting. It should be emphasized that this improved outcome could not be demonstrated in patients with concomitant inhalation injury or in patients outside the 17−30 age group. This suggests that a relatively small number of patients would benefit from early, aggressive surgical treatment. If, as may be the case in patients with extensive injury, there is insufficient healthy skin for autografting, a skin substitute may be used and excision and grafting may proceed in a sequential manner (Burke et al., 1981). Materials which restore the important barrier function of the skin either temporarily or permanently have obvious positive metabolic and microbiological implications. It may be that there is some correlation between survival and rapidity of wound closure (Echinard et al., 1982).

Metabolic support

The increase in metabolic rate that occurs in the postresuscitation phase may approach 100% in patients with cutaneous burns exceeding 50% BSA. This hypermetabolism is associated with increased net protein breakdown, nitrogen loss, lipolysis and accelerated gluconeogenesis and may result rapidly in severe protein−calorie malnutrition. In association with this increased metabolism, there is often a slight increase in core temperature of 1−2°C which appears to result from resetting of the hypothalamic temperature centre. Any attempt to reduce core temperature by changing ambient temperature results in an additional increase in energy expenditure in an attempt to maintain body temperature (Barr et al., 1968). Thus, a low ambient temperature may exaggerate the stress response and result in the production of wasted energy (Wilmore et al., 1975). Maintaining ambient temperature at approximately 30°C has been found to reduce significantly the total energy expenditure, and this practice is standard in many burns units.

In addition to ambient temperature control, early and aggressive nutrition is necessary to prevent malnutrition (Wilmore, 1979). Oxygen consumption studies have demonstrated that if ambient temperature is maintained, BMR seldom exceeds twice the BMR as predicted from the Harris−Benedict formula and approximate energy requirements may be obtained from this formula (Table 91.6).

The choice of substrate to provide this energy is more difficult to rationalize. The marked hepatic gluconeogenesis may be suppressed by the infusion of exogenous glucose, and this should constitute at least 50% of the total caloric intake. Fifteen to twenty percent of calories are given as protein and the remainder as fat. There is recent evidence (Alexander et al., 1980) to suggest that the use of high-protein nutrition (with a non-protein calorie : nitrogen ratio of 100 : 1) is associated with improved immunocompetence. It remains to be seen if this has any impact on outcome on the incidence of infection in adults.

Nutritional support should commence as soon as possible in the postresuscitation phase. Preference is for the enteral route but, as a paralytic ileus accompanies extensive burns frequently, enteral feeds should be withheld until peristalsis returns. If the ileus persists beyond 72 h, consideration should be given to parenteral alimentation.

As a general rule, patients with burns exceeding 20−25% BSA benefit from nutritional support and control of ambient temperature.

Anaesthetic considerations

Following resuscitation, the severely burned patient faces the physiological and psychological trauma of burn-wound closure. Whether this is achieved by prompt excision and grafting or by multiple wound debridements and grafting with reconstructive procedures, it necessarily involves anaesthesia. Some anaesthetic problems are unique to the burn patient (de Campo & Aldrete, 1981).

Table 91.6 The Harris−Benedict formula

Male
Basal metabolic rate $= 66 + (13.7 \times W) + (5 \times H) - (6.8 \times A)$

Female
Basal metabolic rate $= 66 + (9.6 \times W) + (1.7 \times H) - (4.7 \times A)$

W, ideal body weight in kg; H, height in cm; A, age in years.
Total daily caloric requirement $= \text{BMR} \times 1.5$.

Vascular access may be difficult, and as blood loss may be considerable (even with a minor debridement or wound excision), a large-bore, reliable intravenous line must be established prior to surgery.

Monitoring. Cutaneous or oesophageal ECG, non-invasive or invasive arterial pressure measurement, temperature and urine output monitoring should be standard for all but the most minor procedures. Central venous pressure measurement is useful if excessive blood loss is anticipated.

Temperature control. The combination of low ambient temperature, large exposed areas of body surface, infusion of large volumes of cold fluid and lengthy operations sets the scene for hypothermia with deleterious metabolic consequences. The onset of postoperative shivering may result in severe arterial desaturation. As a rule, the ambient temperature should be as high as the theatre staff can tolerate comfortably, and attempts should be made to insulate exposed areas; all intravenous fluids and preparation solutions should be warmed to 37°C and inspired gases fully humidified.

Pharmacological considerations

Suxamethonium

It is well known that suxamethonium is associated with ventricular arrhythmias and cardiac arrest in burn patients, and for this reason its use should be avoided (Tolmie *et al.*, 1967). This abnormal response is a result of hyperkalaemia although why burned patients should exhibit such an exaggerated response is uncertain (Bush *et al.*, 1962). The magnitude of the increase in plasma potassium concentration is related to the dose of suxamethonium administered, the time that has elapsed since injury and on the severity or extent of burn injury. It has been speculated that, as in the case of denervation injury, there is a proliferation of nicotinic acetylcholine receptors over the whole muscle membrane when they are limited normally to the area of the neuromuscular junction. The possibility of a hyperkalaemic response to suxamethonium may persist for up to 2 years after the injury.

Non-depolarizing, neuromuscular-blocking drugs

The observation that burn patients are relatively resistant to the effects of non-depolarizing, neuromuscular-blocking drugs has been confirmed by numerous recent studies (Martyn *et al.*, 1980, 1982). To achieve a given response, both the dose administered and the serum concentration required are increased by a factor of 2–3. Numerous hypotheses have been presented to explain this, but the increase in nicotinic acetylcholine receptor density secondary to disease atrophy and immobilization may best explain this altered response.

Miscellaneous drugs

The clinical impression that analgesics, anxiolytics and hypotensive agents need to be given in large doses to burned patients is not supported as yet by pharmacokinetic studies (Martyn, 1986).

Anaesthetic techniques

Many different anaesthetic techniques have been employed successfully in burn patients. All patients require a detailed airway assessment including the extent of mouth opening and neck movements. Anticipation of any difficulty is a resonable indication for awake, blind, nasal intubation preferably with the help of a fibre-optic instrument. This technique should be mastered by all anaesthetists involved with burn victims (Lamb, 1985). Ketamine has been used widely in burned patients and in low doses (1.5–2 mg/kg i.m.) may provide adequate analgesia and amnesia for minor wound debridements and cleansing. Its administration should be preceded by an antisialogogue, and in this dosage it allows rapid establishment of important activities such as eating.

Halothane remains a widely used volatile agent although its advantage over the available agents relate to its predictability and lack of pungency, which facilitates inhalation induction. The possibility of liver injury with repeated administration may be less important in the burned patient, as evidence for halothane hepatotoxicity is lacking in this group of patients (Martyn, 1986). If the hepatotoxic effects of halothane are mediated immunologically, it may be that the anergic state of the burn patient accounts for this anomaly. Despite this, repeated halothane exposure cannot be recommended.

Complications of thermal injury

Acute renal failure

Severe impairment of renal function is a serious complication of thermal injury and has negative prognostic implications (Cameron & Miller-Jones, 1967).

Acute, oliguric renal failure results invariably from acute tubular necrosis representing one extreme of a spectrum of impaired renal function. Non-oliguric renal failure is a more common problem and implies loss of tubular concentrating ability. Causes of renal failure in the context of thermal injury include persistent hypovolaemia, the presence of urinary pigments (haemoglobin or myoglobin) and Gram-negative sepsis. Any patient with pre-existing renal impairment may be expected to be particularly susceptible to these abnormalities. Monitoring of hourly urine output together with frequent estimation of urine osmolality and sodium concentration allow assessment of glomerular filtration and tubular concentrating ability. Calculation of various derived indices, such as fractional excretion of sodium and osmolal clearance, aid in the differential diagnosis of oliguria.

Haemoglobinuria and myoglobinuria occur classically in patients suffering from high-voltage electrical injury, but any full-thickness burn may result in red blood cell and muscle breakdown with the release of haemoglobin and myoglobin into the circulation. It is probable that these pigments predispose the patient to renal injury especially in the presence of renal hypoperfusion. Treatment of renal failure should be instituted early; although peritoneal dialysis may be adequate to cope with mild fluid overload, it is likely that haemodialysis will be necessary in the hypermetabolic patient.

Hypertension

This is seen commonly after severe burns, especially in children (Faulker et al., 1978). It appears within 2 weeks of injury, and the clinical manifestations range from mild irritability to somnolence progressing to convulsions. It is associated with prolonged elevation of plasma catecholamines and increased plasma renin activity. Although reserpine has been advocated, an angiotensin-converting enzyme inhibitor may be more appropriate.

Burn encepalopathy

Acute CNS dysfunction in the absence of raised systemic arterial pressure may be a major problem in burn patients, and presents as an acute brain syndrome which may progress to seizures and coma (Anton et al., 1972). The exact cause is unclear but metabolic factors (hypoxia, hyponatraemia) or septicaemia may precipitate events.

Gastroduodenal ulceration

Described initially by Curling in 1842, acute erosions of the gastric and duodenal mucosa occur in 86% of patients with major burns, within 72 h of injury (Czaja et al., 1976). Reduction in gastric mucosal blood flow and increased gastric acid output are thought to be aetiological factors. Erosions may be manifest as torrential life-threatening haemorrhage, or insidious, acute gastrointestinal blood loss. The mainstay of treatment lies in prevention with early enteral nutrition and the routine use of H_2-receptor antagonists and antacids. In the hyperdynamic phase of injury, the dose requirement for cimetidine increases substantially as both the total and renal clearance of the drug are elevated. The magnitude of this change is proportional to the size of the burn. As this may result in subtherapeutic plasma concentrations, it has been suggested that after 24 h the dose should be doubled. The pharmacokinetics of ranitidine have not been characterized yet.

Outcome

Survival after thermal injury has improved progressively over the past decade. The size of injury associated with a 50% survival has reached 65%, 66%, 47% and 30% in age groups 0—14 years, 15—40 years, 41—65 years and over 65 years respectively (Lutterman & Curreri, 1987). Such figures emanate from a centre of excellence and are quoted to illustrate the potential value of surgery and intensive care techniques to the burn victim. There remains, however, a small group of patients with severe cutaneous burns (over 90% BSA) combined with inhalation injury who have no reasonable chance of recovery (e.g. self-immolation). Medical technology should not be applied to prolong death and suffering and such patients should be given every measure of pain relief, comfort and hygiene. If upper airway obstruction develops, tracheal intubation is indicated to prevent the distress caused by asphyxia rather than as a life-saving manoeuvre. Such decisions should be taken by senior members of the unit team.

References

Aikawa N., Martyn J.A.J. & Burke J.F. (1978) Pulmonary artery catheterisation and thermodilution cardiac output determination in the management of critically ill burned patients. *American Journal of Surgery* **135**, 811—19.

Aikawa N., Ishibiki K., Naito C. & Abe O. (1982) Individualised fluid resuscitation based on haemodynamic monitoring in the management of extensive burns. *Burns* **8**, 249—55.

Alexander J.W. (1985) Burn care; a speciality in evolution. 1985 Presidential Address, American Burn Association. *Journal of Trauma* **26**, 1–6.

Alexander J.W., Ogle C.K., Stinnett J.D. & MacMillan B.G. (1978) A sequential, prospective analysis of immunologic abnormalities and infection following thermal trauma. *Annals of Surgery* **188**, 809–16.

Alexander J.W., MacMillan B.G. & Stinnett J.D. (1980) Beneficial effects of aggressive protein feeding in severely burned children. *Annals of Surgery* **192**, 503–17.

Anton A.Y., Volpe J.J. & Crawford J.D. (1972) Burn encephalopathy in children. *Pediatrics* **50**, 609–16.

Arturson G. (1985) Fluid therapy of thermal injury. *Acta Anaesthesiologica Scandinavica* **29**, 55–9.

Barr P.-O., Birke G., Liljedahl S.O. & Plantin L.O. (1968) Oxygen consumption studies and water loss during treatment of burns. *Lancet* **i**, 164–8.

Baxter C.R. (1974) Fluid volume and electrolyte changes in the early post burn period. *Clinics in Plastic Surgery* **1**, 693–703.

Brown J. & Ward D.J. (1984) Immediate management of burns in casualty. *British Journal of Hospital Medicine* **31**, 360–8.

Bryan C.P. (1931) Minor Surgery. In *The Papyrus Ebers*, Chapter 12. Appleton, New York.

Bull J.P. (1971) Revised analysis of mortality due to burns. *Lancet* **ii**, 1133–4.

Burke J.F., Bondoc L.L. & Quinby W.C. (1974) Primary burn excision and immediate grafting – a method of shortening illness. *Journal of Trauma* **14**, 389.

Burke J.F., Quinby W.C., Bondoc L.L., Sheely F.M. & Moreno H.C. (1977) The contribution of a bacterially isolated environment to the prevention of infection in seriously burned patients. *Annals of Surgery* **186**, 377–87.

Burke J.F., Yannas I.V., Quinby W.C., Bondoc L.L. & Jung W.K. (1981) Successful use of a physiologically acceptable artificial skin in the treatment of extensive burn injury. *Annals of Surgery* **194**, 413–28.

Bush G.H., Graham H.A.P. & Littlewood A.H.M. (1962) Danger of suxamethonium and endotracheal intubation in anaesthesia for burns. *British Medical Journal* **2**, 1081–5.

Cameron J.S. & Miller-Jones C.M.H. (1967) Renal function and renal failure in badly burned children. *British Journal of Surgery* **54**, 132–41.

Clarke C.J., Reid W.H., Gilmour W.H. & Campbell D. (1986) Mortality probability in victims of fire trauma; a revised equation to include inhalation injury. *British Medical Journal* **292**, 1303–5.

Cope O., Nardi G.L., Quijano M., Rovit R.L., Stanbury J.B. & Wight A. (1953) Metabolic rate and thyroid function following acute thermal trauma in man. *Annals of Surgery* **137**, 165–74.

Curling T.B. (1842) On acute ulceration of the duodenum in cases of burns. *Medic-chir Trans* **25**, 260–81.

Czaja A.J., McAlhamy J.L. & Pruitt B.A. (1976) Acute gastroduodenal disease after thermal injury; an endoscopic evaluation of incidence and natural history. *New England Journal of Medicine* **29**, 925–9.

Davies J.M., Dineen P. & Gallin J.Z. (1980) Neutrophil degranulation and abnormal chemotaxis after thermal injury. *Journal of Immunology* **124**, 1467–71.

de Campo T. & Aldrete J.A. (1981) The anaesthetic management of the severely burned patient. *Intensive Care Medicine* **7**, 55–62.

Demling R.H. (1983a) Fluid resuscitation after major burns. *Journal of the American Medical Association* **260**, 1438–40.

Demling R.H. (1983b) Improved survival after massive burns. *Journal of Trauma* **23**, 179–84.

Demling R.H. (1985) Burns. *New England Journal of Medicine* **313**, 1389–98.

Demling R.H., Kramer G. & Harris B. (1984) Role of thermal injury induced hypoproteinaemia on fluid flux and protein permeability in burned and non-burned tissue. *Surgery* **95**, 136–44.

Douglas C.G., Haldane J.S. & Haldane J.B.S. (1912) The laws of combination of haemoglobin with carbon monoxide and oxygen. *Journal of Physiology* **44**, 275.

Dries D.J. & Waxman K. (1991) Adequate resuscitation of burn patients may not be measured by urine output and vital signs. *Critical Care Medicine* **19**, 327–9.

Echinard C., Sajdel-Sulkowska E. & Burke P. (1982) The beneficial effects of early excision on clinical response and thymic activity after burn injury. *Journal of Trauma* **22**, 560–5.

Faulkner B., Roven S. & De Clement F.A. (1978) Hypertension in children with burns. *Journal of Trauma* **8**, 213–17.

Fein A., Leff A. & Hopewell P.L. (1976) Pathophysiology and management of the complications resulting from fire and the inhaled products of combustion. *Critical Care Medicine* **4**, 144–50.

Harrison H.N., Moncrief J.A. & Duckett J.W. (1964) The relationship between energy metabolism and water loss from vaporisation in severely burned patients. *Surgery* **56**, 203.

Herndon D.N., Barrow R.E., Rutan R.L., Rutan T.C., Desai M. & Abston S. (1989) A comparison of conservation versus early excision. *Annals of Surgery* **209**, 547–53.

Jackson D.MacG. (1983) The William Gissane Lecture 1982. The burn wound; its character, closure and complications. *Burns* **10**, 1–8.

Kien C.L., Young V.R., Rohrbaugh D.K. & Burke J.F. (1978) Increased rates of whole body protein synthesis and breakdown in children recovering from burns. *Annals of Surgery* **187**, 383–91.

Lamb J.D. (1985) Anaesthetic considerations for major thermal injury. *Canadian Anaesthetists' Society Journal* **32**, 84–92.

Lund C.C. & Browder N.C. (1944) Estimation of area of burns. *Surgery, Gynecology and Obstetrics* **79**, 352.

Lutterman A. & Curreri P.W. (1987) Burns and electrical injuries. In *Current Therapy in Critical Care Medicine* (Ed. Parillo J.E.) pp. 314–18. B.C. Decker Inc., Toronto.

McIrvine A.J., O'Mahony J.B., Saporoschetz I. & Memmick J.A. (1982) Depressed immune response in burn patients; use of monoclonal antibodies and functional assays to define the role of suppressor cells. *Annals of Surgery* **196**, 297–301.

Martyn J.A.J. (1986) Clinical pharmacology and drug therapy in the burned patient. *Anesthesiology* **65**, 67–75.

Martyn J.A.J., Szyfelbein S.K., Matteo R.S., Ali H.H. & Savarese J.J. (1980) Increased D-tubocurarine requirement following major thermal injury. *Anesthesiology* **52**, 352–5.

Martyn J.A.J., Matteo R.S., Szyfelbein S.K. & Kaplan R.F. (1982) Unprecedented resistance to the neuromuscular blocking effects of metocurine with persistence of complete recovery in a burned patient. *Anesthesia and Analgesia* **61**, 614–17.

Monafo W.W., Chuntrasakul C. & Agvazian V.H. (1973) Hypertonic sodium solutions in the treatment of burn shock. *American Journal of Surgery* **126**, 778–83.

Moncrief J.A. (1973) Burns. *New England Journal of Medicine* **288**, 444–54.

Moncrief J.A. (1979) Topical antibacterial treatment of the burn wound. In *Burns: A Team Approach* (Eds Artz C.P., Moncrief J.A. & Pruitt B.A.) pp. 250–69. W.B. Saunders, Philadelphia.

Moritz A.R. & Henriques F.C. (1947) Studies of thermal injury II. The relative importance of time and surface temperature in the causation of cutaneous burns. *American Journal of Pathology* **23**, 695–720.

Moritz A.R., Henriques F.C. & MacLean R. (1945) The effects of inhaled heat of the air passages and lung. *American Journal of Pathology* **21**, 311–31.

Moylan J.A., Adib K. & Birnbaum M. (1975) Fibreoptic broncho-scopy following thermal injury. *Surgery, Gynecology and Obstetrics* **140**, 541–3.

Muir I.F.K. (1961) Red cell destruction in burns. *British Journal of Plastic Surgery* **4**, 273.

Muir I.F.K., Barclay T.L. & Settle J.A.D. (1987) The practical management of burns shock. In *Burns and their Management* 3rd edn. pp. 30–5. Butterworths, London.

Neely W.A., Petro A.B., Holloman G.H., Rushton F.W., Turner D.M. & Hardy J.D. (1974) Researches on the cause of burn hypermetabolism. *Annals of Surgery* **179**, 291–4.

Settle J.A.D. (1974) Urine output following severe burns. *Burns* **1**, 23–42.

Smith J.S. & Brandon S. (1973) Morbidity from carbon monoxide poisoning at a 3 year follow-up. *British Medical Journal* **1**, 319–21.

Thomsen M. (1977) Historical landmarks in the treatment of burns. *British Journal of Plastic Surgery* **30**, 212–17.

Tolmie J.D., Joyce J.H. & Mitchell G.D. (1967) Succinylcholine danger in the burned patient. *Anesthesiology* **28**, 467–70.

Traber D.L., Linares H.A., Herndon D.N. & Prien T. (1988) The pathophysiology of inhalation injury — a review. *Burns* **14**, 357–64.

Tranbaugh R.F., Lewis F.R., Christensen J.M. & Elings V.B. (1980) Lung water changes after thermal injury; the effects of crystalloid administration and sepsis. *Annals of Surgery* **192**, 479–88.

Trunkey J.D. (1978) Inhalation injury. *Surgical Clinics of North America* **58**, 1133–40.

Venus B., Matsuda T., Copiozo J.B. & Mathru M. (1981) Prophy-lactic intubation and continuous positive airway pressure in the management of inhalation injury in burn victims. *Critical Care Medicine* **9**, 519.

Wanner A. & Cutchavaree A. (1973) Early recognition of upper airway obstruction following smoke inhalation. *American Review of Respiratory Diseases* **108**, 1421–3.

Wilmore D.W. (1979) Nutrition. In *Burns: A Team Approach* (Eds Artz C.P., Moncrief J.A. & Prutt B.A.) pp. 453–60. W.B. Saunders, Philadelphia.

Wilmore D.W., Long J.M., Mason A.D., Skreen R.W. & Pruitt B.A. (1974) Catecholamines — mediator of the hypermeta-bolic response to thermal injury. *Annals of Surgery* **180**, 653–69.

Wilmore D.W., Mason A.D., Johnson D. & Pruitt B.A. (1975) Effect of ambient temperature on heat production and heat loss in burn patients. *Journal of Applied Physiology* **39**, 593.

Zawacki B.E., Spitzer I.C.W., Mason A.D. & Johns L.A. (1970) Does increased evaporative water loss cause hypermetabol-ism in burn patients? *Annals of Surgery* **171**, 236–40.

Zawacki B.E., Azen S.P., Imbus S.H. & Chang Y.T.C. (1979) Multifactorial probit analysis of mortality in burned patients. *Annals of Surgery* **189**, 1–5.

Zikria B.A., Ferrer J.M. & Floch H.F. (1972) The chemical factor contributing to pulmonary damage in 'smoke poisoning'. *Surgery* **71**, 704–9.

Drug Use in the Intensive Therapy Unit

R. A. NELSON AND M. WOOD

On average, a patient receives between 5 and 10 different medications per hospital admission, and adverse responses develop in approximately 5% of patients. Multiple drug therapy is almost always required in the intensive therapy unit (ITU) and therefore the potential is great for adverse drug interactions or effects to occur. Expenditure on drugs is the second greatest expense in the ITU after nursing salaries. Drugs should be administered to patients in a critical care setting only after considering both current drug therapy and the patient's physiological state, as impairment of renal, hepatic or cardiovascular function may alter patient response to drug therapy. Changes in drug therapy should be kept to a minimum, and dosage adjustments made on the basis of titration to effect or the plasma concentration with the careful observation of response over a period of time.

Pharmacokinetics in the intensive therapy unit (see Chapter 15)

Continuous intravenous infusion regimens

Many drugs are given in the ITU by continuous intravenous infusion or by multiple doses. Obviously, it is important that plasma concentrations are maintained within the therapeutic range to maximize optimal drug effect. The plasma concentration at steady state (C_{ss}) achieved by continuous infusion may be calculated from a knowledge of clearance (Cl) and rate of administration. At steady state:

$$\text{Rate of administration} = \text{rate of elimination}$$
$$\text{Rate of elimination} = Cl \times C_{ss}$$

Thus:

$$\text{Rate of administration} = Cl \times C_{ss}$$

Thus, if we know the desired plasma concentration

(C_{ss}) and the drug clearance, we can calculate the rate of administration required. However, it is usual to administer a loading dose before starting the infusion in order to achieve the therapeutic concentration more rapidly.

The loading dose of a drug is that dose required to raise the plasma drug concentration to the therapeutic range and is equal to the amount of drug in the body at therapeutic plasma concentration. Thus:

$$\text{Amount of drug in the body}$$
$$= \text{plasma concentration}$$
$$\times \text{volume of distribution}$$

The loading dose required to achieve a plasma concentration of C_{ss} is therefore dependent on the volume of distribution, and

$$\text{Loading dose} = \text{volume of distribution} \times C_{ss}$$

Alternatively, loading dose may be expressed in terms of the usual maintenance dosage regimen

$$\text{Loading dose} = \frac{\text{usual maintenance dose}}{\text{usual dosing interval}} \times \frac{t_{\frac{1}{2}}}{0.693}$$

These equations allow the clinician to approximate drug administration for an individual patient, and dosage refinements based on the actual plasma concentration or patient response are required as treatment progresses. One problem in predicting loading dose and rate of administration for an individual patient is that the pharmacokinetic parameters for the patient are different from the 'population' values used to calculate the loading dose and infusion rate. Studies of 'population kinetics' in a large number of patients have been undertaken to ameliorate this problem, but have been able to explain only a small amount of interpatient variability as they do not take into account individual pharmacogenetic differences in drug disposition.

Effect of disease on pharmacokinetics

Patients in the ITU may exhibit marked alterations in drug pharmacokinetics as a result of the abnormal physiological states that exist in these patients. Such alterations are important to recognize in order that appropriate dosage adjustments can be made before the development of drug toxicity is produced by inappropriately high plasma drug concentrations. These disease-induced changes in drug disposition are a result often of reduced drug excretion produced by either alteration in drug metabolism or renal excretion of either the drug itself or its metabolites.

Renal disease

The kidneys are the primary route of excretion for a number of water-soluble drugs and also for the water-soluble metabolites of less polar compounds. Excretion of such compounds (e.g. pancuronium) is reduced in patients with impaired renal function. Impaired renal function may be a result of chronic renal disease or the acute reduction in glomerular filtration seen frequently in the ITU. Administration of the customary dose of renally excreted drug to such patients results in drug accumulation and toxicity. To prevent such toxicity, appropriate dosage adjustments are required. Changes in drug binding in renal disease have been shown for a small number of drugs and may lead to alterations in volume of distribution and therefore an adjustment in the loading dose. However, in the absence of a change in volume of distribution in renal disease, no change is required in the loading dose of drug. As stated previously, the maintenance dose of drug required to achieve a therapeutic concentration of drug in plasma at steady state (C_{ss}) is dependent on the rate of drug clearance. Thus, a dosage reduction is required to maintain the same plasma drug concentration when drug excretion decreases, e.g. in patients with renal failure. Many drugs which are excreted in the kidney are excreted also by other routes, so that:

$$\text{Total clearance} = \text{renal clearance} + \text{non-renal clearance}$$

In renal failure, only the renal clearance is altered predictably, so that adjustment of dosage needs to take into account the proportion of drug which is excreted non-renally (Table 92.1). The renal clearance of a drug excreted by glomerular filtration falls in proportion to the change in the patient's creatinine clearance. If the normal creatinine clearance is taken as 100 ml/min in a patient with renal disease:

Table 92.1 Renal and non-renal clearance of some important drugs used in the ITU. (Data from Wilkinson & Oates, 1987)

Drug	Renal clearance* (ml/min)	Non-renal clearance (ml/min)
Ampicillin	340	12
Carbenicillin	68	10
Digoxin	110	36
Gentamicin	78	3
Kanamycin	60	0
Penicillin G	340	36

* Renal clearance when creatinine clearance = 100 ml/min.

$$\text{Patient's renal drug clearance}$$
$$= \text{normal renal drug clearance}$$
$$\times \frac{\text{patient's creatinine clearance}}{100}$$

Thus,

$$\text{Patient's total drug clearance}$$
$$= \text{normal renal drug clearance}$$
$$\times \frac{\text{patient's creatinine clearance}}{100}$$
$$+ \text{non-renal clearance}$$

Although measurement of creatinine clearance is optimal, this is not always possible and the creatinine clearance (Cl_{cr}) may be calculated from a knowledge of the serum creatinine:

$$Cl_{cr} = \frac{(140 - \text{age}) \times \text{wt (kg)}}{72 \times \text{serum creatinine (mg/100 ml)}}$$

Or:

$$Cl_{cr} = \frac{(140 - \text{age}) \times \text{wt (kg)} \times 1.23}{\text{serum creatinine (μmole)}}$$

The calculated value should be reduced to 85% of this value in females.

Having calculated the appropriate total dose, there are two approaches to making the dosage adjustment. First, the dosage interval may be maintained at that used in patients with normal renal function and the amount of each dose reduced appropriately. Second, the normal dose may be given less frequently. This results in considerable variation between peak and trough plasma concentrations. It should be emphasized that both methods result in the same *average* plasma concentrations.

In addition to the effect of diminished renal function on the clearance of renally excreted drugs, the effects of diminished renal function on the clearance of drug metabolites needs to be considered also, e.g. the principal route of excretion for pethidine is normally by metabolism in the liver. N-demethylation of pethidine yields norpethidine which is then excreted renally. Norpethidine accumulates in renal failure so that the ratio of metabolite : parent drug is approximately four-fold higher in renal failure than in patients with normal renal function. Norpethidine is active pharmacologically with approximately 50% of the potency of pethidine as an analgesic and twice the potency as a convulsant. In patients with renal insufficiency, the accumulation of norpethidine after chronic pethidine dosing may cause excitability, twitching and seizures.

Similarly, the metabolism of morphine produces the glucuronides, morphine-6-glucuronide (M-6-G) and morphine-3-glucuronide (M-3-G), which are in turn renally excreted. The elimination half-life of morphine appears to be unaffected by renal failure, but the metabolic products accumulate, and although M-3-G has little pharmacological effect, M-6-G is a more potent opioid than morphine. Thus, when morphine is administered chronically to patients with diminished renal function, the glucuronide metabolites may accumulate, with possible resultant prolonged sedation and delayed respiratory depression.

The pharmacologically active metabolites of the antiarrhythmic drug encainide also accumulate in renal failure. Because of the accumulation of these active metabolites during chronic encainide administration, the dose of encainide should be reduced in patients with renal disease. Drugs that should be used with dosage adjustments in renal disease include digoxin, pancuronium, pethidine, morphine, gentamicin, kanamycin, cimetidine and lithium, and for many of these drugs monitoring of plasma concentrations is indicated (Table 92.2).

Liver disease

Hepatic disease might be expected to decrease the metabolism and clearance of drugs whose major route of excretion is by hepatic metabolism. Unfortunately, there is no measure of liver function which may be used to predict the decline in hepatic drug metabolism in the same way as creatinine clearance may be used to predict the decrease in drug excretion by the kidney. The situation is complicated further by the fact that the effects of hepatic disease on drug metabolism appear to be dependent on the metabolic pathway by which the drug is metabolized, so that drugs whose principal route of metabolism is by

oxidation are affected more than those which are metabolized by glucuronidation. This has been demonstrated well for the benzodiazepines. The clearances of diazepam and chlordiazepoxide, which undergo oxidation, are decreased in liver disease whilst the clearances of lorazepam and oxazepam which are glucuronidated are unaffected (Table 92.3).

In addition to alterations in drug-metabolizing ability in liver disease, haemodynamic alterations occur also and result from both intra- and extrahepatic shunting of blood. Therefore, following oral administration and entry of drug into the portal circulation, some of the drug bypasses functioning liver tissue to enter the systemic circulation directly. For drugs which are normally highly extracted by the liver, such as propranolol or lignocaine, this portacaval shunting results in a substantial increase in plasma drug concentrations.

Shock, reduced cardiac output and cardiac failure

Drug delivery, both to the organs of excretion, the

Table 92.2 Therapeutic concentrations of some drugs

Drug	Therapeutic range
Carbamazepine	3−10 µg/ml
Clonazepam	20−70 ng/ml
Diazepam	600−1200 ng/ml
Digitoxin	10−20 ng/ml
Digoxin	0.5−2 ng/ml
Ethosuximide	60−100 µg/ml
Lignocaine	4−6 µg/ml
Lithium	0.5−1.3 mmol/litre
Phenobarbitone	10−25 µg/ml
Phenytoin	10−25 µg/ml
Primidone	<10 µg/ml
Procainamide	4−8 µg/ml
Propranolol	50−100 ng/ml
Quinidine	2−5 µg/ml
Theophylline	10−20 µg/ml
Thiocyanate	<100 µg/ml
Valproic acid	50−100 µg/ml

Table 92.3 Effects of route of metabolism on the clearance of benzodiazepines in liver disease

Drug	Initial route of metabolism	Cirrhosis	Hepatitis
Diazepam	Oxidation	Decrease	Decrease
Chlordiazepoxide	Oxidation	Decrease	Decrease
Lorazepam	Glucuronidation	No change	No change
Oxazepam	Glucuronidation	No change	No change

liver and kidney, and to the tissues in which the drug is distributed is dependent on adequate tissue perfusion. In shock or states of low cardiac output, perfusion of certain tissues is reduced in order to maintain perfusion of vital organs. The reduction in renal and hepatic blood flow may result in reduced drug clearance with elevation of drug concentrations during multiple-dose therapy. In addition, because drug concentrations following an initial loading dose are dependent on drug distribution and hence perfusion of the tissues to which drug is distributed, reduced tissue perfusion such as is seen in shock, cardiac failure or other low cardiac-output states may be associated with elevated drug concentrations if the usual loading dose of drug is given. In patients with reduced cardiac output or reduced tissue perfusion, a reduced loading dose of drug should be administered followed by appropriate maintenance dosage adjustment to take account of impaired drug excretion.

The multiple mechanisms altering drug disposition in cardiac failure are illustrated well by lignocaine. Lignocaine is excreted primarily by hepatic metabolism and, being a high-clearance drug, its clearance is influenced principally by hepatic blood flow. The reduction in hepatic blood flow together with reduced hepatic drug metabolizing ability in patients with cardiac failure contributes to reduced drug clearance; if usual doses of lignocaine are administered, increased and potentially toxic plasma lignocaine concentrations are produced. The active and potentially toxic metabolites of lignocaine undergo renal excretion, and because of the reduced glomerular filtration may accumulate to toxic concentrations. Finally, the reduced tissue perfusion results in a reduction in both the initial and steady-state volumes of distribution of lignocaine so that the initial loading dose must be reduced if toxicity is to be avoided. Thus, patients with low cardiac output should receive both a lower loading dose and a reduced maintenance dose of lignocaine. Other drugs are affected in the same way so that appropriate caution needs to be exercised in administering drugs to patients with reduced tissue perfusion in the ITU.

Plasma drug concentration monitoring

For some drugs, dosage may be assessed and monitored by direct measurement of the clinical pharmacological response; for example, reduction in arterial pressure following institution of antihypertensive therapy. However, for many drugs, this is not possible, and the measurement of plasma drug concentrations plays an important role in the individualization of patient drug management; particularly for patients in the ITU with acute and chronic disease states. By titrating drug dosage to maintain plasma concentrations within the 'therapeutic window', we may maximize therapeutic effects and reduce toxicity and unwanted pharmacokinetic drug interactions. The monitoring of therapeutic plasma concentrations is useful especially for drugs that have a narrow therapeutic window and exhibit a large interindividual variation in drug dosage. It is important that drug effect should correlate closely with drug concentration and not a metabolite. In addition, a suitable assay should be available for routine use. Table 92.2. lists the therapeutic drug concentrations for a number of drugs used commonly in the ITU.

Respiratory pharmacology in the intensive therapy unit

Four major groups of drugs are used to treat patients with reversible obstructive airway disease; methylxanthine derivatives such as aminophylline, sympathomimetic bronchodilators such as β_2-agonists, anticholinergic compounds and adrenocorticosteroids.

Pharmacology of bronchodilator drugs

In 1948, Ahlquist suggested that adrenergic receptors should be classified into two types; α and β. Lands subdivided further the β-receptors into β_1- and β_2-receptors: stimulation of β_1-receptors leads to chronotropic and inotropic stimulation and stimulation of β_2-receptors leads to smooth muscle relaxation with peripheral vasodilatation, bronchodilatation and inhibition of histamine or mast-cell mediator release. Thus, for bronchospastic patients in the ITU, bronchodilator drugs with minimal α or β_1 effects would be beneficial. The role of the β_2-receptor in the production of bronchodilatation is shown in Fig. 92.1. Sympathomimetic β_2-agonists stimulate the β_2-adrenergic receptor causing an increase in cyclic adenosine monophosphate (AMP), which acts as the second messenger and initiates a series of events resulting in bronchial smooth muscle relaxation. Decreased concentrations of cyclic AMP lead to bronchoconstriction. Cyclic AMP is then broken down to the inactive 5'-adenosine monophosphate by the enzyme phosphodiesterase. Prostaglandins E_1 and E_2 increase cyclic AMP concentrations but prostaglandin $F_{2\alpha}$ decreases cyclic AMP and causes bronchoconstriction.

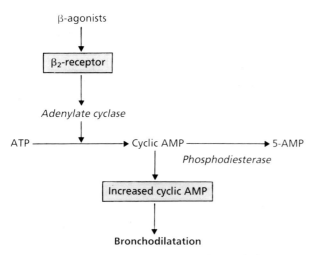

Fig. 92.1 Sympathetic nervous system and control of bronchomotor tone. ATP, adenosine triphosphate; cyclic AMP, cyclic adenosine monophosphate; 5 AMP, 5-adenosine monophosphate.

Cyclic guanosine monophosphate (GMP) is another second messenger which is under the control of the parasympathetic nervous system and causes bronchoconstriction. Stimulation of cholinergic receptors increased cyclic GMP concentrations and increases bronchomotor tone.

The allergic response is a major factor in the production of an asthmatic attack, and mast-cell chemical mediators such as histamine, kinins and slow-releasing substance of anaphylaxis (SRSA) cause bronchial smooth muscle constriction. Cyclic AMP prevents the release of chemical mediators; thus, β-agonists and methylxanthines inhibit mediator-induced bronchospasm.

Table 92.4 lists the smooth muscle receptors of the respiratory tract and the effects resulting from receptor stimulation.

Aminophylline

The solubility of the xanthine compounds is low but is increased by formation of compounds with a wide range of salts; aminophylline is the ethylenediamine salt of theophylline. Theophylline is known to inhibit the enzyme phosphodiesterase, leading to increased concentrations of cyclic AMP which then initiate the physiological response, such as bronchodilatation. However, this effect is produced only at high concentrations, and it is believed now that inhibition of phosphodiesterase may not be the major factor in producing the pharmacological effects of aminophylline. Other mechanisms, such as theophylline-mediated catecholamine release, alterations in intracellular calcium and prostaglandin antagonism may contribute to the clinical effects produced by aminophylline.

The major therapeutic effect of aminophylline is bronchodilatation. Aminophylline is effective optimally in producing bronchodilatation at plasma concentrations of 10–20 mg/litre. Bronchodilatation increases progressively as the serum aminophylline concentration increases, and the use of aminophylline in the ITU is limited by the toxicity rather than plateau or ceiling effects. At levels above 25 mg/litre, 75% of patients exhibit signs of toxicity. The most frequent side-effects include gastrointestinal (anorexia, nausea, vomiting and abdominal discomfort) and CNS (headache, nervousness, anxiety) symptoms. At concentrations of 20–40 mg/litre, cardiac arrhythmias may occur, and at concentrations above 40 mg/litre, seizures or cardiorespiratory arrest may result. The monitoring of serum aminophylline concentrations is the only reliable method of assessing the risk of toxicity and should be undertaken whenever patients with asthma or bronchospastic disease require aminophylline therapy in the ITU. Xanthine derivatives may be given orally and intravenously. Extreme caution should be exercised in patients entering the ITU who have been taking oral theophylline already and in whom systemic therapy is considered. Rapid injection intravenously may cause hypotension. Table 92.5 outlines an infusion regimen for aminophylline.

Theophylline has a mean plasma elimination half-life of approximately 4.5 h in adults and 3.6 h in children. The elimination of theophylline is reduced in premature infants and increases dramatically in childhood. In the late teens, clearance values approach those in adults. Thus, as can be seen in Table 92.5, the loading dose is the same for adults and children but the maintenance infusion rate is increased in children. These are starting-point dosage regimens, and the dose should be titrated to clinical effect and

Table 92.4 Airway smooth muscle receptors

Type	Effect
Adrenergic	
α_1 and α_2	Contraction, bronchoconstriction
β_2	Relaxation, bronchodilatation
Cholinergic	Contraction
Histamine	
H_1	Contraction
H_2	Relaxation

Table 92.5 Aminophylline dosage regimen in the ITU

	Loading dose (mg/kg over 20 min)	Maintenance intravenous infusion $(mg \cdot kg^{-1} \cdot h^{-1})$
Children	6.0	1.10
Adults	6.0	0.90

toxicity, together with monitoring plasma theophylline concentrations. The half-life of theophylline is increased in patients with severe liver disease and pulmonary oedema, and maintenance doses should be reduced for these patients. The half-life of theophylline may also be prolonged in those patients taking concurrent therapy such as cimetidine, or the antibiotic erythromycin and even within a few weeks of receiving a single dose of influenza vaccine. In contrast, theophylline elimination is enhanced in patients receiving phenytoin or barbiturates and also in smokers.

Beta₂-receptor agonist

Sympathomimetic bronchodilators stimulate β_2-adrenergic receptors which leads to an increase in cyclic AMP concentrations and finally bronchodilatation. The endogenous adrenergic agonists, adrenaline and noradrenaline, are potent β-receptor agonists but produce unwanted α-induced haemodynamic effects also. Isoprenaline, a non-selective β_1- and β_2-stimulant, produces bronchodilatation but also stimulation of β_1-receptors, causing positive chronotropic and inotropic effects. More selective β_2-stimulants have replaced isoprenaline in the treatment of bronchospastic disease. However, selective β_2-agonists act also on β_1-receptors to some extent and elicit tachycardia and cardiac arrhythmias if given in high enough doses. Prolonged use of β-receptor agonists leads to 'down regulation' and a reduction in β-receptor number or activity so that desensitization or tolerance develops. This can occur over a period of 1–2 weeks and requires the same period for restoration of normal β-receptor function following termination of drug therapy. When patients are admitted to the ITU for therapy of bronchospasm, they have frequenctly self-administered large doses of β-sympathomimetic agents, and termination of β-receptor agonist therapy with other supportive measures such as steroids and mechanical ventilation may allow the useful re-introduction of sympatho-

mimetic bronchodilator therapy at a later date. Most of the selective β_2-agonists may be administered orally, parenterally or via the respiratory tract as inhaled aerosols or nebulized solutions. Administration by inhalation allows lower doses to be used for the same degree of bronchodilatation and thus minimizes β_1 side-effects. Table 92.6 lists guidelines for drug dosages of the β_2-adrenergic agonists, salbutamol, terbutaline and rimiterol.

Terbutaline is a selective β_2-agonist which may be administered orally, intravenously or by nebulization to treat reversible airway obstruction. Side-effects include β_1 cardiac effects (tachycardia, cardiac arrhythmias), hypokalemia and tachyphylaxis with chronic administration. The hypokalemia results from β_2-receptor stimulation, which causes potassium to be driven into the cells. Duration of action is 4–6 h after inhalation.

Salbutamol is a selective β_2-agonist which reduces airway resistance for 4–6 h. It may be administered by aerosol, nebulizer or intravenously. Cardiac effects are said to be low when the aerosol dose is kept below 400 µg. Side-effects are similar to other selective β_2-agonists and include β_1 cardiac effects and hypokalaemia.

Rimiterol is another selective β_2-agonist that is also effective in reversible airway obstruction. Side-effects and indications are similar to those stated previously. Duration of effect is similar to isoprenaline ($1\frac{1}{2}$–3 h).

Steroids

The mechanism by which steroids act in bronchospastic disease is unknown. They may have multiple actions in reversing asthmatic obstruction (reduction of inflammatory mucosal swelling, direct effects on airway vasculature causing vasoconstriction and reduced capillary permeability). Also, they are useful agents in restoring the responsiveness of asthmatic patients to sympathomimetic agents. Intravenous hydrocortisone may be administered to the patient in status asthmaticus in the ITU in doses of 4 mg/kg 6-hourly, which achieves plasma concentrations around 100–150 mg/100 ml, a concentration considered to be within the therapeutic range. Steroids are useful in improving airflow in patients with chronic obstructive pulmonary disease with acute exacerbations.

Table 92.6 Drug dosage for selective β-agonists in reversible airway obstructive disease

| Drug | Drug dosage and route of administration | | | Duration of action (h) |
	Subcutaneous	Intravenous	Nebulizer	
Terbutaline	0.25–0.5 mg s.c., i.m.	Loading = 250–500 μg Maintenance = 1.5–5.0 μg/min	2–10 mg frequency titrated against response and side-effects	4–6
Salbutamol	8 μg/kg s.c., i.m.	Loading = 250 μg Maintenance = 5–20 μg/min	2.5–5.0 mg frequency titrated against response and side-effects	4–6
Rimiterol			0.6 mg, repeated after 30 min Maximum of 24 doses in 24 h	1.5–3.0

Anticholinergic agents

Ipratropium is a derivative of atropine that is used to treat chronic obstructive pulmonary disease and asthma. Atropine and other anticholinergic drugs cause bronchodilatation by antagonizing the action of acetylcholine at the cholinergic receptor (Table 92.4) and by inhibiting the release of cyclic GMP. Side-effects of ipratropium are those of other anticholinergic drugs, such as dry mouth, blurred vision, palpitations, urinary retention and glaucoma. Ipratropium is a quaternary ammonium compound with low lipid solubility; thus, it is absorbed poorly across cell membranes and when given via the inhalational route, effects are limited to the cholinergic receptors within the lung. Ipratropium bromide may be given via a metered-dose inhaler (36 μg per two inhalations) up to four times daily. It may also be given as a nebulized solution 250 μg to 500 μg 6-hourly if available. It may be a particularly useful adjunct in small children, in whom the response to sympathomimetic agents is variable.

Cardiovascular pharmacology in the intensive therapy unit

Inotropes

Inotropic agents can be divided into three groups: sympathomimetic drugs, the cardiac glycosides and the non-glycoside, non-sympathomimetic agents. The role of inotropic agents is two-fold: to support the failing heart and to improve the performance of the adequate heart in circumstances when a normal cardiac output may not be sufficient for the organism as a whole, for example, during the systemic response to inflammation or trauma (including surgery).

Sympathomimetics

Sympathomimetic drugs mimic the effects of stimulation of the sympathetic nervous system. Noradrenaline, adrenaline and dopamine are endogenous sympathomimetics, whilst isoprenaline is a synthetic catecholamine. Table 92.7 shows the important effects of adrenergic stimulation.

Adrenaline has α and β effects, noradrenaline has predominantly α effects and isoprenaline has predominantly β_1 and β_2 effects. Dopamine has α and β effects depending on dosage and also dopaminergic effects on receptors in the renal and mesenteric beds. Dobutamine has predominantly β_1 effects. Table 92.8 describes the effects of the inotropes, noradrenaline, adrenaline, isoprenaline, dopamine, dobutamine and dopexamine while Table 92.9 gives infusion regimens for these drugs.

Table 92.7 Important effects of adrenergic stimulation

Alpha-receptor stimulation	Beta-receptor stimulation
	Heart; predominantly β_1 Contractility ↑ Rate (sinoatrial node) ↑ Atrioventricular conduction velocity ↑ Refractory period ↓
Vasoconstriction Skin, viscera, gut	*Vasodilatation;* β_2 Skeletal muscle
Mydriasis	*Bronchial relaxation;* β_2
	Uterine relaxation; β_2

↑ Increase; ↓ decrease.

Table 92.8 Comparison of the effects of noradrenaline, adrenaline, isoprenaline, dopamine, dobutamine and dopexamine

Effect	Noradrenaline	Adrenaline	Isoprenaline	Dopamine	Dobutamine	Dopexamine
Heart						
Rate	Slowed (reflex AP increase)	Increased	Increased	Little change or increased	Little change or increased slightly	Increased
Myocardial contractility	Little effect	Increased	Increased	Increased	Increased	Increased
Cardiac output	Little effect or reduced	Increased	Increased	Increased	Increased	Increased
Automaticity	Increased	Much increased	Much increased	Increased	Increased slightly	Little change
Arterial pressure						
Systolic	Rises	Rises	Little change or may fall	Little change or slightly decreased at lower doses	Slightly increased	Little change or may fall
Diastolic	Rises	Falls	Falls	—	Little changed or increased	Falls
Mean	Rises	Rises	Falls	—		Falls
Vascular beds						
Muscle	Constricted	Dilated	Dilated	Dilated or constricted	Dilated	Dilated
Skin/viscera	Constricted	Constricted	Dilated	Dilated*	Dilated	Dilated
Kidney	Constricted	Constricted	Constricted	Dilated	Dilated	Dilated
Coronary blood flow	Increased	Increased	Increased	Increased	Increased	Increased
Total peripheral resistance	Greatly increased	Increased	Decreased	Small increase	Small increase	Decreased
Bronchi	Little effect	Relaxed	Relaxed	—	Relaxed	Relaxed
Uterus (pregnant)	Stimulated	Inhibited	Inhibited	—	Inhibited	—

* Dopamine can cause both relaxation or contraction of vascular smooth muscle, depending on the degree of α- or β-adrenergic receptor stimulation which is dose related. In addition, dopamine stimulates specific dopaminergic receptors causing vasodilatation of renal, mesenteric and coronary vascular beds. AP, arterial pressure.

The cardiac glycosides

Digitalis has been used for over two hundred years, but there still exists controversy over its precise role in the treatment of cardiac disease. In the presence of fast atrial fibrillation there is no doubt of its value, but in sinus rhythm the evidence for efficacy is conflicting. While it has been shown to have a weak chronic inotropic effect, with some heart failure patients worsening following its removal, other studies have shown no such worsening, and some studies have demonstrated no improvement in exercise tolerance

Table 92.9 Inotrope dosage in the ITU

Drug	Dosage ($\mu g \cdot kg^{-1} \cdot min^{-1}$)
Adrenaline	0.01–0.2
Noradrenaline	0.01–0.1
Dopamine	2.0–30.0
Isoprenaline	0.01–0.1
Dobutamine	2.0–30.0
Phenylephrine	0.15–0.7
Dopexamine	0.5–6.0

with digoxin, except in patients with impaired systolic function.

The mechanism of action of digitalis appears to be the inhibition of myocardial Na^+-K^+-ATPase, with consequent elevation of intracellular sodium, that in turn is available for exchange with extracellular calcium. The increased intracellular calcium is responsible for the inotropic effect as well as arrhythmias. In addition to the direct effect on the myocardial cells, digitalis has a parasympathomimetic action, delaying atrioventricular conduction and causing bradycardia.

The pharmacokinetics of digoxin have been described by a two-compartment model with a relatively long initial distribution half-life (35 min) and a clearance of $0.88 \, ml \cdot min^{-1} \cdot kg^{-1}$. Digoxin is almost entirely eliminated by the kidney, with an elimination half-life of 36–42 h. As renal function deteriorates, the fraction eliminated by non-renal mechanisms increases. Digitoxin, in contrast, is metabolized by the liver and has a half-life of 5–7 days.

Because of their long elimination half-lives, digitalis compounds are frequently given with a loading dose. The oral loading dose for digoxin is 10–15 µg/kg, but this is best administered as several divided doses, separated by 3–4 h. Maintenance is then about 0.25 mg/day. Dosage should be reduced in renal failure, and blood concentrations should be measured (Table 92.2). Haemodialysis does not increase digoxin clearance markedly.

Digitoxin is used more rarely. It has the same loading dose as digoxin, and the maintenance dose is 0.1 mg/day. The clearance of digitoxin is reduced in hepatic impairment, and the dose should be adjusted accordingly.

Digitalis compounds should be used with caution in the presence of hypokalaemia, hypomagnesemia, hypercalcaemia, hypoxemia and acid–base disturbances as these can all increase the risk of arrhythmia. Coadministration of amiodarone, verapamil or quinidine increases plasma concentrations and may result in toxicity.

New dopamine analogues — dopexamine

Dopexamine, a dopamine analogue, is a novel symphathomimetic agent that produces both inotropic and vasodilator effects and, in addition, increases renal perfusion. Dopexamine stimulates cardiac β_2-receptors to result in a positive inotropic effect. Because stimulation of cardiac β_1-receptors is minimal, dopexamine produces little direct tachycardia and causes a low incidence of arrhythmias. It is possible that a dopexamine-induced tachycardia that does arise may be mediated via the baroreceptor reflex. It does not appear to stimulate α-adrenoceptors.

Dopaminergic receptors have been divided into two subtypes: DA_1- and DA_2-dopamine receptors. DA_1-receptors are situated on the postsynaptic membrane while DA_2 dopamine receptors are located at the presynaptic sympathetic nerve terminal. Stimulation of DA_1-receptors causes vasodilatation of renal, mesenteric, coronary and cerebral vessels. Renal sodium excretion is increased. Stimulation of presynaptic DA_2-receptor inhibits noradrenaline release. Dopexamine possesses dopaminergic activity and stimulates DA_1- and DA_2-receptors. Thus, dopexamine administration results in vasodilator and renal effects. Renal perfusion is said to reach a maximum at a dopexamine dose of about $4 \, µg \cdot kg^{-1} \cdot min^{-1}$. Dopexamine is also a strong $uptake_1$ inhibitor, i.e. dopexamine inhibits the active reuptake of noradrenaline into the nerve terminal and storage vesicles.

The terminal elimination half-life of dopexamine is 7 min in normal subjects, increasing to 11 min in patients with congestive cardiac failure. It is metabolized by O-methylation and subsequent sulphate conjugation. Elimination of the metabolites is largely renal, but 20% is by the faecal route.

Administration is by infusion, starting at $0.5 \, µg \cdot kg^{-1} \cdot min^{-1}$, increasing by $1 \, µg \cdot kg^{-1} \cdot min^{-1}$ increments to a maximum of $6 \, µg \cdot kg^{-1} \cdot min^{-1}$. Its inotropic effect may be mainly through $uptake_1$ inhibition, causing elevation in myocardial noradrenaline. With its DA_1-receptor activity about one-third that of dopamine and combined with its β_2 effects, dopexamine is a potent vasodilator, and it is this property that contributes largely to its beneficial effects in cardiac failure. Hypotension may be a problem, but this usually responds to adequate cardiac filling volumes. It has been shown to provide renal protection equal to that of dopamine in hepatic transplant patients.

Non-glycoside, non-sympathomimetic agents

These agents comprise the phosphodiesterase III inhibitor class of drugs, the three most widely used being amrinone, milrinone and enoximone. They represent a new class of cardiac inotropic agents, distinct from the catecholamines and cardiac glycosides. They act by inhibition of phosphodiesterase selectively in the myocardium and vascular smooth muscle, with resultant intracellular cyclic AMP elevation (as shown for bronchomotor tone in Fig. 92.1). The increased cyclic AMP concentrations lead to activation of myocardial contractile proteins, thereby increasing myocardial contractility and cardiac output. These drugs reduce both afterload and preload by their relaxant effects on vascular smooth muscle. The overall effect is one of increased inotropy, vasodilatation and enhanced ventricular dilatation. Therefore, amrinone, when given to patients with congestive heart failure, increases cardiac output because of both its inotropic and vasodilatory effects without increase in myocardial oxygen consumption. Pulmonary capillary wedge pressure and total peripheral resistance decrease. Heart rate is generally unchanged, or it may increase slightly.

All three of these drugs may be given intravenously. Long-term studies of their use in chronic heart failure have been disappointing, with increased mortality resulting, possibly from cardiac arrhythmias. In the acute stage, however, they have a beneficial role, being effective in cardiogenic shock, and as a bridging step to cardiac transplantation. The administration of these drugs has also been shown to be of use in the termination of cardiopulmonary bypass.

Because of their effect on afterload, they should be used with caution in the hypotensive patient, but when combined with a pressor agent (e.g. noradrenaline) they may still be useful. Because they elevate cyclic AMP by a different mechanism, they can be used in the presence of beta block, and may be combined with β_1-agonists for increased effect.

Amrinone

Amrinone is a Class III phosphodiesterase inhibitor with an elimination half-life of about 3.6 h. It can be given as a loading dose of 0.75 mg/kg i.v. followed by a maintenance infusion of $5-10\,\mu g \cdot kg^{-1} \cdot min^{-1}$. The loading dose needs to be higher when administered into a cardiopulmonary bypass circuit, up to 1.5 mg/kg. Side-effects include thrombocytopenia, gastrointestinal symptoms such as nausea, vomiting, and abdominal pain and arrhythmias. Amrinone in the oral form is no longer used.

Milrinone

Like amrinone, milrinone is a bipyridine derivative, but it is more potent as an inotrope. It has a similar mechanism of action, and also possesses a vasodilator effect. Elimination half-life is 0.8-1.2 h, but this is increased in renal failure. It does not cause thrombocytopenia.

Enoximone

Enoximone is an imidazole derivative, a Class III phosphodiesterase inhibitor, that is rapidly metabolized to enoximone sulfoxide, with only 1% of the original drug being detectable in the urine. It undergoes substantial first-pass metabolism in the liver. The elimination half-life of the parent compound is 1-2 h in normal subjects, but may be increased to 3-20 h in congestive heart failure. The range of terminal elimination half-lives for enoximone sulfoxide in congestive heart failure has been reported to be between 0.33 and 25.6 h with a large interpatient variability. The sulfoxide is renally excreted, by both glomerular filtration and tubular secretion. Although the metabolite possesses only 14% of the activity of enoximone, it is substantially less bound to plasma proteins, and may therefore be a major contributor to the pharmacodynamic effect of the drug. Retention of the metabolite in patients with acute renal failure in the ITU setting has been described.

It can be administered with a loading dose of 0.5 mg/kg given over several minutes, followed by an infusion of $5\,\mu g \cdot kg^{-1} \cdot min^{-1}$. Higher doses do not provide much greater effect, but increase the drug and sulfoxide concentrations disproportionately, probably because the elimination is saturable.

Other inotropic drugs

Prenalterol is a selective β_1-agonist which may be used as an inotropic agent. The drug increases heart rate slightly. Other haemodynamic effects are predictable: an increase in cardiac output, myocardial contractility, tachyarrhythmias and an increase in total peripheral resistance. Prenalterol may be administered intravenously with doses of 1-5.0 mg given slowly.

Vasodilator therapy in the intensive therapy unit

Vasodilators are used commonly in the ITU to: (i) control arterial pressure; (ii) enhance myocardial function in acute ventricular failure by reducing afterload and thereby decreasing the pressure work of the ventricle; and (iii) for unstable angina and myocardial ischaemia by affecting the factors that determine myocardial oxygen consumption, i.e. heart rate, myocardial contractility and myocardial wall tension. Table 92.10 gives a classification of the hypotensive and vasodilator drugs. Nitroprusside and nitroglycerine are the vasodilators used commonly in the

Table 92.10 Classification of hypotensive and vasodilator drugs according to site of action

---

Decreased central sympathetic activity
Central α_2-receptor agonists
e.g. clonidine, methyldopa
Beta-receptor antagonists
e.g. propranolol, labetalol

Adrenergic receptor antagonists
e.g. phentolamine (α_1 and α_2), prazosin (α_1)

Vasodilators
Arteriolar vasodilators
e.g. hydralazine, minoxidil, diazoxide, pinacidil
Arteriolar and venodilators
e.g. nitroprusside, nitroglycerine

Serotonin antagonists
e.g. ketanserin

Angiotensin-converting enzyme inhibitors
e.g. captopril, enalapril

Calcium antagonists
e.g. nicardipine, nifedipine

Ganglion-blocking agents
e.g. trimetaphan

Prostaglandins
e.g. prostaglandin, prostaglandin E_2

ITU, although other agents may be used in special circumstances.

The mechanism of action of nitroglycerine and other nitrates and nitroprusside has been understood only recently. The nitrate vasodilators act through the production of nitric oxide. Nitric oxide formation activates the soluble guanylate cyclase present in the cytosol of smooth muscle cells which results in cyclic GMP production, activation of a cyclic GMP-dependent protein kinase and eventually, dephosphorylation of myosin light chains. This causes smooth muscle relaxation. Other vasodilators such as histamine appear to act through the same final common pathway.

Nitric oxide may itself have potential as vasodilator therapy. When administered by inhalation in a concentration of about ten parts per million, it has been shown to act as a selective pulmonary vasodilator (its half-life is only a few seconds). This vasodilatation occurs predominantly in the better ventilated areas of the lungs, effectively lowering pulmonary vascular resistance in patients with pulmonary hypertension, with no effect on systemic vascular resistance. It may

prove to be beneficial in the management of the adult respiratory distress syndrome by reducing ventilation: perfusion mismatch and in small children with persistent pulmonary hypertension.

Arteriolar vasodilators such as hydralazine reduce peripheral resistance by a direct vasodilator effect on the arterioles without affecting the venous capacitance vessels to any great extent. The reduction in afterload and absence of effect on venous capacitance vessels result in increased venous return, increased preload and reflex increase in cardiac output. The reduction in arterial pressure activates the baroreceptor reflex and results in increased sympathetic activity, with reflex tachycardia, increased myocardial contractility, increased cardiac output, increased myocardial work and hence increased myocardial oxygen demand. This may precipitate angina or myocardial infarction in patients with ischaemic heart disease. Thus, hydralazine is an unsuitable vasodilator for many patients in the ITU.

Nitroprusside and nitroglycerine are arteriolar and venodilators, but the organic nitrates (nitroglycerine) produce predominantly venous dilatation. Therefore, the degree of afterload reduction is greater with nitroprusside than nitroglycerine. Nitroprusside has variable effects on myocardial oxygen balance. In the patient with severe hypertension, reduction in arterial and venous blood pressure reduces myocardial oxygen demand. However, there is evidence from the laboratory and also from clinical studies that suggests that nitroprusside may shunt coronary blood flow though collaterals away from ischaemic zones. Nitroglycerine may thus be the vasodilator of choice in patients with ischaemic heart disease.

The calcium antagonists nicardipine and nifedipine, which have pronounced vasodilator effects, have been administered as a continuous intravenous infusion to control hypertension in the ITU effectively. Labetalol, an α- and β-blocking agent, may be used to control hypertension also in the ITU when it can be administered intravenously in doses up to 20 mg given slowly over a 2-min period or as a continuous infusion (Table 92.11). The dosage should be reduced initially in the treatment of postoperative hypertension when the residual effects of anaesthetic agents and other drugs may be present.

Phentolamine, an α_1- and α_2-adrenergic blocking agent may be useful occasionally in the ITU, especially for the treatment of pulmonary hypertension. A compensatory reflex increase in heart rate is common. It has a rapid onset of action of 1–2 min and a duration of action of 20 min.

Prostaglandin E_1 or alprostadil is a potent vaso-

Table 92.11 Vasodilator therapy dosage in the ITU

Drug	Dosage ($\mu g \cdot kg^{-1} \cdot min^{-1}$)
Nitroprusside	0.25–5.0
Nitroglycerine	0.25–5.0
Isosorbide	0.8–2.0
Trimetaphan	5.0–30.0
Labetalol	0.03 (2 mg/min)
Diazoxide	1–3 mg/kg i.v. bolus
Phentolamine	0.5–20 (mg i.v. bolus)

dilator that is used widely in the medical management of congenital heart disease to maintain the patency of the ductus arteriosus. However, it may be beneficial as a pulmonary (and systemic) vasodilator in adults. Other drugs that have been used as vasodilators in pulmonary hypertension include hydralazine and diazoxide.

Prostacyclin (PGI_2) is a member of the prostaglandin family formed by the endothelial cells of blood vessels, and is an extremely potent inhibitor of platelet aggregation. Endogenous concentrations are too low to have any systemic effect, so it acts as a local hormone causing vascular smooth muscle relaxation and inhibition of platelet function. As epoprostenol, this compound is now available for infusion. It has been used as a pulmonary vasodilator in adults with pulmonary hypertension and in children following surgery for congenital cardiac lesions where pulmonary hypertension was pre-existing or there remains a risk of right-to-left shunt.

Its action on platelets makes it useful as an alternative to heparin for patients receiving haemofiltration or haemodialysis. It is particularly helpful in patients who develop thrombocytopenia as a complication of heparin therapy, but who need renal replacement therapy to continue.

Administration is by infusion in the range $2-12\,ng \cdot kg^{-1} \cdot min^{-1}$ with $4-5\,ng \cdot kg^{-1} \cdot min^{-1}$ being the usual dose. It may cause hypotension and a decrease in arterial oxygenation has been described, but as the half-life is only 3 min, its effects may be rapidly terminated.

It is important that, whenever vasodilator drugs are used in the ITU, alone or in combination with an inotropic agent, invasive haemodynamic monitoring is carried out and that these drugs are titrated carefully to a clinical effect. Cardiac output, cardiac filling pressures, pulmonary and vascular resistances should be calculated to aid in the selection of particular vasodilator drug according to the site of action and physiological effects pertaining to that agent.

Table 92.11 gives a summary of dosage administration for common vasodilators in the ITU.

Central nervous system pharmacology in the intensive therapy unit

Status epilepticus

Monitoring of drug concentrations in plasma or serum is important to maximize therapeutic benefit while minimizing adverse effects (Table 92.2). It is important to recognize that plasma concentrations are usually measures of total drug in plasma. Many drugs used in the treatment of epilepsy are highly protein bound, and factors that decrease protein binding may cause unexpected toxicity if only total concentrations and not free unbound (pharmacologically active) concentrations are considered when making dosage adjustments.

Diazepam is a valuable agent in the management of status epilepticus. Plasma concentrations of 600–1200 ng/ml are required to suppress seizure discharge. Diazepam should be administered as an intravenous bolus in doses of 0.15–0.25 mg/kg and by infusion of up to 3.0 mg/kg over a 24-h period. Clonazepam, another benzodiazepine, is useful also in the treatment of status epilepticus in doses of 1–3 mg by slow intravenous infusion. Adverse effects for both of these drugs include severe cardiovascular and respiratory depression. In addition, CNS toxicity such as drowsiness, ataxia, dysarthria and sedation occur. Phenytoin may be used also in the treatment of status epilepticus. The recommended dose in adults is 10–15 mg/kg infused over 20–30 min and 100 mg 6–8 hourly.

Status epilepticus is a medical emergency and requires immediate treatment. Anticonvulsants should be given and maintenance anticonvulsant therapy started immediately. However, in addition, to prevent the risk of cerebral hypoxia, an adequate airway and oxygenation should also be established quickly. This requires tracheal intubation, neuromuscular paralysis and ventilation if oxygenation is obviously impaired or the patient is unconscious for more than 15–30 min.

Sedation in the intensive therapy unit

Many patients will require analgesia and/or sedation during their critical illness in the ITU, not only to perform mechanical ventilation more easily, but to decrease anxiety. The pain of surgery, trauma or ITU procedures must be addressed as well as the discomfort of tracheal tubes, urinary catheters and oxygen masks, to name but a few noxious stimuli. The anxiety associated with the illness or interventions (particularly neuromuscular paralysis), is a potent memory for many ex-ITU patients. No drug should take the place of communicating with and reassuring the patient, and a smaller dose of sedative is required if the patient is left undisturbed for a time.

Most physicians working in the UK intensive care units believe that the ideal level of sedation for patients is 'asleep, but easily rousable'. To achieve this aim, any sedative medication must be titrated against response, and this titration is facilitated by the avoidance of neuromuscular paralysis if possible. The use of non-sedating forms of analgesia such as non-steroidal anti-inflammatory drugs or regional block may reduce the use of opioid analgesics.

Sedation in the ITU is not without risk. Oversedation may render the patient at increased risk for pressure sores, deep venous thrombosis and peripheral nerve injury, and may also increase patient risk if disconnection from the ventilator occurs. Although co-operation with controlled ventilation may be enhanced, the patient may not be able to utilize more physiological modes of ventilator support, such as pressure support ventilation. In contrast, undersedation may also be a source of problems. Pain and anxiety cause increased sympathetic nervous system activity with resultant tachycardia, hypertension and increased systemic vascular resistance. This is deleterious to the myocardial oxygen supply/demand balance and may be associated with increased severity of myocardial ischaemia in susceptible patients.

Sedatives administered in the ITU can be classified into the following groups: opioid analgesics, benzodiazepines, intravenous anaesthetic agents and others. Since the introduction of shorter-acting sedative and analgesic drugs, the use of intravenous infusions has become common in the ITU. Table 92.12 gives a summary of dosage regimens for some of the drugs used.

Opioids

To sedate a patient in an ITU setting with non-analgesic sedatives alone, and to leave the patient in pain, may simply result in a more disinhibited, restless patient. Besides their analgesic effects, the opioid analgesics have other potentially useful properties in the patient requiring mechanical ventilation: they are antitussive, cause respiratory depression and produce minimal myocardial depression.

Table 92.12 Dosage regimen of drugs used to provide sedation in the ITU

Drug	Dosage
Pethidine	$0.1-0.3 \, \text{mg} \cdot \text{kg}^{-1} \cdot \text{h}^{-1}$
Midazolam	$0.1-3.0 \, \mu\text{g} \cdot \text{kg}^{-1} \cdot \text{min}^{-1}$ (loading dose 0.1–0.2 mg/kg)
Propofol	$2.0-5.0 \, \text{mg} \cdot \text{kg}^{-1} \cdot \text{h}^{-1}$ (loading dose 1.0–3.0 mg/kg)
Alfentanil	$0.1-2.0 \, \mu\text{g} \cdot \text{kg}^{-1} \cdot \text{min}^{-1}$
Fentanyl	$0.5-1.5 \, \mu\text{g} \cdot \text{kg}^{-1} \cdot \text{min}^{-1}$ (loading dose 50–150 µg)
Morphine	1–3 mg/h (loading dose 2.0–5.0 mg)

Opioids may be administered by mouth, by intramuscular injection, intravenously and by the subarachnoid or extradural route in the ITU. In the ITU, the first two techniques provide unreliable absorption and are usually avoided. When given intravenously, infusions may be employed to avoid peak and trough effects, but bolus dosing may be required to attain therapeutic concentrations early in treatment or before stimulating procedures. In the patient who is conscious, patient-controlled analgesia (PCA) may be useful.

Neuraxial opioids are gaining an increasing popularity in the critically ill, trauma or postsurgical patient. Equal analgesia might be provided with less CNS depression, and opioids may usefully be combined with a local anaesthetic. In addition to analgesia, this may improve respiratory function postoperatively and attenuate the neurohumoral stress response to trauma and pain. Lower-limb blood flow is enhanced by the sympatholytic effect of regional block; this may be of benefit following vascular reconstruction procedures.

Morphine may be administered in the ITU to aid in the management of postoperative pain (Table 92.12). The pharmacokinetics of morphine are altered in patients with renal and liver disease. Morphine is metabolized by glucuronidation to M-3-G and M-6-G. This metabolic pathway is relatively unaffected in liver disease compared with the oxidative pathway of drug metabolism, and consequently, the clearance of morphine is unchanged until cirrhosis becomes severe. However, the excretion of the pharmacologically active metabolite M-6-G is reduced in patients with renal disease, so that, although morphine concentrations may be unaffected, there is delayed excretion of M-6-G.

Pethidine and *Fentanyl* may also be used. Pethidine may cause tachycardia and have cardiac depressant effects. Because of its haemodynamic stability (even in high dose) and apparent short duration of action, fentanyl has acquired popularity in anaesthesia. In the ITU it is less suitable because the apparent short duration of action is related to redistribution to body fat and muscle. High dosage or long-term administration results in accumulation, and thus fentanyl is not an ideal drug for administration by continuous intravenous infusion in the ITU.

Alfentanil is a synthetic opioid, structurally related to fentanyl. The pharmacokinetic profile of alfentanil differs from that of fentanyl. Because alfentanil is less lipid soluble than fentanyl, it has a much smaller volume of distribution. The terminal elimination half-life of alfentanil is very short (1.6h versus 3.1h for fentanyl). These differences result in alfentanil being well suited for use as an analgesic sedative by infusion in the ITU, both in the short and long term. Prolonged sedation with delayed recovery has been described in a patient receiving alfentanil whilst also receiving the antibiotic, erythromycin. Alfentanil is now known to be metabolized by the liver isozyme, cytochrome P4503A4 (see Chapter 9). Drug interactions are likely to occur when two drugs that are metabolized by the same cytochrome P450 enzyme are coadministered. Cytochrome P4503A4 catalyses the *N*-demethylation of erythromycin, which itself has been shown to inhibit alfentanil metabolism. This may be the likely explanation for the side-effects noted in the patient described above. There is evidence that P4503A4 is involved in the metabolism of other drugs commonly administered in the ITU, such as midazolam and lignocaine.

Benzodiazepines

One of the benzodiazepine group of drugs is now commonly administered for the production of prolonged sedation in the ITU. Benzodiazepines are characterized by the production of sedation, amnesia, anticonvulsant activity, muscle relaxation and anxiolysis (see Chapter 3). Their mechanism of action is to facilitate the inhibitory effect of γ-aminobutyric acid (GABA) in the cerebral cortex by binding to specific benzodiazepine receptors that are known to be distributed in the same areas as GABA receptors. In the spinal cord and brainstem they mimic the inhibitory neurotransmitter glycine.

The three most commonly used benzodiazepines in intensive care are diazepam, midazolam and lorazepam. Although *diazepam* is still administered

in the ITU, *midazolam* is now more frequently used by continuous intravenous infusion to provide sedation and amnesia. It is water soluble and has a shorter (though variable) elimination half-life than diazepam. Midazolam is a good amnestic drug and it is this together with its pharmacokinetic profile that have led to its current popularity. Sedative effects in the intensive care patient are seen at concentrations between 50 and 150ng/ml, although much higher concentrations appear to be required for children (in the range of 250ng/ml).

The elimination half-life of midazolam ranges between 1 and 3h in most patients, making it the most rapidly eliminated of the available parenteral benzodiazepines. Volume of distribution is identical to that of diazepam (0.8 to 1.6 litres/kg) and the higher clearance rate of 268–630ml/min accounts for the shorter half-life. Midazolam is metabolized in the liver to the hydroxymidazolam metabolite, which has a lesser sedating effect than its parent compound, and is then rapidly conjugated and eliminated. Midazolam is metabolized by the hepatic enzyme cytochrome P4503A, which exhibits a broad unimodal distribution in the population, giving rise to a wide interindividual variability in patient response. This enzyme is also responsible for the metabolism of alfentanil (see earlier).

Volume of distribution may be increased in certain patient subgroups, producing an increase in the elimination half-life. It is interesting that a three-fold increase in the volume of distribution has been described in a mixed intensive care unit population, producing an increased elimination half-life. In many patients in the ITU, plasma albumin concentrations are decreased, leading to an increased volume of distribution and decreased elimination. Thus, in intensive care, the elimination half-life of midazolam may be prolonged and, in addition, a greater interindividual variability may be noted than seen in normal patients. This may result from changes in protein binding, hepatic and renal disease, aging and also pharmacogenetic factors affecting midazolam metabolism.

Lorazepam is another benzodiazepine drug that may be administered to patients in the ITU. When given intravenously it has a distribution half-life of about 20min and a terminal elimination half-life of 10–22h. It is metabolized in the liver to pharmacologically inactive glucuronides. It has been used in patients with liver disease. Its long terminal elimination half-life and powerful amnestic effects may be useful in the ITU setting.

A new class of specific *benzodiazepine-receptor*

antagonists has recently been described of which *flumazenil* is the first example. Flumazenil undergoes extensive first-pass metabolism and is, therefore, given intravenously. Volume of distribution at steady state is 0.95 litres/kg, with a clearance of 500−1300 ml/min which is hepatic blood flow dependent. The elimination half-life of flumazenil is about 60 min, resulting in a shorter duration of action than that of the drugs it is given to antagonize. Resedation may, therefore, occur.

Administration is usually as small bolus injections of 0.1 mg until the desired effect is achieved. The total dose needed is usually less than 1 mg, and rarely 2 mg may be required. Further bolus doses may need to be given, or an infusion in the range 0.1−0.4 mg/h may be used if resedation is thought likely. Caution should be exercised as seizures have been reported, particularly in patients chronically exposed to benzodiazepines.

Intravenous anaesthetic agents

Most intravenous anaesthetic agents are merely sedative if given at subanaesthetic doses. The barbiturate agents thiopentone and methohexitone are rarely used as sedatives in the ITU because their termination of action following an induction dose is brought about by distribution. Their fat solubility and long elimination half-lives ensure that accumulation occurs if given repeatedly or by infusion. However, thiopentone is still useful for the control of epileptic seizures.

Two agents that were commonly used in the past are now no longer used. It is worthwhile first to consider these two agents because of the cautionary tales they present. *Etomidate* is a carboxylated imidazole derivative that possesses pharmacokinetic parameters (e.g. high plasma clearance) that make the drug suitable for administration by continuous intravenous infusion. It is metabolized by hydrolysis in the liver and only 2% is excreted as unchanged drug. The principal metabolites have no anaesthetic activity. It has a low incidence of allergic reactions and provides cardiovascular stability, even at high doses. Histamine release does not occur. Thus, it has many of the ideal characteristics of a sedative for the ITU. Unfortunately, it became apparent through audit of ITU outcome that the use of etomidate to sedate multiple trauma victims was associated with an increased mortality. The mechanism is a direct effect on adrenocortical function with potent inhibition of steroid synthesis and a reduction in response to exogenous adrenocorticotrophic hormone (ACTH). The effect of etomidate on adrenal function is present even after a single dose for anaesthesia induction. It should no longer be used by continuous intravenous infusion and thus is no longer recommended for intravenous use in the ITU to provide sedation.

Althesin is a mixture of two steroidal agents: alphaxalone and alphadolone. The 3α-hydroxy group on the alphaxalone conferred the greater part of the pharmacological activity but alphadolone was added to increase the solubility of the preparation. Even so, Althesin required the presence of Cremephor-EL as a solubilizing agent. The high incidence of allergic reactions to this solvent led to the withdrawal of Althesin.

Since the recognition of problems associated with these two drugs, agents for sedation of the critically ill have to demonstrate minimal effect on steroidogenesis and their carrier vehicles must be well tolerated.

Propofol is a hindered phenol (2,6,di-isopropyl-phenol) whose pharmacokinetic profile (high plasma clearance $24-33\,ml \cdot kg^{-1} \cdot min^{-1}$) makes it well suited for both prolonged and/or short-term administration. Recovery after propofol is faster than after midazolam and thus may allow for more rapid weaning from the ventilator. The depth of sedation may readily be titrated to patient response. It is poorly soluble in water, and is available as a 1 or 2% solution in a 10% lipid emulsion. For sedation, it is administered as an intravenous infusion without further dilution at a rate of $1.0-5\,mg \cdot kg^{-1} \cdot h^{-1}$. The required dose may be lower if an opioid infusion is also given. Although propofol has a high clearance, the relatively long terminal elimination half-life in some studies suggests that caution should be exercised, as accumulation with possible delayed recovery might occur if propofol is administered for very long periods. However, even after 4 days of infusion, recovery is rapid with response to commands within 10 min of discontinuing infusion.

The pharmacokinetics of long-term propofol infusion (72 h) when used to provide sedation in the ITU have been investigated by Albanese and colleagues (1990). An initial loading dose of 1−3 mg/kg was administered followed by a maintenance propofol infusion at a rate of $3\,mg \cdot kg^{-1} \cdot h^{-1}$; calculated pharmacokinetic values demonstrated a relatively long, terminal elimination half-life (1878 min), a large volume of distribution at steady state and a high total body clearance of 1.57 litres/min. Propofol blood concentrations during sedation were about 2.0 μg/ml. Other studies have shown a blood propofol concentration of about 3.0 μg/ml during sedation, which decreased to 1.0 μg/ml at recovery. It has been suggested that critically ill patients might be particularly sensitive to the cardiovascular depressant effects of propofol.

The use of *inhalation agents* in an ITU setting has limited but interesting application. Nitrous oxide is useful for providing analgesia for painful procedures or physiotherapy, but its use is obviously limited in patients needing a high inspired oxygen concentration. Repeated or prolonged use is associated with megaloblastic bone marrow changes secondary to methionine synthase activity inhibition. Megaloblastic changes have been found in patients exposed to nitrous oxide for 24 h, and also in patients in the ITU exposed to much shorter durations of about 2–6 h. Thus, debilitated patients may be more susceptible. Isoflurane in subanaesthetic doses (0.1–0.6%) is a useful sedative agent, producing satisfactory sedation and a rapid recovery. The potential risks of environmental pollution may limit the applicability of this technique as most ITUs do not possess gas scavenging equipment.

References

Albanese J., Martin C., Lacarelle B., Saux P., Durand A. & Gouin F. (1990) Pharmacokinetics of long-term propofol infusion used for sedation in ICU patients. *Anesthesiology* **73**, 214–17.

Wilkinson G.R. & Oates (1987) In *Harrison's Principles of Internal Medicine* 12th edn. McGraw Hill, New York.

Further reading

Aitkenhead A.R., Willats S.M., Park G.R. *et al.* (1989) Comparison of propofol and midazolam for sedation in critically ill patients. *Lancet* (Sept), 704–9.

Armstrong P.W., Walker D.C., Burton J.R. & Parker J.O. (1975) Vasodilator therapy in acute myocardial infarction: a comparison of sodium nitroprusside and nitroglycerin. *Circulation* **52**, 1118–22.

Bartowski R.R., Goldberg M.E., Larijani G.E. & Boerner T. (1989) Inhibition of alfentanil metabolism by erythromycin. *Clinical Pharmacology and Therapeutics* **46**, 99–102.

Bartowski R.R. & McDonnell T.E. (1990) Prolonged alfentanil effect following erythromycin administration. *Anesthesiology* **73**, 566–8.

Beller J.P., Pottecher T., Lugnier A., Mangin P., Otteni J.C. (1988) Prolonged sedation with propofol in ICU patients: recovery and blood concentration changes during periodic interruptions in infusion. *British Journal of Anaesthesia* **61**, 583–8.

Bennet W.M., Aronoff G.R., Morrison G., Golper T.A., Pulliam J., Wolfson M. & Singer I. (1983) Drug prescribing in renal failure: dosing guidelines for adults. *American Journal of Kidney Disease* **3**, 155–93.

Benotti J.R., Grossman W., Braunwald E., Davolos D.D. & Alousi A.A. (1978) Hemodynamic assessment of amrinone: a new inotropic agent. *New England Journal of Medicine* **299**, 1373–7.

Bion J.F. & Ledingham I.McA. (1987) Sedation in intensive care – a postal survey. *Internal Care Medicine* **13**, 215–16.

Bjornsson T.D. (1986) Nomogram for drug dosage adjustment in patients with renal failure. *Clinical Pharmacokinetics* **11**, 164–70.

Bodenham A., Shelly M.P. & Park G.R. (1988) The altered pharmacokinetics and pharmacodynamics of drugs commonly used in critically ill patients. *Clinical Pharmacokinetics* **14**, 347–73.

Booker P.D., Beechey A. & Lloyd-Thomas A.R. (1986) Sedation of children requiring artificial ventilation using an infusion of midazolam. *British Journal of Anaesthesia* **58**, 1104–8.

Braunwald E. (1977) Vasodilator therapy: a physiologic approach to the treatment of heart failure. *New England Journal of Medicine* **297**, 331–2.

Bredle D.L. & Cain S.M. (1991) Systemic and muscle oxygen uptake/delivery after dopexamine infusion in endotoxic dogs. *Critical Care Medicine* **19**, 198–204.

Burns A.M. & Park G.R. (1991) Prolonged action of enoximone on renal failure. *Anaesthesia* **46**, 864–5.

Campbell G.A., Morgan D.J., Kumar K. & Crankshaw D.P. (1988) Extended blood collection period required to define distribution and elimination kinetics of propofol. *British Journal of Clinical Pharmacology* **26**, 187–90.

Chaudhri S. & Kenny G.N.C. (1992) Sedation after cardiac bypass surgery: comparison of propofol and midazolam in the presence of a computerized closed loop arterial pressure controller. *British Journal of Anaesthesia* **68**, 98–9.

Cohen A.T. & Kelly D.R. (1987) Assessment of alfentanil by intravenous infusion as long-term sedation in intensive care. *Anaesthesia* **42**, 545–8.

Cohn J.N. & Franciosca J.A. (1977) Vasodilator therapy of cardiac failure. *New England Journal of Medicine* **297**, 27–31, 254–8.

Cottrell J.E. & Turndorf H. (1978) Intravenous nitroglycerin. *American Heart Journal* **96**, 550–3.

Dobb G.J. & Murphy D.F. (1985) Sedation and analgesia during intensive care. *Clinical Anaesthesia* **3**, 1055–85.

Fabre J. & Baland L. (1976) Renal failure, drug pharmacokinetics and drug action. *Clinical Pharmacokinetics* **1**, 99–120.

Farina M.L., Bonati M., Iapichine I., Pesenti A., Procaccio F., Boselli L., Langer M., Graziina A. & Tognoni G. (1987) Clinical pharmacological and therapeutic considerations in general intensive care: a review. *Drugs* **34**, 662–94.

Fitton A. & Benfield P. (1990) Dopexamine hydrochloride: a review of its pharmacodynamics and pharmacokinetic properties and therapeutic potential in acute cardiac insufficiency. *Drugs* **39**, 308–30.

Gepts E., Camu F., Cockshot I.D. & Douglas E.J. (1987) Disposition of propofol administered as constant rate intravenous infusions in humans. *Anesthesia and Analgesia* **66**, 1256–63.

Gray P.A., Bodenham A.R. & Park G.R. (1991) A comparison of dopexamine and dopamine to prevent renal impairment in patients undergoing orthoptic liver transplantation. *Anaesthesia* **46**, 638–41.

Grounds R.M., Lalor J.M., Lumley J., Royston D. & Morgan M. (1987) Propofol infusion for sedation in the intensive care unit: preliminary report. *British Medical Journal* **294**, 397–400.

Hakim M., Foulds R., Latimer R.D. & English A.H. (1988)

Dopexamine hydrochloride, a β_2 adrenergic and dopaminergic agonist: hemodynamic effects following cardiac surgery. *European Heart Journal* **9**, 853–8.

Harris C.E., Grounds R.M., Murray A.M., Lumley J., Royston D. & Morgan M. (1990) Propofol for long-term sedation in the intensive care unit. A comparison with papaveretum and midazolam. *Anaesthesia* **45**, 366–72.

Hasselstrom J., Berg U., Lofgren A. & Sawe J. (1989) Long lasting respiratory depression induced by morphine-6-glucuronide? *British Journal of Clinical Pharmacology* **27**, 515–18.

Journois D., Chanu D., Pouard P., Mauriat P. & Safran D. (1991) Assessment of standardized ultrafiltrate production rate using prostacyclin in continuous venovenous hemofiltration. In *Continuous Haemofiltration* vol. 93 (Eds Siebert H.G., Mann H. & Strummroll H.K.) Contributions to Nephrology, pp. 202–4. Karger, Basel.

Kanto J. & Gepts E. (1989) Pharmacokinetic implications for the clinical use of propofol. *Clinical Pharmacokinetics* **17**, 308–26.

Kinsella J.P., Shaffer E., Neish S.R. & Abman S.H. (1992) Low-dose inhalational nitric oxide in persistent pulmonary hypertension of the newborn. *Lancet* **340**, 819–20.

Kong K.L. Walliatts S.M. & Prys-Roberts C. (1989) Isoflurane compared with midazolam for sedation in the intensive care unit. *British Medical Journal* **298**, 1277–9.

Lloyd-Thomas A.R. & Booker P.D. (1986) Infusion of midazolam in paediatric patients after cardiac surgery. *British Journal of Anaesthesia* **58**, 1109–15.

Lowry K.G., Dundee J.W., McClean E., Lyons S.M., Carson I.W. & Orr I.A. (1985) Pharmacokinetics of diazepam and midazolam when used for sedation following cardiopulmonary bypass. *British Journal of Anaesthesia* **57**, 883–5.

Malacrida R., Fritz M.E., Suter P.M. & Crevoisier C. (1991) Pharmacokinetics of midazolam administered by continuous intravenous infusion to intensive care patients. *Critical Care Medicine* **20**, 1123–6.

Mangano D.T., Siliciano D., Hollenberg M., Leung J.M., Browner W.S., Goehner P., Merrick S. & Verrier E. (1992) Postoperative myocardial ischemia: therapeutic trials using intensive analgesia following surgery. *Anesthesiology* **76**, 342–53.

Mason R.A., Newton G.B., Cassel W., Maneksha M.D. & Giron F. (1990) Combined epidural and general anesthesia in aortic surgery. *Journal of Cardiovascular Surgery* **31**, 442–7.

Mathews H.M.L., Carson I.W., Collier P.S., Dundee J.W., Fitzpatrick K., Howard P.J., Lyons S.M. & Orr I.A. (1987) Midazolam sedation following open heart surgery. *British Journal of Anaesthesia* **59**, 557–60.

Mathews H.M.L., Carson I.W., Lyons S.M., Orr I.A., Collier P.S., Howard P.J. & Dundee J.W. (1988) A pharmacokinetic study of midazolam in paediatric patients undergoing cardiac surgery. *British Journal of Anaesthesia* **61**, 302–7.

Millane T.A., Bennett E.D. & Grounds R.M. (1992) Isoflurane and propofol for long-term sedation in the intensive care unit. A cross-over study. *Anaesthesia* **47**, 768–74.

Mitchell P.D., Smith G.W., Wells E. & West P.A. (1987) Inhibition of uptake$_1$ by dopexamine hydrochloride *in vitro*. *British Journal of Pharmacology* **92**, 265–70.

Morgan D.J., Campbell G.A. & Crankshaw D.P. (1990) Pharmacokinetics of propofol when given by intravenous infusion. *British Journal of Pharmacology* **30**, 144–8.

Newman L.H., McDonald J.C., Wallace P.G.M. & Ledingham I.McA. (1987) Propofol infusion for sedation in intensive care. *Anaesthesia* **42**, 929–37.

Osborne R., Joel S., Trew D. & Slevin M. (1988) Analgesic activity of morphine-6-glucuronide. *Lancet* **1**, 828.

Osborne R., Joel S., Trew D. & Slevin M. (1990) Morphine and metabolite behavior after different routes of morphine administration: demonstration of the importance of the active metabolite morphine-6-glucuronide. *Clinical Pharmacology and Therapeutics* **47**, 12–19.

Packer M., Carver J.R., Rodeheffer R.J. *et al.* (For the PROMISE Study Research Group) (1991) Effect of oral milrinone on mortality in severe chronic heart failure. *New England Journal of Medicine* **325**, 1468–75.

Packer M., Gheorghiade M., Young J.B., Constantini P.J., Adams K.F., Cody R.J., Smith L.K., Van Voorhees L., Gourley L.A. & Jolly M.K. (For the RADIANCE Study Research Group) (1993) Withdrawal of digoxin from patients with chronic heart failure treated with angiotensin-converting-enzyme inhibitors. *New England Journal of Medicine* **329**, 1–7.

Paul D., Standifer K.M., Inturrisi C.E. & Pasternak G.W. (1989) Pharmacological characterization of morphine-6β-glucuronide, a very potent morphine metabolite. *Journal of Pharmacology and Experimental Therapeutics* **251**, 477–83.

Pereira-Rosario R., Utamura T. & Perrin J.H. (1988) The interaction of dopexamine with various drugs and excipients in parenteral solutions. *Journal of Pharmaceutics and Pharmacology* **40**, 749–53.

Perucca E., Grimaldi R. & Crema A. (1985) Interpretation of drug levels in acute and chronic disease states. *Clinical Pharmacokinetics* **10**, 498–513.

Ponikvar R., Kandus A., Buturovic J. & Kveder R. (1991) Use of prostacyclin as the only anticoagulant during continuous venovenous hemofiltration. In *Continuous Hemofiltration*, vol. 93 (Eds Sieberth H.G., Mann H. & Stummroll H.K.) Contributions to Nephrology, pp. 218–20. Karger, Basel.

Poole-Wilson P.A. (1990) Drug treatment of heart failure. *Drugs* **39** (Suppl. 4), 25–8.

Prescott L.F. (1972) Mechanisms of renal excretion of drugs with special reference to drugs used by anaesthetists. *British Journal of Anaesthesia* **44**, 246–51.

Roberts R.K., Desmond P.V. & Schenker S. (1979) Drug prescribing in hepatobiliary disease. *Drugs* **17**, 198–12.

Roberts J.D., Lang P., Polaner D.M. & Zapol W.M. (1992) Inhaled nitric oxide in persistent pulmonary hypertension of the newborn. *Lancet* **340**, 818–19.

Rocci M.L. & Wilson H. (1987) The pharmacokinetics and pharmacodynamics of newer inotropic agents. *Clinical Pharmacokinetics* **13**, 91–109.

Rockett B.A. (1985) Kidney function and drug action. *New England Journal of Medicine* **313**, 816–18.

Rubin L.J. Primary pulmonary hypertension: practical therapeutic recommendations. *Drugs* **43**, 37–43.

Rutman H.I., LeJemetel T.H. & Sonnenblick E.H. (1987) New cardiotonic agents: implications for patients with heart failure and ischemic heart disease. *Journal of Cardiothoracic Anaesthesia* **1**, 59–70.

Schlueter D.P. (1986) Ipratropium bromide in asthma. *American Journal of Medicine* **81**, 55–60.

Scott N.B. & Kehlet H. (1988) Regional anaesthesia and surgical morbidity. *British Journal of Surgery* **75**, 299–304.

Sear J.W. (1983) General kinetic and dynamic principles and their application to continuous infusion anaesthesia. *Anaesthesia* **38**, 10–25.

Shapiro J.M., Westphal L.M., White P.F., Sladen R.N. & Rosenthal M.H. (1986) Midazolam infusion for sedation of the intensive care unit: Effect on adrenal function. *Anesthesiology* **64**, 394–8.

Silvasi D.L., Rosen D.A. & Rosen K.R. (1988) Continuous intravenous midazolam infusion for sedation in the pediatric intensive care unit. *Anesthesia and Analgesia* **67**, 286–8.

Smith C.L., Hunter J.M. & Jones R.S. (1987) Vecuronium infusions in patients with renal failure in an ITU. *Anaesthesia* **42**, 387–93.

Stanford G.C. (1991) Use of inotropic agents in critical illness. *Surgical Clinics of North America* **71**, 683–98.

Stephan H., Sonntag H., Henning H. & Yoshimine K. (1990) Cardiovascular and renal hemodynamic effects of dopexamine: comparison with dopamine. *British Journal of Anaesthesia* **65**, 380–7.

Tarr T.J., Jeffrey R.R., Kent A.P. & Cowen M.E. (1990) Use of enoximone in weaning from cardiopulmonary bypass following mitral valve surgery. *Cardiology* **77** (Suppl. 3), 51–7.

Tatham M.E. & Gellert A.R. (1985) The management of acute severe asthma. *Postgraduate Medical Journal* **61**, 599–606.

Vernon M.W., Heel R.C. & Brogden R.N. (1991) Enoximone: a review of its pharmacological properties and therapeutic potential. *Drugs* **42**, 997–1017.

Vincent J.-L., Carlier E., Berre J., Armstead C.W. Jr, Kahn R.J., Coussaert E. & Cantraine F. (1988) Administration of enoximone in cardiogenic shock. *American Journal of Cardiology* **62**, 419–23.

Vree T.B., Shikmoda M., Driessen J.J., Guelen P.J.M., Janssen T.J., Termond E.F.S., van Dalen R., Hafkensheid J.C.M. & Dirksen M.S.C. (1989) Decreased plasma albumin concentration results in increased volume of distribution and decreased elimination of midazolam in intensive care patients. *Clinical Pharmacology and Therapeutics* **46**, 537–44.

Vyas S.J., Apparsundaram S., Ricci A., Amenta F. & Lokhandwala M.F. (1991) Biochemical, autoradiographic and pharmacological evidence for the involvement of tubular DA-1 receptors in the natriuretic response to dopexamine hydrochloride. *Naunyn-Schmiedeberg's Archives of Pharmacology* **343**, 21–30.

Watt I. & Ledingham I.McA. (1984) Mortality amongst multiple trauma patients admitted to an intensive therapy unit. *Anaesthesia* **39**, 973–81.

Webb-Johnson D.C. & Andrews J.L. (1977) Bronchodilator therapy (first of two parts). *New England Journal of Medicine* **297**, 476–82.

Webb-Johnson D.C. & Andrews J.L. (1977) Bronchodilator therapy (second of two parts). *New England Journal of Medicine* **297**, 758–64.

Wilkinson G.R. & Branch R.A. (1984) Effects of hepatic disease on clinical pharmacokinetics. In *Pharmacokinetic Basis for Drug Treatment* (Eds Benet L.Z., Massoud N. & Gambertoglio J.G.). Raven Press, New York.

Wills R.J., Khoo C., Soni P.P. & Patel I.H. (1990) Increased volume of distribution prolongs midazolam half-life. *British Journal of Clinical Pharmacology* **29**, 269–72.

Yate P.M., Thomas D., Short S.M., Sebel P.S. & Morton J. (1986) Comparison of infusions of alfentanil or pethidine for sedation of ventilated patients on the ITU. *British Journal of Anaesthesia* **58**, 1091–9.